# Immunology

# Immunology

## Second Edition

Edited by

## JEAN-FRANÇOIS BACH, M.D., D.Sc.

Professeur of Clinical Immunology
Hôpital Necker, Paris

Foreword by

## ROBERT S. SCHWARTZ, M.D.

Tufts University School of Medicine
Boston

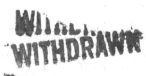

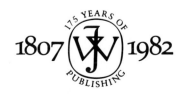

A WILEY MEDICAL PUBLICATION
**JOHN WILEY & SONS**
**New York • Chichester • Brisbane • Toronto • Singapore**

*Cover design by Wanda Lubelska*

Translated and modified from the
original Second French Edition, published
in 1979 by Flammarion under the title
*Immunologie,* ISBN 2-257-20268-6.

**Library of Congress Cataloging in Publication Data:**

Immunologie.   English.
  Immunology.

  (Wiley medical publication)
  Translation of: Immunologie.
  Includes index.
  1. Immunology.   I. Bach, Jean François.
II. Title.   III. Series.   [DNLM: 1. Immunity.
QW 504 I332]
QR181.I4213   1981      599.02′9      81-11503
ISBN 0-471-08044-6                    AACR2

Printed in the United States of America

10  9  8  7  6  5  4  3  2  1

# CONTRIBUTORS

**Stratis Avrameas**   Directeur de Recherches au CNRS, Unité d'Immunocytologie, Institut Pasteur, Paris

**Jean-François Bach**   Professeur Agrégé d'Immunologie clinique, INSERM, U 25, Clinique néphrologique, Hôpital Necker, Paris

**Marie-Anne Bach**   Chargé de Recherches à l'INSERM, Institut Pasteur, Paris

**Jacques Benveniste**   Maître de Recherches à l'INSERM, U 200, Clamart

**André Capron**   Professeur d'Immunologie, Service d'Immunologie et de Biologie parasitaire, Institut Pasteur, Lille

**Claude de Préval**   Chargé de Recherches au CNRS, Centre d'Immunologie, INSERM and CNRS, Marseille

**Robert M. Fauve**   Professeur à l'Institut Pasteur, Unité d'Immunophysiologie cellulaire, Institut Pasteur, Paris

**Claude Griscelli**   Professeur Agrégé de Pédiatrie, INSERM, U 132, Unité d'Immunohématologie, Hôpital des Enfants Malades, Paris

**Philippe H. Lagrange**   Professeur Agrégé de Bactériologie, Institut Pasteur, Paris

**Jean-Paul Lévy**   Professeur d'Hématologie, INSERM, U 152, Laboratoire d'Hématologie, Hôpital Cochin, Paris

**Martine Papiernik**   Chargé de Recherches à l'INSERM, U 25, Clinique néphrologique, Hôpital Necker, Paris

**André P. Peltier**   Maître de Recherches à l'INSERM, U 18, Clinique rhumatologique, Hôpital Lariboisière, Paris

**Jean-Louis Preud'homme** [1] Maître de Recherches à l'INSERM, U 108, Institut de Recherches sur les Maladies du sang, Hôpital Saint-Louis, Paris

**Jean-Pierre Revillard**   Professeur Agrégé d'Immunologie clinique, INSERM, U 80, Département de Néphrologie, Hôpital Édouard Herriot, Lyon

**Félix Reyes**   Professeur Agrégé d'Hématologie, INSERM, U 91, Clinique hématologique, Hôpital Henri Mondor, Créteil

**Charles Salmon**   Professeur d'Immunologie, Centre national de Transfusion sanguine, INSERM, U 76, Hôpital Saint-Antoine, Paris

# FOREWORD TO THE FIRST EDITION

This text was originally published in French by Flammarion. Its general excellence, and in particular its thoroughness and clarity of exposition, immediately marked it as a book worthy of wide distribution. Therefore, this English translation will be greatly appreciated.

As Professor Bach himself notes in the Introduction to the French edition, there is already available a good selection of texts in immunology. In fact, so many are now offered to readers of English that teachers often have difficulty in choosing among them. In the past I have usually recommended two, and sometimes three, different texts because I felt that no one of them satisfied all the needs and questions of my students. I believe that Professor Bach's volume is *the* general text in immunology that will meet the requirements of even the most demanding students and teachers.

The vast and complex subject of immunology is taken up in six sections: the organization and structure of cells relevant to immunity, immunochemistry, types of immune responses, cellular immunology, immunogenetics, and immunopathology. Numerous tables, diagrams, and illustrations enhance the text and imprint upon the reader concepts that often elude words. A good example of the blending of diagrams and words may be seen in the section on the complement system. This is often a very difficult subject for students, but Dr. Peltier has handled the matter skillfully. Another example is the beautifully illustrated chapter on antibody formation at the cellular level. Indeed, Professor Bach has chosen his collaborators well: all of them have made a valuable contribution.

Who should read (and study) this book? Medical students, to be sure. It might be argued that this book is too long or too detailed for many medical students, but of course it is the teacher's responsibility to indicate priorities in the learning process. Graduate students in immunology will find this text invaluable, especially because it deals so competently with topics of medical interest. Physicians in medical and surgical subspecialty training (e.g., hematology, rheumatology, or transplantation surgery) will also find much to interest them. And teachers of immunology will be enlightened by the organization and lucidity of the text. In short, this book should appeal both to beginners and to experienced practitioners of immunology.

I congratulate Professor Bach and his colleagues for their fine addition to the literature.

*Boston, Massachusetts* ROBERT S. SCHWARTZ, M.D.

# PREFACE TO THE SECOND EDITION

Immunology is undergoing a unique technological revolution. For two to three years it has been possible to obtain monoclonal antibodies against defined antigens by means of the hybridoma technique, to maintain and to clone T-cell subsets in long-term cultures using T-cell growth factors, and to clone the genes coding for immunoglobulins. These new approaches have already provided remarkable new information on basic aspects of immunology. Simultaneously, immunopathology has made important progress in such areas as the definition of pathogenetic autoantibodies, the genetics of autoimmunity, and new therapeutic approaches.

This rapid evolution of immunology has justified a new edition of this textbook. It has been updated; new sections have been added, particularly but not exclusively on those new fields mentioned above; and new illustrations have been included. The original goal of this book has been constantly kept in mind: to present a complete and didactic combined approach of basic and clinical immunology.

JEAN-FRANÇOIS BACH, M.D., D.SC.

# PREFACE TO THE FIRST EDITION

Immunology is now considered a major biomedical discipline, on a level with bacteriology or hematology, a branch of which it has been for a long time. Such recognition is justified by the considerable development of immunologic research in the last twenty years.

Several Immunology textbooks have been published in the last decade including the excellent works of Roitt, Weiser; Bellanti; Eisen; Hobart and McConnell; Humphrey and White; and in French, that of Fougereau. However, to our knowledge, no book has simultaneously dealt with immunochemical bases, recent developments in cellular immunology, and modern aspects of immunopathology. This is an ambitious endeavor if one considers the numerous uncertainties persisting in each of these fields, particularly in cellular immunology. While the present knowledge of immunoglobulin structure includes many definitive elements, this is not the case with lymphocyte receptors, theories of B- and T-cell interactions, or tumor rejection. In all these fields data now available may be completely modified in the future. We feel, however, that cellular immunology has reached a stage deserving detailed presentation. It is, in addition, a topic of considerable research, presently even more active than immunochemistry (at least judging by the volume of publications). Clinical immunology has also achieved a certain degree of autonomy, and the time has come to consider it a major clinical discipline based on highly specialized laboratory investigations. We wanted to include clinical immunology in a textbook dealing with basic principles, since it appears more and more that only an excellent knowledge of the theories and techniques of basic immunology will permit immunopathologists to broaden their field of investigation. Conversely, clinical immunology can provide invaluable assistance to basic immunology, as it has already done, for example, with myelomatous immunoglobulins and suppressor T cells.

This book is intended for several types of readers: immunologists, immunology students, nephrologists, hematologists, rheumatologists, immunopathologists, research scientists, and many others who are working in immunology or in related fields.

JEAN-FRANÇOIS BACH, M.D., D.SC.

# ACKNOWLEDGMENTS

I would like to thank Professor Jean Hamburger, who gave me the idea for this book and to whom I owe much. I would also like to thank all those who made the writing of this book possible. First of all the contributors, my wife, and R. S. Swenson, who played a major role in the preparation of the First Edition of the English version. The many friends who agreed to read, reread, and criticize the manuscript deserve many thanks, in particular A. M. Staub, J. Berger, G. Biozzi, J. P. Cartron, L. Degos, M. Fellous, and Necker colleagues C. Carnaud, N. Cashman, J. Charreire, M. Dardenne, M. Digeon, C. Fournier, L. Halbwachs, J. Jacobson, J. Leibowitch, P. Lesavre, J. London, K. Pyke, and F. Tron. I am also grateful for the friendly and efficient collaboration of C. Ollivier and C. Slama for secretarial assistance, M. Netter and M. Lillie for the illustrations, and John Wiley & Sons for the publication of this book.

JEAN-FRANÇOIS BACH, M.D., D.SC.

# CONTENTS

1. INTRODUCTION   1
   *Jean-François Bach*


**PART 1**
**CELLS OF THE IMMUNE SYSTEM**

2. LYMPHOID ORGANS   15
   *Martine Papiernik*

3. LYMPHOID CELLS   38
   *Jean-François Bach and Félix Reyes*

4. B AND T LYMPHOCYTES   60
   *Jean-François Bach*

5. PHAGOCYTES   106
   *Robert M. Fauve*


**PART 2**
**IMMUNOCHEMISTRY**

6. ANTIGENS   129
   *Jean-François Bach*

7. IMMUNOGLOBULINS   163
   *Claude de Préval*

8. COMPLEMENT   252
   *André P. Peltier*

9. ANTIGEN-ANTIBODY REACTIONS   285
   *Jean-François Bach*

**PART 3**
**THE PRINCIPAL TYPES OF IMMUNE**
**RESPONSES**

10.  PHYSIOLOGY OF ANTIBODY PRODUCTION   329
     *Jean-François Bach*

11.  IMMEDIATE HYPERSENSITIVITY   346
     *Jacques Benveniste*

12.  DELAYED HYPERSENSITIVITY   365
     *Jean-Pierre Revillard*

13.  TRANSPLANTATION IMMUNITY AND CYTOTOXICITY
     PHENOMENA   399
     *Jean-François Bach*

14.  ANTITUMOR IMMUNITY   430
     *Jean-Paul Lévy*

15.  NONSPECIFIC IMMUNITY   449
     *Robert M. Fauve*

16.  IMMUNE RESPONSES DIRECTED AGAINST INFECTIOUS
     AND PARASITIC AGENTS   465
     *Philippe H. Lagrange and André Capron*

**PART 4**
**CELLULAR BASES OF ANTIBODY**
**FORMATION**

17.  ANTIBODY FORMATION AT THE CELLULAR LEVEL   505
     *Stratis Avrameas, Jean-François Bach, and Jean-Louis Preud'homme*

18.  CELLULAR INTERACTIONS IN IMMUNE RESPONSES   530
     *Jean-François Bach*

19.  ORIGIN OF ANTIBODY DIVERSITY   556
     *Jean-François Bach*

20.  IMMUNOLOGIC TOLERANCE   575
     *Jean-François Bach*

## PART 5
## IMMUNOGENETICS

21.  INTRODUCTION TO IMMUNOGENETICS 593
     *Charles Salmon*

22.  BLOOD GROUPS 611
     *Charles Salmon*

23.  TRANSPLANTATION IMMUNOGENETICS AND THE MAJOR
     HISTOCOMPATIBILITY COMPLEX 645
     *Jean-François Bach*

24.  GENETIC CONTROL OF IMMUNE RESPONSES 677
     *Jean-François Bach*

## PART 6
## IMMUNOPATHOLOGY

25.  PRINCIPLES OF IMMUNOPATHOLOGY 707
     *Jean-François Bach*

26.  HYPERSENSITIVITY STATES 740
     *Jean-François Bach*

27.  AUTOIMMUNE HEMOLYTIC ANEMIA 770
     *Charles Salmon*

28.  PATHOLOGY OF IMMUNE COMPLEXES AND SYSTEMIC LUPUS
     ERYTHEMATOSUS 794
     *Jean-François Bach*

29.  IMMUNOPATHOLOGY OF GLOMERULONEPHRITIS 829
     *Jean-François Bach*

30.  IMMUNOPROLIFERATIVE DISORDERS 854
     *Jean-Louis Preud'homme*

31.  IMMUNE DEFICIENCY STATES 884
     *Claude Griscelli*

32.  EXTENSION OF THE SCOPE OF IMMUNOPATHOLOGY 914
     *Jean-François Bach*

33.  IMMUNOMANIPULATION 942
     *Jean-François Bach*

APPENDIX
INVESTIGATION OF IMMUNITY IN MAN   967
*Jean-François Bach*

GLOSSARY   977

ABBREVIATIONS USED IN THE TEXT   989

INDEX   993

# Immunology

# Chapter 1

# INTRODUCTION

## Jean-François Bach

Immunology is now a major scientific discipline, but its history is not very old, less than 100 years if one refers to the studies of vaccines by Pasteur, and even less if one considers cellular immunology, which did not really begin until 1950 (Fig. 1.1).

## I.  A FEW DEFINITIONS

The term "immunity" (from the Latin *immunis*, "free of") initially referred to the resistance of individuals to microbial infection. Immunology was then the study of immunity against bacteria. This definition has been widened today to include analogous reactions, specific or nonspecific, to a given antigen which tend to eliminate foreign substances. Immune reactions do not always have favorable effects, as can be seen in hypersensitivity reactions, such as anaphylaxis.

A common feature of the major immune responses is their specificity for antigen. Antigens are substances that react specifically with antibodies or cellular receptors and are capable of stimulating antibody production or cellular reactions. Substances that react with antibodies but are not able by themselves to stimulate antibody production are haptens. The capacity of antigens to provoke an immune response defines their immunogenicity. Antibodies are defined as substances whose production is elicited by administering antigens or haptens coupled to carriers and that are capable of binding specifically to antigens or haptens. One notes the mutual dependence of antigen and antibody definitions. The antigen specificity mentioned above is, indeed, the original element of the immune response. This point becomes obvious after a second stimulation with the same antigen; antibodies or cellular reactions are then produced with greater intensity than during the primary response, whereas a second stimulation by another antigen gives rise to a primary-type immune response. One foresees here the concept of "immunologic memory." Before examining the main types of immune reactions, a brief historical survey should permit a better grasp of the various fields of immunology.

1

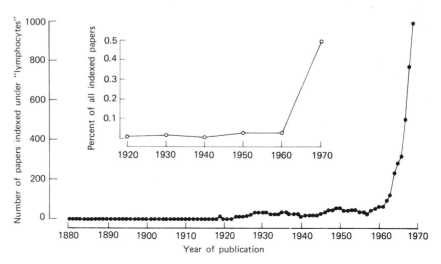

**Fig. 1.1** Historical evolution of the literature on lymphocytes. (From R. A. Good, in Advances in the biosciences, New York, 1972, Pergamon Press, p. 125.)

## II. HISTORICAL SURVEY

The history of immunology may be divided into four main periods. Initially, immunity was the main preoccupation; this was the time of the first vaccines. Next, serology became the main object of investigation after the discovery of antibodies and complement. The third period, contemporary with the development of molecular biology, was that of studies of immunoglobulin structure. The present period examines cellular immunology, a discipline begun by Metchnikoff and Ehrlich at the beginning of this century but studied in depth only since 1950. This classification of immunology into four periods is obviously artificial, and it is clear that each of the above topics still provides very important contributions, even today, including the development of new vaccines, purification of vaccine antigens, homograft and tumor immunity, interferon, phagocytosis, defense against infectious agents, immunoglobulin genetics, and improvement of serologic techniques. This classification is also made artificial by the increasing interdependence of the various branches of immunology: for example, both immunochemists and cellular immunologists are interested in the structure of antigen-binding receptors on the lymphocyte surface.

### IMMUNITY AGAINST INFECTIOUS DISEASES

It has long been known that numerous infectious diseases develop only once in a given individual, but only at the beginning of the eighteenth century was the first vaccination achieved. Vaccination from man to man was introduced in 1721 in England by Lady Montagu, wife of the British Ambassador to Turkey, where vaccination was already commonly performed. However, the method was too direct and included risks of severe reactions and transmission of infections, such as leprosy and syphilis. The method was rationalized by Jenner, who, in 1796, proposed vaccination by a cow-produced vaccine. Vaccination, in the broader sense, was then rapidly developed against diseases other than measles and smallpox. Great progress was achieved under the aegis of Pasteur, who prepared the first antibacterial vaccine by attenuating cholera bacilli after prolonged in vitro culture.

Pasteur also produced a vaccine against rabies by injecting the spinal extract of rabid animals obtained after drying for several days at room temperature. The first and famous vaccination of a young man (Joseph Meister) was performed on July 6, 1885, Pasteur Institutes were founded in Paris and in various European cities for vaccine production.

Several years later, in 1902, the French investigators Portier and Richet discovered a new aspect of the immune response, anaphylaxis. In immunizing dogs with sea anemone toxin, Portier and Richet showed that small amounts of the toxin injected into already sensitized animals induced a lethal syndrome characterized by convulsions and collapse. It was the first demonstration of a noxious effect of the immune response, quite different from the favorable effects already known and exemplified by serotherapeutic successes. About the same time, Metchnikoff discovered macrophage functions, and, under the leadership of Pfeiffer and Von Behring, immunity was shown to be borne by substances present in the serum of hyperimmunized animals. Ehrlich proposed a prophetic theory of the cellular mechanisms of antigen recognition and antibody production. This theory was rapidly forgotten before being reintroduced with little modification 50 years later.

## SEROLOGY

In parallel with the development of vaccinations, the first approaches to the cellular and humoral bases of immunity, initiated by Metchnikoff and Von Behring, became the subject of passionate discourse between supporters of "humoral" and "cellular" theories. However, for many years the humoral aspect was exclusively considered. Agglutination (Gruber, Widal), complement (Bordet), and precipitation (Oudin, Outcherlony) were successively discovered. In 1942, Coons described immunofluorescence, and in 1945 the use of antiglobulins for hemagglutination was discovered by Coombs.

## IMMUNOCHEMISTRY

The biochemical nature of antigens and antibodies was progressively explored between 1922 and 1960. Haptens were discovered in 1921 by Landsteiner. Evidence that low-molecular-weight substances could react with antibodies gave a decided impetus to the biochemical study of antigens. Landsteiner later became famous with his discoveries, at 25-year intervals, of the ABO and Rhesus blood groups, which made blood transfusion possible. At about the same time, Heidelberger described the biochemical basis of the structure of polysaccharide antigens by means of quantitative precipitation. Kabat, a pupil of Heidelberger, showed soon afterward that antibodies migrate in electrophoresis concurrent with γ-globulins. Then began the biochemical characterization of immunoglobulins, which reached its definitive form with Porter and Edelman's work in the 1960s. By use of enzymatic degradation, Porter showed the existence of four polypeptide chains in the immunoglobulin molecule, and Edelman presented the first amino acid sequence of an immunoglobulin light chain. The discovery of IgE and its role in allergy by Ishizaka, Bennich, and Johansson permitted a new approach to the phenomenon of allergy previously described by Prausnitz and Kustner.

## CELLULAR IMMUNOLOGY

The discovery of delayed hypersensitivity is not a recent one. At the end of the last century, Koch first described tuberculin allergy, which is now known to exclusively involve lymphoid cells and not serum antibodies. In fact, however, direct evidence of the major role of lymphocytes in all types of immune responses was not forthcoming until the 1960s, when Gowans showed that it was possible to transfer immunocompetence and immunologic memory to irradiated animals by the use of pure lymphocyte preparations. The role of the thymus was discovered in 1962 by J. Miller, a French-born Australian. At the same time, R. A. Good's group established the role of the bursa of Fabricius of the chicken in the differentiation of antibody-producing cells. Numerous experiments were then performed to dissect lymphocyte populations, in particular at the Walter and Eliza Hall Institute in Melbourne, Australia, under G. Nossal's direction and in Mill Hill Institute in London with J. Humphrey and N. A. Mitchison. The demonstration of the existence of two lymphocyte categories, B and T cells, cooperating in the production of antibodies rapidly followed. The nature of the cells implicated in cellular immunity, in particular cytotoxic cells, was determined by taking advantage of newly developed cell culture techniques that allowed nearly complete in vitro reproduction of the various types of in vivo immune responses. All of these data permitted a reconsideration of theories of antibody formation; the clonal hypothesis of Burnet and Jerne became the subject of passionate controversy. The immunologic tolerance phenomenon was extensively studied after the pioneering work of Medawar. The last 10 years have seen the rapid development of immunogenetics leading to the discovery of immune response genes by B. Benacerraf and H. McDevitt and to the description of the products of the major histocompatibility complex and of their multiple functions.

## III. CLASSIFICATION OF IMMUNE RESPONSES

The polymorphism of immune responses is striking. It is now known that there are multiple cell types that support various immune responses. These cells interact, either synergistically or antagonistically, as, for example, in immune rejection of grafts and tumors. In most cases, a given antigen simultaneously initiates several types of immune responses.

## CELLULAR AND HUMORAL IMMUNITY

The basic and rather ancient differentiation between cellular and humoral immunity remains valid and has recently been confirmed by numerous experimental findings.

Schematically, humoral immunity is mediated by antigen-specific molecules, namely, antibodies, produced at a distance from their site of action. Humoral immunity is easily transferred by serum and less well by cells. Humoral immunity is completely suppressed by neonatal bursectomy in birds and is influenced little by neonatal thymectomy.

Cell-mediated immunity is borne by specifically sensitized cells that come in contact with target tissue and then release locally nonantigen-specific mediators. Cell-mediated immunity is easily transferable by cells but not by serum. It is suppressed by neonatal thymectomy and not by bursectomy. We shall see later that this dichotomy between humoral and cell-mediated immunity is contingent on the differences between B and T lymphocytes.

## GELL AND COOMBS' CLASSIFICATION

Gell and Coombs proposed a simple classification of immune responses into four types. The classification is obviously arbitrary but remains essentially valid, particularly in terms of immunopathology, and for type-I, -III, and -IV reactions, type-II reactions being very heterogeneous and somewhat artifically grouped.

Type-I responses are reactions in which antigens react with antibodies passively bound to cell surfaces. Such interaction releases pharmacologically active mediators from the passively sensitized cells; anaphylaxis is one example.

Type-II responses correspond to cytotoxicity reactions induced by antibodies in the presence of complement. Hemolysis by anti-erythrocyte antibodies illustrates this mechanism. They also include cellular damage or molecular inhibition secondary to the binding of antibodies to antigens borne by certain cells or molecules.

Type-III responses correspond to the lesions induced by immune complexes, soluble or insoluble. Serum sickness and Arthus reactions are the classic examples of this type of hypersensitivity.

Type-IV responses are cell-mediated immune reactions, such as tuberculin allergy and graft or tumor rejection.

### Type-I Reactions (Anaphylactic)

Type I are anaphylactic reactions. Anaphylaxis is acute and often lethal, developing within minutes after injection of an antigen to which the host has already been sensitized. One should note, however, that the term anaphylaxis is sometimes incorrectly applied to type-II or -III reactions. Thus, one speaks of reverse passive anaphylaxis for local or general type-II responses observed after local or systemic injection of anti-Forssman antiserum to guinea pigs. Also, the term aggregate anaphylaxis is applied to type-III Arthus reactions observed in the skin of rabbits or humans subjected to repeated local injections of antigens.

The understanding of the mechanisms of type-I reactions has been considerably enhanced by the knowledge of the nature of anaphylactic antibodies and by the dissection of the events that follow contact between antigen and sensitized cells (as will be examined in detail in chap. 11). Let us mention, however, that anaphylactic antibodies (reagins) have a strong tendency to bind passively to cells ("cytotropic" antibodies), with considerable species specificity (reagins from one species do not bind well to cells from other species). For a long time, reaginic antibodies have been evaluated by the Prausnitz-Kustner phenomenon, which is a passive cutaneous anaphylactic (PCA) reaction. This reaction does not, however, detect only anaphylactic antibodies. In fact, intradermal injection of fairly large amounts of precipitating antibodies followed by intravenous injection of the corresponding antigen causes an inflammatory reaction within a few hours; this reaction is not, however, type I but rather an Arthus phenomenon (see below). An essential difference between Arthus's and anaphylactic reactions is the requirement (in the latter) for a lag time during which reaginic antibodies bind to cells.

In man, reaginic antibodies belong to the immunoglobulin E (IgE) class and in the guinea pig to the IgGl class. The mechanism of anaphylactic reactions is relatively monomorphous. Reaginic antibodies bind to tissue mast cells and to basophils in the peripheral blood. The antigen is bound by the antibodies and causes release of various mediators, including histamine, which produces local edema and contraction of the smooth muscle (hence, asthma in anaphylactic shock). Nonreaginic antibodies may also be cytophilic, but they do not seem able to induce release of vasoactive hormones by mast cells.

Type-I reactions in man include generalized anaphylactic shock, characterized by asthma, widespread urticaria, and vascular collapse, which occur after introduction of an allergen into the circulation of individuals previously sensitized to this allergen. The rupture of hydatic cysts, drug intake (particularly penicillin), and unsuccessful desensitization by, for example, pollen extracts or an insect sting, may cause such shock. Less commonly, the antigen is introduced by inhalations. Local antigen administration to the lung or skin more often induces local anaphylactic reactions, such as hay fever, allergic asthma, or urticaria.

### Type-II Reactions (Cytotoxic)

Type-II reactions are mediated by antibodies directed against cellular antigenic determinants or against antigens or haptens intimately linked to cell membranes. The antibody is generally of the IgG or IgM class and is activated after fixation of complement, which is the effector mechanism of cytotoxic lesions.

Examples of type-II reactions are numerous; post-transfusion hemolysis after administration of incompatible red blood cells is a type-II reaction (however, urticaria or bronchospasm, sometimes observed simultaneously, is a type-I reaction). Type-II reactions against cellular antigens include newborn hemolytic disease, autoimmune experimental orchitis, Masugi's nephritis, and hyperacute homograft rejection. One may also classify as type-II the blastic transformation of lymphocytes that react with anti-Ig or antilymphocyte serum. Lastly, type-II reactions include those in which antibodies are directed against antigens or haptens passively absorbed onto cells. Allergies to some drugs (e.g., Sedormid, quinine or quinidine) are examples of this phenomenon: the drug (antigen) is bound to red blood cells or leukocytes. In fact one may note that type-II reactions include very heterogeneous phenomena, to which one could also add the inhibition of the function of some molecules such as hormonal receptors, enzyme or coagulation factors.

### Type-III Reactions (Immune Complexes)

Antigen-antibody complexes formed with a slight excess of antigen in the presence of complement deposit in various tissues with toxic consequences. Complexes may be formed in the presence of excess antigen when large amounts of antigen circulate and small amounts of antibodies are produced (e.g., serum sickness) or after antibody injection into tissues that contain local high antigen concentrations. Such is the case for the Arthus phenomenon that develops after several hours (hence, the alternative term semidelayed hypersensitivity). The Arthus phenomenon can be produced passively by injecting antibodies intravenously and antigen locally.

The experimental and practical rationale for differentiating between type-I and -III reactions is supported by the therapeutic efficacy of administering antihistamine drugs in type-I reactions, which is not true for those classified as type III (with the exception of reduction in edema), and by suppression of type-III reactions after elimination of platelets or polymorphs or by heparin therapy, all of which have no effect on type-I reactions. Lastly, the intensity of type-III reactions is directly proportional to the titer of precipitating antibodies, which are not involved in type-I reactions.

Examples of type-III reactions are numerous in immunopathology. They include the experimental model of serum sickness disease, acute glomerulonephritis, systemic lupus erythematosus, some drug allergies, and interstitial pneumonia, farmers' lung, or pigeon breeders' disease.

### Type-IV Reactions (Delayed Hypersensitivity)

Type-IV reactions are represented by the model of delayed hypersensitivity observed in tuberculin allergy. The "delay" refers to the time required for expression of the reaction induced by the second stimulation and not the induction of hypersensitivity, which has a time duration of the same order of magnitude as that of other immune responses. Delayed hypersensitivity reactions provoke hypertrophy of paracortical areas of lymph nodes, which contrasts with the cortical hypertrophy and the development of germinal centers observed in type-I, -II, and -III reactions. The use of adjuvants (particularly Freund's) favors the development of delayed hypersensitivity. Delayed hypersensitivity skin reactions develop in several stages. Locally injected antigens may immediately induce a slight nonantigen-specific inflammatory reaction similar to that observed with any high-molecular-weight molecule. It is only after several hours that a mononucleated cell infiltrate develops, essentially originating from the blood. Sensitized cells then release various mediators. One should, however, note that specifically sensitized cells comprise a minority of cells present in the infiltrate. Nonsensitized cells are attracted to the infiltrate by chemotactic mediators. It is important to note that type-IV reactions are only transferable by cell transfusion, which is at variance with type-II and -III reactions, both transferable by serum.

All efforts to isolate from lymphoid cells a humoral mediator that bears antigen-specific information have failed, except perhaps for the work on transfer factor by Lawrence.

Examples of type-IV phenomena in man include skin reactions to tuberculin and to numerous bacterial and fungal antigens. They are also incriminated in the immune rejection of allografts and tumors and in certain autoimmune diseases. It is clear that type-IV reactions should no longer be called "hypersensitivity reactions" but more generally "cell-mediated reactions," even if this term then necessitates further subcategorization, which includes delayed hypersensitivity and reactions mediated by cytotoxic T cells.

## CONCLUSIONS

Gell and Coombs' classification is certainly useful, but, as mentioned above, it is of necessity arbitrary and therefore too limiting. It can be seen that immune responses may often include more than one type of reaction. The interrelationships among various types of hypersensitivity is illustrated by an experiment in which guinea pigs are vaccinated with killed pneumococci on several occasions. If, after priming, the guinea pigs are reinoculated with the same but live bacteria, they are much more resistant to infection by pneumococci. They have developed an immunity to the bacteria. This immunity is borne by antibodies which in the presence of complement leads to enhanced pneumococci removal (type-II reaction).

If, on the other hand, the vaccinated animals receive an intravenous injection of a solution of the polyosidic capsule extracted from the same pneumococcal type, they die from acute anaphylactic shock. These guinea pigs have developed immediate-type sensitivity (type-I reaction).

If the same polyosidic solution is injected intradermally, within 3–4 hr local inflammatory and hemorrhagic lesions follow, which go on to necrosis. This form of hypersensitivity is mechanistically different from anaphylaxis, it is an Arthus reaction (type-III).

If, instead, the same animals receive an intradermal injection of protein extracted from the bacillum body of the pneumococcus, at the injection site an inflammatory reaction appears 12 hr later, which reaches its maximum in 24–48 hr and disappears slowly thereafter. This reaction is a delayed-type hypersensitivity phenomenon, which may thus develop simultaneously with type-I, -III, and -IV reactions in the same animal after a simple vaccination and challenge by various antigen preparations of the same bacteria, using different routes of administration.

The immune responses just described represent various reactions of the organism to invasion by a foreign agent. In the example given, the four types of immune response assess the sensitization of the immunized animal; therefore, the word "allergy," introduced by Von Pirquet, should include all of these forms of immune response. However, one usually restricts its use to situations in which there is hypersensitivity. Such hypersensitivity may have a rapid and even explosive onset, in the case of anaphylaxis or Arthus phenomenon, or, conversely, may develop slowly, as in delayed hypersensitivity reactions.

# IV.  ELEMENTS OF THE IMMUNE SYSTEM

The multiple immune responses mentioned above involve numerous cells and mediators that will be the subject of several of the following chapters; we will limit ourselves here to a simple listing.

## CELLS

### Lymphocytes

Lymphoid cells are the cells responsible for specific immunity (both cellular or humoral) as demonstrated by Gowans' work that showed that it is possible to transfer immunocompetence and even immunologic memory to irradiated animals by injecting purified lymphocytes. One distinguishes two categories of lymphocytes, each of which contains several subpopulations (see p. 61). Schematically, B lymphocytes produce antibodies, and T lymphocytes are responsible for cell-mediated immunity.

### Macrophages and Monocytes

Macrophages and monocytes (the circulating precursors of macrophages) play an important role in the onset, and probably also in the expression, of immune responses. Their true significance has not yet been established, and opinions have indeed fluctuated widely, depending on current experimental findings. Thus, these cells were considered essential at the time of Metchnikoff's work on phagocytosis, merely accessory after the discovery of antibodies and complement, again critically important when Fishman and Adler demonstrated that macrophages could transfer an antigen-specific RNA to lymphocytes, and then repudiated when the RNAs in question were shown to be contaminated with antigens. At present, an intermediate viewpoint has emerged, in which a role for macrophages is accepted but without antigen specificity. Macrophages seem to play a very important role in antigen digestion, in presentation of antigen to lymphocytes, and in some cytotoxicity reactions.

### K Cells

K cells are able to lyse target cells coated with small amounts of IgG (see p. 413). They are as yet poorly defined and may belong either to a new lymphocyte category or to a subpopulation of B lymphocytes or may be immature or atypical monocytes.

### Other Cells

The role of the mast cells and basophils in anaphylactic reaction and that of neutrophils and eosinophils in nonspecific immunity and complement-producing cells (liver cells and macrophages) is now well recognized. At this point we should also mention a newly discovered population of cytotoxic cells known as natural killer (NK) cells.

# MEDIATORS

### Antigen-Specific Mediators

#### ANTIBODIES

Antibody activity is borne by immunoglobulins, which are high-molecular-weight proteins comprised of four polypeptide chains (two light and two heavy chains). There are five classes of immunoglobulins with differing antigenicity, structure, and function.

#### LYMPHOCYTE RECEPTORS FOR ANTIGEN

Receptors for antigen present on the surface of lymphocytes are immunoglobulins in the case of B cells. The nature of T-cell receptors is more controversial. B- or T-cell receptors may exist in the circulation under certain conditions.

#### MEDIATORS SECRETED BY T LYMPHOCYTES

Studies of cellular cooperation between B and T lymphocytes have demonstrated that T lymphocytes produce antigen-specific mediators. Two types of mediators have been distinguished, namely "helper" factors secreted by T cells, which cooperate in a positive manner with B cells, and "suppressor" factors secreted by suppressor T cells.

#### TRANSFER FACTOR

The transfer factor has been described by Lawrence as a low-molecular-weight factor, extractable from leukocytes of sensitized subjects and capable of transferring antigen-specific delayed hypersensitivity. Its biochemical nature and even its existence are controversial, perhaps due to the fact that it is difficult to find in species other than man.

### Nonantigen-Specific Mediators

#### T CELL-PRODUCED MEDIATORS

T cells activated by antigen or nonspecific mitogens produce a large number of nonantigen-specific mediators, even when the stimulating factor is the specific contact between antigen and the recognition receptor. Some of these mediators have been demonstrated in association with delayed hypersensitivity. These mediators include leukocyte migration-inhibitory factor (MIF), chemotactic

**Table 1.1   Some Important Dates**

**Anti-infectious immunity, 1720–1925**

| | | |
|---|---|---|
| 1721 | Lady Montagu | Interhuman vaccination |
| 1798 | Edward Jenner | Bovine vaccination |
| 1880 | Louis Pasteur | Attenuation of chicken cholera bacillus |
| 1884 | Élie Metchnikoff | Discovery of phagocytosis |
| 1885 | Louis Pasteur | Rabies vaccination |
| 1890 | Robert Koch | Koch phenomenon and delayed hypersensitivity reaction |
| 1890 | Emil Behring | Antitoxins |
| 1897 | Paul Ehrlich | Studies on immunity |
| 1902 | Charles Richet and Paul Portier | Anaphylaxis |
| 1903 | Maurice Arthus | Local hypersensitivity |
| 1905 | Clemens Von Pirquet | Serum sickness disease |
| 1932 | Gaston Ramon | Toxoid immunization |
| 1957 | Alick Isaacs | Interferon |

**Serology, 1900–1950**

| | | |
|---|---|---|
| 1896 | Max Gruber and Herbert Durham | Agglutination test |
| 1897 | Rudolf Kraus | Precipitation test |
| 1898 | Jules Bordet | Complement |
| 1901 | Karl Landsteiner | Erythrocyte blood groups |
| 1921 | Carl Prausnitz and Heinz Küstner | Reagins |
| 1940 | Karl Landsteiner and Alexander Wiener | Rhesus antigens |
| 1942 | Albert Coons | Immunofluorescence |
| 1945 | Robert R. A. Coombs | Antiglobulin tests |
| 1946 | Jacques Oudin and Orjän Outcherlony | Immunodiffusion |
| 1948 | George Snell | The H-2 system of histocompatibility |
| 1953 | Pierre Grabar | Immunoelectrophoresis |
| 1958 | Jean Dausset | Human leukocytic antigens |

**Immunochemistry**

| | | |
|---|---|---|
| 1917 | Karl Landsteiner | Haptens |
| 1929 | Michael Heidelberger | Quantitative chemical serology |
| 1938 | Elvin Kabat | Antibodies as $\gamma$-globulins |
| 1956 | Jacques Oudin | Allotypes |
| 1958 | Rodney R. Porter | Immunoglobulin structure |
| 1959 | Gerald M. Edelman | Immunoglobulin sequence |
| 1963 | Jacques Oudin and Henry Kunkel | Idiotypes |

**Cellular immunology**

| | | |
|---|---|---|
| 1942 | Merrill Chase and Karl Landsteiner | Cellular transfer of delayed hypersensitivity |
| 1958 | McFarlane Burnet and Niels Jerne | Clonal selection theory |
| 1958 | Peter Medawar | Tolerance phenomenon |
| 1959 | James Gowans | Lymphocytic function |
| 1962 | Jacques Miller | Effect of neonatal thymectomy |
| 1963 | Baruj Benacerraf and Hugh MacDevitt | Immune response genes |
| 1975 | Cesar Milstein and George Köhler | Hybridomas |
| 1977 | Rolf Zinkernagel | H-2 restriction |

factor, blastogenic factor, and lymphotoxin. Other mediators have been demonstrated in experiments in which B and T cells collaborate to produce antibodies. Some examples are the allogeneic factors produced by T cells activated by allogeneic reactions, skin graft, or graft-versus-host reactions and that are capable of stimulating antibody production by B cells. More recently, the importance of nonantigen-specific T-cell growth factors (interleukin 2) in the T cell help toward B cells or other T cells has been emphasized.

### MEDIATORS PRODUCED BY MACROPHAGES

Macrophages produce a number of soluble substances whose significance is, as yet, poorly understood. Examples are the lymphocyte activating factor (LAF or interleukin-1) and certain factors involved in cellular cooperation, such as the "genetically related factor" (GRF) and the prostaglandins.

### MEDIATORS OF IMMEDIATE-TYPE HYPERSENSITIVITY

Mast cells and basophils, once passively sensitized by reaginic antibodies, release various pharmacologically active mediators, such as histamine, serotonin, slow-reacting substance of anaphylaxis (SRS-A), and platelet-activating factor (PAF), after contact with the antigen.

### OTHER MEDIATORS

Other mediators may be involved in nonspecific immunity. Included in this category are interferons, lysozyme, and especially the complement system with its multiple factors and inhibitors. Here we should also mention thymic hormones, which induce the maturation of T cells, and the factors that stimulate colony formation by granulocytes and macrophages.

# Part 1

# CELLS
# OF THE
# IMMUNE SYSTEM

## Chapter 2

# LYMPHOID ORGANS

## Martine Papiernik

I. INTRODUCTION

II. THYMUS

III. BURSA OF FABRICIUS

IV. BONE MARROW

V. LYMPH NODES AND LYMPHATIC SYSTEM

VI. SPLEEN

VII. TONSILS

VIII. GUT-ASSOCIATED LYMPHOID SYSTEM

IX. CONCLUSIONS: LYMPHOID SYSTEM ORGANIZATION AND THE HOMING PHENOMENON

## I. INTRODUCTION

Lymphoid cells are born, educated, and stored within specialized lymphoid organs. Lymphoid organs have a blood and lymphatic system that facilitates internal cellular movement and makes possible a ubiquitous distribution of the cells involved in immune responses. The lymphoid system includes a set of fixed cells that comprise the network of the lymphoid organ pathways of circulation and a set of mobile cells that are responsible for transporting information and instituting recognition and intervention mechanisms at a distance.

Two organs are called the "central lymphoid organs," because they give rise to the two lymphocyte populations involved in humoral and cell-mediated immunity: B cells (bursa dependent) and T cells (thymus dependent) (see p. 61). The thymus controls the production of T cells; the bursa of Fabricius, at least in birds, produces B cells. The equivalent of the bursa in mammals has not yet been discovered. The origins and development of the thymus and of the bursa of Fabricius (which occur very early in ontogenesis) are independent of antigenic stimulation. Stem cells that colonize the thymus and the bursa originate in the yolk sack and the liver, in fetal life, and in the bone marrow, in adults.

The spleen, lymph nodes, tonsils, and the gut-associated lymphoid system comprise the peripheral lymphoid system. Their development to maturation is conditioned by antigenic stimulation, as indicated by their poor development in germ-free mice (axenic mice).

B and T lymphocytes produced in the central organs migrate to peripheral organs, where they occupy preferential locations. Thus, one finds within lymphoid organs distinct functional compartments with T- or B-cell predominance. The analysis of these compartments may be performed by studying cellular markers specific for one cell type, in the various immunodeficiency states. Thus, the study of the lymphoid organs in athymic nude mice or neonatally thymectomized mice, by comparison with normal mice, allows definition of thymus-dependent and thymus-independent areas (see p. 35).

Some lymphoid cells present in blood or in peripheral lymphoid organs recirculate, that is, return to the peripheral lymphoid organs after passage through the circulatory system. To do this, they use specialized structures within postcapillary venules of lymph nodes and Peyer's patches and sinus walls of the marginal zone of the spleen. From the lymph nodes and Peyer's patches, cells travel to the circulation by means of efferent lymphatic channels and the thoracic duct. Recirculating cells reenter and remain in the white pulp of the spleen. Central lymphoid organs are excluded from recirculation. The recirculating cells are essentially long-lived T cells and prolonged external drainage of the thoracic duct (which includes 70 to 90% of T cells in rodents) or neonatal thymectomy depletes all thymus-dependent areas of peripheral lymphoid organs. However, only a small portion of competent medullary cells in the thymus recirculate between blood and lymph. Thus, superimposed on the morphologic structure of the lymphoid organs, there exists a functional dichotomy of areas where different types of cells implicated in the immune response may preferentially develop as a result of selective migration.


## II.  THYMUS

The thymus is a voluminous, pale-white organ located in the upper anterior mediastinum at the level of origin of the major blood vessels, contiguous to the pericardium. In most species, two lobes originate from two lateral anlagen, which originally migrated to each side of the neck. The final organs are connected to each other across the midline by connective tissue. As mentioned above, the thymus in mammals is the only lymphoid organ that develops in the absence of antigenic stimulation. Axenic animals submitted to minimal antigenic stimulation show normal thymus development, whereas the peripheral lymphoid system remains atrophic. The weight and activity of the thymus are not modified by immunizations, at variance with spleen and lymph nodes.


### ONTOGENESIS (Fig. 2.1)

The thymus arises from an anlage of the third and fourth endodermal pharyngeal pouches. This anlage progressively loses its ties with the pharynx,

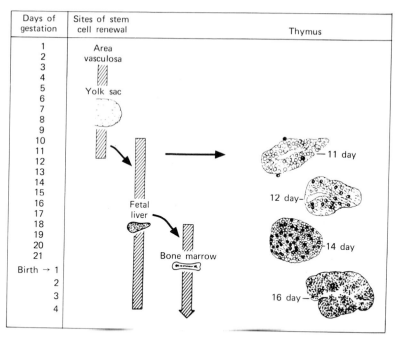

| Days of gestation | Sites of stem cell renewal | Thymus |
|---|---|---|

**Fig. 2.1** Thymic ontogeny in the mouse. (From J. J. Owen, in Ontogeny of acquired immunity, Amsterdam, 1972, Elsevier, p. 45.)

and its central lumen disappears. At this point, the thymus is a small and dense mass of epithelial cells that will next migrate downward to its definitive location in the upper thorax. In man, the thymic and parathyroid primordia are the same, which explains the symptomatology of DiGeorge's syndrome, in which the thymus and cell-mediated immunity are absent, as are the parathyroids. The thymus is the earliest lymphoid organ to appear in birds and in most mammals. The origin of thymic lymphocytes has long been controversial. It was initially believed that lymphocytes appeared locally from the epithelial network. It is now recognized that the thymic epithelial anlage becomes colonized by immigrant blood-borne stem cells that originate elsewhere. This hypothesis was suggested by Owen and Ritter, who, in 1969, showed that 10-day-old embryonic thymuses cultured in vitro never became lymphoid, while 11-day-old thymuses could become lymphoid. These results, which will be discussed later in more detail, indicate that thymic lymphopoiesis in the epithelial primordium is dependent on stem cell migration at the 11th day of gestation. The origin of these stem cells is variable during ontogenesis. They initially come from the yolk sac; when yolk sac hematopoiesis diminishes, cellular influx is produced by fetal liver; finally, the bone marrow becomes the source of stem cells in the adult. In man, the thymus completes its organogenesis during fetal life; at about 20 weeks of gestation, its aspect is that of the mature thymus. The rate of thymus growth, in relation to body weight, reaches a plateau in the third week of gestation and decreases thereafter. However, mouse thymus does not complete its development until after birth.

## STRUCTURE (Fig. 2.2)

Each thymic lobe contains connective tissue septae that support the blood vessels and constitute lobules. Lobule size is relatively fixed (0.5 to 2 mm), despite highly variable thymic size in various species. These lobules are not totally separate from each other, because serial sections reveal narrow parenchymal zones that provide continuity between lobules. Each lobule features a periphery, very rich in lymphocytes, a cortex, and a medulla, which is less abundant in lymphocytes and shows weaker staining.

The thymus is nourished by vessels that arise from the internal thoracic arteries. The arteries branch at interlobular septa and penetrate lobules at the level of the corticomedullary junction. The cortex is vascularized by arterial capillaries with anastomotic arcades; the arterioles join postcapillary venules at the corticomedullary junction. The medulla contains arterioles and venules. Some lymphatics may be seen within the connective tissue, but the parenchyma itself is not penetrated by lymphatic vessels. The thymic parenchyma consists of a network of epithelial cells, which delineate spaces, without interstitial tissue in which lymphocytes accumulate, especially in the cortex.

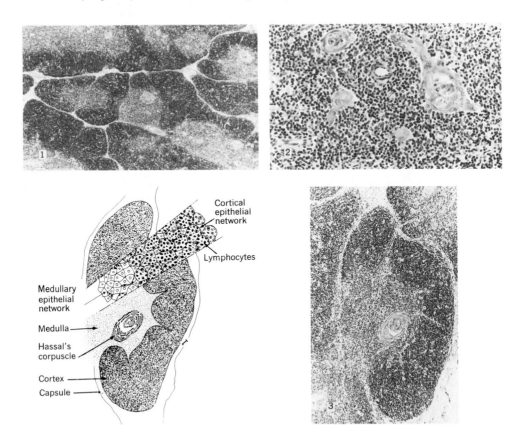

**Fig. 2.2**  Thymus. 1: Child's thymus (18 months). Each lobule contains a dark cortex and a light medulla. 2: Detail of the medulla with Hassal's corpuscles. 3: General scheme and detail of a thymic lobule.

### Epithelial Network of the Thymus

The thymic network is comprised of epithelial cells of endodermal origin (see p. 16). In the cortex, these cells are elongated and have cytoplasmic extensions between lymphocytes. Epithelial cells are larger and more numerous in the medulla. The study of epithelial cells by electron microscopy shows linkage by desmosomes; some of the tonofilaments in the cytoplasm are inserted into the desmosomes. These epithelial cells are contiguous to small numbers of macrophage-type reticular cells of mesenchymal origin. Epithelial cells possess secretory granules in their cytoplasm, which suggests that they may play an important role in the secretion of lymphocyte maturation-inducing thymic factors. This hypothesis has been corroborated by functional studies that show that the thymus or purely epithelial thymoma grafts restore the immunologic competence of neonatally thymectomized mice and by the ability of in vitro cultured epithelial cells to induce the appearance of T-cell markers in thymectomized mouse lymphocytes.

In the medulla, epithelial cells are grouped in round structures called Hassal's corpuscles. In some species, for example, the mouse, corpuscles are, instead, simple aggregates of epithelial cells. Hassal's corpuscles consist of cells piled and coiled on top of one another. Their size is variable, and they may be cystic, with a central eosinophilic substance plus pyknotic cells. Electron microscopy confirms the epithelial nature of the cells that form these corpuscles. Here, too, they are linked together by desmosomes and show cytoplasmic tonofilaments. In the middle of the corpuscle may be seen nuclear pyknosis, a decreased number of intracytoplasmic organelles, and large amounts of keratohyalin, which are characteristics similar to those of skin epithelial cells. The peripheral cells contain microvilli directed toward the corpuscle's center, sometimes thick enough to form a brushlike border. The functional significance of Hassal's corpuscles remains obscure. The presence of active cells with numerous microvilli and the mode of vascularization, which resembles that of endocrine glands, suggests that Hassal's corpuscles may be active organelles rather than degenerative structures. They could conceivably play a role in transferring the humoral products of the thymus to the circulation.

### Thymic Cortex

The thymic cortex is densely infiltrated by lymphocytes of various sizes. Large lymphocytes are less numerous and are mostly located in the subcapsular cortex. Moreover, in this zone, the stem cells penetrate and divide, explaining the high incidence of mitoses. It is interesting to note that small lymphocytes of the superficial cortex have already acquired T cell-specific membrane antigens ($\theta$ and TL antigens in the mouse). The deep cortex stores small lymphocytes. One may also observe cellular destruction in the deep cortex: a large number of cortex-produced lymphocytes die locally.

### Medulla

Very few lymphocytes are present in the medulla; therefore, its epithelial framework is easily visible alongside Hassal's corpuscles. Medullary lymphocytes are the most mature thymic lymphocytes. They include lymphocytes that migrate from cortex to medulla and then leave the thymus (although direct migration of cortical cells into the blood stream has recently been suggested). In mice, medullary lymphocytes differ from cortical lymphocytes by several criteria: they do not bear the TL antigen, they express more H-2 antigen and less θ antigen, they respond to phytohemagglutinin (PHA) and concanavalin A (Con A), and they are capable of inducing the graft-versus-host reaction. They are steroid resistant, which permits their selective isolation after destruction of cortical thymocytes by hydrocortisone treatment.

Lymphocytes leave the thymus by passing between cells of the medullary venule wall. Raviola and Karnovsky have shown that tracers injected into the systemic circulation may be found in the thymic medullary parenchyma. Conversely, cortical arterioles are impermeable to tracers: cortical vessels contribute to the building of a barrier between blood and cortical cells. These data, along with knowledge of the vascular system of thymic lobules, suggest that only medullary cells come into contact with antigens.

It was formerly thought that medullary lymphocytes, which are the most mature lymphocytes in the thymus, were derived from immature cortical thymocytes and were the precursors of peripheral T lymphocytes. However, recent data suggest that the cortical lymphocytes (which are steroid sensitive) and the medullary thymocytes (which are steroid resistant) represent two independently developing cell populations. Both these cell populations appear to be capable of migrating to the peripheral lymphoid organs, where they give rise to distinct subpopulations of T cells. The thymus, unlike peripheral lymphoid organs, does not normally contain lymphoid follicles or germinal centers; these structures are found only in pathologic states, such as lupus erythematosus and myasthenia gravis. In these disease states, they are exclusively present in the medulla, where antigenic stimulation may occur.

## INVOLUTION

The thymus involutes with age. This involution begins at a precocious age; for example, in the mouse, the thymus weight begins to decrease at 6 weeks of age, first rapidly, then more slowly. Thymus atrophy initially occurs in the cortex, which becomes progressively thinner, and the parenchyma is then infiltrated by adipose tissue. In man, thymus involution begins at puberty, as shown by a reduction in the corticomedullary ratio. However, the thymus never completely disappears. Even in old age, one finds, on studying numerous histologic sections, islets of thymic parenchyma that contain a few lymphocytes within the adipose tissue that has invaded the thymus (Fig. 2.3).

## III.  BURSA OF FABRICIUS

The bursa of Fabricius is a lymphoid organ located at the terminal portion of the cloaca in birds. Like the thymus, it is lymphoepithelial. It is also a primary lymphoid organ whose development is independent of exogenous antigenic stimulation.

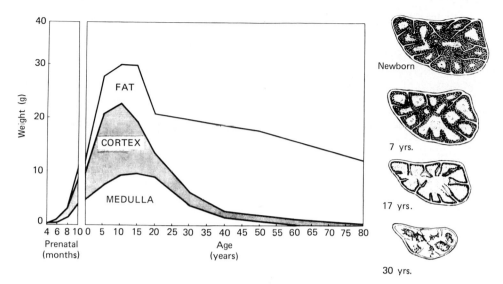

**Fig. 2.3** Thymic involution with age in man. (From J. A. Hammar, Leipzig, 1936, Barth.)

## ONTOGENESIS

The bursa of Fabricius is the second lymphoid organ, after the thymus, to appear in birds. On the fifth day of incubation, it appears as an invagination of the posterior wall of the cloaca. Around the 10th to the 12th days, the epithelial cells that line the "evagination" proliferate into epithelial buds, which arise within the underlying connective tissue. On the 12th to 13th days of incubation, large basophilic cells, the lymphoid stem cells, appear in the epithelial primordium. The origin of bursal lymphocytes is as controversial as the origin of thymocytes. Moore and Owen showed, in parabiotic animals with chromosomal markers, that bursal lymphocytes were not endogenous but represented migrating cells brought to the bursa by the bloodstream, probably originating in the yolk sac.

The bursa of Fabricius is the locus of differentiation of B lymphocytes that produce antibodies. Lymphocyte maturation begins early in ontogenesis. Bursectomy on the 17th day of incubation induces agammaglobulinemia, with absence of germinal centers and plasma cells in peripheral lymphoid organs.

## STRUCTURE (Fig. 2.4)

The bursa of Fabricius is an asymmetric medial organ that opens into the posterior wall of the terminal intestine. It is shaped like a sack and contains a star-shaped lumen that is continuous with the cloacal cavity. Its maximal diameter is 3 cm in the chicken. The mucosa, the musculosa, and the serosa of the bursa are in continuity with the corresponding tissues of the intestine. The epithelial surface, like that of the intestine, consists of cylindrical cells, but the

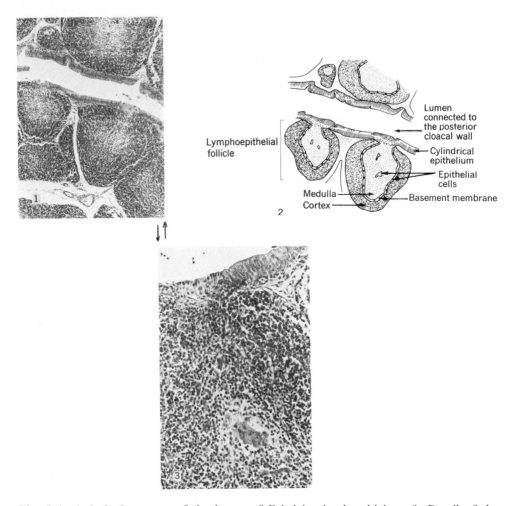

**Fig. 2.4** 1 & 2: Structure of the bursa of Fabricius in the chicken. 3: Detail of the medulla of a lymphoepithelial follicle and of its junction with epithelial coating. Presence of a voluminous aggregate of epithelial cells in the medulla.

bursa has no mucous cells. Lymphoepithelial nodules are present in the lamina propria directly under the epithelium. These nodules contain a light medulla and a dark cortex. The medulla contains epithelial cells that form a continuous area in the periphery, which projects into the epithelial coating. The center of the medulla is less structured; it contains, in addition, epithelial cells and various other types of cells, including large lymphocytes, plasma cells, reticular cells, macrophages, and granulocytes. Unlike the thymus, in which no precise separation exists between cortex and medulla, there is present in the bursa of Fabricius a 100- to 140-nm basement membrane, which separates the medullary epithelium from the cortex. On micrographs, it looks like a central homogeneous zone 15 nm in diameter and is bordered on both sides by an amorphous glycoprotein layer. This membrane is not completely impermeable, because it permits exchange between the two zones of the lymphoepithelial nodule. The cortex consists mostly of small lymphocytes and plasma cells.

## INVOLUTION

Like the thymus, the bursa involutes rapidly with age. At 4 months, a time that corresponds to puberty in the chicken, the bursa begins to atrophy and practically disappears by the end of the first year. Bursal regression is related to increases in testosterone or estrogen levels at puberty. Premature regression occurs after administration of testosterone. If administered in ovo between 5 and 8 days of incubation, testosterone may eliminate bursal development.

## BURSAL EQUIVALENT IN MAMMALS

A bursal equivalent has been sought in mammals for a long time. The equivalent tissue might be responsible for B-cell differentiation. B-cell precursors are found in the mammalian fetal liver and in adult bone marrow. Nothing, however, is known of the microenvironment necessary for B-cell maturation in mammals. Some investigators suggested that the gut associated lymphoid system may be the central B-cell maturation organ. However, there is considerable evidence to the contrary, and no real bursal equivalent is recognized in mammals at this time (see p. 100). In fact, it is apparent that such an equivalent does not exist in mammals in which successively the liver, the spleen and the bone marrow can directly induce B cell differentiation (see p. 100).

# IV.  BONE MARROW

In the strict sense, this structure is not just a lymphoid organ. It has major importance, however, because the bone marrow produces precursor cells of various lymphocyte populations and macrophages in the adult. A single bone marrow cell injection completely restores the lymphoid system of irradiated (but not thymectomized) rats or mice. Bone marrow has a ubiquitous distribution and fills the free spaces inside bones.

## ONTOGENESIS

Bone marrow is initially composed of mesenchymal primitive elements. The precise onset of hematopoiesis varies among bones and species. In man, active zones of hematopoiesis are observed in the clavicle of 10-week-old (43 mm) embryos, whereas hematopoiesis does not occur in the femur until the 14th week (75 mm). Bone marrow reaches full hematopoietic activity only at mid gestation, at which time liver hematopoiesis begins to regress.

## STRUCTURE

Bone marrow represents a complex vascular system within the hematopoietic tissues.

### *Vascular System*

The vascular system consists of an afferent artery, a capillary network, and venous sinuses. The afferent artery perforates the cortical bone and then divides into an arterial capillary network that communicates directly with venous sinuses. These venous sinuses are highly developed: they are bordered by endothelial cells, which may be phagocytic, and have a glycoprotein basement membrane. The basement membrane is coated by a layer of adventitial cells that possess extensions that enter the hematopoietic compartment. Sinus walls are discontinuous, thus allowing cellular exchange between blood and tissue. Venous sinuses open into longitudinal central veins.

### *Hematopoietic Tissue*

Hematopoietic tissue includes all circulating blood cell lines and their precursors: erythroblasts (grouped in islets around one or two reticular cells), granulocytic cells, monocytes, megakaryocytes, and lymphoid cells, including a few plasma cells. Lymphocytes comprise as much as 20% of bone marrow cells, especially in rodents; the number of lymphoid cell precursors is not established, because they are difficult to identify. The proportion of various cells varies, however, according to peripheral needs.

# V.   LYMPH NODES AND LYMPHATIC SYSTEM

Lymph nodes are round, or reniform, lymphoid organs, that consist of a parenchyma infiltrated by lymphocytes and surrounded by a capsule. Nodes may be single but more often are grouped along the pathway of a lymphatic vessel.

## ONTOGENESIS

Embryonic development of lymph nodes is closely linked to the lymphatic system. The lymph node parenchyma develops from the mesenchyma, which surrounds the lymphatic plexus around primitive lymphatic pouches and which is very early infiltrated with stem cells. In man, organized lymph nodes may be recognized in 50-mm embryos (11 to 12 weeks) in axillary and iliac areas; stem cell aggregates may be seen much earlier (in the 30-mm embryo).

## LYMPHATIC VASCULAR SYSTEM AND LYMPH NODE LYMPHATIC CIRCULATION

The blood capillary network is surrounded by a lymphatic network. Lymphatic capillary vessels ending blindly carry lymph from extravascular spaces to the blood. Lymphatic capillaries become channels of a larger diameter that end in large collector vessels, the thoracic duct and the right lymphatic cord, which, in turn, enter large blood vessels in the neck. The capillary wall is very thin, representing only one layer of endothelial cells, the edges of which may overlap. The absence of a basement membrane permits exchange with the interstitial medium. The larger lymphatic vessels have a thicker wall, which contains collagenous and elastic fibers and, sometimes, smooth muscle fibers, and an internal elastic membrane. However, the distribution of different layers is not as well structured as in blood vessels. These lymphatics have valves with the free edge pointing toward the direction of flow, which prevent reflux. Each series of valves is associated with widening of the vascular diameter, thus giving an irregular appearance to the lymphatics. The absence of an organized vessel wall explains why lymph flow is dependent on mobilization by adjoining structures, particularly muscular contractions. The lymph nodes that connect to these vessels receive their lymph by means of vessels that penetrate the capsule. The capsule and the lymph node parenchyma are separated by a peripheral sinus sending out intermediary sinuses along fibrous trabeculae; these intermediary sinuses enter the cortical parenchyma and then branch into medullary sinuses separated by medullary cords. The sinuses enter the efferent lymphatic pathway, which leaves the lymph node at the hilum. The sinus wall is bordered by endothelial cells that rest on a reticular network that is continuous with the parenchyma. Fibers bridge the sinuses and hold star-shaped cells and macrophages. This sinus architecture represents a remarkably efficient filtration and exchange system between lymph node parenchyma and the lymph.

## LYMPH NODE BLOOD SUPPLY

An artery enters the lymph node at the hilum. Its branches follow the fibrous trabeculae, penetrate the medullary cords, and reach the cortex, where they fan out into a terminal capillary at the level of the lymphoid follicle. Postcapillary venules extend from the capillaries into the deep cortex. Their wall consists of endothelial turgescent cuboidal cells without a muscular layer; circulating lymphocytes leave the capillaries, pass between the large cells of postcapillary venules, and also may pass through endothelial cells. Veins exit from the lymph node at the hilum. Similar vessels are found in other lymphoid organs, such as Peyer's patches, tonsils, and the appendix.

## LYMPH NODE PARENCHYMA

The lymph node parenchyma consists of a network of reticular fibers and reticular cells within which motile cells, including lymphocytes, plasma cells, and macrophages, are trapped. The lymph node contains a cortical zone and a lighter and less cellular medullary zone that contains numerous sinuses. Two zones can be distinguished within the cortex: the external cortex, also called the subcapsular cortex, where lymphoid follicles with germinal centers develop, and the deep cortex, also known as the paracortical or diffuse cortex.

### External Cortex

Lymphoid follicles and their germinal centers are located in the external cortex. The follicles without germinal centers are "primary follicles," whereas those with a germinal center are "secondary follicles." Secondary follicles, when correctly oriented, have a polarity directed toward the capsule. Within the germinal center, there are two different zones. The portion close to the capsule is less cellular. The pole opposite from the capsule is denser (darker). In the dark zone, the tightly packed lymphoid cells show numerous mitoses. Various phases of evolution are apparent, including lymphoblasts, large and medium lymphocytes, and young cells of the plasma cell series. Macrophages contain phagocytosed cellular debris. This is the fertile zone of the germinal center. The light zone of the germinal center does not contain cells undergoing mitosis and is progressively replaced by small lymphocytes; the young cells have basophilic cytoplasm in the dark zone. All cells rest on a network of anastomosed dendritic cells. In the periphery, reticular fibers are distributed concentrically and disappear into the germinal center. The germinal center is ringed by lymphocytes, which are particularly numerous on the top of the lighter pole of the center, causing a "cap" appearance, which diminishes closer to the fertile zone (Figs. 2.5 and 2.6).

Follicular cells belong to the B-cell lineage. Follicles are not depleted by thymectomy or by chronic cannulation of the thoracic duct (during which procedures recirculating long-lived lymphocytes are depleted). They show membrane immunoglobulins, by immunofluorescent staining.

In addition to B cells, germinal centers contain occasional T cells. The presence of these T cells is critical for the formation of the germinal center. In artificially T cell-depleted mice (thymectomized, irradiated, and bone marrow reconstituted), and in naturally T cell-deprived nude mice, germinal centers are infrequent or absent (Fig. 2.6).

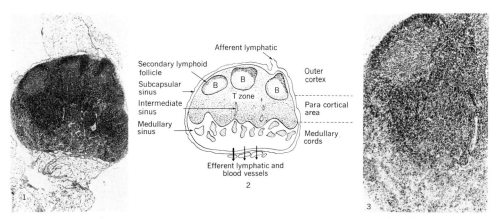

**Fig. 2.5** Lymph nodes. 1 & 2: Structure of a peripheral lymph node in the mouse. 3: Detail of the same lymph node shows three zones: superficial cortex with lymphoid follicles, paracortical area with intermediary sinus, and medullary cords.

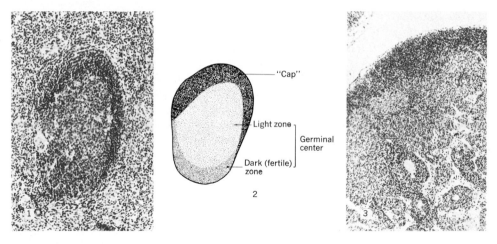

**Fig. 2.6** Germinal centers. 1 & 2: Structure of germinal centers. 3: Nude mouse lymph node. Absence of germinal centers in the cortex. Lymphoid depletion of paracortex (compare with Fig. 2.5).

### Deep Cortex of the Lymph Node

The deep cortex contains postcapillary venules through which lymphocytes travel. This part of the cortex is mostly composed of T lymphocytes. This zone is depleted after neonatal thymectomy or by thoracic duct cannulation. In nude mice, the deep cortex is present but does not contain lymphoid cells.

### Medullary Parenchyma

The medullary parenchyma contains cordlike structures with numerous ramified sinuses and is of mixed cellularity. Macrophages, plasma cells (which migrate into the efferent lymph after immunization), and also T lymphocytes are present in this zone. We shall see later that the paracortical zone is mostly populated by T lymphocytes, whereas lymphoid follicles are essentially thymus independent.

## LYMPH NODE MODIFICATIONS DURING IMMUNIZATION

The relative volume of the above areas within the lymph nodes (including external cortex, deep cortex, and medulla) varies, depending on quiescence or immunologic activity. Immunization alters the relation and absolute size of B and T cell-dependent areas, depending on the type of immune response elicited.

### Cell-Mediated Immunity

The lymph node that drains the skin area of guinea pig and mouse ear after local application of a cell-mediated immunity stimulant, such as oxazolone, undergoes characteristic modifications. Islets of pyroninophilic blast cells are seen in the deep cortex at 24 hr. These cells then proliferate up to day 4, causing an increase in the volume of the deep cortex, while the medulla is compressed. Postcapillary venules show significant changes during the 2 days after immunization. Endothelial cells increase in size, and many lymphocytes cross the capillary wall. Activity diminishes when blast proliferation starts in the deep cortex. Blast cells are still present on day 4 but have completely disappeared by the seventh day, after giving rise to a new population of small lymphocytes. The cortical zone and its follicular crown are very little modified by immunization.

In neonatally thymectomized animals, lymph nodes remain small, and cellular proliferation is not seen in the deep cortex (which is deficient in lymphocytes). Cell-mediated reactions are not always so selective: the changes described above are not unique and are followed, at the beginning of the second week, by a reaction of the thymus-independent zones, with germinal center formation and appearance of immature and mature plasma cells in the medulla.

### Humoral Responses

Immunization by a thymus-independent antigen that gives rise to antibody production, such as polysaccharide, provokes changes mostly in the thymus independent zones of lymph nodes. The injected antigen is very rapidly found in the medulla. It is then taken up by the lymphoid nodules of the superficial cortex in less than 1 hr for a primary immunization and in less than 10 min for a secondary immunization. The antigen is found in the marginal zone of the follicle, linked to reticular cells whose ramified projections penetrate between lymphocytes. The antigen is then attracted toward the follicle's center, where it induces proliferation, starting in the fertile zone of the germinal center. The newly formed cells, which progressively assume the appearance of immature plasma cells, migrate toward the apical light pole of the germinal center between days 5 and 6. Lastly, an influx of mature plasma cells is observed in the medulla. Only few modifications occur in the deep cortex throughout immunization.

## VI.  SPLEEN

The spleen is a voluminous filter placed on blood vessels. It retains particles and cellular debris carried by the circulation, collects antigens, and is the locus of B or T cell-mediated reactions. In some vertebrates, it also plays a role in the formation of granulocytes, erythrocytes, and platelets.

## ONTOGENESIS

The spleen appears initially as a mesenchymal thickening of the left posterior edge of the stomach in 8- to 10-mm human embryos (fifth week). This mesenchymal tissue includes star-shaped cells that will form the reticular web of the spleen; in early mammals, it consists of a capillary network connected to afferent arteries and efferent veins. Irregular spaces, which subsequently become sinuses, appear and make contact with the vascular system. Later on, at variable periods before and after birth perivascular areas are infiltrated with

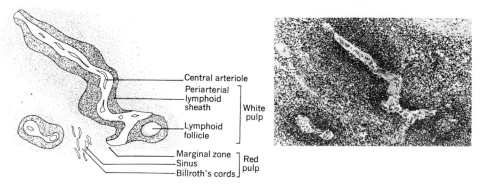

Central arteriole
Periarterial
lymphoid
sheath
White pulp
Lymphoid
follicle

Marginal zone
Sinus
Billroth's cords
Red pulp

**Fig. 2.7**  Human spleen.

circulating lymphoid cells; these cells represent the initial primordium of the white pulp, whose definitive organization is only achieved after birth.

## VASCULARIZATION AND ORGANIZATION (Fig. 2.7)

The splenic capsule sends fibrous trabeculae that penetrate and partition the organ. The capsule and connective tissue walls contain elastic and smooth muscle fibers that, in certain species, play an important role in altering the volume of the organ. Branches of the splenic artery enter the hilum and penetrate the splenic parenchyma along the connective tissue walls. Splenic arteries divide and become surrounded by a lymphoid sheath.

The periarterial lymphoid tissue constitutes the white pulp of the spleen and is visible macroscopically as grey zones, contrasting with the red pulp. On sectioning, the white pulp shows classic malpighian corpuscles. Splenic arteries branch to form "penicillated" arterioles that lose their lymphoid sheath and divide into two or three capillaries that enter the venous sinuses of the red pulp. These venous sinuses are vascular spaces bordered by an endothelium that rests on a fenestrated basement membrane through which important cellular exchanges occur. The sinus wall is in continuity with the reticular tissue of splenic cords (Billroth's cords). Venous sinuses, vessels, and Billroth's cords constitute splenic red pulp. Venous sinuses open into pulp veins that penetrate the fibrous trabeculae and are drained by hilar veins that are tributaries of the splenic vein.

Lymphatic vascularization is little developed and poorly understood. In some mammals, a lymphatic efferent pathway runs along the central arteriole of the white pulp. This pathway may be the immigration route of lymphocytes in these species.

## RED PULP

We have seen that the red pulp contains vessels, venous sinuses, and Billroth's cords. These cords consist of a reticular fiber network that supports the star-shaped cells that cling to the sinus walls. Some of these star-shaped cells are fixed macrophages, which play an important role in eliminating sick cells and particles in the blood. The cellular network thus formed between sinuses contains mobile cells, including, in variable proportions, depending on the functional state of the spleen, numerous macrophages with inner debris, plasma cells, lymphocytes, erythrocytes, and granulocytes. The spleen is a hematopoietic organ in the embryo, and even in the adult for certain mammalian species. In the latter case, it contains erythroblastic islets, young cells of the myeloid lineage, and megakaryocytes. The red pulp also plays a role in the capture of antigens that are initially bound to macrophages in the marginal zone and the rest of the red pulp.

## MARGINAL ZONE

The marginal zone is an intermediate area between the red and white pulps and contains numerous sinuses oriented concentrically around the periarterial zone. Its proximity to the arterial influx explains why cells and/or antigens injected into the systemic circulation are very rapidly accumulated. It contains more lymphocytes and plasma cells than does the red pulp. It contains the zone of exchange with the white pulp. The walls of the marginal sinuses in the marginal zone have the same function as postcapillary venules in lymph nodes. Thus, lymphocytes labeled with tritiated thymidine and injected into the systemic circulation are found in the marginal zone within 15 to 30 min and are present in the periarterial zone of the white pulp within 24 hr. Red pulp and marginal zone contain both B and T lymphocytes (mixed zones).

## WHITE PULP

The white pulp is organized around central arteries. Lymphocytes that surround these arteries are enclosed in a reticular network that constitutes several peripheral layers and thereby isolate this periarterial zone from the marginal zone. The reticular network contains several "windows" that permit cellular and particle exchanges between the periarterial and marginal zones. The periarterial lymphocyte layer is composed essentially of small and medium lymphocytes. The periarterial reticular layer includes lymphoid follicles with their germinal centers distributed excentrically to the central artery. Ramification of this artery ensures the vascularization of the follicles, whose structure is similar to that described above for lymph node follicles. Splenic follicles are oriented in such a way that the light zone of the germinal center and the lymphoid crown are turned toward the red pulp; the fertile zone is oriented toward the central artery.

As in lymph nodes, the white pulp of the spleen contains thymus-dependent and -independent zones. The periarterial thymus-dependent areas are depleted of lymphocytes in neonatally thymectomized mice and in mice thymectomized, irradiated, and bone marrow reconstituted. Conversely, the external lymphoid sheath and follicles are thymus independent.

## MODIFICATIONS OF THE SPLEEN DURING IMMUNIZATION

Antibody production is associated with numerous modifications of splenic red and white pulps. Antigen binding occurs first, almost immediately in the red pulp and in the marginal zone at the level of the dendritic projections of reticular cells. The antigen is very rapidly concentrated in the marginal zone and after 2 hr is found in the white pulp at the periphery of lymphoid follicles. Antigen movements inside the germinal center occur as described (see sect. V.). Within 24 hr, the marginal zone is cleared of antigen, which is then concentrated in the germinal centers. The thymus-dependent periarteriolar zone of the white pulp, however, remains free of antigen. The cellular events that accompany or follow antigen binding in the spleen involve various organ compartments: the appearance of blast cells in the thymus-dependent periarteriolar zone, cellular proliferation and the appearance of young plasma cells in the germinal centers and of intermediate and mature plasma cells in the germinal centers in the marginal zone, and in the red pulp. Cellular events in the white pulp precede those that occur in the red pulp and in the marginal zone. The intensity and rapidity of modifications within the thymus-dependent areas, lymphoid follicles, and their germinal centers vary according to the route of immunization and the primary or secondary nature of the response.

## VII.  TONSILS

Tonsils are lymphoid organs circumferentially placed around the pharynx. In man, the palatine tonsils are located between the columns of the soft palate; lingual tonsils are located at the back of the ventral tongue; tubal tonsils are present adjacent to eustachian tubes; and the pharyngeal tonsils are located on the posterior wall of the pharynx. Taken together, these tonsils constitute Waldeyer's ring. Tonsils are lymphoid aggregates that contain lymphoid follicles with germinal centers identical to those of the lymph nodes. Their light zone is oriented toward the epithelium. Tonsillar tissue is immediately adjacent to malphighian-type epithelium, whose crypts penetrate deeply into the lymphoid tissue. Immunofluorescence studies show that IgA and IgG cells are preferentially located in the mucosa, whereas IgM cells are found in the germinal centers.

## VIII.  GUT-ASSOCIATED LYMPHOID SYSTEM*

### ANATOMY

There are three general localizations of lymphoid cells in the gut: the digestive mucosa itself; lymphoid organs regularly distributed along the small intestine, ending in the vicinity of the appendix (when grouped together within the small

* This section has been authored by D. Guy-Grand.

intestine, these organs constitute Peyer's patches at the antemesenteric edge of the intestine; rodents have nine to 11 Peyer's patches, but in man their number varies according to age, reaching a maximum of approximately 300 at 12 years); and mesenteric lymph nodes that are distributed throughout the mesentery.

### Digestive Mucosa

The intestinal mucosa (Figs. 2.8 and 2.9) includes connective tissue, lamina propria that separates Lieberkühn's glands, which underlie the small bowel villi, and an external epithelium. The lamina propria in adults contains numerous plasma cells and T lymphocytes. Only IgA-type plasma cells are found in the mouse and the rat. In man, plasma cells are mostly IgA, but there are also some IgM and IgG plasma cells. Lymphocytes are distributed among epithelial cells, usually adjacent to the basement membrane. These lymphocytes do not contain surface immunoglobulins detectable by immunofluorescence, and this fact suggests a thymic origin. This suggestion has been confirmed by evidence, in mice, that they bind rabbit anti-T heterospecific antisera.

### Peyer's Patches

Peyer's patches were once considered the bursal equivalent of mammals. They are, in fact, a peripheral lymphoid organ that contains both B and T cells (Fig. 2.8). They make their appearance late in fetal life (man) or only after birth (mouse). In the adult, they consist of lymphoid follicles with very large germinal centers.

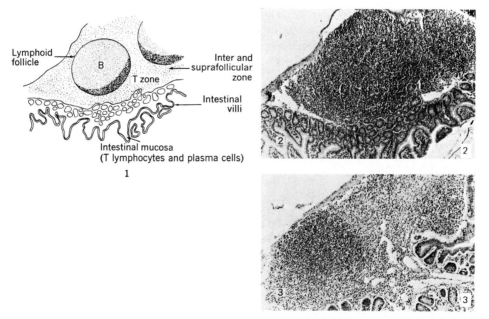

**Fig. 2.8** Peyer's patch in the mouse. 1 & 2: Structure of a Peyer's patch in the normal mouse. 3: Nude mouse Peyer's patch. Absence of germinal centers and lymphoid depletion of inter- and suprafollicular zones.

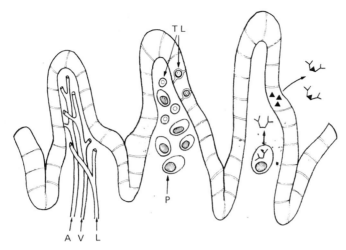

**Fig. 2.9** Intestinal villi. A, artery; V, vein; L, lymphatic; P, plasma cell; TL, T lymphocyte.

As in lymph nodes, the germinal centers contain a few T lymphocytes; however, the great majority are rapidly dividing B cells (it is possible to label them in 1 hr in vitro by adding tritiated thymidine). They are immature cells without plasma cell differentiation. Half of them bear α chains on their surface. Adjacent to the follicles of Peyer's patches, the flattened mucous membrane contains both T and B lymphocytes interspersed among epithelial cells. Follicles are separated by mucosal areas coated with T cell-infiltrated villi. These areas are extremely hypoplastic in nude mice and in neonatally thymectomized mice. A few IgA, IgM, and IgG plasma cells are located at the periphery of the patches.

### Mesenteric Lymph Nodes

Mesenteric lymph nodes have the same structure as other lymph nodes, including a superficial thymus-independent cortex and a deep cortex that contains T cells and a plasma cell-rich medulla. Unlike peripheral (and axillary or popliteal) lymph nodes, mesenteric lymph nodes experience constant antigenic stimulation, as indicated by the number and size of germinal centers found in the superficial cortex and the medulla. Half of these rapidly dividing B cells of mesenteric lymph nodes contain α chains (analogous to Peyer's patches); medullary plasma cells are mostly of the IgA type.

Lymphatic vessels connect the various gut-associated lymphoid organs. The lymph that drains the intestinal wall is collected in centrovillous lymphatic channels that join to form a subserous network, particularly dense at the level of Peyer's patches. This network then gives rise to lymphatic trunks that constitute the efferent vessel of mesenteric lymph nodes. Nearly all gut-produced lymph is thus carried to mesenteric lymph nodes. Efferent vessels of mesenteric nodes form a unique network that opens directly into the thoracic duct. Only the lymph from the lower colon connects to lateroaortic and inguinal nodes. Thus, intestinal lymph, after remaining in the mesenteric nodes, enters the thoracic duct and proceeds to the venous and arterial circulations.


# CYCLE OF IgA-BEARING CELLS

IgA plasma cells in the lamina propria are mature short-lived cells (4- to 5-day half-life in the mouse) that are also secretory. Precursors of these plasma cells, recognized by the presence of α immunoglobulins, are found in germinal centers of Peyer's patches and in mesenteric lymph nodes. It is possible to repopulate IgA plasma cells in irradiated rabbits by injecting cells from Peyer's patches. Proliferation of precursor cells depends on at least two factors: local antigenic stimulation and B- and T-cell collaboration.


## *Precursor Proliferation*

### LOCAL ANTIGENIC STIMULATION

Germinal centers in Peyer's patches and IgA plasma cells (intestine) develop after the appearance of normal intestinal flora (after weaning in the mouse) and are absent in axenic mice. Moreover, only gut immunization induces the appearance of IgA plasma cells in the mouse. In man, antipolio vaccination provokes antibody formation only in the mucous secretion when a living attenuated virus is administered orally.


### NEED FOR B- AND T-CELL COLLABORATION

There are few or no plasma cells in the intestinal mucous membrane of nude mice (there are, however, α precursors). Thymus grafting induces both an increase in T cells in Peyer's patches and the appearance of germinal centers.


## *IgA-Cell Migration*

The IgA cells of the digestive mucosa represent an actively migrating cell population. Transfer experiments and analysis of the cellular content of various lymphoid organs have demonstrated the existence of a true IgA-cell cycle. The precursors leave Peyer's patches by means of lymphatic vessels, undergo a progressive maturation, and transform into IgA-containing mature cells in mesenteric nodes, which then enter the thoracic duct and finally preferentially localize in the intestine and, to a lesser degree, the spleen.

The mechanisms whereby mature IgA cells are attracted to the intestine remains largely hypothetical. Attraction by the antigens of the intestinal flora seems unlikely. It is possible that intestinal receptors for the secretory portion of IgA play a role, but no evidence exists to support this possibility.

T cells appear in the intestinal mucous membrane rather late, after plasma cells. The origin and role of these cells are also unknown.

# IX.  CONCLUSIONS: LYMPHOID SYSTEM ORGANIZATION AND THE HOMING PHENOMENON

The comparative morphologic study of the lymphoid system in normal and thymus-deprived animals and the study of morphologic changes associated with cell-mediated immunity and humoral reactions demonstrate that the peripheral organs contain thymus-dependent and -independent zones. Thymus-dependent zones include the deep cortex of the lymph node (paracortical area), the periarterial lymphoid sheath of the splenic white pulp, and inter- and supra-follicular zones within Peyer's patches. Thymus-independent zones include the follicles of the external cortex of lymph nodes and Peyer's patches, and the follicles of the peripheral zone of the splenic white pulp. Splenic red pulp, particularly the marginal zone and the medulla of lymph nodes, contain predominantly B cells, but they are also areas where B and T cells circulate; these regions are therefore considered to be mixed territories.

The phenomenon of selective migration of B and T lymphocytes to distinct zones of peripheral lymphoid organs is as yet unexplained. This remarkable ability of lymphocytes to recognize and colonize privileged locations was termed "homing," or "ecotaxis," by De Sousa; it has been studied by following the localization in peripheral organs of cells of various origins, after radiolabeling and injection into syngeneic hosts. Thoracic duct and thymic lymphocytes migrate preferentially to thymus-dependent areas. Spleen cells are of heterogeneous composition (B and T cells) and distribute in several B and T peripheral compartments. Lymph node cells essentially migrate to thymus-dependent areas, but a certain proportion of cells migrate to follicles of the external cortex. Bone marrow cells migrate to thymus-independent areas, the red pulp of the spleen and lymph node medullary cords. Some marrow cells, poorly differentiated, return to the bone marrow as myeloid cells.

Several hypotheses have been proposed to explain "homing." Structural differences in the reticular network of the various compartments have been suggested. The looser web seen in thymus-dependent zones might select out a particularly mobile cell type. Chemotaxis, which plays a role in the mobilization of certain cells (like polymorphs), has not been demonstrated for lymphocytes. The property of cellular adherence could also play a role, because thymus-dependent cells, which are nonadherent, show a different mobility than that of thymus-independent cells (which are adherent). A current theory is intervention of membrane receptors that are able to fix lymphocytes onto privileged sites, particularly at the level of endothelial cells of postcapillary venules. It is interesting to note that alteration of surface receptors of thoracic duct lymphocytes by neuraminidase or trypsin prevents normal migration of these cells and their homing into spleen and lymph nodes. Conversely, such treatment augments their nonspecific localization into the liver and lungs. The effects of neuraminidase, which splits off the sialic acid terminals from carbohydrates, indicate that the membrane carbohydrates probably play an important role in the phenomenon of homing. Hepatic cells bear receptors which bind glycoproteins which have lost their sialic acid terminal and the modification of cell migration induced by neuraminidase may be associated with preferential fixation of neuraminidase-treated cells by the hepatocytes. Even if the role of sialic acid residues is not entirely specific, its importance is illustrated by the observation that any virus that is capable of splitting sialic acid may cause profound alterations of lymphocyte migration patterns. Treatment in vitro with trypsin also modifies lymphocyte migration.

Thoracic duct lymphocytes treated in vitro with this enzyme and then reinjected are unable to migrate toward the regional lymph node and recirculate. This block of specific migration toward the lymph node is reversible by incubation at 37°C, and this reversibility implies protein synthesis. Therefore, T lymphocytes in the thoracic duct carry on their surface trypsin-sensitive receptors, which control their ability to traverse the walls of the postcapillary venules of lymph nodes. In contrast, it is interesting to note that the migration of lymphocytes to the spleen is not modified by trypsin and, thus, probably depends on receptors differing from those controlling migration into lymph nodes. A similar mechanism has been advanced for B lymphocytes that are rich in receptors for the Fc fragment of IgG and the third factor of complement. The complement system might also play a role in follicular aggregation of lymphocytes. The "homing" phenomenon, which determines the nature and organization of the peripheral lymphoid system, may, thus, have several mechanisms.

# BIBLIOGRAPHY

BRYANT B. J. Thymic and bursal microenvironments in the context of alternative pathways of immunogenesis. *In* L. Brent and J. Holborow, Eds., Progress in immunology. II. Vol. 3. Amsterdam, 1974, North Holland, p. 5.

COTTIER H., SCHINDLER R., and CONGDON C. C. (Ed.) Germinal centers in immune responses. New York, 1967, Springer.

DYMINSKI J. W, FORBES J., GEBHARDT B., NAKAO Y., KONDA S., and SMITH R. T. Relationship between structure and function of human and mouse thymus cell subpopulations. *In* L. Brent and J. Holborow, Eds., Progress in immunology. II. Vol. 3, Amsterdam, 1974, North Holland, p. 35.

FAHEY K. J. Immunological reactivity in the foetus and the structure of foetal lymphoid tissues. *In* L. Brent and J. Holborow, Eds., Progress in Immunology. II. Vol. 3, Amsterdam, 1974, North Holland, p. 49.

FIORE-DONATI L. and HANNA M. G. (Eds.) Lymphatic tissue and germinal centers in immune response. Adv. Exp. Med. Biol., Vol. 5. New York, 1969, Plenum Press.

HALL J. G. Observations on the migration and localization of lymphoid cells. *In* L. Brent and J. Holborow, Eds., Progress in Immunology. II. Vol. 3, Amsterdam, 1974, North Holland, p. 15.

JANKOVIC B. D. and ISAKOVIC K. (Eds.) Microenvironmental aspects of immunity. Adv. Exp. Med. Biol., Vol. 29. New York, 1973, Plenum Press.

LINDAHL-KIESSLING K., ALM G., and HANNA M. G. (Eds.) Morphological and functional aspects of immunity. New York, 1971, Plenum Press.

METCALF D. and MOORE A. J. S. Haemopoietic cells. Amsterdam, 1971, North Holland.

OWEN J. J. T. Ontogeny of the immune system. *In* L. Brent and J. Holborow, Eds., Progress in immunology. II. Vol. 5, Amsterdam, 1974, North Holland, p. 163.

PARROT D. M. V. and DE SOUSA M. Thymus dependent and thymus-independent populations: origin, migratory pattern and lifespan. Clin. Exp. Immunol., 1971, *8*, 663.

DE SOUSA M. Ecology of thymus dependency. Contemp. Topics Immunobiol., 1973, *2*, 119.

WEISS L. The cells and tissues of the immune system. Structure, functions, interactions. Englewood Cliffs, N.J., 1972, Prentice Hall, 252 p.

WEISSMAN I. L. Development and distribution of Ig-bearing cells. Transpl. Rev., 1975.

## ORIGINAL ARTICLES

CLARK J. L. Jr. Incorporation of sulfate by the mouse thymus; its relation to secretion by medullary epithelial cells and to thymic lymphopoiesis. J. Exp. Med., 1968, *128*, 927.

DAVIES A. J. S., CARTER J. L., LEUCHARS E., WALLIS V., and KOLLER P. C. The Morphology of immune reactions in normal, thymectomized and reconstituted mice. I. The response to sheep erythrocytes. Immunology, 1969, *16*, 57.

GOLDSCHNEIDER F. and McGREGOR D. D. Migration of lymphocytes and thymocytes in the rat. I. The route of migration from blood to spleen and lymph nodes. J. Exp. Med., 1968, *127*, 155.

GOWANS J. L. The recirculation of lymphocytes from blood to lymph in the rat. J. Physiol., London, 1959, *146*, 54.

GUY-GRAND D., GRISCELLI C., and VASSALI P. The gut associated lymphoid system; nature and properties of the large dividing cells. Eur. J. Immunol., 1974, *4*, 435.

JOLLY J. La bourse de Fabricius et les organes lympho-épithéliaux. Arch. Anat. Micr. Morph. Exp., 1915, *16*, 363.

NOSSAL G. J. V., ADA G. L., AUSTIN C. M., and PYE J. Antigens in immunity. VIII. Localization of [125]I labelled antigens in the secondary response. Immunology, 1965, *9*, 349.

PAPIERNIK M. Correlation of lymphocyte transformation and morphology in the human fetal thymus. Blood, 1970, *4*, 470.

RAVIOLA E. and KARNOVSKY M. J. Evidence for a blood-thymus barrier using electron opaque tracers. J. Exp. Med., 1972, *136*, 466.

Chapter 3

# LYMPHOID CELLS

**Jean-François Bach and Félix Reyes**

I.    DEFINITIONS

II.    DEMONSTRATION OF LYMPHOID CELL INTERVEN-
TION IN IMMUNE REACTIONS

III.    LYMPHOCYTE ORIGIN

IV.    LYMPHOCYTE MORPHOLOGY

V.    PHYSICAL PROPERTIES OF LYMPHOCYTES

VI.    LYMPHOCYTE LIFE-SPAN

VII.    LYMPHOCYTE CIRCULATION AND RECIRCULATION

VIII.    LYMPHOBLASTIC TRANSFORMATION

## I. DEFINITIONS

Lymphoid cells are responsible for specific humoral or cell-mediated immunity. They are not, however, usually identified on the basis of these specific functions, but rather on morphologic criteria. Lymphoid cells include lymphocytes, lymphoblasts, and plasma cells. Lymphocytes have a characteristically high nuclear to cytoplasmic ratio; their cytoplasm contains ribosomes and few or no lysosomes. Their size is highly variable; they are usually classified as small, medium, or large. However, classification on the basis of size is merely arbitrary, particularly because there is no correlation between size and function and also because variation in size represents a continuum (as opposed to a trimodal distribution). Lymphoblasts are large cells with a basophilic cytoplasm and a large nucleus. Plasma cells are also large (12 to 16 $\mu$m in diameter in man), either round or oval, and have an excentric nucleus that contains coarse chromatin; the cytoplasm is deeply basophilic and is rich in mitochondria and ergastoplasm.

    It has not been demonstrated that all lymphocytes are immunocompetent. This point is hard to resolve, particularly because the morphologic criteria by which lymphocytes are defined are not very specific. There is no apparent transformation between lymphocytes and other blood cell lineages, including macrophages. On the other hand, the small lymphocyte is not an "end stage" cell, as had been earlier thought. It is now known that under various influences, small lymphocytes may give rise to younger-appearing blastlike cells.

## II.  DEMONSTRATION OF LYMPHOID CELL INTERVENTION IN IMMUNE REACTIONS

Lymphocyte involvement in immunity was suspected after the demonstration that highly purified lymphocyte preparations were able to induce a graft-versus-host (GvH) reaction and were able to transmit immunologic memory, delayed hypersensitivity (DH), or graft immunity to irradiated animals. Gowans' experiments (in 1964) showed that removal of large numbers of lymphocytes (by thoracic duct cannulation in the rat) depressed antibody production; with readministration of "pure" thoracic duct lymphocytes, the immunocompetence of irradiated rats was restored. This finding provided definitive evidence of the exclusive role of lymphocytes in specific immunity. The subsequent introduction of numerous in vitro cellular immunity techniques, including lymphocytotoxicity, macrophage migration inhibition, or the mixed lymphocyte reaction (which will be discussed later), showed an essential role of lymphocytes in all steps of the specific immune response, even though other cells (phagocytes, monocytes, and mast cells) may play an important role in induction or in the nonspecific expression of certain immune responses. The localization of immunoglobulins inside of plasma cells by means of immunofluorescence showed that they were antibody-producing cells; this function is not, however, exclusive to these cells, because lymphocytes have also been shown to produce antibodies.

## III.  LYMPHOCYTE ORIGIN

Lymphocytes originate in primitive hemopoietic stem cells of the bone marrow, as do other blood cells.

### HEMOPOIETIC STEM CELLS

Hemopoietic stem cells give rise to various cell lines (erythrocytes, granulocytes, monocytes, lymphocytes, and platelets). Their capacity to undergo extensive proliferation ensures the production of more differentiated cells and permits constant replacement. The first stem cells found in the fetus are located in the yolk sac and (probably after migration from the yolk sac) are then seen in the liver, the spleen, and finally in the bone marrow, where they persist throughout adult life.

## METHODS FOR STUDYING STEM CELLS

Three techniques allow direct study of hemopoietic stem cells: the in vivo colony technique of Till and McCulloch, Kennedy's technique, which is an adaptation of the preceding technique to immunocompetent cells, and the granulocyte and macrophage in vitro colony technique. The in vivo colony technique described by Till and McCulloch consists of injecting a cell suspension that contains stem cells (colony-forming units, CFUs) into lethally irradiated syngeneic mice. Eight to 10 days later, hemopoietic colonies appear in the spleen and may be quantified by microscopic counting techniques. Microscopy of the colonies shows the presence of erythrocytes and/or granulocytes. Macrophages and lymphocytes are always distributed homogeneously throughout the colonies. The colony technique has been modified by Kennedy to study antibody-producing cell precursors. In this technique, a cell suspension is injected simultaneously with sheep red blood cells into irradiated mice; 8 days later, the spleen is removed and, after sectioning, areas that contain hemolysis plaque-forming cells are enumerated. The in vitro colony technique of Metcalf consists of culturing stem cells in a gel medium. These cells (colony-forming cells, CFC) proliferate under the influence of various factors, including a humoral "colony-stimulating factor" (CSF) for granulocytes and erythropoietin for erythrocytes. These colonies, however, contain only polymorphs and macrophages but no lymphoid cells. B-cell colonies have recently been obtained in the presence of mercaptoethanol by Metcalf, and T-cell colonies in the presence of phytohemagglutinin.

## MULTIPOTENTIALITY OF STEM CELLS

Each hemopoietic stem cell (as assessed by CFUs) can potentially differentiate into one of several blood cell lines. Colonies formed in the spleen of irradiated mice after injection of bone marrow cells may include erythrocytes, lymphocytes, polymorphs, macrophages, and megakaryocytes (even if numerous colonies contain one predominant lineage). The CFUs clonal nature has been demonstrated by use of chromosomal markers, especially radiation-induced chromosomal lesions: all cells from one dividing CFUs bear the same chromosomal marker, which is conclusive evidence of monoclonality when the chromosomal lesion is sufficiently complex to be considered unique. At variance with CFUs, CFCs are not multipotential but already committed to a precise blood-cell lineage.

The factors that determine stem cell differentiation to one or another blood cell lineage, or to simple production of identical daughter cells, remain for the most part unknown. An essential role in conditioning these cells toward specific stem cell differentiation is played by the tissue microenvironment at the time of initial cell differentiation. Humoral factors may also play a role in late phases of cell maturation. We will later analyze the various stages involved in B- and T-lymphocyte maturation.

# IV. LYMPHOCYTE MORPHOLOGY

## INTRODUCTION

The morphology of lymphocytes of different animal species was studied long before the function of these cells had been clearly established. Thus, observations made by light or electron microscopy have been globally applied to different functional classes of lymphocytes. The recent demonstration of lymphocyte duality, namely, T and B cells, has prompted new studies to establish morphologic differences between these two lymphocyte populations (see p. 64). The most classic descriptions are, however, essentially valid, at least for lymphocytes not actually implicated in an active immune response, namely, the small lymphocytes, whether of T or B origin. These descriptions were made by light or electron microscopy by use of ultrathin cell sections. With very few reservations, similar interpretations obtained by different methods have been made when lymphocytes from numerous animal species were studied, and within one given species for cells of different lymphoid tissues; the common feature was a mononucleated cell with a high nuclear to cytoplasmic ratio.

## LIGHT MICROSCOPY

### Smear Examination

On smears of human blood stained by Giemsa, lymphocytes are in majority represented by cells of 7 to 8 μm diameter, that is, "small lymphocytes." Other lymphocytes are larger in size (9 to 15 μm) and are called "medium" or "large" lymphocytes; the latter are sometimes difficult to distinguish from monocytes. The functional significance of the "large" lymphocytes is still imprecise; they probably represent a step in the maturation of some small lymphocytes.

Small lymphocytes, which are more prevalent in blood and the thoracic duct, constitute morphologically a characteristic homogeneous population (Fig. 3.1). The nucleus fills most of the cell, except for a narrow rim of slightly basophilic cytoplasm (blue on Giemsa staining) in which no structures are usually visible. The nucleus is round or vaguely kidney-shaped (reniform) and has a dense appearance due to condensed chromatin deposits; nucleoli are rarely observed.

In large lymphocytes, the area of visible cytoplasm is larger. The cytoplasm is pale and discretely basophilic; one may observe occasional lysosomes, which appear in the form of "azurophilic" red granules. In the nucleus, the chromatin is also lumpy in distribution but is slightly less dense than in small lymphocytes.

### Phase-Contrast Microscopy Examination

The phase-contrast microscopy technique gives supplementary information on cytoplasmic content and permits observation of living, that is, motile cells. In the concavity of the kidney-shaped nucleus of small lymphocytes, a light cytoplasmic zone, called the "centrosome," is seen that contains Golgi's apparatus

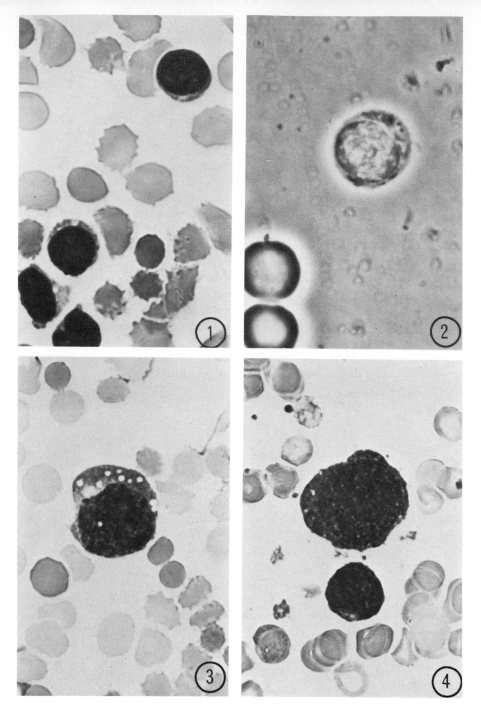

**Fig. 3.1** Immunocyte morphology by light microscopy. I: Small lymphocytes in normal human blood on smears (×900). 2: Small lymphocyte shown by phase-contrast microscopy. At the bottom are two erythrocytes (×1250). 3: T immunoblast obtained in vitro by use of phytohemagglutinin (smears). The cytoplasm, whose grey color on this picture corresponds to the basophilia observed on colored smears, contains numerous vacuoles. Compare size to that of small lymphocytes in 1 (×900). 4: B immunoblast observed in a patient with lymphoma. The appearance of this cell is identical to that obtained in vitro by use of polyclonal mitogen. Intense basophilia gives the immunoblast its dark color, similar to that of the nucleus. At the bottom is a small lymphocyte (×900).

and centrioles. The centrosome is surrounded by numerous mitochondria, which appear as more or less elongated, small black granules. In large lymphocytes, one may also see lysosomes that are difficult to distinguish from mitochondria. In some lymphocytes, study by phase-contrast microscopy reveals a spheric and birefringent inclusion of 0.5 μm diameter, the "Gall body," of unknown significance.

At variance with blood monocytes and polymorphs, lymphocytes are unable to spread or adhere to their glass support. They are, however, able to move and form various patterns, the most remarkable of which is the so-called hand mirror. The posterior cytoplasmic expansion (the mirror handle), called the "uropod," contains the centrosome and mitochondria. It is generally conceded that the uropod is responsible for contact between the motile lymphocyte and other cells. It may therefore represent the "privileged" contact area between lymphocytes and target cells of critical interest in the cytotoxicity phenomenon. It is believed that the uropod membrane corresponds to the area where surface determinants are redistributed and concentrated in the capping phenomenon (see p. 82).

## ELECTRON MICROSCOPY

Electron microscopy has provided much information on the status of intracellular organelles and correlations between cell organization and its functional state. However, this technique can be applied only to a tiny portion of each cell, thus limiting the available information in a given ultrathin section. In most sectional planes, small lymphocytes show a very characteristic aspect that confirms light microscopy data (Fig. 3.2): the nucleus contains numerous lumps of condensed chromatin (or heterochromatin). A small nucleolus is often seen surrounded by heterochromatin (hence, the difficulty in observing it by light microscopy). The nucleus is surrounded by an ergastoplasmic sheet (or perinuclear space) interrupted by nuclear pores located between heterochromatin clumps. In the cytoplasm, there are occasional short ergastoplasmic layers, sometimes edged with ribosomes. Ribosomes composed of cytoplasmic RNA are present mostly as monoribosomes scattered throughout the cytoplasm. Very few polyribosomes (aggregated ribosomes) are present.

The Golgi apparatus is poorly developed, represented only by some saccules and vesicles. A few dense granules, which are lysosomes, may be found in this area. According to the plane of sections, centrioles with radiating microtubules may be seen. Mitochondria are numerous. The large lymphocytes have a comparable structure. It is, in fact, difficult to appreciate the cell size in ultrathin sections. All intermediate sizes between small and large lymphocytes can be observed.

These ultrastructural features, characterized by limited development of organelles involved in protein synthesis (monoribosomes, ergastoplasm) and the dense chromatin pattern, long suggested that lymphocytes were relatively inert (end-stage cells). In fact, these are characteristics of cells involved in antigen recognition; that is, cells that synthesize antigen-specific surface receptors, including surface Ig in B lymphocytes. After the specific antigen recognition

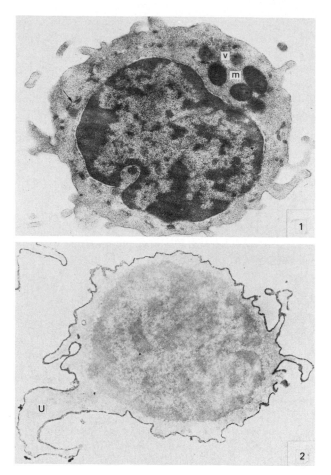

**Fig. 3.2** Small lymphocytes. 1: Section of a human peripheral blood small lymphocyte shown by electron microscopy. The nucleus contains dense blocks of heterochromatin. In addition to the perinuclear space, one observes only short segments of endoplasmic reticulum (arrow). The cytoplasm contains dispersed monoribosomes (m, mitochondria; v, Golgi vesicles) (×11,500). 2: Section of a human peripheral blood lymphocyte fixed in movement shows the classic picture of a "handle mirror" (u, uropod). In addition, this cell bears surface Ig, revealed by peroxidase-coupled antibodies as a fine black line that surrounds the whole microvilli-spiked cell surface. This cell is B lymphocyte. In this experiment, surface Ig redistribution (normally induced by anti-Ig antibody) is not observed because the cell has been previously fixed (×12,000).

step, or after polyclonal stimulation by mitogens, these cells are capable of considerable morphologic change with appearance of intense synthetic activity (see p. 52).

In some cases, electron microscopy of "small lymphocytes" reveals very large amounts of ribosomes and ergastoplasm. These cells are not numerous but are present in blood and the thoracic duct. Their basophilia may be difficult to appreciate on smears because of the small amount of visible cytoplasm. These cells probably correspond to a particular stage in the maturation process of some B lymphocytes.

## RECENT MORPHOLOGIC DATA

Since the demonstration of the dichotomy (B and T cells) of the lymphoid system, there have been various attempts to distinguish between the two cell populations morphologically. The differences observed at the level of intracellular organelles by light and electron microscopy are very slight however.

A denser appearance of cytoplasm has been described in T lymphocytes, along with a higher content of lysosomes and microfibrils (which are contractile filamentous structures that control cellular movements). More recently, examination of human lymphocyte suspensions by scanning electron microscopy has revealed a clear morphologic dichotomy between microvilli-bearing and smooth cells (Figs. 3.2 and 3.3). Immunologic identification of these cells by immunoelectron microscopy showed the villous nature of the B-lymphocyte surfaces, as contrasted with the smooth surface of thymocytes and circulating T lymphocytes. These differences are not, however, absolute. These observations are dependent on some technical conditions (such as collection and handling of cells) and are therefore still controversial.

It seems that the appearances of these cells are greatly influenced by technical considerations and the metabolic state of the cells, whatever their origin. All technical circumstances being equal, however, including a minimum of in vitro manipulation (without cell separation), the B lymphocytes of human peripheral blood still appear to have a microvillous surface. A further source of controversy arises from the studies performed on the lymphocytes of patients suffering from certain lymphoproliferative disorders. We now know that the B lymphocytes in certain lymphatic leukemias do not possess a villous surface structure, probably because they are at a different stage of maturation from those of normal human peripheral blood lymphocytes. These studies underline the erroneous interpretation that may be generated by solely morphologic examination of T and B cells in human proliferative disorders. For normal cells, however, it is interesting to compare the microvillous features of the B-lymphocyte surface with their tendency to adhere to certain substrates, such as nylon fibers (which also retain monocytes and polymorphs).

It has been noted that B and T lymphocytes are not capable of spreading on a glass slide, which is a characteristic feature of phagocytic cells. The absence of phagocytosis (as defined by ingestion of large particles) by lymphocytes does not preclude, however, their property of endocytosis of various macromolecules. A striking example of this property is provided by the membrane behavior of B lymphocytes during membrane Ig redistribution induced by anti-Ig antibodies (capping phenomenon). The ultrastructural observation of this phenomenon shows complexes grouped at a cell pole that are interiorized as pinocytotic vesicles, followed by migration toward the Golgi apparatus region, which is at the level of the uropod in motile lymphocytes. On ultrathin sections, the uropod surface then appears irregular and packed with microvilli.

Cytochemical studies have been performed to search for enzymatic activities

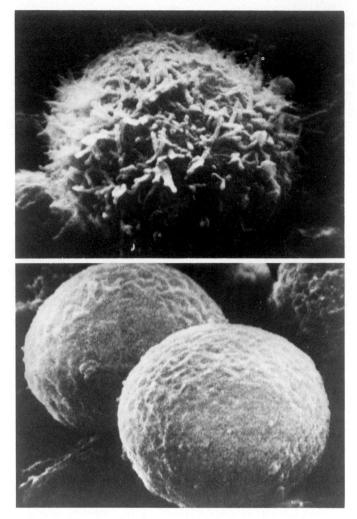

**Fig. 3.3** Rough (*top*) and smooth (*bottom*) lymphocytes seen by scanning microscopy. The controversial interpretation of these pictures is discussed above. (From A. Polliack, N. Lampen, B. D. Clarkson et al., J. Exp. Med. 1973, *138*, 607.)

that might be characteristic of lymphocytes, as is the case for other myeloid cell lines. Various hydrolases and esterases have been demonstrated.

Using standard cytochemical methods, the T cells of acute or chronic leukemias contain granules that stain positively for hydrolases as well as for β-glucuronidase and acid phosphatase. In addition, esterase activity, different from that present in monocytes, is present in normal T lymphocytes in the form of a single inclusion body close to the Golgi region. Finally, the absence of myeloperoxidase and other types of peroxidase activity may help to distinguish lymphocytes from cells of the monocyte-macrophage series (in ordinary light cytochemistry and ultracytochemistry). It is also possible to demonstrate, by a cytochemical reaction, the presence of glycogen particles scattered throughout the cytoplasm of some normal peripheral blood lymphocytes; unless cytochemical methods are employed, these are often confused with ribosomes.

# V.  PHYSICAL PROPERTIES OF LYMPHOCYTES

Lymphocytes have heterogeneous physical properties, but overall these properties are appreciably different from those of other blood cell elements. These characteristics may be used to distinguish lymphocytes and their subpopulations. The physical properties that have been studied most extensively are size, density, adherence, and charge.

## SIZE AND DENSITY

It is possible to separate cells according to size by velocity sedimentation, which involves cellular movement by simple gravity across a gradient of increasing density, utilizing, for example, bovine serum albumin. The gradient's purpose is to minimize turbulence. Cell size may be quantified directly under the microscope by use of automatic counters, such as the "coulter counter."

The cells may also be separated according to density by equilibrium centrifugation in a linear or discontinuous density gradient (by use of bovine serum albumin or Ficoll). The cells are centrifuged until each cell reaches a gradient level whose density matches its own specific gravity. Cell density generally relates to nuclear size; the lighter cells show a lower nuclear to cytoplasmic ratio.

Size and density studies that employ velocity or density gradients have shown significant lymphocyte heterogeneity. In practice, as we shall see later, T-cell subpopulations may be distinguished by these two criteria (p. 79).

## ADHERENCE

Lymphocytes may adhere to glass, plastic, cotton, or nylon. Interestingly (we shall come back to this point), all lymphocyte subpopulations, defined by origin or maturation, do not show identical adherence properties (see p. 79).

## CHARGE

Lymphocytes placed in an electric field migrate at different rates according to the amount of negative charge present on their surface. Lymphocyte electrophoresis may be helpful in separating lymphocyte subpopulations.

## LYMPHOCYTE ISOLATION

Isolation of lymphocytes is the first step in any cellular immunology experiment. In the animal, one may use lymphoid organs, such as thymus, spleen, and lymph node, in which 95% or more of cells are lymphoid. In man, the only practical lymphocyte source is the circulating blood. Isolation of blood lympho-cytes requires elimination of red blood cells, polymorphs, platelets, and mon-ocytes, while at the same time minimizing loss of lymphocytes. Loss of numerous lymphocytes is inevitable and is detrimental not only because of the resultant low yield of cells but also because it may select out certain lymphocyte subpopulations.

The usual method employed to isolate lymphocytes consists of placing blood on a mixture of Ficoll and Triosil, which has a density intermediate between that of lymphocytes and polymorphs. After centrifugation, red blood cells and polymorphs cross the Ficoll, leaving behind a ring of mononucleated cells above the Ficoll. This ring essentially contains lymphocytes and monocytes.

Another method involves sedimenting whole blood, either spontaneously or by addition of dextran or Plasmagel, which selectively accelerates red blood cell sedimentation. A leukocyte layer ("buffy coat") is visible above the red blood cells. Here, one finds polymorphs, monocytes, and lymphocytes. Another method is cell filtration through a nylon or cotton fiber column, which retains all of the polymorphs and monocytes but allows passage of a significant percentage of pure lymphocytes. The disadvantages of this technique are its cumbersome nature, poor yield and, above all, the loss of certain lymphocytic subpopulations that contain most of the B lymphocytes and some of the immature T cells.

## VI. LYMPHOCYTE LIFE-SPAN

A cell life-span is the period between two divisions or between a division and death.

### STUDY METHODS

The best method available for study of life-spans consists of incorporating into cells a radiolabeled precursor (e.g., thymidine) during the S phase of DNA synthesis that precedes mitosis and to follow the labeled cells by autoradiography. Labeling of cells with a long life-span (more than 40 days) is accomplished by injecting tritium-labeled thymidine either by constant perfusion or by multiple injections during an 8- to 15-day period. Lymphoid organs are studied by autoradiography 40 days after the last injection, at which time short-lived labeled cells have disappeared. Labeling of short-lived cells is performed by injecting a tritium label by perfusion or by multiple injections over a 5-day period. Lymphoid organs are collected one day after the last injection. The labeled lymphocytes now include most short-lived lymphocytes (less than 6 days old) and a small percentage of long-lived lymphocytes that divided during the 6-day labeling period. These techniques are technically easy, but bias may be introduced because of reutilization of labeled thymidine originating from dead cells.

## SHORT- AND LONG-LIVED LYMPHOCYTES

In his first studies in the rat, Everett showed that a very high percentage of lymphocytes was short-lived. Labeled lymphocytes are, however, still observed when one lengthens the period between labeling and collection of lymphoid organs up to 270 days. One may therefore distinguish (according to Everett) two lymphocyte populations, short-lived cells (less than 2 weeks, average cell life-span of 4 to 5 days) and long-lived cells, which survive several months. This classification is, in fact, very arbitrary, because a marked heterogeneity exists in lymphocyte life-span, including intermediate life-spans of 5 days to several months.

# VII.  LYMPHOCYTE CIRCULATION AND RECIRCULATION

Lymphoid cells are concentrated in primary lymphoid organs (thymus, bone marrow) and peripheral lymphoid organs (spleen, lymph node). Only a small fraction of these cells circulate in the blood. Nonetheless, these circulating lymphocytes are of particular interest, because they recirculate, that is, leave the blood, go to lymph nodes, enter the lymph, and return to the blood via the thoracic duct, within 14 hr (in the rat). An unexpected finding was the passage of some cells directly across endothelial cells of postcapillary venules within lymph nodes and Peyer's patches. By this circuit, some recirculating lymphocytes return to the lymphatic system. Recirculating lymphocytes may also return to the spleen by crossing the endothelial cells of marginal sinuses. This recirculation potentially has considerable physiologic importance, in that lymphocytes may meet and recognize antigens whatever their localization within the organism (Figs. 3.4 and 3.5).

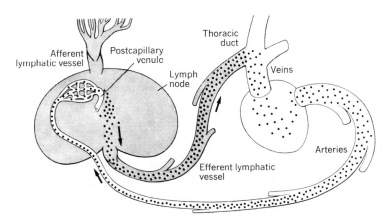

**Fig. 3.4**  Lymphocytic recirculation. (From J. L. Gowans, in R. A. Good and D. W. Fisher, Eds., Immunobiology, Stamford, Conn., 1971, Sinauer, p. 19.)

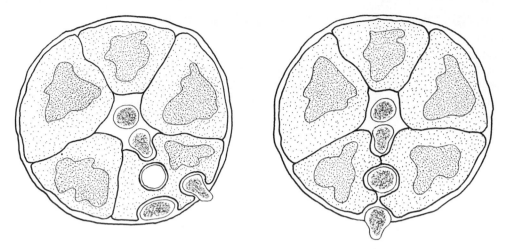

**Fig. 3.5**  Lymphocytic emigration outside postcapillary venules in lymph nodes. It is not known whether lymphocytes cross endothelial cells (*left*) or infiltrate between two adjacent cells (*right*).


## STUDY METHODS

The method most commonly used to study recirculation consists of labeling the cells with $^{51}$Cr or tritiated uridine and reinjecting them into syngeneic recipients. The fate of injected cells may be evaluated by autoradiography or by the total count of each lymphoid organ. It is possible to deplete an animal of recirculating lymphocytes, for example, by thoracic duct cannulation, and to study the effects of this depletion on lymphoid organs.


## RECIRCULATION

Recirculating lymphocytes represent a very small proportion of all lymphocytes and an even smaller percentage of circulating lymphocytes. Recirculating lymphocytes seem to possess special surface receptors that permit interaction with endothelial cells of postcapillary venules. It is interesting to note that this interaction is reversibly inhibited by preincubation of cells with proteolytic and glycolytic enzymes, such as trypsin and neuraminidase. Recirculation is modified by corticosteroids, which seem to prevent the migration of recirculating lymphocytes from blood into lymph nodes, and by *pertussis bacillus* and heparin, which induce, within a few hours, hyperlymphocytosis and lymph-node depopulation, which explain the peripheral lymphocytosis of whooping cough.

Lymphocyte recirculation is also modified by antigenic stimulation. Thus, after intravenous immunization, recirculating lymphocytes are localized to the spleen and, after subcutaneous injection, to regional lymph nodes. Such lymphocytic accumulation contiguous to the antigen site and their very rapid removal from the circulation are not entirely antigen specific but are particularly clear-cut in lymphocytes specific for the injected antigen. Indeed, one or 2 days after injections of sheep red blood cells (SRBC), thoracic duct lymphocytes have a very diminished capacity to transfer anti-SRBC immunity to syngeneic irradiated mice. It is possible that uptake is not specific but that nonantigen-specific lymphocytes are retained for a shorter time close to the antigen site. In addition, it is noteworthy that sensitized lymphocytes, whether lymphoblasts or small lymphocytes, that bear immunologic memory are found in the thoracic duct after antigenic stimulation, although one does not really know whether these cells recirculate.

# VIII.   LYMPHOBLASTIC TRANSFORMATION

## INTRODUCTION

When lymphocytes are incubated with the antigen to which they are sensitized or with nonspecific mitogens, such as PHA, they have the capacity to differentiate and transform into blast cells and to proliferate (Table 3.1). Lymphoblast transformation may be studied in vitro by morphologic or isotopic methods, which involve measuring the incorporation of labeled precursors of DNA, RNA, or proteins whose synthesis is increased during transformation. This remarkable

**Table 3.1   Agents That Induce Lymphocytic Transformation**

Soluble antigens (bacterial, fungal, or viral antigens, pollens, proteins,
     drugs, synthetic polymers of amino acids) in animals sensitized against
     these antigens
Allogeneic cells (mixed-lymphocyte culture)
Phytomitogens (lectins)
     Phytohemagglutinin *(Phaseolus vulgaris)*
     Concanavalin A *(Canavalia ensiformis)*
     Pokeweed mitogen *(Phytolacca americana)*
     Lentil *(Lens culinaris)*
Bacterial products
     Lipopolysaccharide (lipid A)
     Staphylococcal enterotoxin B
     Streptolysin S
     Aggregated tuberculin
     *Nocardia*
Antibodies
     Antilymphocyte
     Anti-immunoglobulin
     Anti-$\beta_2$-microglobulin
     Carbohydrate specific
Antigen-antibody complexes
Miscellaneous
     Sodium metaperiodate
     Heavy metals (zinc, mercury, nickel)
     Proteolytic enzymes (papain)
     $Ca^{2+}$ ionophore A-23187

phenomenon, which proves in itself that small lymphocytes are not end-stage cells, has been the subject of extensive study because it permits study of both antigen and mitogen receptors and the proliferative phase of the immune response. We shall present in detail a description of the morphologic and biochemical events that characterize it.

## MORPHOLOGIC ASPECTS (Fig. 3.6)

The first observations that demonstrated the ability of lymphocytes to transform in vitro under the influence of mitogens were morphologic.

### PHA and Con A Transformation

On stained smears, transformed cells are characterized by increased size (15 to 30 μm in diameter), cytoplasmic basophilia (linked to RNA content), and by the development of vacuoles and numerous lysosomes. These changes are seen as early as the second day of culture and are followed by mitoses that are maximal by 72 hr (Figs. 3.1 and 3.6).

On sections examined by electron microscopy, "large blast cells" have a nucleus that contains very little heterochromatin, limited to a thin marginal layer; it also contains a large nucleolus. The cytoplasm is remarkable in its abundance of ribosomes, grouped in aggregates (polyribosomes). The Golgi apparatus is large; mitochondria are numerous and dilated. In addition, there are a few short ergastoplasmic lamellae. Although these aspects are especially clear-cut after 48 hr of culture, the first changes may be detected earlier. Thus, one may observe within a few hours after PHA addition an augmentation in the size of the nucleous (which corresponds to increased RNA synthesis). The dispersion of nuclear chromatin corresponds to the S phase, that is, DNA synthesis. The increase in cytoplasmic size is present as early as 24 hr. The study of intracytoplasmic organelles shows that transformed cells have acquired, parallel to their lysosome enrichment, properties of endocytosis: one observes numerous pinocytotic vesicles, some of which migrate toward the Golgi region and fuse with lysosomes. In addition, electron microscopy reveals important glycogen aggregates and numerous microfibrils. After the third day, medium and small lymphocytes are present, probably due to division of the transformed cells (Fig. 3.6).

Transformed cells, or "immunoblasts," are remarkably homogeneous. It has been established that, under usual technical conditions, these two lectins preferentially stimulate T lymphocytes of mice and man. For this reason, the ultrastructural aspects just described may be considered characteristic of T immunoblasts. Conversely, different patterns are observed when lymphocytes are stimulated by other mitogens, such as pokeweed, which stimulates both B and T cells.

### Pokeweed Mitogen-Induced Transformation

Morphologic changes induced by pokeweed mitogen have the same kinetics as those described for PHA and Con A. They are also characterized by the presence of large blastlike basophilic cells (Fig. 3.1). Ultrastructural study shows

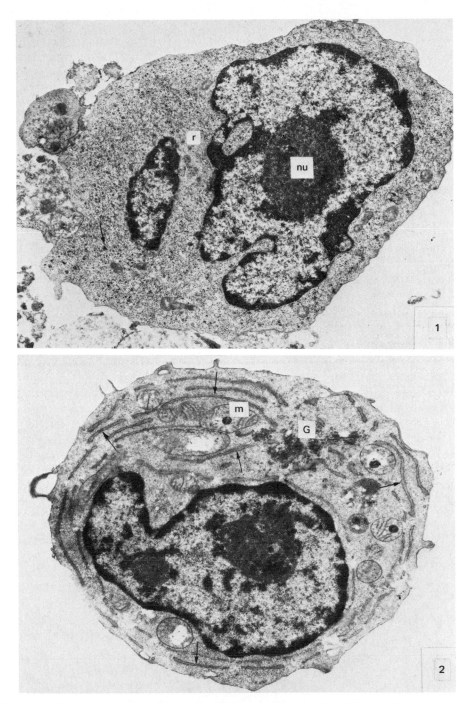

**Fig. 3.6** T and B immunoblasts. 1: T-immunoblast section. The nucleus contains a marginal heterochromatin line and a voluminous nucleolus (nu). Numerous ribosomes (r) (often grouped together) are found in the cytoplasm. One also observes dense glycogen aggregates (arrow). Endoplasmic reticulum lamellae are not numerous ($\times$6750). 2: B immunoblast. On this section, one notes the large mitochondria (m), the importance of the Golgi apparatus (G), and, in particular, the development of endoplasmic reticulum, the lamellae of which are numerous (arrows) ($\times$6750).

two cell types. Some cells have the same characteristics as those observed after PHA or Con A stimulation, whereas others differ by an important development of the ergastoplasm readily apparent in the polyribosome-rich cytoplasm (Fig. 3.6). Hence these cells have already gained the cytoplasmic characteristics of plasma cells; they are considered to be their probable precursors, thus the term "plasmablast" is sometimes used to define them. Similar ultrastructural aspects are also obtained when lymphocytes are cultured in the presence of bacterial lipopolysaccharides (LPS), which selectively stimulate mouse B lymphocytes. Such "plasmablastic" aspects, which probably correspond to an initial step of the B-lymphocyte maturation into plasma cells, have, therefore, for these cells, led to the term "B immunoblasts." Intracytoplasmic immunofluorescence shows that these cells already actively synthesize Ig, particularly IgM, which accumulates in significant amounts in the ergastoplasm (Fig. 3.7). Finally, the B- and T-cell dichotomy corresponds to a morphologic duality of immunoblasts produced after nonspecific mitogen stimulation. However, the LPS model in mice has also shown that the first immunoblasts to be produced are characterized only by a high polyribosome content; endoplasmic reticulum development, as described above, appears as a later event. Therefore early B immunoblasts may have the same ultrastructural features as T immunoblasts. This emphasizes the need for additional immunologic identification for these cells. Such a situation is also found in the studies of some human lymphomas (Fig. 3.8).

Such immunoultrastructural studies have enabled two types of B immunoblasts to be distinguished, one with a poorly developed endoplasmic reticulum, the other with none. In the former, IgM is only detectable in small quantities in the perinuclear space (Fig. 3.8). In contrast, the cytoplasm of the second type of B immunoblast contains IgM distributed in a diffuse fashion among the polyribosomes, and therefore it is not stored in the reticulum for secretory purposes (Fig. 3.9). It is yet undetermined whether these varieties of immunoblasts represent different phases of maturation or are distinct populations.

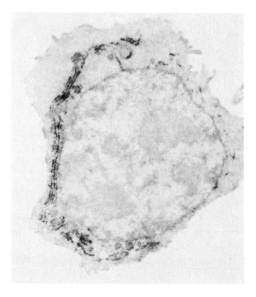

**Fig. 3.7** Cell resulting from pokeweed stimulation. Storage of synthesized IgM is seen in the already developed endoplasmic reticulum. IgM is demonstrated by the use of antibody coupled to plant peroxidase.

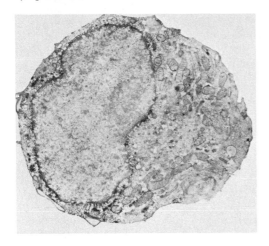

**Fig. 3.8** B immunoblast from a human lymphoma. This large cell does not contain a developed endoplasmic reticulum, but rather dispersed ribosomes. Its B derivation is demonstrated by the detection of immunoglobulin synthesis, which is revealed here by the cytochemical staining of the perinuclear space (an endoplasmic reticulum lamella) in the presence of peroxidase coupled anti-immunoglobulin antibodies ($\times 20,000$).

## BIOCHEMICAL ASPECTS

Most biochemical work that deals with blast transformation concerns PHA stimulation, because this compound facilitates study by the large number of lymphocytes it causes to be transformed. Similar studies are more difficult to perform after antigenic stimulation, because only a small fraction of lymphocytes recognizes the antigen and transforms. After PHA addition, one observes

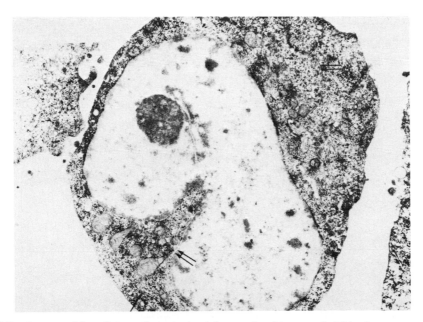

**Fig. 3.9** Immunoblast from a human lymphoma. In this case, IgM is demonstrated to be diffusely present throughout the cytoplasm in association with free polyribosomes or along the occasional lamellae of endoplasmic reticulum (arrows). Note that the lumen of the perivascular space (double arrow) is not stained any more deeply than that of the Golgi apparatus (G).

changes in intralymphocytic levels of cyclic AMP, adenyl cyclase, and cyclic GMP (whose significance is still a matter of controversy), and an increase in calcium influx. One also notes a very rapid increase in lipid turnover, followed by an increase in nucleoprotein phosphorylation (detectable by acridine orange incorporation) and in acetylation of histones. As early as the second hour, there is increased RNA synthesis, particularly in ribosomal RNA. Between 2 and 4 hr after stimulation, protein synthesis increases. At the 36th hour, augmentation of DNA synthesis may be detected, which increases exponentially during the next few days (Fig. 3.10).

## ROLE OF PROLIFERATION

Lymphocyte cultures are generally examined 3 to 7 days after mitogen stimulation. It is always difficult to know the respective roles of transformation and proliferation and that of death of other cells in evaluating blast cell number or DNA incorporation. The existence of proliferation is suggested by the daily exponential increase in lymphoblast numbers and by the augmentation in absolute numbers of cells in culture. By direct demonstration (microcinematographic study), mitosis has been shown to occur about every 12 hr following PHA stimulation, after the second day of culture. Proliferation does not, however, necessarily explain all of the increase in DNA synthesis after the second day. There is a permanent recruitment of new cells, partly under the influence of soluble mediators released by the initially activated lymphocytes. The blastogenic factor is the best known of these mediators. Recent studies have shown that mitogen-induced T cell proliferation was dependent on T cell growth factors (Interleukin 2, see p. 386) produced by mitogen-activated T

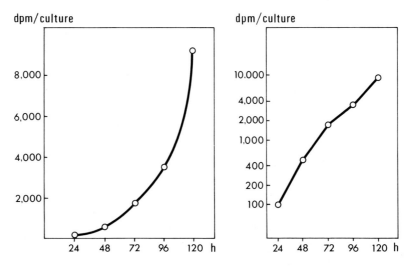

**Fig. 3.10** Incorporation of [14]C-labeled thymidine by human lymphocytes cultured in the presence of tuberculin (purified protein derivative). Experimental values (dpm) are expressed on arithmetic (*left*) and logarithmic (*right*) scales.

cells. Such factors do not induce proliferation in resting small lymphocytes but do so when the cells have been exposed to the mitogen. On the basis of absorption experiments it is assumed that the lectin dependent acquisition of responsiveness to growth factors by resting cells corresponds to the expression of receptors for T cell growth factors. Once the lymphoid cells express such receptors, the presence of the mitogen is no longer needed and the growth factors alone exert their mitogenic activity.

## ROLE OF MACROPHAGES

Highly purified lymphocyte preparations, which contain no monocytes or macrophages, are poorly stimulated in vitro by soluble antigens. They also respond less well to stimulation by allogeneic cells and PHA. Antigen response is normalized by addition of macrophages. It is not clear whether macrophages intervene by presenting antigen to the lymphocytes or whether they act independently of the antigen. The latter has been suggested by substitution of macrophages with the supernatant from macrophage cultures (see chap. 18).

## NATURE OF MITOGEN RECEPTORS

We will not discuss lymphocytic antigen receptors here because they will be dealt with later (see chap. 4). Lectins and heterologous antilymphocytic sera (ALS) receptors are located on the cell surface and are apparently distinct from antigen recognition receptors, both topographically and biochemically. The addition of specific sugars (α-methyl-D-mannoside for Con A) inhibits stimulation, even when added 18 hrs after the mitogen. This is evidence that lectins exert their effects through binding to cell surface saccharide receptors whose structure is similar though not necessarily identical to that of the inhibitory sugars. These saccharide receptors are constituents of glycoproteins and probably also of glycolipids, which serve as important components of cell membranes. Efficient stimulation must provoke receptor cross-linkage, that is multiple bridges that link receptors. Thus, ALS or anti-Ig serum monovalent Fab fragments do not stimulate despite binding to the lymphocyte surface. Insolubilized lectins (the valence of which is increased) would stimulate a larger number of lymphocytes than do soluble lectins; some lymphocyte subpopulations have been claimed to be stimulated only by insolubilized lectins. A final point to be mentioned is that once having bound the mitogen, the receptors undergo redistribution, which concentrates the mitogen at one cell pole (the capping phenomenon).

## REACTIVE CELLS

Various lymphocyte subpopulations do not respond identically to different mitogens. These differences in reactivity are utilized as markers for various subpopulations (see p. 71). The nature and the origin of the cells that respond to the antigen or to allogeneic cells will be discussed later (see p. 73).

## SIGNIFICANCE OF BLAST TRANSFORMATION

Antigen-induced blast transformation is a valuable model for studying antigenic recognition by sensitized lymphocytes; the mixed lymphocyte culture is a unique model of the first phases of allograft reaction. Nonspecific mitogen-induced transformation may represent a useful marker for evaluating various lymphocyte subpopulations. This transformation is not abortive or sterile, because it resembles in many respects antigen-induced stimulation, even beyond the initial differentiation and proliferative phases. It has been demonstrated that nonspecific mitogens may induce true polyclonal activation. Hence, LPS and pokeweed mitogen may stimulate IgM synthesis and secretion, leading to the development of endoplasmic reticulum; Con A may provoke secretion of migration-inhibitory factor and blastogenic factor, and even of suppressor activities on antibody formation. These data suggest that several aspects of lymphocyte response are innate and may be expressed independently of antigenic stimulation, under the influence of binding of various ligands to surface receptors.

## *BIBLIOGRAPHY*

BESSIS M. Cellules du sang normal et pathologique. I vol. Paris, 1972, Masson.

CEBRA J. J., KAMAT R., GEARHART P., ROBERTSON S. M., and TSENG J. The secretory IgA system of the gut. *In* Immunology of the gut. Ciba Foundation Symposium 46, Amsterdam, 1977, Elsevier, p. 5.

COUTINHO A., GRONOWICZ E., MOLLER G., and LEMKE H. Polyclonal B cell activators (PBA). *In* OPPENHEIM J. J. and ROSENSTREICH D. L. Eds., Mitogens in immunobiology, New York, 1976, Academic Press, p. 173.

DOUGLAS S. D. Electron microscopic and functional aspects of human lymphocyte response to mitogens. Transpl. Rev., 1972, *II*, 39.

ELVES M. W. The lymphocytes. London, 1972, Lloyds-Luke, p. 604.

FORD W. L. and GOWANS J. L. The traffic of lymphocytes. Semin. Hemat., 1969, *6*, 67.

GOWANS J. L. and McGREGOR D. D. The immunological activities of lymphocytes. Prog. Allergy, 1965, *9*, I.

GREAVES M. F., OWEN J. J. T., and RAFF M. C. T and B lymphocytes; origin, properties and roles in immune response. Amsterdam, New York, 1973, Exc. Med. American Elsevier, p. 316.

HALL J. Lymphocyte recirculation and the gut: the cellular basis of humoral immunity in the intestine, Blood cells, 1979, *5*, 479.

LING N. R. Lymphocyte stimulation. Amsterdam, 1973, North Holland.

LUCAS D. O. Regulatory mechanisms in lymphocyte activation. Proc. IIth Leuk. Cult., New York, 1977, Academic Press, p. 825.

MARCHALONIS J. J. The lymphocytes: structure and function. Immunological series (M. Dekker ed.) New York, 1977, *5*, 704 pp.

METCALF D., and MOORE M. A. S. Haemopoietic cells. Amsterdam, 1971, North Holland, p. 550.

MÖLLER G. Eds. Lymphocyte activation by mitogens. Transpl. Rev., 1972, *II*.

OSMOND D. The origins, life span and circulation of lymphocytes. Proc. 6th Leuk. Cult. Conf., New York, 1972, Academic Press, p. 3.

OWEN J. J. T. The origins and development of lymphocyte populations. *In* Ontogeny of acquired immunity. Ciba Foundation Symposium. Amsterdam, 1972, Elsevier, North Holland, p. 35.

PARKER C. W., SNIDER D. E., and WEDNER H. J. The role of cyclic nucleotides in lymphocyte activation. *In* L. Brent and J. Holborow, Eds., Progress in immunology. II. Vol. 2, Amsterdam, 1974, North Holland, p. 85.

PAUL W. E. Lymphocyte biology. *In* Clinical Immunology (Parker C. W. ed.) Saunders. Philadelphia, 1980, p. 19.

SELL S. Development of restrictions in the expression of immunoglobulin specificities by lymphoid cells. Transpl. Rev., 1970, *5*, 19.

SHARON N. Cell surface receptors for lectins: markers of murine and human lymphocyte subpopulations. *In* Immunology '80 (M. Fougereau and J. Dausset eds.) Academic Press. New York, 1980, p. 254.

SPRENT J. Migration and life span of lymphocytes. *In* F. Loor and G. Roelants, Eds., B and T cells in immune recognition. New York, 1977, Wiley, p. 59.

VALENTINE F. T. The transformation and proliferation of lymphocytes in vitro. *In* J. P. Revillard, Ed., Cell-mediated immunity. In vitro correlates. Basel, 1971, Karger.

ZUCKER-FRANKLIN D. The ultrastructure of lymphocytes. Semin. Hemat., 1969, *6*, 4.

# ORIGINAL ARTICLES

BIBERFELD P. and MELLSTEDT H. Selective activation of human B lymphocytes by suboptimal doses of pokeweed mitogen (PWM). Exp. Cell. Res., 1974, *89*, 377.

BOYUM A. A one-stage procedure for the isolation of granulocytes and lymphocytes from human blood. Scand. J. Lab. Invest., 1968, *21*, 21.

EVERETT N. B., CAFFREY R. W., and RIEKE W. D. Recirculation of lymphocytes. Ann. N.Y. Acad. Sci., 1964, *113*, 887.

EVERETT N. B. and TYLER R. W. Lymphopoiesis in the thymus and other functional implications. Int. Rev. Cytol., 1967, *22*, 205.

JANOSSY G., SHOHAT M., GREAVES M. F., and DOURSMARSHKIN R. R. Lymphocyte activation. IV. The ultrastructural pattern of the response of mouse T and B cells to mitogenic stimulation in vitro. Immunology, 1972, *21*, 211.

MATTER A., LISOWSKA-BERNSTEIN B., RYSER J. E., LAMELIN J. P., and VASSALI P. Mouse thymus-independent and thymus-derived lymphoid cells. II. Ultrastructural studies. J. Exp. Med., 1972, *136*, 1008.

POLLIACK A., LAMPEN N., CLARKSON B. D., DE HARVEN E., BENTWICH Z., SIEGAL F. P., and KUNKEL H. G. Identification of human B and T lymphocytes by scanning electron microscopy. J. Exp. Med., 1973, *138*, 607.

REYES F., LEJONC J. L., GOURDIN M. F., MANNONI P., and DREYFUS B. The surface morphology of human B lymphocytes as revealed by immunoelectron microscopy. J. Exp. Med., 1975, *141*, 392.

ZATZ M. M. and LANCE E. M. The distribution of chromium-51 labelled lymphoid cells in the mouse. A survey of anatomical compartments. Cell. Immunol., 1970, *1*, 3.

# Chapter 4

# B AND T LYMPHOCYTES

**Jean-François Bach**

I.   INTRODUCTION
II.  THE CONCEPT OF B AND T CELLS
III. B- AND T-CELL MARKERS
IV.  CIRCULATING B AND T CELLS: LIFE-SPAN AND PHYSI-
     CAL PROPERTIES
V.   ANTIGEN RECEPTORS OF B AND T CELLS
VI.  B- AND T-CELL MATURATION

## I.  INTRODUCTION

All small lymphocytes are morphologically alike. Some slight differences between individual lymphocytes are seen on electron microscopy, but these findings are minimal and ill-defined. However, small lymphocytes show heterogeneity in their density, electrophoretic mobility, life-span, "homing" after intravenous injection, and response (in vitro) to mitogen stimulation. And, most important functionally, there are several lymphocyte subsets that act separately or together in various types of immune responses. Two important classes, T and B lymphocytes, may be distinguished. T-lymphocyte maturation depends on the thymus, apparently by direct contact of precursor cells with the thymic epithelium, although a role for thymic humoral influence is probably also operative. B-lymphocyte maturation does not depend on the presence of the thymus but on another central lymphoid organ, the bursa of Fabricius (at least in birds). The expression "B lymphocytes" used for bursa-dependent lymphocytes is fortunate, even though there is no known equivalent of the bursa of Fabricius in mammals, because the "B" can refer to "bone marrow," from which B lymphocytes come. However, this term is not totally satisfactory because T cells may also originate in the bone marrow, and in species other than mouse, bone marrow may contain fairly numerous T cells, particularly in rabbit and man.

# II.   THE CONCEPT OF B AND T CELLS

Long before the role of lymphocytes in immunity was known, it was noted that immune responses against infectious agents were either essentially humoral, mediated by antibodies, or cellular, mediated by the direct action of cells without secretion of antibodies. Similarly, today, one distinguishes between cell-mediated immunity, transferable by lymphoid cells but not by serum and including graft rejection, graft-versus-host reactions, delayed hypersensitivity reactions and cell-mediated immunity against bacterial or viral agents, and humoral immunity, transferable by serum and to a lesser extent by cells, which consists of production of specific antibodies, in particular those responsible for immediate hypersensitivity reactions (anaphylaxis, atopy), and Arthus phenomenon. This dichotomy of immune responses has been corroborated by the complementary effects of neonatal thymectomy and bursectomy.

## THYMECTOMY AND BURSECTOMY EXPERIMENTS

### Adult Thymectomy

Adult thymectomy has few obvious effects on immunity. Lymphocytopenia may be observed in the weeks that follow the operation, but one must wait several months in the mouse and several years in larger animals to see a very slow but progressive diminution of the capacity to reject skin grafts, develop delayed hypersensitivity reactions, and undergo graft-versus-host reactions. This time delay and the relative subtlety of events that follow adult thymectomy explain why the essential role of the thymus in immunity was not discovered until 1961. In fact, we shall see later that adult thymectomy does have effects on the immune system (see p. 545). In particular, it results, within a week, in the disappearance from the spleen of $\theta$-positive cells, which form rosettes with sheep red blood cells and induces, after 4–6 weeks, a diminution in the absolute number of $\theta$ cells and Lyt123$^+$ cells (see p. 65) which are involved in the expression of suppressor effects and regulate the in vitro response to alloantigens.

### Neonatal Thymectomy

When thymectomy is performed within 24 hr after birth, thymectomized animals present a major immune deficiency, including a decreased number of circulating lymphocytes in peripheral blood and thoracic duct, depletion of so-called thymus-dependent areas in lymph nodes and spleen (see p. 35), and, most importantly (as shown by J. Miller in 1961), abnormalities in immune responses, particularly in cell-mediated immunity (skin allograft rejection, graft-versus-host reaction, delayed hypersensitivity), but also in humoral immunity (production of some antibodies). The latter observation permits us to distinguish between thymus-dependent antigens, against which neonatally thymectomized mice show a depressed response (including serum proteins and heterologous red blood cells), and thymus-independent antigens, toward which neonatally thymectomized animals show a normal or even increased response (as in the case of polyvinylpyrrolidone and lipopolysaccharides). All of these abnormalities are corrected by thymus grafting. Neonatal thymectomy is not the only experimental model of T-cell deficiency. Other models of experimental thymic deprivation include the nude mouse, in which a congenital thymus agenesis provides us with the purest model of T-cell absence. Thymectomized, irradiated, and bone-marrow-reconstituted mice are also T-cell deficient particularly if T cells that contaminate the bone marrow inoculum are earlier destroyed by in vitro treatment by an antiserum directed against T cell-specific antigens: in this model, endogenous B and T cells have been destroyed by irradiation and B cells, but not T cells, are replaced.

### In Ovo Bursectomy (in the Chicken)

In ovo bursectomy (ideally in association with irradiation) leads to major abnormalities in immunoglobulin production. In ovo bursectomized chickens have no circulating serum immunoglobulins, and there is no antibody production after stimulation by thymus-dependent or -independent antigens. However, delayed hypersensitivity and skin graft rejection are preserved. Neonatal (or in ovo) injection of testosterone or cyclophosphamide causes atrophy of the bursa of Fabricius and identical (as follows in ovo bursectomy) alterations in immune responses.

### Human Immunodeficiencies

The recognition of human immune deficiencies allowed Good to extrapolate these findings of lymphocyte duality in the mouse to man, by demonstrating clinical syndromes similar to those that follow neonatal thymectomy or bursectomy. Thus, several examples of congenital agammaglobulinemia with no humoral immunity but with normal cell-mediated immunity are recognized. In DiGeorge's syndrome (thymic agenesis), there is normal antibody production but no cell-mediated immunity (see chap. 31).

## CELLULAR COOPERATION

Claman has shown that the injection of thymus or bone marrow cells into irradiated and thymectomized mice does not restore immune competence. However, simultaneous injection of both cell populations gives full restitution, for example, of the immune responses to sheep red blood cells. These classic experiments have been performed by using other antigens and other species with very similar results. They provide additional evidence of the dichotomy of lymphocytes.

## CONCLUSIONS: A FEW UNANSWERED QUESTIONS

The experiments mentioned above demonstrated the existence of two lymphocyte populations: T cells, which require the thymus for maturation and which are essentially responsible for allograft rejection and delayed hypersensitivity reactions, and B cells, which are primarily involved in antibody production. T-

**Table 4.1  Effects of Selective Depletion of B and T Cells**

| | T cells | B cells |
|---|---|---|
| In vivo methods | Neonatal thymectomy<br>Nude mice<br>Adult thymectomy plus irradiation (and reconstitution with bone marrow cells or fetal liver cells*)<br>Treatment with antilymphocyte serum<br>Thoracic duct cannulation | In ovo bursectomy<br>Testosterone or cyclophosphamide in ovo (in birds) |
| In vitro methods | Anti-θ serum<br>Xenogeneic anti-T serum | Xenogeneic anti-B serum<br>Anti-Ig serum (cytotoxicity or filtration on anti-Ig-coated columns) |
| Effects on cellular immunity | | |
| Graft rejection | + | 0 |
| Delayed hypersensitivity | | |
| Graft versus host reaction | | |
| Effects on humoral immunity toward thymus-dependent antigens, such as: | + | + |
| Sheep red blood cells | | |
| Bovine serum albumin | | |
| γ-Globulins | | |
| Effects on humoral immunity toward thymus-independent antigens, such as: | | |
| Polysaccharides | | |
| Polyvinylpyrrolidone | | |
| Polymerized flagellin | 0<br>(or ↗ in certain cases) | + |

* These should be treated with anti-θ serum plus complement to obtain optimum effects.

63

and B-cell precursors in thymus, bone marrow, or bursa of Fabricius are not identifiable as B and T cells per se, although they belong to the B- and T-cell lineages. Therefore, thymus lymphocytes should not be called "T lymphocytes," nor should the term "B lymphocytes" be applied to all bone marrow or bursa of Fabricus lymphocytes, even though some are mature B or T cells.

Complementary experiments, which will be considered subsequently, have shown that only B cells produce the antibodies seen in the serum. Further validation of the existence of two populations of B and T cells is provided by the demonstration of markers and different properties of B and T cells. Several questions, however, remain unanswered: do B and T cells have the same precursor, or do bone marrow stems cells have a precommitted fate before passing through the thymus and the bursa of Fabricius or its mammalian equivalent? What is the specificity of T-cell involvement in antibody production? What is the nature of surface receptors of B and T cells? All are major questions for which definitive answers cannot yet be given.

## III.   B- AND T-CELL MARKERS

We have already noted that B and T cells are difficult to distinguish morphologically. Differences have been seen by scanning electron microscopy (Fig. 3.3): B lymphocytes have been reported to show microvilli not present on T lymphocytes. Unfortunately, these differences remain largely statistical, with many exceptions, which seem to depend on the physical state of the cells. There are, however, differences other than morphologic that delineate B and T lymphocytes. Some are sufficiently clear-cut so as to be considered markers and thereby provide separation methods for B and T cells. These markers can be grouped into three categories; surface antigens, surface receptors, and mitogen responses.

Surface antigens are generally detected by the cytotoxicity test. The lymphocytes are incubated with a specific antiserum and complement, and the percentage of cells killed is evaluated either by use of trypan blue (which stains dead cells) or by measuring $^{51}Cr$ release from previously tagged lymphocytes. Results are expressed as percentage of dead cells or released $^{51}Cr$. Fluorescent antisera (by either the direct or indirect techniques see p. 304) may also be used to detect cells bearing antigenic markers.

Surface receptors can be studied by immunofluorescence by use of anti-receptor antisera, by the rosette test, or by autoradiography when the determinant against the receptor is present, bound to erythrocytes, or is radiolabeled.

Mitogen responses are determined from radiolabeled thymidine uptake following 3 to 5 days of lymphocyte culture in the presence of the mitogen. It is important to examine thymidine uptake at several mitogen concentrations, because optimal concentration varies according to experimental conditions. Results are expressed in absolute units (dpm) of thymidine uptake in the presence of mitogen, from which the isotopic count in the absence of mitogen is subtracted, or as a stimulation index, which is the ratio of the isotope incorporations in the presence and absence of mitogen.

# T-CELL MARKERS (Table 4.3)

## Surface Antigens

### θ ANTIGEN (IN THE MOUSE)

The θ antigen (or Thy-1 by modern terminology) is an alloantigen present on thymocytes, peripheral T cells, cerebral tissue, and epidermis. Its absence on B cells makes it one of the best T-cell markers. There are no, or only a few, θ-bearing lymphocytes in neonatally thymectomized mice or in nude mice. The antigen is genetically controlled by a locus of the 9th chromosome with two alleles: the θ AKR allele or Thy-1$^a$ (present in AKR mice) coding for the specificity Thy-1.1 and the θ C3H allele or Thy-1$^b$ (present in most commonly used strains) coding for the specificity Thy-1.2. Anti-θ sera are prepared by injecting C3H or CBA thymocytes into AKR mice that are histocompatible at the H-2 loci (see chap. 23). Such sera, however, contain contaminating antibodies, including autoantibodies and antiallotype antibodies which are not detectable by the usual cytotoxicity tests with guinea pig complement but may be readily demonstrated by use of rabbit serum or techniques other than cytotoxicity. To avoid such problems, anti-θ sera have been prepared between mice strains congenic at the θ locus, that is, differing only at this locus. Monoclonal antibodies produced by hybridomas have also been prepared.

### OTHER ALLOANTIGENS

The TL antigen is exclusively expressed on cortical thymocytes. It is genetically controlled by four genes located at the Tla locus on the 17th chromosome close to the D extremity of the H-2 locus. The TL antigen is also found on cell surfaces in some spontaneous or induced mouse leukemias, thus its name, "thymus leukemia antigen."

### GIX ANTIGEN

Also expressed by thymocytes and some Gross virus-induced leukemias, this antigen seems to have a significance similar to that of TL antigen.

### LY ANTIGENS

Like the θ antigen, these antigens are not identically represented on the surface of thymocytes and peripheral B and T lymphocytes. Several Ly* systems are now known: Lyt1, Lyt2, Lyt3, Ly4 ... with, apparently, two alleles per locus (Lyt-1$^a$ and Lyt-1$^b$) and thus two phenotypes per system (e.g., Lyt-1.1 and Lyt-1.2). Convergent data indicate that Lyt1, Lyt2, and Lyt3 antigens are not equally distributed on T-cell subsets and Ly4 antigens, as contrasted with Lyt1, Lyt2, or Lyt3 antigens, have been claimed to be found essentially on B cells. Thus most cortical thymocytes are Lyt 123$^+$ and in the normal spleen about 50% lymphoid cells are Lyt 123$^+$ (they are depleted by adult thymectomy and

---

* Recently, according to defined terminology, the symbol Lyt is used to deonote antigens specifically found on T cells, and Lyb for those specifically found on B cells.

**Table 4.2  Comparison of B- and T-Lymphocyte Properties in the Mouse**

| | B lymphocytes | T lymphocytes |
|---|---|---|
| Morphology | No specific features | No specific aspect |
| Differentiation | Under the influence of the bursa of Fabricius in birds and perhaps of its equivalent (unknown) in mammals (depleted in neonatally bursectomized chickens) | Under the influence of the thymus (depleted in neonatally thymectomized and nude mice) |
| Surface antigens | | |
| θ | − | + |
| TL | − | + (only on cortical thymocytes) |
| GIX | − | + (only on cortical thymocytes) |
| Lyt1,2,3 | − | + (with variable expression on T-cell populations) Lyt1,2,3+ = immature T cells Lyt1+ = helper T cells Lyt2,3+ = cytotoxic and suppressor T cells |
| PC | + (only on plasma cells) | − |
| H-2 | + | + |
| Antigen receptors | Ig in large amounts (restricted to one class, one idiotype and one allotype) | Specific receptors for the antigen, probably with a weak density; uncertain nature (Ig variable part?) |
| Other receptors | | |
| Complement (C3b and C3d) | + | − |
| Fc of IgG | ++ | + |
| Sheep red blood cells (in man) | − | + |

| | | |
|---|---|---|
| Proliferative responses | | |
| PHA, Con A | − | + |
| MLC | − | + |
| Pokeweed | + | + |
| LPS | + (in mice) | − |
| Approximate frequency (in each organ, %) | | |
| Blood | 15 | 85 |
| Lymph nodes | 15 | 85 |
| Thoracic duct | 10 | 90 |
| Spleen | 65 | 35 |
| Bone marrow | 10–15 | <3 |
| Thymus | <3 | >97 |
| Traffic | No or little recirculation. Localized in follicles around germinal centers | Recirculation of many T cells. Localized in thymus-dependent areas |
| Life-span | Majority are short-lived but there are also long-lived B cells | Coexistence of short- and long-lived lymphocytes |
| Sensitivity to inactivation in vivo by: | | |
| Irradiation | +++ | ++ |
| Antilymphocyte sera | (+) | +++ |
| Cyclophosphamide (high doses) | +++ | + notably suppressor T cells |
| Azathioprine | + | +++ |
| Functions | | |
| Antibody production | Secretion | Regulatory functions, positive (helper function, carrier specific) and negative (suppressor) |
| Delayed hypersensitivity | No known role | Effector cells |
| Graft and tumor rejection | Production of blocking and cytotoxic antibodies | Effector cytotoxic cells |
| Tolerance | Late and transient | Early and long lasting |

**Table 4.3    Subpopulations of T Lymphocytes as Defined by Lyt Antigens**

|                                                                 | Lyt1,2,3 | Lyt1 | Lyt2,3 |
|-----------------------------------------------------------------|:--------:|:----:|:------:|
| Distribution in lymphoid organs (% T cells)                     |          |      |        |
|   Thymus                                              | 90       | 10   | 10     |
|   Spleen and lymph nodes                              | 50       | 30   | 5–10   |
| Helper and amplifier function                                   |          |      |        |
|   • for antibody production by B cells (primary and   | +        |      |        |
|     secondary responses)                   |          |      |        |
|   • for cytotoxic T-cell production                   | +        |      |        |
|   • for the production of delayed hypersensitivity    | +        |      |        |
|     (monocytes, macrophages)               |          |      |        |
| Suppressor function                                             |          |      |        |
|   for antibody production by B cells                  |          |      |        |
|   • primary response                                  | +        |      | +      |
|   • secondary response                                |          |      | +      |
|   • after polyclonal activation                       |          |      | +      |
|   • during allogenic response (MLC, CML)             | +        |      | +      |
| Cytotoxic T cells                                               |          |      |        |
|   Against allogeneic cells                            |          |      |        |
|     Precursors                             | ±        |      | +      |
|     Cytotoxic cells                        |          |      | +      |
|   Against TNP-modified "self"                         |          |      |        |
|     Precursors                             | +        |      |        |
|     Cytotoxic cells                        |          |      | +      |

After Cantor and Boyse.

thought to be immature T cells), 30 to 35% are Lyt1$^+$ and considered to include most helper T cells and the rest (5 to 10%) are Lyt23$^+$ and considered to include cytotoxic and antigen specific suppressor T cells. Knowledge concerning the Lyt1, 2, and 3 antigens has resulted in the definition of the three subpopulations of T lymphocytes (Lyt123$^+$, Lyt1$^+$, and Lyt23$^+$) whose characteristics are shown in Table 4.3 and discussed on p. 98. Note that recent studies using the sensitive immunofluorescence technique have indicated that Lyt23$^+$ cells also bear a significant amount of Lyt1 antigen. It should also be noted that the Ly4 antigen belongs to B cells (this yet requires confirmation) and, more generally, that some Ly antigens (e.g., the Ly6 antigen) seem to belong to a peripheral T-cell population whose function and state of maturation remain to be elucidated (Tables 4.2 and 4.3).

Qa ANTIGENS

A large but still ill-defined fraction of T cells carry the Qa antigens coded for by 3 closely related loci (Qa-1, Qa-2, Qa-3), mapping close to the Tla locus.

In conclusion, there are many differentiating alloantigens on the surface of thymocytes and T cells not found on B cells, which thereby permit one to delineate "specific" T-lymphocyte markers. The multiplicity of cell alloantigens means that their use as markers must be undertaken with knowledge that a given antiserum may contain contaminating antibodies against several T-lymphocyte markers, which may not necessarily be specific for one cell type.

Xenogeneic antisera prepared against pure B- and T-cell populations, in fact, contain a mixture of anti-B and anti-T antibodies due to the numerous common antigenic determinants of B and T lymphocytes. One may, however, obtain a T-cell-specific antiserum by immunizing, for example, a rabbit with mouse thymocytes and absorbing repeatedly the antiserum by B cell-rich preparations (spleen cells from nude mice or bone marrow cells), to eliminate anti-B antibodies and by applying liver, serum and erythrocytes to the same antisera to eliminate species-specific antibodies. This general technique has the advantage of applicability to man. Here, one can use as a T-antigen source not only thymus cells but also lymphocytes from agammaglobulinemic patients or, oddly enough brain; for a B-antigen source, cells can be obtained from patients with chronic lymphocytic leukemia or DiGeorge's syndrome or continuous lymphoblastoid cell lines that are essentially of B origin. Specific (anti-T-cell) xenogeneic antisera may be used in man; however, it must be recognized that small amounts of contaminating antibodies may be present that have low affinity and are therefore difficult to preabsorb, in addition to contamination by immune complexes due to repeated absorptions. These immune complexes may interfere with in vitro immune reactions.

It is to be hoped that recent progress in knowledge of the chemical structure of these xenoantigens (separated on polyacrylamide gel) and the use of monoclonal antibodies (produced by hybridomas) will facilitate the use of such xenogeneic anti-T cell antibodies. This would allow more precise definition of T-cell subpopulations in man; similar to those that have been discerned in the mouse, such as the Thy-1 and Lyt antigens. In this context should be mentioned the recent use of autoantibodies directed against certain T-cell subpopulations in patients suffering from autoimmune disorders, such as lupus erythematosus and juvenile rheumatoid arthritis, and, especially, the use of monoclonal antibodies against various lymphocyte subsets produced by mouse hybridomas. Various antihuman T-cell monoclonal antibodies have recently become available. They are produced by hybridizing mouse myeloma cells with spleen cells from mice immunized with thymocytes or T cell-enriched peripheral blood lymphocytes. One may distinguish antibodies recognizing most T cells the equivalent of anti-Thy-1 sera) and those specific for T-cell subsets (immature T cells, helper cells, suppressor cells). The identification of the various T-cell subsets is performed by indirect immunofluorescence, using an antimouse Ig-labeled antiserum.

### Surface Receptors

SHEEP ERYTHROCYTE SPONTANEOUS ROSETTES

Fifty percent to 80% of lymphocytes from human peripheral blood form rosettes when mixed with sheep red blood cells (SRBC) (Fig. 4.1). The rosettes are not antigen specific and are not inhibited by anti-immunoglobulin (anti-Ig) sera, which differentiates this phenomenon from rosette formation observed in the mouse, in which cells that produce antierythrocyte antibodies and cells that specifically recognize these antigens are detected (Table 4.4). The "human" spontaneous rosettes necessitate specific technical conditions for their formation in optimal numbers (prolonged incubation at 4°C, gentle resuspension). The same phenomenon is also observed in species other than man, in particular in pig and dog. Interest in the phenomenon is due to its exclusive expression on T cells: the number of rosette-forming lymphocytes is diminished in situations where T cells are decreased (thymic aplasia, B-type chronic lymphatic leukemia) and is increased in agammaglobulinemic blood or in the normal thymus. In addition, the formation of sheep rosettes is inhibited by anti-T-cell sera (and not by anti-B-cell sera), and these rosette-forming cells do not have the B-cell markers that will be discussed later (membrane Ig, complement receptor). In practice, the evaluation of the number of cells that form rosettes with sheep erythrocytes in human blood represents the simplest way of enumerating T lymphocytes in man.

Rosettes possessing the same significance may also be obtained using red cells from rhesus monkeys and, to a lesser extent, with neuraminidase-treated human red cells. Active rosettes may also be obtained by incubation at 37°C, but these represent a subpopulation of T lymphocytes whose significance remains obscure.

RECEPTORS FOR THE Fc FRAGMENTS OF IgG AND IgM

Moretta has recently demonstrated that two subpopulations of human lymphocytes may be distinguished and separated on the basis of the presence

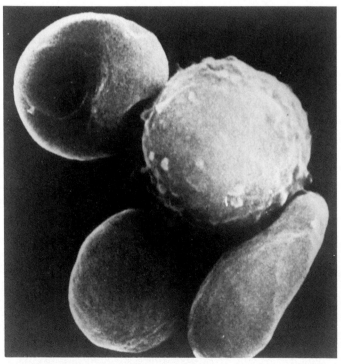

**Fig. 4.1** Human T lymphocytes from a rosette with SRBC. (From P. S. Lin, A. G. Copper, and H. H. Wortis, N. Engl. J. Med. 1973, *289*, 548.)

**Table 4.4 Comparison of Spontaneous Sheep Red Blood Cell Rosettes in the Mouse and in Man**

|  | *Mouse* | *Man* |
|---|---|---|
| Number (%) |  |  |
| Thymus | 0.01 | 95 |
| Blood | 0.05 | 60–80 |
| Spleen | 0.1 | 20–40 |
| Technical parameters |  |  |
| Temperature | Not sensitive to temperature | Number greatly increased at 4°C |
| Formaldehyde erythrocyte treatment | Without effect | Suppresses the phenomenon |
| Contaminating autologous erythrocytes | No role | Marked depletion |
| Inhibition |  |  |
| Anti-Ig serum | + | − |
| Antilymphocyte serum |  |  |
| With complement | + | + |
| Without complement | − | + |
| Significance | Antigen-binding cells (B and T cells and macrophages) | Nonspecific T-cell marker |

of receptors binding Fc fragments of IgM (Tμ cells or T.M) or IgG (Tγ or T.G). About 75% of human T lymphocytes bear Fcμ receptors, much smaller proportions (less than 20%) bearing Fc receptors. Tγ and Tμ cells respond in a similar manner to Concanavalin A (Con A). Importantly, study of the "helper" and "suppressor" T cells, defined by their effect on the polyclonal differentiation of B cells induced by pokeweed mitogen, has shown that helper cells are comprised essentially of Tμ cells, whereas suppressor cells in the same system are mainly Tγ. However, some suppressor cells also seem to have Tγ cell characteristics. A role for the activation of Tγ cells by immune complexes has been suggested. These results have recently been questioned and the relationship of T cells with the null cell population that includes K, NK, and some monocytic cells, is open to speculation.

### Proliferative Responses in Vitro

T cells transform and proliferate in vitro in response to various stimuli (see p. 51), some of which may be used as T-cell markers, because they stimulate only T-cell transformation.

NONSPECIFIC MITOGENS

The specificity of B- and T-cell responses to mitogens has been evaluated by studying pure B- and T-lymphocyte populations: thymocytes, spleen cells depleted in B cells by passage through anti-Ig-coated columns, bursectomized chicken or agammaglobulinemic lymphocytes (T cells); anti-θ serum-treated spleen cells, nude mouse spleen cells, or lymphocytes from DiGeorge's syndrome patients (B cells). For the phytohemagglutinin (PHA) response, the thymic origin of the stimulated cells has been directly demonstrated by A. J. S. Davies by use of a chromosomal marker: thymectomized, irradiated CBA mice were reconstituted with an injection of syngeneic bone marrow cells and a thymus graft from a CBA donor that bore a translocation of the 14th chromosome pair (T6 chromosome). The nature of the mitosing (T-cell) population in response to PHA stimulation could then be recognized by the presence of the T6 chromosome.

Two lectins, PHA and Concanavalin A (Con A), selectively stimulate T cells. However, if mixtures of B and T cells are employed (e.g., normal spleen cells or normal peripheral lymphocytes), T-cell stimulation seems to induce a secondary recruitment of some B cells. Similarly, it has been reported that purified B cells are strongly stimulated by PHA or Con A made insoluble by fixation to glass beads (this observation, however, is controversial). Lastly, all T-cell populations do not respond identically to the two mitogens. Thus, lymph node lymphocytes respond well to both PHA and Con A, whereas thymocytes respond more to Con A stimulation than to PHA. These facts, all of which relate to problems in quantifying transformation, explain why measurements of PHA and Con A responses must be viewed with caution in evaluating T-cell function. The mechanisms by which mitogens selectively act on B and T lymphocytes are obscure. This selective action is not, however, due to differences in lectin receptor concentrations, because PHA and Con A bind similarly on T- and B-cell surfaces.

ANTIGEN-SPECIFIC RESPONSE

Lymphocytes from a sensitized animal have the property of transforming in the presence of the antigen. Both T and B lymphocytes may transform in vitro in the presence of the sensitizing antigen, but T cells respond better. This difference explains why there is fairly good correlation between DNA synthesis in response to an antigen and delayed hypersensitivity against the same antigen and also explains why neonatally bursectomized chickens present good proliferative responses in vitro in the presence of antigen, whereas thymectomized chickens show no or only minimal response. Lastly, for immunization by a hapten-carrier complex, proliferative responses are exclusively directed against the carrier to which the T cells were sensitized. One should be cautious in equating antigen-induced transformation to a T-cell reaction, because B cells may give a significant response. In addition, there are situations where delayed hypersensitivity develops with in vitro production of mediators (such as migration-inhibitory factor) but without in vitro antigen-induced transformation. Some recent work suggests that MIF may, in fact, be secreted by both B and T cells.

MIXED LYMPHOCYTE REACTION (MLR)

Lymphocytes transform in the presence of allogeneic histoincompatible lymphocytes (we will discuss this phenomenon later in Chaps. 13 and 23). For now, we will examine only the origins of responding and stimulating cells, which can be evaluated separately by inactivating populations.

Responding cells are exclusively T cells, as has been proven by the presence of T-cell chromosomal markers in "chimeric" mice (T6 chromosome). The suppression of MLR by neonatal thymectomy or in vitro treatment with anti-θ serum confirms the thymic origin of responding cells. Conversely, neonatal bursectomy in the chicken does not suppress MLR. However, some B cells do proliferate in MLR, probably due to recruitment secondary to blastogenic factors released by activated T cells.

Lymphocytes are apparently not the only cells capable of provoking an MLR. Fibroblasts, macrophages, and epidermal cells also seem to possess this capacity. Among lymphocytes, it has been reported that B lymphocytes stimulate more than do T lymphocytes; these findings are controversial and may depend on experimental conditions. MLRs allow the study of another T-cell parameter, lymphocytotoxicity, because cytotoxic T cells specifically directed against stimulating cells are generated in an MLR (see p. 410). These cytotoxic cells may represent a cell subset different from the proliferating cells but are also exclusively of thymic origin.

**Table 4.5   Markers of Human Lymphocyte Membranes**

|  | T cells | B cells |
|---|---|---|
| Antisera (or monoclonal antibodies) | | |
|     Anti-human T-cell antigens | + | − |
|     Anti-Human B-cell antigens | − | + |
|     Anti-Ig | − | + |
| Viruses | | |
|     EBV | − | + |
|     Measles | + | − |
| E rosettes | | |
|     Sheep | + | − |
|     Man | ± | − |
|     Rhesus monkey | + | − |
|     Mouse | − | + |
| Lectins | | |
|     Helix Pomatia | + | |
|     Peanut agglutinin (PNA) | + | − |
| Complement | | |
|     C3 (C3b, C3d) | − | + |
|     C4b | − | + |
| Immunoglobulins | | |
|     Aggregated IgG | ± | + |
|     Erythrocyte + IgG | + | + |
|     Erythrocyte + IgM | + | − |
| N-acetyl esterase | + | − |

## B-CELL MARKERS

### Surface Antigens

#### ALLOANTIGENS

Several alloantigenic systems have recently been described on B cells such as the Lyb-1, -2, -3, -4, -5, -6 and 7 antigens. One may also mention the existence of a plasma cell-specific antigen (Pcl) in the mouse. This antigen is also found in kidney and liver but not on nonantibody-forming lymphoid cells.

Moreover, it is important to note the existence of Ia antigens in the mouse and DR antigens in man, which are present on B-lymphocyte surfaces but are not expressed on T cells unless they are activated, particularly by alloantigens. Antisera directed against the Ia or DR antigens or against the protein of which these antigens are comprised have been employed to evaluate B-cell function. The lack of absolute specificty of these B-cell antigens and, in particular, their presence on some T lymphocytes and monocytes does, however, urge some caution in their use as B-cell markers.

#### XENOANTIGENS

It is possible to prepare anti-B xenogeneic antisera similar to those described for T cells. B antigens may be obtained in the mouse from the lymph nodes of thymectomized, irradiated, and bone marrow-reconstituted mice (preferably after in vitro treatment of the bone marrow cell inoculum with anti-θ serum to eliminate contaminating T cells) or from nude mouse cells. In man, one may use lymphocytes from patients with chronic leukemia or lymphoblastoid cell lines. The absorptions are performed by use of thymus cells and also liver and red blood cells to eliminate species-specific antibodies. In the mouse, the B antigens thus defined have been termed "mouse bone marrow leukocyte antigen" (MBLA). Plasma cell-specific heteroantigens have also been defined with sera prepared against myeloma cells. Experience shows, however, that, for unknown reasons, specific anti-B xenogeneic antisera are generally more difficult to obtain than anti-T antisera.

### Surface Receptors

Three receptor categories have been demonstrated on the B-cell surface: membrane immunoglobulins, complement receptors, and receptors for the Fc fragment of IgG.

#### MEMBRANE IMMUNOGLOBULINS

Membrane Ig present on lymphocyte surfaces are for the most part antigen-recognizing receptors. However, we shall consider them here only as B-cell markers. A large proportion of lymphocytes, variable as to organ and species, are coated with membrane Ig. These Igs can be visualized by immunofluorescence by use of anti-Ig-labeled antisera, specific for light or heavy chains. Only B lymphyocytes have detectable Ig on their membrane. Ig-bearing lymphocytcs are not found in neonatally bursectomized chickens or in agammaglobulinemic patients, and their proportion in lymphocytes increases after T-cell elimination by in vitro treatment with anti-θ serum. Moreover, their number is normal or increased in neonatally thymectomized mice, nude mice, and children with thymic aplasia. One must, however, interpret with caution the results obtained by immunofluorescence because, as we shall later see, there are also receptors for the Fc IgG fragment on K cells, monocytes, and even on T lymphocytes, which may cause false positive reactions due to passive binding of IgG to the cells. To eliminate this source of error in interpretation, it may be necessary to demonstrate true synthesis of membrane Ig by lymphocytes by showing reappearance of Ig after elimination by proteolytic enzyme treatment (e.g., trypsin) or by using noncomplement fixing Fab or $(Fab')_2$ fragments of immunoglobulins as a fluorescent antibody reagent. Furthermore, it is necessary to discount monocytes and macrophages that may be detected, for example, by the peroxidase reaction or by their ability to ingest latex particles.

B lymphocytes have antigen-specific receptors detectable by autoradiography or by the rosette test. Such antigen binding by B cells is more intense and more stable than for T cells. However, it cannot be considered a B-cell marker, because T cells also bind the antigen.

COMPLEMENT RECEPTORS

Some lymphocytes have receptors for the third component of complement. These receptors may be visualized by rosette formation by use of erythrocytes coated with antibody and complement (EAC). It is necessary to utilize an IgM antibody that does not bind to receptors for the Fc IgG fragment (see below) and subhemolyzing concentrations of complement. There are, in fact, two classes of receptors, one for C3b and the other for C3d, two degradation products of C3. There are also receptors for C1q and C4b. C3 receptors also exist on the surface of phagocytic cells (particularly monocytes and polymorphs), which means that caution must be applied when interpreting the results obtained with the EAC marker. Lymphocytes that bear C3 receptors are, indeed, B lymphocytes, because their percentage is abnormally elevated in nude and neonatally thymectomized mice; they are absent in the thymus, and they are insensitive to the action of anti-θ serum. However, although all complement receptor-bearing lymphocytes may be essentially B cells, not all B cells show these receptors.

**Table 4.6  Examples of Marker Studies of B and T Lymphocytes in Man**

|  | Membrane immuno- globulins (%) | Aggregated immuno- globulin binding (B) (%) | Sheep red blood cells (T) (%) |
|---|---|---|---|
| Normal subjects | 21 | 23 | 70 (60–80) |
| Thymic aplasia | 87 |  | 0.2 |
| Agammaglobulinemia | 0.7 | 12 | 71 |
| Chronic B-type lymphocytic leukemia | 95 | 98 | 5 |
| Sezary syndrome | 3 | 2 | 75 |

RECEPTORS FOR THE Fc FRAGMENT OF IgG

A significant percentage of lymphoid cells shows receptors for the Fc fragment of IgG. These receptors, which are separate from C3 receptors, may be detected by autoradiography or by immunofluorescence with labeled immune complexes, for example, radiolabeled bovine serum albumin (BSA) linked to an anti-BSA antibody, or aggregated IgG labeled with fluorescein. One may also detect them by a rosette technique that employs antierythrocyte antibody-coated target cells (e.g., rhesus positive D erythrocytes coated with anti-D antibodies), the EA (erythrocyte-antibody) rosette test. Noncomplexed or aggregated IgG also binds to the receptors but in a less efficient way than does complexed IgG. In both cases, the presence of complement is not required. Fc receptor-bearing lymphocytes include a large proportion of B cells. The Fc receptor cannot, however, be considered a good B-cell marker, because the Fc receptor is probably not unique and does not implicate only B lymphocytes. There exists a heterogeneous family of receptors that bind aggregated IgG according to the size of aggregates or, for antibody-coated red blood cells, according to the degree of sensitization. Furthermore, monocytes, T cells (in particular when they are activated), and K (killer) cells also show Fc receptors. Lastly, not all B cells have Fc receptors.

### Other Markers

Other markers of B lymphocytes in man have recently been described. In particular the receptor for mouse erythrocytes (mouse erythrocyte rosettes are formed exclusively with B cells) and receptors for the Epstein-Barr virus should be mentioned.

### Mitogen Responses

Mouse B cells are selectively stimulated by lipopolysaccharides (LPS), including *Escherichia coli* endotoxin, aggregated tuberculin (independently of previous sensitization), and anti-Ig sera. Pokeweed mitogen stimulates both B and T cells. In man, only anti-Ig sera can be used as a B-cell marker because, surprisingly, LPS usually does not stimulate human peripheral lymphocytes. Recent reports suggest that *Nocardia* extracts stimulate human peripheral blood B cells. Note also that mitogen-induced B-cell responses are submitted to the dual control of amplifier and suppressor T cells.

## NULL CELLS

Some lymphocytes (2 to 10%, depending on the organ) show neither T- nor B-cell markers. Whether they belong to lymphocytic lines is still disputed by some but is apparently corroborated by electron microscopy (insofar as there are specific criteria to define lymphocytes). These "null" lymphocytes could include a new cell population (K cells) involved in lymphocytotoxicity against IgG-coated target cells (see p. 413). Though some B and T cells seem capable of killing target cells coated with IgG, the majority of the cells implicated in the

**Table 4.7  Effects of Fractionation of Normal Human Leukocytes on B- and T-Cell Markers and on the K-Cell Population**

| | Ficoll (%) | Ficoll plus nylon (%) | Ficoll plus nylon plus E-rosette depletion |
|---|---|---|---|
| Lymphocytes | 65–90 | 97–100 | 97–100 |
| Monocytes | 5–20 | <2 | <2 |
| E rosettes (T cells) | 72 ± 2 | 90 ± 1 | 30–40 |
| EAC rosettes } B cells | 12 ± 0.9 | 0.6 ± 0.2 | <3 |
| Ig +cells } | 18 ± 1.8 | 3 ± 0.2 | <4 |
| EA rosettes | 26 ± 1.5 | 20 ± 2 | 50–70 |
| ADCC (K cells; mean cytotoxic index) | 9 ± 1.1 | 29 ± 2 | 50 ± 4 |

* Nylon column filtration removes the majority of B cells and monocytes, E-rosette depletion on a Ficoll gradient removes mostly T lymphocytes. K cells and a subpopulation of EA rosettes are not altered by these two treatments (ADCC = antibody-dependent cell-mediated cytotoxicity.)
After Feketé, Fournier, Descamps, and Bach.

phenomenon of antibody-dependent cell-mediated cytotoxicity (ADCC), the K cells, only appear to carry Fc receptors. Null cells, defined by the absence of membrane IgG and failure to form rosettes with sheep red blood cells, represent a heterogenous population that also includes precusors of B and T cells, which do not yet express B- or T-cell markers. The null lymphocytes are, in fact, increased in number in neonatally thymectomized mice and in nude mice as well as in children with clinical immunodeficiency in whom a dissociation between cell markers may be present (e.g., the presence of Fc and complement receptors with an absence of surface immunoglobulins). The problem has recently been complicated by the observation that low affinity E rosette-forming cells might include a small minority of non-T cells and that, reciprocally, it is difficult to prove that 100% T cells form E rosettes.

# IV.  CIRCULATING B AND T CELLS: LIFE-SPAN AND PHYSICAL PROPERTIES

We have reviewed several properties of B and T cells that may be used for nonoverlapping markers of cell categories. There are also additional properties of B and T cells that do not differentiate sufficiently between the respective populations and, therefore, do not provide useful markers, but they are of considerable help in understanding B- and T-cell physiology.

## CIRCULATION AND RECIRCULATION

Most recirculating lymphocytes are of thymic origin. Thoracic duct lymphocytes (80 to 90% of which bear the θ antigen in the mouse) labeled with thymidine and reinjected into syngeneic hosts home selectively (autoradiography) to thymusdependent areas of lymph nodes and spleen. The same histologic sites are selectively depleted by thoracic duct cannulation. Neonatal thymectomy and antilymphocyte serum (ALS) (which, in vivo, selectively eliminates T cells; see chap. 33) considerably decrease the output of thoracic duct lymphocytes and lower the percentage of lymph node cells that have the capacity to home back to lymph nodes. However, some T cells do not seem to recirculate. Thus, cortical thymocytes do not recirculate, whereas some medullary cells (TL negative and corticoresistant) do, and they also migrate to lymph nodes after injection into a syngeneic host. There are few B cells present in the thoracic duct, but the majority of them do not return to lymph nodes after syngeneic host injection. However, a small population of recirculating B cells return (home) to thymus-independent areas of lymph nodes and spleen. These data concern largely the mouse and the rat, and extrapolation to man would be premature at this time.

## LIFE-SPAN

We have previously noted (see p. 49) that lymphocytes can be classified on the basis of life-span (defined on p. 48), for example short-lived (1 to 6 days) versus long-lived lymphocytes (several months). A high percentage of T lymphocytes is long-lived, as shown by their diminution after neonatal thymectomy or ALS treatment. There are also, however, long-lived B lymphocytes. Thus, in nude mice or thymectomized, irradiated, and bone marrow-reconstituted mice (deprived of T cells), more than 70% of thoracic duct lymphocytes are still long-lived. It is usually believed that there is no clear predominance of T cells among long-lived cells and that B and T cells are probably similarly distributed with respect to percentage among short- and long-lived lymphocytes, even though long-lived T cells seem to have, on the average, a longer life-span than do long-lived B cells.

Of course, a short or long life-span for individual B and T cells does not necessarily imply a short or long life-span of the entire lymphocyte population. One could propose that relatively short-lived cells give rise to identical daughter cells that maintain the population and its properties. Therefore, it is not necessary to imagine that all B- and T-cell functions that persist after adult bursectomy or thymectomy are exclusively borne by long-lived cells. The functions they express may just as well be borne by rapidly dividing cells, independently of the thymus or of the bursa of Fabricius. Finally, it is noteworthy that in the thymus, the majority of cells are short-lived, except for a few medullary cells. Similarly, almost all bone marrow lymphocytes are short-lived.

## PHYSICAL PROPERTIES OF B AND T CELLS: APPLICATION TO SEPARATION

B and T cells show certain differences in physical properties that allow them to be separated.

### Size

B and T cells are of heterogeneous size and without clear differences. Activation of B or T cells induces an increase in the cell size.

### Density

The density of B and T cells is also heterogeneous. The less dense lymphocyte population isolated by a BSA gradient is deficient in θ-positive cells and enriched in T-cell precursors in the mouse. The B-cell percentage is, however, analogous to that of the initial preparation. Medullary thymocytes, which are immunocompetent, are less dense than immature cortical thymocytes, thus raising the possibility of separating these two lymphocyte populations by centrifugation on a density gradient.

### Adherence

B lymphocytes are more adherent to glass, plastic, and nylon than are T lymphocytes; therefore, B lymphocytes may be depleted by filtration (nylon column at 37°C). Filtration will indeed retain the majority of Ig-and complement-receptor-bearing lymphocytes. This method of separating B lymphocytes has a drawback, however, of eliminating numerous T cells, including most immature ones. In general, immunoblasts are more adherent than are quiescent small lymphocytes.

### Charge

Electrophoresis separates out several lymphocyte subsets. The more mobile lymphocytes (with the most negative charge) are essentially of thymic origin, whereas B cells (MBLA positive and antibody secreting) are less mobile. Preparative electrophoretic procedures have been used to separate B and T cells.

## B- AND T-LYMPHOCYTE SEPARATION

Several methods are now available that separate B- and T-cell populations by means of destruction or inactivation of one of the two populations or by means of physical separation.

### Obtaining Purified T Cells

Relatively pure T cells are found in the thymus (in particular, the pool of steroid-resistant thymocytes) and in neonatally bursectomized chickens. One may eliminate B cells present in the lymphoid organs of normal animals by treatment with an anti-B serum (anti-MBLA in the mouse) or by passing the cells through nylon columns or glass beads, Degalan or Sephadex columns, each of which have been coated with anti-IgG antibody or antigen-antibody complexes.

### Obtaining Purified B Cells

Relatively pure B cells are found in the bursa of Fabricius in the chicken, in the spleen of nude and neonatally thymectomized mice, or in thymectomized, irradiated, and bone marrow-reconstituted mice. One may eliminate the T cells present in lymphoid organs of normal animals by treatment with anti-T serum (anti-θ serum in the mouse, heterologous anti-T serum in man) or in man by rosette formation with SRBC, followed by centrifugation on a density gradient that selectively eliminates "rosetting" T cells.

### Fluorescent Cell Separator

An electronic system has recently been employed to separate cells according to their size and fluorescent intensity after immunofluorescent marking. Microdrops of the cell suspension are prepared in such a manner as to contain only a single cell. The microdrops pass in front of a laser beam and the cells are analyzed by means of a histogram. Simultaneously, the microdrops are separated according to their size and surface fluorescence.

## V.  ANTIGEN RECEPTORS OF B AND T CELLS

Specific antigen recognition by lymphocytes is a function of membrane surface receptors. Receptors are molecules that combine specifically with another class of molecules. Determination of the nature of specificity of lymphocyte receptors is essential to understand immunologic diversity thus the considerable number of studies (often contradictory) concerning this topic. Five main approaches have been used with variable success.

1.  Direct demonstration of receptors by antiserum, labeled with fluorescein or with an isotope, directed against the receptor antigenic determinants. The demonstration by immunofluorescence of Ig on B lymphocyte surface constituted very significant process in this regard.

2.  Biochemical analysis of membranes after labeling their molecules by radiolabeled iodine in the presence of lactoperoxidase. Membranes are solubilized and fractionated according to specific radioactivity.

3.  Study of antigen binding to lymphocyte surfaces by use of particulate antigens like red blood cells (which then form rosettes) or radiolabeled antigens detected by autoradiography.

4.  Elimination of lymphocyte subsets that react specifically with a given antigen by contact on immunoadsorbent of the antigen (antigen-coated column, cellular monolayers, rosette depletion, incubation with heavily labeled antigens). The suppression of specific cell retention by incubation with various antisera allows the study of the antigenicity of recognition receptors.

5.  Study of the inhibition of in vitro (or in vivo) activities of B and T cells by various antisera directed against the receptors (for example, anti-Ig sera).

All of these approaches are associated with methodologic uncertainties concerning the specificity of the antisera, the possibility of passive fixation of receptors on the lymphocyte surface, and the always present risk that the structure under study is not the receptor in question but rather a structure in proximity.

## B-CELL RECEPTORS: MEMBRANE IMMUNOGLOBULINS

### Demonstration of Surface Immunoglobulins on B Cells

The presence of membrane Ig and B cells is shown by binding of fluorescent anti-Ig antisera to lymphocytes (Fig. 4.2). Thus in human blood, 15 to 20% of lymphocytes are labeled with antilight-chain sera, 5 to 20% by anti-$\mu$ sera, 1 to 7% by anti-$\gamma$ sera, 5 to 10% by anti-$\delta$ sera, and less than 5% by anti-$\alpha$ sera. Note that IgD-bearing lymphocytes generally also bear IgM. The exclusive B-cell origin of Ig-bearing lymphocytes has been discussed earlier (see p. 74).

Ig secretion by lymphocytes as opposed to passive fixation is shown by trypsinization, which abolishes membrane Ig, followed by reappearance of Ig 2 hr later (37°C). One sees in newborn rabbit the paternal allotype on the lymphocyte surface and, later, circulating Ig that bears the same allotype. Lastly, some patients with agammaglobulinemia, nonetheless, show Ig-bearing lymphocytes (see chap. 31).

### Biochemical Nature of Membrane Immunoglobulins: Class, Allotypic, and Idiotypic Restrictions

The two classes of light chains and all heavy-chain classes are expressed on lymphocyte surfaces. Each lymphocyte contains antigenic patterns of both heavy

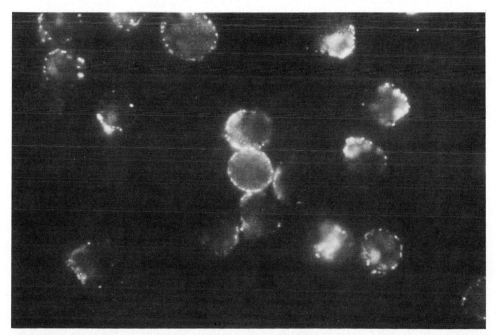

**Fig. 4.2** Membrane immunoglobulins on a B-lymphocyte surface (from J. L. Preud'homme).

chains and light chains, which suggests that receptors are complete immuno-globulins. Allotypic determinants of the variable portion (in rabbit) and of the constant part (in rabbit and mouse) have also been demonstrated for surface Ig. The relative proportions of separate Ig classes vary according to organ and species. In the mouse and man, the majority of cells bear κ chains. For heavy chains unlike serum Ig, the μ chain predominates; IgM is apparently monomeric (7S to 8S) on the lymphocyte surface. These data, obtained by immunofluoresc-ence, have been confirmed both by autoradiography and by extraction of membranes previously labeled with radioactive iodine in the presence of lactoperoxidase. A given lymphocyte does not possess both κ and λ chains and, in general, has only one heavy-chain class. A small percentage of lymphocytes may contain both μ and γ chains (especially in the first few days after immunization) or, simultaneously, different heavy-chain subclasses. However, at some time after immunization, B lymphocytes express only one class of heavy chain (with the exception of the μ-δ association mentioned above). There is also allotypic restriction, except for the first few days after immunization (days 3 to 8). Lastly, there is idiotypic restriction, which correlates with the antigen specificity restriction. Note that IgM and IgD on B cells share the same light chain and probably the same variable part (shared idiotypes and antibody activity).

### Position of Membrane Immunoglobulins: Movement and Turnover

One might assume that the variable portion of receptor molecules with antigen specificity is exposed on the lymphocyte surface because receptors specifically bind to antigen. In fact, it seems that most parts of the molecule are exposed, as suggested by data obtained by iodination-extraction, immunoflu-orescence, and inhibition of antigen binding by anti-Ig antibodies.

Ig, like other surface receptors or antigens, is mobile within the membrane. One may provoke its movement by incubating lymphocytes with anti-Ig anti-bodies ("capping phenomenon"). Three distinct phenomena may be serially observed after incubation of lymphocytes with an anti-Ig serum labeled with fluorescein or ferritin (Fig. 4.3).

1. Patch formation corresponds to passive aggregation of surface Ig, probably induced by Ig "cross-linking" with divalent anti-Ig antibodies (mon-ovalent antibodies do not produce this phenomenon).

2. "Cap" formation corresponds to Ig movement toward the cell pole, that is, uropod, located at the level of the Golgi apparatus. At variance with the previous phenomenon, this phenomenon is active; it is observed only at 37°C and is suppressed by metabolic inhibitors, such as sodium azide.

3. Polar Ig pinocytosis leads to "cap" disappearance. If the cells are washed and reincubated at 37°C for 6 to 20 hr, Ig reappears on the entire surface of the cell membrane. Membrane Ig turnover is very rapid; the estimated half-life is only a few hours (3 to 10 hr).

Ig capping analogous to that just described (under the influence of anti-Ig sera) is also observed in the presence of multivalent antigens. Thus, flagellin or hemocyanin induce capping of antigen-binding receptors. Interestingly, re-gardless of whether capping is induced by anti-Ig sera or antigens, one observes

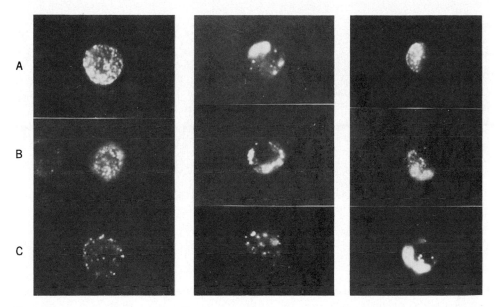

**Fig. 4.3** Capping induced by fluorescent anti-Ig antisera in B lymphocytes. (From J. L. Preud'homme.)

a redistribution of both antigen-binding receptors (detected by autoradiography) and of Ig (detected by labeled anti-Ig sera).

The capping phenomenon, which is linked to cell membrane fluidity (Fig. 4.4), is not limited to immunoglobulin antigen receptors. Similar phenomena have been described for θ, H-2, and HLA antigens on the lymphocyte surface and also for IgE on basophils and H-2 antigens on fibroblasts. One should note that in some of these settings, the antireceptor antibody cannot induce capping by itself but requires the addition on an anti-Ig divalent antibody that binds to the antireceptor antibody before capping is induced.

The biologic significance of these observations is unclear. One might anticipate a relation to facilitation and tolerance, where antibodies might modify graft cell antigenicity, and in activation of lymphocytes by antigens. This hypothesis may also explain the phenomenon of antigenic modulation (as described for TL, Ig, and H-2 antigens), in which lymphocytes may lose the expression of some of their surface antigens after contact with the corresponding antibody.

### Specificity of Membrane Immunoglobulins for the Antigen

The specificity of surface receptors for antigen may be studied by antigen binding to the lymphocyte surface by use of visible antigens, such as red blood cells (which give rosettes), or radiolabeled compounds (detected by autoradiography). It is also possible to use antigens with biologic activity (like some enzymes or bacteriophages) to reveal antigen binding by means of biologic activity (reaction of enzymes with the substrate for peroxidase or galactosidase, bacteriolysis for bacteriophages). Before any immunization, 0.1 to 1 per 1000 B

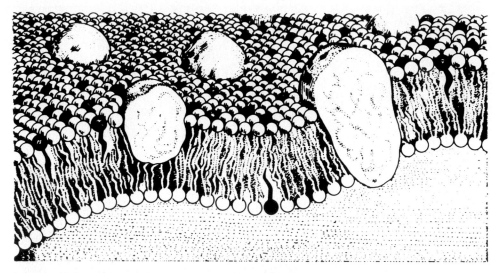

**Fig. 4.4** Structure of cellular plasma membranes according to Singer. In the bilayer sea of lipids (shaded) and cholesterol (solid), the globular proteins float as icebergs, with their hydrophilic ends protruding from the membrane and their hydrophobic ends embedded in the bilayer. (From S. J. Singer, Hosp. Pract. 1973, *8*, 31.)

lymphocytes bind sheep erythrocytes or radiolabeled flagellin. This binding is specific because one lymphocyte binds only one antigen. This number increases after immunization by a factor of 5 to 100, and this increase is antigen specific; it is not observed for other nonrelated antigens. Receptors detected by immunofluorescent anti-Ig antisera are, indeed, antigen receptors, because antigen-induced receptor redistribution also provokes Ig capping (assessed by immunofluorescence) and, reciprocally, anti-Ig sera-induced Ig redistribution provokes capping of antigen-binding receptors (as assessed by autoradiography). Paradoxically, plasma cells that secrete the largest amounts of antibodies do not always bind antigens at the membrane, and conversely, most antigen binding cells do not secrete large amounts of antibodies.

Antigen receptors detected by in vitro binding techniques do include receptors involved in in vivo antigen recognition. This statement is supported by the finding that elimination of antigen-binding cells by "suicide" with a heavily labeled antigen that lethally irradiates the cells that bind this antigen (Ada) or by cell centrifugation after rosette formation (Bach) produces tolerance to the antigen in question. Similar results have been obtained by Wigzell after passage of cells through glassbead columns coated with antigen. "Passed" cells are tolerant to the antigen bound on the column.

Antigen-binding cells are specific for the antigen. However, especially in the nonimmunized animal, there is a wide heterogeneity of cell avidity for binding a given antigen. This heterogeneity probably explains why in both the rosette test and autoradiography one sees an increase in the number of antigen-binding cells with antigen concentration. The avidity of immunocytes for antigen increases after immunization. It is difficult, however, to know if the global increase in avidity is linked to an increase in the number of receptors, of affinity, or to both mechanisms.

## T-CELL RECEPTORS

T-cell involvement in specific immunity suggests that T cells have antigen-specific receptors on their surface. However, the nature and specificity of these receptors remains a matter of considerable controversy. The crucial point is whether T-cell receptors are immunoglobulins or related substances.

### Discussion of the Immunoglobulin Nature of T-Cell Receptors

Attempts to directly show Ig (by immunofluorescence) on the T-cell surface have essentially been unsuccessful, although occasionally positive results have been claimed. Similar findings apropos Ig extraction from T cells have been noted. Marchalonis has reported the presence of significant amounts of 7S IgM in T-lymphocyte membranes extracted after iodination in the presence of lactoperoxidase, but this finding has not been confirmed by Uhr, Vitetta, and others. The differences in findings cannot be explained by quantitative considerations, because the quantity of Ig in T cells has been reported to be similar to that in B cells. Implantation of Ig within the T-cell membrane might be involved, but, as we shall see, inhibition of antigen binding on T cells with anti-Ig sera indicates that receptors are freely exposed on the T-cell surface (at the level of the antigen binding sites). Furthermore, attempts to "expose" Ig by treatment with proteases, neuraminidase, or phospholipases have not increased detectable Ig. T-cell receptors might conceivably be released by T cells on contact with anti-Ig serum; however, metabolic inhibitors that should depress this phenomenon do not increase the amount of Ig detectable on the lymphocyte surface.

Another approach consists of inhibiting in vitro and in vivo T-cell activities by anti-Ig sera. Antilight-chain and anti-μ chain sera inhibit labeled hemocyanin binding or SRBC rosette formation by θ-positive lymphocytes in the spleen and thymus. In these two systems, anti-Ig sera at noninhibiting doses produce capping of antigen-binding receptors. Some authors have not succeeded in demonstrating the presence of antigen-binding receptors on the T-cell surface. However, technical reasons probably explain this failure, because T-cell receptors are much less numerous than B-cell receptors, and antigen binding is much more difficult to demonstrate. This is also perhaps the explanation of why neonatally bursectomized chickens immunized with SRBC do not form rosettes. This finding might also be explained by an involvement of an Ig secreted by B cells that binds to the T-cell surface (receptors for the Fc fragment of IgG after T-cell activation), but one would not then understand why antigen-binding T cells are antigen specific: any one T cell binds only one antigen.

Inhibition of T-cell functions by anti-Ig sera has, in general, much less clear effects on MLR, GvH, and lymphocytotoxicity, except for occasional positive experiments. Most authors report negative data. It is interesting to note that these reactions are easily inhibited by alloantisera against histocompatibility antigens and by anti-idiotypic antibodies as we shall see now.

Binz and Wigzell have shown that anti-idiotypic antibodies (see p. 209) produced in (Lewis xDA) $F_1$ rats immunized against Lewis anti-DA antibodies or against Lewis T cells react with both T and B lymphocytes of Lewis rats, which possess receptors for the transplantation antigen of DA rats. These antibodies, which bind to 1% of B lymphocytes and 5% to 7% of T lymphocytes, specifically inhibit anti-DA-mixed lymphocyte reaction and the graft versus host response as well as delay the rejection of skin grafts. Therefore, T lymphocytes appear to express certain idiotypes found in conventional serum antibodies. However, although the idiotype-bearing receptors, or B cells, are 7S–8S IgM molecules, those of T cells are polypeptide chains of about 70,000 daltons, which may exist as dimers and which neither react with conventional anti-Ig antibodies (including antilight-chain antibodies) nor with antibodies directed against transplantation antigens. In addition, these idiotypes are inherited and linked to a heavy-chain Ig allotype, which suggests that the idiotype–bearing receptors on T cells are coded for in the H-chain variable region (V$\kappa$) gene pool. These receptors do not seem to be directly associated with other polypeptides of different molecular weight. The simplest view is that simple or dimeric IgH chains have a previously undescribed constant region and serve as receptors for antigens on T lymphocytes.

The findings reported by Eichmann and Rajewsky are consistent with this view. These authors used anti-idiotype antibodies raised in guinea pigs against an A/J mouse strain antibody specific for streptococcal group A carbohydrates. A small dose of these antibodies (of the IgG1 fraction) sensitizes A/J mice against group A streptococci: sensitization occurs in both T-helper cells and B cells, which indicates that B and T cells use the same inherited $V_H$ genes for responding to group A streptococcal carbohydrates. Moreover, only those anti-idiotype antisera that recognize idiotypes genetically linked to H chain alone are able to stimulate both T and B cells in vivo, whereas those that react with idiotypes that require light (L) chains for their expression can only stimulate B cells. It should also be noted that, in the same system, injection of IgG2 antibodies induced the generation of suppressor T cells and hence a specific suppression of the immune response. Results that confirm the presence of idiotypic receptors have been obtained in the mouse for delayed hypersensitivity responses against phosphorylcholine and in the rabbit for ribonuclease-binding T cells (Cazenave).

### T-Cell Receptors, Histocompatibility Loci, and Ir Genes

Alloantisera directed against histocompatibility antigens inhibit blast transformation of T cells in the presence of antigen, antigen binding by T cells, and the MLR. Because of the presence of Ir genes within the histocompatibility complex (see chap. 24), McDevitt and Benacerraf have proposed that T-cell receptors may be Ir gene products or substances controlled by Ir gene products. It remains, however, to be determined whether the relationships between Ir genes and H-2 loci are fortuitous or have a functional basis. Another more likely possibility is that the T-cell receptor is a complex of a (classic or new) Ig associated with a histocompatibility antigen molecule. Lastly Ir gene expression may be associated with the presentation of antigen as a complex formed with Ir gene products (Ia antigens); for example, on macrophage surface (see below).

### Specificity of T-Cell Receptors for Antigen

The other side of the T-cell recognition puzzle concerns the target antigens that T cells see. T cells, as seen above, bind antigen to their surface. The possibility of a passive absorption of receptors onto the T-lymphocyte surface cannot be completely excluded but seems unlikely because of the existence of receptor synthesis by T cells after their elimination secondary to capping and of antigen-binding specificity. The percentage of antigen-binding cells (for example, for sheep erythrocytes or hemocyanin) depends to a large extent on experimental conditions but is generally of the order of 0.1 prior to immunization and of 0.5 to 1.0 after immunization. These receptors are antigen specific; one cell binds only one antigen. Receptors that bind antigen in vitro include the T cells that recognize the antigen in vivo; incubation of thymic cells with a radiolabeled antigen induces the binding to the surface of a small percentage of thymocytes (autoradiography) and causes a specific inability of these thymic cells to interact with normal bone marrow cells for subsequent antibody production directed against this antigen. Moreover, it is possible to eliminate immune cytotoxic T cells directed against transplantation antigens of a given specificity by adherence to a monolayer of allogeneic cells of the same specificity.

There is increasing evidence that T cells only respond maximally to conventional antigens when they see them in association with antigens coded for by the major histocompatibility complex (MHC). Thus, in order for cytotoxic T cells to respond optimally to haptens, viral or minor histocompatibility antigens on mouse target cell surfaces, they must see them in association with H-2D or H-2K gene products; primed T cells that proliferate in response to antigen-coated "macrophages" in vitro recognize antigens in association with the Ia antigens of the macrophage; helper T cells seem to see antigens in association with Ia antigens and T cells responsible for delayed hypersensitivity see some antigens (foreign gamma globulins, for example) in association with Ia antigens, and others (such as dinitrofluorobenzene) in association with H-2D or H-2K gene products. This restriction, initially described by Zinkernagel and Doherty in lymphocyte choriomeningitis, may explain a number of experimental results that were previously thought to be examples of "syngeneic preference" in which it was thought that T cells and macrophages or T cells and B cells must be syngeneic for the I-region determinants to be able to cooperate.

It is not known whether the "antigenic" determinants of the major histocompatibility complex must be physically associated with the surface of the target cell or macrophage or if they are present in the form of a free complex. Neither has it been established whether T cells recognize a single glycoprotein determinant of the major histocompatibility complex that has been modified by antigens (modified "self") or recognize separately through two distinct receptors, the MHC product and conventional antigens. Binz and Wigzell have reported that about 5% of rat T cells are labeled with anti-idiotypic receptors, as described

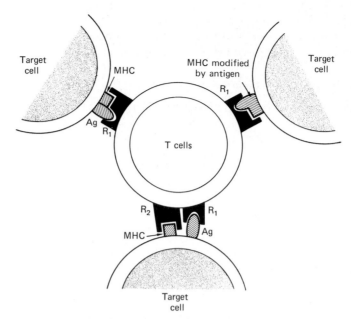

**Fig. 4.5**   Three models explaining syngeneic restriction (after Zinkernagel). Upper left: Single receptor that recognizes a complex of conventional antigen and a major histocompatibility product (MHC). Upper right: Single receptor recognizing modified "self." Below: Two receptors, one recognizing conventional antigen, the other an MHC product.

above, and we have seen that these antibodies essentially react with the products of the $V_H$ genes of Ig, recognizing the determinants of the DA major histocompatibility complex. It seems therefore that the genetic pools of the heavy-chain variable regions and the hypothetical "second" receptor of T cells may be strongly implicated in the genetic control of MHC recognition. We shall return (chap. 24) to the phenomenon of syngeneic restriction, discussing in particular the condition under which it occurs in the fetal thymus during development.

## VI.   B- AND T-CELL MATURATION

The discrete changes occurring during T-lymphocyte maturation, whose remarkable functional diversity has been mentioned, have been and remain the object of intensive research and passionate discussion. The outcome of such arguments is of tremendous importance in theoretical immunology because of the opportunity that it opens to enable detailed studies of the states of differentiation of a cell with such diverse functions. Such arguments are of equal significance for clinical immunology since knowledge of this maturation process may enable the development of therapeutic maneuvers in numerous pathologic states in which abnormalities of lymphocyte differentiation play an important etiological role.

Earlier, we introduced the concept of lymphocyte differentiation from hemopoietic stem cells. The present question is how lymphocyte precursors give rise to mature and immunocompetent lymphocytes. We will examine B and T cells separately, but we will also consider the possible differentiation of pluripotent stem cells into pre-B and pre-T cells before their passage through the thymus and the bursa of Fabricius (or its equivalent). Several studies have suggested that cells are predestined to mature into B or T cells before their respective passage through the thymus or bursa of Fabricius-existence of common xenoantigens on brain and T cells, presence of small quantities of θ antigen on a significant proportion of lymphocytes from nude mice, augmentation or even induction of θ antigen expression on immature lymphocytes by thymic hormones and other products that elevate intralymphocyte levels of cyclic AMP. However, other data favor the chance migration of lymphoid stem cells toward the thymus or bursa of Fabricius, possibly under the influence of chemotactic factors.

# T LYMPHOCYTES

Knowledge of T-cell maturation derives not only from experiments that bear on thymic function in the adult animal but also to a large extent from thymic phylogeny and ontogeny. The existence of long-lived T cells and the fact that thymectomy, when performed more than 24 hr after birth, has no longer a spectacular effect on immunity indicate the importance of T-lymphocyte production in the fetus.

## T-Lymphocyte Ontogeny

### THYMUS ONTOGENY

The thymus is the first lymphoid organ to appear in the embryo, arising from the third and fourth pharyngeal pouches. In the mouse, the thymic anlage appears on the 10th day of gestation. There are then only two cell types, an epithelium and a mesenchyme. However, as early as the 11th day one notes the presence of basophilic cells, which are probably lymphocyte precursors. These cells are more numerous on the 12th day when the thymic primordium migrates to the anterior mediastinum, where it appears on the 13th to 14th days as a bilobed vascular organ engaged in active lymphopoiesis. Recent data have shown that it is at this stage of development that the thymic epithelium acquires the expression of Ia antigens. The thymus more closely resembles the adult gland and progressively increases in size until birth. A parallel development is observed in the chicken, with the appearance of the epithelial primordium on the sixth day of embryonic life and of lymphocytes on the 12th day.

It had long been thought that lymphocytes issued directly from epithelial cells; however, it is now very clear from parabiosis and transfer experiments (Moore and Owen) with chromatin markers in chicken and quail (Le Douarin) that the epithelial primordium is, in fact, colonized by mesenchymatous cells derived from the blood. The mesenchymatous cells differentiate into lymphocytes under the influence of the thymic epithelial microenvironment. Thus, when one grafts an epithelial primordium from an 8-day fetus onto the chorioallantoidian membrane of 10-day embryos, the thymocytes that populate the graft 8 to 9 days later are all of host type, whereas if the graft is taken from a 10- to 12-day embryo, the grafted thymus is mainly populated, 8 to 9 days later, by graft-derived lymphocytes. Moreover, thymus explants from 10-day-old mouse fetuses cultivated in vitro do not produce lymphocytes, whereas 12-day explants, which contain the basophilic cells mentioned earlier, generate lymphocytes.

N. Le Douarin came to identical conclusions following experiments with similar grafts in the quail and chicken. The nuclei of lymphocytes from Japanese quail may be distinguished from those of chicken lymphocytes by the appearance of their chromatin under ordinary light microscopy. Those nuclei derived either from the chicken or the quail in interspecies embryonic grafts can therefore be recognized. Thymic rudiments from the quail were transplanted into 3-day-old chicken embryos. When the graft originated from 9-day-old quail embryos, at which age the thymus is purely endodermal (i.e., epithelial) and not yet infiltrated by blood-born cells, examination of the thymus at 12 days revealed that it only contained lymphocytes of the host (i.e., of chicken origin). Conversely, when a complete quail thymic rudiment, containing epithelium and blood-born cells and removed at 5-6 days of incubation, was grafted, the lymphocytes examined on day 12 were composed of a mixture of quail and chicken cells. These results confirm that the lymphocytes cannot be directly derived from the epithelium. It should also be noted that, in the same experimental quail-chicken system, when the graft was taken from an embryo after the 6th day of development and implanted into an embryonic chicken, all the thymic cells examined on day 12 were derived from the quail. This suggests that chicken precursor cells were unable to colonize the thymic primordium. In other words, it seems as though once it becomes saturated, the thymus is unable to receive new precursors.

The cells that colonize the epithelial primordium are present in yolk sac and liver; the liver does not produce them at the beginning of fetal life but is itself colonized by yolk sac cells. The large basophilic cells observed in the thymic primordium are most likely lymphocyte precursors. Experimental verification of this hypothesis was shown when hemopoietic embryonic cells, labeled with radioactive thymidine, were injected into 8- to 9-day chicken embryos (before the appearance of lymphocytes in the thymic primordium). Twenty-four hours later, numerous labeled cells were observed in the primordium, and 48 hr later, true-labeled lymphocytes were visible.

Fetal thymocytes are not immunocompetent, yet they are observed to fix certain antigens onto their membranes and are capable of proliferating in response to PHA at 14 to 16 weeks of gestation in man. Not until birth or even some days after does the capacity to develop GvH reaction or B-cell cooperation begin to appear.

DIFFERENTIATION STAGES

The steps of lymphocyte maturation in ontogeny may be followed in mice and in chickens by the appearance of T-lymphocyte markers and by immuno-

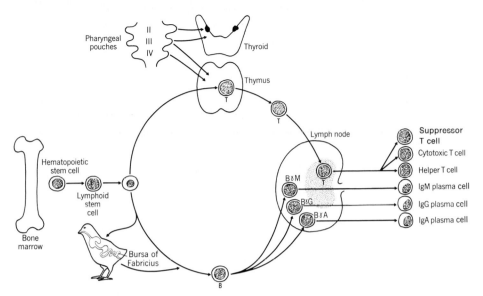

**Fig. 4.6**  B- and T-lymphocyte maturation.

competence development. The cells of the 14-day-old primordium are still θ and TL negative. However, after 2 days of in vitro culture of dissociated thymic cells collected from 14-day-old fetuses, one sees a few TL-or θ-positive cells, and after 4 days of culture, the majority of cells have become TL and θ positive. Similarly, in vivo, θ-positive cells are seen around day 16. At variance with in vitro experiments, these latter studies do not reveal whether θ-positive cells issue from cells that were θ negative the day before or have just recently migrated to the thymus.

Stutman's experiments produced new and important information with respect to functional T-cell maturation. The capacity of various cell types to restore immunocompetence in neonatally thymectomized mice at 45 days was studied. At this age, thymus grafts do not restore immunocompetence, probably because of the absence of precursor cells. A good restoration was obtained with 14-day-old embryo cells, for example, liver cells in the presence of a free thymus graft; however, the same cells were without effect when the thymus was grafted into a Millipore chamber or when thymoma was grafted, two situations in which only humoral function of the thymus is present. Conversely, neonatal liver cells or neonatal spleen cells restored immunologic competence in thymectomized mice in association with the same thymic graft placed into a Millipore chamber or with an epithelial thymoma graft. This finding indicates a difference in maturation of 14-day-old embryo T-cell precursors and newborn cells. Fourteen-day-old embryo cells are capable of migrating toward the thymus, a finding that supports Stutman's hypothesis, namely, that precursor differentiation between day 14 and birth occurs under the direct influence of the thymus, thus the term "post-thymic" cells, given to some newborn spleen, bone marrow, or liver cells. As yet another illustration of this hypothesis, thymus grafting in a Millipore chamber restores immunocompetence of neonatally thymectomized mice as long as the graft is performed before post-thymic cells have disappeared

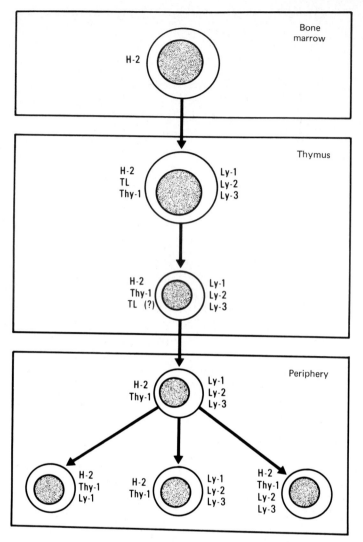

**Fig. 4.7**  Variation of differentiation antigens during T-cell maturation.

(30-45 days). This same graft is without effect in nude mice, which have never possessed a functional thymus and therefore have no post-thymic cells. These post-thymic cells, whose characteristics are listed in Table 4.8 seem to differentiate into mature T cells in the peripheral lymphoid organs under the influence of thymic hormones. In this model, post-thymic cells are Lyt 123$^+$ and give rise to Lyt 1$^+$ and Lyt 23$^+$ cells described on p. 65.

Immunocompetence of T cells is not found at birth in the mouse; one must wait 2 to 4 weeks before detecting the capacity to reject allografts or to produce antibodies directed against thymus-dependent antigens. This slow maturation is due in part to the existence of an extrathymic maturation (see p. 65). In the human, however, fetal cells respond in an MLR as early as the 10th week of gestation and to PHA stimulation as early as the 14th week.

### T-Lymphocyte Production in the Adult

T lymphocytes are produced in the adult, with precursor cells originating in bone marrow. This fact has been shown by grafting thymuses that contain the T6 chromosomal marker into irradiated thymectomized mice that were reconstituted with bone marrow cells deficient in the T6 marker. In a first phase after grafting, thymic cells and a small percentage of peripheral lymph node and spleen cells that respond to PHA bear the T6 marker, thus indicating the existence of T-cell migration from the thymus. Two to 3 weeks later, T lymphocytes without the T6 marker are seen in the thymus and in the periphery demonstrating continuous formation of lymphocytes by the adult thymus. T-cell release by the thymus is also evident from migration of thymocytes, labeled in situ by thymidine. However, numerous (more than 95% in some studies) thymocytes die locally.

Recent studies suggest that T cells that leave the thymus arise from only a small proportion of the corticosteroid-resistant medulla, which contain a high percentage of long-lived immunocompetent cells. Numerous cells that have recently migrated from the thymus (followed by thymidine incorporation techniques) into the peripheral lymphoid organs are corticosteroid sensitive and are derived from the thymic cortex.

The thymus atrophies with age. This process begins as early as 3 months in the mouse and by the 10th year in man. Linked to this atrophy, but differing with respect to time because of long-lived lymphocytes, there is a decrease in immunocompetence after the 18th month of life in the mouse and after 60 years in man.

### Factors in T-Lymphocyte Differentiation

The thymus contains epithelial cells and lymphocytes. We have discussed the primordial role of the epithelium in differentiating stem cells coming from the yolk sac and, later, from the fetal liver. This essential role of the epithelium is maintained in adults, because neonatally thymectomized mice regain immunocompetence after grafting of an adult thymus that was rendered purely epithelial by in vitro incubation or irradiation or by incubation in a Millipore chamber in an intermediate host. Two nonmutually exclusive hypotheses may be envisaged to explain the mechanism of this differentiating action of thymic epithelium. The first hypothesis attributes the critical role to contact between epithelial cells and bone marrow precursors; secondly, it may be postulated that there are local or distant effects of humoral factors secreted by the thymic epithelium.

CELLULAR THEORY (EPITHELIAL MICROENVIRONMENT)

Differentiation of thymic cell precursors after direct contact with the epithelial network would be analogous to hemopoietic stem cell differentiation of erythrocyte or granulocyte precursors after contact with the spleen or bone marrow microenvironment. The apparent necessity for T cells to pass through the thymus, which is suggested by thymic graft experiments, is compatible with this hypothesis, as are the visibly close contacts between epithelial tissue and

**Table 4.8  Principal Characteristics of the Different Stages in the Maturation of T Lymphocytes in the Mouse (After Stutman)**

| Biological characteristics | Prethymic cells (or prothymocytes) | Precursor cells (post-thymic) | Mature T cells |
|---|---|---|---|
| **Distribution** | | | |
| Embryo (14 days) | Yolk-sac, liver, blood | Liver | |
| Newborn | Liver | Spleen, liver | |
| Adult | Bone marrow | Spleen bone marrow | Spleen, thymus, lymph nodes |
| **Ontogenesis** | | | |
| Date of appearance in fetus | 9th day | 15th day | After birth |
| **Circulation** | | | |
| Migration | Spleen, thymus | Spleen | Lymph nodes |
| Recirculation | No | No | Yes |
| Immune competence | No | Regulatory function (especially suppressor) | Yes |
| **Reconstitution of thymectomized mice** | | | |
| Alone | No | No | Yes |
| After thymic graft | Yes | Yes | Yes |
| After humoral thymic factors only | No | Yes | Yes |

94

**Presence after various types of thymus deprivation:**

| | | | |
|---|---|---|---|
| Neonatal thymectomy | Yes | Yes[+] | No |
| Adult thymectomy | Yes | Yes[+] | Yes |
| Nude mice | Yes | No | No |
| Mice treated with ALS | Yes | Yes | No |
| Cortico-steroid-treated mice | Yes(?) | No | Yes |
| **Differentiation antigens** | | | |
| θ (Thy-1) | +/− | + | + |
| TL | − | +/− | − |
| Lyt | − | $123^+$ | $1^+,23^+123^+$ |
| **Other markers** | | | |
| Membrane Ig | − | − | − |
| Fc | − | − | ± |
| TdT | −(?) | + | − |
| Peanut agglutinin | +(?) | + | − |
| **Other properties** | | | |
| Life-span | ? | 30–60 days | Usually low |
| Density (BSA gradient) | Low | Low | High |
| Adherence to nylon | No | Yes | No |
| Degree of proliferation | Low(?) | High | Low |

[+] In the 30 to 40 days following thymectomy.

95

lymphocytes on electron microscopy. The observation that a free (intact) thymus graft is necessary to induce differentiation of 14-day-old embryonic cells, while humoral function suffices for differentiation of newborn spleen cells, suggests that the microenvironment theory is particularly crucial during the first maturation phases. In this context, it should be noted that the studies of Zinkernagel described on p. 692 demonstrate how, during the period of contact with thymic epithelium, T cells acquire the specificity for autologous MHC antigens and at the same time develop their capacity to recognize conventional antigens.

### HUMORAL THEORY (THYMIC HORMONES)

It is possible to restore immunocompetence in neonatally thymectomized mice by placing a thymus graft in a cell-impermeable chamber. Equivalent results may be obtained by injecting thymic extracts, although, for obvious reasons (quantity), the extracts are prepared in species other than the mouse. Therefore, one might argue a contributory role of nonspecific stimulation of immunity by heterologous proteins contained in thymic extracts. Additional evidence for a humoral function of the thymus is provided by the fact that neonatally thymectomized mice gain immunocompetence during gestation, probably due to hormonal secretion by the fetal thymus. The involvement of humoral thymic factors, which is implicit in these experiments, is corroborated by the presence of secretion grains in the thymic epithelium, visible on electron microscopy.

For almost 10 years, several groups have attempted to determine the structure of thymic hormones. At present, there is no consensus of opinion about their structure and it is not difficult to suppose that eventually the answer will indicate that several hormones exist, each producing effects at different stages of lymphocyte differentiation.

A. Goldstein and A. White have obtained from calf thymus a preparation, thymosin, which contains a number of peptides. A. Goldstein has reported the amino acid sequence of a peptide known as thymosin α1 with a molecular weight of about 3,000. He has proposed a hypothesis suggesting that the thymic hormones are in fact a group of products (thymosin α1 being one of them) whose biologic effects are manifold. This theory is interesting in the theoretical overview of the immune system. It leads to the concept of the existence of several products with different effects at several stages of maturation.

G. Goldstein has approached the problem from a different angle. He isolated a protein that inhibits neuromuscular conduction in the guinea pig: the amino acid sequence of this peptide was determined and an active fragment was synthesized. This peptide, initially named "thymin" and then "thymopoietin" was found to induce T-cell membrane markers on T-cell precursors. Various functional activities have been found to be attributable to this factor, following either in vitro or in vivo treatment.

Trainin, in Israel, has also isolated from calf thymus a "thymic humoral factor" of low molecular weight (less than 3,000) that possesses several biologic activities. In particular, it has been found capable of inducing MLR and GvH reactivity. Its amino acid sequence has not yet been described.

Facteur thymique sérique (FTS) has been isolated, as its name suggests, from serum by our group at the Hôpital Necker (Fig. 4.8). Its thymic dependence is demonstrated by the fact that it disappears from the serum after thymectomy and reappears following a thymic graft. Its presence in the thymus epithelium has recently been shown by use of immunofluorescence. Serum FTS levels are age-dependent and diminish in parallel with thymic weight. Its mode of action is as yet unknown but seems to exert its effect by means of the intervention of cyclic nucleotides as do many of the other factors cited above. FTS has been isolated through its capacity to induce the appearance of $\theta$ antigen on precursor cells in the bone marrow. It has also been found to induce a number of functional changes in T lymphocytes both in vitro and in vivo and to bind to high affinity receptors.

FTS is a nonapeptide (<Glu-Ala-Lys-Ser-Gln-Gly-Gly-Ser-Asn). It has now been synthesized and the synthetic product is as biologically active as the natural product, which has been isolated from serum (0.01 pg/ml $- 10^{-14}$ M in vitro and 0.1 ng in vivo). Several analogues have also been synthesized, demonstrating that only a part of the molecule is biologically active. Comparative studies of the amino acid sequence of FTS, $\alpha 1$ thymosin, and thymopoietin demonstrate that these are quite different entities. Only further studies will reveal whether or not FTS is identical or similar to thymosin other than $\alpha_1$ or Trainin's factor. FTS may in fact represent the circulating form of one of these products.

CONCLUSIONS

Insufficient evidence is now at hand. Contact with the thymic microenvironment appears to be necessary for the first differentiation phases. One or several thymic hormones may then be implicated, active locally (thymus gland) or peripherally, analogous to the respective roles of erythropoietin and the "colony-stimulating factor" for erythrocytes and polymorphs. It is possible that the first maturation phase is also under the influence of humoral factors that act at high concentrations within the thymus gland. Recent data also suggest that T-cell growth factors (Interleukin 2, see p. 386) produced by medullary Lyt1$^+$ thymocytes could also intervene in promoting intrathymic T-cell differentiation. Thus, nude mouse spleen cells can generate cytotoxic T cells in the presence of Interleukin 2.

### Extrathymic Maturation

T-LYMPHOCYTE HETEROGENEITY

All T cells are not equal. Within the thymus, one may already distinguish two cell populations: one in the cortex, TL and $\theta$ positive, destroyed by hydrocortisone injection and immunologically incompetent; the other in the medulla, $\theta$ positive (but containing less $\theta$ antigen than that contained by the cortical population), TL negative, hydrocortisone resistant, and immunocompetent. All thymus cells that bind antigen, respond to PHA and in an MLR, are capable of inducing a GVH, and that cooperate with B cells in antibody production belong to the second (medullary) population. On a quantitative level, it is interesting to note that a 5-mg hydrocortisone acetate injection

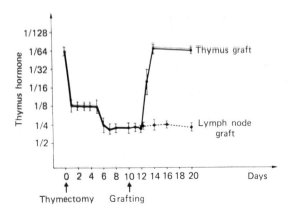

**Fig. 4.8** Effects of adult thymectomy and thymus grafting on the serum level of thymic hormone in the adult mouse (After J. F. Bach and M. Dardenne, 1972.)

destroys 95% of thymic lymphocytes in the mouse but increases the PHA reactivity of the remaining lymphocytes about twentyfold (as evaluated for a constant cell number).

Additionally, spleen and lymph node T cells are not all identical. Thus, adult thymectomy leads within a few weeks to a decreased number of θ and Lyt 123-positive lymphocytes in the spleen without an effect on the number of θ-positve lymph node cells. Moreover, adult thymectomy leads to a decrease in the spleen cell response to PHA and allogeneic cells and probably to the loss of certain suppressor T-cell function as assessed by enhanced production of antibodies against thymus-independent antigens.

Finally, a synergy has been demonstrated between thymic or splenic lymphocytes and lymph node or blood lymphocytes in vitro in cell-mediated lymphocytotoxicity and in vivo in GvH reaction. There appears, then, to be two T-lymphocyte populations: one predominates in the spleen and thymus, bears Lyt123 antigens, and is short-lived, or perhaps is permanently dependent on the thymus, possibly by means of a thymic hormone; the second predominates in lymph nodes, bears Lyt1 or Lyt23 antigens, is long-lived, recirculates, and is thymus independent after differentiation in that organ. The second population is not exclusive to lymph nodes but is also found in thymus and spleen, although in a numerical minority as compared to the first population. One should finally mention that populations of suppressor T cells are found in large number in thymus and spleen in the adult and in the newborn spleen and that antigen-specific suppressor T cells have been reported to bear Lyt23 antigens.

REAPPEARANCE OF IMMUNOCOMPETENCE IN THYMECTOMIZED MICE AFTER
THYMUS GRAFTING

Several weeks elapse before the reappearance of the PHA response or skin allograft rejection capacity in thymectomized, irradiated, and bone-marrow-reconstituted mice subsequently grafted with thymus. However, if one removes the newly grafted thymus after 8 days, before the reappearance of immunocompetence, immunocompetence develops 4 or 5 weeks later, which suggests a role of slow extrathymic maturation.

It appears, from our analysis of these data, that there is an extrathymic maturation of the long-lived recirculating T cells present in lymph nodes. Possibly, although less well documented, there is also extrathymic maturation of short-lived T cells of the spleen. One might postulate that the spleen T-cell population (not recirculating) includes precursors of recirculating long-lived lymph node T cells; alternatively, these two cell types may be parallel lineages of a common precursor. Suppressor T cells might represent a third lineage or might belong, in part, to the noncirculating spleen cell population.

# B LYMPHOCYTES

There is much less knowledge of B-lymphocyte maturation than of T cells, which is easily explained by our ignorance as to the B-cell differentiating organ in mammals. The bursa of Fabricius in birds has as yet no known equivalent in mammals.

## B-Lymphocyte Ontogeny

### ONTOGENY OF THE BURSA OF FABRICIUS

The bursal primordium appears in the chicken embryo on day 4 as an epithelial evagination of the dorsal wall of the cloaca. The first lymphoid cells appear on day 13, as an infiltrate in the epithelial buds. At this stage, they are large, morphologically undifferentiated cells, with a deeply basophilic cytoplasm, analogous to the first lymphoid cells that appear in the thymus (see p. 89). True lymphocytes are observed as early as the 15th or 16th day. Just before birth, a few foci of granulopoiesis appear simultaneously with lymphoid follicles (a cortex and a medulla composed of a reticuloepithelial network infiltrated with lymphocytes).

The origin of bursal lymphocytes has been the object of lively discussion similar to that summarized earlier relative to thymic lymphocytes. Some authors advanced the hypothesis of local transformation of epithelial cells into lymphoid cells. It has now been proven, however, by transfer experiments and grafting experiments with chromatin markers in quail and chicken, analogous to those described for thymus, that precursor cells originate in yolk sac and the mesenchyme, travel through the blood, and infiltrate the epithelium, where they differentiate.

Despite the importance of the bursa of Fabricius in the generation of antibody-producing cells, the bursa itself contains very few of these lymphocytes. It is, however, the first site where, in the embryo, IgM-synthesizing cells may be found (between days 14 and 18): this period occurs soon after infiltration of the organ by stem cells. IgG-synthesizing cells are found only at birth, and even then, one must wait about 8 days to see Ig synthesis in the spleen. The bursa also contains, as early as the 14th day, an important quantity of flagellin-binding cells, this phenomenon may, however, represent passive binding of maternal cytophilic antibodies.

SEARCH FOR A MAMMALIAN EQUIVALENT OF THE BURSA OF FABRICIUS

Numerous studies have attempted to locate a mammalian equivalent of the bursa of Fabricius. Lymphoid organs of the gut, tonsils, and Peyer's patches have been serially examined because of an ontogenic development analogous to that of the bursa, and becaue of the deficiency of humoral immunity after ablation of these organs (at least when associated with irradiation and injection of fetal liver cells). In fact, these analogies with the bursa are more apparent than real. The organs in question, unlike the bursa, contain T cells that respond to PHA and are $\theta$ positive in the mouse; additionally, they contain antibody-producing cells after immunization and are thus more similar in that regard to the secondary peripheral lymphoid organs than to the bursa of Fabricius. As in the bursa, lymphocytes are detected very early, before birth, in these organs, but, in contrast with the bursa, these cells do not synthesize Ig. The absence of Peyer's patches in human agammaglobulinemias might be secondary to B-cell deficiency rather than primary. Finally, even though one cannot exclude the possibility that gut lymphoid organs have some functions of primary lymphoid organs (analogous to the bursa), these functions have not really been demonstrated and are associated with the function of secondary lymphoid organs analogous to lymph nodes. One may also note that lymphoid gut-associated formations other than the bursa exist in birds. Some authors have suggested that bone marrow could be both the site of stem cell production and the bursa equivalent. The early presence of Ig-bearing lymphocytes in the spleen and fetal liver also suggests that these organs might be the primitive differentiation sites for B cells in the fetus. If mouse fetal liver is removed 5 days before B lymphocytes appear in the intact animal and is placed in organ culture, Ig-bearing cells appear after 7 days of culture as they would have done in vivo (Owen, Cooper and Raff). B lymphocytes bearing IgM can first be found in the liver of human fetuses at 9 weeks gestation.

DIFFERENTIATION PHASES

We have already mentioned the appearance of lymphocytes containing cytoplasmic IgM (pre-B cells) and surface IgM as early as day 14 in fetal life in the chicken bursa of Fabricius (16th–17th day in the mouse and 9th week in man), IgG appearing later at the time of birth and IgA even later. The question remains, however, whether IgG- and IgM-bearing cells are two independent lines or whether they issue one from another, as is the case after immunization (IgM to IgG switch; see p. 538). The latter possibility is suggested by data that show that injection of anti-μ serum on fetal day 13 in chickens that are subsequently bursectomized (too late to induce an agammaglobulinemia) prevents both IgM and IgG production. Analogous experiments have been performed in mice, where injections of anti-μ sera at birth block the ultimate production of not only IgM but also of IgG and IgA. The observation of numerous cells in the bursa that contain both IgG and IgM and the observation that bursectomy performed 2 days before birth prevents IgG production without altering IgM production are in the same vein. One might postulate that some IgM cells have already left the bursa and that the IgM-IgG differentiation does not occur only outside the bursa. The failure of Ig synthesis to increase

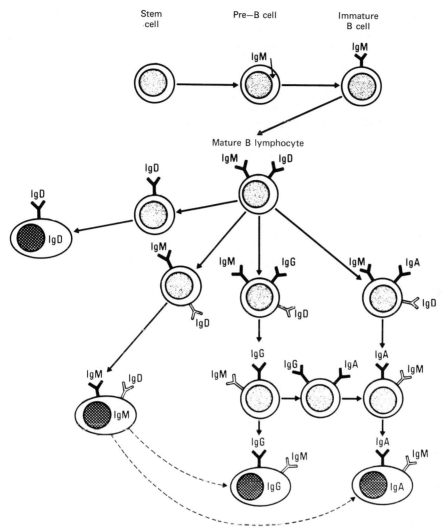

**Fig. 4.9** Maturation model for B cells (after J. L. Preud'homme and M. Seligmann). Dotted arrows and open immunoglobulins refer to hypothetical features that require confirmation.

in bursal cells after injection of antigen indicates that bursal Ig production is independent of antigenic stimulation. An important role of mitoses in creating B-lymphocyte clones has been suggested, especially because antigen receptors are found on bursal lymphocyte surfaces. Let us mention also the recent discovery in mouse and man of IgD-bearing cells early in bursal development. IgD and IgM often coexist in one cell early in development; however, IgM is the first Ig to appear in fetal ontogeny.

In parallel with the appearance of the different classes of Ig, B lymphocytes develop their different antibody specificities. This occurs sequentially, among the first to appear being IgM-producing lymphocytes. This conclusion is derived from sequential studies of lymphocytes that bind several antigens such as hemocyanin (T, G)-A––L or sheep red blood cells and of B cells producing antibodies after in vitro stimulation. This diversity appears very early in ontogenesis, probably at the pre-B cell stage (as defined by the presence of cytoplasmic Ig), which excludes the intervention of these antigens at the origin of its generation.

The ontogenic appearance of receptors other than membrane Ig on the B-cell surface has been the subject of many recent studies. Fc and C3 receptors seem to appear before Ig, as suggested by agammaglobulinemia with the presence of Fc receptors and the absence of membrane Ig. Detailed studies have serially followed the appearance of surface Ig in the chicken embryo. Ig appears as soon as the 10th day and thereafter increases in amount. In normal mammals, bone marrow lymphocytes contain variable amounts of membrane Ig; the youngest cells (labeled with tritiated thymidine) contain the least Ig.

### Factors in B-Cell Differentiation

The mechanisms of induction of B-cell differentiation under the influence of the bursa of Fabricius are unknown. Restoration of antibody production in neonatally bursectomized chickens after grafting of a bursa of Fabricius in a Millipore chamber suggests a humoral action, but the specificity of these experiments has been criticized, especially because of the possibility of the presence of bacteria in the grafts, which was not excluded and which could nonspecifically stimulate function of the few remaining B cells. Identical experiments with uncontaminated embryonic bursas have been negative. One might also suggest a role of direct stem cell contact with the epithelial microenvironment. Thus, one finds, again, two nonmutually exclusive humoral and cellular hypotheses similar to those discussed in the analysis of T-cell differentiation.

## BIBLIOGRAPHY

AIUTI F. and WIGZELL H. Thymus, thymic hormones and T lymphocytes. London, 1980, Academic Press, 445 p.

BACH J. F. and CARNAUD C. Thymic factors. Progr. Allergy, 1976, *21*, 342.

BEKKUM D. W. VAN. The biological activity of thymic hormones. Rotterdam, 1975, Kooyker, 271 p.

BINZ H. and WIGZELL H. Antigen binding, idiotypic T lymphocyte receptors. Contemp. Topics Immunobiology. New York, 1977, Plenum, 113.

CANTOR H. and BOYSE E. A. Regulation of cellular and humoral immune responses by T cell subclasses. *In* Cold Spring Harbor symposia on quantitative biology, 1977, Cold Spring Harbor Laboratory, vol. 41, p. 23.

CANTOR H. and WEISSMAN I. Development and function of subpopulations of thymocytes and T lymphocytes. Progr. Allergy, 1976, *20*, I.

CHESS L. and SCHLOSSMAN S. F. Human lymphocyte subpopulations. Adv. Immunol., 1978, *25*, 213.

COOPER M. D., KEARNEY J. F., LAWTON A. R., ABNEY E. R., PARKHOUSE R. M. E., PREUD'HOMME J. L., and SELIGMANN M. Generation of immunoglobulin class diversity in B cells: a discussion with emphasis on IgD development. Ann. Immunol. 1976, *127c*, 5–73.

COOPER M. D. and LAWTON A. R. III. B-cell generation and maturation. *In* L. Brent and J. Holborow, Eds., Progress in Immunology. II, Vol. 5, Amsterdam, 1974, North Holland, p. 175.

DAVIE J. M. and PAUL W. E. Antigen-binding receptors on lymphocytes. Contemp. Topics Immunobiol., 1974, 3, 171.

DAVIES A. J. S. The thymus and the cellular basis of immunity. Transpl. Rev., 1969, 1, 43.

DAVIES A. J. S. and CARTER R. L. (Eds) Thymus dependency. Contemp. Top. Immunobiol. 1973, 2.

DICKLER H. B. Lymphocyte receptors for immunoglobulin. Adv. Immunol., 1976, 24, 167.

DWYER J. M. Identifying and enumerating human T and B lymphocytes. Progr. Allergy, 1976, 21, 178.

EICHMANN K. Expression and function of idiotypes on lymphocytes. Adv. Immunol., 1978, 26, 195.

FAUCI A. S. and BALLIEUX R. Antibody production in man: in vitro synthesis and clinical implication. New York, Academic Press, 1979, 398 pp.

FRIEDMAN H. (Ed.) Thymus factors in immunity. Ann, N.Y. Acad. Sci. (special no.), 1975, 149.

FRIEDMAN H. Subcellular factors in immunity. Ann. N.Y., Acad. Sci., 1979, 332.

GOTTLIEB P. D. Biochemical properties of non immunoglobulin, non MHC lymphocyte surface components. In Immunology 80 (M. Fougereau and J. Dausset [eds]) New York, 1980, Academic Press, 209.

GREAVES M. F., OWEN J. J. T., and RAFF M. C. T and B lymphocytes. Origin, properties and roles in immune responses. Amsterdam, 1973, Excerpta Media, 316 p.

HAYWARD A. and GREAVES M. F. Human T and B lymphocyte populations in blood. In R. A. Thompson, Ed., Recent advances in clinical immunology. Edinburgh, 1977, Churchill-Livingstone, p. 149.

JANEWAY C. A., WIGZELL H., and BINZ H. Two different $V_H$ gene products make up the T cell receptors. Scand. J. Immunol. 1976, 5, 994.

KATZ D. H. Lymphocyte differentiation, recognition and regulation. New York, 1977, Academic Press, 749 p.

LEDOUARIN N. and JOTEREAU F. V. Homing of lymphoid stem cells to the thymus and the bursa of Fabricius studied in avian embryo chimaeras. In Immunology 80 (M. Fougereau and J. Dausset [eds]) New York, 1980, Academic Press, 285.

LOOR F. Structure and dynamics of the lymphocyte surface. in F. Loor and G. Roelants, Eds., B and T cells in immune recognition. New York, 1977, Wiley, p. 153.

LOOR F. and ROELANTS G. B and T cells in immune recognition. New York, 1977, Wiley, 504 p.

MACKENZIE I. F. and POTTER T. Murine lymphocyte surface antigens. Adv. Immunol., 1979, 27, 151.

MARCHALONIS J. J. The lymphocytes: structure and function. Immunological series. Vol. 5, New York, 1977, M. Dekker, 704 pp.

MÖLLER G. (Ed.) Activation of antibody synthesis in human B lymphocytes. Immunol. Rev., 1979, 45.

MÖLLER G. (Ed.) Lymphocyte activation by mitogens. Transpl. Rev., 1972, 11.

MÖLLER G. (Ed.) Subpopulation of B-lymphocytes. Transpl. Rev., 1975, 24.

MORETTA L. MINGARI M. C., MORETTA A., HAYNES B. F., and FAUCI A. S. T cell Fc receptors as markers of function human lymphocyte subsets. In Immunology 80 (M. Fougereau and J. Dausset [eds]) New York, 1980, Academic Press, 223.

OWEN J. J. T. B cell development. In Immunology 80 (M. Fougereau and J. Dausset [eds]) New York, 1980, Academic Press, 303.

PREUD'HOMME J. L. and SELIGMANN M. Surface immunoglobulins on human lymphoid cells. In R. S. Schwartz, Ed., Progress in clinical immunology. New York, 1974, Grune & Stratton, p. 121.

RAFF M. C. Cell surface immunology. Sci. Amer., 1976, 234, 30.

REINHERZ E. L. and SCHLOSSMAN S. F. The differentiation and function of human T lymphocytes. Cell., 1980, 19, 821.

SELIGMANN M., PREUD'HOMME J. L., and KOURILSKY F. M. Membrane receptors of lymphocytes. Amsterdam, 1975, North Holland.

SOLOMON J. B. and HORTON J. D. (Eds.) Developmental immunobiology. Amsterdam, 1977, Elsevier.

STUTMAN O. Two main features of T cell development: thymus traffic and post-thymic maturation. Contemp. Topics Immunobiol., 1977, 7, 1.

STUTMAN O. Intrathymic and extrathymic T cell maturation. Immunol. Rev., 1978, 42, 138.

WEISSMAN I., BAIRD S., GARDNER R. L., PAPAIOANNOU V. E., and RASCHKE W. Normal and neoplastic maturation of T-lineage lymphocytes. In Cold Spring Harbor symposia on quantitative biology 1977. Cold Spring Harbor Laboratory, vol. 41.

WIGZELL H. and BINZ H. Lymphocyte receptors. In Immunology 80 (M. Fougereau and J. Dausset [eds]) New York, 1980, Academic Press, 94.

WORTIS H. H. Immunological studies of nude mice. Contemp. Topics Immunobiology, 1974, 3, 243.

ZINKERNAGEL R. M. T cell differentiation and T cell restriction. In Immunology 80 (M. Fougereau and J. Dausset [eds]) New York, 1980, Academic Press, 338.

## ORIGINAL ARTICLES

BACH J. F. Evaluation of T-cells and thymic serum factors in man using the rosette technique. Transpl. Rev., 1973, 16, 196.

BACH J. F., BACH M. A., BLANOT D., BRICAS E., CHARREIRE J., DARDENNE M., FOURNIER C., and PLEAU J. M. Thymic serum factor. Bull. Inst. Pasteur, 1978, 76, 325.

BHAN A. K., REINHERZ E. L., POPPEME S., MacCLUSKEY R. T., and SCHLOSSMAN S. F. Location of T cell and major histocompatibility complex antigens in the human thymus. J. Exp. Med., 1980, 152, 771.

BINZ H., FRISCHKNECHT H., SHEN F. W., and WIGZELL H. Idiotypic determinants on T cell subpopulations. J. Exp. Med., 1979, 149, 910.

BINZ H. and WIGZELL H. Shared idiotypic determinants on B and T lymphocytes reactive against the same antigenic determinants (I and II). J. Exp. Med., 1975, 142,, 197 and 218.

CANTOR H. and BOYSE E. A. Functional subclasses of T lymphocytes bearing different Ly antigens (I and II). J. Exp. Med., 1975, 141, 1376 and 1390.

COOPER M. D., LAWTON A. R., and KINCADE P. W. A two-stage model for the development of antibody-producing cells. Clin. Exp. Immunol., 1972, 11, 143.

EICHMANN K. and RAJEWSKY K. Induction of B and T cell immunity by anti-idiotypic antibody. Eur. J. Immunol., 1975, 5, 661.

EVANS R. L., BREARD J. M., LAZARUS H., SCHLOSSMAN S. F., and CHESS L. Detection, isolation and functionnal characterization of two human T cell subclasses bearing unique differentiation antigens. J. Exp. Med., 1977, 145, 221.

GILLIS S., UNION N. A., BAKER P. E., and SMITH K. A. The in vitro generation and sustained culture of nude mouse cytolytic T lymphocytes. J. Exp. Med., 1979, 149, 1460.

GOLDSCHNEIDER I., GREGOIRE K. E., BARTON R. W., and BOLLUM F. Demonstration of terminal deoxynucleotidyl transferase in thymocytes by immunofluorescence. Proc. Nat. Acad. Sci. USA, 1977, 74, 734.

GREAVES M. and JANOSSY G. Elicitation of selective T and B lymphocyte response by cell surface binding ligands. Transpl. Rev., 1972, 11, 87.

KRETH H. W. and HERZENBERG L. A. Fluorescence-activated cell sorting of human T and B lymphocytes. I. Direct evidence that lymphocytes with a high density of membrane-bound immunoglobulins are direct precursors of plasmocytes. Cell. Immunol., 1974, 12, 396.

LAWTON A. R. and COOPER M. D. Modification of B lymphocyte differentiation by anti-immuno-globulins. Contemp. Topics Immunobiology, 1974, 3, 193.

LE DOUARIN N. M. and JOTEREAU F. Tracing of cells of the avian thymus through embryonic life in interspecific chimeras. J. Exp. Med., 1975, 142, 17.

MATHIESON B. J., SHARROW S. O., CAMPBELL P. S., and ASOFSKY R. An Lyt differentiated thymocyte subpopulation detected by flow microfluorometry. Nature, 1979, *277*, 478.

MORETTA L., WEBB S. R., GROSSI C. E., LYDYARD P. M., and COOPER M. D. Functional analysis of two human T cell subpopulations: help and suppression of B cell response by T cell bearing receptors for IgM or IgG. J. Exp. Med., 1977, *146*, 184.

PARROTT D. M. V. and DE SOUSA M. Thymus-dependent and thymus-independent populations: origin, migratory patterns and lifespan. Clin. Exp. Immunol., 1971, *8*, 663.

ROELANTS G. E. Quantification of antigen-specific T and B lymphocytes in mouse spleen. Nature, New Biol, 1972, *236*, 252.

TAYLOR R. B., DUFFUS W. P. H., RAFF M. C., and de PETRIS S., Redistribution and pinocytosis of lymphocyte surface Ig molecules induced by anti-Ig antibody. Nature, New Biol., 1971, *233*, 225.

WEKERLE H., KETELSEN U. P., and ERNST M. Thymic nurse cells. Lymphoepithelial cell complexes in murine thymuses: morphological and serological characterization. J. Exp. Med., 1980, *151*, 925.

ZINKERNAGEL R. F., CALLAHAN G., KLEIN J., and DENNERT G. Cytotoxic T cells learn specificty for self H-2 during differentiation in the thymus. Nature, 1978, *271*, 251.

# Chapter 5

# PHAGOCYTES

## Robert M. Fauve

I.   ORIGIN
II.   MORPHOLOGY
III.   STUDY METHODS
IV.   FUNCTIONS
V.   CONCLUSIONS

Phagocytes are cells capable of incorporating and, under certain conditions, of digesting inert or living particles. These cells include polymorphs and mononuclear cells, both monocytes and macrophages.

Since 1882, when Elie Metchnikoff discovered the importance of these cells in the resistance of organisms to infectious diseases, it has been shown that the function of phagocytic cells, especially macrophages, is not limited to destruction of infectious agents but also includes numerous immune functions.

## I.   ORIGIN

Polymorphs, monocytes, and macrophages originate from bone marrow stem cells (Fig. 5.1). In bone marrow cell cultures, macrophage and polymorph clones appear. The quantity of clones produced may be augmented by addition of a serum substance, colony-stimulating factor (CSF). CSF production is increased in inflammatory states and by infection. However, the mechanisms by which preferential monocytosis or polymorph leukocytosis occurs are unknown, despite numerous studies.

### POLYMORPHS

One may distinguish between a proliferation period that lasts 6 days, during which time the stem cells give rise, successively, to myeloblasts, progranulocytes,

106

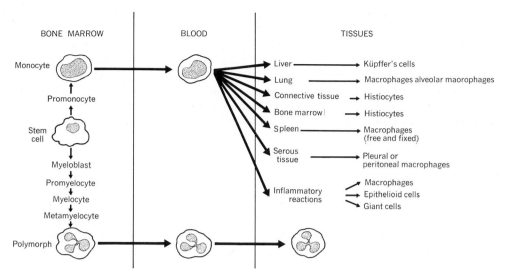

**Fig. 5.1** Origin of phagocytic cells.

myelocytes, and metamyelocytes, and a maturation period, which also lasts 6 days, during which time metamyelocytes transform into polymorphs. Neutrophil, eosinophil, and basophil polymorphs are distinguished on the basis of the staining characteristic of the granules they contain. Mature polymorphs exit from the blood vessels by diapedesis into inflamed areas (see chap. 15). In the extravascular spaces, polymorphs survive only a few days. In man, $10^{11}$ polymorphs disappear each day, largely into the gut and other mucosal surfaces.

## MONOCYTES AND MACROPHAGES

The bone marrow origin of monocytes and macrophages is now universally accepted, but it is not yet known whether the promonocyte is the only intermediary between stem cell and monocyte. However, there is no doubt that monocytes are the precursors of mononuclear phagocytic cells found in the tissues. These cells differentiate from monocytes that have crossed blood vessels by diapedesis, as in the case of alveolar macrophages found in lungs, histiocytes in the connective tissue, and peritoneal, pleural, and lymph node macrophages. Other monocytes are fixed along liver or spleen sinusoids, giving rise to liver Küpffer cells and to splenic macrophages. Unlike polymorphs, which are rapidly lysed after diapedesis, monocytes may persist in the tissues for a long time. When monocytes leave the vessels, they undergo, within a few days, an increase in size and in lysosome content. Under special conditions (see chap. 15), such as the presence of foreign substances that are difficult to resorb (e.g., mycobacteria, oil or mineral adjuvants), macrophages may transform themselves into giant cells and epithelioid cells. Macrophage life-span has especially been studied in the mouse: it is 20 to 40 days for peritoneal macrophages, 60 days for Küpffer cells, and 50 days for alveolar macrophages. In the rabbit, it has been possible to observe, in vivo after diapedesis, the transformation of a monocyte into a macrophage and its survival in connective tissue of the ear for 140 days. Generally speaking, macrophages do not divide, at least in tissues. However, under certain conditions, an important proliferation may be observed; thus, after subcutaneous injection of Freund's complete adjuvant, there is initially a monocyte immigration, maturation into macrophages, and then cessation of diapedesis. At this point, macrophages may proliferate for at least 3 months.

## II.   MORPHOLOGY

It is easy to differentiate between polymorphs, with a fragmented or "lobular" nucleus connected by nuclear filaments, and monocytes or macrophages, the nucleus of which is homogeneous and oval or kidney-shaped. These cells have other distinguishing features.

### HYALOPLASM

Very clear differences between polymorphs and mononuclear phagocytes are striking when the living cells are observed under a phase-contrast microscope, or better yet, with scanning microscopy (Figs. 5.2 and 5.3). Polymorphs have

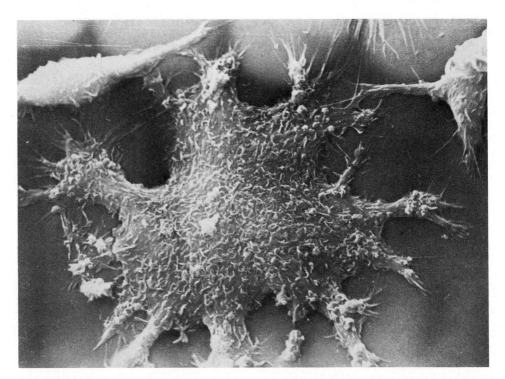

**Fig. 5.2**  Mouse peritoneal macrophage. (Electron micrograph courtesy of L. G. Chevance.)

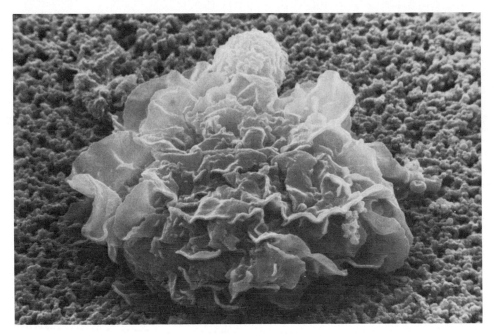

**Fig. 5.3** Mouse peritoneal macrophage. (Electron micrograph courtesy of L. G. Chevance.)

pseudopods, which are cellular extensions. Macrophages manifest characteristic cell membrane movements (waves). These waves are due to a continuous emission of hyaloplasmic veils that may cover half or more of the cell diameter. These "veils" are emitted not only at the point of contact with the substrate but overlay the entire cell surface. Their number and development are considerably increased when the macrophages have become "activated."

## CYTOPLASMIC ORGANELLES

### Mitochondria

At variance with polymorphs, which contain few or no mitochondria, monocytes and macrophages possess mitochondria of variable size.

### Endoplasmic Reticulum

Although practically absent in polymorphs, the endoplasmic reticulum is present in varying quantities in mononuclear phagocytes. Ribosomes may be quite profuse in macrophages when found in inflammatory foci or immunostimulated animals.

### Golgi Complex

Practically nonexistent in polymorphs, the Golgi complex is fairly prominent in monocytes and macrophages.

### Lysosomes

Lysosomes are particularly numerous and of various size in polymorphs, constituting polymorph granules. In monocytes, these organelles are rare. In macrophages, their number varies with the immune situation and degree of macrophage activation. In phagocytic cells, the lysosomes contain numerous enzymes and other substances, including cationic proteins, such as lactoferrin. It has been shown that various substances are absorbed by macrophages by means of pinocytic vacuoles formed by hyaloplasmic membrane invaginations. These vacuoles are then transferred to the perinuclear zone. Proteins and proteolytic enzymes that originate in the endoplasmic reticulum cisternae are transferred to the vesicles derived from the Golgi complex, which are called primary lysosomes. Primary lysosomes fuse with pinocytic vacuoles to form secondary lysosomes. These secondary lysosomes may again fuse with pinocytic vacuoles or, as we shall see, with a phagocytic vacuole to become a phagosome.

### Retractile Structures

Tubules and filaments have been recently demonstrated in macrophages. They play a role in cell motility, since it has been shown that cytochalasin-

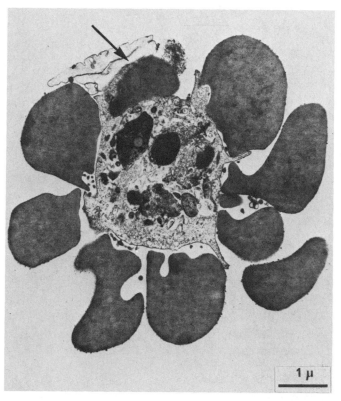

**Fig. 5.4** Mouse spleen macrophage forming a rosette with SRBC. One may note phagocytosis occurring at the top of the figure. (From F. Reyes and J. F. Bach, Cell. Immunol. 1971, 2, 182.)

induced alteration of the microfilaments can modify the orientation of cellular organelles and suppress membrane movements.

### Other Intracytoplasmic Organelles

Phagocytic cells obtained from inflammatory exudates very often contain vacuoles of variable size. These organelles include not only pinocytic vacuoles but also larger phagocytic vacuoles. In many cases, the phagocytic material is still present, and after staining (May-Grünwald-Giemsa), the inside of the vacuole may appear eosinophilic. In polymorphs, one also finds important amounts of glycogen by electron microscopy.

In summary, phagocytic cells are characterized by a large quantity of lysosomes, pinocytic and phagocytic vacuoles, and numerous membrane extensions.

## III. STUDY METHODS

It is easy to obtain phagocytic cells from animals, but not from man, which explains why most studies of phagocytosis have been performed in the former.

### IN VIVO

The only method that permits in vivo observation of macrophages or polymorphs consists of creating an inflammatory focus under conditions in which its development may be followed under the microscope. One can, for instance, perforate a rabbit's ear and fix to each side of the ear a glass or transparent plastic slide. If the distance between the two slides does not exceed 20 μm, it is possible to see, first, the healing of the wound and, ultimately, the neovascularization of the connective tissue. Inflammation can then be provoked; it is now possible to observe diapedesis of polymorphs and monocytes and to follow transformation of the latter into macrophages. By this means, the same (one) macrophage has been followed for as long as 140 days.

It is also possible to study some macrophage functions, especially uptake of foreign particles (Fig. 5.5), by measuring the rate of blood elimination of carbon or radioactive particles. This method, introduced by Biozzi, Benacerraf, and Halpern, consists of injecting mice intravenously with a carbon suspension and collecting, at regular intervals, the blood from orbital venous sinuses. Under these conditions, the carbon particles are mainly ingested by macrophages of the spleen, liver, and lung, and also, to a certain degree, by those of the bone marrow and adrenal glands. Photocolorimetry of the samples collected at various times gives the carbon content in systemic blood. It has been shown that elimination of the carbon particles is exponential. A phagocytic index, $K$, can be calculated as follows:

$$K = \frac{\log C_0 - \log C_t}{t}$$

where $C_0$ and $C_t$ are serial blood carbon concentrations. This formula does not

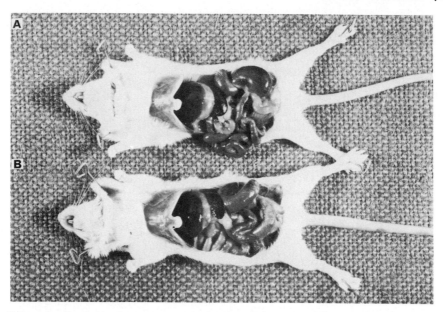

**Fig. 5.5** Distribution of intravenous carbon particles in the phagocyte system. Two hours after intravenous injection of carbon particles, particles are trapped by the hepatic and splenic macrophages in the mouse. (*a*): normal mouse; (*b*): mouse injected with carbon particles intravenously.

take into account variations in carbon removal due to alterations in liver or spleen weight that may change after immunostimulating treatments or that relate to age or animal strain. To take these parameters into account, one expresses the results by a corrected phagocytic index:

$$\alpha = \sqrt[3]{K \; \frac{W_A}{W_L + W_S}}$$

where $K$ is the phagocytic index, $W_A$ represents the animal's weight, $W_L$ is the liver weight, and $W_S$ denotes spleen weight.

This technique examines the ability of macrophages to ingest, not their ability to destroy ingested material. Such an estimation may be performed by intravenous injection with bacteria that are known to be easily ingested and insensitive to serum bactericidal factors. Like carbon particles, the bacteria rapidly disappear from the blood; 2 hr after injection, 90% of bacteria are found in liver and spleen macrophages. At variable intervals, between 0 and 3 hr postinjection, spleen and liver are collected and their bacterial contents are measured. The difference between the number of organ-localized bacteria at 1 and 3 hr after injection expresses the relative propensity of the liver and spleen macrophages to ingest bacteria. This method is particularly useful in studying the bactericidal potency conferred by immunization against bacteria that proliferate in the macrophages of normal animals.

# IN VITRO

In vitro methods of studying polymorph or macrophage functions may be applied immediately after cell collection or, for macrophages, after variable times of in vitro survival.

## *Obtaining Materials*

Polymorphs can be obtained from blood or from inflammatory exudates. Macrophages may be obtained not only from the same sources but also from organs, organ fragments, and natural body cavities.

### BLOOD

One of the oldest methods involves collecting the buffy coat after blood sedimentation, either spontaneous or accelerated by means of polyvinylpyrrolidone or lectins. Of these "buffy" leukocytes, only polymorphs and monocytes adhere to the glass walls; the other cells are eliminated by washing. After a 3-day incubation at 37°C, only monocytes that have transformed into macrophages persist. It is also possible to obtain monocytes directly by centrifugation of heparinized blood in the presence of a concentrated albumin solution or gradients of high-molecular-weight substances.

### INFLAMMATORY EXUDATES

The injection of protein or glycogen into the peritoneal or pleural cavities produces an inflammatory exudate within a few hours. Twenty-four hours later, the exudate contains mostly neutrophils; 4 days later, essentially only macrophages are found. One must, however, recognize that macrophages obtained by these methods are not all functionally identical. The frequent use of oil and culture medium for bacteria (such as thioglycollate medium) induces the production of exudates that contain macrophages that have incorporated oil or agarose particles. It has been shown that these inflammatory agents may produce metabolic and functional changes in phagocytic cells. For example, the bactericidal potency of macrophages obtained after agarose injection is much higher than that of macrophages obtained after mineral oil injecton.

Rebuck's technique is often used in man. After skin abrasion with a needle, a sterile glass slide is applied to the skin and maintained for variable periods of time. The inflammatory reaction thus provoked features exudation, which is rapidly followed by polymorph and mononuclear cell diapedesis. About 10 hr later, the majority cells are polymorphs. After 4 days, the majority of cells are macrophages. In man, another technique involves the application to the skin of a blistering agent (cantharidin) and removal of cells from the blister at varying times after application of the agent. This technique has demonstrated that a diminished inflammatory response is elicited in patients suffering from malignant disease (F. G. Lacour).

### ORGANS OR ORGAN FRAGMENTS

It is an old observation that liver or spleen fragments from newborn animals placed into a nutritive medium are rapidly surrounded by very mobile macrophages. This phenomenon makes possible the isolation of liver macrophages by two different methods. The first one (described by Rous) consists of injecting animals intravenously with very fine iron carbonyl particles. The liver is then perfused, and the perfusion liquid is placed into a magnetic field that retains the Küpffer cells that ingested magnetic particles. Another method, described recently (Garvey), is also applicable to spleen macrophages. It involves fragmenting tissues and incubating them successively in collagenase and trypsin. The cells obtained are put into culture, and an early washing separates out macrophages by means of their glass adherence property. A method for obtaining lung alveolar macrophages (described by Myrvik) consists of rinsing the lungs with physiologic medium introduced into the trachea. After repeated washings, the liquid contains a suspension of macrophages detached from lung alveoli.

Lastly, it is possible to separate spleen macrophages from other cells by cutting the spleen into small pieces and incubating spleen cells in petri dishes. After 1 or 2 hr of incubation, followed by repeated washings, spleen macrophages are separated by their adherence property from other spleen cells.

### Culture

Numerous techniques can be used to obtain macrophages in culture. Macrophages must be maintained in an enriched synthetic medium, such as Parker's or Eagle's, that contains 10 to 15% fetal serum with a pH of 6.8 to 7.2. Serum may be replaced by 2% albumin. At variance with some cell lines that may be maintained in suspension, macrophages can only be kept alive in vitro as long as they adhere to a supporting surface. It is rare, under usual conditions, to observe a significant in vitro proliferation of peritoneal macrophages taken from adult animals. It is possible to observe a certain degree of macrophage proliferation when they are cultured in media that contain supernatants of fibroblast cultures (Virolainen) or chronic inflammatory exudates (Fauve).

At variance with the majority of cell types, macrophages cannot be separated by use of trypsin or calcium chelator. When one wants to recover macrophages from a culture, it is necessary to culture them on either collagen or coagulated serum. In this setting, collagenase or trypsin may be used to detach cells from their "support." For polymorphs, it is not possible to maintain viability in vitro for more than 24 hr. The media described above for macrophages can be used for short periods of time, as in the case of macrophages; polymorph functions must not be studied in cells in suspension but only when cells are fixed to culture recipients. Recently, macrophage lines have been more readily established following their transformation by oncogenic viruses (e.g., SV40, polyoma virus).

## IV.  FUNCTIONS

In addition to phagocytosis (which is discussed later in further detail), phagocytic cells, particularly macrophages, have several other functions.

# NONIMMUNOLOGIC

### Lipid Metabolism

With $^{14}$C-labeled fat, it has been shown that macrophages, especially Küpffer cells, ingest and degrade chylomicrons. Macrophages also participate in fatty acid and cholesterol syntheses. It has been shown in experimental arteriosclerosis that macrophages localized in the aortic walls synthesize a significant amount of the cholesterol present in the atheromatous lesion.

### Protein and Carbohydrate Metabolism

Because of their high content of hydrolytic enzymes, macrophages are able to degrade proteins (globulins, albumin) and polysaccharides. Protein degradation is variable and relates to the type of macrophage present. This variability may explain why one antigen is destroyed by certain macrophages but not by others. It has also been shown that rat and mouse peritoneal macrophages can synthesize transferrin and $\beta_1C$ plus $\beta_1E$ globulins. In addition, liver macrophages may synthesize antihemophilic globulin, prothrombin, and proconvertin.

### Other Functions

The "detoxification" function of macrophages is very important. It has long been known that alveolar macrophages are capable of incorporating atmospheric dust. Macrophages are also involved in liver glycuroconjugation. They play a central role in healing processes: macrophages eliminate necrotic cells and foreign bodies from inflammatory foci. Lastly, their role is important to erythropoiesis, because they carry iron to erythrocytic precursors.

# IMMUNOLOGIC

The intervention of macrophages and polymorphs in immunologic reactions by means of phagocytosis is well established. Macrophages are implicated also in interferon and antibody syntheses, delayed hypersensitivity, and tumor immunity. In this chapter, we shall only examine those aspects relating to pinocytosis and phagocytosis.

Pinocytosis is the process whereby particles less than 10 nm are ingested by the phagocytic cells; it may also be accomplished by other cellular elements such as platelets.

Phagocytosis is characterized by the ingestion and eventual digestion of larger particles greater than 10 nm in diameter. Such particles may be inert (e.g., aggregates, silica crystals) or living (e.g. cells, viruses, bacteria, parasites). The classic three phases in phagocytosis are as follows (Figs. 5.6 and 5.7): an adhesion phase, during which the phagocytic cell comes in contact with the particle; an incorporation phase, during which the particle is absorbed into the cytoplasm; and a third phase, which features alternative possibilities that depend on the functional state of the cell and the nature of the ingested material. The latter may be digested or persist. In the latter circumstance, living microorganisms may proliferate inside the cytoplasm of macrophages.

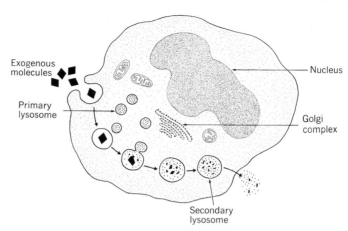

**Fig. 5.6**  Phagocytosis.

### Adhesion Phase (Attachment)

To make contact with the material to be phagocytased, phagocytic cells must be able to move. This movement is possible only if the cell forms pseudopods (polymorphs) or cytoplasmic veils (macrophages). The adhesion of phagocytic cells to particles is the consequence of various interactions between cellular and extracellular factors. It depends also on the nature of the particles being ingested.

CELLULAR FACTORS

Cellular factors are relatively hard to study, because it is always difficult to distinguish between purely cellular factors and the various substances present in the "halo" of the cell surface. All results must be interpreted strictly in relation to the techniques used. We shall see later that the factors that determine adhesion of a particle to phagocytic cells are very different when the cells are in suspension from those that apply when the cells are adherent to a surface. It is known that the characteristic movements of the membranes of macrophages are not present when the cells are in suspension. Thus, although it is technically easier to quantify the results when phagocytic cells are in suspension, this experimental condition is very artificial and bears little resemblance to cells that have adhered in vivo.

It has been believed that contact between phagocytes and particles might depend on their respective electric charges (Fenn). Phagocytes and bacteria are electronegative, but whether this charge is uniformly distributed is not known. Pethica has shown that on a theoretical basis, two electronegatively charged cells can come in contact if their respective global electric charge differs and if they adhere to each other through the intermediary of membrane extensions of radius less than 0.1 μm. Such conditions are easily met by macrophage membrane expansion or polymorph pseudopods, thus explaining why these cells easily ingest electronegative corpuscles.

Several authors, including Berken, Benacerraf, and Howard, have examined the macrophage surface for potential receptors responsible for the binding of cytophilic antibody, which would permit sheep erythrocyte adhesion to guinea pig macrophages. Reducing agents (mercaptoethanol), enzymatic inhibitors (FlNa, 2,4-dinitrophenol), and enzymes (trypsin, papain, lipase, hyaluronidase, and neuraminidase) have no effect on the antibody binding. However, substances that react with either free sulfhydryl groups (iodoacetamide, p-chloromercurylbenzoate) or with sulfhydryl and amide groups (formaldehyde,

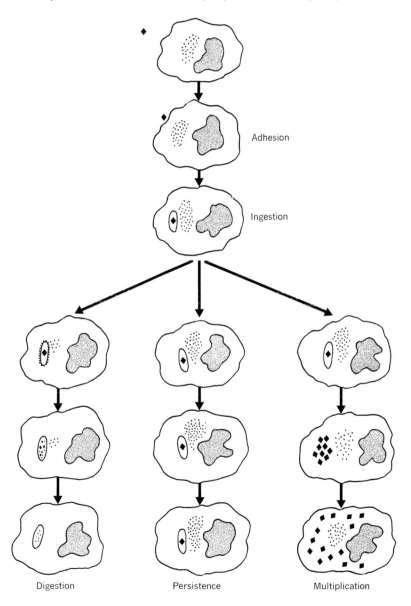

**Fig. 5.7** Fate of bacteria after phagocytosis.

isothiocyanate) and oxidizing agents (periodate, nitrite) are capable of inhibiting binding to cytophilic antibodies. These authors believe that sulfhydryl groups play an important role at the level of macrophage membranes.

Huber, studying erythrocytes sensitized with IgG-class anti-RhD antibodies, has shown IgG-specific receptors on the surface of human monocytes and spleen and liver macrophages. These monocyte receptors have since been shown to be specific for IgG1 and IgG3 subclasses (Abramson).

Phagocytic cell metabolism is another important factor, because it controls the continuous movement of the cellular membrane. It is obvious that the more vigorous these movements are, the greater the possibility of contact occurring between phagocytes and particles. Perhaps, an increase in metabolism explains the considerably higher capacity of macrophagic ingestion in animals pretreated with estrogens, endotoxin, lecithin, or some lymphokines.

EXTRACELLULAR FACTORS

Temperature plays an important role in the adhesion phenomenon. The optimal value coincides with the normal body temperature of the phagocyte donor; pH does not seem to be important, because adhesion and subsequent particle ingestion may occur over a fairly wide range, 6.5 to 7.2. The ionic strength of the medium is also important. An increase in ionic strength leads to decreased adhesion; conversely, a decrease in ionic strength causes enhanced adhesion.

Modifications of the extracellular medium may alter adhesion. Divalent cations play an important role; it is known that in the presence of a calcium chelator, the medium totally suppresses adhesion. Some lipids, like triolein, may augment adhesion, but others may decrease it. Some complement fractions favor adhesion, but this is probably true only in the case of polymorphs. It has been shown by McCutcheon and Vaughan that macrophages may perform phagocytosis without complement, especially when they are maintained in vitro in the absence of serum globulin and when they adhere strongly to a surface. However, even under these conditions, one cannot totally exclude a role of some complement components, because it has been shown that macrophages are able to synthesize $\beta_1C$ and $\beta_1E$ globulins.

Antibodies play an important role in the phagocytosis of both bacteria (as opsonins) and viruses, but this phenomenon appears to be less important for macrophages than for polymorphs. In vivo, in the absence of bacteria-opsonizing globulins (axenic animals or newborn pigs), peritoneal and subcutaneous macrophages ingest pathogenic and virulent bacteria.

Furthermore, it has been shown by Wardlaw and Howard that macrophages from the perfused liver are able to phagocytose *Staphylococcus aureus, Bacillus cereus, Corynebacterium murium,* and *Streptococcus pyogenes* more efficiently in the absence of serum; *Escherichia coli, Pseudomonas pyocyanea,* and *Proteus mirabilis* can also be eliminated in the absence of normal serum. One concludes from all this information that bacteria do not require the presence of antibody to be phagocytosed. However, in particular, for pyogenic bacteria, the addition of antibody considerably enhances phagocytosis. In vitro, macrophages kept in suspension are unable to phagocytose some bacteria (*Salmonella typhimurium* smooth, *Klebsiella pneumoniae*) in the absence of specific opsonins. Conversely, if the same macrophages are maintained, not in suspension but on a surface (glass slide), bacterial phagocytosis occurs. For some bacteria, such as *Listeria monocytogenes* and *Mycobacterium tuberculosis,* the presence of a specific antiserum does not significantly modify the adhesion of macrophages to these bacteria. This particular aspect of phagocytosis by cells adhering to a surface is termed "surface phagocytosis."

If, indeed, specific antibodies have an adjunctive effect on the adhesion phase, they no longer seem as indispensable as previously thought. Moreover, macrophages seem to require less serum protein factors than do polymorphs. It is of interest to consider what portion of the molecule binds to the phagocytic cells to facilitate adhesion. Berken and Benacerraf and, more recently, Huber have shown that the Fc fragment of antibody is responsible for this binding. Abramson has additionally demonstrated that for IgG, the N-terminal part of the Fc fragment is implicated and that the binding occurs only when the disulfide bridge that links the two heavy chains is intact.

Nonspecific opsonins have been little studied in the case of macrophages, and it is unwise to extrapolate to macrophages from findings obtained by studying polymorphs. The only information now available concerns the degree of ingestion, which depends on previous adhesion, when macrophages of peritoneal cavities are stimulated by various substances. It is, however, difficult to dissociate the role of extracellular substances from that of the cell itself. As far as polymorphs are concerned, results must be interpreted with caution because of the particular experimental conditions utilized in these studies.

The adhesion of particles to phagocytes greatly depends on the physico-chemical nature of the particles. Here again, it is perhaps too easy to explain adhesion and preferential ingestion of certain particles on the basis of the respective electric charges. It is likely that the surface electric charge does play a role in the initial contact between particle and the phagocytic cell, but a definite conclusion on this point cannot now be stated. It is known that certain substances present on the particle surface may considerably diminish or even inhibit adhesion. One very striking example is that of pneumococcal polysaccharides, which act to suppress phagocytosis of pneumococci by phagocytic cells. Analogous observations are seen for M proteins of streptococci and for smooth walls of salmonellae. It is possible to inhibit phagocytosis of certain bacteria by resuspending them in mucin and to significantly modify particle adhesion by heating or treatment with certain basic polypeptides. An adverse effect of certain detergents has also been demonstrated, both in vivo and in vitro.

A description of the adhesion phenomenon must naturally include a description of erythrophagocytosis. Vaughan has observed that even though macrophages (in suspension) cannot usually phagocytose red cells in absence of the specific antibody, the antibody is not needed for phagocytosis of aged red blood cells. This finding indicates that splenic macrophages do not need opsonins to remove aged erythrocytes from the circulation. It would be important to know the factor(s) on the surface of young erythrocytes that inhibit their phagocytosis by macrophages of the reticuloendothelial system.

The problem of recognition of "nonself" by phagocytes is probably relevant to adhesion. Data on this subject have essentially been obtained with macrophages. Is a given macrophage able by itself to recognize a foreign cell? Experiments on this subject (in particular, those of Perkins and Leonard) have shown that when red blood cells of various species are incubated with mouse macrophages in the presence of mouse serum, the greater the phylogenetic differences, the greater the phagocytosis. Similar experiments and findings have been performed with human macrophages. Recognition does not occur in the absence of serum factors. Therefore, macrophages must recognize foreign cells with the help of serum constituents.

### Ingestion Phase

Ingestion refers to the penetration of inert or living particles in the cytoplasm of the phagocyte. Ingestion is associated with an "invagination" of the macrophage membrane, which then contains the ingested particle. The periphery of this "invagination" next fuses to form a "phagocytic vacuole," also called a "phagosome."

It is known that this phagocytosis phase is dependent on the metabolism of the phagocytic cell. Karnovsky has shown that ingestion is temperature dependent and that it occurs within pH limits of 6 to 8. Ingestion is associated with energy consumption due to a change in macrophage metabolism that occurs during ingestion. One must, however, distinguish between different metabolic mechanisms in alveolar and peritoneal macrophages. In the guinea pig, alveolar macrophages expend energy provided by oxidative phosphorylation; for peritoneal macrophages, energy is provided by glycolysis. The penetration of the particle into the cell results from the mechanical effects of the action of microfilaments and microtubules as shown by the administration of a number of inhibitors (colchicine, cytochalasin B, etc.). It is not yet possible to dissect the cascade of events that follows the adhesion of the substrate particle to the phagocytic membrane and that serves as the signal for phagocytosis. There is a correlation between cyclic AMP concentrations and phagocytosis: increased concentrations of intracellular cyclic AMP coincides with the inhibition of endocytosis (effects of $PGE_1$ theophylline and dibutyryl cAMP). Ongoing studies are attempting a more precise definition of the composition of phagosome membranes. It is, however, known that sites that facilitate the transport of certain substances disappear during the invagination of the plasma membrane.

### Intracytoplasmic Fate of the Ingested Particles

Depending on the nature of the ingested particle and the origin and function of phagocytic cells, there are three possible end points. The particle may be digested, may simply persist, or may proliferate inside the phagocyte (Fig. 5.7).

DIGESTION

When a living or inert particle enters a phagocytic vacuole, lysosomes come into contact and release their contents. From phase-contrast and electron microscopy, it is now known that, initially, adhesion occurs between lysosome walls and phagocytic vacuole (Hirsch and Cohn). Lysosome and vacuole walls then fuse. The free communication between the lysosome and the phagocytic vacuole allows lysosomal enzymes to make contact with the ingested particle.

Several factors seem to be responsible for fusion of lysosome walls and phagocytic vacuoles. The low pH within the phagocytic vacuole and changes in the peripheral wall tension of the membrane may play particularly important roles. One readily sees that in the case of biodegradable materials, digestion may occur after contact of the particle with numerous enzymes contained in the phagocytic lysosomes (aminopeptidase, succino-dehydrogenase, acid phosphatase, cathepsin, lysozyme, glucuronidase, ribonuclease, deoxyribonuclease, arylsulfatase, lipase, cytochrome $c$ oxidase, cholesterol esterase, galactosidase). Some authors also believe that there are, in addition, bactericidal or bacteriostatic substances in lysosomes. Amano, Gershon, and Ramseier have found isolated substances, chemically poorly defined, that exert a marked bactericidal action. One should note, however, that these results have not yet been confirmed and that the bactericidal activity reported by these authors does not correspond to that observed in macrophages. It is generally believed that bacterial death may occur within minutes after ingestion: the intravacuolar environment cannot alone explain why bacteria are killed inside the macrophage, at least in relation to pH and enzymatic content.

Even though we do not yet know how macrophages kill bacteria, some information is available for polymorphs. It is known (Iyer and Klebanoff) that the bactericidal effect of polymorphs is due to hydrogen peroxide; when glucose is oxidized by the hexose monophosphate shunt, NADPH (nicotinamide-adenine dinucleotide phosphate) is transformed into NADP by NADPH oxidase:

$$2NADPH + O_2 \rightarrow H_2O_2 + 2NADP$$
$$\uparrow$$
$$NADPH \text{ oxidase.}$$

NADH oxidase also promotes transformation of NADH to NAD with release of $H_2O_2$ and NAD:

$$2NADH + O_2 \rightarrow 2NAD + H_2O_2$$
$$\uparrow$$
$$NADH \text{ oxidase.}$$

The bactericidal effect of $H_2O_2$ is enhanced by the activity of myeloperoxidase contained in polymorphs. Klebanoff has shown that the bactericidal effect was also enhanced by certain halogens, such as iodine, that were present in significant quantities in polymorphs. It has also been shown that the $H_2O_2$ + halogen + myeloperoxidase system is bactericidal at concentrations lower than are necessary when each constituent acts alone or together. Recent studies have shown that free radicals may offer some explanation for the bacteriologic abilities of polymorphs and macrophages (Weiss et al.).

In the minutes following their contact with microorganisms, polymorphs release superoxide anions ($O_2^-$), which, in the presence of the superoxide dismutase in their cytoplasm, combine with hydrogen to form $H_2O_2$:

$$2\ O_2^- + 2H^+ \rightarrow O_2 + H_2O_2$$

It is interesting to note that polymorphs from patients with chronic granulomatosis (see p. 904) concomitantly cannot produce $O_2^-$ and kill bacteria.

Recent studies have confirmed that monocytes and macrophages are also able to produce $O_2^-$ and $H_2O_2$ according to the same mechanism. Murray and Cohn have reported that intra-macrophage lysis of certain parasites such as *Toxoplasma gondii* is due to the formation of oxygen free radicals: the hydroxide radical OH. and the oxygen singlet $^1O_2$, which derive from the interaction of $O_2^-$ with $H_2O_2$ according to Haber-Weiss' reaction:

$$O_2^- + H_2O_2 \rightarrow {}^1O_2 + O\ H. + O\ H^-$$

The intracellular presence of oxygen free radicals can be detected by chemiluminiscence: oxygen radicals are electronically instable and their return to a stable state is associated with photon production. Sensitive detection of chemiluminescence is achieved in liquid scintillation counters or photometers (after addition of an amplifying agent: 5-amino-2, 3 dihydro-1, 4 phtalazine-dione or luminol). This bioluminescence phenomenon which occurs in the seconds following polymorph contact with microorganisms or inert particles, is strongly diminished in presence of superoxide dismutase and not seen in chronic granulomatosis.

PERSISTENCE

This phenomenon is seen whenever the particle cannot be digested by phagocytic cells, despite the presence of lysosomal enzymes. Thus, part of atmospheric dust (carbon, silica, asbestos) may persist throughout the entire lifespan of macrophages. Such persistence is observed not only for inert particles; intact bacteria, parasites, and probably viruses may also persist within the phagocyte cytoplasm. This persistence, more precisely an equilibrium between certain microorganisms and macrophages, has important consequences and, in particular, may relate to the origin of latent infection. Another important consequence of persistence of microorganisms inside macrophages relates to therapy. It is well known that intracellular microorganisms are not only protected from the humoral defense mechanisms of the organism but also from antibiotics. For example, salmonella, brucella, tubercle bacillus, or *Listeria monocytogenes* may persist within macrophages, even when the macrophages are placed into a medium that contains antibiotic concentrations 10 times higher than that shown to inhibit bacteria in vitro. The significance of this observation in clinical infection is obvious. This observation explains why infections should be treated rapidly, by use of high antibiotic doses. It also explains, at least in part, why such infections as brucellosis and tuberculosis often become chronic and difficult to cure.

MULTIPLICATION

This phenomenon is seen in the case of macrophages infected by virulent mycobacteria, salmonella, listeria, brucella, pasteurella, some staphylococci, and streptococci. Certain parasites, such as toxoplasma, histoplasma, fungal agents, including *Candida guilliermondi,* and numerous viruses can also multiply inside macrophages. Multiplication is the basis of another aspect of virulence of the microorganism within the phagocytic cell. It is known that some microbes, like pneumococci, are virulent because they are not ingested by phagocytic cells (protected by their polysaccharides). Here the virulence is manifested by the ability of these bacteria, once ingested, to proliferate inside the macrophages. One should note, in addition, that the virulence of salmonellae also relates to their difficult intake (due to the smooth aspect of the bacterial wall) plus their ability to proliferate within the phagocytic cells. These observations underscore the complexity of anti-salmonella immunity.

One wonders why some microorganisms are able to multiply within the cytoplasm of macrophages, which at other times possess a remarkable bactericidal potency. Some have suggested that substances necessary for microorganism multiplication are present within macrophages, namely, erythritol in the case of brucella growth. However, if, indeed, such substances favor the growth of certain bacteria, extrapolation from the culture tube to the macrophage cannot fully be accepted, because this phenomenon relates to the cytotropism of only certain bacteria. In fact, as we have already discussed, when bacteria are enclosed within the phagocytic vacuole, unfavorable conditions for growth are present due to the high concentration of hydrolytic enzymes and especially the acid pH. It is obvious that some bacteria are still able to multiply under these conditions; possibly, the ingested bacteria do not come into contact with lysosomal enzymes, or perhaps the vacuolar pH is not always acid. The first possibility can be excluded, particularly for listeria. The second hypothesis remains to be tested. In experiments performed with mouse peritoneal macrophages, it has been observed that bacteria apparently able to multiply within macrophages (*Mycobacterium tuberculosis* $H_{37}RV$, *L. monocytogene*, *Brucella melitensis*) are, indeed, ingested. This ingestion is not, however, followed by disappearance of all lysosomes. The phagocytic vacuole is therefore not readily seen. Conversely, bacteria incapable of multiplying inside the macrophage (*Bacillus anthracis*, *S. typhimurium* smooth, *Kl. pneumoniae*) are seen within large phagocytic vacuoles, and their ingestion is followed by disappearance of lysosomes. These observations led Fauve to propose that bacterial multiplication inside of macrophages was made possible by inhibiting the release of lysosomal contents. This hypothesis, recently confirmed, explains why certain bacteria may multiply inside macrophage cytoplasm. It seems obvious that because they are not vulnerable to the lytic action of lysosomal enzymes or to the low pH, some bacteria may multiply within the phagocytic vacuole (which has been observed with electron microscopy). In addition, inhibition of release of lysosomal contents into a phagocytic vacuole may also explain why ingested bacteria are shielded from antibiotics that are contained in secondary lysosomes; Bonventre has shown that antibiotics present in the extracellular medium penetrate the macrophage by pinocytosis and then are present in lysosomes. Another consequence of intracellular multiplication is that metabolic products of some bacteria diffuse into the cytoplasm, eventually resulting in macrophage necrosis. This phenomenon has been well demonstrated during phagocytosis of *M. tuberculosis* and *Listeria*; the metabolic cytolysin may lyse lysosomes once the membrane of the phagocytic vacuole has been lysed. Recently, Goren has shown that the fusion of phagocytic vacuoles with lysosomes may be inhibited by the sulphates present in *M. tuberculosis*. On the other hand, the use of certain detergents or suramine facilitates the fusion of lysosomes with the phagocytic vacuoles (D'Arcy Hart).

Less well studied have been the factors that influence virus multiplication or nonmultiplication within macrophages. Multiplication has been observed for such viruses as murine hepatitis and ectromelia; as with bacteria, nonpathogenic or less virulent viruses are destroyed, whereas virulent viruses multiply. The multiplication of the virus inside macrophàges may have great importance to certain viral infections. In the case of ectromelia or murine hepatitis, virus multiplication in Küpffer cells may produce lesions of the liver parenchyma.

It has been shown by Hirsch that eosinophil polymorphs can also phago-cytose bacteria. It is noteworthy that eosinophils are heavily represented within exudates of allergic reactions. In vitro, eosinophils are attracted to antigen-antibody complexes, especially in the presence of antigen excess. Eosinophils ingest the antigen-antibody complexes, then degranulation occurs. Because the granules contain substances capable of blocking the physiologic action of histamine, serotonin, and bradykinin, it is possible that eosinophils not only protect the tissues and the host by phagocytosing antigen-antibody complexes but also diminish the effects of mediators of the inflammatory reaction.

Phagocytosis may be depressed in certain immunodeficiency states (septic familial granulomatosis, Chediak-Higashi syndrome). Phagocytosis may be decreased by some immunodepressants (corticosteroids, cyclophosphamide, ionizing radiation). However, these agents alter not only the mechanism of phagocytosis but also production of phagocytic cells.

Phagocytosis may be stimulated by a recruitment of phagocytic cells at the sites of inflammatory foci or by activation of phagocytic cells, particularly after injection of various immunostimulants (BCG [Bacillus Calmette-Guérin], bac-terial endotoxins, synthetic polynucleotides, bacterial extracts).

## V.  CONCLUSIONS

Phagocytic cells act to remove altered and dead cells and play an important role in the metabolism of the living organism. Through phagocytosis they eliminate a large number of pathogenic agents from the organism. To these well-recognized concepts of macrophage functions are now added a number of other important functions that will be dealt with later (see chaps. 16 and 18).

After antigen-trapping, macrophages are implicated in the immune re-sponse at several other levels. Through their ability to catabolize antigens, they contribute to the avoidance of a tolerant state. Certain macrophages play an essential role in the presentation of antigens to lymphocytes. As will be seen later, for certain antigens it is probably at the macrophage surface that the phenomenon of syngeneic restriction takes place, since antigen recognition can only be accomplished if the macrophage and the lymphocyte bear identical histocompatibility antigens (see chap. 24). This genetic restriction is also seen at the stage of the efferent arc of the immune response. In the mouse, the importance of the H-2 complex and, particularly, that of the I-A region in the recruitment of macrophages at the site of a delayed hypersensitivity response has been readily shown. At the same time, the same constraints are observed when a sensitized lymphocyte in contact with its sensitizing antigen induces an increase in the bactericidal activity of macrophages.

Lymphocyte-macrophage interactions are not solely limited to the transfer of antigenic information. It is now recognized that macrophages are necessary for the activation of B cells and T cells in vitro, playing an important trophic role in this context. An adequate delayed hypersensitivity response can only develop in vivo if a sufficient number of macrophages are present at the site of the response (see p. 371).

This cooperation between lymphocytes and macrophages is also seen in antitumor immune responses. Macrophages may be revealed to be cytostatic or cytotoxic in the presence of certain factors synthesized by sensitized lymphocytes. More recently, the same observations have been made in the course of graft immunity.

# BIBLIOGRAPHY

BELLANTI J. A. and DAYTON D. S. (Eds.) The phagocytic cells in host resistance. New York, 1975, Raven Press.

CARR I. The macrophage; a review of ultrastructure and function. New York, 1973, Academic Press.

FLOREY L. (Ed.) General Pathology. London, 1970, Lloyd-Luke.

GOREN M. B. Phagocytes lysosomes: interactions with infectious agents, phagosomes and experimental pertubations in function. Ann. Rev. Microb., 1977, 31, 507.

METCALF D. and MOORE M. A. S. Haematopoietic cells. In Neuberger and Tatum, Eds., Frontiers of biology. Vol. 24, Amsterdam, 1971, North Holland.

NELSON D. S. (Ed.) Immunobiology of the macrophage. New York, 1976, Academic Press.

NELSON D. S. (Ed.) Macrophages and immunity. Amsterdam, 1969, North Holland.

STUART A. E. (Ed.) The reticulo-endothelial system. Edinburgh, 1970, Livingstone.

UNANUE E. R. The regulatory role of macrophages in antigenic stimulation. Adv. Immunol., 1972, 15, 95.

VAN FURTH R. (Ed.) Mononuclear phagocytes. Oxford, 1970, Blackwell.

VAN FURTH R. (Ed.) Mononuclear phagocytes in immunity, infection and pathology. Oxford, 1975, Blackwell.

VERNON-ROBERTS B. The macrophage. Cambridge, 1972, University Press.

WAGNER W. H. and HAHN H. (Eds.) Activation of macrophages. 2nd Workshop Conference Hoechst. Amsterdam, 1974, Excerpta Médica.

WILLIAMS R. C. and FUDENBERG H. H. (Eds.) Phagocytic mechanisms in health and disease. New York, 1972, Intercontinental Medical Book.

ZWEIFACH B. W., GRANT L., and McCLUSKEY R. T. (Eds.) The inflammatory process. Vol. 1. New York, 1974, Academic Press.

## ORIGINAL ARTICLES

BAINTON D. F. Neutrophil granules. Brit. J. Haemat., 1975, 29, 17.

COX J. P. and KARNOVSKY M. L. The depression of phagocytosis by exogenous cyclic nucleotides, prostaglandins and theophylline. J. Cell. Biol., 1973, 59, 480.

Goren M. B., D'Arcy Hart P., Young M. R., and Armstrong J. A. Prevention of phagosome-lysosome fusion in cultured macrophages by sulfatides of *Mycobacterium tuberculosis*. Proc. Nat. Acad. Sci., USA, 1976, *73*, 2510.

Griffin F. M. Jr., Griffin J. A., Leider J. E., and Silverstein S. C. Studies on the mechanism of phagocytosis. I. Requirements for circumferential attachment of particle-bound ligands to specific receptors on the macrophage plasma membrane. J. Exp. Med., 1975, *142*, 1263.

Griffin F. M. Jr., Griffin J. A., and Silverstein S. C. Studies on the mechanism of phagocytosis. II. The interaction of macrophages with anti-immunoglobulin IgG-coated bone marrow-derived lymphocytes. J. Exp. Med., 1976, *144*, 788.

Karnovsky M. L. The biological basis of the functions of polymorphonuclear leucocytes and macrophages. *In* L. Brent and J. Holborow, Eds., Progress in immunology. Amsterdam, 1974, North Holland, p. 83.

Lajtha L. G. Haemopoietic stem cells. Brit. J. Haemat., 1975, *29*, 529.

Lobuglio A. F., Cotran S., and Jandl J. H. Red cells coated with immunoglobulin G. Binding and sphering by mononuclear cells in man. Science, 1967, *158*, 1582.

Silverstein S. C., Steinman R. M., and Cohn Z. A. Endocytosis. Ann. Rev. Biochem., 1977, *46*, 669.

Stiffel C., Mouton D., and Biozzi G. Kinetics of the phagocytic function of reticuloendothelial macrophage in vivo. *In* R. Van Furth, Ed., Mononuclear phagocytes. Oxford, 1970, Blackwell.

Van Furth R. The kinetics and functions of polymorphonuclear and mononuclear phagocytes. *In* L. Brent and J. Holborow, Eds., Progress in immunology. Amsterdam, 1974, North Holland, p. 73.

Van Furth R. and Cohn Z. A. The origin and kinetics of mononuclear phagocytes. J. Exp. Med., 1968, *128*, 415.

Ward P. A. Leukotaxis and leukotactic disorders. A review. Am. J. Path., 1974, *77*, 520.

# Part 2

# IMMUNOCHEMISTRY

## Chapter 6

# ANTIGENS

### Jean-François Bach

I.   INTRODUCTION
II.  HAPTENS
III. PROTEIN ANTIGENS
IV.  POLYOSIDIC ANTIGENS
V.   OTHER ANTIGENS
VI.  INFLUENCE OF IMMUNOGENICITY ON THE TYPE OF
     IMMUNE RESPONSE

# I.  INTRODUCTION

## DEFINITIONS

Antigens are usually defined as substrates capable of stimulating the production of antibodies that will react specifically with said antigens. This definition is incomplete, however, because antigens may provoke responses other than the production of antibodies, such as delayed hypersensitivity and tolerance. In a wider sense, antigens may be defined as molecules that induce an immune response, that is, trigger a complex biologic process that includes the proliferation of lymphoid cells and synthesis by said lymphoid cells of recognition molecules (either antibodies or cellular receptors), which have the property of specifically combining, in vivo or in vitro, with the inducing antigen. Antigen molecules generally have several determinants whose configuration is complementary to the antibody site of the corresponding Ig.

## ANTIGENICITY AND IMMUNOGENICITY: CONCEPT OF HAPTEN

The definition of antigen, like that of antibody, has two aspects: one concerns the initiation of antibody production, the other involves the antigenic reaction

The author thanks Dr. A. M. Staub for reviewing this chapter.

with the antibody. Some molecules, called haptens, react with antibodies but are themselves unable to induce their production. Dinitrophenol (DNP), for example, reacts specifically with anti-DNP antibodies in the same manner in which bovine serum albumin reacts with anti-BSA antibodies. However, unlike BSA, DNP does not induce the formation of anti-DNP antibodies when injected intraperitoneally into mice and guinea pigs, even in the presence of an adjuvant. In order to obtain antibodies, it is necessary first to bind DNP covalently to a larger antigenic molecule (carrier). Substances capable of stimulating antibody production are called immunogens. A third class of substances, to be defined later, has the ability to induce tolerance rather than antibody production. These substances are called tolerogens. However, their autonomy with regard to immunogens is a relative one; some molecules are immunogens or tolerogens, depending upon dose or route of administration.

A final term, proantigen, is sometimes used to define substances of low molecular weight that are capable of becoming immunogenic after coupling with a protein, for example, after fixation to a host protein when subsequently injected. Unlike haptens, proantigens, which essentially induce delayed hypersensitivity reactions, cannot bind to T cell-specific receptors, unless there has been prior "complexing" with the autologous protein. Iodine, mercury, nickel, formaldehyde, iodoform, mercaptan, picryl chloride, dinitrochlorobenzene, and even some resins or sterols may, under certain circumstances, behave like proantigens.

## FACTORS THAT CONTROL IMMUNOGENICITY

Quantity, class, subclass, and affinity of antibodies produced against a given antigen as well as the presence or absence of cell-mediated immunity depend not only on the chemical structure of said antigen but also on the conditions of immunization and on certain genetic factors characteristic of the host.

### Antigen Dose

The nature and quantity of antibodies produced during immunization depend on the quantity of antigen injected. As a rule, a low antigen dose induces the formation of small amounts of antibodies with high affinity and specificity. These antibodies include those responsible for immediate hypersensitivity (IgG1 in guinea pigs and IgE in man). The administration of low antigen doses tends to stimulate T cells; thus, immunologic memory may be induced by doses that do not produce detectable antibody production, and cell-mediated immunity may be produced without circulating antibodies. Finally, it is important to recognize the considerable variations in minimal antigen doses needed to elicit antibody production, within and between different species ($10^{-4}$ g for BSA, $10^{-14}$ g for endotoxin in rodents).

### Administration Route

Also, the route of antigen administration greatly affects the nature of the immune response. The parenteral route, often used, allows rapid contact between the antigen and immunocompetent cells within regional lymph nodes (intradermal, subcutaneous, or intramuscular immunizations) or within the spleen (intravenous immunizations). Important variations in immunization may be observed, depending on the route of administration. For example, poly-D,L-alanine, long regarded as being nonimmunogenic in rabbits, is, in fact, immunogenic in 80% of them when injected intradermally at various points. The digestive route, used for the administration of certain vaccines, may involve the risk of denaturation. The respiratory route is particularly important in allergology (see chap. 26).

### Association of Immunogens, Secondary Responses, Adjuvants

Simultaneous administration of several antigens may have synergistic effects on antibody production. Conversely, administration of two antigens at 2- to 3-day intervals may depress the response to the second antigen; this phenomenon, is called antigenic competition (see p. 343).

The quantity, quality, and specificity of antibodies change after repeated immunizations by the same antigen. Thus, antibodies produced in large amounts after a booster injection are essentially high-affinity IgG. Paradoxically, the injection of a second antigen, only slightly different from the first but with common antigenic determinants may trigger an anamnestic response stronger to the first than to the second antigen (the phenomenon of "original antigenic sin," see p. 336). Adjuvants increase the intensity of immune responses by stimulating either macrophages or B and T cells. However, all adjuvants do not similarly stimulate cell-mediated immunity and antibody production (see chap. 33).

### Genetic Factors

Immune responses to a given antigen vary according to species. Mice develop delayed hypersensitivity reactions with relative difficulty, whereas these reactions are easily obtained in guinea pigs.

In addition, within a species, some animals may respond to an antigen, whereas others are refractory. The genetic factors that control such variations in response have been extensively studied. This information has led to the concept of immune response genes (see chap. 24). Briefly, there exists a series of antigen-specific Ir genes that control the production of antibodies against a given antigen. These Ir genes have been located close to the genes that code for transplantation antigens within the major histocompatibility complex. Parallel to antigen-specific genetic regulation of recognition, there is non-specific genetic regulation of antibody production levels (see chap. 24).

### Detection Methods

Antibody definition and specificity studies obviously depend on the methods used to detect them. A serum that appears to be specific for one antigen in one test may be shown to contain antibodies of several specificities in another test. Some tests exclusively detect certain antibody classes or categories; one example is immunodiffusion, which detects precipitating antibodies only. Hence the importance of techniques that are not based on the biological activity of antibodies. One such example is the Farr assay, which directly measures antigen-antibody binding. Some polypeptidic antigens are detectable only by such techniques. For practical reasons, however, we often prefer to use immuno-diffusion, which allows simultaneous analysis of antigen or antibody mixtures. However, its lack of sensitivity and the focus on precipitating antibodies must be taken into account when interpreting the results.

The specificity of an immune reaction is governed by the molecular steric complementary nature of antigen and antibody. Most natural antigens are macromolecules and contain several (different or identical) antigenic sites, hence the considerable complexity of antigen analysis and the possibility of cross-reactions of some antibodies with molecules showing identical or similar antigenic determinants.

### Cross-Reactions, Absorptions (Table 6.1)

The immunologist often has to deal with mixtures of antigens and anti-bodies. All cells contain numerous categories of antigenically distinct molecules. For example, a bacterium may contain flagellar, somatic, and capsular antigens, and any antiserum prepared against this bacterium will contain a mixture of antibodies against these different antigenic constituents, some of which may be common to several bacteria. The same reasoning may apply at the molecular level, because a macromolecular antigen always contains several determinants. Immunization of an animal to an antigenic molecule, however pure and isolated, will cause antibody formation toward all of these determinants, some of which may be found in antigens from different molecular species. In any case whether antigen molecules are common to two antigenic preparations, or determinants common to two antigen molecules or still determinants very similar but not strictly identical, cross-reactions may occur. Antisera may be rendered specific for a given antigenic determinant by absorption. Absorptions may be performed by incubation of antisera with cells, bacteria, or insoluble antigens. It is interesting to note that "reciprocal cross-reactions" are frequent but not obligatory. For example, rabbit immunization with BSA triggers the production of antibodies that also react against ovalbumin; similarly, immunization with

**Table 6.1   Cross-Reactions Between Precipitating Antibodies Directed Against Corneal Antigens from Different Species**

| Antiserum produced against cornea from: | Tested against corneal extracts from: | | | |
|---|---|---|---|---|
| | Sheep | Pig | Chicken | Fish |
| Sheep | + ++ | +++ | + | − |
| Pig | +++ | +++ | + | − |
| Chicken | + | ++ | ++++ | − |
| Fish | − | − | ++ | ++++ |

After K. Landsteiner.

ovalbumin triggers the production of anti-BSA antibodies. On the other hand, an antiserum produced against 2-aminobenzoic acid will react strongly with 2-aminobenzene sulfonic acid, but the reciprocal reaction does not occur.

### Species Specificity, Organ Specificity

Antigens may be classified as xenoantigens, alloantigens, or autoantigens. Xenoantigens are antigens present in all individuals of one or several species different from the species of the immunized subject. However, administration of xenogeneic preparations may introduce, in addition to xenoantigens, alloantigens and even autoantigens because of common or similar determinants among antigens of different species. The administration of extracts from xenogeneic organs is a method frequently used to obtain autoantibody production. Alloantigens (formerly called isoantigens) are antigens unequally distributed among individuals of one given species that bring about the formation of antibodies in an individual who does not possess the test antigen. Alloantigens, less commonly than xenoantigens, may promote the production of autoantibodies. Autoantigens are antigens present in the cells of a given animal or subject.

Natural proteins have a certain species specificity that is more apparent when antisera are produced between distant species. In more closely related species, however, numerous cross-reactions may occur between antibodies directed against one given protein in the different species. These cross-reactions are often increased by protein denaturation. Some antigens, called heterophil, are present in numerous remote species, including vegetable ones. An example of this type is the Forssman antigen, which is present on erythrocytes of numerous species (dog, sheep, goat, guinea pig, horse), as well as in certain microorganisms, but is absent in man (except in subjects of A and AB blood groups), rabbit, and ox.

Functional differences among molecules are generally associated with structural differences. It is therefore not surprising that albumin and serum globulins within one species are antigenically further apart than albumins from different species. In fact, even relatively distant species, such as man and ox, have antigenically very similar albumins. More generally speaking, these remarks can also be applied to the concept of organ-specific (more precisely cell-specific) antigens, which are often common to several species. Usually, two different organs possess both common and private antigens. Among the latter, some are found exclusively in the organ in question and will be regarded as organ-specific within the limits of the techniques of detection. Organ-specific antigens are defined by antisera prepared against a given organ and are absorbed by other organs. T lymphocyte specific antigens (described on p. 65) are examples of organ-specific antigens.

The notion of alloantigens primarily applies to antigens of erythrocytes, leukocytes, platelets, and some serum proteins (in particular, Ig). However, this concept is expected to apply to organ antigens, as already suggested by some data concerning pancreas and colon (alloantigen groups in the human colon have been described).

## MAIN ANTIGEN CATEGORIES

Antigens include substances as structurally diverse as proteins, polysaccharides, lipids, and nucleic acids. Their molecular weight varies from several million to a few thousand daltons and, in some cases, to less than 1,000 daltons. On the basis of origin, four types of immunogens can be recognized: haptens, active only when coupled to a carrier; natural immunogens found in nature, particularly in animal tissues; artificial immunogens, obtained by chemical modification of natural immunogens; and synthetic immunogens, artificially created.

Artificial antigens are natural immunogens to which one or several new molecules have been bound, generally by covalent bonds. Artificial antigens used most often are polypeptidyl proteins, which consist of proteins to which polypeptides have been coupled through an intermediary, like lysine amido groups of polypeptides. Often these polypeptides contain only one repetitive amino acid. Rather than fixing an already formed polypeptide to the protein, one may directly polymerize the N-carboxyl anhydride of the α-amino acid to the protein, as is the case for the production of synthetic poly-α-amino acids. It is interesting to note that these biochemical changes usually do not alter the biologic activity of the protein.

# II.   HAPTENS

The word "hapten" (from the Greek "haptein" "to grasp") was introduced by Landsteiner in 1921 to describe an alcoholic extract of horse kidney that was not by itself immunogenic in rabbits, but was able to combine with the antibodies produced by rabbits immunized with a kidney tissue homogenate. However, the alcoholic extract was subsequently shown to be capable of inducing antibody production after covalent binding to a carrier.

## CARRIER COUPLING

Numerous molecules, especially proteins and polysaccharides (in the mouse), may be coupled covalently to a hapten to act as a carrier. For this purpose, haptens may also be bound to erythrocytes, bacteriophages, artificial or synthetic macromolecules, and even to insoluble carriers. The hapten should possess one or several reactive groups that permit binding (covalent bonds) to carrier functional groups, under physicochemical conditions that maintain the integrity of the hapten structure, and as much as possible, of the carrier protein.

In some cases, binding of hapten to carrier requires mere contact (this is the case for nitrophenyl derivatives); most often, however, a coupling agent is required. When the hapten itself does not possess any reactive group, it may be introduced through a previous reaction. Thus, in order to couple steroids without carboxyl function to proteins, their alcohol function may be transformed into hemisuccinate, which introduces a carboxyl group.

### Carrier Choice

Proteins are the most commonly used carriers. They are easily prepared in large amounts, are water soluble, resist denaturation relatively well, and are very immunogenic. The latter property is not essential, because even nonimmunogenic autologous carriers can be utilized, toward which no immune response is seen. Albumins and heterologous γ globulins are commonly used carrier proteins. Particulate carriers, such as erythrocytes and bacteriophages, may also be utilized; however, carrier sites are then poorly defined. The degree of substitution, defined by the number of hapten molecules bound per carrier molecule, is a critical parameter for obtaining a good carrier effect. Landsteiner observed that, in the case of serum albumin, a maximum effect was obtained when there were 10 hapten groups per carrier molecule.

Of particular interest among the carriers are also the synthetic amino acid copolymers and the agarose particles (such as Sepharose 2B, activated by cyanogen bromide, and Sepharose CH and AH, which carry acidic and amido functions and contain galactose polyosidic chains). These particles are often utilized to make immunoadsorbents.

### Coupling Techniques

Generally, the hapten is bound to reactive functions, such as amino, carboxylic or thiol groups, or to certain carbon atoms of some amino acid side chains, such as lysine, or aromatic and heterocyclic residues. Coupling is accomplished by the use of conjugation agents that achieve a stable, covalent bond between hapten and one or several reactive groups, identical or not, of the carrier. The use of a particular technique depends primarily on the nature of those functional groups present on the hapten molecule. We shall now examine the most important coupling techniques, which are widely used in immunology, independently of the preparation of carrier-hapten conjugates, for antibody or antigen labeling (by fluorescein, iodine, or ferritin), and in immunoadsorbent preparation.

#### COUPLING OF DIAZOTATED COMPOUNDS

Certain haptens contain functional "azo" groups ($-N{=}N-$) that may be used, after their transformation into diazonium salts, to bind to amino acids, such as tyrosine, histidine, or lysine.

The transformation of the hapten into a diazonium salt may require treatment with nitrous acid at low temperature if the hapten has an aromatic or heterocyclic structure. If not, the hapten must be previously fixed to a molecule that has one or the other of these structures.

The coupling reaction itself consists of electron substitutions.

If the molar concentration of diazonium salts is of the same order as that of Tyr, His, and Lys residues in the protein, the reaction essentially gives a conjugate with monosubstituted Tyr and His and disubstituted Lys residues. If the number of diazonium salt moles is higher than that of Tyr, His, and Lys residues, one obtains disubstituted derivatives for all amino acids and even fixation onto Arg and Trp. The carrier effect is usually optimal when 15 to 30 hapten molecules are coupled to each carrier molecule.

The diazotation method has the advantage of causing minimal denaturation and producing colored derivatives, thus permitting simple spectrophotometric titration of the haptenic content of the conjugate. It has, however, the drawback of binding haptens to several different functional groups of the carrier; thus, the conjugate may be somewhat heterogeneous.

COUPLING BY FORMATION OF AMIDE (CO—NH) AND ISOTHIOCYANATE
(CS—NH) BONDS

CO—NH and CS—NH bonds permit fixation of proteins to haptens that possess nucleophilic reactive groups (for example, $NH_2$, SH, or OH) or to haptens that have a high affinity for nucleophilic groups. Hapten $NH_2$ groups bind to carrier COOH groups, or vice versa.

Several reagents may be used to produce coupling:

*Carbodiimides.*   N—N' disubstituted carbodiimides have a general formula RN=C=NR', where R and R' are aryl and alkyl groups. The coupling reaction may be summarized as follows:

$$R'COOH + R''NH_2 + RN{=}C{=}NR \longrightarrow R'CO{-}NHR'' + RNH{-}CO{-}NHR.$$
hapten       carrier      carbodiimide       conjugate

This coupling method has been applied to peptides, hormones, certain drugs (like aspirin), prostaglandins, cyclic adenosine monophosphate, nucleotides, phenols, and sugars.

*Isocyanates (RN=C=O) and Isothiocyanates (RN=C=S).*   The coupling reaction consists of binding the hapten to the $NH_2$ groups of the carrier by amide (CO—NH) or isothiocyanate bond (CS—NH).

$$RN{=}C{=}O + NH_2{-}Prot \longrightarrow R{-}NH{-}CO{-}NH{-}NH{-}Prot$$
isocyanate                      conjugate

or

$$RN{=}C{=}S + NH_2{-}Prot \longrightarrow R{-}NH{-}CS{-}NH{-}Prot$$
isothiocyanate                  conjugate

The most utilized coupling reagent is toluene 2,4-diisocyanate (TDIC).

This reagent binds through one of the two isocyanate groups to a protein and can bind, through its second isocyanate group, to a second protein. Thus, two proteins may be conjugated, such as BSA and myoglobin or insulin, Ig and ferritin or fluorescein, as well as various proteins on red blood cells for the purpose of passive hemagglutination reactions.

*Mixed Anhydride.*   Mixed anhydride permits the coupling to proteins of haptens with a carboxyl function (either spontaneously present or secondarily bound). The reaction consists of binding the haptenic COOH group to the protein by formation of a peptidic CO—NH bond on an $NH_2$ function of the carrier in the presence of tributylamine. This method is used to join proteins or to bind them to erythrocytes or to couple steroids and polypeptides to proteins.

DIRECT BINDING

Nitrophenylated derivatives bind directly and covalently to proteins by nucleophilic substitution on the $\epsilon$-$NH_2$ group of lysine or the $\alpha$-$NH_2$ of the terminal amino acids, as well as on cysteine SH groups. DNP and trinitrophenyl (TNP) may thus be bound directly to $\gamma$-globulins or albumin. Similarly, picryl chloride binds directly to skin proteins and brings about delayed hypersensitivity reactions.

dinitrophenol (DNP)   trinitrophenol (TNP)   picryl chloride   fluoro 2—4 dinitro—benzene

*Halogens.*   Halogens, which have a high affinity for benzyl nuclei, may bind to protein tyrosine residues and, to a lesser degree, to histidine and cysteine. Iodine is most often used because it is least electrophilic. Chloride and bromide may also be used but require the use of catalysts, and the absence of light. Protein iodination is used to modify the antigenicity of certain proteins and especially to label proteins (by [131]I or [125]I).

*Penicillin.*   The penicillin molecule combines directly with the $NH_2$ and SH groups of proteins by forming amide bonds (penicilloyl-protein conjugates) or disulfide bridges (penicillanic acid-protein conjugate). These reactions are also observed in vivo and are the cause of allergic reactions to penicillin.

CONCLUSIONS

There are numerous possibilities for coupling haptens to a carrier. It should be noted, however, that in each of the systems described above, haptens bind to some degree to groups other than those for which the carrier has been chosen. We shall see later that haptenic groups may form different determinants according to their binding site, hence the risk of obtaining, with certain conjugates, an antiserum that recognizes several specificities.

## METHODS FOR OBTAINING ANTIHAPTEN ANTIBODY

The hapten-carrier conjugate is separated from nonconjugated haptens and secondary reaction products by dialysis or chromatography. Subcutaneous or intradermal (or rarely intravenous) immunization provokes simultaneous production of antihapten and anticarrier antibodies. The addition of Freund's complete adjuvant and the use of repeated immunizing injections are usually needed to obtain antibodies of high titer, specificity and affinity. Antibodies are purified by means of filtration through an insoluble immunoadsorbent of the conjugate, followed by elution at low pH. The use of immunoadsorbents which consist of conjugates of both the hapten and of a carrier other than that used for immunization, produces pure antihapten antibodies devoid of any anticarrier antibodies.

## METHODS FOR STUDYING ANTIBODY-HAPTEN REACTIONS

Hapten-antibody reactions observe the general laws of antigen-antibody reactions and as a matter of fact, they constitute the ideal model. They may be studied by various techniques, which may be physical (equilibrium dialysis, fluorescence quenching, ultracentrifugation), immunochemical (precipitation, precipitation inhibition), serological (inhibition of passive hemagglutination, bacteriophage inactivation, or radioimmunological. In all of these reactions, except for precipitation, the hapten is used alone without conjugation to the carrier. In fact, monovalent haptens do not bring about precipitation, because each molecule binds to only one of two antibody sites, and the complexes so formed remain soluble. Aggregation of several identical monovalent haptens may, however, produce precipitation. This applies, for example, to the triazoic derivative of resorcinol and to certain bivalent haptens, like di-DNP lysine.

## MOLECULAR BASIS OF HAPTEN SPECIFICITY

Knowledge of the structure of numerous haptens has brought about a better understanding of the chemical basis of antigenic specificity.

### Contribution of the Carrier Microenvironment to the Antigenic Determinant: Notion of Haptenic Group

Very often, the complementary nature (specificity) of an antibody and of the hapten (used for its production) may be no better than with slightly different haptens, as is the case with conjugates of the hapten and an amino acid. This preliminary observation has led to the concept of "haptenic group," a structure thought to be larger than the hapten molecule, which may include several carrier atoms contiguous to the hapten. In this hypothesis, the antibody reacts with both the hapten and its carrier microenvironment. In some cases, however, especially when the hapten is large or when the hapten molecule extends over a relatively long distance outside the carrier (as with long aliphatic chains), the antibody may react only with part of the hapten or haptenic group.

Let us consider one such example: $p$-aminobenzoic acid (PAB) is coupled to a carrier, bovine $\gamma$ globulin (BGG), by diazotation of PAB followed by coupling of diazoic acid to BGG.

The antiserum obtained after immunization (by the BGG-PAB conjugate) is precipitated by BGG alone, and by BGG-PAB conjugate, but not by a heterologous protein unrelated to BGG (for example, ovalbumin). The antisera, however, may be precipitated by ovalbumin if the latter molecule is coupled to PAB acid (OA-PAB) but not if it is coupled to another substitute, such as azobenzene arsonate. Finally, incubation of the antiserum with nonconjugated PAB acid inhibits the precipitation of the ovalbumin-PAB conjugate by the serum. It is interesting to note that inhibition is more intense with certain analogs than with PAB itself (Fig. 6.1). This fact supports the concept of haptenic group mentioned above. In some cases, such antibodies may have a greater affinity for a similar, though different, antigen than that used for the initial immunization. These are known as heteroclitic antibodies. For example, C57BL/6 mice produce heteroclitic antibodies against acetylated 4-hydroxy-5-nitrophenyl determinants.

Similarly, if DNP inhibits the precipitation of PAB conjugates by an antiserum produced against the BGG-PAB conjugate, DNP-aminocaproate or DNP-lysine is more inhibitory than DNP. This is particularly interesting in light of the hypothesis that the carrier microenvironment contributes to the haptenic group. According to this hypothesis, lysine would participate at the combination site with the antibody by bridging the hapten and the polypeptide chains of the carrier.

### Determinants of the Hapten Alone

The hapten alone may control the determinant. Thus, BSA coupled to polyalanine (D,L or DL), brings about distinct antipolyalanine antibodies without cross-reactions. Study of the reaction inhibition by haptens of different size shows that inhibition is maximum with the pentamer, although significant inhibition is obtained with a dimer. The dimensions of the site have been calculated on the basis of five residues and have been shown to be $2.5 \times 1.1 \times 0.65$ nm. The minimum inhibition produced by poly-L-Ala-$\epsilon$-aminocaproate suggests that, in this particular case, the side chain of the amino-acyl residue, which links the hapten to the peptidic chain, contributes little to haptenic specificity and implies that the hapten alone comprises the antigenic site.

### Determinants Carried by Portions of the Hapten

As we have seen above, in some cases the determinant is confined to a portion of the molecule, usually the part most distant from the site where the

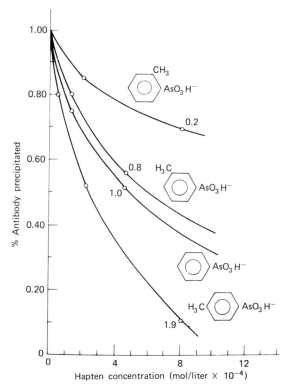

**Fig. 6.1** Haptenic inhibition of the precipitation reaction. Several haptens related to *p*-azobenzene arsonate inhibit the precipitation of an antiserum directed against that hapten by a protein-*p*-azobenzene arsonate conjugate. The hapten with a methyl group (CH$_3$) in the para position is the most inhibitory ($K$ = 1.9). It is more inhibitory than haptens with methyl groups in meta or ortho positions. (From D. Pressman, Advan. Biol. Med. Phys. 1953, *3*, 99.)

molecule attaches to the carrier. Thus, antidigoxin antibodies obtained after immunization by a conjugate (in which digoxin was coupled by its glucidic part) are directed essentially against the steroid located at the end of the molecule, as indicated by (1) the weak antidigoxin antibody reactivity when digitoxin contains the same sugar but a different steroid, (2) their strong reactivity, quasioptimal, with deslanoid, which contains the same steroid but a different sugar, and (3) good reactivity with digitoxigenin, or aglycone, which does not contain sugar.

### Multiplicity and Heterogeneity of Antihapten Antibodies

An antihapten serum often contains several antibodies directed against various parts of the haptenic group as well as against the whole group. This is often complicated by the fact that the hapten may contain several determinants, the number of which defines hapten valence.

In short, for a given monovalent hapten, immunization by a hapten-carrier conjugate may produce three antibody categories: (1) anticarrier antibodies, totally absorbed by the carrier; (2) antihapten antibodies, reacting with the conjugate of the hapten and of the carrier protein used for immunization as well as with the conjugates of the hapten and of any other protein; (3) residual antibodies, found after absorption by the carrier and by a conjugate of the hapten with a carrier other than that used for immunization. Those antibodies which precipitate only the conjugate of the hapten and of the initial carrier are called "antilink" antibodies, because they are, a priori, directed against a determinant located in the contact zone between hapten and carrier. It is interesting to note that these antibodies are inhibited by large free hapten excess, which underscores the essential role of the structures in the hapten itself.

In addition, we should point out that "heteroligating" antibodies directed against two haptens bound to the same carrier are not observed. The absence of such antibodies has been demonstrated for ovalbumin simultaneously conjugated to arsanilic acid and iodine haptens.

### Molecular Basis of Hapten Immunologic Specificity

Chemical modifications of hapten molecules have variable effects on specificity. At times, minor changes may lead to great modifications in specificity, while major chemical alterations may change their specificity only slightly. Finally, if there is a relatively close complementarity between hapten and antibody, it is far from being absolute, as if in the classic Ehrlich representation of key and lock, the lock (antibody) were of simpler structure than the key (antigen).

Chemical substitution of some simple haptenic groups has allowed analysis of the nature of immunoreactive sites. Charged groups seem to be essential for specificity, whereas neutral groups make a smaller contribution. In addition, optical isomers may bring about completely different antibodies, which tells us that specificity of a haptenic determinant depends on both the chemical composition of the molecule and on its spatial orientation.

Cross-reactions observed between an antiserum and various haptens may be due to the existence of similar or identical determinants on these haptens. In the former case, the determinant shows a strong reaction with the antibody exhibiting cross-reaction, but precipitation is inhibited at lower concentrations with the homologous hapten than with the heterologous hapten. However, the heterologous hapten (bound to a carrier) in sufficient concentrations may completely absorb the antibody.

In conclusion, on the basis of these data, the antigenic determinant or epitope (as opposed to paratope, i.e., the antibody) may be defined as the smallest structural unit recognized by an antibody, the antigenic pattern as the largest structure recognized by a given antibody population (Table 6.2).

## III. PROTEIN ANTIGENS

All polypeptides with sufficient molecular weight (as a rule higher than 1000 daltons) and, a fortiori, all proteins are immunogenic but in various degrees.

**Table 6.2   A Few Definitions**

An antigen is a category of molecules (a molecular species) defined by its antigenic specificity

An antigenic specificity is the property of a given antigen to combine with a (usually heterogeneous) given population of antibody

An antigenic pattern is the structure or a set of structures of the antigen that participate in its combination with a given antibody population. The terms "antigenic specificity" and "antigenic pattern" are often used almost synonimously. The expression "antigenic site" used by some authors may lead to confusion, and the term "site" should probably be reserved for antibodies (antibody site)

An antigenic determinant is a structure present on the antigen molecule's surface, capable of binding to an antibody molecule, and a single one. In his new terminology, Jerne speaks of the epitope as opposed to paratope (antibody)

After J. Oudin

According to the intensity of the induced immune response, there are strong or weak antigens: albumins are generally strong antigens, whereas small peptides are weak antigens. Protein modifications by physical (heat) or chemical treatments that produce conformational change may sometimes modify or diminish immunogenicity. Enzymatic hydrolysis may also alter to varying degrees protein immunogenicity. However, formaldehyde, which abolishes biologic activities of proteins (in particular, those of polypeptidic toxins, by transforming them into anatoxins), does not modify their immunogenicity.

## METHODOLOGIC APPROACHES

For many years, the main biochemical approach to protein antigenicity consisted of modifying proteins by various chemical treatments and then studying the specificity of these altered antigens. The results were often difficult to interpret, because the chemical modifications were often complex, affecting several antigenic sites simultaneously. The use of protein fragments, obtained by enzymatic digestion, has been shown to be very helpful. Very often each fragment (isolable by chromatography) has only one or two determinants, and it is possible to determine its amino acid sequence. The application of these methods to four materials will now be surveyed: silk fibrillar protein, lysozyme, ribonuclease, and human albumin.

## NATURAL PROTEINS

### *Silk Fibrillar Protein (Example of Application of Hydrolysis Techniques)*

Silk fibrillar protein (SFP) is a linear protein consisting of a single polypeptide chain with a molecular weight of about 50,000 to 60,000 daltons. Landsteiner had already shown in 1942 that partial acid hydrolysis produced several peptides of seven to 62 amino acids (AA). The anti-SFP-SFP antibody precipitation may be inhibited by these peptides, which shows that some have retained a determinant from the native molecule. Intact SFP precipitation may be inhibited by up to 50% with a decapeptide and by 40% with an octapeptide. When one removes the C-terminal residue of the octapeptide (a tyrosine), the residual hexapeptide induces no more than 20% inhibition. These results indicate that the antigenic determinant of SFP consists of about eight to 12 AA (i.e., 2.7 to 4.4 nm in chain length) and that tyrosine plays a special role in its immunologic activity. However, precipitation inhibition was only obtained at very high molarities and one must recognize that even the largest of these inhibitory peptides represent only a part of the antigenic pattern. In addition, these experiments did not exclude the existence of determinants not borne by hydrolysis-derived peptides nor of determinants that bring about primarily production of nonprecipitating antibodies, which as a result remained undetected in precipitation experiments.

### Lysozyme (of Special Interest Because of Known Primary and Spatial Structure) (Fig. 6.2)

Lysozyme is a protein that consists of a single polypeptide chain (129 AA) with a molecular weight of 14,500 and includes several basic AA. Both its sequence and its secondary and tertiary structures are known. Two major antigenic determinants have been demonstrated. Studies by Sela showed that the first of these determinants comprises the region containing residues 57 to 107 (including the "loop" peptide, made up of residues 64 to 80). This

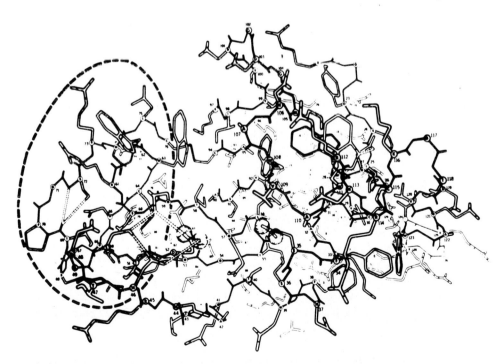

**Fig. 6.2** Lysozyme structure (the "loop peptide" is limited by the dotted line). (From R. Arnon, in L. Brent and J. Holborow, Eds., Progress in immunology II, Vol. 2, Amsterdam, 1974, North Holland, p. 8.)

determinant is able to absorb 12% of antibodies produced against the whole molecule. The second determinant, which may absorb as much as 50% of antibodies, includes AA 7 to 27 and 122 to 129. In addition, it should be noted that after reduction and alkylation, lysozyme no longer has the same antigenicity because the antibodies directed against native lysozyme do not react with denatured lysozyme, or vice versa. The same does not apply, however, to cell-mediated immunity reactions, and not, in a wider sense, to T cells that show significant cross-reactions against native and denatured lysozymes.

### Ribonuclease (Example of Application of Hydrolysis and Biochemical Treatments)

Ribonuclease (RNase) is a protein of low molecular weight (about 14,000 daltons, 124 AA). Its complete amino acid sequence has been elucidated and its synthesis made possible. RNase is hydrolyzed between residues 20 and 21 by subtilisin, with release of a 20-AA peptide (the S peptide) and a 104-AA polypeptide (the S protein), both of which inhibit precipitation of anti-RNase antibodies by RNase. Neither of these two polypeptides is biologically active, but added together, they may reassociate to produce the initial molecule. The S peptide does not precipitate anti-RNase antibodies, but the S protein does, although to a lesser degree than RNase itself. The reassociation of the S peptide and the S protein produces a molecule that precipitates antibodies just like the initial molecule. This phenomenon emphasizes the importance of secondary and tertiary structures for the expression of antigenicity.

On the other hand, while removal of the valine residue of the C-terminal extremity of RNase (by carboxypeptidase) does not modify immunologic activity, removal of the four C-terminal AA (121 to 124) decreases it significantly. Breakage of all four disulfide bridges causes loss of immunologic activity, and rupture of two of the bridges causes a significant decrease in activity. Deamination and guanidination also decrease immunologic activity. These results, when taken together, indicate that the RNase molecule has at least two determinants, one containing disulfide bridges and terminating in a lysine, and the other possessing one or more disulfide bridges and a portion of the 120 to 123 amino acid chain.

Another chemical modification has permitted Brown to further elucidate the role of secondary structure. Oxidized by performic acid, RNase provokes the formation of antibodies that react against oxidized RNase but not against native RNase. Enzymatic degradation of oxidized RNase provides, unlike native RNase, peptides that are strongly immunoactive, such as peptides 38 to 61 and 105 to 124. These peptides react with different antibodies and provide precipitation inhibition (higher than 50%) of those antibodies directed against the native RNase. Study of oxidized RNase shows that it is possible to obtain inhibitory peptides and that there are, in fact, determinants in a range of 20 to 25 amino acids.

### Human Serum Albumin (Problem of a Protein with a Not Completely Known Structure)

Degradation of human albumin by proteolytic enzymes, such as pepsin, chymotrypsin, and trypsin, creates fragments that precipitate differently antialbumin antibodies. Each of these fragments still contains several of the original determinants since they precipitate antialbumin antisera. Lapresle has, however, isolated two fragments that react with antialbumin sera without precipitation. The first of these fragments (called the inhibitor) has a molecular weight of 11,000 daltons and includes 89 AA; it was obtained through degradation of serum albumin by rabbit cathepsin D. Although it does not itself precipitate antialbumin antibodies, the fragment strongly inhibits precipitation of antibodies by intact albumin. The amount of inhibitor necessary to obtain 50% of maximum inhibition corresponds to an inhibitor/albumin molar ratio of 1. The second fragment, F1, with a molecular weight of 6600 daltons and 53 AA, obtained through tryptic digestion of the inhibitor, combines with only part of the antibodies that react with the inhibitor. Ultracentrifugation has shown that with an antibody excess, the immune complexes formed with the inhibitor are of the Ab2-Ag type, whereas those formed with the F1 fragment are of the Ab-Ag type, thus showing that the inhibitor is bivalent and the F1 fragment is monovalent.

### Conclusions

The above data, as well as others not discussed here, allow some general conclusions to be drawn as to the chemical basis of protein antigenicity.

Fibrillar proteins have 12 to 25 AA determinants, but smaller peptides (8 to 12 AA) have a significant, although weaker, inhibitory capacity, which suggests that protein antigenic determinants include about 20 AA or that about 20 AA are necessary to maintain a 10 to 12 AA determinant in an adequate configuration. Globular proteins have a more complex structure. Their antigenicity is linked to a protein conformation that results from their secondary, tertiary, and possibly quaternary structures. Their determinants correspond to 10- to 20-AA structures. Contrary to previous opinion, no specific role can be attributed to any given AA. Tyrosine-deficient peptides, for example, prepared from oxidized ribonuclease or human albumin may thus be immunoactive.

It should be noted also that total molecular weight plays an important role

**Table 6.3 Correlation Between Antigenic Molecular Weight and Valence**

| Antigen | Molecular weight | Approximate molar antibody/ antigen ratio of precipitate in extreme antibody excess* |
|---|---|---|
| Pancreatic bovine ribonuclease | 13,600 | 3 |
| Chicken ovalbumin | 42,000 | 5 |
| Horse serum albumin | 69,000 | 6 |
| Human γ globulin | 160,000 | 7 |
| Horse apoferritin | 465,000 | 26 |
| Thyroglobulin | 700,000 | 40 |
| Tomato bushy stunt virus | 8,000,000 | 90 |
| Tobacco mosaic virus | 40,000,000 | 650 |

* Because antibody molecules are at least bivalent, valences of antigens are higher than antibody/ antigen ratios.
After Kabat.

in immunogenicity; the smallest immunogens in the absence of the carrier have a molecular weight of less than 1000 daltons (e.g., vasopressin and oxytocin). The role of aggregates is also very important, since albumins and Ig are only immunogenic when aggregated (these molecules become tolerogen when aggregates are removed through ultracentrifugation; see p. 577).

## MODIFIED PROTEINS: POLYPEPTIDYL PROTEINS

Important information about the chemical basis of protein immunogenicity has been obtained by studying natural proteins coupled to synthetic polypeptides. It is necessary to differentiate between those cases in which the carrier protein is already immunogenic and those in which it is only slightly so or not at all.

### Cases Where the Protein is Spontaneously Immunogenic

Protein immunogenicity is maintained after polypeptide coupling; the conjugate produces antibodies directed against the initial protein. In addition, antibodies are produced against the polypeptide (the protein serving then as the carrier if the polypeptide is not by itself immunogenic), and antilink antibodies are formed against the new specificities created in the contact area between the protein and the grafted polypeptide.

### Cases Where the Protein Is Slightly, or Not at All, Immunogenic

Gelatin is an extremely weak immunogen. Sela has shown that grafting of chains of tyrosine, tryptophan, phenylalanine, or cyclohexylamine makes it highly immunogenic in the guinea pig and rabbit. A moderate increase in immunogenicity is also obtained using cysteine, but alanine, glutamic acid, serine, lysine, and proline have no effect. This enhancement of immunogenicity has been attributed to increased rigidity of molecular determinant sites, which Haurowitz previously suggested as the necessary condition for immunogenicity. An increase in rigidity would be linked to the creation of side chains of aromatic amino acids or cyclohexane nuclei or, using cysteine, to the formation of disulfide bridges. A similar enhancement has been observed after pepsinogen tyrosilation. It is interesting to note that, with regard to gelatin, a mere 2% binding rate of L-tyrosine induces the appearance of antigelatin antibodies, whereas a 10% binding rate leads to the production of antityrosine antibodies that are also precipitated by heterologous proteins, other than gelatin, coupled to tyrosine or tyrosine-rich copolymers.

## SYNTHETIC POLYPEPTIDES

The study of immunogenic potency of synthetic polypeptides has contributed significantly to our knowledge of antigen patterns and protein immunogenicity. Indeed, it is possible to select their AA composition and spatial arrangement, their molecular weight, electric charge, or molecular conformation, and then evaluate their effect on antigenic specificity. Those synthetic antigens used most often are synthetic (L, D or LD) AA polymers produced from one, two, or three different amino acids (Fig. 6.3). Homopolymers are formed with only one amino acid, whereas copolymers are formed by adding two, three, or more AA. Synthesis is brought about through polymerization of N-carboxyamino acid anhydrides which does not change optical D or L configuration. One may deal with linear homopolymers (cross-linked or branched), linear copolymers (with random or alternating sequences), and branched copolymers with multiple chains, including a main linear chain to which lateral chains are attached. Copolymers are often heterogeneous with regard to residue sequence and chain length. For this reason, some authors have attempted to produce copolymers of ordered sequence. Several examples of synthetic polypeptides are described in chapter 24.

### Role of Global Amino Acid Composition

Homopolymers composed of one AA type are usually not immunogenic, with a few exceptions: homopolymers poly-L-Pro, poly-L-Glu, poly-L-Arg, and poly-L-Lys are immunogenic in selected guinea pig and rabbit strains. Poly-L-Lys and its derivatives have been used by Benacerraf to study the genetic regulation of immune responses in the guinea pig (see chap. 24). Copolymers of two AA are not always immunogenic, especially in mouse and man. Copolymers with three or more AA, however, have good immunogenic potency in all species. Their immunogenicity is particularly high when they contain one aromatic amino acid, although this functional group is not an essential requirement for immunogenicity. In conclusion, it appears that a certain degree of molecular complexity is necessary in order for a synthetic polypeptide to be immunogenic.

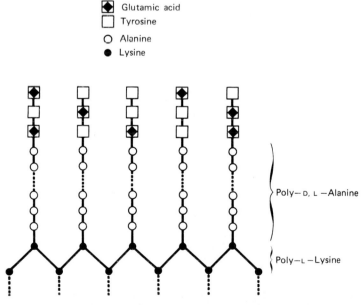

**Fig. 6.3** (T,G)-A--L. Poly-L-(tyrosine, glutamic acid)-poly-D,L-alanine--poly-L-lysine (see Table 24.1).

### Role of the Spatial Position of Certain Groups

It is possible to study the role of spatial position of certain AA by comparing the immunogenicity of polypeptides with identical central chain and lateral chains of the same composition but with different AA sequences. Sela has shown that a reversal of two AA is sufficient to modify immunogenicity significantly. Accessibility of the determinants is necessary, since an inward positioning of critical AA causes a significant loss in immunogenicity. Figure 6.4 shows an example, in which the Tyr-Glu dipeptide is immunogenic only when located on spaced chains or at the end of close lateral chains. Further evidence of the essential role of determinant accessibility is the adjunction of immunogenic groups (for example, Tyr, Glu) to an inactive polymer, thus making it immunogenic, and conversely, the coupling of nonimmunogenic groups (poly-Ala, for example) to an immunogenic copolymer, inducing loss of its immunogenicity.

### Role of Molecular Conformation

Secondary and tertiary structures of synthetic polypeptides have little influence on their immunogenicity but may greatly modify their antigenic specificity. Thus, the copolymer with a repetitive Tyr-Ala-Glu sequence produces antibodies of different specificity, according to its being helicoidal or linear, for a comparable immunogenic potency.

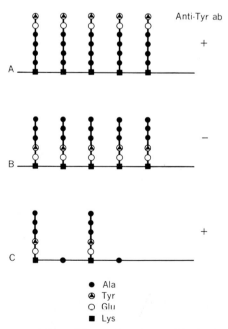

**Fig. 6.4** Role of the spatial position of amino acids in immunogenicity of synthetic polypeptides. The Tyr-Glu dipeptide is only immunogenic when it is located at the end of close lateral chains or on spaced chains.

**Table 6.4 Antigenicity of Synthetic Polypeptides**

| | *Antigenic polypeptides* | *Molecular weight* | *Nonantigenic polypeptides* | *Molecular weight* |
|---|---|---|---|---|
| Rabbit | ALA$^{60}$ Glu$^{40}$ | 30,000 | Ala$^{40}$ Glu$^{60}$ | 47,000 |
| | Glu$^{58}$ Lys$^{42}$ | 3,7000 | Glu$^{50}$ Lys$^{50}$ | 42,000 |
| | Glu$^{50}$ Tyr$^{50}$ | 12,000 | D-Glu$^{55}$ D-Tyr$^{45}$ | 13,000 |
| | Ala$^{38}$ Glu$^{52}$ Tyr$^{10}$ | 4000 | | |
| | Glu$^{80}$ Leu$^{20}$ | 89,000 | | |
| Guinea pig | Ala$^{60}$ Glu$^{40}$ | 35,000 | Ala$^{10}$ Glu$^{90}$ | 75,000 |
| | Glu$^{80}$ Leu$^{20}$ | 89,000 | D-Glu$^{55}$ D-Tyr$^{45}$ | 13,400 |
| | Glu$^{50}$ Tyr$^{50}$ | 12,000 | | |
| | Ala$^{38}$ Glu$^{52}$ Tyr$^{10}$ | 4100 | | |
| Mouse | Ala$^{30}$ Glu$^{42}$ Lys$^{28}$ | 62,000 | Ala$^{40}$ Glu$^{60}$ | 33,000 |
| Human | Ala$^{35}$ Glu$^{36}$ Lys$^{24}$ Tyr$^{5}$ | 35,000 | Glu$^{60}$ Lys$^{40}$ | 80,000 |
| | Ala$^{5}$ Glu$^{57}$ Lys$^{38}$ | 50,000 | | |
| | Glu$^{58}$ Lys$^{38}$ Tyr$^{4}$ | 94,000 | | |

After J. J. Barrett.

### Role of Electric Charge

Neutral polypeptides without electric charge may be immunogenic. Thus, electric charge is not essential for immunogenic potency. However, Sela has shown the existence of an inverse relationship between overall electric charge of an antigen and that of the corresponding antibody.

### Role of Amino Acid Optical Configuration

All synthetic polypeptides used in the preceding experiments were L-amino acid polymers. Nonetheless, it is possible to synthesize immunogenic D-amino acid polymers, but their immunogenicity is then decreased and depends closely on the dose administered to the animal, whereas L-polyamino acid immunogenicity is virtually independent of dose. Excessive doses of D-polyamino acids (e.g., more than 1 μg in mice) produce immune paralysis, which explains previous inability to provoke immunization through the use of these products. Similarly, macromolecules that contain up to 95% L-AA but with lateral chains terminated by 5% D-AA are just as poorly immunogenic as 100% D-AA polymers. Conversely, the presence of L forms at the end of the chain renders D-AA polymers highly immunogenic. Immune response to D-polyamino acids has other peculiarities: slow antigen degradation, weak responses, and absence of secondary response after booster injection. D-Polyamino acids are poor immunogens and powerful tolerogens.

There is another difference between L- and D-polyamino acids: L-poly-AA bring about thymus-dependent responses, whereas D-poly-AA produce thymus-independent responses. Sela has shown that among the four possible enantiomers, LL, LD, DL, and DD, of *p*-(Tyr,Glu)-*p*(Lys) copolymers, the response is thymus dependent only for the LL form and is thymus independent for the three other forms, which are weak immunogens with slow catabolism. Within one polymer, the *p*-(L-Phe,L-Glu)-*p*-(D-Pro)-*p*-(D-Lys), the response to the external portion (L) is thymus dependent, whereas that to the internal part (D) is thymus independ-ent. Finally, antibodies obtained with L or D forms are, as a rule, specific with respect to optical form. As a result, there is no cross-reactivity between $p$-(D-Tyr,D-Glu,D-Lys) and $p$-(L-Tyr,L-Glu,L-Lys).

### Role of Molecular Weight

In general, synthetic polypeptides are good immunogens when their molecular weight is higher than 4000 daltons. In this case, their immunogenicity can be as strong as that of much larger molecules. However, molecules of smaller size (500 to 1000 daltons) may also be immunogenic and produce both antibodies and delayed hypersensitivity. This applies to oligotyrosine peptides (hexa- and even tripeptide) and to oligolysine peptides and their DNP deriva-tives: oligolysines are immunogenic after eight AA, DNP derivatives after seven AA.

### Comparison of Immunogenic and Antibody-Binding Sites

We have indicated earlier that some polypeptides are not immunogenic because their "immunoactive" region is not accessible. Nonetheless, some of these polypeptides may react with antibodies produced against immunogenic substances that are chemically related. As a result, antibody-binding sites, strictly speaking, are not necessarily immunogenic sites.

## GENERAL CONCLUSIONS ON THE CHEMICAL BASES OF ANTIGENIC SPECIFICITY AND PROTEIN IMMUNOGENICITY

The above data concerning specific examples enable us to formulate some general conclusions. A certain diversity of structure and sufficient molecular weight (500 to 1,000 daltons) are necessary for immunogenicity (homopolymers are, as a rule, not immunogenic). Exposure and accessibility of antigenic determinants on the molecule surface are necessary for full expression. There are usually several antigenic determinants within the same molecule. Specificity closely depends upon primary structure; a single AA difference may alter it significantly. Nonetheless, secondary, tertiary, and quaternary structures are also important. The size of the antigenic determinant may vary, but is generally small (10 to 20 AA).

Substances that are poorly metabolized are also poorly immunogenic and often thymus independent.

The charge on the entire antigen molecule seems to play a more important role than that of the antigenic determinant, as indicated by the acid or basic nature of anti-$p$-azobenzene arsonate antibodies, depending on whether the hapten is coupled to poly-L-lysyl ribonuclease (basic conjugate) or to rabbit serum albumin (acidic conjugate).

In view of all these observations it appears that the relationship between immunogenicity and primary molecular structure does not conform to any strict rules. Changing several amino acids may not modify immunogenicity, whereas even a minor alteration in a single amino acid (e.g., the alteration of a single

**Table 6.5  Effects of Certain Amino Acid Substitutions on the Antigenicity of Bradykinin, Studied by Radio-immunoassay Using an Antiserum Produced Against Polysylbradykinin (i.e., Bradykinin Coupled to Polylysine at Its N-Terminal in the Presence of Toluene-di-isocyanate)**

| Amino Acids | Antigenicity (% activity of natural peptide) |
|---|---|
| Arg - Pro - Pro - Gly - Phe - Ser - Pro - Phe - Arg | |
| Ac Arg ———————————————————————————— | 160 |
| NO$_2$ Arg ——————————————————— NO$_2$ Arg | 130 |
| ———————————————————————— | 6 |
| ———————————————————— D Arg | 77 |
| —— D Pro ————————————————— | 7 |
| ——— D Pro ———————————————— | <1 |
| ——————————————————————— Arg | 16 |
| ————————————— Phe ——————————— | 14 |

After Kabat.

radical) may suffice to produce significant diminution or even the disappearance of antigenicity. Table 6-5 demonstrates the effects of changing one amino acid at several points in the sequence of the bradykinin molecule on the antigenicity of this peptide. It can be seen that by simply changing the second or third residue for its dextrorotary form practically eliminates its antigenicity and that the second, third, fourth, and fifth residues appear to play a particularly important role, despite their proximity to the N-terminal end on which is branched the polylysine used for the immunization. It is equally interesting to note that, in this particular case, the integrity of the peptide is necessary for its immunogenicity, although this is unusual for peptides of more than 9 or 10 amino acids. In general, amino acid substitution produces clearer effects, the more the shape of the peptide becomes modified.

# IV.  POLYOSIDIC ANTIGENS

The study of polyosides has long played an important role in understanding the chemical basis of antigenic specificity because of their relative structural simplicity, and because of the negligible role of secondary or tertiary structures (as we have seen, they complicate the study of protein antigens).

## POLYOSIDIC STRUCTURE

### Simple Polyosides

Polyosides are molecules obtained through polymerization of sugars (hexose, pentose, heptose, and, less frequently, sugars with eight or nine carbon atoms). The osidic unit may be replaced by alcohols of three or five carbon atoms (glycerol or ribitol). Hydroxyl groups of these sugars can be substituted by methyl, acetyl, amine or acetylamine, or they can be reduced (deoxy sugars) or oxidized (uronic acid). To these variants one may add the existence of D and L isomers and of anomeric alpha and beta positions of the sugars involved in a given bond. Oligosides contain up to 10 or 12 sugar units (in nature, oligosides are generally associated with lipids or proteins). Polyosides usually contain more than 12 sugars.

Polyosides can be classified into several categories according to their structure. They include branched polyosides (e.g., dextrans and levans), linear polyosides (e.g., pneumococcal polyosides, or the Vi antigen of salmonella), and branched polyosides (e.g., pneumococci and streptococci polyosides as well as teichoic acids). Dextrans and levans are made up of a great number of identical sugar units (glucose or fructose) linked similarly (I → 4, I → 6), except at their junction point. Their molecular weight may reach several tens of millions of daltons. This is, however, an average value since dextrans and levans are polydispersed molecules. Partial hydrolysis produces fragments of different size. Type-III pneumococcus polysaccharide (S III) is a cellobiuronic acid polymer. Simple polyosides may be immunogenic in man and mouse, independently of any protein contamination, when their molecular weight is higher than 100,000 daltons, but great variations in response occur among species (polyosides are not particularly immunogenic in the rabbit). Precipitating antibodies persist in man at high levels and over long periods (sometimes becoming almost homogeneous) because of decreased antigen catabolism. We shall see later that simple polyosides with repetitive functional groups are generally thymus-independent antigens; that is, they may induce antibody synthesis in neonatally thymectomized animals.

### Complex Polyosides and Glycoproteins

These include lipopolysaccharides of enterobacteria, as well as glycoproteins, in particular those of blood group substances and lectins.

## CHEMICAL BASES OF POLYOSIDE ANTIGENIC SPECIFICITY

Although polyosides usually have several antigenic determinants, it is possible to study the bond between one of these determinants and its corresponding antibody. To do this, antibodies are selected by differential absorption or precipitation, or polyosides are used in which certain determinants have been selectively destroyed.

### Position of Determinants on the Polyosidic Chain

Most polyosides induce the synthesis of numerous antibodies, some of which cross-react with polyosides other than that used for immunization. However, some antibodies seem to react exclusively against the homologous polyoside. The fact that A and B specificities of blood groups, present in AB-group subjects, are coprecipitated by anti-A as well as by anti-B sera suggests that the same polyoside molecule bears both A and B specificities. Analogous results have been obtained by Staub, who has shown the existence of several distinct antigenic determinants on salmonella polyoidic chains, findings that suggest the hypothesis of an immunodominant sugar.

## CONCEPT OF IMMUNODOMINANT SUGAR

When inhibiting the precipitation of an antibody directed against one determinant by different sugars, one generally observes that all sugar units of the polyoside are inhibitory (with a few exceptions) but that for equal quantities, one sugar inhibits better than the others: the latter sugar is called the immunodominant sugar. Immunodominant sugars tend to be located at the end of lateral chains, like glucose in Salmonella factor 1. However, occasionally, immunodominant sugars are located inside a chain, such as glucuronic acid in pneumococcal S III polysaccharide. More generally, the immunodominant determinant is the main point of contact of the antigenic determinant and the antibody's combining site; in other words, it is the group that contributes most of the energy toward the binding of the antigen to the antibody.

## DETERMINANT SIZE

Kabat has systematically compared the capacity of oligosides of increasing size to inhibit antipolyoside antibodies. Inhibition increases until the hexoses are reached and then remains constant, which indicates that the determinant consists of six sugars. However, for any given polyoside, the inhibition by oligosides of different size may vary considerably depending on the antisera used; therefore, the adaptation of all antibodies directed against one single six sugar determinant is not invariably perfect. Kabat formulated the existence of not one type of antibody but an antibody family whose sites are complementary for oligosides of different size. It was also possible to isolate antibodies optimally inhibited by di-, tri-, or pentoses. However, the dimensions of the oligoside which corresponds to minimal-size antibody site remained to be determined. In this regard, the study of Salmonella polyosides proved to be particularly useful: it showed that two polyosides with identical glucose lateral chains, not fixed to the same galactose carbons produced no cross-reaction. This result, as well as others observed with *Escherichia coli* polyosides, showed that rabbit antibodies could be adapted to multiple diosides but not to one single dose. This finding explains why, as soon as two sugars are linked identically, a cross-reaction may be detectable, even when the remaining oligoside differs. It also explains why it is impossible to obtain (rabbit) antipolyoside antibodies by injecting an immunodominant sugar linked to a protein, even though such antibodies do result from the administration of diosides or even one single acetylated sugar.

All of these data have been obtained in rabbits, and it seems that a different situation applies to the goat. In the goat, the antibodies produced against a single sugar, colitose, agglutinate 0 55 and 0 III *E. coli* and are precipitated by the corresponding polyosides. This is one example of antibodies adapted to only one sugar or even less than one. It should be noted that horses react like goats, and guinea pigs like rabbits.

NUMBER OF ANTIBODY FAMILIES THAT CORRESPOND TO ONE
IMMUNODOMINANT OLIGOSACCHARIDE

The same immunodominant sugar may contribute to several specificities. Thus, the short glucose lateral chain of the C4 polyoside of salmonella produces two distinct antibody families, one of which corresponds to oligosides located on the right side of the glucose, the other to those on the left side.

NUMBER OF SUGARS THAT PLAY THE ROLE OF IMMUNODOMINANT

All sugars in a polyoside do not necessarily play a role in polyoside immunogenicity. For example, rhamnose of E2 Salmonella polyoside does not seem to be involved in the immunogenicity of this polyoside in rabbits (after binding to a carrier) even though it may be a factor in the horse. In other words, within a given species, all diosidic bonds do not always produce antibodies. *Salmonella Newington* polyoside could theoretically trigger the production of a large number of antibodies, however, the actual number of specificities obtained in the rabbit is much lower than the theoretical estimate. This can be explained as follows: (1) some structures may be common to both the polyoside, and to certain autoantigens of the animal, especially erythrocyte autoantigens; (2) unstable structures may be destroyed before stimulation of antibody production occurs; and (3) there may be antigenic competition between various structures with different immunogenic potencies. Thus, when a short branched chain is present on the principal chain, the great majority of antibodies are directed against the lateral chain. MacCarthy's studies, for example, have shown this to be true for D-group streptococcal polyosides. These have a main chain of glycerol teichoic acid with lateral di- and triglucose chains. Antistreptococcal D sera do not react with polyglycerol alone (the main chain). Conversely, the sera produced against polyglycerol alone, which contain exclusively antibodies directed against the main chain, react with streptococcal D sera. One calls this phenomenon nonreciprocal cross-reaction. (4) All antibodies do not necessarily bind to the polyoside when determinants are locked inside a large molecule because of steric hindrance. This applies in particular to some salmonella polyosides. Similarly, if very long lateral chains are present, only those sites located at the end of the long chains bind to the antibodies. This explains the electron microscopy findings of Sands, who made labeled antibodies (ferritin) react with *E. coli*: an antibody halo is observed at a distance from the bacteria. These phenomena of steric hindrance explain why it is possible, in certain cases, to obtain antibodies that do not react with the polyoside used for immunization but which bind to another polyoside possessing identical, but more accessible determinants.

### Genetic Alterations of Polyosides

We have shown that antigenic specificity of polyosides is controlled by the individual sugar bonds; specific sites are borne by oligosides with five or six sugars. It is assumed that any modification of diosidic bonds or changes in one sugar may modify immunogenicity, that is, may induce the appearance or disappearance of certain specificities. These changes may occur in bacteria during mutation, conversion, or conjugation.

# V.  OTHER ANTIGENS

## LIPIDS

Pure lipids are not immunogenic. However, when coupled to proteins, they may act like haptens. For example, one may obtain antilecithin, anticephalin, or anticholesterol antibodies. Some glycolipids, such as cardiolipin (used in the Bordet-Wassermann reaction for syphilis diagnosis) may become immunogenic after binding to a carrier.

## NUCLEIC ACIDS

The immunogenicity of nucleic acids has long been questioned and contradictory findings reported. Attempts at the experimental production of antibodies often failed, and there were considerable difficulties for in vitro study: highly charged nucleic acids bring about nonspecific interactions with numerous serum proteins, which were often confused with immunologic reactions, when in fact, it is possible to obtain antibodies by coupling nucleic acid to a carrier. One illustration of this method is methylated serum albumin, which produces electrostatic interactions with nucleic acids without covalent bonds, thus eliminating the risk of denaturation. The injection of such conjugates (within which nucleic acid is protected from nuclease action) in the presence of Freund's complete adjuvant (rabbit) produces antibodies directed against DNA, RNA, synthetic polynucleotides, or oligonucleotides of four or even three residues. Other methods of conjugation (carbodiimide treatment or diazotation) may be used for oligonucleotides in which covalent bonds do not lead to denaturation.

Strict specificity of antinucleic acid antibodies for the immunizing antigen is unusual. Generally speaking, specificity depends on the particular nature of the nucleotide.

In addition, there are base-specific antibodies, and antibodies whose specificity depends on their sugar content.

It should be noted that it is also possible to obtain antibodies against nucleic acids by immunization with phage lysates (whose proteins serve as carriers) and ribosomal preparations. Native antinucleic acid antibodies, such as anti-DNA antibodies, are commonly seen in sera of patients suffering from systemic lupus erythematosus or other autoimmune diseases (see chap. 28).

# VI.  INFLUENCE OF IMMUNOGENICITY ON THE TYPE OF IMMUNE RESPONSE

Basically, we have discussed humoral antibody responses so far. One wonders whether the basis of antigenic specificity in delayed hypersensitivity reactions follows the same principles as those mentioned earlier with regard to antibodies. In a wider sense, one wonders whether T lymphocytes responsible for cell-mediated immunity as well as for the helper effects, in fact recognize antigenic patterns different from those recognized by antibody producing B lymphocytes. In this chapter, we will limit our discussion to the problem of delayed hypersensitivity, while chapter 24 will examine transplantation antigens, which may induce either antibody production or a cell-mediated immunity reaction.

## IMMUNOGENICITY AND DELAYED HYPERSENSITIVITY

Delayed hypersensitivity (DH) reactions may be studied through one of several in vivo (skin reactions) or in vitro techniques (inhibition of macrophage migration, thymidine incorporation in the presence of antigen). Schlossman has done extensive studies on the immunogenicity of DNP conjugates with L-lysine polymers. In this system, the smallest antigen capable of inducing antibodies as well as DH (in the guinea pig) is α-DNP-hepta-L-lysine, in which DNP is bound to the amino terminal nitrogen of a seven-residue L-lysine polymer. Conjugates of DNP with homopolymers of more than seven lysines are all immunogenic. The addition of a single lysine to α-DNP-hexa-L-lysine, itself not immunogenic for either antibody formation or DH, renders it immunogenic for both antibody formation and DH. Lysine homopolymers (without DNP) are immunogenic if they contain more than eight residues. Also, the α, DNP-Lys-9 conjugate loses its immunogenicity if a D-lysine is introduced into the middle of the L-lysine sequence (e.g., the $L_4DL_4$ sequence), while its location at one of the extremities does not suppress immunogenicity ($L_7DL$ or $LDL_7$). Collectively, these data suggest that oligolysine recognition is more important than hapten position or the type of bonding to oligolysine.

While conditions of immunogenicity, necessary to stimulate antibody formation or induce a DH reaction are identical, the products that combine with antibodies or reveal DH in vivo or in vitro are different, as shown in Table 6.6. Conjugates of DNP and three to six lysine homopolymers, when injected intradermally, produce an Arthus reaction without DH. However, the ability to inhibit the precipitating activity of anti-DNP-lysine antibodies increases with the size of the lysine polymer, reaching a maximum at seven lysines, and acting as though the α,DNP-Lys-7 were the largest determinant with which the antibody reacted. It is interesting to note that the Lys-8-10 homopolymer without DNP has a lesser capacity to inhibit the antibody than DNP-Lys-9, which suggests that DNP plays an immunodominant role. Conversely, and paradoxically, Lys-8-10 induces thymidine incorporation when it is mixed with guinea pig lymphocytes sensitized against DNP-Lys-8, while DNP-Lys-3-6 or DNP-Lys-9 (L4DL4) are without effect.

It has been reported that the conjugate of azobenzene arsonate and tyrosine (5ABA-tyrosine), with a molecular weight of 409, stimulates DH reactions in the guinea pig but does not bring about antibody production.

Azobenzene arsenate may induce a delayed hypersensitivity reaction when it is coupled to a high-molecular-weight protein and also when it is conjugated with a simple N-chloroacctylatcd tyrosine (ABA-T). ABA-T induces a pure delayed hypersensitivity response with the production of little or no antibody. This DH response is manifested in a proliferative response specific to the antigen, skin reactions, and leukocyte-migration inhibition. At the same time,

**Table 6.6 Immunogenicity of Dinitrophenyl-Oligolysines and of Oligolysines**

|  | Humoral and cellular responses |
|---|---|
| α, DNP-Lys 3 | No |
| α, DNP-Lys 4 | No |
| α, DNP-Lys 5 | No |
| α, DNP-Lys 6 | No |
| α, DNP-Lys 7 | Yes |
| α, DNP-Lys 8 | Yes |
| α, DNP-Lys 9 | Yes |
| α, DNP-Lys>9 | Yes |
| α, DNP-Lys 9 (L$_4$DL$_4$) | No |
| α, DNP-Lys 9 (L$_7$DL) | Yes |
| α, DNP-Lys 9 (LDL$_7$) | Yes |
| 5, ε, DNP-Lys 9 | Yes |
| 9, ε, DNP-Lys 9 | Yes |
| Lys 3–6 | No |
| Lys 8–10 | Yes |

After Schlossman.

animals sensitized with ABA-T possess specific memory for the carrier in the production of antibodies against ABA-T hapten conjugate. In addition, they possess amplifier and suppressor cells for the DH response directed against ABA-T. At first sight, it might be thought that ABA-T functions in a similar manner to DNCB by binding to skin proteins. In fact, ABA-T exhibits little or no binding to proteins. In addition, strong DH skin reactions may be elicited in animals sensitized against ABA-T by numerous conjugates of ABA and proteins without the reaction so induced having any specificity whatsoever for

**Table 6.7 Reactions Induced in Vivo and in Vitro by Various Polymers of Lysine and DNP in Guinea Pigs Immunized by DNP-Lys 9**

|  | In vivo reactions after intradermal injection | | In vitro reactions | |
|---|---|---|---|---|
|  | Arthus | Delayed hypersensitivity | Thymidine incorporation | Migration-inhibitory factor secretion |
| α, DNP-Lys 3 | Yes | No | No | No |
| α, DNP-Lys 4 | Yes | No | No | No |
| α, DNP-Lys 5 | Yes | No | No | No |
| α, DNP-Lys 6 | Yes | No | No | No |
| α, DNP-Lys 7 | Yes | Yes | Yes | Yes |
| α, DNP-Lys 8 | Yes | Yes | Yes | Yes |
| α, DNP-Lys 9 | Yes | Yes | Yes | Yes |
| α, DNP-L$_4$DL$_4$ | Yes | No | No | No |

After Schlossman.

the proteins used for the coupling, thus differing from what is observed in contact hypersensitivity.

In conclusion, similar or identical determinants are responsible for antibody production and the development of DH reaction, at least in the DNP-Lys system. Conversely, the same does not apply to stimulation; the binding between T cells and antigen seems to require recognition of a determinant equivalent to that recognized by B lymphocytes, but the determinant that reacts with the antibodies is of a smaller size than that of the immunogenic determinant. In addition, T cells are able to recognize precisely those various polypeptides that induce a DH with high discrimination potency, similar to that of B cells.

## THYMUS-DEPENDENT AND THYMUS-INDEPENDENT ANTIGENS

Thymus-dependent antigens are those in which antibody production requires T-cell participation. Examples are serum proteins and heterologous red blood cells. Thymus-independent antigens are those in which antibody production needs no T-cell participation and may thus occur in nude or neonatally thymectomized mice. These antigens include polysaccharides, such as endotoxin lipopolysaccharides, pneumococcal polysaccharides, and polyvinylpyrrolidone. Antibody production against thymus-independent antigens may, however, be sensitive to suppressor T-cell action (see p. 546). In addition, thymus-independent antigens are often B-cell mitogens and activators of the complement alternative pathway, which has led to various interesting hypotheses regarding B lymphocyte stimulation (see p. 544).

From a chemical point of view, thymus-independent antigens are characterized by the repetitive nature of their determinants (or epitopes) and by their slow degradation (we have discussed earlier the thymus-independent D-amino acid synthetic polypeptides). Flagellin has been the subject of interesting biochemical studies regarding antigen thymus dependence. Flagellin extracted from *Salmonella adelaide* is a proteic antigen that has two forms, a polymerized flagellin (molecular weight of several million daltons) and a monomeric form (40,000 daltons). The study of various chemical alterations of the flagellin molecule has demonstrated an inverse relationship between the ability to stimulate antibody production and production of DH. In addition, acetoacetylated forms are capable of inducing a tolerance to further injections of monomeric flagellin. The monomer is thymus dependent, whereas the polymer is thymus independent.

**Table 6.8   Thymus-Dependency of Antigens**

Thymus-dependent antigens
   Heterologous serum proteins, synthetic polypeptides of L-amino acids, heterologous erythrocytes, monomeric flagellin
Thymus-independent antigens
   S-III pneumococcal polysaccharide, lipopolysaccharides, polyvinylpyrrolidone, synthetic polymers of D-amino acids, polymerized flagellin, dextrans, levans

**Table 6.9 Thymus-Independent Antigens**

| Antigen | Abbreviation | Composition of monomer | Average molecular weight (polydisperse) | Average number of monomeric units | Loss of immunogenicity with polymer size (monomeric) units |
|---|---|---|---|---|---|
| Pneumococcal polysaccharide | S-III | Cellobiuronic acid (glucose-glucuronic acid) | 200,000 | 560 | 10 |
| Native levan | LE | Fructose | 20,000,000 | 111,000 | 55 |
| E. coli lipopolysaccharide | LPS | Oligosaccharide side-chain determinants on LPS core | 10,000,000 | Not known | Not known |
| Polyvinylpyrrolidone | PVP | $-CH_2-CH$ ... $H_2C-C=O$ / $N$ / $H_2C-CH_2$ | 360,000 | 3200 | 90 |
| Polymerized flagellin | POL | Protein | 10,000,000 | 300 | <1 |

After Basten and Howard.

## ANTIGENIC DETERMINANTS RECOGNIZED BY HELPER AND SUPPRESSOR T CELLS

Studies by Michison's group have shown that the presence of at least two distinct antigenic determinants are necessary for antibody production. Thus, in glucagon (a polypeptide consisting of 29 amino acids), it is possible to identify an amino-terminal fragment, which contains the main haptenic determinant recognized by antibodies, and a carboxy-terminal fragment, which includes the carrier determinant responsible for T-cell responses. Comparison of the humoral responses against artificial molecules whose haptenic site (e.g., DNP) and carrier site (e.g., L-tyrosin-azobenzene-$p$-arsenate) are separated by a variable number of intercalated molecules (such as 6-aminocaproic acid) has shown that a certain alignment of two sites is necessary to obtain an optimal antibody response against the hapten. It is also of interest that the two determinants may be represented by the same group so that they are both readily accessible, the same determinants serving for the stimulation of helper T cells and B cells. Finally, it should be remembered that ABA-tyrosine induces an exclusive T-cell type of immunity. Only bifunctional compounds may induce antibody production.

The situation is even more complicated if one considers the sites that may induce suppressor T cells. Effectively, it has been shown that nonimmunogenic compounds may induce production of suppressor T cells, which inhibit cellular or humoral responses against chemically related immunogens. Thus, the injection of polyvinylpyrrolidone (molecular weight 10,000), or of GT (a synthetic polypeptide), which are not immunogenic, suppresses, at least in certain mouse strains, the antibody response against related immunogenic products (PVP of molecular weight 36,000 or GT coupled to methyl BSA). Furthermore, Sercarz has shown that on the β-galactosidase and lysozyme molecules there exist determinants that induce suppressor T-cell production (not, apparently, helper T cells), such determinants being quite distinct from those determinants that induce helper T cells (not suppressor T cells). These observations suggest that helper T cells and suppressor T cells possess, at least in part, different repertoires. The recognition of a single determinant by suppressor T cells seems sufficient to elicit suppression of humoral responses, whereas the helper effect seems to require the intervention of several determinants of the molecule that are distinct from those recognized by the suppressor cells.

In conclusion, interesting and, doubtless, significant differences exist with regard to the recognition and activation of different subpopulations of lymphocytes and the repertoire of antigenic specificities recognized by B lymphocytes, helper T lymphocytes, and suppressor T lymphocytes. However, the molecular and cellular basis for these differences are, as yet, ill understood.

## BIBLIOGRAPHY

ADORINI L., HARVEY M. A., RUZYCKA-JACKSON D., MILLER A. and SERCARZ E. E. Differential major histocompatibility complex-related activation of idistypic suppressor T cells. Suppressor T cells crop-reactive to two distantly related lysozymes are not induced by one of them. J. Exp. Med. 1980. *152*, 521.

ARNON R. Conformation and physico-chemical factors influencing antigenicity. *In* L. Brent and J. Holborow, Eds., Progress in immunology. II. Vol. 2, Amsterdam, 1974, North Holland, p. 5.

BENJAMINI E., MICHAELI D., and YOUNG J. D. Antigenic determinants of proteins of defined sequences. Contemp. Top. Microbiol. Immunol., 1972, *58*, 85.

BOREK F. Immunogenicity. Physico-chemical and biological aspects. Amsterdam, 1972, Elsevier, North Holland.

BULLOCK W. W. ABA-T determinant regulation of delayed hypersensitivity. Immunol. Rev., 1978, *39*, 3.

BUTLER V. P. and BEISER S. M. Antibodies to small molecules: biological and clinical applications. Adv. Immunol., 1973, *132*, 77.

CISAR J., KABAT E. A., DORNER M. M., and LIAO J. Binding properties of immunoglobulins combining sites specific for terminal or non-terminal antigenic determinants in dextran. J. Exp. Med., 1975, *142*, 435.

FELDMANN M., HOWARD J. G., and DESAYMARD C. Role of antigen structure in the discrimination between tolerance and immunity by B cells. Transpl. Rev., 1975, *23*, 78.

GILL T. J. Polypeptides as models for the tertiary structure of proteins. *In* H. Peters, Ed., Protides of the biological fluids. New York, 1969, Pergamon Press, p. 21.

GOODMAN J. W. Immunochemical specificity. Recent advances. Immunochemistry, 1969, *6*, 139.

GOODMAN J. W. Antigenic determinants and antibody combining sites. *In* M. Sela, Ed., Antigens III, New York, 1974, Academic Press, p. 127.

GOODMAN J. W., BELLONE C. J. HANES D., and NITECKI D. E. Antigen structural requirements for lymphocyte triggering and cell cooperation. *In* L. Brent and J. Holborow, Eds., Progress in immunology. II. Vol. 2, Amsterdam, 1974, North Holland, p. 27.

GOODMAN J. W., FONG S., LEWIS G. K., KAMIN R., NITECKI D. E., and DER BALIAN G. Antigen structure and lymphocyte activation. Immunol. Rev., 1978, *39*, 36.

KABAT E. A. Structural concepts in immunology and immunochemistry. New York, 1968, Holt, Rinehart & Winston.

KABAT E. A. Heterogencity and structure of antibody-combining sites. Ann. N.Y. Acad. Sci., 1970, *169*, 43.

LANDSTEINER K. The specificity of serological reactions. Harvard University Press, 1945.

NISONOFF A., TUNG A., and CAPRA J. D. Factors determining immune responsiveness at the level of B-cells. *In* L. Brent and J. Holborow, Eds., Progress in immunology. II. Vol. 2, Amsterdam, 1974, North Holland, p. 17.

NOSSAL G. J. V. and ADA G. L. Antigens, lymphoid cells and the immune response. New York, 1971, Academic Press.

PARISH C. R. Functional aspects of antigen structure in terms of tolerance and immunity. *In* L. Brent and J. Holborow, Eds., Progress in immunology. II. Vol. 2, Amsterdam, 1974, North Holland, p. 39.

REICHLIN M. Aminoacid substitution and the antigenicity of glycoproteins. Adv. Immunol., 1975, *20*, 71.

RUDE E. Structure and immunogenicity of synthetic antigens. Angew Chem. Intern., 1970, *9*, 206.

SCHLOSSMAN S. F. Antigen recognition: the specificity of T-cells involved in the cellular immune response. Transpl. Rev., 1972, *10*, 97.

SELA M. Antigenicity: some molecular aspects. Science, 1969, *166*, 1365.

SELA M. (Ed.) The antigens. New York, 1974, Academic Press.

SELA M. and MOZES E. The role of antigenic structure in B-lymphocyte activation. Transpl. Rev., 1975, *23*, 189.

SERCARZ E. E., VOWELL R. L., TURKIN D., MILLER A., ARANEO B. A., and ADORINI L. Different functional specificity repertoires for suppressor and helper T cells. Immunol. Rev., 1978, *39*, 108.

THOMPSON K., HARRIS M., BENJAMINI E., MITCHELL G., and NOBLE M. Cellular and humoral immunity. A distinction in antigenic recognition. Natur. New Biol. 1972, *238*, 20.

WEIR D. M. Handbook of experimental immunology, ed. 2. Oxford, 1973, Blackwell Scient. Publ.

# Chapter 7

# IMMUNOGLOBULINS

## Claude de Préval

I. FUNCTIONAL DUALITY OF IMMUNOGLOBULINS

II. MODELS FOR IMMUNOGLOBULIN STUDIES

III. A STRUCTURAL MODEL FOR IMMUNOGLOBULINS: THE IgG

IV. ANTIBODY FUNCTION OF IgG

V. LEVELS OF IMMUNOGLOBULIN HETEROGENEITY

VI. IMMUNOGLOBULIN METABOLISM

VII. PHYLOGENY AND ONTOGENY OF IMMUNOGLOBULINS

VIII. ORGANISATION AND EXPRESSION OF IMMUNOGLOBULIN GENES

IX. GENETIC DETERMINISM OF IMMUNOGLOBULINS

Given the proper circumstances, the injection of an antigen into an animal produces a specific antiserum that reacts selectively with the antigen. This antiserum contains proteins that are responsible for this recognition, and that are said to possess an "antibody function." This functional criterion is used to designate these proteins as "antibodies" or, in a wider sense, as "immunoglobulins" (Ig).

Initially, it appears as if the injection of antigen Ag1 induced the synthesis of antibody Ab1, antigen Ag2 induced the synthesis of antibody Ab2, and antigen Agn produced the synthesis of antibody Abn. The purpose of this chapter is to analyze the difference between antibody Ab1 and Ab2, in other words, to study the structural basis of antibody functions. A definition of antibody molecule should include the four following elements: a given antibody molecule is synthesized by a given *clone* of lymphocytes, its synthesis is *specifically induced* or *paralyzed* by the corresponding antigen, depending on those conditions as referred to in chapter 20.

# I.  FUNCTIONAL DUALITY OF IMMUNOGLOBULINS

Antibody molecules have two independent functions.

### Recognition Function

The specificity of antigen recognition by antisera was described in the beginning of this century by Behring, Ehrlich, and Landsteiner. This specificity is very precise, since, for example, antibodies are able to discriminate on a given protein between the side chain of a leucine and the side chain of a valine (see p. 148). These two amino acids differ only in that one methylene group is added.

### Effector Functions

Analysis of the immune response shows that, independent of their capacity for specific recognition, immunoglobulins are capable of other functions, including complement fixation, binding to certain cells, and placental transfer. These phenomena are called effector functions.

Two antibody populations directed against bacteria may either agglutinate or lyse them. Only in the latter case are antibodies able to bind complement, directly responsible for cytolysis.

Immediate hypersensitivity reactions may be induced by various antigens, thus involving immunoglobulins of different specificities. However, all antibodies involved in this type of immune response share a common capacity to bind to mastocytes, basophils or blood platelets (see p. 353).

Some antibody populations cross the placental barrier, thereby conferring to the fetus (and to the newborn) a passive immunity, which protects the new organism prior to development of its own defense mechanisms.

Recent findings of biochemistry and molecular biology show that this functional duality reflects a structural duality (Fig. 7.1). However, this conclusion presents us with an apparent paradoxical situation: while the number of effector functions is small and therefore the number of effector sites limited, the number

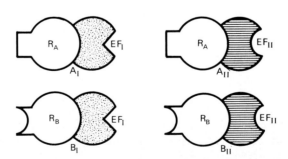

**Fig. 7.1**  Functional duality of immunoglobulins. Each immunoglobulin molecule has a pole that recognizes the antigen (R), and a pole that features various effector functions (EF). Two antibody molecules (AI and AII) may recognize the same antigen, but the nature of their effector functions may be different, and vice versa (AI and BI). (After M. Fougereau, Elements d'immunologie fondamentale, Paris, 1975, Masson, p. 9.)

of recognition sites (antibody sites) is infinitely higher ($10^8$). Ig structure must be sufficiently stable in order to explain the conservation of effector sites as well as the conservation of the physicochemical properties of these antibodies, while at the same time, they must allow various molecules to be sufficiently different in order for all antibody sites to be formed. Genetically speaking, it is even more difficult to understand how these contradictory requirements have allowed the emergence of such a specific protein family. Indeed, selection of the recognition function, that is, of structural Ig variability, appears to run counter to the selection of molecular stability required to assure the conservation of effector functions. It is interesting to note that until now only the immune system has raised such problems of structure and molecular evolution. Therefore, a fundamental purpose for a structural analysis of Ig lies in the study of their genetic determinism.

# II.  MODELS FOR IMMUNOGLOBULIN STUDIES

The main difficulty in studying Ig is their heterogeneity, the origin of which is twofold: the complexity of antigen structure and of the functions of the immune system.

The above diagram, in which injection of antigen Ag1 induces synthesis of antibody Ab1, is incorrect at the molecular level. Antigens contain in most cases, a great number of determinants (see p. 150). If antigen Ag1 has $n$ determinants, it will trigger the formation of $n$ antibodies capable of recognizing it. However, antibody heterogeneity does not reflect antigen heterogeneity only. In fact, several different Ig molecules may recognize the same antigenic determinant (see p. 289). Therefore, the antigen-antibody recognition system is said to be partially degenerate.

According to the clonal theory (described on p. 561) this heterogeneity, observed at the molecular level, reflects the heterogeneity of antibody-producing cells. Indeed, all cells from one clone are thought to synthesize the same Ig. One antigen stimulates several clones, some of which synthesize antibodies directed against the same antigenic determinant. If such a mechanism is applied to all antigens encountered by an organism, one has some idea as to the complexity of chemical structures in an Ig population.

### Immunoglobulin Isolation

ISOLATION OF Ig FRACTION OF SERUM

It has been known for 40 years that antibodies are serum proteins. When analyzing serum through moving boundary electrophoresis, Kabat and Tiselius observed four main families of serum proteins: albumin and $\alpha$, $\beta$ and $\gamma$ globulins (Fig. 7.2). Antibodies were mostly found in the $\gamma$-globulin fraction, to a lesser extent in $\beta$ globulins. Ig are still being isolated on the basis of their net charge, either through zone electrophoresis using an inert solid support (starch or Pevikon) or through ion exchange chromatography using an anionic resin such as DEAE-cellulose. This technique makes use of the fact that at neutral pH and at low ionic strength, only the $\gamma$-globulin fraction (or at least most of it) is not

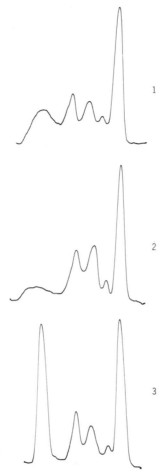

**Fig. 7.2**  Paper electrophoresis of one normal serum and two myeloma sera. When comparing the serum profiles of patients 2 and 3, note the different position of monoclonal Ig peaks as well as their narrowness and their symmetry, both signs of their homogeneity. (1 : normal serum, 2 : β-myeloma, 3 : γ-myeloma).

retained by the resin. Other proteins can also be eluted if the ionic strength of the elution buffer is gradually increased. This technique becomes more practical when chromatographing an Ig-enriched fraction through differential precipitation of serum proteins by means of neutral salt (ammonium sulfate or sodium sulfate).

These protein preparations can be purified even further on the basis of molecular weight by means of molecular sieving, using different kinds of gels.

These methods make it possible to separate antibodies of 150,000 molecular weight, from heavier antibodies, that is, macroglobulins, and possibly, from non-Ig proteins (transferrins in particular), which could otherwise contaminate the preparations.

A combination of salt precipitation, DEAE-cellulose chromatography (or zone electrophoresis), and possibly gel filtration enables the isolation of Ig preparations that are pure enough to allow a study of their physicochemical properties.

ISOLATION OF SPECIFIC ANTIBODIES

Preparations of specific antibodies are required in order to study the thermodynamic parameters of antigen-antibody reactions. The purification principle is based on the fact that antigen-antibody combinations are reversible because noncovalent bonds are involved:

$$Ag + Ab \xrightleftharpoons{K_A} Ag - Ab \qquad 10^5 \leq K_A \leq 10^{12} \text{ mole}^{-1} \text{ (see p. 286)}$$

Antibodies in the antiserum are precipitated by the antigen. This precipitate, isolated through centrifugation, can be dissociated by nonspecific means, that is, using low or high pH, using a buffer of high ionic strength, or using concentrated urea. Antigen and antibody are then separated through gel filtration, electrophoresis, or other method. The antigen-antibody precipitate can also be dissociated in a specific way when an anti-hapten antibody is involved. For example, a precipitate of anti-DNP—DNP-HSA* can be dissociated by an excess of free hapten, such as DNP-lysine or DNP-glycine. The antibody-hapten complex is then dissociated as described above.

This method of specific isolation of antibodies may be applied to all types of antigens by using two-phase physical systems. Antibodies are kept in solution while antigens are made insoluble (immunoadsorbents) through polymerization with bifunctional chemicals (carbodiimide, ethyl-chloroformate, or glutaraldehyde). Antiserum antibodies are then adsorbed to polymerized antigens and may subsequently be eluted by applying a buffer of low pH or high ionic strength. Another variant of the same technique consists of fixing covalently the antigens to a solid support, such as agarose beads (Sepharose), with cyanogen bromide, or to acrylamide beads (Biogel) with glutaraldehyde. Adsorption and elution operations are identical with those used for insolubilized antigens.

ANTIBODIES WITH LIMITED HETEROGENEITY

As suggested earlier, antibody preparations homogeneous at the molecular level have not yet been obtained. Numerous attempts have been made to obtain antibodies of limited heterogeneity.

The simplest approach is to limit as much as possible the number of antigenic determinants borne by the antigen. By fixing angiotensin molecules (octapeptides), to a poly-lysine chain, Haber obtained antibodies which were homogeneous with respect to their association constant.

Another method described by Krause consists of injecting rabbits repeatedly with pneumococcal or streptococcal walls or with polysaccharides extracted from these walls and containing the essential antigenic fraction. Some animals respond with a high titer of restricted heterogeneity antibodies. Homogeneity

* DNP = Dinitrophenol; DNP-HSA = Dinitrophenyl Human Serum Albumin

of these antibodies can be increased even further by subjecting these sera to affinity chromatography using an immunoadsorbent made from the immuno-dominant sugar of the polysaccharide. Such antibody preparations of limited heterogeneity are very useful for the study of the detailed structure of antibody molecules.

### LYMPHOCYTE CLONING

In vitro cloning of normal B lymphocytes has not yet been accomplished despite progress in cell fractionation and cell culture techniques. However, clones have been isolated in vivo in mice. Williamson and Askonas irradiated mice in order to inactivate their lymphocytes, then restored these animals with a small number of educated lymphocytes taken from mice that had been primed by dinitrophenylated bovine $\gamma$ globulins. One booster injection of these recon-stituted mice triggered production of anti-DNP antibodies of limited hetero-geneity, thus demonstrating the presence of a major lymphocyte clone derived from the transplanted cells. Through a series of lymphocyte transfers to irradiated animals of the same strain, this clone was maintained for more than one year, producing identical antibodies throughout this period of time.

### MALIGNANT CLONAL TRANSFORMATION: MYELOMA AND BENCE-JONES PROTEINS

In vivo clones can be observed during malignant transformation of anti-body-forming cells. The cancer cell then produces a clone that rapidly prolif-erates in the organism to the point of becoming predominant. This clone synthesizes immunoglobulins that become predominant in the bloodstream, their concentrations sometimes reaching 10 g/liter. These proteins are perfectly homogeneous from a chemical point of view because they all originate in cells which express the same genetic information.

*Human Myeloma.* Multiple myeloma or plasmacytoma is a cancer of white bone marrow cells, involving B-cell-derived plasma cells (see chap. 4). When the serum of a myeloma patient is subjected to zone electrophoresis (Fig. 7.2), a large, narrow peak of Ig as well as a significant decrease of other protein levels, can be observed. The sharpness of this peak underscores the homogeneity of the predominant serum Ig. When comparing a large number of sera from similarly affected subjects, positions of the peaks are found to vary from one patient to another, and can occur in all areas where normal Ig migrate. In some cases the patient's urine contains proteins that are antigenically related to the myeloma Ig. This biological subunit of the myeloma Ig is the "Bence-Jones" protein (see chap. 30).

*Inducible Myeloma in Mice and Rats.* Potter and Fahey have been able to induce plasmacytoma in mice (1960) by injecting mineral oil into the peritoneal cavity, thus producing either ascitic or solid tumors. They are transplantable within the strain in which they have been induced and provide an almost inexhaustible source of monoclonal Ig. More recently, transplantable plasma-cytomas have also been described in rats (Bazin).

*Myeloma in Other Species.* Myeloma is a disease that appears to affect numerous higher animal species. Several cases of feline and canine myeloma have been studied.

Myeloma proteins synthesized under pathologic conditions do not at all differ from normal Ig. It has therefore been possible to extrapolate with quasi-certainty all information gained from myeloma protein analysis to normal Ig. This is why the term monoclonal Ig is now preferred over the old term paraprotein. Myeloma proteins are choice materials for the study of the chemical structure of Ig. However, there is a significant limitation in that antibody activity of these Ig remains unknown in most cases, even though it has been possible to describe myeloma proteins with antibody function, such as antinucleotide, anti-DNP, antiphosphorylcholine, anti-Ig, or anti-dextran (see chap. 30).

### Establishment of Permanent Lines or Transformed Lymphocytes: Hybridomas

Since 1976 a new approach has been developed for the production of lymphocyte clones with a given physiologic function. The principle of this approach relies on two facts:

1. Malignant cells possess the property of intense proliferation and are thus relatively easy to maintain in culture.

2. Malignant transformation is an individually acquired characteristic of certain cells in a given population and is transmissible by means of mitotic division.

For example, to obtain a clone of lymphocytes that secrete antibodies of a given specificity, one must attempt to transform some cells in a heterogeneous lymphocyte population (such as immune spleen cells from a mouse); then, the malignant cells are selected on the basis of their capacity to multiply in culture in certain media. Among these cells there are cells that can be further subselected, cells that have retained their capacity to secrete the desired antibody (which can be found in the culture supernatant).

The transformation of the effector lymphocytes may be accomplished in two ways:

1. The lymphocytes may be transformed by a virus. In man, the Epstein-Barr virus exclusively transforms B lymphocytes. In G. Klein's laboratory it has been found that, using peripheral blood lymphocytes from immune human donors, it is possible to clone, in vitro, transformed lymphocytes that secrete antihapten antibodies.

2. Normal cells may be "hybridized" with a cell belonging to an already-transformed cell line. The normal cell carries the information necessary for the expression of its effector function, such as the synthesis of a given antibody. The other cell contains the information required for the expression of the malignant characteristics. In such experiments, the two cell populations are mixed in the presence of an agent, such as Sendaï virus or polyethylene glycol which facilitates the fusion of the two types of cell membranes. The cell mixture is then transferred to a culture medium that selectively enables the survival of the hybrid cells to the exclusion of the nonfused parental cells. Normal cells die quite quickly in culture and, in general, tumor cells are chosen that have an enzyme deficiency, which necessitates special culture conditions. The transformed cell lines used in these experiments are usually obtained from lympho-

cytic tumors, such as myelomas or lymphomas. Kohler and Milstein were the first to employ successfully these cellular fusion techniques in the myeloma × antibody-secreting B plasmocyte system. Subsequently, several workers have also successfully fused lymphomas with helper or suppressor T cells. The term, hybridoma, has been chosen to designate the permanent cell lines thus obtained. It should be noted that following the first division of hybrid cells, certain chromosomes originating from one of the parental cells may be expelled. Such cells, which possess incomplete sets of chromosomes, are extremely useful to geneticists for gene localization or for the study of the regulation of the biosynthesis of antibodies or of certain differentiation antigens.

### Classification Criteria: Notion of Isotype

Initially, Ig were classified according to their physicochemical properties (molecular weight, sedimentation coefficient, electrophoretic mobility), and their antigenic characteristics (immunoglobulins synthesized by one organism and injected into a different organism are recognized as being foreign). Later, the chemical basis of these criteria was studied through the analysis of primary and tertiary structures of certain Ig.

On the basis of these general criteria, all individuals within a given species have in common various Ig categories, called *isotypes*. In man, for example, it has been possible to identify 10 isotypes in 5 *classes*, that is, IgG, IgM, IgA, IgD, and IgE. They are identified on the basis of their molecular weight, among other criteria. (This 1972 WHO International nomenclature replaces the former designations γG, γM, γA, γD and γE.)

## III.  A STRUCTURAL MODEL FOR IMMUNOGLOBULINS: THE IgG

IgG are the predominant serum Ig. With a molecular weight of 150,000 daltons and sedimentation coefficient of 6.7S, they are also the smallest.

### Multichain Structure

As early as 1950–1955, Putnam and Porter were able to analyze the number of amino-terminal residues of IgG. However, because of the heterogeneity of Ig, these studies did not allow an accurate evaluation of the number of chains that form these molecules.

Between 1959 and 1964 numerous authors contributed to the discovery of IgG structure, among them R. R. Porter and G. M. Edelman, who received the 1972 Nobel Prize for Medicine. Their individual approach was different. Porter attempted to isolate IgG fragments containing a biologic function through enzymatic cleavage, while Edelman searched for the existence of biosynthetic subunits by attempting to dissociate IgG molecule components through breakage of disulfide bridges and of noncovalent bonds.

In 1959, Porter was able to cleave rabbit IgG through papain hydrolysis and to separate three fragments I, II, and III through ion exchange chromatography using a cationic resin column (carboxymethyl-cellulose). Fragments I and II have the same antigenicity but do not cross-react with fragment III. Fragments I and II possess each an antibody combining site. They are now called "Fab fragments" (antigen-binding fragments). Fragments I and II do not represent two distinct fragments of the same Ig molecule; instead, they derive from two different kinds of IgG with slightly different net charge. Fragment III does not bind the antigen but has effector functions (complement fixation, cell binding, etc.). In addition, it can crystallize, hence its name, "Fc fragment." A similar cleavage performed on human IgG enabled Edelman to separate through electrophoresis two fractions without common antigenic determinants. These were equivalent to the two types of fragments from rabbit IgG. These studies have shown that a single IgG molecule has two identical antibody-binding sites.

In 1959, Edelman showed that upon reduction of the disulfide bridges, the molecular weight of IgG measured in 8M urea decreased by one third. He then separated two subunits in a dissociating buffer through chromatography using carboxymethyl cellulose, thus identifying "light chains" (L chains, molecular weight 23,000) and "heavy chains" (H chains, molecular weight 50,000). A mild reduction in a nondissociating buffer opens the disulfide bonds between H and L chains. However, these chains can only be separated in the presence of urea or at low pH, thus indicating that the chains are also held together by strong noncovalent bonds. Fleischmann et al. adapted molecular sieving on Sephadex to the study of H and L chains and were able to quantify the relative proportion (by weight) of the two chains: 66% heavy chains against 33% light chains. IgG heavy chains (γ chains) are all antigenically related, but IgG light chains are of two antigenic types, κ or λ.

When taken together, these various data led to the formulation of a topological model:

—molecules have two identical antibody sites associated with even numbers of polypeptide chains; as a result, they must be symmetrical;

—each molecule of 150,000 molecular weight includes two γ heavy chains (molecular weight 50,000) and two light chains (molecular weight 23,000) of the same type, either κ or λ;

—papain cleavage leads to the release of two Fab fragments (molecular weight 50,000) and one Fc fragment (molecular weight 50,000);

—all light chain antigenic determinants are borne by the Fab fragment;

—some heavy chain antigenic determinants are found on the Fc fragment;

—the Fab fragment contains all L chains, which implies that, because of their higher molecular weight, H chains are shared by Fab and Fc fragments;

—light chains are linked to heavy chains by means of one disulfide bridge, while heavy chains are linked together by a variable number of disulfide bridges.

These data led to the proposal by Porter and Edelman of an IgG model (Fig. 7.3 shows the topological model by Porter). The amino-terminal portion of those heavy chains included in the Fab fragment is called "Fd" fragment.

### Structural Duality of IgG

The analysis of Ig primary structure produced its first results in 1965; by establishing chemical proof of the structural duality of Ig, these studies soon

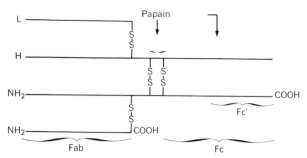

**Fig. 7.3** Topological model of Porter (1962). Papain cleaves the immunoglobulin in three main fragments: two identical Fab fragments and one Fc fragment (the Fc' fragment may be obtained in lower concentration).

allowed a more complete understanding of the many results that had been obtained through different techniques. At the same time, these studies provided a unique research model, not only to immunologists but also to geneticists and molecular biologists.

METHODOLOGY

Complete sequence studies can only be done with homogeneous Ig preparations. We have seen earlier that this requirement is met when using monoclonal Ig synthesized by myeloma or hybridoma or when using antibodies of limited heterogeneity under certain precautionary conditions. However, some authors have studied the sequence of heterogeneous Ig preparations. Analysis then becomes significantly more difficult, and even though predominant amino acids may be accurately located in each position, an interpretation of the results becomes much more delicate.

Another difficulty encountered when doing sequence studies is due to the large size of Ig, even though the isolation of H and L chains and of Fab and Fc fragments simplifies the analysis.

As a rule, sequence studies begin with the cleavage of molecules into large fragments, using cyanogen bromide, which hydrolyzes polypeptide chains on the carboxylic side of the methionyl residues, of which there are only few in the protein (Fig. 7.4). These fragments are then in turn cleaved by proteolytic enzymes (trypsin, chymotrypsin, pepsin, subtilisin, thermolysin, etc.) The order of the peptides after two or several different hydrolyses is derived from patterns of mutual overlapping. Peptide isolation and purification require molecular sieving and/or ionic exchange chromatography followed by electrophoresis and/ or chromatography on paper or thin layer gels. Recent progress in high pressure liquid chromatography (HPLC) makes this task much easier. Peptides are then degraded sequentially according to the Edman method: The peptide is dissolved in an aqueous solution. Phenylisothiocyanate (PITC) is added, thereby binding to the free amino function of the peptide terminal residue. This modified amino acid is then detached from the rest of the peptide through acid hydrolysis, which releases a new peptide containing one amino acid less.

The operation can be repeated as needed in order to obtain a complete degradation of the initial peptide. The modified amino acid released at each step is extracted in an organic solvent and identified through techniques of thin-layer chromatography, gas chromatography, HPLC, or ion exchange chromatography.

Edman and Begg have introduced the automation of the degradation method. Automatic sequences degrade between 35 and 50 amino acids (manual techniques can recurrently degrade no more than 10 to 20 amino acids using about 1 to 5 nanomole of peptide per step). The introduction of automation has brought about a change in techniques used by biochemists. Rather than isolating numerous small peptides, they now attempt to gather large fragments through specific cleavages, often after chemical modification of amino acid side chains in order to avoid or favor specific hydrolysis.

Close to 100 grams of protein were required in order to determine the first complete sequences of immunoglobulins with manual techniques. The complete sequence of murine monoclonal IgG MOPC 173 by Fougereau's group required the sera of about 25,000 plasmacytoma-bearing mice.

A new microtechnology is making rapid progress in several laboratories. Its goal is to sequence protein under the picomole level ($10^{-9}$ mg). Techniques vary but continue to be based upon the principle of Edman degradation.

Sequence analysis can be performed in two ways:

In order to study a functional resemblance or difference, a position-by-position comparison of amino acids is made; indeed, in the event of permutation, the function of the side chain may be maintained (e.g., Asp/Glu, Tyr/Phe, Leu/Val, Thr/Ser substitutions). The positions of some amino acids, which play a crucial role in the spatial structure (Gly, Pro, Trp, or Cys), can also be compared.

In order to trace a common genetic origin, it is more appropriate to compare at each position those codons that correspond to amino acids (the last

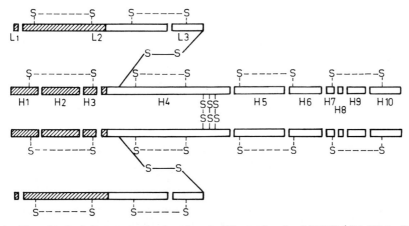

**Fig. 7.4** Topological diagram of a murine IgG2a molecule, MOPC 173. This diagram shows the position of those fragments obtained after cleavage of the molecule using cyanogen bromide, as well as the arrangement of interchain and intrachain disulfide bridges. (After A. Bourgois and M. Fougereau, Eur. J. Biochem., 1970, *12*, 558; C. de Préval and M. Fougereau, Eur. J. Biochem. 1972, *24*, 446.)

possible codon base is always chosen in order to maximize homology). Fitch has proposed that the homology of two sequences be expressed by the average minimum number of mutations required per codon to pass from one sequence to another. He has calculated that homology is significant if less than an average of 1.3 mutations per codon are required to pass from one sequence to another. An example of this type of comparison is given in Table 7.1.

VARIABLE AND CONSTANT REGIONS

In 1962, Gally and Edelman showed that Bence-Jones proteins were Ig light chains of the κ or λ type. The first κ chain sequence was identified by Putnam in 1965. The same year, Hilschmann reported the analysis results for two human κ chains. These showed that both chains had the same length (212 residues), that the carboxy-terminal halves of both chains (residues 108 to 212) were identical, with one exception to be discussed later (permuation Val/Leu at position 191), and that the amino-terminal halves (residues 1 to 107) differed significantly in many positions.

Similar observations made with regard to λ light chains have shown that they are of equivalent length and have a variable half on the aminoterminal side (about 100 residues), as well as a constant half. Gamma chains have approximately 440 amino acids. This number includes a variable region of 110 amino acids at the amino terminal; the rest of the sequence is constant. These segments of 110 residues at the amino-terminal part of the chains are called variable or "V" regions. If needed, the origin of the V region is indicated by a second letter (e.g., $V_L$, $V_H$ or $V_κ$, $V_λ$, $V_γ$, . . . ). The same holds true for the constant part of the chains, called "C" regions ($C_L$, $C_H$, or $C_κ$, $C_λ$, $C_γ$, . . . ).

The sequence of a $V_κ$ region is clearly different from that of a $V_λ$ or $V_H$ region. This shows that variability is not distributed randomly among these 110 amino acids. There are, in fact, hypervariable zones, where differences are concentrated, adjoining more constant zones where three types of regions can be recognized: $V_κ$, $V_λ$, or $V_H$. The detailed structure of these regions will be discussed later. The concept of V and C regions had led to the unique notion in molecular biology that a polypeptide chain can be synthesized by two different genes.

This structural duality brings satisfactory chemical evidence to support the functional duality of Ig: variable regions could very well support recognition functions, while constant regions could be responsible for effector functions.

## Conformation and Spatial Structure of IgG

CONCEPT OF DOMAIN

Sequence studies show that κ or λ L chains contain two intrachain disulfide bonds, one in each amino or carboxy-terminal half of the polypeptide. These bridges form two roughly symmetrical loops of about 60 residues each. The γ H chain has four intrachain disulfide bridges distributed regularly over four adjacent segments (two in the Fd fragment, two in the Fc fragment). Each segment forms a loop of about 60 residues as in the case of light chains (Fig. 7.4).

# Table 7.1 Sample of Sequence Comparison Using the Fitch Method and Involving 10 Residues of Two Heavy Chains

| | 79 | | | | | | | | | 88 |
|---|---|---|---|---|---|---|---|---|---|---|
| MOPC 173 (mouse) | Leu | Tyr | Leu | Gln | Met | Ser | Lys | Val | Arg | Ser |
| VIN (human) | Leu | Tyr | Leu | Asn | Met | Asn | Ser | Leu | Arg | Pro |
| Codons MOPC 173 | CUX | UAX | CUX | CAX | AUG | AGX | AAX | GUX | CGX | UCX |
| Codons VIN | CUX | UAX | CUX | AAX' | AUG | AAX | UCX | CUX | CGX | CCX |
| Minimum mutations required | 0 | 0 | 0 | 2 | 0 | 1 | 2 | 1 | 0 | 1 |

Total number of compared codons: 10

Minimum total number of mutations required to transfer from one sequence to another: 7

Minimum average number of mutations required to transfer from one sequence to another: MR = 0.7

Hill et al. have identified internal homologies in the primary structure of the Fc fragment of rabbit γ chains, between the two amino and carboxy-terminal halves. In addition, homologies are also found when comparing these regions with both halves of the light chains. Hill interpreted these results as being an indication of a single ancestral gene coding for about 110 amino acids, which would have evolved through a series of duplications.

This hypothesis was confirmed when Edelman's group determined the complete sequence of a human IgG molecule. A comparison of the different segments of 110 residues identified two types of internal homologies: those with respect to $V_H$ and $V_L$ variable regions, and those with respect to constant regions, including the $C_L$ region, the constant half of the Fd fragment, and both halves of the Fc fragment (Fig. 7.5). An analysis of the complete sequence of a murine IgG has enabled this concept to apply to immunoglobulins of other species (Fig. 7.6). It is important to note that a stronger homology can be observed between regions with equivalent functions, $V_H$ and $V_L$ (antibody function) and $C_H$ and $C_L$ (effector functions) than within one single polypeptide chain ($V_L$ and $C_L$ or $V_H$ and $C_H$). This demonstrates that the divergence of V from C genes occurred prior to the divergence of $C_L/C_H$ genes or $V_L/V_H$ genes. Evolution would seem to have selected, independently from each other, those structures that are responsible for both antibody and effector functions, although they are both present on the same molecule.

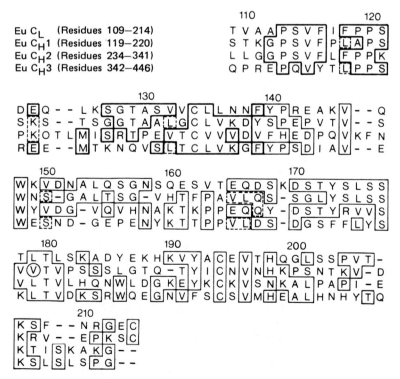

**Fig. 7.5** Internal homologies of a human IgG1 immunoglobulin (Eu) (see code: Fig. 7.20). (After G. M. Edelman et al., Proc. Nat. Acad. Sci., U.S.A., 1969, *63*, 78.)

**Heavy chain**

10  20
Glu-Val-Lys-Leu-Leu-Glu-Ser-Gly-Gly-Pro-Leu-Val-Gln-Leu-Gly-Gly-Ser-Leu-Lys-Leu-
30  40
Ser-Cys-Ala-Ala-Ser-Gly-Phe-Asp-Phe-Ser-Arg-Tyr-Trp-Met-Ser-Trp-Val-Arg-Gln-Ala-
50  60
Pro-Gly-Lys-Gly-Leu-Glu-Trp-Ile-Gly-Glu-Ile-Asp-Pro-Asn-Ser-Ser-Thr-Ile-Asn-Tyr-
70  80
Thr-Pro-Ser-Leu-Lys-Asp-Lys-Phe-Ile-Ile-Ser-Arg-Asn-Asp-Ala-Lys-Asn-Thr-Leu-Tyr-
90  100
Leu-Gln-Met-Ser-Lys-Val-Arg-Ser-Glu-Asp-Thr-Ala-Leu-Tyr-Tyr-Cys-Ala-Arg-Ser-Pro-
110  120
Tyr-Tyr-Ala-Met-Asp-Tyr-Trp-Gly-Gln-Gly-Thr-Ser-Val-Thr-Val-Ser-Ser-Ala-Lys-Thr-
130  140
Thr-Ala-Pro-Ser-Val-Tyr-Pro-Leu-Ala-Pro-Val-Cys-Gly-Asp-Thr-Thr-Gly-Ser-Ser-Val-
150  160
Thr-Leu-Gly-Cys-Leu-Val-Lys-Gly-Tyr-Phe-Pro-Glu-Pro-Val-Thr-Leu-Thr-Trp-Asn-Ser-
170  180
Gly-Ser-Leu-Ser-Ser-Gly-Val-His-Thr-Phe-Pro-Ala-Val-Leu-Gln-Ser-Asp-Leu-Tyr-
190  200
Ser-Ser-Val-Thr-Val-Thr-Val-Thr-Ser-Ser-Ser-Thr-Trp-Pro-Ser-Gln-Ser-Ile-Thr-Asn-
210  220
Cys-Asn-Val-Ala-His-Pro-Ala-Ser-Ser-Thr-Lys-Val-Asp-Lys-Lys-Ile-Glu-Pro-Arg-Gly-
230  240
Pro-Thr-Ile-Lys-Pro-Cys-Cys-Pro-Pro-Lys-Cys-Pro-Ala-Pro-Asn-Leu-Leu-Gly-Gly-Pro-
250  260
Ser-Val-Phe-Ile-Phe-Pro-Val-Lys-Ile-Lys-Asn-Pro-Leu-Met-Ile-Ser-Leu-Ser-Pro-Ile-
270  280
Val-Thr-Cys-Val-Val-Val-Asp-Val-Ser-Glu-Asp-Asp-Pro-Asp-Val-Gln-Ile-Ser-Trp-Phe-
290  300
Val-Asp-Asn-Val-Glu-Val-His-Gln-Ala-Gln-Thr-Thr-His-Thr-Arg-Gln-Asn-Tyr-Asx-Ser-
310  320
Thr-Leu-Arg-Val-Val-Ser-Ala-Leu-Pro-Ile-Gln-His-Gln-Asn-Trp-Met-Ser-Gly-Lys-Glu-
330  340
Phe-Lys-Cys-Lys-Val-Asn-Asn-Lys-Asp-Leu-Pro-Ala-Pro-Ile-Glu-Arg-Thr-Ile-Ser-Lys-
350  360
Pro-Lys-Gly-Ser-Val-Arg-Ala-Pro-Gln-Val-Tyr-Val-Leu-Pro-Pro-Pro-Glx-Glx-Met-Thr-
370  380
Lys-Lys-Glu-Val-Thr-Leu-Thr-Cys-Met-Val-Thr-Asn-Phe-Met-Pro-Glu-Asp-Ile-Tyr-Val-
390  400
Glu-Trp-Thr-Asn-Asn-Gly-Lys-Thr-Glu-Leu-Asn-Tyr-Lys-Asn-Thr-Gln-Pro-Val-Leu-Asp-
410  420
Ser-Asp-Gly-Ser-Tyr-Phe-Met-Tyr-Ser-Lys-Leu-Arg-Val-Glu-Lys-Lys-Asn-Trp-Val-Glu-
430  440
Arg-Asn-Ser-Tyr-Ser-Cys-Ser-Val-Val-His-Gln-Gly-Leu-His-Asn-His-(Val,Ser)Thr-Lys-
447
Ser-Phe-Ser-Arg-Thr-Pro-Gly

**Light chain**

10  20
Asp-Ile-Gln-Met-Thr-Gln-Thr-Thr-Ser-Ser-Leu-Ser-Ala-Ser-Leu-Gly-Asp-Arg-Val-Thr-
30  40
Ile-Ser-Cys-Ser-Ala-Ser-Gln-Ser-Ile-Gly-Asn-Tyr(Leu,Asx,Trp)Tyr-Gln-Gln-Lys-Pro-
50  60
Asp-Gly-Thr-Val-Lys-Leu-Leu-Ile-Tyr-Tyr-Thr-Ser-Ser-Leu-His-Ser-Gly-Val-Pro-Ser-
70  80
Arg-Phe-Ser-Gly-Ser-Gly-Ser-Gly-Thr-Asp-Tyr-Ser-Leu-Thr-Ile-Ser-Asx-Leu-Glx-Pro-
90  100
Glx-Asx-Ile-Ala-Thr-Tyr-Tyr-Cys-Gln-Gln-Tyr-Ser-Lys-Leu-Pro-Arg-Thr-Phe-Gly-Gly-
110  120
Gly-Thr-Lys-Leu-Glu-Ile-Lys-Arg-Ala-Asx-Ala-Ala-Pro-Thr-Val-Ser-Ile-Phe-Pro-Pro-
130  140
Ser-Ser-Glx-Glx-Leu-Thr-Ser-Gly-Gly-Ala-Ser-Val-Val-Cys-Phe-Leu-Asn-Asn-Phe-Tyr-
150  160
Pro-Lys-Asp-Ile-Asn-Val-Lys-Trp-Lys-Ile-Asp-Gly-Ser-Glu-Arg-Gln-Asx-Gly-Val-Leu-
170  180
Asx-Ser-Asx-Thr-Glx-Trp-Asp-Ser-Lys-Asp Ser-Thr-Tyr-Ser-Met-Ser-Ser-Thr-Leu-Thr-
190  200
Leu-Thr-Lys-Asp-Glu-Tyr-Glu-Arg-His-Asn-Ser-Tyr-Thr-Cys-Glu-Ala-Thr-His-Lys-Thr-
210  214
Ser-Thr-Ser-Pro-Ile-Val-Lys-Ser-Phe-Asn-Arg-Asn-Glu-Cys

**Fig. 7.6** Complete sequence of a murine IgG2a immunoglobulin (MOPC 173). (After M. Fougereau et al., 1975.)

**Table 7.2    Proteolytic Fragments of IgG**

| Fragment | Domains | Enzyme |
|----------|---------|--------|
| Fab | $V_L$, $C_L$, $V_H$, $C_H1$ | Papain, trypsin |
| Fc | $(C_H2, C_H3)_2$ | Papain, trypsin |
| Fd | $V_H$, $C_H1$ | Papain |
| Fab' | $V_L$, $C_L$, $V_H$, $C_H1$ | Pepsin |
| Fab" | $V_L$, $C_L$, $V_H$, $C_H1$ | Cyanogen bromide |
| Fc' | $C_H3$ | Papain, pepsin |
|  |  | Subtilisin |
| Facb | $(V_L, C_L, V_H, C_H1, C_H2)_2$ | Plasmin |
| Fb(s) | $C_H1$, $C_L$ | Subtilisin |
| Fv | $V_H$, $V_L$ | Pepsin |
|  | $V_L$, $C_L$ | Pepsin, trypsin, papain |
|  | $V_H$ | Papain |
|  | $C_H2$ | (CNBr) |
|  |  | Trypsin |

See Fig. 7.7 for the molecular diagram of these fragments.
After W. E. Gall and R. d'Eustachio, Biochem., 1972, **11**, 4621.

These observations led Edelman to further develop Hill's hypothesis (1970): each homology region (the 110 residues segment)—$V_L$, $C_L$, $V_H$, $C_H1$, $C_H2$, $C_H3$,—would fold in similar fashion to form a compact "domain," stabilized by a disulfide bond, and linked to neighboring domain(s) by less tightly folded stretches of the polypeptide chains. The thermodynamic independence of the domains (the fact that each one can fold independently of its neighbors) would allow their independent evolution, and each domain would contribute to at least one biologic function. This would explain how selection can cause one single immunoglobulin molecule to have several different functions.

The domain hypothesis has been confirmed by chemical analyses: one can cleave the IgG molecule between each homology region, as shown in Table 7.2 and Fig. 7.7, then recover certain IgG biological functions on isolated fragments.

During their studies, Givol and colleagues demonstrated that the antibody combining site is formed by the combination of $V_H$ and $V_L$ domains: one fragment containing these two variable regions (the Fv fragment; Fig. 7.7) has been isolated after cleavage of the monoclonal IgA MOPC 315* and shows the same anti-DNP activity as the native molecule. The $C_H2$ domain contains the complement fixation site, while the $C_H3$ domain is responsible for fixation of cytophilic IgG to mastocytes and macrophages. However, the structure of the corresponding effector sites in each domain is not yet known.

The accuracy of the domain hypothesis has also been demonstrated by the analysis of x-ray diffraction of Fab fragment, Fab' fragment and Bence-Jones protein dimer crystals. In 1972, Poljak's group showed on the basis of a diffraction pattern to a 0.6 nm resolution, that the Fab fragment contained four globular regions, each located within a $4 \times 2.5 \times 2.5$ nm parallelepiped.

* Human myeloma proteins are identified by letters taken from the patient's name; murine proteins are identified by a conventional code.

Domains in the homologous position on a pair of H and L chains, $C_H1 - C_L$ and $V_H - V_L$, interact more strongly than adjacent domains on each chain (Fig. 7.8). Finally, studies of L-chain denaturation at equilibrium and analysis of its kinetics, show that each $C_L$ and $V_L$ domain can unfold and refold independently of one another.

INTERNAL STRUCTURE OF DOMAINS

Studies using optical rotatory diffusion (ORD) or circular dichroism (CD) and x-ray diffraction point out that IgG, their chains and fragments contain

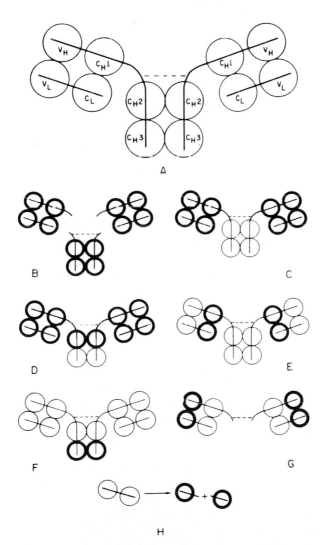

**Fig. 7.7** Diagram of the various proteolytic fragments isolated from IgG. A: Model of the intact molecule and its various domains. Isolated proteolytic fragments are shown in heavy lines; B: top, Fab fragments, bottom, Fc fragment; C: Fab'; D: Fabc; E: Fb(s); F-Fc'; G: Fv; H: $V_L$ and $C_L$ separated from light chains. (After W. E. Gall and R. d'Eustachio, Biochem., 1972, *11*, 4621.)

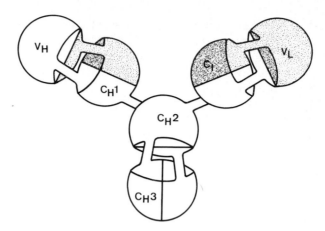

**Fig. 7.8** Diagram of an IgG molecule. The drawing of this model has been based upon analysis results of X-ray diffraction by Fab' fragment crystals of a human IgG, to a resolution of 0.6 nm. (After R. J. Poljak, Nature, Lond., 1972, *235*, 137.)

few if any α helices within the domains (similar studies of other classes of Ig have led to the same conclusion).

The presence in each domain of β-pleated sheets linked by hydrogen bonds is compatible with studies of CD spectra as well as theoretical considerations based upon the analysis of H and L chain primary structure. The region of CD spectra characteristic of β sheets does not vary much when the chains are separated, or even when $V_L$ and $C_L$ domains are analyzed independently. This suggests that domain internal structure is not greatly altered by the interaction between a given domain and the complementary one ($V_H - V_L$ or $C_H1 - C_L$ ...).

The results of Poljak's x-ray analysis of the Fab' fragment to a 0.2 nm resolution clearly show that the four homology regions ($V_H$, $V_L$, $C_H1$ and $C_L$) have very similar three-dimensional structures, a finding that concurs with the above spectroscopic data.

The carbon chain is folded into two β pleated sheets, made up of 2 or 3 antiparallel loops, hydrogen bonded in several places (Fig. 7.9). The $V_H$ region, slightly longer than the other homology regions, forms a small supplementary loop, which does not alter the general structure of the domain. The intrachain disulfide bond links the two β-pleated sheets in a direction approximately perpendicular to their planes. It is always located close to a tryptophanyl residue found in the primary structure, about 15 residues after the first cysteine. In order to reduce the intrachain disulfide bonds, the polypeptide chain must first be denatured in concentrated urea or guanidine, unlike the interchain bridges, which are directly accessible in nondenaturing buffers. The residues located in invariable positions within the V regions are involved in interdomain and intradomain interactions, whereas the residues in hypervariable positions are found in very close or in direct contact with the solvent.

The above structure is entirely compatible with the presence of a few supplementary disulfide bridges found in the $C_H1$ domain of rabbit γ chains, in the $V_H$ region of "Daw" monoclonal human IgG, and between the $V_L$ and $C_L$ domains of rabbit $\kappa$B chains.

GENERAL CONFORMATION AND FLEXIBILITY OF IgG

Even though biochemists have been able to separate all IgG domains, it must be emphasized that the molecular region located between the Fab and Fc fragments is by far the most accessible for proteolysis. This region, in the middle of the $\gamma$ chains, contains about 15 residues, including several prolines and those accessible cysteines involved in interchain bridges. Since as early as 1955, x-ray diffusion studies of IgG solutions showed that IgG molecules were elongated rather than globular; the question has been raised whether this "hinge region" might contribute to a possible flexibility of the molecule. Physical experiments have been done in order to determine whether IgG behavior in

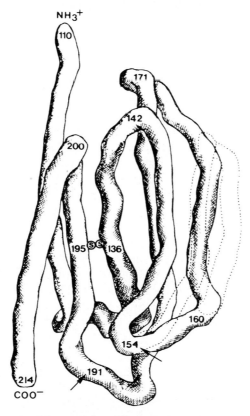

**Fig. 7.9** Diagram of polypeptide chain folds of the $C_L$ region showing the basic spatial structure of immunoglobulin domains. Full lines indicate the structure of $C_L$ and $C_H$1 constant domains. Numbers indicate the location of residues on $C_\lambda$. Dotted lines show the supplementary loop, which is characteristic of $V_L$ and $V_H$ regions. Arrows indicate the location of antigenic markers, to be discussed on p. 191. (From R. J. Poljak et al., Proc. Nat. Acad. Sci. U.S.A., 1973, *70*, 3305.)

solution was more compatible with that of rigid or flexible molecules. Such experiments are based on the measurement of one or more physical parameters related to Brownian motion, which depends, among other factors, upon the shape of the molecules.

Three methodologies stand out:

When Ig are oriented in an electric or hydrodynamic field, light undergoes a double refraction, thus making the solution birefringent. When the field is interrupted, the time of rotational relaxation can be calculated by measuring the decay time of anisotropy of the refractive index of the solution. These measures of the Kerr effect, or of flow birefringence, make it possible to obtain relaxation times that relate mainly to the movement of the longitudinal axis of the proteins.

Movements of IgG molecules can also be followed by observing fluorescent chromophores which have been bound covalently (DNS groups or fluorescein isothiocyanate). Ig rotation brings about a time difference between the decay of the two polarized components of the fluorescence emitted by the solution after excitation. It becomes thus possible to measure relaxation times for rotation and deformation of IgG molecules.

Finally, the principles of x-ray diffusion by Ig solutions have already been referred to earlier.

With the recent progress in electronics, these studies, most of them done 10 to 15 years ago, have regained significance, even though an exhaustive interpretation of the data is not yet possible at the present time due to the theoretical and technological difficulties. Most authors, however, agree that the IgG molecule model is elongated, flexible and Y- or T-shaped. Both Fab fragments may form angles that are more or less open, but they cannot move close enough as to allow them to interact, thus requiring a minimum angle of 80° to 95° between Fab fragments in solution. Electron microscopy studies on these molecules done in a high vacuum are consistent with the concept of a Y- or T-shaped model (see Figs. 7.7 and 7.8).

The axes of the domains of each polypeptide, which is part of the Fab fragment, do not run parallel with one another. Studies of the "New" molecule by Poljak show light chains that form an angle of 100° to 110° in the middle between both domains. The same is true with regard to the Fd fragment, where the main axes of $V_H$ and $C_H1$ domains form a smaller angle of 80° to 95°. In the Fab fragment of another Ig studied by Segal et al., these angles were shown to be slightly wider.

### Carbohydrate Moiety

IgG contain within the Fc fragment a carbohydrate moiety located on the $C_H2$ domain (Fig. 7.6). In some cases, sugars have also been found on the Fab fragment or on Bence-Jones proteins.

The structures of these glucidic fractions, generally formed by a branched oligosaccharide, vary from one IgG molecule to another. Sugar units (galactose, galactosamine, mannose, fucose) are attached to the IgG molecule when travelling from the endoplasmic reticulum to the Golgi apparatus; this process involves membrane transglycosidases that do not seem to be specific for immunoglobulins. Some authors have suggested that the addition of sugars might be involved in processes of active transmembrane transportation and secretion; however, Bence-Jones proteins without oligosaccharides can be observed to be secreted regularly by plasma cells: the role of these carbohydrate groups has not yet been elucidated.

# IV.  ANTIBODY FUNCTION OF IgG

## Antibody Specificity Depends upon its Primary Structure

In 1940, Pauling suggested that all antibody molecules have the same chemical structure and only acquire specificity in the presence of the antigen through direct molding. However, recent biochemical data refute all such "instructionist theories."

### ANALYSIS OF AMINO ACID COMPOSITION OF ANTIBODIES WITH DIFFERENT SPECIFICITIES

Between 1964 and 1967, M. Koshland studied the amino acid composition of rabbit antibodies directed against haptens that do not cross-react: phenylarsonate with negative charge, ammonium phenyltrimethyl with positive charge, and neutral β-phenyl lactoside. Even though the amino acid compositions remained very similar, variations with respect to six different residues were observed. Antibodies directed against the positively charged hapten were more acidic. Conversely, antibodies directed against the negatively charged hapten were more basic. Some changes in the neutral residues were also observed. These differences in amino acid composition have been related to the structure of the antibody site, since they are found in association with, for example, antiarsonate and antilactoside antibodies from various animals. Koshland attempted to locate more precisely these differences on IgG molecules and concluded that they are located on heavy chains and on the Fab fragment, hence also on the Fd fragment. This observation concurs with the presence of the $V_H$ region in the amino-terminal half of this fragment.

### RENATURATION OF ANTI-RNase FAB FRAGMENTS

Studies by Anfinsen have demonstrated that the information which controls enzyme tertiary structure is entirely contained in the primary structure. Studies similar to those by Anfinsen were done by Haber on anti-RNase antibody Fab fragments. In the absence of antigen, Fab fragments are totally reduced and denatured in 10 M urea or 6 M guanidine. Their structure resembles that of a random coil. After the removal of denaturing and reducing agents through dialysis, disulfide bridges can reoxidize and fragments can renature. Recovery of antibody activity (evaluated through antigen binding) was found to be between 20% and 50% of the initial activity, which is remarkable considering the heterogeneity of antibodies. Thus, the presence of antigen is not necessary for the formation of specific antibody sites. This experiment dismissed all "instructionist theories."

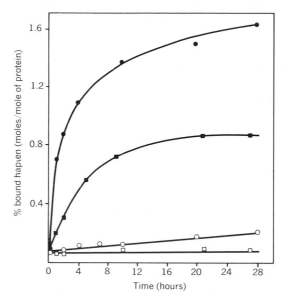

**Fig. 7.11** Comparison of fixation kinetics of both DNP-derived reagents, BADL and BADE, on anti-DNP antibodies and on normal IgG. Reagent/protein molar ratio / 2/1; ● BADE with antibodies; ○ BADE with IgG; ■ BADL with antibodies; □ BADL with IgG. (After Y. Weinstein et al., BBRC, 1969, *35*, 694.)

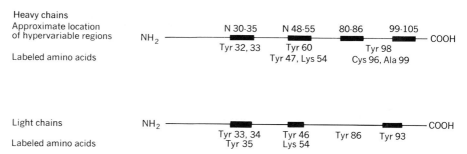

**Fig. 7.12** Main residues affinity-labeled on heavy and light chains. The position of labeled residues is compared with that of hypervariable regions of heavy and light chains. (Residue numbers are approximate, since most of them have been given on the basis of homology with other sequences.)

The main types of reagents used as haptens in affinity labeling experiments are:

*Diazonium derivatives:* Phenylarsonatediazonium fluoroborate; carboxymethyldiazonium fluoroborate; p-nitrophenyldiazonium fluoroborate; 2,4 dinitrophenyldiazonium fluoroborate; m-nitrobenzenediazonium fluoroborate (MNBDF).

*Bromoacetyl derivatives:* α-N-bromoacetyl, N-DNP-lysine (BADL); N-bromoacetyl, N-DNP-ethylenediamine (BADE); bromoacetyl-L-ormithine (BADO); and derivatives of variable length with an active group at both ends.

*Photosensitive derivatives:* Arylnitrenes: 4 azido-2-nitrophenyl (NAP) diazoketone DNP-glycyldiazoketone.

methodologic reservations: (1) the majority of reactive groups coupled to haptens cause selective labeling of certain amino acids; (2) peptides from the hypervariable zone containing labeled residues may become lost during purification due to their dilution, while peptides containing amino acids from conserved positions are easily isolated due to their high concentrations; and (3) without a precise picture of the antibody site-hapten complex, it is difficult to distinguish amino acids directly involved in a chemical bonding with the antigenic determinant from amino acids close to the binding site.

The use of bromoacetylated derivatives by Givol's group, in studies of the structure of anti-DNP sites, has enabled a comparison of the analysis of specific antibody and monoclonal Ig sites sharing the same antibody activity. Figure 7.11 shows that, in a given antibody population, 1.6 BADE groups and 0.9 BADL groups per protein molecule are found. These data reflect the heterogeneity of the antibody population but do not indicate whether the site is shared or modulated. However, with respect to murine immunoglobulin MOPC 315, both reagents bind with the same efficiency. 0.75 BADE groups are found per heavy chain and 0.75 BADL groups per light chain (Fig. 7.13). This finding implies that both chains participate in the active site.

From the conceptual point of view, two significant findings have resulted from affinity labeling experiments:

1. Labeled amino acids belong to both H and L chains, which support the shared-site hypothesis.

2. All residues that have been identified are located in the $V_H$ and $V_L$

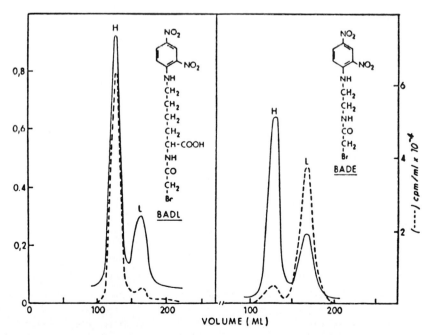

**Fig. 7.13** Affinity labeling of the MOPC 315 protein. Separation of heavy and light chains after [14]C-BADL (left) and [14]C-BADE (right) labeling. (From J. Haïmovich et al., Proc. Nat. Acad. Sci. U.S.A., 1970, *67*, 1656.)

regions, both in hypervariable and in more conserved regions (Tyr 30–33, Trp 35, Cys 96). Therefore antibody-combining sites possess an individual structure, which reflects their individual specificity, while they also share a common overall organization, which reflects the conformational stability of the Fv fragment.

MODEL PROPOSED BY VALENTINE AND GREEN

The first topological location of antibody sites on the Ig surface was obtained by the electron microscopy studies of Valentine and Green. These authors used bis-N-DNP octamethylene diamine (Fig. 7.14), a divalent hapten of minimum length able to bind two anti-DNP antibody IgG molecules. Using an appropriate hapten-to-antibody ratio, they observed, through electron microscopy, rings of three to five IgG molecules, their Fab fragments linked two by two to the hapten (Fig. 7.14). When these preparations are subjected to hydrolysis with pepsin, the globules at each angle disappear, indicating that they are Fc fragments.

It is interesting to note, from a methodological point of view, that the 60° angles between Fab fragments, as shown in Fig. 7.14, are narrower than those for IgG in solution. Similarly, fragment dimensions are slightly smaller than those calculated through x-ray diffusion analysis of IgG solutions.

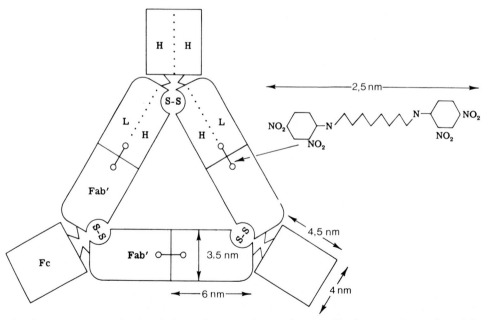

**Fig. 7.14** Structural model derived from the antigen-antibody complexes found by Valentine and Green using electron microscopy. The Fab fragments of two different antibody molecules are linked together two by two by their extremities by means of the bifunctional hapten bis-N-DNP-octamethylene diamine. (After R. C. Valentine and N. M. Green, J. Mol. Biol. 1967, 27, 615.)

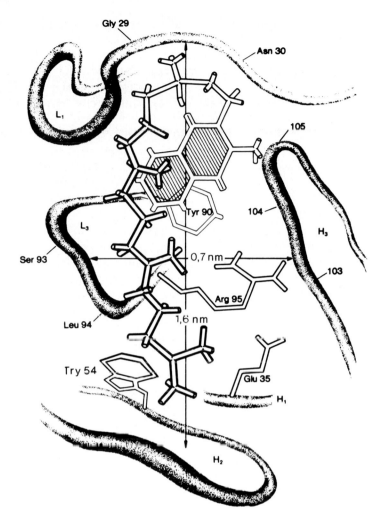

**Fig. 7.15** Diagram of hydroxylated vitamin K1 in the antibody site of the "New" IgG. L1 and L3, H1, H2 and H3 indicate positions of hypervariable regions in L and H chains. (From L. M. Amzel et al., Proc. Nat. Acad. Sci., U.S.A., 1974, *71*, 1427.)

X-RAY ANALYSIS OF THE ANTIBODY SITE

Two examples of Fab-hapten complexes have been subjected to x-ray analysis. They were made from the "New" human monoclonal Ig with antihydroxylated vitamin K1 activity (Poljak's group) and from monoclonal murine Ig McPC 603 with antiphosphorylcholine activity (Segal et al.).

These studies confirmed that the active site is located at the extremity of the Fab fragments. This finding agrees with Valentine and Green's model. The walls of both antibody sites are formed by residues that belong to the hypervariable regions of both polypeptide chains: $L_1$, $L_3$ and $H_1$, $H_2$, and $H_3$ (Figs. 7.12 and 7.15). We shall see that, when sequences are compared, it is sometimes necessary to take into account amino acid insertions in certain hypervariable regions in order to maximize homology. McPC 603 is an example of such a case. Its $L_1$, $H_2$, and $H_3$ regions are longer than those of the "New" molecules, and H and L polypeptide chains form loops that give the antibody site its structure. With regard to McPC 603, the polypeptide chains are longer and protrude towards the outside, forming a wider and deeper cavity. The "New" site is only a slight groove on the protein surface between H and L chains, whereas the McPC 603 site is a deep V-shaped furrow with asymmetric walls. The length, outside width, and depth of the "New" site are $1.6 \times 0.7 \times 0.6$ nm respectively, those of the McPC 603 site are $2 \times 1.5 \times 1.2$ nm. The dimensions of full-length hexose used by Kabat to fill antidextran antibody sites ($3.4 \times 1.2 \times 0.7$ nm), give some idea as to the maximum size of an antibody site.

A comparison of chemical forces involved in the interactions of both protein-hapten systems referred to above, shows that in each case, several hydrogen bonds and van der Waals forces are involved. In addition, phosphorylcholine, which has two negative charges and one positive charge at pH 7, establishes strong electrostatic bonds with one lysine, one arginine, and one glutamic acid. The phosphate group of the hapten is found inside the McPC 603 site cavity, whereas the choline is directed towards the outside. Since the hapten does not fill the entire site, one may wonder whether the complementary antigenic determinant of this active site is not, in fact, larger than this small hapten.

With regard to vitamin K1 derivative, there is a close interaction between the methylnaphthoquinone aromatic ring and the side chain of light-chain tyrosine 90 (the tyrosine residue already identified by affinity labeling experiments). Figure 7.15 shows that the quinone moiety is also in contact with H104 and H105 residues; the phytyl chain is in contact with L93, L94, H54, H57, and H63 residues.

## V.   LEVELS OF IMMUNOGLOBULIN HETEROGENEITY

The fact that immunoglobulin chains are encoded by two different genes implies that antibody heterogeneity occurs at least at two levels. Furthermore, each C or V locus can be polymorphic—in other words, can exist under different allelic forms. This introduces a third level of heterogeneity, which is superimposed on the two previous ones. These three levels were clearly distinguished during analysis of immunoglobulin antigenicity: according to the terminology introduced by Oudin, specificities that are uniform in all individuals of the same species are called "isotypic specificities," thus defining isotypes; specificities that are peculiar to antibodies directed against a given antigen (or specificities that are peculiar to each myeloma protein) are called "idiotypic specificities," thus defining idiotypes; specificities that are different in different groups of individuals of the same species are called "allotypic specificities," thus defining allotypes.

The chemical nature of heavy chains varies according to the immunoglobulin classes, whereas light chains are ubiquitous. For example, in man and mouse, five classes of Ig have been described, IgG, IgM, IgA, IgD and IgE, defined by their 5 heavy chains, $\gamma$, $\mu$, $\alpha$, $\delta$, and $\epsilon$. The purpose of analysis of the various isotypes is twofold: from a genetic viewpoint, it will enable us to determine the number of C genes coding for the different isotypes, and from a physiologic viewpoint, it will provide information as to the structure and function of immunoglobulin effector sites.

The multichain structure of IgG is common to all immunoglobulins. In some cases, the symmetrical structural unit $H_2L_2$ described above, is polymerized in such a way that the antibody molecules may be described by the general formula $(H_2L_2)n$, in which n varies from 1 to 5 (Table 7.3).

## CONSTANT REGIONS: ISOTYPY

### Light Chains

Two types of light chains, designated $\kappa$ and $\lambda$, have been described in man. They have no common antigenic determinant and their primary structures are very different. Nonetheless, sufficient homologies can be found in order to show a clearly common origin (as referred to earlier). Both light chain types are found in each Ig class, but only one type is present per single molecule. Thus, the formula for IgG molecule is either $(\kappa\gamma)2$ or $(\lambda\gamma)2$.

Two different antigenic markers have been found on $\lambda$ chains, Kern+/Kern− and Oz+/Oz−. Chain sequence analysis shows that they correspond to two point permutations of amino acids. The Kern factor is related to the substitution in position 154 (Gly/Ser), the Oz factor to the substitution in position 190 (Lys/Arg) (Fig. 7.9). Since these four amino acids are found in the $\lambda$ chains of all individuals, it can be concluded that these variants are not encoded by alleles. The association Gly 154, Lys 190 (Kern$^+$ Oz$^+$) has never been found on the same chain; therefore it was assumed that there should be three $C_\lambda$ isotypes in man encoded by three different cistrons. However, when Leder group analyzed the germline DNA coding for the human $\lambda$ locus, 4 $C_\lambda$ genes were found to be present, including one coding for the Kern$^+$, Oz$^+$ chain.

Kappa chains represent 66% of human Ig light chains. Two types of light chains that have a structure analogous to that of human light chains have been found in several other species. In mice, $\kappa$ chains represent roughly 97% of light chains, $\lambda$ chains account for approximately 3%. The sequence of mouse myeloma proteins would indicate that there are two $C_\lambda$ isotypes within this species. One of them is represented by the $\lambda$ chain of the IgA MOPC 315 and is extremely rare in all mice strains, except in motheaten mutants. When the mouse $\lambda$ locus was studied, a third $\lambda$ gene $C_{\lambda III}$ was found. Until now, this chain has never been described on an Ig molecule. In rabbits, the $\kappa/\lambda$ ratio is 4/1 (80%/20%), but $\kappa$ chains divide into subtypes $\kappa A$ and $\kappa B$, which correspond to the product of two different genes. The predominant $\kappa B$ chains have an additional intrachain disulfide bridge linking $V_L$ and $C_L$ domains.

**Table 7.3  Characteristics of Human Immunoglobulin in Chains**

| Chain type | L chains | | H chains | | | | |
|---|---|---|---|---|---|---|---|
| | $\kappa$ | $\lambda$ | $\gamma$ | $\alpha$ | $\eta$ | $\delta$ | $\epsilon$ |
| Chain molecular weight | 23,000 | 23,000 | 50,000 | 50,000 | 58,000 | 56,000 | 61,000 |
| Isotypes where chains are present | ubiquitous | | IgG | IgA | IgM | IgD | IgE |
| Molecular formula of isotypes | | | $L_2\gamma_2$ | $L_2\alpha_2$ or $(L_2\alpha_2)_2$SC,J* | $(L_2\mu_2)_5$J* | $L_2\delta_2$ | $L_2\epsilon_2$ |
| Molecular weight of various Ig isotypes | | | 150,000 | 152,000 or 385,000 | 900,000 | 175,000 | 190,000 |
| Isotype variants | | $\lambda$1 to $\lambda$3 | IgG1 to IgG4 | IgA1 to IgA2 | IgM1 to IgM2 | — | — |
| Variability subgroups | $V_\kappa$1 to $V_\kappa$III | $V_\lambda$1 to $V_\lambda$V | | | $V_H$1 to $V_H$III | | — |
| Main allotypes | Inv 1,2,3 | | Gm(I $\rightarrow$ 2,3)Am 1,2 | | — | | — |

* J: J chain; SC: secretory component.

### IgM Immunoglobulins

IgM have a molecular weight of about 900,000 and a sedimentation coefficient of 19S (as a result, they are sometimes referred to as macroglobulins). These molecules are pentameres of the formula $(L_2\mu_2)_5$. In a nondissociating buffer, it is possible to obtain IgM subunits (molecular weight 180,000; 7.8S) through a reversible reduction of the molecule. These subunits can in turn be reduced in order to separate L chains from $\mu$ chains with a molecular weight of 58,000 (plus 5% to 10% carbohydrates). As in the case of IgG molecules, limited proteolysis studies have contributed to the proposal of a topological model for these Ig. Papain and pepsin allow separation of Fab$\mu$ or (Fab'$\mu$)2 fragments. Tryptic digestion releases a pentameric (Fc$\mu$)5 fragment (molecular weight 340,000). A mild reduction of this fragment makes it possible to obtain the monomeric Fc$\mu$ fragment. This indicates that the five IgM subunits are linked between one another by disulfide bridges at the level of the carboxy-terminal part of their $\mu$ chains.

Electron microscopy reveals starlike patterns with five branches distributed evenly around a central ring (Fig. 7.16). Some electron micrographs show that these branches may have orientations that are different from one another, and that they may be on a plane different from that of the central ring. It is clear that pentameric subunits are Y-shaped, thus matching the relative positions of Fab and Fc fragments in IgG. The distance between the center of the ring and

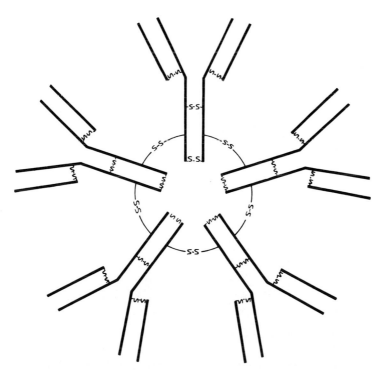

**Fig. 7.16**   Structural diagram of the pentameric IgM molecule.

the connecting points for the subunits is 8 to 10 nm. The length of each branch is 6 to 8 nm.

The problem of the number of IgM antibody sites has not yet been resolved satisfactorily. Using certain antigens, 10 hapten moles can be bound per IgM mole, but other results suggest a pentavalent molecule. On specific IgM of rabbits, five high-affinity sites in addition to five more sites of low affinity have been found. While the hypothesis of two penatavalent antibody populations with different sites can be rejected, no structural data are able to predict an asymmetry for the two Fab fragments of the same subunit. As a result, the question of possible interactions between these fragments within the complete molecule remains unsolved.

In 1973, Putman's and Hilschmann's groups reported independently the complete primary structure of two $\mu$ chains. In addition to the $V_H$ domain, the $\mu$ chain contains four constant domains, $C_\mu 1$, $C_\mu 2$, $C_\mu 3$, and $C_\mu 4$, as suggested by its molecular weight (Fig. 7.17). Internal homologies are found between these domains as well as those of the $\gamma$ chains. The best $\gamma/\mu$ homologies are found between $C_\gamma 1$ and $C_\mu 1$, $C_\gamma 2$ and $C_\mu 3$, and $C_\gamma 3$ and $C_\mu 4$ regions (this amounts to approximately 40% homology when a few deletions are taken into account, Fig. 7.18). Consequently, it appears that the $\gamma$ chain has lost the domain that corresponds to $C_\mu 2$, and that this domain has been replaced by the hinge region of 15 to 20 amino acids, which contains the interchain disulfide bridges (Fig. 7.18).

Five carbohydrate groups of different size are bound to the $\mu$ chain (Fig. 7.17). There are two inter-$\mu$-chain disulfide bridges within a subunit and one intersubunit bridge, probably located between the $C_\mu 3$ domains. In addition, a J chain has been found to be associated with the pentamer. It has an approximate molecular weight of 20,000 and is very acid and rich in cysteines. It is believed to play a role in subunit polymerization.

IgM appear at the very beginning of immune response, as early as the third day, reaching maximum serum levels between the 5th and 6th day. By the 10th day they disappear, to be replaced by IgG (see chap. 10). While IgM do not cross the placental barrier, they are capable of binding complement.

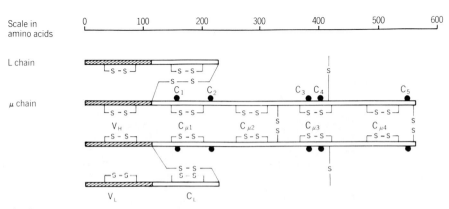

**Fig. 7.17** Structural diagram of the monomeric IgM subunit. •C1 to C5: carbohydrate patterns.

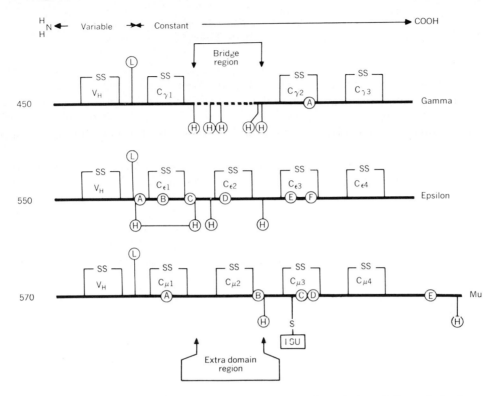

**Fig. 7.18** Topological domain comparison of γ, ε and μ chains. A F: carbohydrate units; ISU: intersubunit disulfide bridge of μ chains. (After H. Bennich et al., *In* L. Brent and J. Holborow, Eds., *Progress in Immunology, II*, Vol. I, Amsterdam, 1974, North Holland, p. 49.)

### IgA Immunoglobulins

IgA are found in the serum and secretions (colostrum in particular, intestinal or bronchial mucus, tears, etc.). They consist of two L and two α heavy chains. Though the monomeric form, $L_2\alpha_2$ with a molecular weight of 152,000 and 7S, is predominant in human serum, dimers or forms with greater polymerization levels are also found. The dimer (11S) is the most common form of IgA in secretions of all species in which it has been found. Disulfide bridges link the $L_2\alpha_2$ units to a J chain, as well as to another chain, which remains largely unknown and which is referred to as "secretory component" (SC). Here, the molecular formula is $(L_2\alpha_2)_2$-J-SC. As a rule, disulfide bridges link α chains, but in certain IgA molecules, a disulfide bridge links both L chains, while noncovalent interactions alone are responsible for H-L links.

Alpha chains have a molecular weight of about 50,000, plus 5% to 10% carbohydrates, which suggests that they are composed of three $C_\alpha$ domains. Fabα, Fcα, and (Fab′α)2 fragments can be obtained through enzymatic cleavage. The sequence of an α chain has been identified in its entirely by Putman et al. The strongest homology between μ and α chains has been found within their last domains (50% to 60% homology).

Electron microscopy studies of human and murine IgA molecules indicate that they are Y-shaped. Dimers have been found in the shape of two Ys, which are rigidly linked together along the same axis at the terminal carboxyl end of the heavy chain. The four Fab fragments are oriented, two by two, in opposite directions. When linked, both Fc fragments form a 12.5 nm long axis, while each Fab fragment forms a 7-nm-long arm whose orientation may be different from that of the Fc fragments. The position of the J chain could not be determined in this study.

Electron micrographs of human or rabbit secretory IgA reveal only one Y, while showing three arms of identical size. When interpreting these pictures, Svehag and Blouth suggested that the two monomeric IgA are superimposed, thereby hiding the secretory component.

High concentrations of IgA are found in the colostrum of mammals, whose placenta does not allow the passage of IgG molecules across the placental barrier. These IgA provide the newborn with antibodies, which will protect him for the period during which he does not yet synthesize his own immunoglobulins in sufficient quantities.

### IgD Immunoglobulins

A decade ago, Rowe described IgD immunoglobulins when studying a myeloma Ig. They are present in small amounts in the serum, and very little is known as yet of their role and structure.

IgD molecules are monomeric. Their sedimentation constant is 6.2S, but their molecular weight is higher than that of IgG or IgA (175,000 to 180,000): IgD structure must therefore be less compact than that of other Ig classes, which might explain their greater sensitivity to proteolysis. The molecular weight of the human $\delta$ chain ranges from 55,000 to 59,000 plus 5% to 10% carbohydrates. Only one disulfide bridge links the heavy chains together. In rodent species, it was found that the $\delta$ chains are smaller and lack the $C_\delta 2$ domain (this recent evolution is reminiscent of the IgG/IgM comparison reported above).

Recent observations suggest that IgD might play a receptor role on lymphocyte membranes; however, their effector functions are unknown.

### IgE Immunoglobulins

Among serum immunoglobulins, IgE are found in lowest concentrations. They are monomeric; the molecular weight of the $\epsilon$ chain is 61,000 plus 11—12% oligosaccharides spread over five positions within the constant region. IgE can be cleaved enzymatically like other Ig classes. The primary structure of an $\epsilon$ chain has been determined in its entirety by Bennich et al.; it include 537 amino acids and five intrachain disulfide bridges, one in the $V_H$ region and one in each constant domain, $C_\epsilon 1$ through $C_\epsilon 4$ (Fig. 7.18).

IgE are characterized by their ability to bind to autologous cells. This function is borne by one of the two last domains of the heavy chain, probably the $C_\epsilon 4$ domain, which features the strongest homology with the $C_\gamma 3$ domain.

**Table 7.4  Physicochemical and Physiological Properties of Human Immunoglobulins**

| WHO term | IgG | IgA | IgM | IgD | IgE |
|---|---|---|---|---|---|
| Former name | 7S | $\gamma A$, $\gamma_2 A$ | 19S, $\gamma M$, $\beta_2 M$ | — | Reagin |
| Percentage of total Ig | 75–85 | 5–10 | 5–10 | 1 | 1 |
| Concentration (mg/ml of serum) | 12.1 | 2.5 | 0.93 | 0.023 | 0.003 |
| Molecular weight | 150,000 | 150,000–170,000 | 900,000 | 175,000 | 190,000 |
| $S_{20}$ (sedimentation coefficient) | 6–7S | 7–11S | 19S | 6.1S | 8.2S |
| Carbohydrates (%) | 2.5 | 5–10 | 5–10 | 5–10 | 11.5 |
| Sulfhydryl resistant | Good | Intermediate | Poor | Good | — |
| Molecular structure | $\kappa_2\gamma_2$ or $\lambda_2\gamma_2$ | $\kappa_2\kappa_2$ or $\lambda_2\alpha_2$ | $(\kappa_2\mu_2)_5$ or $(\lambda_2\mu_2)_5$ | $\kappa_2\delta_2$ or $\lambda_2\delta_2$ | $\kappa_2\epsilon_2$ or $\lambda_2\epsilon_2$ |
| Associated paraproteinemia | $\gamma$G myeloma | $\gamma$A myeloma | Waldenström's macroglobulinemia | $\gamma$D myeloma | $\gamma$E or ND myeloma |
| Appearance after immunization | Last | Intermediate | First | — | Early |
| Appearance of production in newborns | Last | Intermediate | First | — | — |

**Table 7.5  Biologic Functions of Human Immunoglobulins**

|  | IgG | | | | IgA | IgM | IgD | IgE |
|---|---|---|---|---|---|---|---|---|
|  | I | 2 | 3 | 4 |  |  |  |  |
| Placental transfer | + | + | + | + | − | − | − | − |
| Reaginic activity | − | − | − | − | − | − | − | + |
| Binding to monocytes | + | − | + | − | − | − | − | − |
| Complement fixation |  |  |  |  |  |  |  |  |
|    Classic pathway | + | ± | + | − | − | + | − | − |
|    Alternative pathway | + | + | + | ? | + | + | − | + |

It is interesting to note that cytophilic IgG bind to macrophages and mastocytes of animals from different species through this very $C_\gamma3$ domain.

Despite their low concentrations in the serum, IgE play an important role in immunopathology, inasmuch as they support immediate hypersensitivity reactions such as anaphylactic shock, asthma, hay fever, and urticaria (see chap. 26). IgE bind to basophils as well as skin mastocytes. Through a mechanism that is not yet understood, antigen fixation triggers the release of several mediators (see chap. 11).

### Subclasses

Analysis of antibody heterogeneity has shown that immunoglobulins carrying determinants that are characteristic of one class can also carry certain determinants that identify the so-called "subclasses." Among human immunoglobulins, for example, four subclasses IgG1 through IgG4 have been found, identified by their heavy chains $\gamma1$ through $\gamma4$. From a genetic point of view (analysis of C gene heterogeneity), the use of both terms, class and subclass, is unjustified since there is no supplementary level of heterogeneity. These two terms are now consolidated in one single designation: isotype. From a conceptual point of view, there is no difference between $C_\gamma1, C_\gamma4, C_\mu, C_\alpha$ genes, and so on. By the same token, however, a comparison of homology levels of various isotypes is significant for the analysis of C gene evolution, as referred to on p. 000 (Ig phylogeny). A comparison of Fc fragments of human $\gamma1$ and $\gamma4$ shows only 24 different residues, whereas equivalent domains of Ig from different classes generally have no more than a 40% homology. However, it is not these substitutions that best characterize the different isotypes from a chemical point of view, but rather the distribution of interchain disulfide bridges (Fig. 7.19) as well as the sequence around the cysteines involved in H—H disulfide bonds. The fact that the hinge region is also the heavy chain zone which is most specific for each isotype (Fig. 7.19) has been utilized by Milstein's group in proposing a chemical method of classifying human IgG. This method is based on electrophoretic mobility of peptides carrying cysteines that are involved in interchain bonds, which were previously labeled with [14]C iodoacetic acid. For reasons that are still unknown, the selective pressure on which $C_H$ gene evolution depends is clearly not the same for this hinge region as it is for other domains.

Rocca-Serra et al. have shown recently that, within the $C_H1$ domain, two other isotype specific regions enable to distinguish clearly between murine IgG1 and IgG2a immunoglobulins (Fig. 7.20).

The analysis of peptide maps has established the existence of two IgM isotypes. There are two known IgA isotypes, IgA1, and IgA2. Fig. 7.19 shows the respective positions of their interchain disulfide bridges. Antigenic differences that were found when using an anti-IgD antiserum, seem to indicate the existence of several IgD isotypes. In every animal species studied so far, a similar heterogeneity of $C_L$ and $C_H$ isotypes has been found, for example, rabbit κA and κB chains as referred to earlier, or IgG1, IgG2a, IgG2b, and IgG3 of mice.

## VARIABLE REGIONS: IDIOTYPY

We have seen earlier that the variable regions of heavy and light chains, irrespective of their isotypes, are composed of about 110 amino acids in terminal position. Certain common characteristics of these V regions can be described. Sequence differences are mainly due to point permutations of amino acids. In numerous instances, there is a conservation of physicochemical properties of those residues found in modified positions. Most of these variations correspond

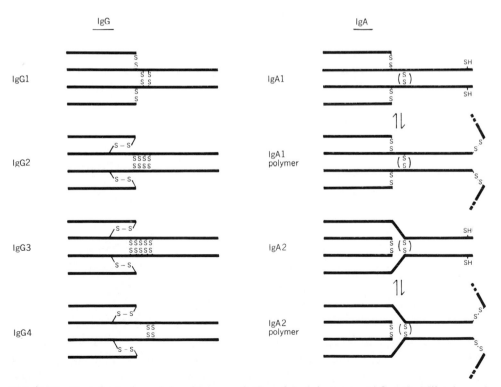

**Fig. 7.19** Topological models of human IgG and IgA isotypes. (After C. Milstein and J. R. L. Pink.)

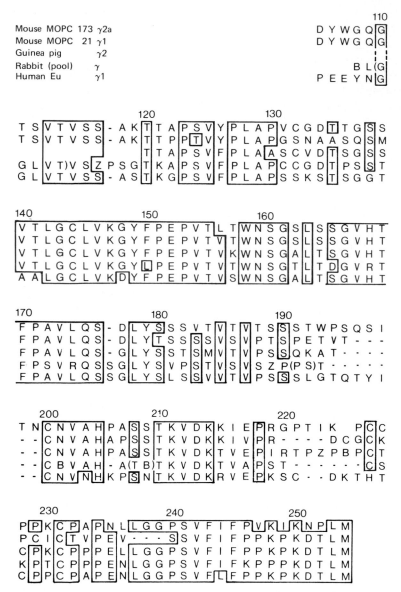

**Fig. 7.20** Sequence comparison of various γ isotypes between residues 110 and 250. Note sequence differences in regions 130–140 and 190–200. (From J. Rocca-Serra, M. Millili and M. Fougereau, Eur. J. Biochem., 1975, *59*, 511.) Key: A: Ala; B: Asx; C: Cys; D: Asp; E: Glu; F: Phe; G: Gly; H: His; I: Ile; K: Lys; L: Leu; M: Met; N: Asn; P: Pro; Q: Gln; R: Arg; S: Ser; T: Thr; V: Val; W: Trp; Y: Tyr; Z: Glx.

to a single base change per codon within the DNA. The size of the variable regions is not always the same: when different sequences are compared, it is often necessary to insert or delete 3 to 6 residues in order to avoid misalignment of homologous positions.

Kabat and Wu have done a systematic analysis of all published sequences.

They defined the variability for each position, using the following ratio:

$$v = \frac{\text{number of different amino acids}}{\text{frequency of the most common amino acid}}$$

Two results of such analysis are shown in Fig. 7.21.

### Two Categories of Variable Positions

We have stressed that, a priori, we expect to find amino acids of two different functions in the V domains: some to be the complementary determining residues, and some to build the overall structure of the V regions. A comparative analysis of the sequences allows to describe two categories of positions: one in which clustered residues are hypervariable, and other positions which represent a far less variable framework. However, within the less variable framework there exist two kinds of positions: some are completely invariable, and some show linked groups of residues that allow a grouping of the more homologous V sequences.

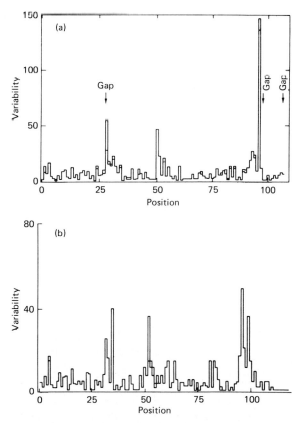

**Fig. 7.21** Variability of human $V_L$(a) and $V_H$(b) regions using the Kabat and Wu method. (From E. A. Kabat and T. T. Wu, Ann. N. Y. Acad. Sci., 1971, *190*, 392.)

Fig. 7.21 clearly shows several zones with high concentrations of variability: within the light chains (Fig. 7.21a), three hypervariable zones $L_1$ to $L_3$ located in positions 25–34, 55–60, 89–97; within the heavy chains (Figs. 7.21b and 7.22), four hypervariable zones $H_1$ to $H_4$ in positions 31–35, 50–65, 81–87 and 95–102. We have seen earlier (p. 185) that amino acids within these regions are in contact with their specific antigenic ligand and can be marked by affinity labeling. Consequently, amino acids which are located in these positions are good candidates for being the complementary determining residues.

Conserved regions between all $V_\kappa$, $V_\lambda$, and $V_H$ chains have been found, particularly in positions 1–8, 36–47, 90–98, and 103–111 within the heavy chains (Fig. 7.22). Due to their presence in the main folds of the polypeptide chain as well as their involvement in interdomain or intradomain interactions, these regions play a significant structural role with respect to the $F_V$ fragment.

Milstein classified human $V_\kappa$ sequences in three subgroups, $V_\kappa I$, $V_\kappa II$, and $V_\kappa III$, according to their homology (1967). The homology between chains belonging to a single subgroup is greater than that of chains belonging to two different subgroups. This observation will be dealt with in some detail because of its great significance with regard to the discussion of the origins of antibody diversity.

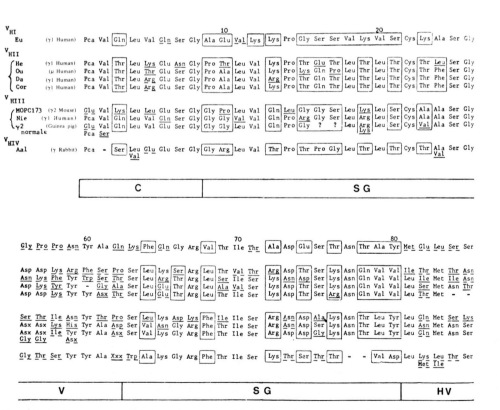

**Fig. 7.22** Sequence of $V_H$ subgroups. Note the interspecific homology found in subgroup $V_H III$. C: conserved region; SG: subgroup specific region; HV: hypervariable region; $V_H SG$ specific residues are boxed. (From A. Bourgois, thesis dissertation, 1974.)

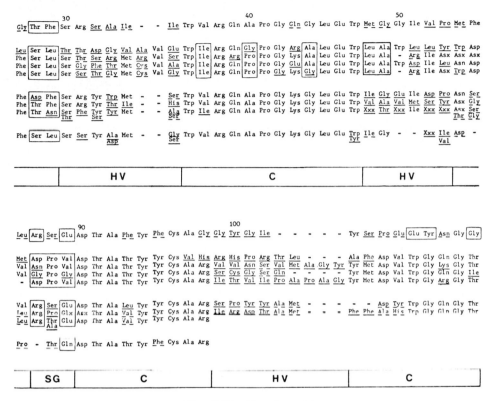

**Fig. 7.22**  (Continued.)

### Variability Subgroups

Subgroup-specific residues are not uniformly distributed within the variable sequence. For each subgroup, it is possible to define a "basic sequence" on the basis of the most common amino acid in each position (Fig. 7.23).

*V$_\kappa$ Variability Subgroups.*  Individual sequences of κ chains within a given subgroup differ from basic sequences only by a very small number of permutations, while chains from different subgroups may show as much as a 40% difference (Fig. 7.23). Since residues 1-27 of the V$_\kappa$ region are subgroup specific, Fougereau was able to propose chemical typing of subgroups based upon the isolation of peptides that contain cysteine 23, labeled by [14]C iodoacetate. This method has been used to analyze a very large number of κ chains; in 90% of them, one of the three characteristic peptides was found, thus confirming the validity of Milstein's classification. In addition, antigenic differences enabled the production of antisubgroup sera in various laboratories.

An analysis of Ig κ chains from normal sera shows that amino acids that are characteristic for all three V$_\kappa$ subgroups can be found in the same sample. This indicates that cistrons that code for regions V$_\kappa$I, V$_\kappa$II, and V$_\kappa$III are not alleles of the same locus but rather different genes (these results are ample justification for the use of myeloma proteins as models for Ig analysis).

In mice the spectrum of the variability of the κ-chains almost follows that of all the L chains because only 3% of antibody molecules carry λ chains.

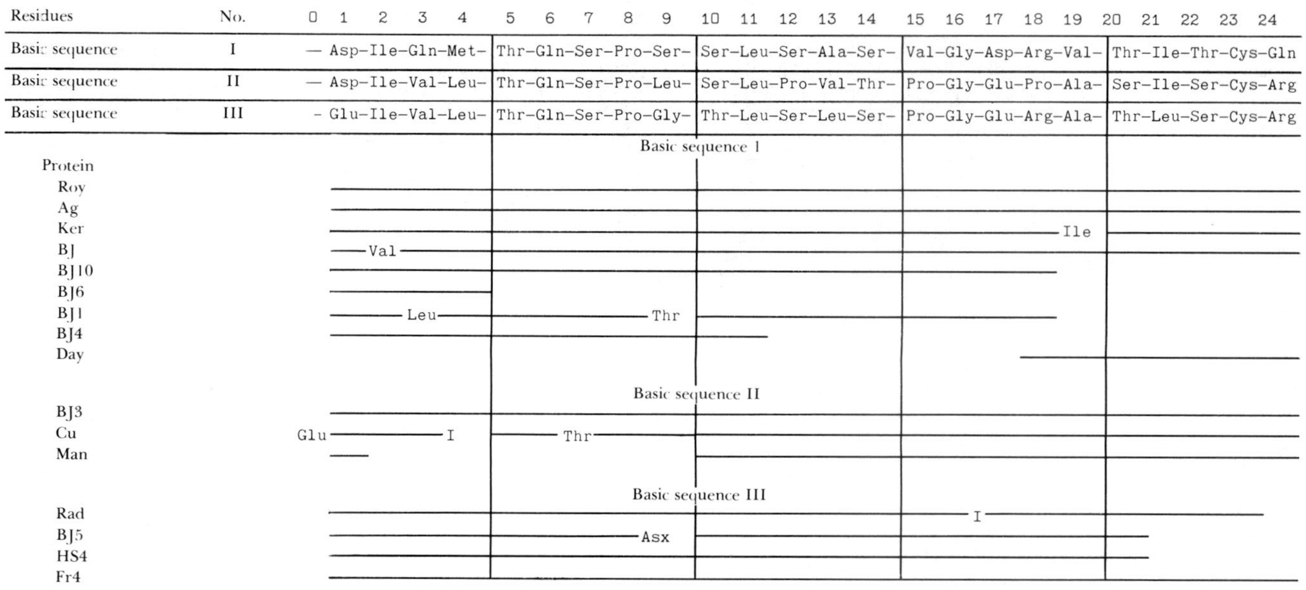

**Fig. 7.23** Human $V_\kappa$ variability subgroups. Classification proposed in 1967 by C. Milstein, who grouped all published $V_\kappa$ sequences into three variability subgroups based upon their homology. For each subgroup, a basic sequence can be arrived at on the basis of the most common amino acid in each position. Uninterrupted lines indicate a structure that is identical with the basic sequence shown at the top; amino acids that have been inserted indicate a difference. (From C. Milstein, Nature, Lond., 1967, *216*, 330.)

| Residues | No. | 0 | 1 | 2 | 3 | 4 | 5 | 6 | 7 | 8 | 9 | 10 | 11 | 12 | 13 | 14 | 15 | 16 | 17 | 18 | 19 | 20 | 21 | 22 | 23 | 24 |
|---|---|---|---|---|---|---|---|---|---|---|---|---|---|---|---|---|---|---|---|---|---|---|---|---|---|---|
| Basic sequence | I | — | Asp | Ile | Gln | Met- | Thr | Gln | Ser | Pro | Ser- | Ser | Leu | Ser | Ala | Ser- | Val | Gly | Asp | Arg | Val- | Thr | Ile | Thr | Cys | Gln |
| Basic sequence | II | — | Asp | Ile | Val | Leu- | Thr | Gln | Ser | Pro | Leu- | Ser | Leu | Pro | Val | Thr- | Pro | Gly | Glu | Pro | Ala- | Ser | Ile | Ser | Cys | Arg |
| Basic sequence | III | — | Glu | Ile | Val | Leu- | Thr | Gln | Ser | Pro | Gly- | Thr | Leu | Ser | Leu | Ser- | Pro | Gly | Glu | Arg | Ala- | Thr | Leu | Ser | Cys | Arg |

*Basic sequence I* — Proteins: Roy, Ag, Ker (Ile at 19), BJ (Val at 3), BJ10, BJ6, BJ1 (Leu at 3, Thr at 9), BJ4, Day

*Basic sequence II* — Proteins: BJ3, Cu (Glu at 1, I at 4), Man (Thr at 6)

*Basic sequence III* — Proteins: Rad (I at 16), BJ5 (Asx at 9), HS4, Fr4

Conversely, in man, to obtain a complete picture of the $V_L$ regions, it is necessary to consider the overall situation of the $V_\kappa$ and $V_\lambda$ regions. Thus, unlike the relatively simple classification of human $V_\kappa$ regions, the classification of murine $V_\kappa$ sequences is much more difficult. Potter has proposed that sequences that do not differ by more than three positions between residues 1–23 should be placed in the same "group." Thus, in 1978, after 64 sequences of the $V_\kappa$ region described in the BALB/c strain, 26 groups may be defined and, after 31 sequences of the V region described in the NZB strain, 14 groups may be defined. There appears to be no strain-specific difference between the $V_\kappa$ region of these two strains of mice, and statistical analysis of all this data suggests the existence of about 50 groups in the $V_\kappa$ region in this species. However, as with human variable regions, there are associated residues conserved within certain sequences over those of the 1–23 region. This allows the subdivision of the groups into subgroups when considering the whole framework of the variable regions. Hence, in the group designated "$V_\kappa 21$," 22 complete sequences have been determined in Weigert and Hood's laboratories. These workers, on the basis of homologies found between residues 23 and 98, have divided this protein group into 6 subgroups comprised of 2–5 sequences and designated $V_\kappa 21$A to F. In addition, it is possible that several other $V_\kappa 21$ subgroups exist since several sequences are not classed within subgroups A–F (Fig. 7.24). Some antisera obtained against two $\kappa$ chains of the groups serve to distinguish the individual $V_\kappa 21$ proteins from one another on the basis of their cross-reactivity.

$V_\lambda$ *Variability Subgroups.* Unlike $\kappa$ chains, human $\lambda$ chains do not permit a simple classification. Also, the number of sequences that have been published is more limited. At least five subgroups, $V_\lambda$I to $V_\lambda$V, can be distinguished. Since chains that belong to different subgroups are not of identical length, it is necessary when comparing $\lambda$ chains to introduce a few deletions in order to avoid misalignment of homologous sequences.

Twelve out of 18 murine $V_\lambda$ regions, which have been sequenced in part or in their entirety, appear to be identical; the others differ by one to three positions within the hypervariable zone. This suggests that there is only one $V_\lambda$ framework. However, this analysis does not include the $V_\lambda$ MOPC 315 sequence which is linked to another isotype $C_\lambda$II. as referred to earlier (p. 191).

Rabbit $\lambda$ chains have some variability, but it has been studied very little.

$V_H$ *Variability Subgroups.* Sequences of all known $V_H$ regions are sufficiently alike to form a group that can be easily distinguished from $V_\lambda$ or $V_\kappa$ chains, independently of the $C_H$ region with which they were associated. Sequences can be classified into three variability subgroups, $V_H$I, $V_H$II, and $V_H$III (Fig. 7.22), randomly associated with various isotypes, $C_\gamma$, $C_\mu$, $C_\delta$, $C_\alpha$, $C_\epsilon$. A comparison of variable regions within one $V_H$ subgroup shows a homology of about 75%, whereas two $V_H$ regions belonging to two different subgroups show a homology of only 50%.

Statistical analysis of known mouse $V_H$ sequences are indicative of a complex situation. On the basis of partial sequence studies, Prastad has suggested that there are at least four different $V_H$ subgroups within this species, one of them being very homologous to the $V_H$III human subgroup. This observation, first made by Bourgois and Fougereau, shows that the process which led to the

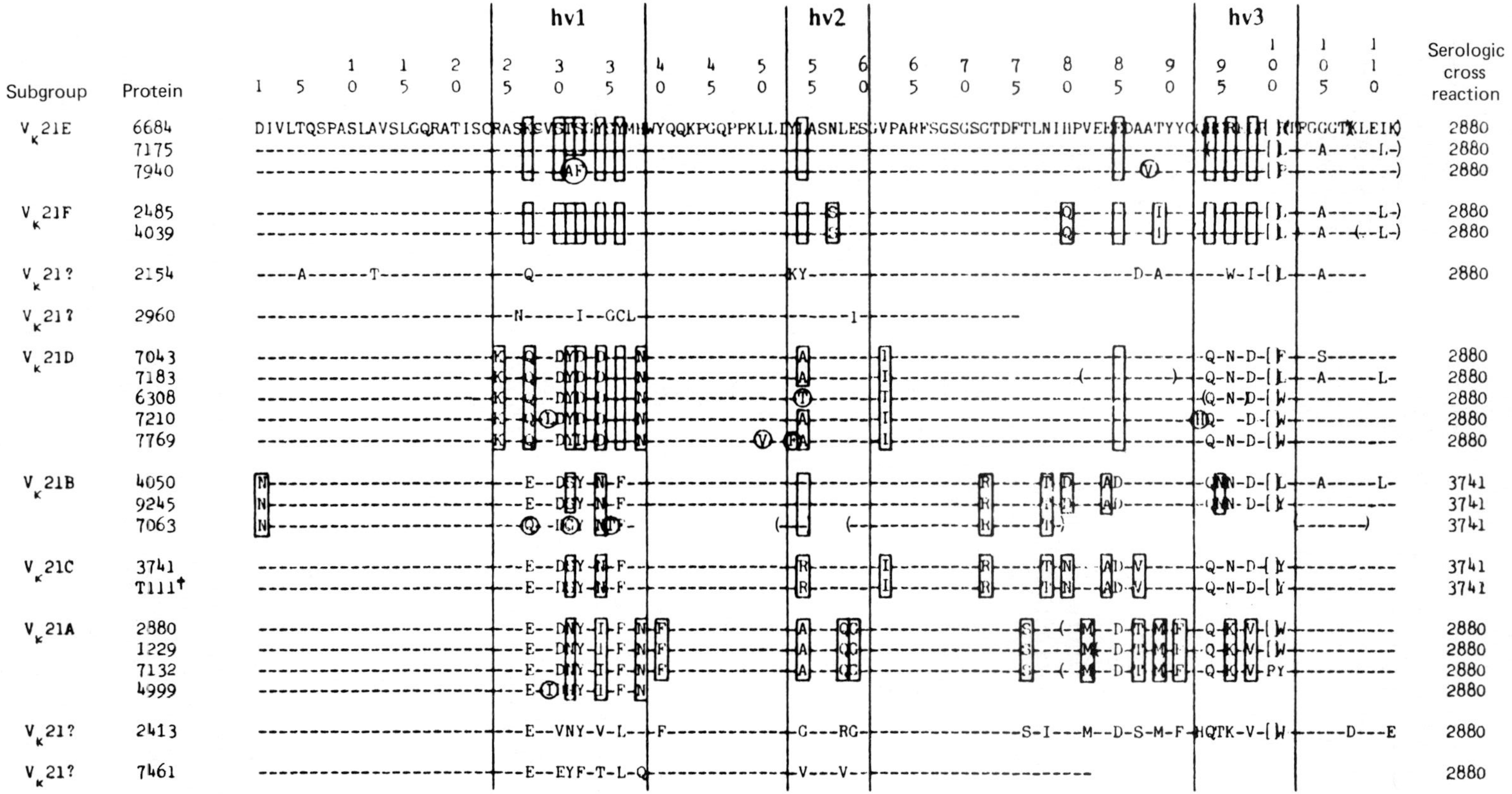

**Fig. 7.24** Amino acid sequences in the V region of the murine group $V_\kappa 21$. The sequences are divided into subgroups designated $V_\kappa 21$ A to $V_\kappa 21$ F. Some potential supplementary subgroups are indicated by a question mark. The specific subgroup residues are framed. Variable residues in the same subgroup are enclosed in circles. hv1, hv2, and hv3 and indicate the three hypervariable regions. Serological cross-reactions are shown on the right. (After M. Weigert et al., Nature, 1978, 276, 785.)

emergence of V genes in mice is different for $V_H$ and $V_\kappa$ gene sets. Indeed, in this $V_L$ system, no particular homology has been found with $V_\kappa$ subgroups of another species. Subsequently, this very $V_H$III variability subgroup has been found in several other species (Kehoe, Capra). This suggests that the ancestral gene of the present $V_H$III region existed prior to species differentiation.

To date, published sequences of rabbit heavy chains do not show such a clear homology with sequences of one of the human $V_H$ regions. Some authors have advanced a resemblance with the $V_H$II subgroup, whereas others have proposed a fourth $V_H$ subgroup (Fig. 7.22). Since the rabbit has no myeloma proteins, our understanding of its immunoglobulin primary structure moves ahead at a slower pace. However, several homogeneous antibodies are now under study.

### Phylogenetically Associated Residues

It is not possible to identify an animal by the position of certain "species-specific" amino acids in its $V_H$ sequence. However, a systematic analysis of partial $V_H$III sequences in various species allows for a more flexible concept, that of "phylogenetically associated residues" (Table 7.6). The genetic significance of this notion will be discussed later.

### Partial Evaluation of Structural Analysis

CONCEPT OF TRANSLOCATION GROUP

The structure of Ig light and heavy chains has led us to analyze independently constant as well as variable regions. We have been able to identify three cistron groups that code for constant ($C_\kappa$, $C_\lambda$, and $C_H$) regions as well as three other cistron groups that code for variable ($V_\kappa$, $V_\lambda$, and $V_H$) regions. Diversi

**Table 7.6  Phylogenetically Associated Residues in Several Positions of $V_H$III Sequences among Various Species**

| Species | 1 | 2 | 3 | 10 | 19 | 21 | 23 | 38 |
|---|---|---|---|---|---|---|---|---|
| Man | Glu | Val | Gln | Gly | Arg | Ser | Ala | Val |
| Dog | Glu | Val | Gln | Asp | Arg | Ser | Val | Val |
| Cat | Asp | Val | Gln | Asp | Arg | Thr | Val | Val |
| Guinea pig | Glu | Val | Gln | Gly | Arg | Ser | Val | Ile |
| Pig | Glu | Glu | Gln | Gly | | Ser | Val | |
| Mouse | Glu | Val | Lys | Gly | Lys | Ser | Ala | Val |
| Rat | Glu | Val | Gln | Gly | Lys | Ser | | |
| Opossum | Glu | Ile | Gly | Asp | | | | |
| Mink | Glu | Val | Gln | Asp | Arg | Ser | Ala | |
| Pigeon | Ala | Ile | Gln | Gly | Arg | Val | Gly | |
| Goose | Ala | Ile | Gln | Val | Arg | Val | Gly | |
| Duck | Ala | Ala | Thr | Gly | Arg | Val | Gly | |
| Turkey | Ala | Val | Gln | Gly | Arg | Val | Gly | |
| Chicken | Ala | Val | Thr | Gly | Arg | Val | Gly | |

From J. M. Kehoe and J. D. Capra, Contemporary Topics in Immunology, vol. 3, G. L. Ada, ed., New York; Plenum Publishing Corporation, 1974, p. 143.

fication of these V and C regions into variability subgroups and isotypes indicates that the number of V and C genes coding for the κ, λ, and H chains is not necessarily identical. This separation of V and C genes and the require-ment for their association have led to the fact that cistrons that are necessary for Ig synthesis are being regarded as three translocation groups (Fig. 7.25). A more precise understanding of the relationship between V and C genes requires genetic studies of their specific markers (the idiotype and allotype determinants) as we shall see later.

ORIGIN OF VARIABILITY PROBLEMS AND HYPOTHESES

Structure peculiarities of variable regions soon raised questions among immunochemists, who offered their theories as to the genetic origin of specific Ig diversification. We have seen that amino acid permutations are not distributed randomly along the variable region sequence; there are hypervariable zones within a framework of more conserved zones, which are either invariable or subgroup-specific.

However, even within these frameworks, certain variations do occur. In order to explain their origin, two theories have been offered. (1) There are as many genes as there are different framework sequences. This amounts to

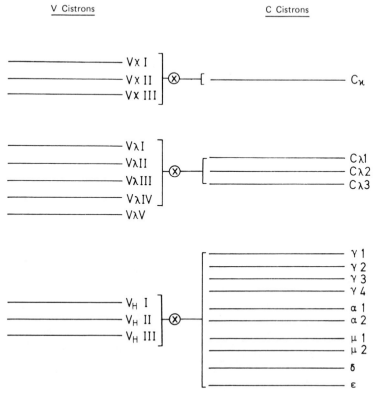

**Fig. 7.25** The three translocation groups in man, identified on the basis of the minimum number of genes that code for immunoglobulins.

theorizing that chains from one identical variability subgroup are synthesized by a gene family that appeared in the recent past and evolved over a short period of time, since diversification of their respective structures has not been significant. This hypothesis would require approximately 100 cistrons per $V_\kappa$, $V_\lambda$, and $V_H$ system. It should be stressed that according to this hypothesis, the concept of subgroup does not correspond to the notion of genetic unit, but it is analogous to the concept of subclass, as discussed above. (2) Variations are explained by V gene polymorphism and by a few somatic mutations.

The structure of hypervariable regions can also be explained from a germinal or somatic viewpoint. (1) There are as many genes in the germinal line as there are different sequences in variable regions, thus requiring about $10^3$ to $10^4$ cistrons for each V system. (2) The accumulation of mutations occurs through a somatic process during ontogenesis of lymphoid cells. For such a mechanism to explain all sequence variations found in relatively conserved zones as well as in hypervariable zones, the number of V cistrons in the germinal line would have to be equal to the minimum number of variability subgroups. This is the only hypothesis where the concept of subgroup corresponds with that of genetic unit.

An intermediate hypothesis can also be proposed. According to this theory, the structure of hypervariable regions would be acquired through somatic mutation, while restricted variability of the framework would be of germinal origin. This hypothesis would require approximately 100 genes per V system.

In short, there are three types of explanation for Ig diversity: (1) purely somatic hypotheses, requiring a small number of genes; (2) purely germinal hypotheses, requiring a large number of genes (about $10^4$ per V system); and (3) mixed hypotheses, whereby a somatic mechanism explains hypervariability only (about 100 genes per V system).

As a result, the selection of one of these various hypotheses depends on the number of genes involved in Ig synthesis. It is therefore absolutely essential to be able to determine precisely this gene count. This was facilitated through immunochemical analysis, which allowed the study of the segregation of genetic markers in variable regions and the identification of their relationships with constant regions.

### Immunoglobulin Idiotypy

We have seen earlier that Ig may act as antigens when injected into an animal that considers them as being nonself. This very property is utilized when preparing anti-isotype antibodies through immunization between different species. Immunizations within the same species have revealed allelic variants of these isotypes (see allotypes). They have also demonstrated the appearance on Ig of new antigenic specificities that are detectable only after injection of an antigen and that are linked to the synthesis of specific antibodies.

DEMONSTRATION OF IDIOTYPE SPECIFICITIES

The concept of idiotype is due to Oudin, who conducted the first experiment in rabbits (1963). Independently, Kunkel reported similar results in studies of human myeloma proteins during that same year. Two rabbits, A and B, are chosen; these rabbits are genetically as similar as possible in order to simplify the analysis. Rabbit A is bled before any immunization; this bleeding (Ao) is to be a control at the end of the experiment. Rabbit A is then injected with an antigen (*Salmonella typhi* in Oudin's initial experiment; see Fig. 7.26). This animal will synthesize anti-*S. typhi* antibodies, which will be collected in bleeding A1. An agglutinate (*S. typhi*—anti-*S. typhi* antibodies) is prepared and injected into rabbit B; precipitation reactions are then conducted, as described in Fig. 7.26. Rabbit B serum contains antibodies specifically directed against the immunizing antibodies which it received (rabbit A anti-*S. typhi* antibodies). Rabbit B serum does not react with A serum collected before immunization nor does it react with anti-*S. typhi* serum of other rabbits. The synthesis by rabbit A of anti-*S. typhi* antibodies must have induced the appearance of new antigenic determinants in its serum. Rabbit B antiserum is called anti-idiotypic serum. It recognizes A1 idiotypes, that is, anti-*S. typhi* antibody molecules from rabbit A, which are themselves defined by their idiotypic specificity, that is, by their particular antigenic determinants. The term "*S. typhi* idiotypic system" refers to all immunizing anti-*S. typhi* antibodies and anti-idiotype antibodies that recognize

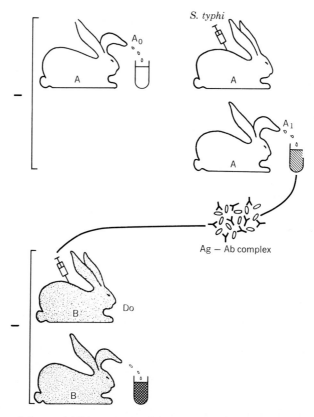

**Fig. 7.26** Protocol for anti-idiotypic immunization. Rabbit A is immunized with *S. typhi*. Rabbit B with the same allotypic formula as A, is then immunized with an agglutinate of *S. typhi*—rabbit A anti-*S.typhi* antibodies. Rabbit B produces "anti-idiotype" antibodies that are precipitated by serum $A_1$, but not by serum $A_0$ collected before immunization.

them. The precipitation reaction described in Fig. 7.26 is called a "homologous reaction," according to the terminology of Landsteiner.

If one attempted to bring about a precipitation reaction between this anti-idiotypic B serum and an anti-*S. typhi* antiserum from a rabbit other than A, there would be a "heterologous reaction" (Landsteiner). As we shall see, such reactions have been described in other systems, particularly with antibodies of restricted heterogeneity synthesized against pneumococcal or streptococcal polysaccharides in rabbits.

Heteroimmunization may also be used to obtain anti-idiotype sera (for example, by injecting a rabbit with human immunizing antibodies). All antibodies directed against the nonidiotype determinants must then be extracted from the anti-idiotypic serum. An elegant technique has been developed for the guinea pig: before receiving immunizing rabbit antibodies and through the injection of normal rabbit Ig, the guinea pigs are made tolerant to those determinants that are common to all rabbit antibody populations. They then synthesize anti-idiotype antibodies only.

Idiotypy studies have largely been done with mice, and this for two reasons: (1) heterologous reactions can be observed rather easily between mice of the same strain, and (2) various idiotype crossreactions have been described between sera raised against myeloma proteins with antibody activity and antibodies from immune sera with identical specificity within the same mouse strain (myeloma proteins have "individual determinants," thus constituting a particular case of idiotypy).

LOCATION OF IDIOTYPE DETERMINANTS

The very fact that idiotype specificities are linked to antibody function suggests that idiotype determinants are located in variable regions. Fab fragments do in fact carry these determinants; in some systems, isolated L or H chains can be recognized by anti-idiotype antibodies. However, the best evidence was furnished when the Fv fragment of the MOPC 315 murine protein was isolated (see Fig. 7.7 and Table 7.2), because this very fragment contains the individual antigenic determinants of the protein.

In antihapten antibody systems, it has been possible to achieve total or partial inhibition by the hapten of anti-idiotype antibodies binding to the idiotype. From these studies, it can be concluded that some idiotype determinants are, indeed, associated with the antibody site but that this location is not exclusive.

EVOLUTION OF IDIOTYPES DURING IMMUNE RESPONSE

Long ago, it was shown that antibodies produced during immune response saw their heterogeneity and average affinity increase with time (see p. 339). We know now that with time, the population of idiotypes evolves as well. Indeed, one can observe the disappearance or appearance of new idiotype specificities, even if the reappearance of the same anti-*S. typhi* idiotype is found in a rabbit after a two year interval. In addition, changes in the molecular distribution of idiotype specificities are found. A demonstration of identical determinants on specific IgM and IgG molecules, which appear sequentially during immune response (Oudin and Bordenave), concurs with the fact that $V_H$ regions associate with various $C_H$ regions (we shall discuss other immunochemical evidence of such V—C transfer). In this connection, the very same individual determinants have been found on monoclonal IgM and IgG2 molecules of one human myeloma: an analysis of both $V_H$ sequences showed them to be identical. Other examples of redistribution of idiotype specificities are not understood as well.

These observations, as well as the rarity of heterologous reactions, emphasize the heterogeneity of antibody populations and show once again that several different molecules can recognize a single antigenic determinant.

GENETIC TRANSMISSION OF IDIOTYPE SPECIFICITIES

The study of variable region markers is essential for the analysis of the genetic origin of variability. Idiotype determinants provide the necessary instrument for this analysis, especially in species and systems that allow easy observation of heterologous reactions. However, it must be stressed that there are significant methodological difficulties associated with the use of anti-idiotype antisera. We have seen that several types of zones can be distinguished in variable regions. Idiotype determinants have been shown to be related to both the combining site, thus involving hypervariable residues, and to other positions, thus involving framework residues. Depending upon whether an anti-idiotypic serum recognizes one pattern or the other (or both), one may expect to find different genetic results, which could be erroneously interpreted as evidence of the presence or absence of a somatic mechanism in variability generation.

If the origin of hypervariable regions is somatic, hereditary transmission should not be observed. Inheritance of idiotypes has been researched in rabbits and in mice by using an antigenic system that enables to demonstrate heterologous reactions. Thus far, findings have proven to be rather different, depending upon the system under study.

While studying idiotypy of the anti-*Salmonella abortus equi* system in rabbits, Oudin and Bordenave observed that heterologous reactions were more frequent within a family than in randomly chosen animals. However, back-crosses did not increase the frequency of such heterologous reactions.

It is also known that the ability of some rabbits to synthesize antibodies of limited heterogeneity depends upon genetic factors. Eichmann and Kindt used such antistreptococcal antibodies when studying three generations of one family with an exceptionally significant proportion of homogeneous antibodies and found complete as well as incomplete heterologous reactions. In order to explain incomplete reactions, one could suppose that a single polypeptide chain had been recognized by the anti-idiotypic serum, whereas determinants from both chains had been recognized in complete reactions. This finding is consistent with hereditary transmission. When using type-VIII pneumococcal polysaccharide, however, which also induces antibodies of limited heterogeneity, no such heterologous reaction could be demonstrated for three generations by Wingfield et al.

The fact that, for a given antigenic system, the frequency of heterologous reactions within certain inbred mice strains is rather significant indicates that there is a genetic effect on the determinism of those idiotype specificities that are responsible for these heterologous reactions.

Sher and Cohn showed that individual determinants borne by BALB/c myeloma Ig with antiphosphorylcholine (PC) activity could be found on anti-PC antibodies induced in the same strain. Crosses and back-crosses using mice of other strains that do not possess this idiotype have indeed shown a dominant inheritance involving one gene linked to the $C_H$ genes and another gene linked to the H-2 gene complex. According to the authors, these observations support the hypothesis that suggests that the V regions of murine anti-PC antibodies are specified by germline genes selected for their significant survival value for the species. However, among lymphocytes synthesizing anti-PC antibodies, 30% produced molecules of different idiotypes, thus indicating that this example of genetic inheritance of V genes does not rule out the existence of a possible somatic process of variability.

Idiotypic inheritance of anti-$p$-azo-phenylarsenate (ARS) antihapten antibodies has been described in A/J mice (Nisonoff's group). In these experiments anti-idiotype sera used as a probe were not raised against a myeloma protein but against individual sera. Twenty percent to 70% of cross-reactions were reported with individual sera. Only in the single case of anti-$\alpha$ (1–3) dextran (DEX) BALB/c antibodies were 100% of idiotypic cross-reaction seen between individual sera. In the case of BALB/c anti-$\alpha$ (1–3) dextran (DEX) antibodies, more than 70% of idiotypic cross-reaction among individual sera is seen in the primary response. The common idiotypic determinant, named IdX, is present on the three myeloma proteins which possess anti-dextran activity (J 558, MOPC104E, U102). These myeloma proteins and anti-$\alpha$ (1–3) dextran antibodies all share the $\lambda$1 light chain, whose presence is necessary for the expression of the common idiotype IdX. In addition, each myeloma protein possesses an individual idiotypic specificity "IdI" which is present on a very small fraction of the polyclonal anti-DEX antibody population. Precise structural correlations for IdX and IdI have been defined when a series of monoclonal antibodies produced by anti-DEX hybridoma were analysed in Davies and Hood's laboratories. Because $\lambda$ chains are identical, idiotypic variability is encoded only within the heavy chains. Expression of the IdX determinant was associated with the presence of two residues and/or carbohydrate in the second hypervariable region in position 54 (Asn) and 55 (plus carbohydrate). Two individual idiotypes correlate with a pair of aminoacids in the third hypervariable region, in positions 100 and 101; i.e., M104E IdI Tyr-Asp, and J558 IdI, Arg-Tyr.

Studies on the light chain idiotypes of inulin-binding myeloma proteins restrict the location of an IdI and IdX determinants to a few aminoacids each. Similar analyses were undertaken in the antigalactan and the antilevan systems where IdX determinants were found to be common to specific antibodies and to several myeloma proteins, whereas IdI determinants were shared by very few molecules.

The finding of IdX determinants suggests the presence of germline genes which code for specific antibodies (this point will be discussed in more detail (p. 236). However, as we shall see, experiments on idiotypic suppression show that when a given idiotype cannot be expressed, new specific antibodies with different V regions may appear.

GENETIC MAPPING OF MURINE $V_H$ GENES

The description of 7 idiotype systems available now for genetic mapping of murine heavy chains is another major result of the study of idiotype inheritance. These systems are the following:

(1) the T15 marker corresponds to the individual specificity of a BALB/c antiphosphorylcholine IgA$\kappa$ myeloma protein (TEPC 15); (2) the J558 marker corresponds to the individual specificity of a BALB/c anti-$\alpha$(1–3) dextran IgA$\lambda$ myeloma protein; (3) the S117 marker corresponds to the individual specificity of another BALB/c anti-N acetyl glucosamine IgA$\kappa$ myeloma protein; (4) the A5A marker corresponds to the idiotype of anti-group A streptococcal carbohydrate antibodies produced by a clone of spleen cells transferred in vivo in A/J mice; (5) the ARS marker corresponds to the idiotype of anti-$p$-azo-phenylarsonate antibodies raised in individual A/J mice; (6), and (7) the NP marker and the BNrP marker are not defined by antisera but by the cross-reaction pattern of the antibodies directed against derivatives of the 4-hydroxyphenyl-acetic acid. The relative affinity of anti-NP or anti-BNrP for a series of other structurally related haptens allows the definition of a "fine specificity index" (FSI), which acts like a genetic trait.

For each system, the strain distribution of the marker was studied on the appropriate antibodies. With a very few exceptions, the markers follow exactly the distribution of the $C_H$ alleles (called the Ig-1 alleles) of the reference strain. This suggests that the idiotype is specified by a gene closely linked to the Ig-1 locus. This has been confirmed by three genetic approaches: (1) Breeding experiments: they show a dominant mendelian Ig-linked segregation. These experiments also allow the isolation of recombinants (see below). (2) The analysis of congenic strains: on the same background (BALB/c) different Ig-1 alleles, or different H-2 haplotypes are introduced by successive back-crossing. The distribution of the markers follows, once again, the distribution of the Ig-1 alleles. (3) Analysis of recombinant inbred (RI) strains of mice: different strains were developed from brother-sister crosses of BALB/c and C57BL/6 mice (Bailey's CXB strains) or AKR and C57L. (Taylor's AKXL strains), each line sharing a different combination of genes, especially of Ig-1 alleles and H-2 haplotypes. Again, an idiotypic linkage to the $C_H$ locus was found.

When taken together, these results show that $V_H$ and $C_H$ genes are closely linked. The relative order of some of these genes is known because in the course of the breeding experiments 3 new groups of linkages were observed in recombinant mice. Crossovers have taken place between the NBrP and the T15 loci (the BAB14 recombinant), between the J558 and the Ig-1 loci (the CBF 5 recombinant) and between the A5A and the ARS loci (the BB♂ 7 recombinant). It had been shown independently that the Ig-1 locus is linked to the Pre locus coding for prealbumin alleles. As a result, a preliminary map can be proposed, such as the following diagram by K. Eichmann.

| A5A | ARS<br>J558 | T15 | Ig-1 | Pre |
|-----|-------------|-----|------|-----|
|     | NP<br>NBrP<br>S117 |  | Ig-2<br>Ig-3<br>Ig-4 |  |

Vertical bars indicate positions in which crossovers have been observed, except for the one between T15 and Ig-1, which is assumed. The order of genes is based upon the assumption that all $V_H$ genes cluster to one side of the $C_H$ genes. Analysis of the percentage of recombinants enables to establish a scale for this map: 9% recombinants were reported between Ig-1 and Pre, 0.4% between J558 and Ig-1, and 3.2% between A5A and Ig-1. Recent findings of Barstad et al. and Capra et al. would suggest a correlation between the $V_H$ subloci and the $V_H$ subgroup-specific sequences.

### IDIOTYPIC SUPPRESSION

Several authors have attempted to prevent the synthesis of Ig that bear certain idiotype determinants by injecting animals with anti-idiotypic serum prior to immunization with the corresponding antigen. These experiments, which utilize systems in which idiotype specificities are transmitted in a hereditary manner, have produced two types of results.

Cosenza and Köhler studied the phosphorylcholine (PC) system in BALB/c mice. The injection of pneumococcal cell walls produced anti-PC antibodies, which were then precipitated by a serum directed against the individual specificities of anti-PC myeloma protein. Injection of this anti-idiotypic serum prior to immunization of mice with pneumococcal walls prevented the appearance of anti-PC circulating antibodies. Also, a total in vitro suppression in a culture of spleen cells of these very same BALB/c mice can be observed.

In A/J mice, Hart obtained different results with the antiphenylarsonate system. Injection of anti-idiotypic serum in this system suppresses the production of Ig that bear those specificities recognized by the anti-idiotypic serum; however, the immune response is not suppressed, and the level of antihapten antibodies does not vary. If these antibodies are used to obtain a new anti-idiotypic antiserum, which is injected along with the first anti-idiotypic antiserum, a third antibody population appears. It contains new idiotype specificities that are different from those recognized by the first two antisera. These experiments confirm the significant heterogeneity of antibodies directed against a single hapten within a give mouse strain.

Bordenave studied the anti-*Salmonella abortus equi* (S.A.E.) system in the rabbit. Since there is no apparent hereditary transmission of idiotype specificities, the entire experiment must be carried out with the same rabbit. Anti-*Salmonella* antibodies obtained after a first immunization are used to produce an anti-idiotypic antiserum. The rabbit, which was immunized with S.A.E. prior to booster injection, is then injected six months later with these antibodies. The production of anti-S.A.E. antibodies is the same as that obtained in control animals. However, like the experiments of Hart et al., this experiment does not reveal the specificities recognized by the anti-idiotypic serum.

### IDIOTYPY OF ANTIBODIES WITH DIFFERENT SPECIFICITY AGAINST THE SAME ANTIGEN

When an animal is simultaneously injected with different antigens, no idiotypic cross-reaction can be found between the corresponding antibodies. Nevertheless, the study of anti-*S. typhi* antibodies led Oudin to wonder whether antibodies directed against different determinants of the same antigen molecule might not have the same idiotype specificities. In addition, there is the failure to detect through gel precipitation more than six or seven different idiotypes within a given serum; this number is small, even though some antibodies may not be detected. These facts led to the systematic search for evidence of identity in idiotype specificities for antibodies directed against different determinants. Cazenave and Oudin studied three systems using protein antigens.

*Ovalbumin System.* The same idiotype specificities have been located on antiovalbumin antibodies, whether or not they are precipitable, and even on nonspecific IgG which have no known antibody function and which appear after ovalbumin immunization.

*Fibrinogen System.* Human fibrinogen can be cleaved by plasmin into two fragments, D, and E, without any common antigenic determinant. Cazenave and Oudin injected a rabbit with complete fibrinogen and separated its anti-D and anti-E antibodies. These antibodies did not cross-react but shared the same idiotype determinants (although their molecular distribution was slightly different).

*Human Serum Albumin System.* The human serum albumin system is similar to the previous one. Lapresle showed that using cathepsin D, albumin fragments without common antigenic determinant could be obtained (see p. 144). When using the complete molecule, anti-albumin antisera contain antibodies directed against the three fragments, which, once again, bear the same idiotype determinants.

These results are completely different from what can be observed when two antigens are simultaneously injected. These unexpected results (which Jerne called the "Oudin-Cazenave paradox") are poorly understood. One can postulate that the antigen molecule is recognized as a whole at the beginning of antigenic stimulation. However this is in contradiction with the clonal theory (see chap. 19) which says that lymphocytes are precommitted to recognize a single antigenic determinant. Obviously the idiotypic marker shared by the two populations of antibodies of different specificities should not be present on the combining sites. Jerne rephrased the problem when he described his "network theory" (see chap. 19), but no clear explanation has been found yet.

### IDIOTYPY OF T-CELL RECEPTORS

In Rajewsky's laboratory, it was shown that guinea pig serum directed against A/J antibodies which recognize group A streptococcal carbohydrate, or directed against BALB/c myeloma protein which bind the same antigen, stimulate B precursor cells as well as T helper cells when injected into mice of the appropriate strain. In Wigzell's laboratory, it was shown that in rats, anti-idiotype antibodies raised against specific antigen-binding T-cell receptors which bind a rat histocompatibility antigen can react with IgG antibodies sharing the same specificity. Furthermore, this antireceptor-idiotype can be used to stain B and T cells, or, in combination with complement, to kill the relevant T cells involved in the specific MLC or GvH reactions. These experiments (see p. 86) suggest that T-cell receptors share the same (or part of the same) V regions as the immunoglobulins that are present on the B-cell surface or in the plasma.

Recently, anti-idiotype sera were also used to investigate the cellular mechanism of suppression. These important data will be discussed in greater detail in chapter 18.

# V- AND C-REGION POLYMORPHISM: ALLOTYPY

About twenty years ago, the polymorphism of genes that code for immuno-globulins was described, independently from one another, by Oudin in rabbits and Grubb in man. Within the same animal species and upon proper immu-nization, some individuals can recognize immunoglobulin determinants of other individuals as being nonself. These specificities are called "allotype markers" in contrast to isotype markers, which are common to all individuals of the same species. Using antiallotype antisera, the hereditary transmission of these spec-ificities can be studied. They segregate in a simple mendelian manner, like codominant alleles of the same autosomal locus.

Allotype specificities have been described for heavy as well as for light chains, for constant regions, and occasionally, for variable regions. The discovery of the $V_H - C_H$ linkage (see above) became possible because $C_H$ markers, the allotype determinants, were available.

## Allotypy of Rabbit Immunoglobulins

In his initial experiment, which demonstrated rabbit allotypy, Oudin immunized an animal with an antigen-antibody precipitate from an antiserum provided by another rabbit. Antiallotype antibodies can also be prepared from animals of different species, but it is necessary then to eliminate from the antiserum those antibodies directed against isotype determinants.

Gel analysis of the precipitation zones formed by a combination of antial-lotype antibodies and of serum Ig from various rabbits has revealed six main allotype specificities. Oudin noted that these specificities correspond to two groups of three specificities and that a single rabbit never exhibited more than two specificities of the same group. In other words, these two groups represent two series of three alleles that belong to two distinct loci controlling two types of allotypic specificity. They were designated Aa1, Aa2, and Aa3 for the allotype specificities of the a series and Ab4, Ab5, and Ab6 for the allotype specificities of the b series. We shall see that a-series specificities are borne by the heavy chains and that those of the b series are carried by light chains.

### LIGHT-CHAIN ALLOTYPES

*Location of b-Series Specificities on κ Chains.*   In addition to specificities b4, b5, and b6, specificity b9 has been found. All of these specificities are located on κ chains, as well on κA as on κB. Immunologic studies suggest that several allotype determinants are present on the same light chain. Recent analyses in Hood's laboratory of the $C_κ$ sequences of homozygous b4 and b9 rabbits have shown that the corresponding C-gene sequences differ by 33 bases and 3 nucleotide gaps out of 330 positions. The origin of these complex allelic differences remains speculative.

*Location of C-Series Specificities on λ Chains: Allotypic Suppression.*   C7 and C21 specificities have been described for rabbit λ chains. In order to study the location of these determinants, some authors have attempted to increase the λ chain concentration by using the "allotypic suppression" technique described by Dray (1962). An example of this technique is to inject a homozygous b5 pregnant rabbit or its homozygous newborn with an anti-b5 serum. The b5 chains disappear from the offspring serum or remain at an extremely low level, whereas the total concentration of light chains does not vary because of increased synthesis of "b-negative" chains, that is, of $\lambda$ chains (we shall discuss this phenomenon again in chap. 18, p. 548, in connection with suppressor T cells). As a result, it was possible to show that C7 and C21 specificities are probably located in $C_\lambda$ regions; however, the precise number of $\lambda$ isotypes is not known. $V\lambda$ regions are very variable and have not been studied sufficiently; it is not known whether they possess allotypes.

### HEAVY-CHAIN ALLOTYPES

*Location of A-Series Specificities on $V_H$ regions.*    Studies of amino acid composition of $\gamma$ chains by M. Koshland and sequence studies have enabled the location of the a allotypes in $V_H$ regions. We have already emphasized the difficulties involved in analyzing a mixture of polypeptide chains. This observation is particularly significant when studying rabbit $V_H$ regions, because it is extremely difficult to determine what is due to allotypes or to possible subgroups or simply to variability. Porter's group found several variable positions associated with allotype specificities in the 34 amino-terminal residues (regions 15–18 and 27–29, in particular). In addition, differences associated with Aa1 and Aa3 specificities have been described in residues 80–85. However, when examining antibody chains of limited heterogeneity, Jaton did not confirm some of these correlations, particularly those for residues 80–85. These discrepancies illustrate the difficulties encountered when interpreting this complex system.

The multiplicity of IgG antigenic determinants that are precipitated by antiallotype antisera agrees with the multiplicity of substitutions in sequences. Two nonprecipitating anti-Aa1 sera, for example, may yield a mixture which precipitates Aa1 allotypes.

*Notion of Variants of Allotype Specificities.*    As early as 1960, Oudin reported that anti-a2 antisera were able to detect two distinct a2 families of molecules (i.e., a'2 and a''2), which appeared to have the same genetic determinism and which were always in the same relative concentration in all the tested sera. Recent studies in different laboratories (Cazenave, Dray, Mage) have yielded this very observation through the analysis of cross-reactions between the patterns of the a series. Cross-reactions of the a1 specificity with some anti-a3 sera, for example, allowed Brezin to describe six variants of this specificity. Each specificity of the a or b series is a family of variants, which always occurs together in a given serum; thus, a and b loci are complex loci composed of several cistrons (Fig. 7.28).

*The Todd Phenomenon.*    In 1963, when the concept of variable and constant regions had not yet been proposed, allotypy of the a series brought a major contribution to the understanding of the structural basis of antibody diversity. Todd showed that allotypes of this series were found on both IgG and IgM molecules. This observation, later extended to IgA and IgM, seemed paradoxical at first because these allotype markers were borne by isotype-specific chains. The "Todd phenomenon" was the first demonstration that the pool of $V_H$ regions could associate at random with the various $C_H$ regions.

Allotypic suppression experiments, analogous to thhose described above for the b series, were performed with the a series. When studying $a^-$ chains, Kim and Dray found two other sets of specificities $x^{32}/x^{32-}$ and $y^{33}/y^{33-}$, which are encoded by two independent $V_H$ loci called x and y.

*Location of Specificities of Other Series in $C_H$ Regions.* Several allotypes of constant regions have been found on $C_\gamma$ regions: the d locus corresponds to A11 and A12 specificities (Thr/Ser permutations in position 229), and the e locus corresponds to A14 and A15 specificities (Thr/Ala permutations in position 309). Two other specificities, A8 and A10, could be linked to the structure of the carbohydrate moiety of the molecule, as well as a third specificity, Xg, found independently of the previous ones.

Two allotypes, n81 and n82, located on $\mu$ chains have been described by Dray. Certain data suggest that the n locus might have other alleles for which no reagents are yet available. Other specificities (Ms) have been described by Kellus et al., but the possibility of their relationship with specificities of the n locus has not yet been examined.

Two loci, f and g, associated with two subclasses have been described on $\alpha$ chains; the f locus has three alleles, specificities f71, f72, and f73, and the g locus has two alleles, specificities g74 and g75.

### PROBLEMS LINKED TO ALLOTYPIC EXPRESSION AND GENETICS

*Allelic Exclusion.* In a heterozygous animal, there is never a hybrid Ig that bears two specificities of the same locus on its heavy or light chains. This phenomenon, first described in 1963 by Dray and Nisonoff for $b_4$ $b_5$ rabbit IgG (Fig. 7.27), also applies to other loci. As a result, an animal that is genetically $a_1a_2$, $b_4b_5$ can only have the following allotypes:

$$a_1a_1, b_4b_4 \quad a_1a_1, b_5b_5 \quad a_2a_2, b_4b_4 \quad a_2a_2, b_5b_5$$

Through immunofluorescence techniques it has also been shown that plasma cells do not synthesize more than one allotypic specificity per locus (see pp. 82 and 562). This allelic exclusion, or functional haploidy, supports the clonal theory, according to which one cell synthesizes only one Ig type.

*Genetic Linkage and Recombinations.* Studies of allotypic inheritance within various rabbit families have shown that specificities of the a, b, and c series are not linked and segregate independently. It is possible that these three loci are borne by different chromosomes.

Conversely, the d, e, n, f, and g loci, which code for the $C_H$ regions, are linked with one another and with the a locus. The $V_H$ region loci, a, x, and y, are also associated. As a result, there is a set of $V_H$-$C_H$ genes that are linked together on the same chromosome. Such a system forms what is called a "translocation group." Results obtained with light chains suggest the existence of two other translocation groups in the rabbit genome (Fig. 7.28).

Some rare cases of recombination have been described in $C_H$ loci with a recombination frequency of 0.4%. The distance between variable and constant genes can be compared with that separating the first and second subloci of the H-2 region in the mouse (1.4% recombination) and the HLA region in man (0.8% recombination).

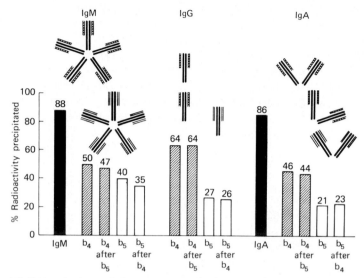

**Fig. 7.27**  Allelic exclusion of the b locus on IgM, IgG and IgA. All immunoglobulins come from rabbits which are b4b5 heterozygous at he κ locus. In the initial experiment of Dray and Nisonoff (1963), 97% to 99% of the $^{125}$I-IgG are precipitable by a goat antirabbit IgG antiserum; 64% are precipitable by an anti-b4 serum and 27% are precipitable by an anti-b5 serum. Specific precipitation of an allotype does not modify the proportion of the other allotype still present in the supernatant. In other words, there is no individual b4b5 molecule. IgM or IgA yield the same result. (From R. G. Mage et al., *In* B. Amos, Ed., Progress in immunology, New York,1971, Academic Press, p. 47.)

## Allotypy of Human Immunoglobulins

Generally speaking, human allotypes cannot be detected by means of precipitation reactions because of the small number of determinants that define allotype specificities. This explains why passive hemagglutination inhibition is frequently used. The specificities that have been described are located exclusively on the constant regions of light and heavy chains.

### INV MARKERS OF κ CHAINS

In Ropartz's and Steinberg's laboratories the alleles of a locus coding for the $C_κ$ regions have been described. The probe into the structural basis of these allotype determinants is an interesting example of analysis, in that it requires immuno-chemical data as well as knowledge of the primary and tertiary structures of light chains. The Inv(1) and Inv(3) specificities represent two alleles, but among caucasians, L chains with Inv(1) specificity are associated in 98% of cases with another specificity, Inv(2). A comparative analysis of the sequences of Inv(1,2) and Inv(3) chains has shown a Leu/Val substitution at position 191, which corresponds to a single base difference in the DNA. When analyzing a rare κ chain, Inv(1, -2, -3), C. Milstein found at position 153 a Val/Ala difference with the sequence of Inv(1,2) chains; this substitution also corresponds to a single base change per codon. The three known allotypes are as follows:

| Inv | Residues | |
|---|---|---|
| | 153 | 191 |
| 1,2,-3 | Ala | Leu |
| -1,-2,3 | Ala | Val |
| 1,-2,-3 | Val | Leu |

A fourth possible sequence, Val, Val, has not been described. The three-dimensional structure of several $C_\lambda$ domains is known; the amino acids that form the Kern and Oz markers, at positions 154 and 190 respectively, are located at the outside angles of the polypeptide chain (Fig. 7.9). The side chains of residues in homologous positions $\kappa 153$ and $\kappa 191$ could thus be separated by a distance of 4 nm.

The anti-Inv(1) antiserum recognizes the Leu 191 residue independently of the residue at position 153.

The anti-Inv(2) antiserum recognizes neither the Leu 191 nor the Ala 153 residue but recognizes the complete set Ala,Leu (153,191).

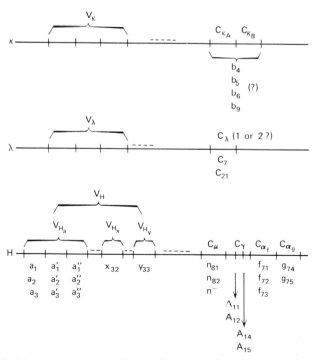

**Fig. 7.28** Tentative arrangement of the three translocation groups in rabbits. V-C genetic linkage has only been found in the case of heavy chains, since no markers have been located on $V_\kappa$ or $V_\lambda$ regions. $a_1$, $a_1'$, $a_1''$, etc., indicate variants of the a series; however, their total number is not shown. (After M. Fougereau, Elements d'immunologie fondamentale, Paris, 1975. Masson, p. 122.)

The anti-Inv(3) antiserum could recognize the Val 191 residue, but one cannot dismiss the possibility that it also recognizes the complete Ala,Val (153,191) set; in this respect, the allotype of the Val 153 and Val 191 κ chains would have to be known, assuming that the corresponding gene would exist.

There is no known allotype on human λ chains.

## HEAVY-CHAIN MARKERS

The first series of markers to be described was that of the Gm system (Grubb); each γ isotype bears a series of Gm specificities, which segregate like a simple mendelian trait. These markers correspond to a limited number of substitutions, for example:

| γ1 chain | 214 | Arg/Lys | Gm(4)/Gm($-$4) |
|---|---|---|---|
|  | 356–358 | Asp-Glu-Leu Glu-Glu-Met | Gm(1)/Gm($-$1) |
| γ3 chain | 296 | Phe/Tyr | Gm(5)/Gm(21) |
| γ4 chain | 309–311 | Val-Leu-His | Gm(4a)/Gm(4b) |
|  | 309–310 | Val/His |  |

In addition, with the $IgA_2$ isotype, allotype specificities have been described on the α2 heavy chain: Am(1)/Am($-$1).

### PROBLEMS ASSOCIATED WITH ALLOTYPE GENETICS

*Translocation Groups.* Genes which code for γ1, γ2, and γ3 and for α2 chains are closely linked. The γ4 gene is also thought to belong to this group, but a definitive, experimental proof has not yet been furnished. Structural genes of heavy chains (Gm markers) are linked to structural genes of α-1-antitrypsin (Pi markers). There is no link between Gm and Inv factors. These data confirm the theory of three independent translocation groups, as shown in Fig. 7.29.

*Recombinations.* One of the most important arguments in favor of linkage of $C_\gamma 1$-$C_\gamma 3$ genes is based upon serum analysis of an individual living in a closed religious community (Steinberg). The Fab fragments of his immunoglobulins share the γ3 chain markers, while the Fc fragments share the γ1 chain markers. In other words, a recombination between $C_\gamma 1$ and $C_\gamma 3$ genes has occurred. Another hybrid case, γ2-γ4, has been reported. Two conclusions may be drawn:

It is possible to propose the following probable order of $C_H$ genes on the chromosome: γ1, γ3, γ2, γ4, and α2.

There is only one copy of each $C_H$ gene on a given chromosome. If there were several copies of the same genes, normal γ1 and γ3 chains would have been found in the serum studied by Steinberg.

The low incidence of recombinations confirms these conclusions. These arguments are important when determining the number of genes necessary for antibody synthesis.

Certain cases of collective inheritance of markers which would normally be allelic, for example, specificities Gm(1,2,17) and Gm(-1,3), can be explained by

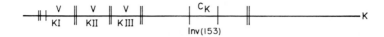

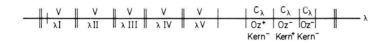

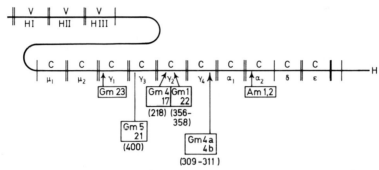

**Fig. 7.29** Tentative arrangement of the three human translocation groups. It shows the position of certain allotype specificities of the heavy chains (numbers in parentheses indicate the position of the corresponding amino acid substitutions). Each subgroup is shown by a single cistron. This represents the minimum number of genes required for V region synthesis. However, it must be noted that a subgroup in such a diagram may represent a family of related cistrons. (After J. E. Gally, *In* M. Sela, Ed., The antigens, New York, 1973, Academic Press.)

assuming that after unequal recombination, a chromosome possesses two copies of the same gene, in this case γ1. Similarly, total absence of certain Gm specificities in some individuals could be explained by the loss of a gene, which is due to this very mechanism of unequal crossing over.

*Allotypy: Structural or Regulatory Genes?* Rivat, Gilbert, and Ropartz (1970) cultured lymphocytes in vitro from individuals with known allotypes. They then searched for Gm factors on Ig excreted in the culture medium. In several cases, Gm specificities, which had not been detected on serum Ig, were found in the cultures. The authors explained this unexpected result by theorizing that an individual possesses all of the information necessary for synthesizing all Gm markers; the apparent Mendelian segregation of allotypes would be due to the polymorphism of regulatory genes.

More recent findings by Strosberg would confirm this hypothesis: after hyperimmunization of a heterozygous rabbit, b4b5a1a3, the specificities b4b5b6 and a1a2a3 were found in its serum. The hypothesis of regulatory gene allelism more easily explains the origin of multiple amino acid interchanges found between polypeptide chains of different allotype (i.e., b4 and b9 rabbit κ chains).

However, this does not explain the allelic exclusion; instead, the problem has now shifted to another set of genes, and new constraints are imposed upon any other explanation of this phenomenon. The superimposing of a double gene polymorphism at regulatory and structural loci is also possible.

### Allotypy of Mouse Immunoglobulin

Eight different isotypes have been described in mice: IgG1, IgG2a, IgG2b, IgG3, IgA, IgM, IgD and IgE. The constant regions of heavy chains $\gamma$2a, $\gamma$2b, $\alpha$, and $\gamma$1 have eleven, six, five and three alleles, respectively. The genes, which code for these four $C_H$ regions, are closely linked on the same chromosome. In 1976, two series of allotypes, encoded by the $\delta$ and $\mu$ loci, have been described. Certain allotype specificities have been selected in inbred strains. Eleven linkage groups have been described for $C_H$ regions. No case of recombination of these allelic series through interbreeding of mice of different strains has ever been reported. However, a few rare cases of recombination have been observed between wild mice living in different regions.

Formal genetic analysis in vivo has not yet enabled the localization of $C_H$ genes into any known linkage group. However, it is recognized that an association exists between the Ig-1-locus coding for the $C_H$ regions and two other loci, one of which codes for prealbumin, whereas the other controls the anti-sheep red blood cell response (Biozzis). Observing the segregation of parental chromosomes during the study of somatic genetics in murine hybridomas, Hengartner and his colleagues (1978) demonstrated that the genes coding for the $C_H$ and C$\kappa$ regions lay within chromosomes 12 and 6 respectively.

No allotypic marker has been described for the $V_H$ and $C_\kappa$ region. On the other hand, structural differences in the $V_\kappa$ region have been observed for normal immunoglobulin light chains (Gottlieb) or specific antibodies (De Preval). These biochemical markers are found only in certain species of mice and are genetically linked to the chromosome 6 at the Ly 3 locus, which codes for T-cell differentiation antigens. Thus, it is possible that a degree of polymorphism exists at the locus that codes for the $V_\kappa$ genes.

There is no known allotype in mice for $\lambda$1 or $\lambda$2 light chains. The presence of two $\lambda$ translocation groups, $V_\lambda$I-$C_\lambda$1 and $V_\lambda$II-$C_\lambda$2, now seems to best describe our genetic and structural knowledge of these chains (Geckeler).


# VI.   IMMUNOGLOBULIN METABOLISM

Ig metabolism has been largely studied using immunoglobulin molecules that are radiolabeled (e.g., by $^{125}$I) and whose isotype is known. A summary of the results of these studies is found in Table 7.7. Ig have a metabolism similar to that of other plasma proteins, with an increase in catabolism during hyperthermia. There are, however, significant differences among the isotypes. IgG has a halflife that is ten times that of IgE (22.5 and 2.5 days). The knowledge of a given Ig serum level does not enable a ready assessment of its synthesis rate. The relationship between degradation rate and serum concentration depends upon the Ig class. Degradation of IgG increases at higher serum concentrations,

**Table 7.7    Metabolic Characteristics of Human Immunoglobulins**

| Properties | IgG | IgA | IgM | IgD | IgE |
|---|---|---|---|---|---|
| Serum concentration (mg/ml) | 12.1 | 2.5 | 0.93 | 0.023 | 0.0003 |
| Half-life (days) | 22.5 | 5.8 | 5.1 | 2.8 | 2.5 |
| Intravascular percentage | 45.0 | 42.0 | 80.0 | 75.0 | 51.0 |
| Rate of synthesis (mg/kg of body weight per day) | 33.0 | 24.0 | 6.7 | 0.4 | 0.016 |
| Catabolism rate (percent of intravascular pool breakdown per day) | 6.7 | 25.0 | 18.0 | 37.0 | 89.0 |

IgG1, IgG2, and IgG4 have the same half-life (23 days) but that of IgG3 is shorter (8 to 9 days). The half-life of IgG is 5 to 6 days in the rabbit, 7 days in the rat, and 7 to 9 days in the guinea pig. After Waldmann.

thus insuring a sort of autoregulation of IgG serum levels with catabolism decreasing at lower serum concentrations. However, this relationship is not a rule; IgA and IgM degradation is not affected by serum concentrations; IgD and IgE catabolism increases when serum concentrations are lower. The study of metabolism of Ig fragments shows that Fab fragments and light chains have a very short halflife (less than 24 hr) while Fc fragments have a lifespan comparable to that of intact IgG. Finally, it is interesting to note that more than half of the IgG and IgA molecules are extravascular, whereas IgM, IgD, and IgE molecules are largely intravascular. (These differences cannot be explained by mere differences in molecular weight).

## VII.  PHYLOGENY AND ONTOGENY OF IMMUNOGLOBULINS

We have seen that the evolution of Ig probably occurred through serial gene duplications. As a result, a certain number of domains emerged, probably selected for their distinct functions. It is possible even today to study Ig molecular evolution in primitive species. Such a "horizontal" comparison might be able to reveal the significant stages of "vertical" evolution (appearance of antibody function and of multichain structure, evolution of domains, etc.)

Certain invertebrates have inducible agglutinins or antibacterial substances, but these molecules are not really analogous to Ig (i.e., they are nonspecific and their production cannot be paralyzed). However, reactions that are analogous to those of cell-mediated immunity in mammals have been described in certain invertebrates, including xenograft or allograft rejection. This suggests that T cell-linked immunity emerged prior to B cell-mediated immunity (Fig. 7.30).

All vertebrates reject allografts and have circulating lymphocytes and circulating antibodies. The development of the immune system is seen as progressive among vertebrate classes. Cyclostomes (hagfish, lamprey) synthesize antibodies, but complement fixation on antigen-antibody complexes does not appear until the emergence of elasmobranches (dogfish, shark). Classes which are more advanced than cyclostomes begin to show thymus and spleen primordia (Table 7.8).

**Table 7.8  Emergence of the Characteristics of the Immune System in Vertebrates**

| Class | Lympho-cyte | Plasma cell | Thymus | Spleen | Lymph node | Bursa of Fabricius | Anti-bodies | Allograft rejection |
|---|---|---|---|---|---|---|---|---|
| Tunicates* | + (?)† | – | – | – | – | – | ? | + (?) |
| Cyclostomes | | | | | | | | |
|   Lamprey | + | – | Prim‡ | Prim | – | – | + | + |
|   Hagfish | + | – | ND§ | ND | – | – | + | + |
| Elasmobranchs | | | | | | | | |
|   Primitive | + | – | + | + | – | – | + | + |
|   Advanced | + | + | + | + | – | – | + | + |
| Holosteans (bowfin) | + | + | + | + | – | – | + | + |
| Chondrosteans (paddlefish) | + | + | + | + | – | – | + | + |
| Teleostei | + | + | + | + | – | – | + | + |
| Dipnoi | + | (+) | + | + | – | – | + | + |
| Amphibians | | | | | | | | |
|   Urodeles | + | + | + | + | – | – | + | + |
|   Anurans | + | + | + | + | + (?) | – | + | + |
| Reptiles | + | + | + | + | + (?) | + (?) | + | + |
| Aves | + | + | + | + | + (?) | + | + | + |
| Mammals | | | | | | | | |
|   Prototheria | + | + | + | + | + (?) | + (Eq.)¶ | + | + |
|   Metatheria | + | + | + | + | + | + (Eq.) | + | + |
|   Eutheria | + | + | + | + | + | + (Eq.) | + | + |

* Tunicates represent a protochord subphylum of chordates. All other groups represent vertebrate classes.
† Structures have been described but their exact homology with lymphoid structures is not clearly established.
‡ Primitive.
§ Not detected.
¶ Presence of lymphoid structure that might serve as an equivalent.
From J. J. Marchalonis and R. E. Cone, Aust. J. Exp. Biol. Med. Sci. 1973, 51, 461.

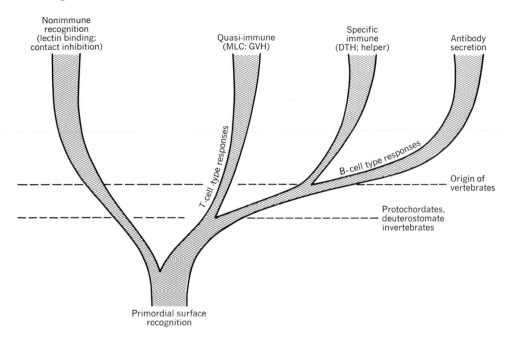

**Fig. 7.30** Emergence of cells involved in immune reactions. (After J. J. Marchalonis, *In* L. Brent and J. Holborow, Eds., Progress in immunology, II, Vol. 2, Amsterdam, 1974, North Holland, p. 249.)

### Evolution of Variable Regions

Even in the most primitive vertebrates circulating antibodies have very heterogeneous variable regions. The study of known partial sequences indicates that the variability mechanism was already established in phyla, which diverged 300 million years ago. The primary structure of $V_L$ regions in both elasmo-branches (shark) and primates (man) shows homologies in the aminoterminal region. It is clear that homologies exist among the $V_H$ regions of various vertebrate species, including elasmobranches (paddlefish and shark). These results seem to suggest that the emergence of Ig is due to their most basic characteristic, namely their recognition function.

Analysis of $V_H III$ subgroups shows that their structure is particularly conserved among various species. As we have seen, this finding allowed Bourgois to propose, on the basis of intra-$V_H$ homologies, that the size of the Ig ancestral gene was half of that of a V cistron. Structural considerations suggest, however, that according to this hypothesis, only a dimer could have had an immunological function.

### Evolution of Constant Regions

Cyclostome antibodies have a multichain structure, 2L + 2H. The size of the single heavy chain is similar to that of human $\mu$ chains. Between the two chains or between $L_2\mu_2$ subunits of lamprey, disulfide bridges have not been found. With elasmobranches, in which a single IgM-like class is also found, there appear interchain and intersubunit disulfide bridges, in addition to a J-like chain. The level of polymerization $(L_2\mu_2)n$ varies with vertebrate class but remains constant within a given class. These $\mu$-like heavy chains, made up of one variable domain and four constant domains, have been found in all vertebrates studied so far.

With the emergence of dipnoies, there appear several antigenically distinct classes, 19S and 5.7S. The $\gamma$-like heavy chains seem to have only two constant domains and one variable domain. A homologous H chain is found in reptiles (tortoise) and birds (duck), but this chain does not seem to exist in mammals (even though a similar chain type might exist in the rabbit).

Amphibians, reptiles, and birds synthesize multiple classes of immunoglobulins that contain identical L chains but class-specific H chains. However, their $\gamma$-like heavy chains differ in a number of properties from the mammalian $\gamma$ chains. The $C_\gamma$ gene found in all three existant groups of mammals (Protherians, Metatherians and Eutherians) should have emerged only in the therapside line of reptiles, which was ancestral to all three mammalian lines.

We have seen that the structural relationship is not equal among all the isotypes. Division of classes into subclasses (see p. 198) reflects the larger homologies of some C regions (e.g., the human chains $\gamma1$ to $\gamma4$ or $\lambda$ Kern$\pm$/ Oz$\pm$).

These homologies are greater among subclasses of a single species than among subclasses of different species. Therefore, duplications that produced these subclasses must be recent and must have emerged after speciation.

### Problems Associated with the Origin of Histocompatibility Antigens

The structure of histocompatibility antigens (see chap. 25) shows striking analogies with the structure of Ig. Both are membrane-bound macromolecules. They are symmetric multichain proteins made up of domains of about 100 amino acids, including an intrachain disulfide bridge. Peterson et al. were first to suggest (Fig. 7.31) that HLA antigens in man and H-2 antigens in mice consist of two chains, one which contains a single constant domain, the $\beta_2$-microglobulin, and the other which contains three domains, one of which bearing carbohydrate moiety and at least one other being highly polymorphic, thus explaining various histocompatibility specificities. The primary sequence of human $\beta_2$microglobulin shows clear homologies with the $C_H3$ domain of IgG1. The complete sequence of HLA-A and HLA-B heavy chains are known (Strominger et al.) as the complete sequence of one H-$2^k$ heavy chain (Nathenson et al.). These three polypeptides show striking homologies (some stretches show 80–95% homology, while the others show at least 50%). Thus, human and mouse histocompatibility antigens have a common structural ancestor and have not evolved very much after speciation. However, homology of each of these three chains with IgG regions is very weak. If one considers the domains of HLA heavy chains, only the third one shows some degree of homology with Ig $C_H$ domains. The first two domains do not present any homology with Ig molecules nor with any other known human proteins. Thus, if the ancestral genes coding for human Ig and HLA domains were related, it would imply that the first two HLA domains evolved very rapidly under selective forces which

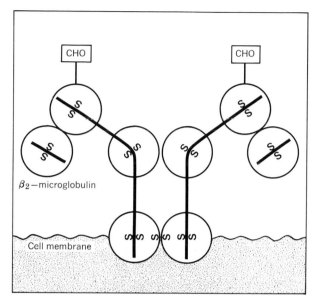

**Fig. 7.31** Molecular structure of HLA antigens. Note the striking homology between this multichain models of histocompatibility antigens and the multichain model of IgC. The heavy chain contains three domains, at least one of which must vary from one antigenic type to the other. The light chain referred to as $\beta_2$-microglobulin, is constant for all antigens of the same species. (After P. A. Peterson.)

did not influence the evolution of $C_H$ genes. In summary, the homology between $\beta_2$-microglobulin, HLA and $C_H$ domains, whatever its actual degree, argues in favor of a common origin of major histocompatibility antigens and Ig; the first system would provide "self" markers, and the second would preserve their integrity.

Figure 7.32 summarizes the emergence of the various chains related to the Ig system.

### Immunoglobulin Ontogeny

Ig production has not matured at birth. At the end of fetal life, there are lymphocytes which bear membrane Ig, such as IgM and IgD (see p. 000). However, no IgG production is yet detectable, and IgM and IgA levels are still very low. The high IgG serum levels found during the first weeks of life are of maternal origin (Table 7.9). IgG are not produced until 2 months after birth, that is, after the disappearance of maternal IgG. Toward the age of 3 months, there is a period of a few weeks during which IgG serum levels are very low (Fig. 7.33). IgM production is the first to reach adult levels, followed by IgG, and much later by IgA and IgE (Table 7.10). It is interesting to note that the increase in production of these various Igs is affected by infections, as shown by the slow development of Ig production in axenic animals and, conversely, the excessively rapid Ig production in children infected in utero.

**Table 7.9  Concentrations of Different Immunoglobulin Classes According to Age**

| Age | IgG (mg/100 ml) | IgA (mg/100 ml) | IgM (mg/100 ml) | IgD (mg/100 ml) | IgE (units/ml)* |
|---|---|---|---|---|---|
| Newborn | 1359 ± 268 | — | 10 ± 5 | — | 1,6 (0.7–3.4)† |
| 6 months | 453 ± 203 | 16 ± 9 | 54 ± 20 | — | 16 (4.2–60) |
| 5 to 6 years | 960 ± 311 | 101 ± 62 | 76 ± 34 | 1.1 ± 0.7 | 65 (21–198) |
| 13 to 15 years | 1470 ± 386 | 133 ± 87 | 84 ± 30 | 3.6 ± 3.7 | 86 (12–618) |

* It has been recommended that IgE concentrations be expressed in international units (IU), defined in relation to a standard OMS reference preparation from the World Health Organziation (one unit corresponds approximately to 2 ng).
† 95% confidence level.
After Outcherlony and Nilsson.

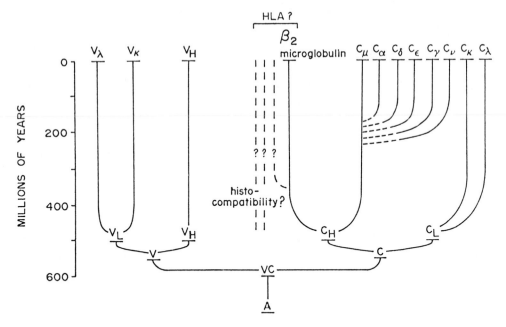

**Fig. 7.32** Hypothetical diagram of the evaluation of cistrons coding for polypeptide chains.

This diagram, adapted from Marchalonis incorporates the theory of Bourgois, who suggests that an ancestral gene coding for half a domain existed. It also incorporates the conclusion of Peterson, who assumes that $\beta_2$-microglobulin and $C_H$ domains have a common origin. The origin of histocompatibility antigens is still speculative.

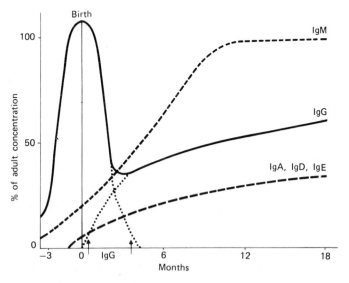

**Fig. 7.33** Evolution of immunoglobulin serum levels in the human fetus and newborn. (After I. Roitt, Essential Immunology, Oxford, 1973, Blackwell, p. 56.)

**Table 7.10   Transmission of Various Classes of Maternal Antibodies of Offspring in Various Species**

| Species | Route of transmission | Class of antibody transmitted | Principal period of transmission | Contribution to antimicrobial defense |
|---|---|---|---|---|
| Man | Placenta | Mostly IgG | Last trimester | ++++ |
| | Intestine (colostrum) | IgA | First few days of life | Probably affords some protection to gastrointestinal tract |
| Rat | Yolk sac | IgG | — | ++ |
| | Intestine (colostrum and milk) | ? | 20 Days | +++ |
| Cow | Placenta | None | — | − |
| | Intestine (colostrum) | All? | First 24 to 48 hr | ++++ |
| Pig | Placenta | None | — | − |
| | Intestine (colostrum) | All? | First 24 hr | ++++ |
| Chicken | Yolk sac | All? | Last 4 days before hatching | ++++ |

# VIII.   ORGANISATION AND EXPRESSION OF IMMUNOGLOBULIN GENES

Recent progress in the sphere of molecular biology and genetic engineering has opened an entirely new chapter in the physiology and genetics of eukaryotes. Two examples will serve to show briefly the type of strategy employed in the cloning of murine DNA fragments containing V or C genes.

Tonegawa and his coworkers, using a restriction enzyme, cleaved DNA from embryonic cells or plasmocytomas. The fragments were then separated according to their size by agarose electrophoresis. Those fragments which were able to hybridize with a messenger RNA purified from a myeloma cell were inserted into a phage DNA opened by means of the restriction enzyme previously used. Leder and coworkers have extracted and purified from a myeloma cell a messenger RNA which they have been able to use to synthesize the complementary DNA using a reverse transcriptase. Subsequently, at each end of double-stranded cDNA were attached short synthetic nucleotide sequences corresponding to the recognition sites for a restriction enzyme. The cDNA thus prepared was inserted into a plasmid by means of the selected restriction enzyme.

These DNA fragments were then amplified, permitting determination of their sequences. Once characterized, they could serve as a probe to enable the analysis of other DNA fragments or could be used to study the reiteration of the V and C genes in the total cellular DNA.

These studies have already given a number of significant results.

Light and heavy chains are synthesized as a single entity in the cytoplasm, and colinearity with the corresponding mRNA species (Fig. 7.34) has been found. However, it was shown that these chains are encoded by sequence of nucleotides (the exons) which are interrupted by nontranslated region (the introns). This is general to all eukaryotic genes but contrasts with the gene-protein colinearity which has been demonstrated for prokaryotes.

## THE V GENES

$V_H$, $V_\kappa$, and $V_\lambda$ genes are found in the genomic DNA on 3 separate clusters, confirming the conclusions of linkage analysis described earlier.

### V genes are Encoded by Several DNA Segments

In the embryo, the DNA sequence coding for the variable region of λ chains is interrupted before the end of the third hypervariable region, around the position corresponding to residue 99. The sequence coding for the dozen aminoacids representing the end of the variable region is found some distance away from the V segment, and 1.2 kilobases (kb) from the C segment. This area is known as the "junction sequence" or "J" sequence. The same type of organisation holds true for the $V_\kappa$ and $V_H$ genes. It has been shown that murine and human genomes include a large set of V genes and on the 3' side to these and the 5' side to the C genes, a limited cluster of J genes. BALB/c and NZB mice possess 5 $J_\kappa$ segments (one of which, $J_3$, has never been found to code for a J polypeptidic region), and probably 4 $J_H$ segments.

When the $V_H$ gene of the IgA myeloma protein S 107 was studied, it was found, by L. Hood and his collegues, that the corresponding $V_H$ germline gene codes for residues 1 to 101 and the $J_H$ gene for residues 107 to 123. These segments do not specify an extremely variable stretch of up to seven aminoacids preceding the $J_H$ segment. Hence the authors have postulated the existence of a new series of DNA segments called "D" for diversity. In Tonegawa's laboratory, 9 contiguous D gene-segments were found between the $V_H$ and $J_H$ loci. The V–D distance is still unknown but D and J sequences were found on a restriction fragment of approximately 50 Kb.

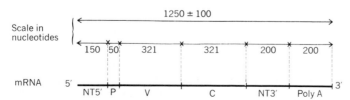

**Fig. 7.34** Structure of messenger RNA of the murine κ chain synthesized by the MOPC 21 tumor. NT 5' and NT 3': nontranslated sequence at the 5' and 3' ends. P: sequence coding for amino acids found in the precursor of the MOPC 21 chain. V and C: the number of nucleotides, is derived from the primary structure of κ chains. (From C. Milstein et al., Nature, Lond., 1974, *252*, 354.)

### V Genes are Created by Somatic Recombination

Restriction enzyme mapping was used to compare embryonic DNA with plasmocytoma DNA. It was seen that the relative positions of the V, J, and C segments differ in the two cells (Fig. 7.35). At the embryonic stage, the V and J regions are clearly separated whereas in the secreting plasmocyte they are joined. However, the introns which may be present in the V or C regions are still present and the J–C intervening sequence is not altered.

One can see that the V–J joining mechanism is a capital event in the development of lymphocytes. For molecular biologists, these DNA rearrangements offer a unique model for studying cellular differentiation.

### Somatic Diversity is Introduced by Combinatorial Junction

When B cell matures, one $V_L$ and one $V_H$ segments are randomly linked to any one of the corresponding $J_L$ and $J_H$ segments. The combinatorial assortment of different $V_\kappa$ with the four $J_\kappa$ segments would give a four-fold increase in the total number of $V_\kappa$ regions. Furthermore, additional variation

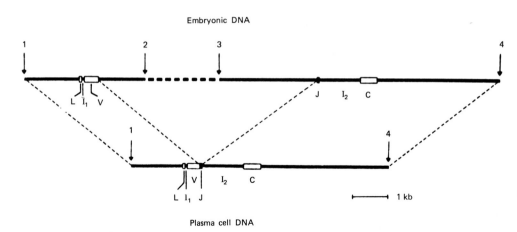

**Fig. 7.35** Arrangement of Mouse $\lambda_1$ Gene Sequences in Embryos and $\lambda_1$ chain-Producing Plasma Cells. In embryo DNA, a full $\lambda_1$ gene sequence consists of two parts that lie on two separate Eco Rl fragments. On one of these fragments, the coding sequence is further split into two parts, one for most of the leader peptides (L) and the other for the rest of the leader peptides plus the variable region peptides (V). The two coding sequences are separated by a 93 nucleotide long intervening sequence ($I_1$). On the second Eco Rl fragment, the coding sequence is also split into two parts by a 1250 base long intervening sequence ($I_2$). The two parts are for the constant region peptides (C) and approximately 13 residue peptides near the junction of the variable and constant regions (J). The relative orientation of and the distance between the two Eco Rl fragments are unknown. In the DNA of a $\lambda_1$ chain-producing myeloma (H 2020), the $\lambda_1$ gene sequence is rearranged as a result of one (or more) recombination(s) that involves sequences in the two embryonic Eco Rl fragments. One recombination takes place at the ends of the V and the J sequences and brings the two sequences into direct contact. The limits of the corresponding sequences in the embryo and the myeloma DNAs are indicated by thin dotted lines. (From C. Brack et al.; Cell, 1978, *15*, 1.)

is introduced at the first $J_\kappa$ codon (residue 96) by alternative recombination within the codon. For example, recombination between $V_\kappa$ MOPC 41 and $J_\kappa 1$ may give rise to three known aminoacid sequences, or recombination with $J_\kappa 2$ may give rise to another known sequence:

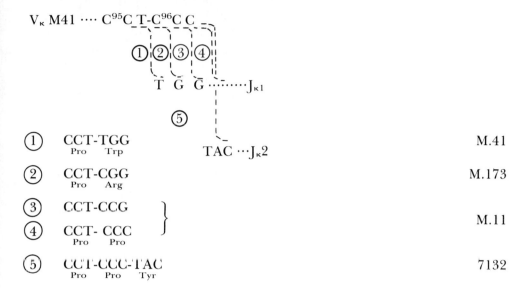

| | | |
|---|---|---|
| ① | CCT-TGG<br>Pro   Trp | M.41 |
| ② | CCT-CGG<br>Pro   Arg | M.173 |
| ③ | CCT-CCG | } M.11 |
| ④ | CCT- CCC<br>Pro   Pro | |
| ⑤ | CCT-CCC-TAC<br>Pro  Pro  Tyr | 7132 |

The 5 $J_\kappa$ segments share on their 5′ flanking regions two signal sequences which are probably involved in the V–J junction (Fig. 7.36): an heptanucleotide palindrome C-A-C-T-G-T-G was found adjacent to each of the first J codon, together with a T rich sequence about 20 nucleotides to its 5′ side. These structures are complementary to inverted repeats next to the germ line V regions on the 3′ side. Their associations are visualized as a stem-like structure (Fig. 7.36) bringing V and J coding sequences in contact when the intervening V and J segments are deleted. In situ hybridization experiments clearly indicate that such deletions occur.

Variability may also be introduced on the $J_H$ regions by alternative recombination which can eliminate the first one or two $J_H$ codons and hence strikingly reduce the length of the last hypervariable region. Base substitutions were also found to alter individual $J_H$ aminoacids.

We have seen above that in germline DNA several D genes are present close to the $J_H$ locus. A D gene is made of three clusters of heptanucleotides separated by intervening sequences of 12 nucleotides each. The basic frame of the heptanucleotides is T-A-$\frac{T}{C}$-G-G-T-A on which a few variations are found.

The three clusters are called L (left), C (Core) and R (right). $L_1C_1R_1$ is adjacent to $L_2C_2R_2$, and so on. The primary structure of the D segments found in proteins vary very much in length; one can reconstruct all these sequences by recombinations of the heptanucleotides. These sequences are made of one C segment and a variable number of L and/or R segments; i.e.: $L_1C_1R_1$, $L_1C_1R_1R_2$, $L_3L_2C_2R_2$, etc... Hence several recombinations generating variability can take place already at the level of the D segment.

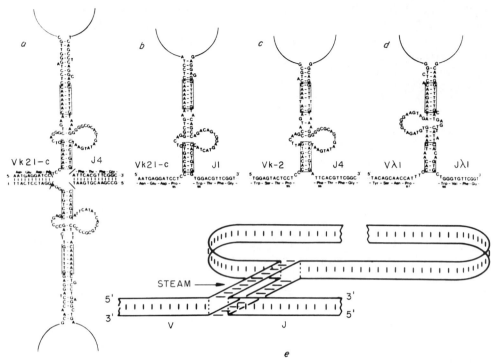

**Fig. 7.36** Inverted repeat stem structures. Inverted repeat stem structures formed between 3'-non-coding regions of embryonic V DNAs and 5'-flanking regions of J DNAs. *a*, V$_\kappa$21-C and J4; *b*, V$_\kappa$21-C and J1; *c*, V$_{\kappa-2}$ and J4; *d* V$_{\lambda I}$ and J$\lambda$I. Except for *a*, sequences for antisense strand have been omitted. Conserved base pairs in the stem, $\frac{CACTGTG}{GTGACAC}$ and $\frac{GTTTTTG}{CAAAAAC}$, are surrounded. Oblique lines in *a* indicate the cleavage sites by a putive recombinase. (From Sakano, et al., Nature, *280*:288, 1979.) (e) is a three-dimensional representation of the hypothetical stem intermediate. V- and J-coding sequences interact with their opposite strands in a normal DNA duplex, but the inverted repeat adjacent to the V gene is drawn as a stem interacting with its complement located on the same strand, presumably many thousands of bases away adjacent to a J sequence. (From Max, et al., Proc. Natl. Acad. Sci. (USA), *76*:3450, 1979.)

### Are the IdX and IdI Idiotypic Determinants Germline or Somatic Markers?

We have seen previously (see p. 214) that monoclonal antidextran antibodies share an IdX determinant made by aminoacids of the second hypervariable region of heavy chains, hence encoded by genes within the V$_H$ gene cluster. The comparison of germline and rearranged V$_H$ sequences would allow formerly to conclude about the germinal origin of this IdX marker.

In addition, some anti dextran antibody molecules carry an IdI determinant which involves the V$_H$ residues 100–101. These positions are extremely variable as shown by sequence data and by the very low frequency of a given IdI within the total antibody population. These two aminoacids may result from the insertion of a D segment. The origin of the IdI determinants would be more difficult to access because of the structure of the D gene segments. The finding of a given IdI in a few BALB/c mice, even in very low amount, indicates that the same pattern of somatic recombinations may have taken place in different clones of dextran specific lymphocytes.

### A Basis for the "Expansion-Contraction" Hypothesis

Flanking sequences may also contribute to generate somatic diversity. A significant observation has been made by Leder and his colleagues in the course of their study on the DNA coding for the $V_\kappa$ region of MOPC 41 and MOPC 149. The nucleotide sequences coding for these two V regions are sufficiently different to prevent their hybridization under the conditions used. However, a strong homology exists in the nontranslated segments adjacent to $V_\kappa$-MOPC 41 and $_\kappa$-MOPC 149, bearing on at least 3000 pairs of bases (i.e. almost nine times the length of the V-region sequence). These authors have proposed the hypothesis that this strong homology between the nontranslated regions favors unequal crossingovers and permits recombination between different variable regions. Such recombinations may bring about the loss or the multiplication of a whole set of V genes in an animal population (see p. 247: the "Expansion-Contraction" Hypothesis). It should be pointed out however that this result is not general, and several other flanking regions of V gene segments do not show such an homology.

## THE C GENES

### One Domain, One Exon

The sequences of genomic DNA coding for mouse γ1, γ2b, γ2a, γ3, α and μ chains are known and those of δ and ε genes are currently under study. Each domain, and the hinge region when there is one, is encoded by an independent exon, which is separated from its neighbour(s) by introns of various sizes (about 60 to 400 bases long). For example, see the top line of Figure 7.38.

Sequence studies of the human λ locus show a new isotypic $C_\lambda$ gene, so far undetected at the protein level (see p. 191.). Analysis of the mouse λ locus demonstrated the presence on DNA of three related C genes, $C_{\lambda1}$, $C_{\lambda11}$ and $C_{\lambda111}$; each one however is part of a separate translocation system, $V_{\lambda1}$-$C_{\lambda1}$, $V_{\lambda11}$-$C_{\lambda11}$, and $V_{\lambda111}$-$C_{\lambda111}$ (but mouse immunoglobulins L chains corresponding to the latter combination were never found).

### The Switch Mechanism Involves DNA Deletions

Among several possible mechanisms for the isotype switch which occurs in a lymphocyte clone, Honjo and Kataoka proposed a deletion model: deletion of DNA shifts the active $V_H$ gene, associated first with $C_\mu$, to another $C_H$ gene. There is now a general agreement, based on various experimental results, that this model is correct. Furthermore the same type of mechanism seems to account for $J_H$ joining and $C_H$ switch. But it should be stressed that signal sequences involved in the V–J junctions are different from signal sequences involved in VJ–C switches. Figure 7.37 summarizes the different steps of

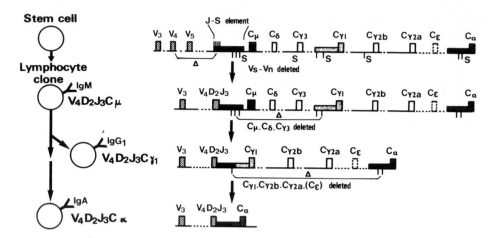

**Fig. 7.37** Mechanism by which a lymphocyte clone switches from expression of one $C_H$ gene to another while maintaining the same V region. The germline H chain locus is shown at the top, and below, the H chain locus in a lymphocyte clone that first expresses IgM and subsequently switches to IgG1 and to IgA. Both V/J joining and $C_H$ switching are mediated by an ~ 6 kb segment of DNA located 5' to the $C_\mu$ gene and designated here as the J–S element. Joining of a particular $V_H$ and $D_H$ gene to one of the four $J_H$ genes towards the 5' end of the J–S element leads to $\mu$ expression. Subsequent deletions attach the expressed $V_H D_H J_H$ gene to the 5' flanking region of another $C_H$ gene. These switch steps occur by recombination between switch sites (S) located within the J–S element and 5' to other $C_H$ genes; the number of switch sites associated with each $C_H$ gene is unknown. Thus an active $\alpha$ gene, for example, is a mosaic of separate $V_H$, $D_H$ J–S and $C_\alpha$ elements. Owing to the deletions, the DNA in each lymphocyte is distinctive, for at least one allele. (Adams J. M., Immunol., Today, *1*:10, 1980.)

lymphocyte activation: the first step would bring together, for example, $V_{H4}$, $D_2$, $J_{H3}$. This would lead to formation of an active $\mu$ gene. Then, interestingly enough, a large segment of the $J_H$–$C_\mu$ intervening sequence shifts with the active V region elements. This segment ends at a switch site "S" which will recombine with another switch site within the flanking region 5' to another $C_H$ gene.

In Figure 7.37, two examples are given: relocation of the active $V_4 D_2 J_3$ gene together with much of the J–S element near $C_\delta 1$ leads to IgG1 expression; if such a switch occurs near the $C_\alpha$ segment, the lymphocyte synthezises IgA molecules. It is known that J–S elements contain more than one switch site and there is suggestive evidence that switching can occur in more than one position with respect to the $C_H$ to be subsequently expressed.

In the example of Figure 7.37, it should be stressed that the DNA segment $J_4$ located between $J_3$ and $C_\mu$ is not deleted. The first RNA transcript within the nucleus will copy all the DNA sequence, including this $J_4$ segment and the untranslated sequences. Then RNA splicing pathways will delete, most probably in several steps, the $J_4$ copy, the untranslated segments between J and C and the introns present within the V and C genes, leading finally an mRNA molecule where all the coding sequences are contiguous from the leader sequence to the last C domain (Fig. 7.34). Using mouse plasmocytomas which have each undertaken a different switch, cross-hybridization experiments between their DNAs and individual cDNA probes coding for the various heavy chain isotypes allows one to propose the following gene order: $\mu$, $\delta$, $\delta3$, $\delta1$, $\delta2b$, $\delta2a$, $\epsilon$ and $\alpha$. The deletion model described above seems verified for physiological switches in B cells. However exceptions were noticed when studying myeloma cells maintained in culture: some switches occurring in selected mutant cells can be explained only by the general mechanism of chromatid recombinations.

### RNA Splicing Pathways Control the Discrimination Between Membrane Bound and Secreted Ig

Biochemical evidence argues in favor of structural differences between secreted IgM (IgMs) and membrane IgM (IgMm) which seems to have a longer $\mu_m$ chain containing an hydrophobic segment at its C-terminal end. However, there is strong evidence that only a single copy of $C_\mu$ gene exists per haploid mouse genome. It has been recently demonstrated that there is indeed only one $C_\mu$ gene but that two $\mu$-mRNA species differing at their 3' end are produced at the posttranscriptional level by alternative processing pathways. Figure 7.38 shows that contiguous to the segment coding for the $C_\mu4$ domain is a segment specific for the $\mu_s$ C-terminal sequence and the $\mu_s$-mRNA 3' non-coding region, while 1.6 kb away are gene segments for the $\mu_m$ C-terminal sequence and the $\mu_m$-mRNA non-coding region. The $\mu_m$-RNA possesses an extra segment coding for 21 aminoacids. This polypeptide segment contains a long stretch of

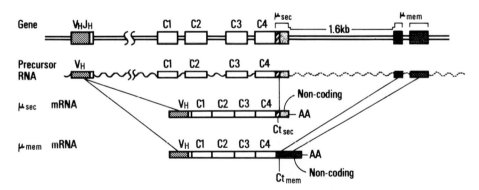

**Fig. 7.38** Distinctive $\mu$ mRNA species encoding secreted (sec) and membrane (mem) $\mu$ polypeptides are generated from a single $C_\mu$ gene by alternative modes of RNA splicing. The 3' terminal portion of the $\mu_{sec}$ mRNA is derived from sequences contiguous with the coding segment (exon) for the fourth $C_\mu$ domain (C4), wheras the 3' terminal portion of the $\mu_{mem}$ mRNA is derived from two exons located about 1.6 kb further downstream. Hence each mRNA species encodes a distinct carboxy-terminal peptide ($C^t$), as well as having a distinct 3' non-coding segment. (The more distal $\mu_{mem}$ exon includes two codons for the $\mu_{mem}$ peptide). Both mRNA species may be derived by alternative modes of RNA splicing from a common nuclear precursor RNA species which spans the $\mu_{mem}$ exons. Alternatively, the $\mu_{sec}$ mRNA may be derived from a shorter transcript which only spans the $\mu_{sec}$ exons. (Schema drawn by Adams J. M., Immunol. Today, 1:10, 1980; from data of Att F. W., et al., Cell, 20:293 (1980); Rogers J., et al. ibid, p. 303; Early P., et al., ibid, p. 313.)

hydrophobic residues involved in the anchorage of the $\mu_m$ chain within the membrane lipid bilayer.

Such exons coding for anchorage polypeptides exist 3′ to the last domain of other heavy chains. This is demonstrated for $C_{\gamma 1}$, $C_{\gamma 2b}$, and $C_{\gamma 2a}$ genes. Therefore this alternative mode of RNA splicing is a general feature of heavy chain synthesis.

### The Simultaneous Expression of $\mu$ and $\delta$ Heavy Chains.

Since deletion is an irreversible event, the V–C translocation discussed above is likely to represent an irreversible commitment of the B cell and its progeny. A clone that has switched from $\mu$ to $\gamma$ cannot revert to the $\mu$ synthesis once the $\mu$-mRNA has been degraded. So, to account for the simultaneous expression of IgM and IgD on the membrane of lymphocytes (see p. 81), recent data suggest that a single nuclear transcript bearing the V, $\mu$, and $\delta$ sequences is made and then spliced in two different ways to generate $\mu$ and $\delta$ mRNAs sharing the same $V_H$ region.

The various RNA splicing pathways of this single nuclear transcript can give rise to 4 different mRNA molecules coding respectively for the IgMm, IgMs, IgDm and IgDs molecules. The single transcript and the 4 types of messenger RNAs have indeed been characterized in several laboratories.

Other cases of lymphocytes secreting two isotypes could be explained either by long lived mRNAs or, perhaps, by a deletion that brings two $C_H$ genes into such proximity that it creates a single transcriptional unit.

### Toward the Understanding of Allelic Exclusion

To approach the problem of allelic exclusion, and the related problem of $\kappa/\lambda$ discrimination, several laboratories have investigated whether the gene rearrangements have taken place on a single or both parental chromosomes. Conflicting results have been obtained so far: in some B cell lines a single chromosome has undergone a V–C recombination, in many other cases both chromosomes are rearranged, and in some tumor lines one allele has clearly rearranged in an aberrant fashion. The use of untransformed cells may bring new insights on this problem: rearrangements were analyzed in lymphocytes from $F_1$ animals possesing two different $C_H$ allogroups. It appears that rearrangements occur randomly on both chromosomes until a functional V–C junction is reached. Rearrangements then stop and biosynthesis can begin. The mechanism which stops the rearrangements when a functional gene is generated is still unknown.

## IX.   GENETIC DETERMINISM OF IMMUNOGLOBULINS

The results of structural and genetic analyses of Ig enable us to examine much deeper the problem of their genetic determinism. First, we will recall those findings which enable us to estimate the number of C and V genes; then, we will examine to what extent the various theories of variability origin take into account the various observations of this chapter.

## Evaluation of the Number of Cistrons Necessary for Antibody Synthesis

The minimum number of cistrons necessary for Ig synthesis can be calculated on the basis of the number of isotypes and variability subgroups. The presence of allotype markers, which allows the study of gene transmission, enables a more precise count. Two studies with respect to the minimum number of genes were presented earlier when we defined translocation groups in man and rabbits (see p. 222; Figs. 7.28 and 7.29).

### A COMPARISON OF V AND C GENE EVOLUTION

The ongoing evolution of isotypes is illustrated by the recent duplication of human $C_\lambda$ genes, and by the fact that the number of $C_H$ subclasses is not the same in each species. Isotype differences of various $C_H$ regions can be compared to what is known about the evolution of nonimmunoglobulin proteins, such as globins. All immunologists agree with the proposal of Dreyer and Bennett (1965) that in the genome of the various animal species, there is only one cistron per constant region because of the rare recombination rate of their allotypes.

As far as variable regions are concerned, it would seem that recent duplications leading to the emergence of new subgroups occurred after the divergence of the various species, just like they did with respect to C regions. It seems as if each species developed differently its very own set of variable regions. In man, for example, the $V_\kappa$ system is rather simple, but in mice this system is much more complex; the opposite is true for $V_\lambda$ systems. In addition, $V_\kappa/V_\lambda$ ratios are different for any given species.

Similar observations have been made for $V_H$ regions: whereas the three subgroups $V_H I$, $V_H II$, and $V_H III$ are found in comparable proportions (36%, 25%, and 39%, respectively) in man, only the $V_H III$ subgroup appears to exist in cats and dogs.

Each from a different point of view, Milstein and Hood suggested that each species developed or restricted certain parts of the genetic information that it initially contained. This is the so-called "expansion-contraction" mechanism.

### PROBLEMS ASSOCIATED WITH GENE REITERATION IN DNA

For some years now, RNA-DNA hybridization techniques have been used to evaluate the number of genes coding for light and heavy chains on the basis of messenger RNA isolated from myeloma cells. Two techniques may be used for studying DNA-RNA hybridization.

1. mRNA or cDNA are purified and labelled with a radioactive isotope. The kinetics of their reassociation in the presence of a large excess of unlabeled denatured cellular DNA is then followed. To measure the percentage of hybridization, the duplexes are purified to eliminate the single strands and their radioactivity is then counted.

The amount of hybridization is proportionate with the initial concentration of DNA, Co, and with the DNA and RNA incubation time, t: the product of these two values is called "Cot." The plot of the hybridization percentage as a function of the Cot logarithm shows a "transition curve," whose inflection point (Cot 1/2) is proportionate with cistron redundancy: (1) The greater the number of gene copies (i.e., the greater the concentration), the smaller the Cot 1/2. (2) The fewer gene copies are present, the higher the Cot 1/2; in other words, DNA concentration or incubation time must be increased in order to obtain the same hybridization.

2. The quantity of mRNA or cDNA necessary to saturate a given quantity of denatured cellular DNA may be determined.

These two techniques do not lead to the same conclusions. Under the conditions employed for kinetic measurements, a minimum estimate is reached since hybridization between the most complementary nucleotide sequences is favored at the expense of less homologous sequences. This is why molecular biologists prefer to base their calculations on saturation curves; in effect, the sequences of cellular DNA, which possess a restricted homology with that of the radioactive probe, are able to hybridize without competition. Figure 7.39 presents the results of a study of the kinetics of hybridization between the cellular DNA and mRNA of the $\kappa$ chain of MOPC 41 and the $\lambda$ chain of MOPC 104 E. This experiment shows that the reiterative frequency of $V_{\lambda 1}$ and $V_{\kappa}$ segments of MOPC 41 $V_{\lambda 1}$ are of the same order, that is, less than five copies per haploid genome. Taking account of the structure of $\lambda 1$ chains, discussed on p. 191, the finding that $V_{\lambda}1$ and $V_{\kappa}$ segments have the same reiterative frequency provides a forceful argument in favor of a single gene for the framework of each variable region (i.e., for each V sequence considered without its three hypervariable regions). A saturation hybridization experiment between the cloned $\kappa$ MPC II-cDNA and embryonic DNA is shown in Figure 7.40. The calculation provided by these curves indicates the presence of two to three

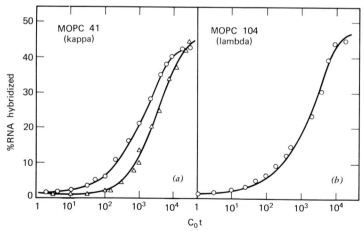

**Fig. 7.39** Kinetics of DNA-mRNA hybridization. Purified and [125]I labeled L chain mRNA from MOPC 41 (A) and from MOPC 104 (B) are hybridized with their respective sonicated DNAO—O. GS hemoglobin [125]I mRNA is hybridized with MOPC41 DNA△—△. (From B. Mach et al., Proc. 10th FEBS meeting, G. Bernardi, F. Gros, Eds., North Holland/American Elsevier, 1975, *38*, 299.)

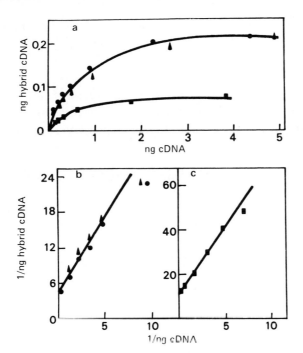

**Fig. 7.40** Saturation hybridization experiments between murine embryonic DNA and molecules of cDNA cloned from MPC II.

The two cDNAs used are composed either of the $C_\kappa$ + $V_\kappa$ sequence or the $C_\kappa$ sequence alone. The two probes are marked with $^{125}I$; 0.448 mg of embryonic DNA is hybridized with increasing quantities of cloned cDNA. The final value of Cot in these reactions is $5.4 \times 10^4$ mol $1^{-1}$S.

(a) saturation curves obtained with complete DNA (▲ and ● represent two separate experiments) and with cDNA-$C_\kappa$ (■); (b and c) represent reciprocal saturation curves obtained respectively with complete DNA and with cDNA-$C_\kappa$ (the intersection of these curves with the ordinate axis allows the calculation of the quantity of DNA hybridized for the theoretical addition of an infinite quantity of cDNA. (After O. Valbuena et al., Nature, 1978, *276*, 780.)

copies for $C_\kappa$ segments and 8 to 11 copies for $V_\kappa$ segments. Similar experiments performed with four mRNAs of four κ chains belonging to the $V_\kappa 21$ group suggest a mean reiteration of 7 $V_\kappa$ segments per group in a murine haploid genome.

### Origin of Immunoglobulin Diversity

We have seen that three different hypotheses can be offered to explain the origin of Ig diversity: a germinal hypothesis, requiring a large number of genes; a somatic hypothesis, requiring a minimum number of genes; and mixed hypotheses, which favor a somatic variability mechanism for hypervariable regions only. The general principles and implications of these hypotheses were formulated between 1970 and 1975. However, new information (the genetics of numerous idiotypes and, especially, DNA analysis) has allowed a more precise definition of the bases of the current theories. We shall quickly examine the initial propositions before proceeding to see which arguments have been strengthened by the partial knowledge of DNA structure.

All immunologists now recognize V gene/C gene dichotomy. No one any longer supports the theory of the presence of a large number of associated V-C cistrons, according to which these would be copied $10^3$ and $10^4$ times on a given chromosome. The absence of recombination among C region allotypes excludes such a possibility.

Hood and Talmage classified all known sequences according to phylogenetic trees and theorized that within Ig there are as many V genes as there are V sequences. They estimated that 0.2% of cellular DNA would be required for these cistrons. This rate is not negligible since only a small percentage of the genome may contain structural genes (Crick).

In addition, it must be explained how "phylogenetically associated" amino acids are maintained and how allotypes of the a series have appeared on a great number of genes at the same time in rabbits.

Supporters of this theory suggest that an "expansion-contraction" mechanism accounts for the great and rapid duplication of certain particular genes within a given animal species. However, this theory of a very redundant system does not explain why markers, such as the Aa allotypes, are found to be homozygous in numerous individuals, unless one theorizes that there is a special process that does not allow recombination. However, we have seen previously that many translocations take place within the Ig loci.

Germline theories favor the argument of nonrecombination of constant regions in order to explain the small number of C genes. However, the following example clearly shows that conservation of V regions is equivalent to that of C regions. Fig. 7.41 compares the Fc fragments of a murine IgG2a, a rabbit IgG, and a human IgG. Figure 7.42 shows the sequence of variable regions of the $V_H III$ subgroups in three different species (mouse, guinea pig, and man). The conservation, and therefore the selective pressure, seems to have been the same for variable $V_H III$ domains and for $C_H 2$ and $C_H 3$ domains (Table 7.11) (When excluding the complementary determining residues from the comparison of fig. 7.41 and 7.42, the V regions would appear to be even more conserved than the C regions!). The above hypothesis with regard to constant regions should also apply to variable regions, which would then favor the existence of a small number of V genes.

The objections against the germline concept of the origin of antibody diversity do not rule it out: the simplicity of this theory is attractive, in that it requires no particular mechanism to account for variability.

Unlike the previous theory, this hypothesis favors a very small number of germline genes. Variability occurs through somatic mutations (Milstein, Cohn). This proposition is based on the fact that all the substitutions within the same variability subgroup correspond to a change of a single base per codon, and occur in the vast majority in the hypervariable regions.

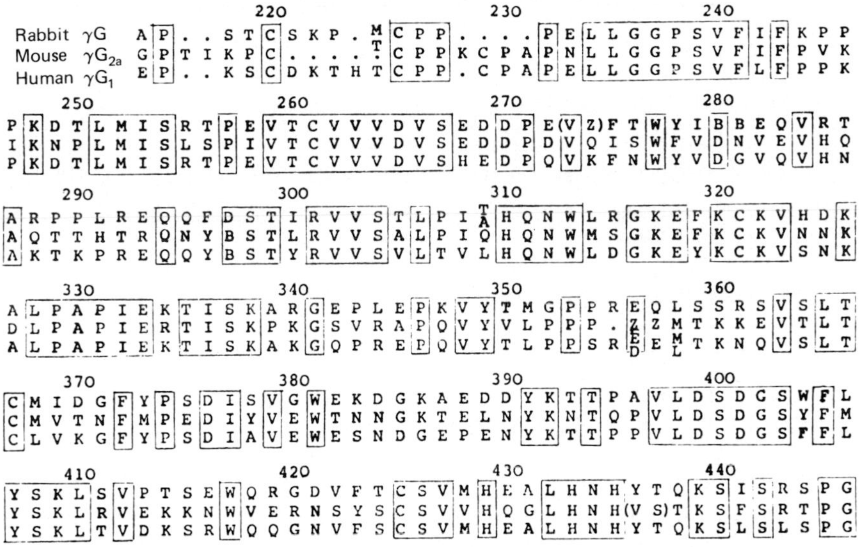

```
                    220              230            240
Rabbit  γG   A P . . S T C S K P . M C P P . . . . P E L L G G P S V F I F K P P
Mouse   γG2a G P T I K P C . . . . T C P P K C P A P N L L G G P S V F L F P V K
Human   γG1  E P . . K S C D K T H T C P P . C P A P E L L G G P S V F L F P P K

      250           260            270            280
P K D T L M I S R T P E V T C V V V D V S E D D P E(V Z)F T W Y I B B E Q V R T
I K N P L M I S L S P I V T C V V V D V S E D D P D V Q I S W F V D N V E V H Q
P K D T L M I S R T P E V T C V V V D V S H E D P Q V K F N W Y V D G V Q V H N

      290           300            310            320
A R P P L R E Q Q F D S T I R V V S T L P I T/A H Q N W L R G K E F K C K V H D K
A Q T T H T R Q N Y B S T L R V V S A L P I Q H Q N W M S G K E F K C K V N N K
A K T K P R E Q Q Y B S T Y R V V S V L T V L H Q N W L D G K E Y K C K V S N K

      330           340            350            360
A L P A P I E K T I S K A R G E P L E P K V Y T M G P P R E Q L S S R S V S L T
D L P A P I E R T I S K P K G S V R A P Q V Y V L P P P . Z/E Z M T K K E V T L T
A L P A P I E K T I S K A K G Q P R E P Q V Y T L P P S R D/E E M/L T K N Q V S L T

      370           380            390            400
C M I D G F Y P S D I S V G W E K D G K A E D D Y K T T P A V L D S D G S W F L
C M V T N F M P E D I Y V E W T N N G K T E L N Y K N T Q P V L D S D G S Y F M
C L V K G F Y P S D I A V E W E S N D G E P E N Y K T T P P V L D S D G S F F L

      410           420            430            440
Y S K L S V P T S E W Q R G D V F T C S V M H E A L H N H Y T Q K S I S R S P G
Y S K L R V E K K N W V E R N S Y S C S V V H Q G L H N H(V S)T K S F S R T P G
Y S K L T V D K S R W Q Q G N V F S C S V M H E A L H N H Y T Q K S L S L S P G
```

**Fig. 7.41** A comparison of the sequence of Fc fragments of rabbit IgG, of a murine IgG2a and of a human IgG1. (From A. Bourgois et al., Eur. J. Biochem., 1974, *43*, 330.)

Objections against the germinal theory with respect to (1) the presence of Aa allotypes in variable regions; (2) the absence of their recombination; (3) the existence of phylogenetically associated residues; and (4) the parallel evolution of $V_H$ and $C_H$ regions, do not apply to this hypothesis. However, we have also seen that distribution of variability does not occur randomly. There remains a problem of selection.

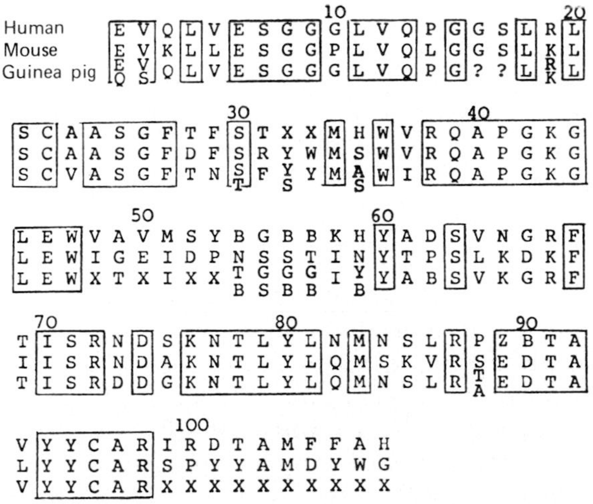

```
                         10                20
Human       E V Q L V E S G G G L V Q P G G S L R L
Mouse       E V K L L E S G G P L V Q L G G S L K L
Guinea pig  E/Q V/S Q L V E S G G G L V Q P G ? ? L R/K L

                30              40
S C A A S G F T F S T X X M H W V R Q A P G K G
S C A A S G F D F S R Y W M S W V R Q A P G K G
S C V A S G F T N S/T F Y/S Y M A/S W I R Q A P G K G

          50              60
L E W V A V M S Y B G B B K H Y A D S V N G R F
L E W I G E I D P N S S T I N Y T P S L K D K F
L E W X T X I X X T/B G/S G/B G/B I Y/B Y/B A B S V K G R F

  70            80            90
T I S R N D S K N T L Y L N M N S L R P Z B T A
I I S R N D A K N T L Y L Q M S K V R S E D T A
T I S R D D G K N T L Y L Q M N S L R T/A E D T A

          100
V Y Y C A R I R D T A M F F A H
L Y Y C A R S P Y Y A M D Y W G
V Y Y C A R X X X X X X X X X X X
```

**Fig. 7.42** Sequence comparison of $V_H$ III subgroup variable regions in heavy chains of humans, mice, and guinea pigs. (From A. Bourgois et al., Eur. J. Biochem., 1974, *43*, 330.)

**Table 7.11   Interspecific Identities of $V_H III$, $C_H 2$ and $C_H 3$ Regions***

| Domain | Number of residues | Identical positions among three species | Additional identical positions between two species | | |
| --- | --- | --- | --- | --- | --- |
| | | | Human/rabbit or human/ guinea pig | Human/ mouse | Mouse/rabbit or mouse/ guinea pig |
| $C_H 2$ | 107 (232–338) | 63 | 18 | 9 | 7 |
| $C_H 3$ | 108 (339–446) | 46 | 25 | 17 | 7 |
| $V_H III$ | 108 (1–108) | 58 | 17 | 7 | 7 |

* These results are derived from the analysis of sequences presented in Figs. 7.38 and 7.39. From A. Bourgois et al., Eur. J. Biochem. 1974, *43*, 330.

M. Cohn proposed a mechanism of positive selection by the antigen. A selection of clones which mutate and which produce antibodies with a high affinity for the antigen would occur during the immune response. These clones would multiply more rapidly and thereby mutate more rapidly, thus enabling the antigen to reselect cells which produce even more efficient antibodies. This process would lead to the exclusive selection of clones that produce high-affinity antibodies. Such an explanation requires that a great variety of antigens be in contact with the immune system and remain in contact throughout its development.

N. K. Jerne proposed a negative selection mechanism in which all antibody-producing cells would possess receptors directed against histocompatibility antigens. Survival of these clones during ontogeny would be linked to their ability to mutate and to become tolerant to their own histocompatibility antigens, while at the same time acquiring new specificities. This hypothesis becomes a possibility only if the mutation rate is $10^{-5}$ per division and if renewal in the thymus amounts to $\frac{1}{4}$ of the cells per day. It must also be noted that if selection involves complementary determining residues only, the diversity of the framework can no longer be explained. It must be assumed then that the germinal line contains genes that account for this variability. This assumption is the basis for the mixed hypotheses described below.

MIXED HYPOTHESES: SOMATIC RECOMBINATIONS

Limited variability of the framework is explained by the presence in the germinal line of a certain number of germline genes in each subgroup system. These genes may have appeared in the course of evolution through tandem duplication and each may have been subject to a certain number of mutations. On the other hand, hypervariable regions would have acquired their diversity through a process of somatic mutation or recombination.

Gally and Edelman emphasized the fact that unequal crossingover between homologous DNA sequences may increase or decrease the size of any family of duplicated genes. This mechanism explains both the coevolution of V regions belonging to the same subgroup and the accumulation of a few point mutations.

During ontogeny, a large number of new cistrons could be generated through a series of somatic recombinations, which are due to unequal crossingover. It is clear that the greater the number of germ-line genes, the more this very hypothesis will be subject to objections against germinal theories with respect to the conservation of stable regions. However, the presence of several $V_H$ cistrons in the germinal line could account for the Aa allotype variants, even though the minimum number of gene copies required in order for recombinations to prevent conservation of these allotype markers, is not known.

The above authors pointed out that their hypothesis proposes the same molecular recombination mechanism (an unequal crossingover) to explain both V-C translocation and the generation of variability. Even though the accumulation of mutations in the germinal line does not appear to be sequential, this could be due to the fact that recombinations mix genes at a very rapid rate and that they erase all traces of their evolution.

The propositions of Gally and Edelman proved to be quite remarkable; their concept of the role of somatic recombinations could well be verified considering the first results of the analysis of DNA structure. Not only does it give rise to a V-C junction (with its various aspects, $V\text{-}C_\delta,\text{-}C_\mu,\text{-}C_{\delta 1} \dots$ ) but also the supplementary V-J linkage that may generate some sequence variability during lymphocyte maturation.

Weigert and Hood have attempted to show the role that the V-J association (called the "combinatory junction") may play if the J segment participates in the structure of the third hypervariable region. The analysis of the amino acid sequence of mouse $V_\kappa$ region together with the reiteration frequency of the $V_\kappa$ genes in the same species leads to an estimate of seven V genes in each $V_\kappa$ group. Statistical analysis of the amino acid sequences in this species results in an estimated number of 50 $V_\kappa$ groups and 200 $V_H$ genes. The size of these figures allows an understanding of the frequency of hereditary transmission of certain idiotypes that cannot be explained by the presence of only some tens of genes per translocon. These numbers suggest a minimum of 350 $V_\kappa$ genes that may be associated at random with 200 $V_H$ genes in order to constitute $7 \times 10^4$ molecules of antibody. If this were the case, then more than 90% of the variability would have to be of somatic origin. However, if each $V_\kappa$ segment can associate with 4-5 $J_\kappa$ segments in two or three ways and each $V_H$ may associate with a similar number of $J_H$ segments, then the number of possible antibodies becomes $7 \times 10^6$. Moreover, this combinatory junction mechanisms may form identical V regions in the same strain. Considering the pool of D-regions, this number could even be increased. If these calculations were accurate, only a factor of 2 to 4 due to another somatic event would bring the number of antibody combining sites to above $10^7$. Moreover this combinatory junction mechanism may form identical V regions in the same strain. Such a mechanism was evoked to explain the sharing of an IdI determinant between two different monoclonal antidextran antibodies (p. 213). This is also possibly the situation in the mouse anti-NP response and with certain other haptens in the guinea-pig.

Kabat has also suggested that somatic recombination is the basic mechanism that generates variability in antibodies. His evidence is based on a complete statistical analysis of all the variable sequences described in all animal species.

Based on homologies found either at the level of the three hypervariable regions or at the level of the four other regions that separate them, Kabat suggests that germinal DNA contains a large series of "minigenes" that code independently for the seven segments and that are assembled very early in the process of ontogenesis in a very large number of combinations. This hypothesis is in agreement with many experimental findings, such as the hereditary transmission of idiotypic specificities and the observation of an identical hypervariable sequence in two variable regions presenting numerous substitutions along the rest of their sequence. The existence of D and J regions corresponds partly to this hypothesis, but no evidence for independence of other framework or hypervariable regions was found. In addition, no early gene rearrangements between germline and embryonic cells could be documented.

TOWARD A GENERAL AGREEMENT ON THE THREE SOURCES OF ANTIBODY DIVERSITY

The controversy about the origin of antibody diversity is almost out of date after 1980. Indeed studies at the DNA level has produced enough information to begin to make sense of the complexity of immunoglobulin variability. cDNA probes coding for V regions of specific antihapten antibodies are used to isolate the germline DNA segments which can cross hybridize with them. The comparison of cDNA sequences and germline DNA sequences give new insight on the somatic events occuring during lymphocyte differentiation. Three main systems are actively studied: anti-PC, anti-NP and anti-ARS antibodies (see p. 214). The phosphorylcholine system summarizes the main conclusions: as of 1980, 28 $V_H$ sequences of anti-PC antibodies have been determined at the protein level or at the cDNA level. These $V_H$ regions are associated either with $\mu$, $\gamma$ or $\alpha$ chains. The first striking observation is that the $V_H$ variability increases from segments linked to $C_\mu$ to segments linked to $C_\gamma$ and finally to segments linked to $C_\alpha$.

The same observation holds true for the $V_L$ regions of these antibodies, thus excluding that accumulation of mutations in $V_H$ segments is due to repetitive switches. When germline $V_H$ genes were isolated through hybridization with $V_H^{PC}$ cDNA probes, only four genes were counted: the first codes exactly for the prototype $V_H^{PC}$ sequences without any mutation; the second is a pseudogene (a gene which cannot be transcribed because it contains a stop-codon within an exon); and the last two segments are real genes, but their sequences do not correspond to any of the 28 known PC specific sequences. Futhermore, their structure is such that one should derive all the 28 $V_H$ regions from the single germline sequence of the first gene segment. Somatic recombinations described in section VIII cannot explain all the variability of this $V_H$ set; hence somatic mutations should have occurred during the lymphocyte life on CDR positions as well as on framework positions.

In conclusion, the generation of antibody diversity can be visualized as coming from 3 different sources:

1. A large series of germline genes ($V_\kappa J_\kappa$, $V_\lambda J_\lambda$, $V_H D J_H$).
2. An amplification mechanism due to somatic recombinations
3. Somatic mutations occurring within framework, CDR, J or D segments.

The next question which remains is to determine which somatic mutations are neutral, which are counterselected and which are positively selected. Comparisons of the three dimensional structures of antibodies should help to answer this question.

The above discussion of the genetic determination of Ig is based on the analysis of antibody structure. Further discussion of Ig genetic determination will follow on p. 567 after we have analyzed the process of intracellular synthesis of Ig and the phenotypic expression of Ig by lymphocytes (p. 562).

# BIBLIOGRAPHY

ANDREWS D. W. and CAPRA J. D. Structure and function of immunoglobulins. In: Clinical Immunology (Parker D. W. ed.) Saunders. Philadelphia. 1980:1.

Antibodies. Cold Spring Harbor Symp. Quant. Biol. 1967, Vol. 32.

CAPRA J. D. and KEHOE M. Hypervariable regions, idiotypy and antibody combining sites. Adv. Immunology, 1975, *20*, 1.

CATHOU R. E. and DORRINGTON K. J. *In* G. D. Fasman and S. N. Timasheff, Eds., Subunits in Biological Systems, Part C. Biological Macromolecules Series, New York, 1974, Dekker

COHN M. A rationale for ordering the data on antibody diversification. *In* L. Brent and J. Holborow, Eds., Progress in immunology. II. Amsterdam, 1974, North Holland, p. 261.

EDELMAN G. M. Antibody structure and molecular immunology. Science, 1973, *180*, 830.

GALLY J. A. Structure of immunoglobulins. *In* M. Sela, Ed., The antigens. New York, 1974, Academic Press, p. 161.

GECKLER W. R., BLOMBERG B., DE PREVAL C., and COHN M. On the genetic dissection of a specific humoral immune response to (1,3) dextran. Cold Spring Harbor Symp. Quant. Biol., 1976, *41*, 743.

HOOD L., CAMPBELL J. H., and ELGIN S. C. F. The organization, expression and evolution of antibody genes and other multigene families. Ann. Rev. Genet., 1975, *9*, 305.

Immune System: genetics and regulation. ICN-UCLA Symposium. E. Sercarz, L. A. Herzenberg, and C. F. Fox, Eds., New York, 1977, Academic Press.

JERNE N. K. The somatic generation of immune recognition. Eur. J. Immunol. 1971, *1*, 1.

KABAT E. A. Structural concepts in immunology and immunochemistry, 2nd ed., New York, 1976, Holt, Rinehart & Winston.

KENNETT R. M., McKEARN T. J., and BECHTOL K. B. Monoclonal antibodies hybridomas: a new dimension in biological analyses. Plenum Press New York, 1980:423 pp.

LEDER P., MAX E., and SEIDMAN J. The organization of immunoglobulin genes and the origin of their diversity. In: Immunology 80 (M. Fougereau and J. Dausset eds.) Acad. Press. New York, 1980, 34.

LITMAN G. W., and GOOD R. A. Immunoglobulins. Comprehensive Immunology. Vol. 5, Plenum Press. New York, 381 p.

MAGE R., LIEBERMAN R., POTTER M., and TERRY W. D. Immunoglobulin allotype. *In* M. Sela, Ed., The antigens. New York, 1974, Academic Press, p. 299.

MILSTEIN C., CLARK M. R., GALFRE G., and CUELLO A. C. Monoclonal antibodies from hybrid myelomas. In Immunology 80 (M. Fougereau and J. Dausset eds.) Acad. Press. New York, 1980, 34.

NISONOFF A., HOPPER J. E., and SPRING S. B. The antibody molecule. New York, 1975, Academic Press.

NISONOFF A., and GREENE M. I. Regulation through idiotypic determinants of the immune response to the p-azophenylarsonate hapten in strain A mice. In: Immunology 80 (M. Fougereau and J. Dausset eds.) Acad. Press. New York, 1980, 57.

Origin and expression of antibody diversity, molecular and cellular aspects. Réunion de Carry-le-Rouet, Ann. Immunol. (Institut Pasteur), 1976, *127c*, vol. 3–4.

Origins of lymphocyte diversity. Cold Spring Harbor Symp. Quant. Biol., 1977, Vol. 41.

OUDIN J. Idiotypy of antibodies. *In* M. Sela, Ed., The antigens, New York, 1974, Academic Press, p. 277.

PORTER R. R. Structural studies of immunoglobulins, Science, 1973, *180*, 713.

WEIGERT M., and RIBLET R. The genetic control of antibody variable regions in the mouse. Springer Seminar Immunopath., 1978, 1, 139.

## ORIGINAL ARTICLES

BREZIN C. and CAZENAVE P. A. Allotypes of the a series and their variants in rabbit immunoglobulins. Ann. Immunol. (Inst. Pasteur), 1976, *127c*, 333.

BRACK C., HIRAMA M., LENHARD-SCHULLER R., and TONEGAWA S. A complete immunoglobulin gene is created by somatic recombination. Cell, 1978, *15*, 1.

DAVIS M. M., CALAME K., EARLY P. W., LIVANT D. L., JOHO R., WEISSMAN I., HOOD L. A. An immunoglobulin heavy chain gene is formed by at least two recombinational events. Nature 1980. *283*, 733.

DAVIS M. M., KIM S. D., and HOOD L. E. DNA sequences mediating class switching in α immunoglobulins. Science 1980. *209*, 1360.

DRAY S. Effect of maternal iso-antibodies on the quantitative expression of two allelic genes controlling γ globulin allotypic specificies. Nature 1965, *813*, 195.

EARLY P. W., HUANG H. V., DAVIS M. M., CALAME K. and HOOD L. E. An immunoglobulin heavy chain variable region gene is generated from three segments of DNA, $V_H$, $D_H$ and $J_H$. Cell 1980. *19*, 981.

EDELMAN G. M., CUNNINGHAM B. A., GALL W. E., GOTTLIEB P. D., RUTISHAUSER U., and WAXDAL M. J. The covalent structure of an entire immunoglobulin molecule. Proc. Nat. Acad. Sci., U.S.A., 1969, *63*, 78.

EICHMANN K. and KINDT T. J. The inheritance of individual antigenic specificities of rabbit antibodies to streptococcal carbohydrate. J. Exp. Med., 1971, *134*, 532.

FOUGEREAU M., BOURGOIS A., and PRÉVAL C. de Conservation parallèle des régions V et C des immunoglobulines: implications génétiques et fonctionnelles. Ann. Immunol. (Inst. Pasteur), 1974, *125c*, 343.

HART D. A., PAWLAK L. L., and NISONOFF A. Nature of anti-hapten antibodies after immune suppression of a set of cross-reactive idiotypic sepcificities. Eur. J. Immunol., 1973, *3*, 44.

INBAR D., HOCHMAN J., and GIVOL D. Localization of antibody combining sites with the variable portions of heavy and light chains. Biochemistry, 1973, *12*, 1130.

OUDIN J. and MICHEL M. Idiotypy of rabbit antibodies. I. Comparison of idiotypy of antibodies against *S. typhi* with that of antibodies against other bacteria in the same rabbit, or antibodies against *S. typhi* in various rabbits. J. Exp. Med., 1969, *130*, 595. II. Comparison of idiotypy of various kinds of antibodies formed in the same rabbit against *S. typhi*. J. Exp. Med., 1969, *130*, 619.

POLJAK R. J., ANZEL L. M., CHEN B. L., PHIZACKERLEY R. P., and SAUL F. The three-dimensional structure of the Fab' fragment of a human myeloma immunoglobulin at 2,0 Å resolution. Proc. Nat. Acad. Sci., U.S.A., 1974, *71*, 3440.

RIBLET R., BLOMBERG B., WEIGER M., LIEBERMAN R., TAYLOR B. A., and POTTER M. Genetics of mouse antibody. I. Linkage of the dextran response locus $V_H$ Dex to allotype. Eur. J. Immunol. 1975, *5*, 775.

RIBLET R., WEIGERT M., and MÄKELA O. Genetics of mouse antibodies. II. Recombination between $V_H$ genes and allotype. Eur. J. Immunol., 1975, *5*, 778.

ROGERS J., EARLY P., CATER C., CALAME K., BOND M., HOOD L., and WASS R. Two mRNAs can be produced from a single immunoglobulin μ gene by alternative RNA processing pathways. Cell 1980. *20*, 312.

SAKANO H., ROGERS J. H., HÜPPI K., BRACK C., TRAUNECKER A., MAKI R., WALL R., and TONEGAWA S. Domains and the hinge region of an immunoglobulin heavy chain are encoded in separated DNA segments. Nature, 1979, *277*, 785.

SAKANO H., MAKI R., KUROSAWA Y., ROEDER W., and TONEGAWA S. Two types of somatic recombination are necessary for the generation of complete immunoglobulin heavy chain genes. Nature 1980. *286*, 676.

SCHILLING J. G., CLEVINGER B., DAVIE J., and HOOD L. Aminoacid sequence of homogeneous antibodies to dextran and DNA rearrangements in heavy chain V-region gene segments. Nature 1980. *283*, 35.

SEGAL D., PADLAN E. A., COHEN G. H., RUDIKOFF S., and POTTER M. Three-dimensional structure of phosphorylcholine-binding mouse immunoglobulin Fab and the nature of the antigen-binding site. Proc. Nat. Acad. Sci., U.S.A., 1974, *71*, 4298.

SEIDMAN J. G., MAX E. E., and LEDER P. A K immunoglobulin gene is formed by site specific recombination without further somatic mutation. Nature 1979. *280*, 370.

TONEGAWA S., HOZUMI N., MATTHYSSENS G., and SCHULLER R. Somatic changes in the content and context of immunoglobulin genes. Cold Spring Harbor Symp. Quant. Biol., 1976, *41*, 877.

VALBUENA O., MARCU K. B., WEIGERT M., and PERY R. P. Multiplicity of germline genes specifying a group of related mouse chains, with implication for the generation of immunoglobulin diversity. Nature 1978, *276*, 780.

WEIGERT M., GATMAITAN L., LOH E., SCHILLING J., and HOOD L. Rearrangement of genetic information may produce immunoglobulin diversity. Nature 1978, *276*, 785.

YASITA Y. and HONJO T. Deletion of immunoglobulin heavy chain genes from expressed allelic chromosome. Nature 1980. *286*, 851.

## Chapter 8

# COMPLEMENT

## André P. Peltier

I.   INTRODUCTION
II.   COMPLEMENT REACTION
III.   ELEMENTARY BIOLOGIC ACTIVITIES OF COMPLEMENT
IV.   SYNTHESIS OF COMPLEMENT COMPONENTS
V.   COMPLEMENT AND HYPERSENSITIVITY
VI.   GENETICS OF COMPLEMENT

## *I.   INTRODUCTION*

Complement is a complex biologic system made of an as yet undetermined number of components that are serum globulins. The sequential activation of these components follows two main pathways, the classical and the alternative, which join to form a common terminal trunk. Activation of this system may have an immunologic basis (antigen-antibody reaction) or be nonimmunologic (e.g., contact with an endotoxin). Activation leads to the appearance of a series of biologic events that indicate the probable importance of complement as a mediator of numerous pathophysiologic phenomena.

## *II.   COMPLEMENT REACTION*

### CLASSICAL ACTIVATION PATHWAY

Most data regarding complement activation by the classical pathway are based on study of immunohemolysis reactions during which erythrocytes (E) sensitized by antired blood cell antibodies (A) are hemolyzed by complement (C).

The immunohemolysis reaction has the considerable advantage over other cytolytic reactions of complement to use as target cells, the erythrocytes, which are easily obtained in large amounts, are homogeneous, are rich in surface antigens capable of reacting with specific antibodies produced in laboratory animals, and whose lysis leads to hemoglobin release that can be precisely measured by use of spectrophotometry.

The classical pathway of activation involves, successively, nine components (C1, C4, C2, C3, C5, C6, C7, C8 and C9), which may be grouped into three functional units: C1 or recognition unit; C4, C2, and C3 or activation unit; and C5, C6, C7, C8, C9, or membrane attack unit.

### Recognition Phase: C1 Binding and Activation

C1, the heaviest of complement components, is a macromolecular complex composed of three proteins, C1q, C1r, and C1s, linked by calcium ions. A fourth subcomponent of C1 named C1t, has been described by Assimeh et al. According to these authors, C1t may contribute to the stability of macromolecular C1, but would not be necessary for C1 hemolytic activity. On the other hand, Gigli considers C1t as a contaminant of C1 preparations. Structural similarities between C1t and P component of amyloid substance have been established. C1t, C Reactive Protein and the P component belong to the pentraxin group.

C1q, with a molecular weight of 400,000, is the largest subcomponent. It contains much glycin and hydroxylisine, these contents plus a large amount of carbohydrate and equimolecular concentrations of glucose and galactose make C1q bear resemblance to structural glycoproteins, particularly collagen. The C1q molecule is made up of 18 polypeptide chains grouped three by three into six subunits, each of which comprises a globulin portion and a collagen-type portion. In this latter portion, the six subunits are coupled to one another and their three polypeptide chains are wound around one another in a triple helix comparable with that of collagen itself. In the globulin portions the six subunits are independent of one another. The collagen portion of the C1q molecule bears six sites with which the subunits become attached to the corresponding Fc sites of IgG and IgM. The C1q molecule is therefore hexavalent and capable of precipitating immune complexes (or soluble aggregates of IgG) with which it reacts in a liquid phase or gel medium. It has been established that C1q reacts with IgG1 and IgG3, to a lesser degree with IgG2, and not at all with IgG4, IgA, IgE, and IgD.

The site of C1q fixation on IgM molecules is probably localized at the amino-terminal end of the $C_H4$ domain. The amino acid sequence of this portion of the $C_H4$ domain, moreover, has a very strong homology with human $\beta_2$-microglobulin, which also binds efficiently to C1. This portion is homologous to the $C_\lambda3$ IgG domain; however, paradoxically, it has been suggested that the $C_\gamma2$ domain of IgG contains its C1 binding site.

C1q does not react with an Ig molecule unless the latter has previously undergone structural changes that make available the C1q fixation site. These structural changes are induced by the reaction of an IgM or IgG antibody molecule with its specific antigen (formation of antigen-antibody complex) or when IgG molecules are aggregated as, for example, by heating. Only precipitating antigen-antibody complexes, or soluble complexes in slight antigen excess, bind complement.

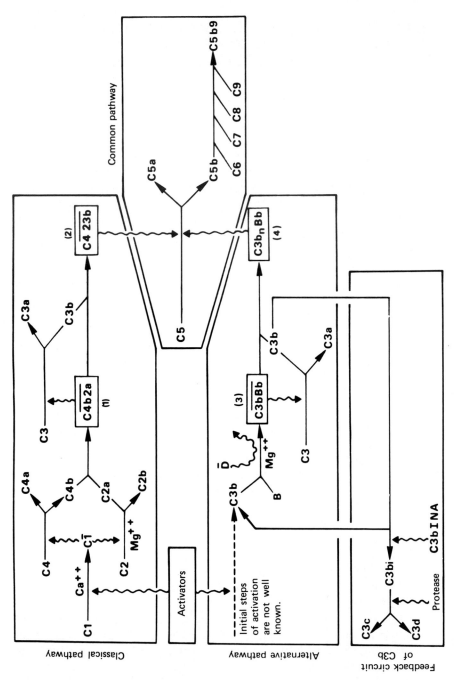

**Fig. 8.1** Schematic representation of the complement system with the classic and alternative pathways of activation, the common trunk, and the C3b feedback circuit (amplification cycle). (1) C3 convertase of the classic pathway, (2) C5 convertase of the classic pathway, (3) C3 convertase of the alternative pathway, (4) C5 convertase of the alternative pathway. "Curly" arrows indicate enzymatic activities or reactions that are

One IgM hemolysin molecule is sufficient to form a hemolytic site on the surface of a red blood cell, but two adjacent IgG hemolysin molecules ("IgG doublet") are required. This requirement may explain why certain antired blood cell antibodies are not hemolytic—if the number of red blood cell antigenic sites to which IgG antibodies specifically bind is low, the site density on the cell surface will be insufficient for doublet formation. Such is the case, for example, with IgG anti-Rh antibodies (5000 to 30,000 antigenic RhD sites per red blood cell) versus 1,000,000 A antigenic sites (see p. 606).

C1 reaction with EA (or with the antibody portion of any complement-fixing immune complex) has two time phases. In the first phase, C1q, after binding to the antibody by its globular portion, undergoes allosteric modifications. These changes subsequently affect C1r, in which the proenzyme is activated to form an enzyme; in the second phase, C1r enzymatically cleaves the single C1s polypeptide chain into two fragments of unequal size, the smaller of which (33,000 daltons) is endowed with esterasic properties. The reaction may be schematized as follows (the bar above the symbol indicates component activation):

$$EA + C1 \xrightarrow[Ca^{2+}]{} EAC1 \tag{1}$$

$$EAC1 \xrightarrow[Ca^{2+}]{} EAC\bar{1} \tag{2}$$

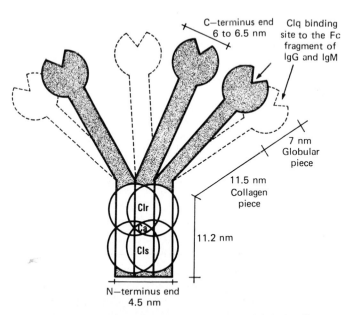

**Fig. 8.2** Schematic representation of the C1q molecule with its "collagen" part, in which each of the six monomers (or subunits) is made of three polypeptide chains wound into a triple helix, and its globulin part, in which the three chains are situated in a poorly defined tertiary arrangement. The "collagen" part is sensitive to collagenase digestion but resistant to pepsin treatment. The globulin part has the reverse properties; C1r and C1s probably attach to the N-terminal end of the collagen part.

or, in more detail:

$$EA + C1qrs \xrightarrow[Ca^{2+}]{} EAC1qrs$$

$$EAC1qrs \xrightarrow[Ca^{2+}]{} EAC1q\bar{r}s$$

$$EAC1q\bar{r}s \xrightarrow[Ca^{2+}]{} EAC1q\overline{rs} + \text{a large C1s polypeptidic fragment.}$$

In addition to IgM and IgG, C1q is capable of reacting with certain polyanions, including DNA, other polynucleotides, lipopolysaccharides of gram-negative bacteria, certain polysaccharides (dextran), chondroitin-sulfates, and CRP (C reactive protein). The pathophysiologic significance of the latter reactions has not been determined.

### *Activation Phase*

FORMATION OF THE $C\overline{4b2a}$ C3-CONVERTASE

The formation of the $C\overline{4b2a}$ convertase is the result of action of C1 esterase (C1$\bar{s}$) on C4 and C2 components.

$$EAC\bar{1} + C4 \left\langle \begin{array}{l} EAC\bar{1}4b + C4a \\ C4i \text{ (or L)} \end{array} \right. \tag{3}$$

$$EAC\bar{1}4b + C2 \left\langle \begin{array}{l} EA\overline{1}4b2a + C2b \\ C2i \text{ (or C)} \end{array} \right. \tag{4}$$

This reaction develops in two time phases; C1$\bar{s}$ cleaves C4 into two fragments: C4b is the heavier of the two (molecular weight 130,000) and binds to specific receptors present on the erythrocyte surface; while C4a is a polypeptide of unknown function.

When C4b and C2a fragments are present in the fluid phase, they are rapidly inactivated (C4i and C2i).

C4b molecules may also directly bind to the hemolysin molecule and be hemolytically active, that is, play a further role in complement activation, leading finally to hemolysis.

C2 is adsorbed onto C4b, already bound to the erythrocyte wall; adsorption occurs only in the presence of $Mg^{2+}$ ions. Immediately after, C2 is cleaved by C1$\bar{s}$ molecule; only the heaviest of its two fragments (C2a, molecular weight, 84,000) remains fastened to C4b, together forming the $C\overline{4b2a}$ convertase. C2a is the subunit that bears the enzymatic site of this bimolecular convertase.

$C\overline{4b2a}$ is very labile; its half-life at 4°C is several hours, but it is less than 10 min at 37°C. After this step, C2a detaches from C4b and loses all hemolytic activity. This "decay" reaction may be schematized as follows:

$$EAC\overline{14b2a} \rightarrow EAC\bar{1}4b + C2ai \tag{5}$$

Once reformed, the EAC$\bar{1}$4b complex has all of the properties of the initial complex and may react with new C2 molecules to form (in the presence of $Mg^{2+}$) a new labile EAC$\overline{14b2a}$ complex.

Oxidation of C2 by iodine increases by 10-fold its hemolytic activity. Convertases formed with $C2^{oxy}$ are much more stable than $\overline{C4b2a}$ convertases.

## $\overline{C42}$ CONVERTASE INTERACTS WITH C3 TO FORM A $\overline{C423}$ C5 CONVERTASE

$\overline{C42}$ convertase has an enzymatic activity of unidentified nature that acts on C3 ($\beta_1$C globulin) to cleave it into two fragments, C3a (molecular weight 8,700) with anaphylatoxinic, and chemotactic properties, and C3b (molecular weight 223,000), which binds to specific receptors of the cell membrane. If these receptors are not available, C3b in the liquid phase is rapidly inactivated (C3i or $\beta_1$G). A single $\overline{C42}$ convertase site because of its enzymatic action binds several hundred C3b molecules.

$$EAC\overline{14b2a} + C3 \begin{cases} EAC\overline{14b2a3b} + C3a \\ C3i \end{cases} \tag{6}$$

A high proportion of bound C3b molecules are hemolytically inactive but possess important immunologic properties, such as immunoadherence and opsonization. Hemolytic activity is possessed only by C3b molecules that bind on $EA\overline{1}$ $\overline{42}$ sites, Forming $EAC\overline{1}$ 423 sites, which thus express a C5 convertase activity. Hence, C3b deposited in proximity to $EAC\overline{142}$ is capable of binding to and inducing a conformational change in C5. C5 bound to C3b therefore becomes susceptible to proteolysis by C5 convertase, which therefore comprises three subunits $\overline{C4b2a3b}$.

### Membrane Attack Phase: Formation of the C56789 Complex

The attack process requires the presence of a membrane surface complex composed of the last five complement components (C5 to C9) and C5 convertases of the classical and alternative pathways. Two main mechanisms have been proposed for the formation of this complex.

#### FORMATION BY SUCCESSIVE STEPS

Under experimental conditions, the C5-7 complex may be formed stepwise, and the cellular intermediates $EAC\overline{14235}$, $EAC\overline{142356}$, and $EAC\overline{1423567}$ are detected; C5 convertases cleave C5 into two fragments: C5a (molecular weight 15,000). like C3a, has anaphylatoxinic and chemotactic properties; C5b (molecular weight 170,000) may either directly enter the liquid phase and be rapidly inactivated (C5bi) or remain in contact with the convertase, subsequently reacting with C6 to form the C5b6 stable complex (see below). If C5b does not react with C6, it is rapidly inactivated (C5bi) despite a brief period of contact with the convertase before detaching into the liquid phase. This two-phase "decay" reaction of $EA\overline{14235}$ may be written as follows:

$$\underset{\text{active site}}{EAC\overline{1}\,\overline{4235}b} \rightarrow \underset{\text{inactive site}}{EAC\overline{1}\,\overline{4235}bi} \rightarrow \underset{\text{liquid phase}}{EAC\overline{1}\,\overline{423}} + C5bi$$

Because of the "decay" reaction, C2 and C5 are limiting factors in the complementary reaction, thus the concept of "T max," according to which, the

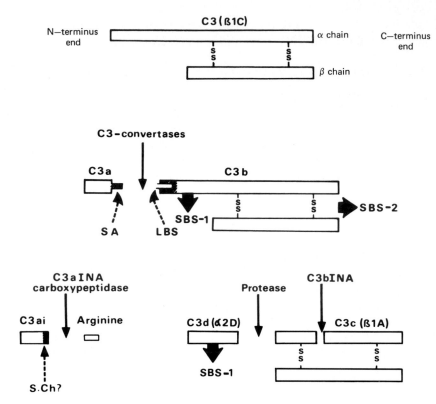

**Fig. 8.3** Successive stages in the activation and cleavage of C3. *First stage:* the native molecule of C3 (or β1C) is cleaved by the C3-convertases of the classical pathway or by C3a (C3-anaphylotoxin) and C3b in the alternative pathway. C3a becomes attached, by its anaphylotoxin sites, to the membranes of mastocytes, basophilic polynuclears, endothelial cells, or smooth muscle fibers. It is then inactivated by C3aINA (C3 anaphylotoxin inhibitor), which acts by detaching an arginine residue from its N-terminal end. The C3a molecule is thus inactivated (C3ai), while apparently retaining its chemotactic properties (ChS: chemotactic site). C3b "acquires" three active sites: LBS (labile binding site) allows the molecule to bind to the "receptor" sites of cellular membranes and immune complexes, this binding allows the C3b to intervene following the complement activation reactions: SBS-1 and SBS-2 are capable of reacting with the receptor sites of cellular membranes (red cells, B and K cells, leukocytes), this reaction resulting in the phenomena of immunoadherence and opsonization. *Second stage:* C3b is split by C3bINA (or KAF) into C3bi, then degraded into C3c and C3d by unidentified plasma proteases. This cleavage is accompanied by the disappearance of SBS-2, the C3c (β1A) having no biologic activity, whereas SBS-1, present on C3d (α2D) is retained.

cellular intermediates EAC$\overline{142}$ and EAC$\overline{14235}$b are optimally firmed during a short incubation time (e.g., 5 min. for EAC$\overline{142}$).

As previously noted, the C5b6 complex is very stable. C6 seems to stabilize the active form of C5 and the C5b6 complex remains hemolytically active, even in the liquid phase. C7 binding to this complex creates a trimolecular complex

**Table 8.1 Principal Physical and Serologic Properties of the Components of Complement**

| | Component | | Electrophoretic Mobility | Molecular Weight | Concentration in Normal Human Serum | | |
| --- | --- | --- | --- | --- | --- | --- | --- |
| | Current Designation | Synonyms | | | Protein μg/ml | Molar* | Hemolytic (CH 50/ml)** |
| Classical pathway | C1 | | | | | | 100,000–200,000 |
| | C1q | | $\gamma$2 | 400,000 | 190 | 28 | |
| | C1r | | $\beta$ | 168,000 | | | |
| | C1s | | $\alpha$2 | 80,000 | 30 | 15 | |
| | C4 | | $\beta$1 | 240,000 | 430 | 125 | 100,000–200,000 |
| | C2 | | $\beta$2 | 170,000 | 30 | 15 | 1,000–2,000 |
| | C3 | | $\beta$1 | 180,000 | 1,300 | 390 | 3,000–6,000 |
| Alternative pathway | Factor B | PA, C3PA, GBG | $\beta$1 | 100,000 | 225 | 135 | |
| | Factor D | PAase, C3PAase, GBGase | $\alpha$ | 24,000 | | | |
| | C3 | HSF, Factor A | $\beta$1 | 180,000 | 1,300 | 390 | |
| | Properdin | | $\gamma$ | 223,000 | 20 | 6 | |
| Common trunk | C5 | | $\beta$1 | 185,000 | 75 | 8 | 600–24,000 |
| | C6 | | $\beta$2 | 126,000 | 60 | 29 | 3,000–12,000 |
| | C7 | | $\beta$2 | | | | |
| | C8 | | $\gamma$2 | 150,000 | 30 | 12 | 60,000–65,000 |
| | C9 | | $\alpha$ | 79,000 | 1 | 1 | 40,000–64,000 |
| Regulatory proteins | C1s INH | C1 esterase inhibitor $\alpha$2-neuraminidase-glycoprotein | $\alpha$2 | 90,000 | 180 | 120 | |
| | C3b INA | KAF | $\beta$2 | 80,000 | 25 | 15 | |
| | $\beta$1 H | C3bINA accelerator | $\beta$1 | 150,000 | 133 | 60 | |
| | C3 NeF | Nephritic factor | $\gamma$ | 150,000 | Absent or traces (?) | | |
| | AI | Anaphylotoxin inhibitor | $\alpha$ | 810,000 | Absent or traces (?) | | |

HSF = hydrazine-sensitive factor, GGG = glycine-rich $\alpha$-globulin, GBG = glycine-rich $\beta$-globulin, GAG = glycine-rich $\gamma$-globulin.

* In molecules/ml $\times 10^3$.

** Using 0.5 ml of EAC per $1.5 \times 10^8$ cells/ml.

that is rapidly inactivated in the liquid phase but is capable of binding strongly to cell membranes. C8 binding to the C5b67 complex definitively alters the membrane and provokes a slow lysis of the cell, which is much accelerated by C9 binding.

ONE-STEP FORMATION

Independently of any activation in the native state, circulating (serum) C5, C6, C7, C8, and C9 have an affinity for each other, forming a reversibly soluble decamolecular complex (molecular weight $1.04 \times 10^6$) in which C5 reacts with C6, C7, C8, and C9 according to the following scheme:

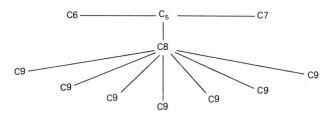

Activation of C5 by C5 convertases cleaves C5 into C5a and C5b and induces conformational changes in C5b that permit an irreversible adsorption of C6 and C7 onto C5. The trimolecular C567 complex realizes a critical molecular arrangement that permits binding of C8 and C9. The C567 portion of the complex is then capable of combining with membrane receptors and penetrating the inner hydrophobic medium of the membrane, in which it now proceeds to rearrange the microenvironment and induce functional changes in the membrane. The C5-9 complex can bind to membrane receptor sites only during a very brief period (less than 0.1 sec). If binding does not occur, the complex remains in the liquid phase and becomes hemolytically inactive. It has no activities other than the cytolytic function.

A circle of 8 to 10-nm diameter that contains a dark center is observed on electron microscopy and probably corresponds to the molecular rearrangement induced by the C5-9 complex within the erythrocyte membrane. Similar situations can be demonstrated in all cellular membranes during development of a complementary reaction. These circles occur in lymphocytes, platelets, bacteria, viruses, mycoplasmas, tumor cells, and even in artificial bilayer lipid membranes (liposomes). It has been suggested that these circles may be holes in the membrane created by the C5-9 complex, establishing a communication between the intra- and extracellular media. This belief is not certain, however, because identical lesions have been observed in lymphoid cell membranes transformed by the Moloney virus that had been incubated with specific antibodies and complement in the S, G2, and M phases of their cellular cycle, at which time total resistance to the hemolytic action of complement is present.

Irrespective of this finding, it is clear that changes induced by the C5-9 complex make the membrane semipermeable, permitting by a Donnan effect the passage of extracellular water and salts into the intracellular milieu. The cell now swells and bursts (cytolysis). If the binding of a single C5-9 complex suffices to create the local membrane "lesion" that provokes cell lysis ("one-hit hypothesis"), it is most likely that under physiologic conditions, especially because of the enzymatic nature of some of the steps of the complement reaction, red blood cell lysis results from multiple lesions that are simultaneously created on the membrane ("multihit reaction").

## ALTERNATIVE PATHWAY OF ACTIVATION

As in the classical pathway, the alternative pathway includes a series of component parts, the activation of which leads to the production of several convertases that react with both C3 and C5.

### Alternative Pathway Activators

The alternative pathway may be activated by immunologic substances (Ig aggregates and, by inference, immune complexes in whose formation immunoglobulins also participate) and also by nonimmunologic substances (polysaccharides of the inulin type, gram-negative bacterial endotoxins, yeast walls, zymosan, cobra venom factor).

Of the human Ig, IgA was formerly believed to be the only Ig capable of activating the alternative pathway. Recently, Frank and colleagues have reported that some IgG1, 2, 3, and 4 and also IgM and IgE molecules may have the same effect.

In the guinea pig, Osler has shown that $\gamma_1$ and $\gamma_2$ are activators of the alternative pathway, whereas only $\gamma_2$ activates the classical pathway. The activation site of the alternative pathway is present on the $F(ab')_2 - 5S$ portion of $\gamma_1$ molecules. Interpretation and extrapolation of the latter results should now be reevaluated because of new knowledge regarding retroactive C3b feedback. C3b formation induced by the activation of the classical pathway could lead to factor-B recruitment, independently of alternative pathway intervention.

According to Alper and colleagues, cobra venom factor (CoF) inducing C3 cleavage and activation of the terminal C5-9 components by the alternative pathway would be cobra C3, modified in such a way as human C3b and therefore capable of activating the alternative pathway.

### Components of the Alternative Pathway

At least six components are implicated in the activation of the alternative pathway of which five components truly belong to the alternative pathway (factors B and D, properdin, $\beta 1H$, and C3bINA), whereas the remaining component, C3, is also involved in the function of the classical pathway. Magnesium ions, but not calcium ions, are essential for the function of the alternative pathway.

Factor B (C3PA, GBG, or glycin-rich glycoprotein) is a $\beta_1$ globulin (molecular weight of about 100,000) that is thermolabile at 50°C for 10 min. Its concentration in normal human serum is relatively high (100 to 200 µg/ml).

Factor D (C3PAase, PAase GBGase) is a globulin (molecular weight 25,000), the active site of which is a serine esterase. Its specific function consists of cleaving factor B into two fragments.

Properdin is a γ globulin (molecular weight 223,000) with an isoelectric point higher than 9.5 that contains four apparently identical subunits, each of 45,000 molecular weight. Properdin activity is linked to its ability to react with C3b and to delay the decay (inactivation) of C3b-dependent convertase. Properdin seems therefore to play a stabilizing role for this convertase.

β1H is a β-globulin of molecular weight 150,000, which is able to dissociate the C3/C5 alternate convertases and to accelerate the inactivation of C3b by C3bINA.

C3bINA (KAF, C3b inactivator) is a β-globulin of molecular weight 90,000, which cleaves C3b into inactivated C3b (C3bi).

### Activation of the Alternative Pathway

Two certain facts dominate our current knowledge of the alternative pathway. These are the existence of two active convertases, one acting on C3, C3 convertase $\overline{\text{C3bBb}}$, the other acting on C5, C5 convertase $\overline{\text{C3bnBb}}$. These convertases are to some degree the equivalents for the alternative pathway of the convertases of the classical pathway and are active on the same components, that is $\overline{\text{C4b2a}}$ convertase acts on C3 and $\overline{\text{C4b2a3b}}$ on C5.

On the other hand, there is a great deal of uncertainty about the processes leading up to the formation of C3 convertase $\overline{\text{C3bBb}}$. Some workers have suggested that the formation of this convertase is preceded by the initial stages of activation involving particular components that are comparable with those of the initial stages of activation of the classical pathway. A component that is evoked at the beginning of this activation has been described ("initiating factor"), but the very existence of this factor is under considerable doubt. The whole problem revolves around the mechanism whereby the first molecules of C3b are formed, these being necessary for the formation of C3b convertase $\overline{\text{C3bBb}}$. Several hypotheses will be presented here. These C3b molecules may be provided by a minute activation of the classical pathway; this seems to occur during the dissolution of immune complexes by complement (see below). Present evidence indicates that C3b may be covalently linked to target particles through a ester bond. The initial C3 deposition from the fluid phase seems to be a random event, low levels C3b deposition occurring on host cells and foreign particles alike.

### C3-CONVERTASE $\overline{\text{C3bBb}}$

The formation of this convertase requires the presence of C3b, factor B, activated factor D ($\bar{\text{D}}$), and $\text{Mg}^{++}$ ions. Factor B binds to C3b to form a bimolecular complex, C3bB, in which B is cleaved under the influence of factor D in the presence of $\text{Mg}^{++}$ ions. The $\overline{\text{C3bBb}}$ complex then acquires enzymatic properties, which render it capable of acting on C3, cleaving it into C3a and C3b. The mode of activation of factor D into $\bar{\text{D}}$ remains to be clarified. It is known that $\bar{\text{D}}$ possesses the properties of a serine-esterase and that it has been related, from the functional point of view, to the subcomponent C1s of C1. It has been suggested that $\bar{\text{D}}$ is nothing more than a fragment of activated prothrombin. It does not appear that the cleavage of factor B is essential for the acquisition of its enzymatic properties. One of the most striking features of the convertase is the fact that one of its main constituents is actually one of the products of its action on its substrate, C3. This fact is an important consideration in the understanding of the C3 amplification cycle (see below).

The central position of this convertase is again exemplified by the multiplicity of regulatory proteins that control its function; in this regard, certain proteins (properdin and nephritic factor) have a stabilizing effect on C3-convertase C3bBb and thus facilitate its action, whereas others (β1H and C3bINA) have the reverse action.

Properdin appears to attach to the C3b convertase couple and protects it from the activity of C3bINA, whereas the nephritic factor, which is an IgG, is an autoantibody specific for a conformational antigenic determinant of convertase. β1H dissociates factor B from C3b, possibly as a result of a competition reaction between factor B and β1H for a different but very adjacent receptor "site" present on the C3b molecule. C3bINA splits C3b into inactivated C3b (C3bi). C3bi is then degraded into C3c and C3d as a result of the action of unidentified plasma proteases. β1H has been called C3bINA accelerator since it permits C3bINA to react with C3b itself, detaching factor B from C3b.

It should be noted that all these reactions, particularly those involving C3bINA and β1H, occur in the liquid phase and at the surfaces of nonactivating particles. On the other hand, they are much less efficient and do not occur at all when the convertase is formed at the surface of an activating particle, such as zymosan or bacteria. On such particles, bound C3b is not accessible to β1H and thus unavailable for inactivation by C3bINA. The C3b molecules escape from control and are then capable of activating the C3b feedback circuit.

### C3b FEEDBACK CIRCUIT (AMPLIFICATION CYCLE)

After the cleavage of C3 by C3-convertase C3bBb, the first molecules of C3b appear. There exist two possible theoretical destinations for these latter molecules. Either they participate in the formation of C5-convertase (C3b$_n$Bb) or they may bind new molecules of factor B and contribute to the formation of an unlimited number of C3 convertases C3bBb. In the absence of any appropriate regulation, uncontrolled function of this feedback circuit leads to an excessive consumption of C3, which may result in almost complete depletion of the animal's C3. In fact, under physiologic conditions, C3bINA splits the newly formed C3b molecules into C3bi (β1A), with the effect of interrupting the cycle. Uncontrolled function of the cycle has been described under two circumstances: congenital absence of C3bINA and membranoproliferative glomerulonephritis. In the absence of C3bINA, newly formed C3b is not cleaved and results in the accumulation of an excessive and unusable quantity of C3 convertase C3bBb. In membranoproliferative glomerulonephritis, the abnormal stabilization of this convertase by nephritic factor leads to the formation of large quantities of C3b and undoubtedly exceeds the capacities of C3bINA. In these two cases, the end result is the formation of excessive quantities of C3b and C3 convertase C3bBb.

### C5 CONVERTASE C3b$_n$Bb

At least one part of the C3b molecules resulting from the cleavage of C3 by C3 convertase C3bBb may be integrated into this convertase, which is transformed into C3b$_n$Bb; these C3b molecules bind C5 and render it susceptible to enzymatic cleavage by C5 convertase. The mechanism of formation of C5 convertase in the alternative pathway is reminiscent of that of the formation of C5 convertase in the classical pathway. This latter, in effect, results from the addition of a C3b molecule to C3 convertase $\overline{C4b2a}$, this addition allosterically modifies C5 and permits its cleavage by C5b and C5a.

# III.  ELEMENTARY BIOLOGIC ACTIVITIES OF COMPLEMENT

The development of the complement reaction leads to the appearance of a series of biologic activities that undoubtedly play a major role in numerous inflammatory phenomena, whether immunologic in origin (e.g., antigen-antibody reaction) or nonimmunologic (e.g., the response to gram-negative bacterial endotoxins).

Some of these activities are directly dependent on the intervention of an unmodified component (e.g., the precipitation of immune complexes by C1q), whereas others are dependent on the action of a cleavage fragment of a component (e.g., the anaphylotoxinic activity of C3a and C5a), and still others involve the intervention of a multimolecular complex that combines several components with one another (e.g., the cytolytic action of the C56789 or C5–9 complexes).

Table 8.2 is a relatively incomplete list of those biologic activities that have been divided (perhaps artificially) into activities occurring on immune complexes, activities concerning vessels and smooth muscle fibers, actions on cells, and, finally, other actions.

## ACTION ON IMMUNE COMPLEXES (IC)

### Precipitation of Immune Complexes and Aggregated IgG by C1q

In vitro, the reaction of C1q with immune complexes is utilized for detecting IC in biologic fluids, whether performed by gel precipitation (Ouchterlony's method) or by precipitation in liquid medium of radiolabeled C1q in the presence or absence of polyethylene glycol (PEG).

It has not yet been demonstrated that IC precipitation by C1q plays an in vivo role. However, it has been shown in systemic lupus erythematosus that C1q is necessary for the formation of mixed polyclonal cryoglobulin, which in addition to C1q, contains IgG, IgM, $\alpha_2M$ and, occasionally, C3 and C4. Cryoprecipitate formation is abolished by heating serum to 56°C for 30 min. The significance of C1q reactivity with certain polyanions (DNA, lipopolysaccharides) remains to be determined; it has been shown that such reactivity is capable of activating C3 through the classical pathway. One possibility is that C1q may react in vivo with circulating DNA, especially when the concentration of the former is very much increased under such conditions as inflammatory processes or corticosteroid treatment.

**Table 8.2  Biologic Activities of Complement**

| Biologic activity | Components (s) |
|---|---|
| *On immune complexes* | |
| Aggregation | C1q |
| Solubilization | C3b |
| *On vessels and smooth muscle fibers* | |
| Increased vascular permeability and smooth muscle contraction | C2 kinin, C3a, C5a |
| *On cells* | |
| Polymorphonuclear and macrophage chemotaxis | C3a, C5a |
| Increased polymorph mobility | Ba |
| Inhibition of macrophage migration and spreading | Bb |
| Mobilization of medullary leukocytes | C3c |
| Aggregation and margination of circulating polymorphs and neutropenia (in vivo) | C5a |
| Polymorph aggregation (in vitro) | C5a |
| Protease secretion by macrophages | C3b |
| Liberation of lysosomal enzymes from polymorphs | C5a |
| Immunoadherence | C4b, C3b |
| Opsonization | C3b |
| Stimulation of B lymphocytes | C3b |
| Histamine release by platelets | C3, C1–6, C1–9 |
| Cytolysis | C8, C9 |
| Modulation of the immune response | C3b, C4b, C3d |
| *On the formation of immunoconglutinin* | C3b |
| *On coagulation* | |
| Platelet-dependent mechanism (rabbit only) | C6 |
| *On viruses* | |
| Neutralization of Herpes virus | C1 + C4 |
| Lysis of cells infected with oncogenic viruses | C1q, C9 |

### Solubilization of Immune Complexes

In the presence of fresh normal serum solubilization of insoluble immune complexes occurs. This solubilization, which results in the liberation into the serum of small-sized complexes, involves the action of complement. It is probable that following the binding of C1q to IgG in the complexes, a slight activation of the classical pathway results in the formation of C3b, which binds onto the complexes and allows the formation of C3 convertase $\overline{C3bBb}$. It is the cleavage of a large number of C3 molecules by this convertase, with the appearance of large quantities of C3b, that is directly responsible for the solubilization of immune complexes. The action of the terminal components of complement (C5 to C9) is not necessary for this effect since it occurs equally readily in the presence of sera deficient in C6, as in the presence of normal sera.

This activity is without doubt of considerable importance in the immune complex diseases in which, after modifying the size of the complexes, it also must, "ipso facto", change their destiny (for example, tissue deposits) and pathogenicity. In patients who are deficient in the early components of the classical pathway (C2, for example), this activity is defective and alters the behavior of the individual with regard to the immune complexes that he may eventually form, thus giving rise to the unusual frequency of immune complex diseases, particularly systemic lupus erythematosus.

## ACTION ON CAPILLARY PERMEABILITY AND SMOOTH MUSCLE FIBERS

### Kinin Activity: C2-Derived Polypeptide

C2, after exposure of C1s to trypsin, releases a polypeptide of a molecular weight of 5000 that, by subcutaneous injection, provokes an immediate increase in capillary permeability not blocked by antihistamines. This peptide might be directly responsible for the increase in vascular permeability seen in angioneurotic hereditary edema.

### Anaphylatoxins (AT): C3a and C5a

Anaphylatoxins are produced by fresh normal serum incubated at 37°C in the presence of immune complexes or colloidal substances (dextran, yeast, gram-negative bacterial endotoxins, cobra venom factor). After intravenous injection into an animal, they provoke lethal shock (anaphylatoxinic shock); placed subcutaneously, an immediate erythema is seen.

Normal human serum releases two anaphylatoxins, C3a (molecular weight 8700) and C5a (molecular weight 17,500), both thermostable at 56°C for 30 min but thermolabile at 65°C. C3a and C5a are disconnected from the main polypeptidic chain of the original molecules (C3 and C5) by breakage of the peptide bond that links the carboxyl group of a basic amino acid (arginine, in the case of C3a) to the main chain fragment. Severance of this bond may be provoked by trypsin, plasmin, and by the trypsinic action of C3 and C5 convertases in the classical and alternative pathways. Additionnally there is, in man an anaphylatoxinic inhibitor (AI) of molecular weight 320,000, which is a thermolabile α globulin that partially inactivates bradykinin. One AI molecule inactivates approximately 500 C3a molecules at 20°C in 2 min. Inactivation follows cleavage of a peptide bond located between the carboxyl group of the carboxy terminal base amino acid and the remaining AT molecule. AI is probably analogous to the carboxypeptidase B described by Erdos. Anaphylatoxinic activities of normal human serum can only develop when AI is absent.

Anaphylatoxins induce an increase in capillary permeability and contraction of smooth muscle fibers by direct or indirect action. The indirect mechanism is accomplished by degradation of basophils and mastocytes, with subsequent release of histamine, serotonin, and heparin. Systemic in vivo AT injection provokes an anaphylatoxinic shock comparable to the anaphylactic shock seen with lung emphysema, featuring bronchial spasma, coronary constriction, erythema, urticaria, and a diffuse increase in capillary permeability; the onset is immediate. Repeated AT injections in guinea pigs render them refractory not only to AT itself but also to anaphylactic shock because of depletion of histamine reserves (particularly pulmonary sources). This represents the tachyphylaxy phenomenon.

In vitro AT application onto guinea pig smooth muscles renders them refractory to further application of AT. Tachyphylaxy is specific for the particular AT utilized. One should note that C5a is a thousandfold more active than C3a in vivo (human skin) and 300 times more active in vitro. AT intervenes only in reactions due to immune complexes but not in those that invoke cytotropic anaphylaxis (using IgE).

### Histamine Release

We have already mentioned the histamine-releasing activity on basophils and mastocytes induced by C3a and C5a (AT). Other mechanisms of complement-induced histamine release have been described, including treatment of rat mastocytes with an antirat anti-$\gamma$-globulin serum and incubation with Cq to C5 components. Similarly, rabbit platelets mixed with particles that possess C3b on their surface and soluble immune complexes, including C1 to C9 components, also release their histamine.

## ACTION ON CELLS

Complement may act on a number of different cells in various ways. Probably most of these activities, at least in their initial stages, involve a reaction between an activator component (or the cleavage product a component) and a specific surface receptor on the target cell, the component being either free or bound, for example to an immune complex. It is known that a number of cells possess complement receptors: C3b receptors on macrophages, polymorphs, B lymphocytes, C1q receptors on B lymphocytes, platelets, and so on.

The main effects of complement on cells are shown in Table 8.2. It can be seen that a great number of these activities involve phagocytic cells that may be mobilized from medullary reserves, attracted to sites where activated complement exists (immune complex deposits, for example), immobilized in this site and stimulated to express phagocytic activity.

### Chemotaxis: C3a, C5a, and C5b67

Three chemotactic factors are derived from complement:

C3a: the chemotactic site is probably different from the AT site because extensive treatment of C3a by trypsin destroys AT but not the chemotactic site;

C5a is more active than C3a;

the $\overline{C5b67}$ complex, which is produced under the influence of C5 convertases of the classical and alternative pathways. One recalls that the $\overline{C5b67}$ complex released in the liquid phase is hemolytically inactive despite chemotactic activity. The circulating C567 complex is not, however, chemotactic.

Normal sera contain in very small amounts chemotactic inhibitors that some pathologic sera contain at fourfold to fivefold higher concentrations (particularly in subjects with Bruton-type agammaglobulinemia and Hodgkin's disease). These inhibitors react with chemotactic factors whether they originate from complement or from other materials (collagen, starch grains, lymphokines, bacterial polyosides).

According to Wissler, AT are not by themselves chemotactic but become so after combination with a crystallizable polypeptide, cocytotaxin ("AT + cocytotaxin").

### Polymorph Lysosome Intracellular Mobilization: C5a

In addition to the chemotactic function, C5a manifests subcellular functions. C5a is capable, independently of phagocytosis, of inducing fusion of polymorph lysosome grains with the cell membrane. The net result is to release the polymorph enzymatic contents outside of the cell. C5a, here, acts indirectly after contact with specific receptors on the cell membrane; this contact provokes an increase in the cellular cyclic guanosine monophosphate level, which leads, in turn, to the assembly of microtubules that regulate intracellular movements of some organelles, particularly lysosomal granules.

### Immunoadherence: C3b and C4b

Nelson was the first to establish that "antigen-antibody complement complexes" are capable of adhering to membranes of both primate red blood cells and to platelets in other species. The immunoadherence reaction occurs essentially through the intermediary of C3b but also by means of C4b. Numerous cells, particularly B lymphocytes, polymorphs, monocycles, macrophages, and red blood cells, bear receptor sites for complement components. Immunoadherence plays an important role in phagocytosis, because it allows contact between immune complexes and the cell membrane. In addition, immune complex phagocytosis requires an interplay between membrane receptors for both C3b and IgG Fc.

Because it is the very earliest phase of phagocytosis, immunoadherence may also play an important role in transport of immune complexes by lymphocytes to strategic areas of the immune response, such as lymphoid follicles; this phenomenon may also facilitate B-lymphocyte binding in areas where immune complexes are deposited (tissues). Recently, it has been suggested that there may exist C1q receptors on B lymphocytes. B lymphocytes and erythrocytes possess specific receptors for C3d ($\alpha_2$D).

### Opsonization or Phagocytosis Enhancement: C3b

The opsonizing activity of complement may follow activation of either the classical or alternative pathway.

Concerning the classical pathway. Gigli and Nelson have shown that after incubation of polymorphs and IgM antibody sensitized red blood cells (EAIgM), addition of C1, C4, and C2 components does not enhance phagocytosis; however, addition of C1, C4, C2, and C3 considerably augments the reaction, whereas further addition of C5 to C9 terminal components is without effect.

Concerning the alternative pathway, it has been shown that C2-deficient human sera may show normal opsonizing activity toward colibacilli, Proteus, *Staphyloccus aureus,* and pneumococci. This activity disappears when serum is treated with cobra venom factor or inulin. Moreover, human serum that has been depleted of C1q by immunoadsorption has a normal opsonizing activity toward colibacilli. This activity is, however, destroyed by heating serum to 50°C for 30 min, which also inactivates C3PA. The addition of C3PA to heated serum restores opsonizing capacity. The opsonizing action of the alternative pathway follows complement activation by antibodies (antipneumococcal antibodies or gram-positive bacterial specific antibodies); alternatively, the activation may be direct, for example, after contact with gram-negative bacterial endotoxins. Jasin demonstrated that sera that show no trace of antibodies or γ globulins maintain their normal opsonizing activity toward colibacilli.

In all cases, complement opsonization requires C3b, for which specific receptor sites exist on numerous cells, particularly phagocytes (monocytes and polymorphs).

## CONGLUTININ AND IMMUNOCONGLUTININ

Conglutinin is a nonimmunoglobulinic protein (molecular weight 750,000), present in the serum of certain ruminants, that aggregates immune complexes by binding to complement. Immunoconglutinins are IgM or IgG iso- or autoantibodies directed against the C3 and C4 antigenic determinants revealed by the C3 and C4 reaction with immune complexes. These antibodies occur during various immunizations, infections, connective tissue diseases, and autoimmune diseases. Conglutinin may inhibit immunoadherence reactions, and under certain conditions, augment complement binding by immune complexes.

## RELATIONSHIPS OF COMPLEMENT TO OTHER BIOLOGIC SYSTEMS

Numerous examples of interplay between complement and other biologic systems, such as the kinins or hemostatic processes (platelets, coagulation, fibrinolysis) have been shown to exist. Many of these relationships have been defined in vitro, but whether or not they are active in vivo remains to be determined.

Activation of the classical pathway may result in activation of the intrinsic coagulation system (contact system) and fibrinolysis. The plasmin thus formed cleaves C1, which gives rise to C1s, which, in turn, activates C4 and C2. Such a mechanism has been proposed to explain the C1s activation responsible for the attacks in familial angioneurotic edema in patients with a congenital deficiency of C1 esterase inhibitor.

In vitro, plasmin has also been shown to be capable of cleaving C3 into C3b and C3a and then C3b into C3c and C3d. Equally, thrombin may also cleave C3, but the molecular site at which this cleavage occurs is different from that brought about by the C3 convertase of the alternative and classical pathways.

In man, immune complexes and aggregated IgG are capable of reacting with platelets. It is highly likely that the mechanism of this reaction is very complex and involves receptor sites for both the Fc part of IgG and complement.

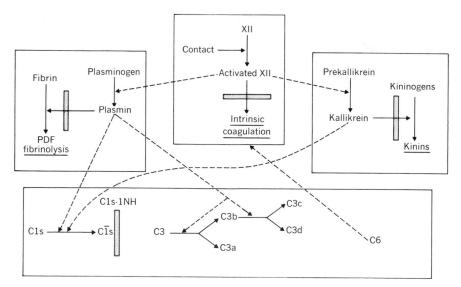

**Fig. 8.4** Relationships among the complement, coagulation, kinin, and fibrinogen systems. Dotted lines indicate C1 esterase inhibitor.

Wautier et al. have shown that only C1 is commonly associated with gel-filtered platelets (GFP). This requires whole C1. After treatment with EDTA only, C1s remains present on the surface of the platelet. This fact, coupled with other experimental arguments, suggest that C1s is the subcomponent of C1, which serves as the attachment portion for C1 onto platelets.

In the rabbit, it has been demonstrated that an intravenous injection of endotoxin or immune complexes initiates a consumption of platelets that results in thrombopenia and a localized or disseminated intravascular coagulation. This consumption of platelets results from an immune complex (or endotoxin)-platelet reaction that requires complement. Under the influence of either one or the other of these agents, complement becomes activated by the classical pathway in the case of immune complexes or by the alternative pathway in the case of endotoxin. This results in the formation of a stable complex, C5b6, which binds to the platelet surface and brings about the release of platelet factor III, either by simple release or by "active lysis." In turn, platelet factor III induces coagulation. C6 is indispensable to this reaction, and this is the basis of the coagulopathy seen in rabbits that are C6-deficient.

### Complement and Kinins

Factor XII and, in particular, its prealbumin fragments (released by pepsin) convert prekallikrein into kallikrein, which, in turn, cleaves kinnogen into kinin; the latter reaction releases a so-called KF fragment that augments C1 action on C4 and C2. The inhibitor of C1 esterase (C1sINH) inhibits not only C1s but also factor XII, plasmin, and kallikrein. We have noted above that C2 cleavage by C1 esterase releases a polypeptide with kinin-like action.

# IV.  SYNTHESIS OF COMPLEMENT COMPONENTS

Numerous techniques have been applied to the study of the cellular site of complement components, in particular, those of in vitro cell culture. Apparently, several types of cells are involved in this synthesis, macrophages and monocytes being one of the main sites of synthesis of these components. The major findings obtained to date in man are listed in Table 8.3.

In the normal individual, the maintenance of relatively constant plasma levels of each component (although the level of each component is quite different) suggests that a regulatory mechanism for their synthesis exists. All attempts to identify humoral regulatorly substances have, to date, been unsuccessful. Only the lymphokines have been demonstrated to have a stimulatory activity on the C2 synthesis by human peripheral monocytes in culture and on C1 synthesis by splenic macrophages in the guinea pig. The simultaneous and appropriate elevation in the different components in the course of the hyper-complementemias suggests, however, that such a mechanism exists. In the course of some consumption hypocomplementemias in man (systemic lupus erythematosus, glomerulonephritis) there occurs a diminished rate of C3 synthesis, which, added to the consumption, contributes even further to the hypocomplementemia.

# V.  COMPLEMENT AND HYPERSENSITIVITY

The multitude of biologic activities that results from activation of the complement system defines an important role for this system in various inflammatory phenomena, irrespective of whether they are immunologically initiated.

Complement plays no apparent role in cytotropic anaphylaxis (associated with the IgE-basophil-mastocyte system) but does have a determinant role in immune complex reactions. Here, complement is activated by complement-fixing Ig, present in either immune complexes or Ig aggregates. Such activation leads to the release of anaphylatoxins and histamine, which react, in turn, with smooth muscle fibers, and increases capillary permeability. The increase in capillary permeability induced by such activation may play a major role in promoting deposition of immune complexes into the subendothelium of vessel walls.

Table 8.3  Cellular Sites of Synthesis of Certain Complement Components

|  | C1 | C4 | C2 | C3 | C9 | C1 INH |
|---|---|---|---|---|---|---|
| Liver (hepatocytes ?) |  | + | + | + | + | + |
| Macrophages | + | + | + |  |  |  |
| Circulating monocytes |  |  | + | + |  |  |
| Ileal epithelial cells | + |  |  |  |  |  |
| Gall bladder epithelium | + |  |  |  |  |  |
| Fibroblasts | + |  |  |  |  |  |

## ARTHUS' PHENOMENON

Complement is necessary for initiating activation of Arthus's phenomenon. Immunohistologic study of early lesions demonstrates superimposition of antigen, antibody, and C3. Its role is corroborated by evidence that Arthus's phenomenon does not develop in decomplemented animals. (Decomplementation is achieved in guinea pigs by treatment with anti-C3 antibody; rats or rabbits are C3 depleted by cobra venom factor; guinea pigs are given the anti-C4 factor from shark serum or levopimaric acid, which produces a C1, C2, C5, C6, and C7 depletion). However, congenitally C4-deficient guinea pigs and C5-deficient mice may develop a normal Arthus's phenomenon. This may be explained by substitution of the alternative pathway for the classical pathway in C3 activation (which appears to be necessary for the development of this phenomenon, whereas C5 and further components would not be necessary). In sensitized animals without complement, which do not develop Arthus's phenomenon, subcutaneous injection of antigen, although not eliciting Arthus's phenomenon, is followed by deposition of antigen-antibody complexes (but obviously not complement) in vessel walls.

Complement intervenes in the genesis of Arthus phenomenon by modifying the local capillary permeability, which favors exudation, edema, and erythrodiapedesis, by attracting locally polymorphs by chemotaxis, and by favoring phagocytosis of immune complexes through its opsonizing properties. This phagocytosis releases locally acid proteases and other hydrolytic lysosomal enzymes that contribute to destructive local lesions that involve vessel basement membranes and adjacent interstitial tissue. This crucial role of polymorphs is evidenced by the absence of Arthus's phenomenon in animals made neutropenic by nitrogen mustard or antileukocyte serum.

## SERUM SICKNESS DISEASE

During the acute phase of serum sickness, at the moment of immune antigen elimination, a transient decrease in serum complement level occurs concomitantly with the appearance of superimposable deposits of antigen, Ig, and complement demonstrable by immunofluorescence. These deposits are located under and between endothelial cells, along the basement membrane, within the internal elastic lamina, and also on the epithelial side of the glomerular basement membrane, where fluorescence reveals a characteristic granular appearance (see chap. 29).

In rabbits treated with cobra venom factor, in which a chronic decrease in total complement occurs, along with the complete disappearance of C3, the arterial lesions are different. The vessel intima is thicker, and lesions are longer-lived; there is a more definitive endothelial cell proliferation and mononuclear cell infiltration. On the other hand, no polymorph influx occurs, and the necrotic lesions usually seen in serum sickness disease, which result from lysosomal enzyme release during phagocytosis, are not observed. Paradoxically, there occur no clinical, histologic, or immunologic changes characteristic of glomerulonephritis. The mechanism by which complement interacts in the genesis of serum sickness (lesions) is comparable to that described for Arthus's phenomenon.

## OTHER EXPERIMENTAL MODELS

The role of complement in the Shwartzman phenomenon will be discussed on p. 363. It should be emphasized that the associated hemodynamic effects (in particular, hypotension) are eliminated by previous decomplementation. Decomplementation may intervene directly or may exhaust reserves of other chemical mediators (massive degranulation of basophils and of perivascular mastocytes).

Localized and systemic Forssman's vasculitis also require complement, because these reactions do not occur in guinea pigs that are congenitally complement deficient or in which complement is depleted by pretreatment with levopimaric acid or anti-C4 factor of shark serum. The latter finding indicates that complement activation in Forssman's vasculitis proceeds through the classical pathway.

Experimental results with respect to Masugi's nephritis (see chap. 29) are less clear-cut. The heterologous phase of glomerulonephritis (GN) may be produced by antibasement membrane antibodies that do not fix complement (duck antibodies). On the other hand, if one utilizes complement-binding antibodies to produce the disease, GN does not develop if the complement-binding sites of these antibodies are previously destroyed in vitro by pepsin or papain or when prior decomplementation by cobra venom factor is performed. The role of complement in the autologous phase remains controversial.

A role for complement in delayed hypersensitivity or in rejection of solid tissue grafts (nonlymphohematopoietic) has not yet been demonstrated.

## HUMAN PATHOLOGY: INVESTIGATION OF THE COMPLEMENT SYSTEM

Study of the human complement system may vary from the very simple measurement of total complement (CH50) to very sophisticated techniques, such as in vivo metabolic studies with radiolabeled components.

### Total Complement

Measurement of total circulating complement (hemolytic complement, CH50) gives important overall information that permits classification of sera as "normo-, hyper-, or hypocomplementemic." The results are expressed in "hemolytic 50 units," per milliliter of serum or biologic liquid ($UH_{50}$/ml or $CH_{50}$/ml).

Numerous techniques for quantifying have been described. The absolute value of $UH_{50}$ may vary considerably among techniques. Therefore interpretation of results must take into account the normal values (means and standard deviations) established for each method.

### Complement Components

Two general techniques for quantifying may be performed.

Hemolytic activity is procedurally cumbersome, and reproducibility is often disappointing. This technique utilizes dilutions of the biologic fluid that contains the test component, appropriate cellular intermediates, such as sheep red blood cells and earlier complement component(s), and a source that contains other complement components in excess. The degree of hemolysis obtained is directly proportional to the concentration of the complement component under study. The results are expressed in stoichiometric terms: $UH_{50}/ml$, or as a percentage of normal concentration. These methods of measurement have the advantage of considering only the native component fraction present in the biologic liquid that is hemolytically active.

Weight quantifying is performed by radial immunodiffusion (Mancini) or by Laurell rocket immunoelectrophoresis (see p. 317). Thus, its use is feasible only when strictly monospecific anticomponent sera are available. Results are expressed as weight per volume (mg of protein/100 ml of serum) or as the percentage of the normal level. These techniques are relatively easy to perform but have a drawback, in that they indifferently quantify the active (native) components and the inactive components, which may have been consumed irreversibly in vivo, for example, by an antigen-antibody-complement reaction. Therefore the quantifying of hemolytic activity correlates better with endogenous immunologic reactions that occur in the organism. Finally it is possible to describe the complete complement profile of an individual, which may be of interest both for diagnosis and for follow-up. The quantity of native C3 may also be determined by immunoadherence techniques, because C3b is mostly implicated in this type of reaction. Recent data, however, indicate that C4b also has an intrinsic immunoadherence activity.

### Anticomplementary Activity

Anticomplementary activity is defined as "substances" present in a biologic fluid capable of binding and thus consuming complement. These substances have a variable nature and mode of action. They may be antigen-antibody complexes, aggregated $\gamma$ globulins, monoclonal paraproteins, or less-defined substances, including the nephritic factor or cryoglobulins. It is apparent that many of these substances include a component of immunologic nature that, by its capacity to bind complement, is responsible for most of the anticomplementary activity. Anticomplementary activity is demonstrated in a biologic fluid by incubating an appropriate volume of the biologic fluid previously cleared of its own complement (by 56°C heating for 30 min) with fresh serum, as the source of complement. The action of anticomplementary substances on fresh serum complement is then recognized by either the resultant decrease in serum hemolytic activity or by the appearance of C3 conversion products, such as C3c ($\beta_1A$) and C3d ($\alpha_2D$).

In some pathologic biologic fluids, one observes a significant inverse relationship between the decrease in the level of endogenous complement and the amount of anticomplementary activity.

### Conversion Products of Complement Components

The activation of complement in the organism may generate conversion products of certain complement components. The presence of these products may be qualitatively detected by immunoelectrophoresis or may be quantified by two-dimensional electrophoresis, according to Laurell's technique. For example, synovial fluid in rheumatoid arthritis may contain appreciable amounts of $\beta_1 A$ and $\alpha_2 D$, the concentration of which is inversely proportional to the total complement level in the fluid and to the titer of rheumatoid factor in the serum. Similarly, in membranoproliferative GN (see chap. 29), one often finds $\alpha_2 D$ in the serum and on the red blood cell surface.

### Tissue and Cellular Complement Deposits

Immunofluorescence may reveal the presence of deposits of complement components in certain tissues. These deposits may occur alone, as do C3 glomerular deposits in certain membranoproliferative GN, or may be associated topographically with superimposable Ig deposits. The former may represent local and direct binding of complement. The latter might be associated with local immune complex deposition, as in glomerular and vascular lesions of circulating immune complex diseases, or might represent complement fixation onto antitissue antibodies themselves bound to specific antigens, as in lung and kidney lesions of Goodpasture's syndrome (or Masugi's experimental GN).

One may compare these tissue deposits of complement components with the presence of C3 (demonstrable by Coombs's complement test) on the surface of red blood cells in some patients with hemolytic autoimmune anemia due to IgG or IgM anti-red cell antibodies. The consequence of complement binding onto the red blood cell surface is not always the same: intravascular hemolysis occurs if complement activation reaches C9; extravascular hemolysis may follow if activation reaches C3 and leads to the formation of EAC3b, whose destruction in reticuloendothelial cells is related to C3b immunoadherence and opsonization activities; red blood cell recirculation occurs when C3bINA cleaves C3b, leaving on the red blood cell surface only C3d, which has no biologic significance.

### Metabolic Studies

Clearance studies can be performed with labeled complement components with the requirement that native and highly purified products be used. These products are injected systemically (intravenously) or locally (intrasynovially, for example), and one estimates rates of synthesis or catabolism of individual components. Studies in normal subjects have shown that approximately half of the circulating serum pool of C3, C4, C1q, and C5 components is renewed daily, thus indicating an extraordinarily fast turnover of these particular globulins.

# INTERPRETATION OF PATHOLOGIC RESULTS IN MAN

## *Hypercomplementemia*

Hypercomplementemia is very common. It is seen in most inflammatory, infectious, and malignant diseases. The elevation in total complement is variable, generally two to three times normal values. The increased total complement level is associated with elevation of most complement components, especially C4, C3, and C9. The pathophysiologic significance of hypercomplementemia is not clear; it may represent stimulation of reticuloendothelial cells that produce most complement components (in particular, macrophages) or byproducts released into the plasma by inflammatory reactions. One sees, generally, a direct and significant correlation between increased levels of complement and non-specific biologic signs of inflammation, including increased $\alpha_2$ globulins, decreased albumin, and an accelerated sedimentation rate.

## *Hypocomplementemia*

Hypocomplementemia is much less commonly seen and may be due to one or more of three mechanisms (Table 8.4): increased consumption, increased catabolism, and decreased production of one or more complement components.

### CONSUMPTION HYPOCOMPLEMENTEMIA

This mechanism is most frequently seen. Complement consumption reflects activation of the classical pathway, alternative pathway, or both. Other phenomena may be causative, including the cleaving action of certain enzymes on one or another complement components (Table 8.4).

Rather than mention all of the diseases that may be associated with hypocomplementemia, we will discuss here two important examples.

The hypocomplementemia that may be seen in systemic lupus erythematosus is representative of other consumption hypocomplementemias and reflects activation of the classical pathway. The degree of hypocomplementemia varies and relates to the disease severity, the extent of organ lesions, and to the evolution of the disease process.

Hypocomplementemia is especially marked in forms of the disease in which skin and renal lesions, autoimmune hemolytic anemia, leukopenia, and thrombocytopenia are seen. The decrease in total complement level is associated with decreased levels of C1q, C1s, C4, C2, and C3, whereas C5 and C9 levels usually remain normal. Repetitive measurements of complement levels in acute disease show that the C4 level is the first to decrease, followed by reduction in levels of C3, total complement, C1q, and, in nephritis, C9. At termination of the acute flare up, restoration of normal values occurs in reverse order, that is, C1q, C3, CH50, and C4: elevated rates of synthesis may coincide (as in inflammatory diseases), but increased catabolic rates predominate in most cases of hypocomplementemia. In this disease state, complement-binding immune complexes can be detected by various techniques and are the most likely cause of consumption hypocomplementemia.

The hypocomplementemia observed in membranoproliferative GN is due

**Table 8.4    Principal Causes of Consumption Hypocomplementemias**

| Biological fluids | Clinical diagnosis | Activation CP | Pathway-involved AP |
|---|---|---|---|
| Serum | Poststreptococcal glomerulonephritis | + | ± |
| | Chronic membranoproliferative glomerulonephritis | 0 | + |
| | Disseminated lupus erythematosus | + | ± |
| | Subacute bacterial endocarditis with glomerulonephritis | + | 0 |
| | Serum sickness | + | 0 |
| | Autoimmune hemolytic anemia | + | 0 |
| | Mixed cryoglobulinemia | + | 0 |
| | Gram-negative endotoxin shock | + | + |
| | Infected arteriovenous shunts | + | 0 |
| | Prodromal phase of viral hepatitis | + | 0 |
| | Homograft rejection | + | 0 |
| | Hereditary angioneurotic edema due to C1INH deficiency | + | 0 |
| | Malaria | + | 0 |
| | Hemorrhagic shock of dengue fever | + | 0 |
| | Rare cases of rheumatoid arthritis, myasthenia gravis, lymphosarcoma, myeloma, macroglobulinemia, multiple sclerosis | + | 0 |
| Synovial, pleural, and pericardial fluids | Rheumatoid arthritis | + | 0 |
| | Disseminated lupus erythematosus | + | 0 |

to alternative pathway activation. Serum C1, C4, and C2 levels are normal; however, serum C3 is considerably decreased. Properdin levels are also depressed in 50% of cases; the glomeruli may contain properdin, C3, and often Ig deposits all superimposed on one another; at the same time, the serum contains C3d and substances (nephritic factor) capable of inducing C3PA (factor B) conversion and cleavage of C3 into C3c and C3d.

COMPLEMENT LOSS

When other serum proteins are lost by various mechanisms, a nonspecific decrease in complement components may be observed. A most typical case is that of large surface area burns. Urinary losses of complement may also contribute to hypocomplementemia of certain glomerular diseases.

SYNTHESIS DEFICIENCIES

*Hepatic Insufficiency.*    Decreased amounts of total complement and some of its components (particularly C4, C2, and C3) are frequently seen in severe hepatic failure, irrespective of etiology (cirrhosis, alcoholic and nonalcoholic, active chronic hepatitis, severe acute viral hepatitis). In these cases, there is an associated decrease in parameters of liver synthetic function (e.g., cholesterol, albumin, coagulation factors).

*Malnutrition.* In certain dietary deficiencies, for example, kwashiorkor, many complement components (C1q, C1s, C5, C6, C8, C9, and C3PA, but not C4) are decreased. These decreases reflect a complex pathogeny that involves decreased synthesis because of insufficient protein intake and infections. This hypocomplementemia is rapidly corrected after restoration of adequate nutrition.

CONGENITAL DEFICIENCIES

These will be discussed with a consideration of the genetics of complement.

### Biologic Fluids Other Than Serum

Study of the complement system in biologic fluids other than serum may be of great interest.

In rheumatoid arthritis (RA) and systemic lupus erythematosus, synovial fluid complement activity is often depressed or even absent. This decrease in complement activity is associated with decreased levels of the various components of the classical pathway and C3PA (factor B), an anticomplementary activity that is inversely related to the level of total complement, and the presence of C3 conversion products. One also notes Ig and C3 deposits together on synovial membranes, in cartilage, and in cells suspended in synovial liquid. There is, finally, local hypercatabolism of radiolabeled C3 (intraarticular injection). All of these elements, in addition to the presence of Ig complexes in the synovial liquid, indicate that RA is probably a localized form of immune complex disease (see chap. 28).

In other inflammatory arthritis, particularly Reiter's and Behçet's syndromes, and in infectious and metabolic arthritis, complement activity is generally high in the synovium; these variations are apparently related to increased permeability of the synovial membrane to serum proteins and, therefore, to complement proteins.

A decrease in complement activity has also been noted in pleural and pericardial effusions, in rheumatoid arthritis, and systemic lupus erythematosus. Here, again, decrements are associated with a decrease in various components of the classical pathway.

Total complement is not present in normal cerebrospinal fluid, but C4 is easily quantitated by hemolytic assays. The component level is decreased in either absolute or relative terms in systemic lupus erythematosus that has meningoencephalic manifestations and, conversely, is elevated in multiple sclerosis, where its variations correlate with the concentration of cerebrospinal fluid proteins.

In the fluid within bullae (dermatitis), the concentrations of total complement and its various components parallel levels of other serum proteins. However, in pemphigus, there is a striking contrast between the relatively high content of protein in bullae and decreased complement activity, probably due to local complement consumption, which suggests an immunologic origin for this disease.

# VI.  GENETICS OF COMPLEMENT

Knowledge of this sphere has arisen from two main sources, namely the study of genetic deficiencies of complement components and that of the polymorphism or allotypy of certain components.

## CONGENITAL DEFICIENCIES

Congenital deficiencies of complement components have been described in man and in several animal species.

### In Animals

In animals it was hoped that valuable information concerning the role of complement in physiologic and pathologic conditions might be obtained.

C4 deficiency in the guinea pig is well tolerated, and there is no abnormality directly linked. The animals are healthy and breed normally. Immunologic Arthus-type reactions, passive cutaneous anaphylaxis, delayed hypersensitivity, and other inflammatory nonspecific reactions due to foreign bodies are within normal limits. The only abnormality defined to date involves the antibody response to low doses of certain antigens and clearance rates of sensitized red blood cells.

C5 deficiency in the mouse is associated with diminished passive cutaneous reactions and a decreased response to *Corynebacterium kutschei* infection and with an abnormal susceptibility to chemical (carcinogen-induced) leukemia. These animals are additionally susceptible to the lethal action of *Plasmodium berghei* and have a limited ability to reject certain sarcoma grafts.

C6 deficiency in the rabbit is associated with numerous immunologic abnormalities: incapacity of the serum to kill gram-negative bacteria and generate the chemotactic activity normally due to C567, diminution of delayed hypersensitivity reactions to tuberculin, and delay in homograft rejection. Associated with these immunologic abnormalities are a low reproductive capacity and the coagulation abnormalities already mentioned.

All of these deficiencies are transmitted by an autosomal recessive gene.

### In Man

In man, the first case of a congenital deficiency of a complement component was described by Klemperer and his colleagues in 1966. This occurred in a healthy man. Since then, the literature on the subject has rapidly expanded to the point where it is now one of the most significant immunodeficiency states and has, at the same time, posed new questions about the pathogenesis of the connective tissue disorders, especially disseminated lupus erythematosus. The deficiency may be homozygous, in which case the subject is totally deficient in the complement component under consideration, or the patient may be heterozygous, the serum level is about 50% of normal for that particular component.

Deficiencies of all the components of the classical pathway, with the exception of C9, have been described, the most frequent being deficiencies of C2 and C7. In a series of over 20,000 sera studies for complement components in the seroimmunology laboratory of the Viggo Petersen Centre, at least 6 cases of homozygous deficiency of C2, 3 cases of homozygous deficiency of C7, 2 cases of homozygous deficiency of C6, and several cases of C1 esterase deficiency were detected. No deficiency in alternative pathway components were described (factor B and D, properdin). It has been suggested that the absent function of the alternative pathway is a lethal condition because of the major role that it plays in the defense against infection at the preimmune stage, that is, before the appearance of antibodies.

The true frequency of homozygous deficiencies in the general population is difficult to establish. Hassig and his colleagues, studying 41,082 sera received

**Table 8.5   Homozygous Deficiencies of Complement Components**

| Deficiency | Number of Cases | Associated Clinical Manifestations | Susceptility to Infection | Link with MHC* |
|---|---|---|---|---|
| C1q | | Never occurs alone but always in association with agammaglobulinemia | + | |
| C1r | 3 | DLE* like syndrome (2 cases) Glomerulonephritis (1 case) | + | |
| C1s | 5 | DLE (1 case) DLE-type syndrome (2 cases) Normal subject (2 cases) | | |
| C4 | 2 | DLE (1 case) DLE-type syndrome (1 case) | | |
| C2 | 40 | DLE (10 cases) Discoid lupus (4 cases) Schönlein-Henoch purpura (4 cases) Dermatomyositis (1 case) Vasculitis (1 case) (frequent) Glomerulonephritis (several cases) Hodgkin's disease (1 case) Variable immune deficiency (1 case) Normal subject (15 cases) | + | + |
| C3 | 5 | Susceptibility to infection by common organisms | + | |
| C5 | 3 | DLE (1 case) Susceptibility to infection (1 case) Recurrent gonococcal septicemia (1 case) | | |
| C6 | 4 | Gonococcal septicemia (1 case) Recurrent or isolated meningococcal meningitis (3 cases) | | |

**Table 8.5    Continued**

| Deficiency | Number of Cases | Associated Clinical Manifestations | Susceptibility to Infection | Link with MHC* |
|---|---|---|---|---|
| C7 | 10 | Transient polyarthritis (1 case) Chronic seronegative arthritis (1 case) Pelvispondylitis (1 case) Raynaud's syndrome, sclerodactyly, Telangiectasia (1 case) Purpura (1 case) Pyelonephritis (1 case) Normal subjects (4 cases with mixed C6–C7 deficiencies) | | |
| C8 | 8 | DLE (1 case) Xeroderma pigmentosum (3 cases in the same family) Gonococcal septicemia (1 case) Diagnosis unclear (1 case) Thalassemia (1 case) Gonococcal + streptococcal endocarditis (1 case) | | |
| C1   INH** | Several hundreds | Hereditary angioneurotic edema in most cases. Complicated by: DLE (1 case) Chronic discoid lupus (4 cases) | | |
| KAF (C3b inactivator)** | | Klinefelter's syndrome + susceptibility to infections. | | |

* MHC: Major histocompatibility complex (HLA system).
** Autosomal dominant heterozygotic defeciency. DLE = Disseminated lupus erythematosus

from the Swiss army, found 14 deficient sera, a frequency of just over 3%, which is very close to the frequency observed by the authors in a population of patients. Naturally, the frequency of heterozygous deficiencies is much higher. For C2, Glass et al. have estimated the frequency to be on the order of 12% in a population of 509 blood donors.

From the genetic point of view, the majority of these deficiencies seem to be transmitted by a codominant or recessive autosomal gene, a subject with a homozygous deficiency having parents who are both heterozygotically deficient. C1-esterase-inhibitor deficiency, which is responsible for hereditary angioneurotic edema, is transmitted by means of an autosomal dominant gene; people who suffer from the angioneurotic edema are all heterozygotically deficient.

No case of C1 deficiency (that is C1q-C1r-C1s complex) has been described. In contrast, partial deficiencies of C1q and complete deficiencies of C1r and C1s have been reported. C1q deficiencies are of interest because they never arise in isolation but are always associated with a significant immunoglobulin deficiency (Bruton-type hypogammaglobulinemia, sporadic agammaglobulinemia, Swiss-type infantile lymphopenic agammaglobulinemia). C1r and C1s deficiencies are rare. In eight cases, five were associated with disseminated lupus erythematosus or related syndromes, one arose owing to complicated glomerulonephritis, and the remaining two were otherwise normal.

C4 deficiencies also appear to be rare since only two cases have been described, one being a young woman suffering from disseminated lupus erythematosus, the other a male infant with a lupuslike syndrome.

Homozygous C2 deficiency is without doubt the most frequent deficiency. The frequency of the gene coding for the C2 deficiency has been estimated at 1%. Over 60 cases of homozygous C2 deficiency have been reported. Of these reported cases, 60% are complicated by clinical manifestations, of which the most frequent are disseminated lupus erythematosus, discoid lupus, and Henoch-Schönlein purpura. Very often in ill patients, there is also a markedly increased susceptibility to common infections (otitis, sinusitis, bronchopneumonia, etc.). C2 deficiency is much more frequent in women than in men, and the incidence of lupuslike syndromes is much more common in deficient women than in deficient men.

Heterozygous deficiencies of C2 appear with equal frequency, unlike other heterozygotic deficiencies, which are not accompanied by any particular pathologic processes. Heterozygous patients seem to suffer from a significantly higher incidence of inflammatory rheumatic disorders (especially juvenile polyarthritis and disseminated lupus erythematosus).

Homozygous C3 deficiency is rare, but all the reported cases are characterized by a dramatic susceptibility to infection by common organisms, which gives rise to a clinical picture that is comparable with that of the more severe agammaglobulinemias. This is an expression of the central position of C3 in the complement system and explains the multiple functions of this component and its cleavage products, that is, chemotaxis, immunoadherence, opsonization, and so on.

Among the other deficiencies, one of the most remarkable is C6 deficiency, which apparently predisposes to infection by the *Neisseria* group of bacteria. Of the four cases reported in the literature, three were detected as a result of meningococcal meningitis and the other during a gonococcal septicemia.

On the basis of the first reported case of complement deficiency, it was concluded that deficiencies of the early components (C1, C4, C2) predisposed mainly to the development of inflammatory and connective-tissue disorders, whereas deficiencies in the later components (C3 to C9) predisposed to early infections. Further experience has not confirmed this impression because lupus type inflammatory disorders may be associated with deficiencies of C5, C8, and C1 esterase inhibitor. In the latter case, it may be that the chronic depletion of C4 and, to a lesser degree, C2, which results from the uncontrolled consumption of these components by C1s, create a truly acquired secondary deficiency of these components that favors the development of disseminated lupus erythematosus, as in the congenital deficiency of these same two components.

In addition to these clinical problems, several other questions are raised by the existence of homozygotic deficiencies.

*Inconsistent Susceptibility to Infection.* If complement really plays the central role with which it has been attributed in the defences against infection, it is rather surprising that not all the homozygous deficiencies with a complete absence of total complement are complicated by susceptibility to infection. There are several possible explanations for this:

1. Complement is, of course, far from being the only barrier in the defence against infection and, for example, among the opsonins, beside those that are complement-dependent (C3b), there are others, such as IgG, that play a preponderant role, which is sometimes synergistic with that of complement.

2. A homozygous deficiency only interrupts part of the function of the complement system. In the case of C2 deficiency, for example, the alternative pathway and the common trunk function normally and, equally important, biologic activities may appear, such as C3b, C3a, C5a, and C567. In the case of C6 deficiency, the classical and alternative pathways function normally and only the end-stages of the common trunk are missing.

3. It might also be supposed that a normal gene, such as an immune-response gene, may be associated with the abnormal deficient gene. This might occur in the case of a deficiency gene that is situated within, or very close to, the major histocompatibility complex (genes C2 and C4).

*Mechanisms of Appearance of Inflammatory Disorders and Connective Tissue Diseases.* The frequency of disorders associated with complement deficiencies may appear paradoxical because of the determining role that has been ascribed to complement and its activation in the pathogenesis of such disorders. Here, again, there are several possible explanations:

1. Complement appears to be indispensable for the normal elimination of immune complexes from the organism (precipitating action of C1q, solubilizing action of C3b, opsonization, etc). It is therefore conceivable that, in the case of deficiency, the organism is no longer capable of behaving normally toward immune complexes whose formation results in persistent infections (e.g., the slow viruses), which are themselves favored by the deficiency.

2. It might also be suggested that the deficiency gene (C2, C4) is situated on chromosome 6 in association with one or several HLA genes that predispose to the disorder.

## POLYMORPHISM OF COMPLEMENT COMPONENTS

In man, an allotypy or polymorphism has been demonstrated for several components of complement, particularly C3, factor B, and C6. Polymorphism of C3, C2, and C7 is also probable. The polymorphism of factor B is dependent on genes situated on a locus that is very close to that of the C2 gene and is, therefore, close to the HLA locus on chromosome 6.

Comparable data have been obtained in animals. In the mouse, the S region of the H-2 complex or the gene(s) control the level of total complement, that of the protein Ss (C4) and that of the C1, C4, C2, and C3 components. In the chicken, the serum levels of total complement also depend on genes that are associated with the major histocompatibility complex represented by blood group B. Finally, in the rhesus monkey, the polymorphism of factor B is bound to different immunologic systems localized on the RhLA complex, which is the equivalent, in this animal, to the major histocompatibility complex.

It is difficult to escape the thought that the presence of the immune-response genes and those coding for the synthesis of complement components, which are only a short distance from the MHC on the same chromosome (chromosome 6 in man), is of major evolutional and functional significance.

## *BIBLIOGRAPHY*

AGNELLO V. Complement deficiency states. Medicine, 1978, 57, 1.

ALPER C. A. and ROSEN F. S. Human complement deficiencies. In: Mechanisms of Immunopathology (Cohen S., Ward P. A. and McCluskey R. T. eds.). John Wiley & Sons, New York, 1979, 289.

ATKINSON J. P. and FRANK M. M. Complement. In: Clinical Immunology (Parker C. W. ed.) Saunders, Philadelphia., 1980, 219.

COLTEN H. R. Biosynthesis of complement. Adv. Immunol. 1976, 22, 67.

GÖTZE O. and MÜLLER-EBERHARD H. J. The $C_3$ activator system: an alternate pathway of complement activation. J. Exp. Med., 1971, 134, 90s.

GÖTZE O. and MÜLLER-EBERHARD H. J. The role of properdin in the alternate pathway of complement activation. J. Exp. Med., 1974, 139, 44.

GÖTZE O. and MÜLLER-EBERHARD H. J. The alternative pathway of complement activation. Adv. Immunol., 1976, 24, 1.

HAUPTMANN G., GROSSHANS E., HEID E., MAYER S., and BASSET A. Lupus érythémateux aigü avec déficit complet de la fraction C4 du complément. Nouv. Presse Méd., 1974, 3, 881.

HUGLI T. E. and MÜLLER-EBERHARD H. J. Anaphylatoxins C3a and C5a. Adv. Immunol., 1978, 26, 1.

MAYER M. The complement system. Sci. Amer., 1973, 229, 54.

MEDICUS G., SCHREIBER D., GÖTZE O., and MÜLLER-EBERHARD H. J. A molecular concept of the properdin pathway. Proc. Natl. Acad. Sci. USA, 1976, 73, 612.

MÜLLER-EBERHARD H. J. Complement. Ann. Rev. Biochem., 1975, 44, 697.

MÜLLER-EBERHARD H. J. and SCHREIBER R. S. Molecular biology and chemistry of the alternative pathway of complement. Adv. Immunol., 1980, 29, 1.

MÜLLER-EBERHARD H. J. Complement reaction pathways. In: Immunology 80 (M. Fougereau and J. Dausset eds.) Acad. Press New York, 1980:1001.

NICOL P. A. and LACHMANN P. J. The alternate pathway of complement activation. The role of C3 and its inactivator (KAF). Immunology, 1973, 24, 259.

PORTER R. R. and REID K. The biochemistry of complement. Nature, 1978, 275, 699.

RAUM D., DONALDSON V. H., ALPER C. A., and ROSEN F. S. Genetics of complement and complement deficiencies. In Immunology 80. (M. Fougereau and J. Dausset eds.). Acad. Press New York, 1980:1244.

RAUM D., GLASS D., CARPENTER C. B., ALPER C. A., and SCHUR P. H. The chromosomal order of genes controlling the major histocompatibility complex, properdin, factor B and deficiency of the second component of complement. J. Clin. Invest., 1976, 58, 1240.

ROSS G. D. Analysis of the different types of leukocyte membrane complement receptors and their interaction with the complement system. J. Immunol. Methods., 1980, 37, 197.

WHALEY K. and RUDDY S. Modulation of the alternative complement pathway of β1H globulin. J. Exp. Med., 1976, 44, 1147.

## ORIGINAL ARTICLE

PANGBURN M. K. and MÜLLER-EBERHARD H. J. Relation of a putative thioester bond in C3 to activation of the alternative pathway and the binding of C3b to biological targets of complement. J. Exp. Med., 1980, 152, 1101.

# Chapter 9

# ANTIGEN-ANTIBODY REACTIONS
# Introduction to Serology

**Jean-François Bach**

I. REACTIONS OF ANTIBODIES WITH HAPTENS
II. REACTIONS OF ANTIBODIES WITH MACROMOLECULES
III. DIRECT BINDING TESTS
IV. IMMUNOPRECIPITATION
V. ANTIGEN-ANTIBODY REACTIONS USING CELLULAR OR PARTICULATE ANTIGENS
VI. CONCLUSIONS

The combination of antibodies with corresponding antigens is the basis of most immunologic reactions, both for serum antibodies and for lymphocyte membrane receptors. Study of the antigen-antibody reaction is complicated by the fact that most antigens are macromolecules and that, even when their structure is known, the nature, number, and localization of the various functional groups present on each molecule are difficult to assess. For this reason, haptens with a limited number of determinants are used to study antigen-antibody reactions. Extrapolation to more complex molecules is then attempted. This approach is warranted, because although antigens and haptens differ in their immunogenicity, that is their capacity to stimulate antibody production, they share the ability to combine with antibodies, which is our present interest. In practice, one may generalize the discussion with the use of the term "ligand" to indicate either antigen or hapten.

The author thanks Dr. J. P. Cartron for reviewing this chapter.

285

# I.   REACTIONS OF ANTIBODIES WITH HAPTENS

Antibodies specific for simple haptens may be obtained with a fair degree of purity quite easily. Haptens are coupled to carrier proteins for the purpose of immunization or are utilized directly, as for oligosaccharides or polysaccharides that contain the hapten in their sequence. The antibodies thus obtained are purified by passage of the antiserum through an immunoadsorbent that contains the hapten, followed by elution of specific antibodies.

## ANTIBODY VALENCE AND AFFINITY

In the classic example, a hapten (or ligand) with only one functional group is bound reversibly to the specific antibody site. For a given antibody concentration, as increasing amounts of hapten are mixed with antibody, the concentration of bound hapten progressively increases until all antibody sites are occupied. When saturation is achieved, the number of bound hapten molecules equals the number of antibody sites. The number of sites on each antibody molecule defines the antibody's valence. If one supposes that binding sites are identical for all antibody molecules of the antiserum and that they react independently of each other, the reaction may be represented as follows:

$$A + H \underset{k'}{\overset{k}{\rightleftharpoons}} AH,$$

where A is the antibody site, H is the haptenic site, and $k$ and $k'$ are the rate constants for association and dissociation of the antibody-hapten (AH) complex

   If one assumes the hypothesis of identity and functional independence of the sites, at equilibrium the mass action law is written:

$$[A][H]k = [AH]k'$$

or

$$\frac{[AH]}{[A][H]} = \frac{k}{k'} = K.$$

The ratio $K = k/k'$ is the intrinsic association constant of the reaction. It quantifies the stability of the hapten-antibody complex or, more precisely, the intrinsic affinity of the antibody site for the hapten. The brackets correspond to respective concentrations of antibody sites occupied by the hapten [AH], of free antibody sites [A], and of free haptenic sites [H]. One notes that the units of the $K$ ratio are concentration divided by concentration squared; therefore, its dimensions are the reciprocal of concentration, most often in units of liters per mole. Increased intrinsic affinity of the complex is associated a larger $K$ value.

# AFFINITY MEASUREMENT

If in the preceding equation $K = [AH]/[A][H]$, one knows the total concentration of antibodies present in the reaction, $[A] + [AH]$, which is the sum of bound and free antibody concentrations, and also the concentration of hapten, $[H] + [AH]$, the sum of bound and free hapten; to calculate $K$, it is sufficient to determine $[A]$, $[H]$, or $[AH]$ at equilibrium. Of these three parameters, the easiest to measure is usually $[H]$, the free hapten concentration. Several methods allow separation of free and bound hapten. The most used method is equilibrium dialysis, which is satisfactory, because it does not alter the equilibrium previously reached by the antigen-antibody reaction, as may theoretically happen when immunoglobulin is precipitated by concentrated saline solutions. Other methods include Ig precipitation by ammonium sulfate or polyethylene glycol, inhibition of precipitation by hapten addition, ultracentrifugation, and fluorescence quenching. Equilibrium dialysis will be dealt with in more detail, because the principles of this method are also applicable in other settings.

# EQUILIBRIUM DIALYSIS

The technique is based on the fact that free hapten, H, of low molecular weight is dialyzable, whereas antibody-hapten complex, AH, is not. Antibodies and hapten are placed into two compartments separated by a membrane. The hapten of low molecular weight diffuses freely across the dialysis membrane, whereas the antibody molecules, whether free or complexed with the hapten, do not cross the membrane (Fig. 9.1). At equilibrium, the hapten concentration is higher in the compartment that contains the antibodies, because the free hapten is in equal concentration on both sides of the membrane. Figure 9.1 shows the evolution of hapten concentrations on both sides of the membrane. In the absence of antibodies, both concentrations are the same at the time of equilibrium. In the presence of antibodies, the difference between concentrations in the two chambers corresponds to hapten that is bound to antibodies. In theory, a difference in concentrations between the two chambers might exist independently of binding to a specific antibody because of Donnan's effect of negatively charged proteins. This phenomenon may be excluded by adding a sufficient concentration of salt to the medium, that is, 0.15 M sodium chloride. Obviously, Donnan's effect does not pertain to electronegative haptens. It is noteworthy that the same equilibrium is obtained when the antibody and the hapten are initially placed in one chamber or in separate chambers, which provides good evidence for the reversibility of antibody-hapten binding.

Simple measurement of the total hapten concentration on both sides of the dialysis membrane permits measurement of the association constant, $K$. If $c$ represents the free hapten concentration (measured experimentally in such units as moles per liter in the antibody-free chamber), $r$ is the average number of hapten molecules bound per antibody molecule at equilibrium, $M$ is the antibody concentration (mole/liter), and if $n$ equals the maximum number of

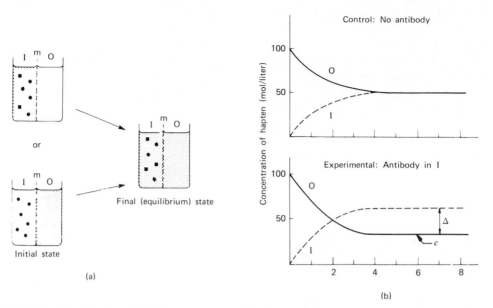

**Fig. 9.1** Equilibrium dialysis. (a) Low-molecular-weight haptens (small dots) diffuse freely between compartments I and O, but antibody molecules (large dots) cannot diffuse. At equilibrium, the hapten concentration is higher in I due to binding by antibody. (b) Changes in haptenic concentrations with time. Equilibrium is reached in about 4 hr. In the experiment represented here, the hapten had been initially placed in compartment O. (c) Free hapten concentration at equilibrium; $\Delta$ that of antibody-bound hapten. (From H. N. Eisen, Immunology. An introduction to molecular and cellular principles of the immune responses, ed. 2. New York, 1974, Harper & Row, p. 361.)

hapten molecules that each antibody molecule can bind (i.e., antibody valence),

$$K = \frac{[AH]}{[A][H]} = \frac{Mr}{M(n-r) \times c} = \frac{r}{(n-r)c}$$

where $c$ is an experimental value (mole/liter), $n$ is a constant, and $r$ equals an average number of sites experimentally determined by $Mr.$ the preceding equation can be expressed by Scatchard's representation:

$$\frac{r}{c} = Kn - Kr, \quad \text{or} \quad r = Knc - Krc, \quad \text{or} \quad r(l + Kc) = Knc,$$

or, by rearrangement,

$$\frac{l}{r} = \frac{l + Kc}{Knc},$$

alternatively,

$$\frac{l}{r} = \frac{l}{nK} \times \frac{l}{c} + \frac{l}{n} \text{ (Klotz's representation)}.$$

The experimental values measured in moles per liter, are the free hapten concentration in the chamber without antibodies [H], $c$; the total hapten concentration in the chamber that contains the antibodies [AH] + [H], ($Mr$ + $c$), and $M$, which permits us to calculate $r$.

Measurements may be repeated at several haptenic concentrations for a fixed antibody concentration. The equation $r/c = Kn - Kr$ states that the curve that represents $r/c$ values as a function of $r$ is a straight line; the intersection with the abscissa corresponds to the number of antibody sites (i.e., antibody valence); the slope of the equation is the reciprocal of the $K$ association constant (if the hypothesis of identity and independence of antibody sites is correct) (Fig. 9.2). In fact, when the free hapten concentration $c$ is very high (in large haptenic excess close to saturation of the antibody site), the $r/c$ ratio approaches zero, and $r$ is nearly equal to $n$, because $r/c = Kn - Kr$. This means that the number of hapten molecules linked to each antibody molecule approximates the total number of sites per antibody molecule, that is, valence. By Scatchard's analysis, linearity of the curve or lack of it also allows an estimation of antibody homogeneity in a given experimental situation.

Experimental observations confirm the theoretical prediction. As shown in Figure 9.2, curve $r/c = f(r)$, is, indeed, linear or nearly so for high $r/c$ values. The intersection point of this line with the abscissa ($r/c = 0$) gives an $r$ value of 2 for IgG, which is known to have two binding sites, and generally $r = 5$ for IgM (see p. 194). One may also note from the family of curves present in Fig. 9.2 that high-affinity antibodies (hyperimmunization) show a straight line with a steeper slope than do antibodies of low affinity obtained after short immunization with high antigen doses. Experimentally, $K$ values range between $10^6$ and $10^{12}$ liter/mole, depending on antibody affinity.

## AFFINITY HETEROGENEITY: AVERAGE AFFINITY

The $r/c = f(r)$ curve is not linear in the majority of experimental situations (Fig. 9.2), which indicates that most antisera contain antibodies with sites that are not independent or not identical. The bivalence of IgG molecules is not in question, because the same types of curves are seen with monovalent IgG fragments prepared by enzymatic digestion. This excludes potential interactions between free and occupied sites on the IgG molecule. In fact, the nonlinear nature of the curves is explained by the heterogeneity of antibody affinity. The only homogeneous antibodies are those directed against certain polysaccharides and myelomatous antibodies. The affinity of these antibodies is sufficiently homogeneous so that the curves $r/c = f(r)$ are straight lines. With these exceptions, the term "antibody" used in the singular represents most often a heterogeneous molecule population that has in common the capacity to bind one given hapten or antigen. In the usual case of affinity heterogeneity, an average intrinsic association constant $K_0$ is defined, which is the average of the association constants for various antibodies.

Antibody heterogeneity may be quantified if one hypothesizes that association constants of the various antibodies are normally distributed (with a gaussian distribution) around the $K_0$ average. This is done by Sips' equation:

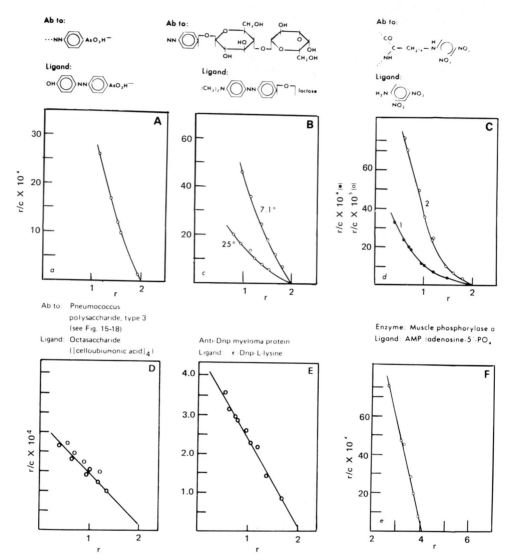

**Fig. 9.2** Specific binding of various haptens to antibodies, plotted according to the equation $r/c = f(r)$. In all cases, extrapolation of the curves to the abscissa indicates that there are two sites per antibody molecule (it is an IgG). Note that the affinity is higher at 7° than at 25°C (B), that the affinity of antidinitroaniline antibodies differs more than thirtyfold (C), and that curves are generally not linear, except for homogeneous antibodies, such as antipolysaccharide antibodies (D) or myelomatous antibodies (E). The curve of binding of muscle phosphorylase to its substrate, which involves four binding sites, is presented for comparison (F). (From H. N. Eisen, Immunology. An introduction to molecular and cellular principles of the immune responses, ed. 2. New York, 1974, Harper & Row, p. 363.)

$r/(n - r) = (Kc)^a$, where $a$ is a dispersion index of association constants similar to the standard deviation of normal distributions (when antibodies are homogeneous, $a = 1$). Sips' equation may be written:

$$\log \frac{r}{n - r} = a \log K + a \log c.$$

$\log r(n - r)$ is thus a linear function of $\log c$.

For $r = n/2$, $\log Kc = 0$, $Kc = 1$, and, finally, $K_0 = 1/c$, which shows that the average intrinsic association constant is independent of $a$.

The average intrinsic association constant is highly variable for different antigen-antibody systems. It is usually of the order of $10^5$ to $10^7$. One must understand that when multiple sites are present, the actual affinity may be much higher than the intrinsic affinity, because the valence augments the stability of the complex by cooperation between sites. This cooperation applies particularly to antigen molecules that have numerous determinants. This phenomenon of monogamous binding may increase $10^3$- to $10^5$-fold the effective association constant. Thus, the association constant of antidinitrophenyl (anti-DNP) antibodies is 100,000 times higher for DNP bound repetitively to bacteriophages than for the monovalent hapten derivative DNP-lysine ($10^2$ to $10^7$). Monogamous binding decreases greatly the risk of dissociation. This fact probably explains the remarkable biologic activity in vivo of very low amounts of antisera directed against viruses and bacteria, which often bear repetitive determinants.

Affinities of the various antibodies present in a given serum are not always distributed in a gaussian way. In some cases, the antibodies may show marked homogeneity. In a case described by Nisonoff, a rabbit anti-*p*-azobenzoate antibody was obtained in crystallized form. The presence of a limited number of molecular species may sometimes explain the observed heterogeneity. Analysis of Sips' curves obtained with an anti-DNP rabbit antibody, and with a wide spectrum of free hapten concentrations by Werblin and Siskind, has shown very limited antibody heterogeneity, in some cases or, at least, no gaussian distribution.

The affinity of IgG antibodies for monovalent haptens is generally higher than is that of IgM antibodies for the same specificity. Similarly, IgG affinity for antigenic erythrocyte sites is more than 100 times greater than the affinity of Fab fragments (3.5 S) produced by enzymatic cleavage of native IgG with papain. This difference in affinity could be due to binding of 7S molecules on red blood cells by their two antibody sites. The intrinsic affinity of an isolated antibody-combining site is usually much lower than the functional affinity measured with the entire molecule. Thus, in the system cited above, one may compare intrinsic and functional affinities of IgG and IgM anti-DNP antibodies to DNP-lysine and to a preparation of DNP coupled to phage $\phi \times 174$. The functional affinity of anti-DNP IgG measured by phage neutralization is $10^3$ times higher than the intrinsic affinity measured with the monovalent ligand. In the IgM case, the ratio is of the order of $10^6$. This difference probably reflects the higher valence of IgM molecules and their capacity to form multiple bonds with structures of sufficient density of antigenic determinants as discussed earlier.

# SPECIFICITY AND AFFINITY

Immunologic reactions derive their uniqueness from their specificity; specificity essentially defines antigens and antibodies. We have seen that even a purified antiserum contains usually a mixture of antibodies of variable affinity. The specificity of an antibody is linked to the ability of this antibody to discriminate between antigenic determinants of similar but different structures, by binding with different affinities; the greater the affinity difference of an antibody for two given haptens, the higher the specificity of the antibody for the hapten of higher affinity (see Fig. 6.1). This is reminiscent of the early Landsteiner definition of specificity: "a disproportional action of several related antibodies toward related haptens." The high affinity antibodies sometimes seem less specific than do low-affinity antibodies when the antibodies are present in low concentrations, because they combine less well with the homologous hapten, but, in fact, the affinity difference between haptens is essential, more so even than are the absolute affinity values and even more so than the binding intensity. In practice, antibody *specificity* is generally defined in relation to an antigen or hapten family (the antibody affinity for several antigens or haptens is measured). Antibody *affinity* is, in general, defined with respect to an antibody family (one compares the average affinity of several antisera for a given hapten).

# PHYSICOCHEMICAL BASIS OF HAPTEN-ANTIBODY BINDING

The forces that link antibodies to haptens or to antigens are not fundamentally different from those that govern the various interactions between proteins or between enzymes and substrates. The nature of these forces and the thermo-dynamics of the reactions in question are thus similar to those of interactions between proteins. They are exclusively noncovalent forces and therefore relatively weak and highly dependent on steric complementarity between antigen and antibody sites.

### Forces Involved in Antigen-Antibody Reactions

The forces that link antigens and antibodies are of four types: van der Waals forces, electrostatic forces (or coulombian forces), hydrogen bonds, and hydrophobic bonds. Their intensity is variable: van der Waals forces are the weakest, of the order of 0.5 kcal/mole versus 2 to 5 kcal/mole for electrostatic forces or hydrogen bonds. They are, in any case, of lesser strength than covalent forces, which reach 50 to 150 kcal/mole. It is important to note that these forces are at least decreased proportionally to the reciprocal of the increasing distance between antigen and antibody molecules. They are stronger at shorter distances, that is, when the two structures are complementary. Increased stability of the antigen-antibody combination is seen when the contact area widens. The theoretical distance between antigen and antibody sites may also be influenced by the flexibility of the antibody molecule, which may allow certain residues to approach closer to the contact area with the antigen.

### VAN DER WAALS FORCES

These forces are linked to the electron movement within molecules and lead to the rapid formation of electric fields that polarize surrounding molecules. The presence of electric fields within one molecule (dipole formation) changes the distribution of electrons in the other molecule, and the two dipoles then attract each other. The interactional energies are inversely proportional to the sixth power of interatomic distances. These relatively weak forces are functional only for closely complementary antigens and antibodies and in these cases are very efficient.

### ELECTROSTATIC FORCES

Electrostatic (or coulombian) forces are those exerted between two ionic groups of opposite charge, for example, the amino ($NH_3{}^+$) group of a protein lysine and the carboxyl group (COO—) of aspartate from another protein.

### HYDROGEN BONDS

These bonds are of weak energy (0.5 to 2 kcal/mole) between electropositive (hydrogen) and electronegative atoms (oxygen or nitrogen). Interactional energies are inversely proportional to the sixth power of the distance between the atoms. The stability of these bonds depends on the presence of water molecules; they are augmented by decreased temperature.

### HYDROPHOBIC BONDS (STABILIZING INTERACTIONS BETWEEN NONPOLAR GROUPS IN WATER) (FIG. 9.3)

Certain amino acids of Ig chains tend to repel solvent water molecules and do not establish hydrogen bonds in aqueous solution. This phenomenon is seen with aromatic amino acids, such as valine and leucine. However, when two of these amino acids come in close contact, after a diminution in the number of neighboring water molecules, there is an energetic increment that augments the bond stability. The energetic increment is higher as the distance between two amino acids decreases. In contrast to hydrogen bonds, the hydrophobic bonds between antigen and antibody are more stable at higher temperature.

### CONCLUSIONS

Once the antigen (or hapten) and the antibody have made contact, several links form between molecules; the different forces discussed above may be involved to varying degrees. The nature of the bonds indicates that binding between antigen and antibody is reversible under thermal agitation of molecules due to heating; the bond is more stable when structures are more complementary.

## Influence of Physicochemical Conditions on Antigen-Antibody Reactions

### EFFECTS OF pH AND IONIC STRENGTH

Antigen-antibody reactions are affected by the existing physicochemical conditions. The effect of these conditions on association constants depends on the nature of the forces involved. Thus, the binding of *p*-aminobenzoate and antibenzoate antibodies decreases from 0.1 to 1 M NaCl. Conversely, pH change does not affect the binding of antibodies to nonionized haptens, for example, the binding of 2,4-dinitroaniline to anti-DNP antibodies. One therefore postulates that the benzoate $COO^-$ group interacts with a positively charged antibody site, whereas ionic interactions have little influence on the binding of antibody to neutral DNP. These effects of low pH and high molarity are used to eluate antibodies from immunoadsorbent columns. One should note, however, that the effects of pH and molarity changes may not be restricted to the reactive sites of antigen or antibody but may alter all of the molecule.

EFFECTS OF TEMPERATURE

The binding forces between antigens and antibodies vary with temperature, which affects the rate of the antigen-antibody reaction. This rate may be optimal at 37°C, especially for some "secondary" reactions, for example, precipitation or complement fixation. The association constant is not necessarily higher, but the reaction occurs more rapidly at 37° than at 4°C. Some reactions occur more rapidly at 4°C. In other cases, the speed of association is no different at 4° and 40°C.

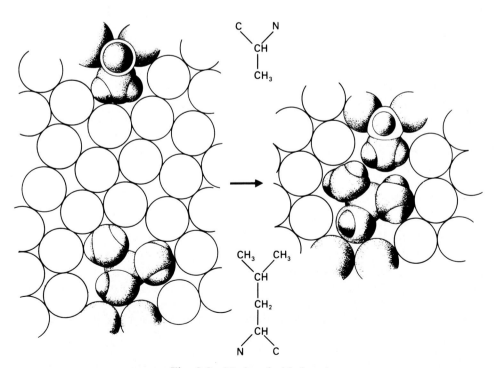

**Fig. 9.3** Hydrophobic bond.

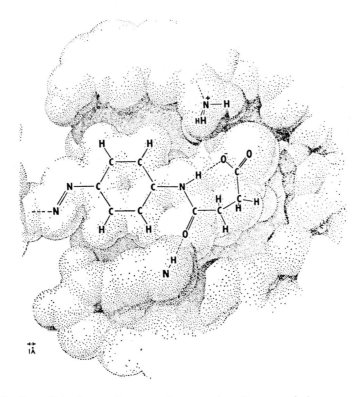

**Fig. 9.4** Binding of the haptenic group *p*-azosuccinonilate coupled to a protein with its specific antibody. (From L. Pauling, Endeavour, 1948, 7, 43.)

THERMODYNAMICS

The formation of an antigen-antibody complex causes a loss of free energy, $\Delta F^0$, proportional to the logarithm of the average association constant:

$$F^0 = -R \times T \times \ln K_0$$

where $R$ is the constant of perfect gas (1.987 cal/mole), $T$ equals the absolute temperature, $\ln K_0$ represents the Neper logarithm of the association constant, and $\Delta F^0$ is the variation of standard energy ($p = 1$ atm; $T = 293$), that is the energy gain or loss (calories) observed when 1 mole of antibody reacts with 1 mole of hapten. $\Delta F^0$ values vary from 6000 to 11,000 cal for association constants of the order of $10^5$ to $10^9$ $M^{-1}$, at 20° or 30°C.

KINETICS

Kinetics of antibody-hapten reactions are generally studied with low hapten concentrations under conditions such that reactions are slow enough to be measured. It is also possible, using a special apparatus, to measure variations in free hapten concentrations at microsecond intervals, thus permitting utilization of higher hapten concentrations. Finally, relaxation methods may be used, in which antibody and hapten are brought to equilibrium, and then equilibrium is modified by change in temperature, pressure, or electric field, and the return to original equilibrium is examined.

The association reaction between a small hapten and an antibody is very rapid, no more than 10 times less than simple diffusion ($10^8$ liter/mole/sec). Reactions between whole proteins and antibodies are also rapid, but they are 10 to 100 times slower than those that occur between simple haptens and antibodies. It is important to recognize that association kinetics of haptens and antibodies are only slightly dependent on the intrinsic association constants; therefore, affinity differences are linked primarily to variations in dissociation rates.

## II. REACTIONS OF ANTIBODIES WITH MACROMOLECULES

All complexes of antibodies and monovalent haptens are soluble. Macromolecular antigens, however, may show precipitation in the presence of certain antibodies. The precipitation reaction has broad biologic significance, because practically all antibodies are precipitating under certain conditions. For this reason, in addition to its historic interest, we will discuss precipitation reactions in detail, making a distinction between theoretical considerations (which essentially concern liquid precipitation) and practical applications (which usually utilize gel precipitation). Before discussing precipitation, we will review the major theoretical aspects of reactions between antibodies and macromolecular antigens, extrapolating insofar as is possible from the data on haptens reported above.

### VALENCE AND COMPLEXITY OF PROTEIN AND POLYSACCHARIDIC ANTIGENS

Macromolecules, as indicated in chapter 6, present multiple antigenic determinants. The number of determinants per molecule is often unknown. These determinants may be identical and repetitive (for example, for polysaccharides) or may be different (as for proteins). In both instances, the practical result is that antigen is complex and multivalent. Extrapolation of the data obtained from study of haptens to macromolecular antigens is therefore of limited usefulness.

### AFFINITY AND AVIDITY

Because most antigens are multivalent, it is generally impossible to define the intrinsic association constant $K$ for a given antibody. In fact, association forces of antibody and antigen molecules do not depend only on association constants but also relate to the number of bonds per antigen molecule. We have seen earlier that the monogamous binding phenomenon, in which several sites of a given antibody molecule react with two closely related determinants of the same antigen molecule, may increase by $10^5$ times the intrinsic association constant of an antibody for a homologous monovalent ligand. For a given complex antigen, the number of functional groups is usually unknown, and even purified antisera contain a mixture of antibodies. Finally, nonspecific factors, such as ionic strength, may also interfere. This fact explains why one often, in practice, utilizes the term "avidity," which simply refers in a semiquantitative way to the ability of an antiserum to exert certain biologic functions that relate directly to binding to specific antigens, such as agglutination or viral neutralization, reserving the term "affinity" for intrinsic association constants.

Measuring affinity for antibodies directed against macromolecular antigens is obviously more difficult than for antihapten antibodies. One may employ Scatchard's analysis and Sips' equation, as has been previously described for antihapten antibodies. However, one must be aware of the limits of these methods, in which numerous nonverified hypotheses are involved. An approximation of affinity may be obtained by examining concentrations of bound antigen at different antigen to antibody ratios (the curve being steeper for high affinity antibodies), by diluting the mixture of antiserum and antigen (which reduces free antigen and antibody concentrations and leads to dissociation) or by adding cold antigen to the complexes formed by antibodies and labeled antigen. The sera with the lowest affinity show the earliest dissociation. The precipitation curve also gives information because the curve is steeper for high-affinity antibodies. Differences in avidity between antisera may be due to (1) differences in the average intrinsic affinity constant of antibodies, (2) varying "specificity," that is, antisera that contain differing proportions of antibodies directed against the various functional groups on the antigen, (3) different proportions of antibody molecules that give rise to the monogamous binding phenomenon, and (4) different numbers of combination sites, (IgM contain five or 10 sites (see p. 194) per molecule and therefore are of higher affinity than IgG, with two sites).

## MODIFICATION OF THE ANTIGEN BY ANTIBODY

The combination of an antibody with an antigen may, in certain cases, induce important changes in the conformation of the antigen. Thus, when metmyoglobulin is added to an antiapomyoglobulin antiserum, ferrous iron is released from the antigen and the antigen-antibody complex no longer contains any heme (a phenomena which does not occur in metmyoglobulin-anti metmyoglobulin complexes). It may, therefore, be concluded that the interaction with antiapomyoglobulin antibodies has induced a modification in the metmyoglobulin that results in the destruction of the heme-binding region. It would be important to know whether this effect is directly due to an action on the antigenic determinant involved in the binding of heme or represents a secondary allosteric modification owing to a reaction with a determinant some distance from the heme. Other examples of the conformational changes of antigenic determinants on contact with antibody sites are now known, particularly for the penicillinases, ribonucleases, and β-galactosidases. Thus, linkage with antibodies may increase the enzymatic activity of these enzymes up to tenfold or even increase their resistance to heating, extreme pH changes, urea, or proteases. In the case of the β-galactosidases, it has been shown that inactive mutants may acquire an enzymatic activity after reacting with antibodies raised against the natural enzyme. From this it may be deduced that the effect of the antibody is directed toward its catalytic activity rather than toward the site of substrate binding.

The concept that antibody binding may modify antigen structure seems quite general. It has been directly confirmed by studies of circular dichroism and optic rotatory dispersion, notably for arsenilic derivatives and TNP- and DNP-lysine conjugates.

## CLASSIFICATION OF ANTIGEN-ANTIBODY REACTIONS

Numerous methods have been described to detect and to measure interactions between antibodies and antigens. These methods belong to three categories (Table 9.1).

### Primary Methods

These methods involve the primary interactions between antigen and antibody, independently of biochemical and biologic phenomena that may follow. Primary reactions depend only on the quantity and affinity of antibodies. The proportion of antigen bound for a given antibody concentration is very sensitive to changes in antigen concentration when the antibody is of high affinity but much less sensitive when antibodies are of low affinity. Conversely, the absolute amount of bound antigen is more variable with respect to antigen concentration for low-affinity than for high-affinity antibodies. This difference indicates that primary-type reactions simultaneously evaluate antibody quantity and affinity, thus the interest in each case of studying several antigen concentrations.

**Table 9.1   Antigen-Antibody Reactions**

*Primary reactions*
  Farr test (ammonium sulfate, polyethylene glycol, anti-Ig sera)
  Equilibrium dialysis
  Fluorescence quenching
  Immunofluorescence
  Radioimmunologic dosage
*Secondary reactions (in vitro)*
  Precipitation
  Agglutination
  Neutralization (toxins, virus, phages)
  Complement-dependent reactions (cytolysis, phagocytosis, chemotaxis)
*Tertiary reactions (in vivo)*
  Intravascular hemolysis
  Anaphylaxis (anaphylactic shock, passive cutaneous anaphylaxis)
  Arthus' reaction

### Secondary Methods

These methods relate to phenomena that are the direct (but not obligatory) consequence of primary interactions. Precipitation is one example: some antibodies give rise to precipitates, but not all antibodies are precipitating, at least under certain technical conditions. Similarly, IgM molecules may be very easily detected by agglutination reactions, whereas the agglutination reaction is 50 to 500 times less sensitive for IgG. Complement fixation and hemolysis, which require Clq binding, ignore noncomplement-fixing antibodies, like IgA and IgE. Secondary methods do not necesarily indicate the entire amount of antibody present in an antiserum. These methods are, nonetheless, very useful in studying heterogeneous antibody mixtures. They may even be used for quantifying in well-defined systems.

### Tertiary Methods

These methods examine the in vivo (biologic) consequences of primary interactions. Their complexity is even greater than that of secondary methods. In addition to the variables inherent in the primary and secondary reactions, other parameters specific to the individual, such as complement level or cellular receptors for IgG Fc fragments, must be considered. The limitations concerning secondary reactions thus also apply to tertiary reactions.

## III.  DIRECT BINDING TESTS

Primary binding tests have common features. They require the utilization of purified antigen or antibody. Methods used to measure antigen and antibody concentrations must be quantitative and sensitive. They usually utilize isotopic or fluorescent labeling. They all involve the separation of soluble antigen-antibody complexes from free antigen or antibody molecules (Table 9.2).

## METHODS THAT EMPLOY PRECIPITATION OF ANTIGEN-ANTIBODY COMPLEXES

Under certain conditions immune complexes may precipitate, whereas antigen alone does not. Thus, 50% ammonium sulfate precipitates Ig (whether free or complexed) without precipitating bovine serum albumin (BSA). The use of labeled BSA allows one to easily measure the proportion of bound BSA at different dilutions of anti-BSA antiserum. This statement describes the Farr test, which is performed at various ratios of labeled antigen and antiserum. It is of practical importance to know that the addition of ammonium sulfate does not itself alter the proportion of labeled BSA bound to antibody, which means that association or dissociation of immune complexes is not affected. Results of the Farr test are expressed as the percentage of bound antigen at a given antiserum dilution or, better yet, by the antiserum dilution that gives 33% precipitation, which is the dilution that corresponds to antigen excess and soluble immune complexes. This method has very wide application. It is

**Table 9.2    Quantitative Methods That Allow Dosage of Antibodies, Based on the Direct Binding Between Antigen and Antibody**

Methods that depend on the separation of bound and free antigen by precipitation of the antigen-antibody complex
    Ammonium sulfate
    Polyethylene glycol (mol wt 6000)
    Heterologous anti-Ig serum
Methods that depend on fluorometric measurement
    Fluorescence quenching
    Fluorescence augmentation
    Fluorescence polarization
Methods that depend on differences in size of bound and free antigen molecules
    Equilibrium dialysis
    Ultracentrifugation
    Gel filtration
Methods that depend on differential electrophoretic mobility of bound and free antigen
    Paper or acetate electrophoresis
    Polyacrylamide gel electrophoresis
Radioimmunologic assays

commonly used for albumin, the M protein of streptococci, somatic antigens of gram-negative bacteria, and DNA. If antigen alone is precipitated by ammonium sulfate, polyethylene glycol (PEG) may be substituted, as may anti-Ig sera (coprecipitation), which precipitate Ig but not antigen. For example, polyvinyl-pyrrolidone is precipitated by 50% ammonium sulfate but not by 20% PEG. The sensitivity of the coprecipitation method is similar to that using ammonium sulfate, except for "early" IgM antibodies of low avidity. In the latter case, coprecipitation is less sensitive (due to cross-reactions of the test antibody with antigens present in the anti-Ig antiserum, nonprecipitated IgM, or incomplete prevention of complex dissociation by anti-Ig antibodies). In addition, coprecipitation is obviously more expensive than ammonium sulfate.

## FLUOROMETRIC METHODS

### *Fluorescence Quenching*

Most proteins emit fluorescent energy in the ultraviolet spectrum. This energy is decreased when certain molecules are bound to the proteins. Fluorescence is due to phenylalanine, tyrosine, alanine and especially tryptophan, which emit at 345 nm. Ig molecules fluoresce. Their excitation is maximal at 290 nm, and the emitted fluorescence has a wavelength of 345 nm. Ig interaction with a hapten diminishes Ig fluorescence, because the hapten absorbs part of the energy, which is then either absorbed or emitted at another wavelength. In either case, emitted fluorescence at 345 nm is diminished. In practice, one measures the extinction of fluorescence after addition of several hapten concentrations (Fig. 9.5).

The main advantage of the technique is its rapidity, simplicity, and the minimal amounts of material consumed. In addition, nondialyzable haptens may be examined. Its limitations relate to the necessity of using purified antigen and antibody preparations. This purity is required because Ig fluorescence represents only a small portion of total serum fluorescence. In addition, it is necessary that the absorption spectrum of hapten overlap that of Ig. Furthermore, numerous haptens and sugars do not modify Ig fluorescence and can therefore not be studied by this method.

### Fluorescence Augmentation

Some molecules that do not fluoresce in aqueous solution do so after binding to certain proteins. Thus, when a fluorescent antigen is incubated in vitro with an antibody, its fluorescence (measured at 345 nm) may significantly increase (the physical basis of this increase is not completely understood). This method is little used, even though it is simple, sensitive, quantitative, and without a requirement for pure antibody preparations. It should be noted, however, that only antigens that show an increase in fluorescence may be studied with this method.

### Fluorescence Polarization

The degree of polarization of the light emitted by fluorescent molecules (excited by polarized light) depends on the size of the molecule. Small molecules with little rotational movement give minimal polarization. If, however, the fluorescent molecule is bound to a large particle, like an antibody, its rotational movement is restricted, and light polarization increases. Thus, the proportion of antigen molecules bound to antibody may be evaluated by measuring fluorescence polarization. This method can be applied only to small antigens and haptens, the fluorescence spectrum of which (natural or modified by the

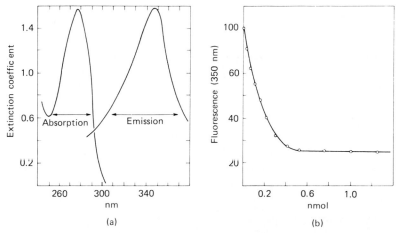

**Fig. 9.5** Fluorescence quenching. (a) Absorption and emission spectra of purified anti-DNP antibodies. By convention, the maximum emission is considered equal to the maximal absorption (although, in fact, only 20% of the energy absorbed by antibodies gives a fluorescent emission). (b) Diminution of antibody fluorescence after binding to ε-DNP-lysine. (From S. F. Velick et al., Proc. Nat. Acad. Sci. USA, 1960, *46*, 1970.)

introduction of fluorescent substitutes) is different from that of Ig. It is a simple, rapid, and sensitive technique; it gives information about the association constant and antibody heterogeneity and eventually on the kinetics of the antigen-antibody reaction. Here also, purified antibodies must be used.

## METHODS BASED ON SIZE DIFFERENCES BETWEEN BOUND AND FREE ANTIGEN

### Equilibrium Dialysis

This method has been presented in detail in connection with haptens (see p. 287). It is applicable to antigens of a molecular weight less than 10,000 daltons.

### Ultracentrifugation

Antibody-antigen complexes sediment more rapidly by ultracentrifugation than do free antigen molecules. By use of radiolabeled antigen, one may obtain bound and free antigen at different sedimentation levels that correspond to various antigen-antibody ratios. The dilution of antiserum associated with a given ratio of free to bound antigen can be evaluated. Unfortunately, this technique is not too precise and is not easily applied to mixtures of IgG and IgM antibodies or to antigens larger than 7S IgG molecules.

### Gel Filtration

Antigen-antibody complexes travel more rapidly in Sephadex than do free antigen molecules and may thus be separated. This method has been used in measuring antiinsulin antibodies.

### Other Methods

Electrophoretic methods (on paper, acetate, or polyacrylamide gel) are based on the differential electrophoretic migration of free antigen (e.g., BSA or diphtheria toxoid) and the immune complex. By use of labeled antigens, one may then calculate the percentage of free or bound antigen (radio counts are determined in several sections of paper or gel).

Another technique consists of measuring the reactivity of a purified labeled antiserum in the presence of a nonlabeled antigen. This method has been used to quantify erythrocyte rhesus antigens after elution of red blood cell antiserum (see p. 534). At the present time, the precision of this technique has not been established.

## RADIOIMMUNOASSAYS

Radioimmunoassays were initially developed as sensitive and specific methods for measuring levels of circulating hormones. The method depends on the binding of a radiolabeled hormone to a standard antiserum of high specificity and avidity for the hormone in question. Admixture of the two reagents produces soluble immune complexes that may be dissociated by unlabeled hormone. The displacement of labeled hormone at different concentrations of unlabeled hormone is determined and a standard curve is established by plotting the ratio of bound to free hormone as a function of added unlabeled hormone concentration. An analogous curve is then prepared by use of the reference standard (cold hormone) and the test serum. By comparing the curves the serum level of the hormone in question can be calculated (Fig. 9.6).

The methodologic problems posed by radioimmunoassays are similar to those discussed previously for the Farr test, particularly in separating bound and free antigen. Separation may be facilitated by taking advantage of the phenomenon of spontaneous binding of some antigens to inert surfaces (paper or glass). Antigen-antibody complexes, in contrast with free antigen, do not bind to these surfaces and are therefore recoverable. Examples of this separation include the adsorbance of insulin onto paper; certain peptide hormones (insulin, growth hormone, parathormone, and ACTH) adsorb onto glass, talc, silica, or Fuller's earth. Similarly, some compounds, such as insulin, bind to carbon. For example, silica earth is added to tubes that contain a mixture of antibodies, antigens, and immune complexes. The mixture is agitated, the tubes centrifuged, and the supernatant decanted. The radioactivity that remains in the tube is that of the free hormone bound on silica earth. Conversely, techniques have been developed in which the antibody (not the antigen) is bound onto inert particles. It is possible to bind antigrowth hormone antibody to polystyrene or polypropylene tubes or to Sephadex derived beads without destroying antibody activity. The antigen may then bind to the antibodies fixed onto the tube walls or onto Sephadex beads (see Fig. 26.1).

Generally speaking, radioimmunoassays are rapid, easily reproducible, very precise, and sensitive methods. Their only limitations relate to the difficulty of obtaining certain reagents, such as labeled hormones, and antisera directed against antigens or haptens of small size, and also to the risk of cross-reaction

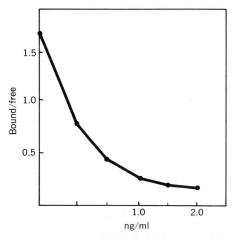

**Fig. 9.6** Radioimmunoassay. Standard curve for the evaluation of a peptide hormone.

between serum antigens and the test hormone. This risk is diminished, but not eliminated, by using very pure antibodies and hormones.

## IMMUNOFLUORESCENCE

Immunofluorescence, discovered by Coons in 1941, consists of detecting antigenic determinants present in cells or tissues by application of a specific antiserum previously made immunofluorescent by the binding of fluorochrome. After washing the preparation, only the antibodies specific for an antigen present in the preparation remain bound and may be detected after illumination by ultraviolet light (see Figs. 29.1 and 29.2).

Fluorochromes are substances that emit a higher-wavelength (530 nm) light than the excitor light (490 nm). The two products most commonly used are fluorescein isothiocyanate (green fluorescence) and rhodamine isothiocyanate (orange fluorescence). Ig labeling must preserve antibody activity. Purified antibodies are combined with fluorochrome: the fluorochrome excess is eliminated by dialysis or filtration on Sephadex gel. The reading requires a microscope illuminated by ultraviolet light emitted by a mercury vapor lamp. The initial filter (excitator) eliminates the visible rays and allows ultraviolet light to pass. A second filter (stopping filter) placed between the objective and the ocular eliminates ultraviolet light and allows passage only of fluorescent light.

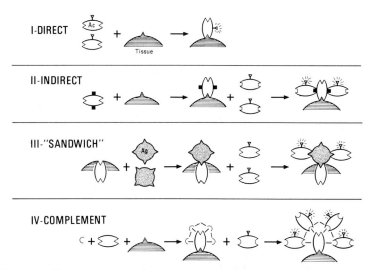

**Fig. 9.7** Immunofluorescence techniques. I. Direct technique. Specific antibody is labeled with fluorescent compound. II. Indirect technique. Unlabeled antibody is reacted with tissue antigen. Fluorescein-labeled antibody directed against immunoglobulin of the species that has given specific antiserum reveals its binding. III. Sandwich technique. This method is used to identify antibody in tissue sections. Antigen is added to tissue, and its fixation is revealed by labeled antiserum specific to that antigen. IV. Complement technique. The reaction of the specific antibody with tissue leads to binding of complement, secondarily added to the preparation. Complement is revealed by labeled antiserum directed against a complement factor. (After S. Sell.)

In practice, one may label directly the antigen-specific antibody. Direct immunofluorescence is most commonly used in studying tissue sections. One may also initially bind the nonlabeled antibody onto the structures studied and then detect binding by addition of heterologous fluorescent anti-Ig serum (indirect immunofluorescence). A third technique consists of adding the specific antibody and complement and then detecting complement binding (thus, antibody binding) by addition of a fluorescent anticomplement serum (Fig. 9.7). Immunofluorescence methods are widely used in virology, bacteriology, parasitology, and immunopathology for detecting circulating antibodies to human tissue antigen (e.g., antibodies to nuclear mitochondria, glomerular basement membrane, gastric cells or smooth muscle).

## IMMUNOENZYMATIC TECHNIQUES

If an enzyme, such as peroxidase or alkaline phosphatase, is coupled to an antibody, it can still react with its substrate; this allows it to be visualized on cells or tissue sections by either light or electon microscopy, or its concentration may be measured by spectrophotometry. Using this phenomenon, it has been possible to establish immunoenzymatic techniques based on the same principle as those of the radiommunoassays, in which either antigen or antibody concentrations may be measured by immunoenzymology.

# IV.  IMMUNOPRECIPITATION

When a specific antiserum and the antigen are placed into a small diameter tube, a precipitate forms at the interface of the two solutions. The ring test may be used for qualitative immunologic studies. It represents the simplest example of the immunoprecipitation phenomenon, the theoretical and practical applications of which have played a considerable role in immunology.

## LIQUID PRECIPITATION

Immunoprecipitation was discovered in 1897, but widespread application awaited the introduction of quantitative methods by Heidelberger in 1933. Heidelberger initially showed that a major antigen of the pneumococcal capsule was a polysaccharide. Conceptually this discovery was important because it established the immunogenicity of nonprotein substances (polysaccharides). Even more importantly, the nonprotein nature of the antigen, for the first time, permitted separate measurement of antigens and antibodies within an immune complex.

### Description of the Quantitative Precipitation Reaction (Fig. 9.8)

If the capsular antigen or type-III pneumococci (SSS III) and the antiserum produced by a rabbit immunized against this antigen are mixed together, a precipitate is observed at certain antigen to antibody ratios. The reaction is

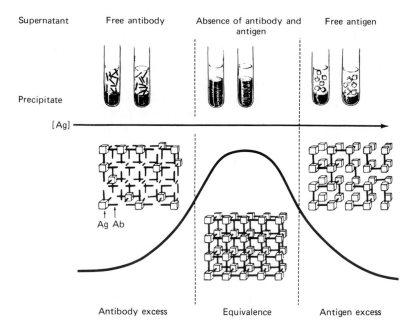

**Fig. 9.8** Quantitative precipitation. Increasing amounts of antigen are added to a constant amount of antibody. The supernatant may contain free antibodies in excess (*left*) or free antigen in excess (*right*). The supernatant does not contain antigen or antibody at equivalence (*middle*). (From J. A. Bellanti, Immunology, Philadelphia, 1971, Saunders, p. 137.)

specific, because no precipitate forms when the antiserum is replaced by rabbit serum collected before immunization, or if another antigen is substituted for SSS-III antigen. After repeated washing, analysis of the precipitate reveals the presence of only proteins and polysaccharides. After elution of antigen, proteins appear to be Ig entirely precipitable by type-III polysaccharide. The eluted polysaccharides can once again be precipitated by an antipneumococcal antiserum. Thus, all protein present, measured by Kjeldahl technique, in the precipitate are antibodies (with the minor exception of complement traces).

When antigen concentration is increased, keeping antibody concentration constant, the amount of precipitated proteins increases, reaching a maximum value and thereafter paradoxically decreasing. The existence of an optimal quantity of precipitate for a very precise antigen to antibody ratio may be simply explained by the hypothesis that the number of antibody sites occupied by the antigen is regularly augmented until a maximum, when a lattice is formed. Once saturation is reached, the additional antigen produces partial lattice dissociation. We shall examine later the theoretical basis for the prozone phenomenon. These early observations concerning saccharidic antigens have general application to protein antigens.

PROZONE PHENOMENON

The content of free antigen or antibody in supernatant may be very easily analyzed after centrifugation and elimination of precipitate. At this point, one may simply add new antigen to detect free antibody or, alternatively, add fresh antibody to detect free antigen. If antigen or antibody are homogeneous, that is, do not comprise a mixture with different specificities, it is noted that none of the tubes contain both free antigen and antibody. One finds free antibody in the ascendant zone (antibody excess), free antigen in the descendant zone (antigen excess), but neither free antigen nor antibody at maximum precipitation (equivalence zone). It is, however, noteworthy, that in certain cases of nonprecipitating antibodies, the maximum precipitate is obtained in slight antigen excess (the antigen is, then, detected in the supernatant). However, most often, antigen and antiserum are not homogeneous, and therefore several precipitation systems develop simultaneously. In these settings, there is no true equivalence, because each system has its own equivalence zone, and most supernatants contain both antigens and antibodies (the excess antigen zone of one system overlaps the antibody-excess zone of another). The antigen to antibody ratio in the precipitate varies proportionally to the quantity of antigen added in the antibody-excess zone. At great antibody excess, the ratio exceeds unity, which indicates that several antibody molecules may combine with one multivalent antigen molecule. In antigen excess, the ratio diminishes, approaching a plateau ratio slightly greater than unity (Table 9.4).

### Lattice Theory

Antigen multivalence suggests that precipitation may represent aggregation of antigen-antibody complexes, each antigen molecule being linked to more than one antibody molecule or, reciprocally, each antibody molecule being linked to more than one antigen molecule. When the size of aggregates exceeds a specified threshold, they spontaneously become insoluble. This hypothesis implies that antibodies are multivalent, as has been demonstrated by equilibrium dialysis. The lattice theory explains variations in the antibody to antigen ratio observed in the precipitates that were long at variance with the dogma of fixed composition of chemical compounds. In large antigen excess, the antibody to antigen ratio approaches unity, defining complexes of linear structure and regular antigen-antibody sequences (Fig. 9.9). In antigen excess, complexes have antibody to antigen ratios of less than 1:0.75 [$AB_3Ag_4$] in weak antigen excess, a ratio of 0.67 [$Ab_2Ag_3$] with great antigen excess, and 0.5 [$AbAg_2$] in very high antigen excess. These ratios apply to bivalent antibody molecules. The formation of the latter small complexes, which do not precipitate, explains the disappearance in antigen excess of precipitate formed at equivalence. Consequently, when antibody to antigen ratios are very high, antibody valence (in antigen excess) may be estimated and/or minimal antigen valence (in antibody excess) approximated. Analysis is complicated by the fact that antigen molecules often include several different antigenic determinants that may cause (synergistic) interaction between several precipitating systems. A small antigen with two determinants, X and Y, may not precipitate in the presence of one or the other anti-X or anti-Y determinants but requires the presence of both antibodies. An antigen molecule may be multivalent toward certain antibodies but monovalent toward others.

**Table 9.3    Main Radioimmunoassays**

Assays that use an antibody as the reagent

| Peptide hormones | Nonhormonal substances |
|---|---|
| Insulin | Intrinsic factor |
| Growth hormone | cAMP, cGMP, cIMP, cUMP |
| Adrenocorticotrophic hormone (ACTH) | Australia antigen (and antibody) |
| Parathyroid hormone | C1 esterase |
| Glucagon | Fructose 1,6-diphosphatase |
| Thyroid-stimulating hormone | Carcinoembryonic antigen |
| Luteinizing hormone | Rheumatoid factor |
| Placental lactogen | IgG, IgA, IgM, IgE |
| Proinsulin | Neurophysin |
| Secretin | Thyroid-binding globulin |
| Vasopressin | $\alpha$-Fetoprotein |
| Angiotensin | Plasmin |
| Oxytocin | Ferritin |
| Bradykinin | Prothrombin |
| Thyroglobulin | Tetanus antibody |
| $\alpha$-MSH | Botulic toxin |
| $\beta$-MSH | Staphylococcal enterotoxin |
| Gastrin | A and B fibrinopeptides |
| Calcitonin | Fibrin |
| Proinsulin C-peptide | Fibrin degradation products |
| PZ-CCK | |
| T3, T4 | Drugs |
| Prostaglandins | Amphetamines |
| Erythropoietin | Barbiturates |
| | Digoxin, digitoxin |
| Nonpeptide hormones | D-Tubocurarine |
| Testosterone | Hydantoin |
| Estradiol | Lysergic acid diethylamide |
| Adosterone | Medroxyprogesterone |
| Estrone | Methylprednisolone |
| Dihydrotestosterone | Morphine |
| | Penicillin |
| | Phenothiazines |
| | Vitamin A |

Nonimmune assay systems that use a substrate different from antibody but that also use saturation analysis

| Hormones | Specific reagent |
|---|---|
| Thyroxin | |
| Cortisol | |
| Corticosterone | |
| Cortisone | Specific plasma-binding proteins |
| 11-Deoxycortisol | |
| Progesterone | |
| Testosterone | |
| ACTH | |
| Nonhormonal substances | Specific reagent |
| Vitamin $B_{12}$ | Intrinsic factor |
| Folic acid | FA reductase |
| Cyclic AMP and GMP | Kinase protein |
| Messenger RNA | Complementary DNA |

**Table 9.4   Precipitation Reactions with Protein Antigens**

| Tube number | Chicken ovalbumin (CO) added (mg)* | Total protein precipitated (mg) | Precipitated antibody evaluated by weight difference (mg) | Supernatant | Antibody/antigen in the precipitate | |
|---|---|---|---|---|---|---|
| | | | | | Weight ratio | Molar ratio |
| 1 | 0.057 | 0.975 | 0.918 | Antibody excess | 16.1 | 4.0 |
| 2 | 0.250 | 3.29 | 3.04 | Antibody excess | 12.1 | 3.0 |
| 3 | 0.312 | 3.95 | 3.64 | Antibody excess | 11.7 | 2.9 |
| 4 | 0.463 | 4.96 | 4.50 | No antibody or CO | 9.7 | 2.4 |
| 5 | 0.513 | 5.19 | 4.68 | No antibody or CO | 9.1 | 2.3 |
| 6 | 0.562 | 5.16 | 4.60 | CO excess | 8.2 | 2.1 |
| 7 | 0.775 | 4.56 | 3.79 | CO excess | 4.9 | 1.2 |
| 8 | 1.22 | 2.58 | — | CO excess | — | — |
| 9 | 3.06 | 0.262 | — | CO excess | — | — |

* Addition of increasing quantity of an antigen to a fixed quantity of antibody. Each tube, contains 1 ml of an antiserum obtained from rabbits repeatedly injected with crystalline chicken ovalbumin.

After M. Heidelberger and F. E. Kendall, J. Exp. Med. 1935, **62**, 697.

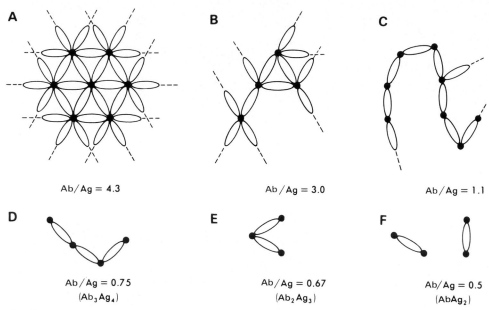

**Fig. 9.9** Hypothetical structure of immune complexes. The numbers refer to antibody to antigen molar ratios. (A) Complexes observed in antibody excess; (B) complexes at equivalence; (C–F) complexes at various antigenic concentrations. (From N. H. Eisen, Immunology. An introduction to molecular and cellular principles of the immune responses, ed. 2. New York, 1974, Harper & Row, p. 374.)

### Nonspecific Factors in Precipitation

The precipitation reaction has two phases: a rapid phase (a few minutes) that coincides with formation of soluble complexes. This phase is followed by a slow phase during which aggregates of complexes form visible precipitates, which may take several days to reach maximal size. The rapid phase corresponds to lattice formation. The second (slow) phase features a progressive association of antibody molecules that come into close contact and then form tight ionic bonds between groups with different charges. The decrease in complex solubility is explained by augmentation of aggregate volumes and decrease in surface charge density. This theory is supported by the decrease in precipitation seen when ionic strength is decreased; conversely, precipitation is augmented when negative charge of antibody is increased by acetylation of free amino groups (the latter does not alter the formation of soluble complexes).

### Nonprecipitating Antibodies

The existence of nonprecipitating antibodies had been suspected because of differences in the amount of precipitate seen when identical concentrations of antibodies were added to reactions in various ways. As an example, if one adds to an antiserum one-tenth of the amount of antigen that gives equivalence, a precipitate forms. Additional precipitate forms when new antigen is repeatedly added. The sum of all precipitated antibodies is much lower than the amount of antibodies directly precipitated in the equivalence zone: the difference represents nonprecipitating antibodies, that is, molecules that do not in themselves precipitate but are included in complexes that contain precipitating antibodies of the same specificity. It was previously thought that these nonprecipitating antibodies were monovalent. They are, however, multivalent but of low affinity. High antigen concentrations must be added to obtain precipitation, thus the formation in antigen excess of soluble complexes.

Let us also note that certain high-affinity antibodies may not precipitate, because they preferentially combine with two determinants of the same antigen molecules to form cyclic complexes. This phenomenon may take place when the determinants are closely repetitive on an antigen surface (e.g., in certain hapten-protein conjugates and for polysaccharides located on the surface of bacteria, viruses, or red blood cells) (Fig. 9.10). Some antibodies may, then, block precipitation of antigens by other antibodies. Because of the relative inflexibility of antibody molecules, monogamous binding develops and prevents the binding of one antibody molecule to two antigen molecules. Nonetheless, monogamous binding considerably increases the association constant (see p. 291).

### Precipitation Reversibility

Precipitates already formed are dissociated by adding fresh antigen (antigen excess). The reversibility is linked to transformation of large complexes into smaller ones. One apparent exception of this phenomenon, the Danysz phenomenon, deserves mention: when diphtheria toxin and antitoxin antibodies are mixed in equivalence, neutralization of the toxic activity depends on how mixing is performed. If toxin and antiserum are added simultaneously, neutralization is complete. But, if the toxin is added on two or three occasions at approximately 30-min intervals, neutralization is incomplete. This observation

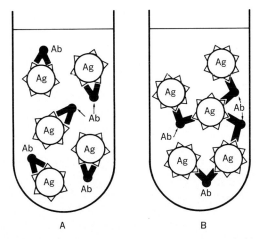

A          B

**Fig. 9.10** Monogamous binding. An IgG antibody molecule may bind by its two sites to the determinants of the same antigen molecule (A), which very much increases solidity of the binding but prevents formation of the lattice normally observed (B).

is explained by formation of indissociable complexes that contain more antibody than antigen molecules, which leaves insufficient antibodies to neutralize the toxin secondarily added. In fact, all complexes are dissociable, even though some contain high-affinity antibodies with a very slow dissociation rate (more than 30 min, and even sometimes several days). Complex reversibility may also be demonstrated by displacing antigen in the presence of large free antigen excess. The apparent irreversibility of complexes is particularly noteworthy for viral and antiviral antibody complexes, even at high dilution (which lowers free antigen and anibody concentrations), probably because of the increase in association constants that relates to the phenomenon of monogamous binding (vide supra).

### *Flocculation*

The precipitation curve, which expresses the amount of precipitate as a function of the antigen concentration, does not always have the aspects presented in Fig. 9.8. In some cases, particularly with horse sera, the formation of insoluble aggregates (precipitation) is only observed after addition of relatively large amounts of antigen. Here, antibody excess inhibits precipitation, as opposed to the more usual inhibition by antigen excess. Precipitation is observed in a very narrow range of antigen to antibody ratios. This phenomenon is called flocculation (Fig. 9.11). Flocculation is observed with certain horse sera, particularly antisera directed against diphtheria toxoid or streptococcal toxins. This property is not species specific, because horse sera directed against proteins or polysaccharides may give precipitation curves of the usual form. In addition, certain human sera may give flocculation with thyroglobulin. Flocculation mechanisms are linked to particular properties of antibodies rather than of antigens, because an antigen that flocculates with one antiserum will not show

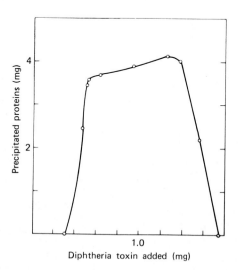

**Fig. 9.11**  Flocculation reaction. Increasing amounts of diphtheria toxin are added to constant amounts of antitoxin sera. (From A. M. Pappenheimer and E. S. Robinson, J. Immunol., 1937, *32*, 191.)

the same response with other antisera. Flocculation mechanisms are not completely understood. They may be provoked by formation of particularly soluble complexes due to high-affinity nonprecipitating antibodies (by the mechanism of, for example, monogamous binding). Only after these antibodies are saturated can the remaining antibodies precipitate the antigen. Flocculation is sometimes used to quantify antitoxin: the intense precipitation observed when one varies the ratio of antigen and antibody concentrations allows a macroscopic titration that is more precise than classic immunoprecipitation. Ramon's technique uses varying antibody concentrations, and Dean and Webb's technique employs varying concentrations of antigen.

## GEL PRECIPITATION

### Introduction

Immunoprecipitation is of great historical importance because of the considerable expansion in knowledge it has produced, as suggested in the preceding discussion. A very wide spectrum of techniques of immunologic analysis have derived from it. The discovery of gel precipitation represented the critical stimulus. We shall first examine general rules of gel immunodiffusion before reviewing major applications, including plate immunodiffusion, radial immunodiffusion, counterelectrophoresis, and immunoelectrophoresis, all ingenious refinements on the initial technique of gel immunoprecipitation in tubes described by Oudin. When one antigen and one antibody are introduced into gelified medium at different loci, they each diffuse, and a precipitate forms at the meeting point, if the ratio of antigen to antibody concentration is adequate. Depending on the support structure, one uses tube and plate immunodiffusions (Fig. 9.12).

### Tube Immunodiffusion (Oudin)

The first gel immunoprecipitation technique was described by Oudin at the Pasteur Institute in 1946. The technique consists of placing agar gel into a glass tube that contains an antiserum, allowing solidification of the gel at 20°C, and then adding an antigen solution. The tube is kept vertical. The antigen spreads by simple diffusion throughout the gel, creating a concentration gradient (which decreases from top to bottom). When an adequate antigen concentration is achieved, a precipitate forms at the progression front of the antigen. In fact, the precipitate extends from the progression front to the zone in which the antigen concentration is excessive. In large antigen excess, the precipitate redissolves into soluble complexes, just as in liquid medium. It is observed that the precipitate line progresses toward the tube bottom, the progression front creating a stable precipitate as rapidly as the antigen concentration becomes sufficient. The upper portions of the precipitate resolve when the antigen concentration becomes too high. The distance traversed by the precipitate line depends on time (the distance covered is proportional to the square root of time), on the coefficient of antigen diffusion in gel, which essentially relates to molecular weight and shape of the molecule, and on antigen concentration in the upper reservoir.

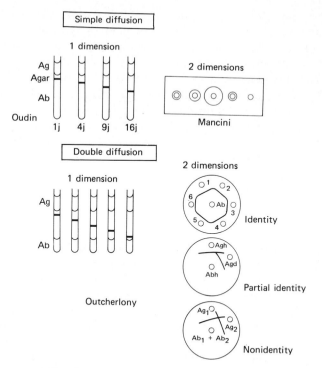

**Fig. 9.12**   Immunodiffusion techniques.

The two last factors mentioned explain that when several antigens diffuse simultaneously in a gelified medium that contains antibodies directed toward each of them, precipitates are not superimposed, each one migrating at its own speed. Obviously, it is possible that two distinct antigens have a similar migration speed and give rise to precipitates that cannot be differentiated. Finally, the number of lines permits estimation of the minimal number of antigens (or antibodies) present in the test solution.

It is possible to apply the tube immunodiffusion technique to determine antigen concentration under standardized conditions, because migration speed depends only on antigen concentration. One may, then, measure antigen and antibody concentrations in the precipitate by means of optical density (photometry). This immunodiffusion technique (tube) may be modified in several ways. Antigen may be incorporated into the gel and antibody added to the reservoir. This modification allows the study of flocculation, which, unlike precipitation, is inhibited by antibody excess. Another widely utilized modification is double immunodiffusion in tubes. In this technique, the gel that contains the antiserum is covered by gel without antiserum, and, on top of these two gels, either free antigen solution or agar-incorporated antigen is added. In this sytem, antigen and antibody diffuse toward each other in the neutral (gel) zone. Precipitates are formed at the point where antigen and antibody concentrations correspond to equivalence. The precipitate is then immobilized, and its intensity is augmented by accumulation of antigen and antibody molecules. Antigens and antibodies continue to react without a change in concentration ratio, at least for two reservoirs filled with amounts of antigen and antibody close to equivalence. In other situations, the precipitate slowly migrates away from the reservoir in which antigen or antibody is in excess.

### Plate Immunodiffusion (Outcherlony)

The use of glass plates to substitute for immunoprecipitation in tubes represented major technical progress. Tubes are replaced by plates that contain wells. Antigen and antibody solutions placed into separate wells diffuse freely in gel and give rise to precipitates at equivalence. If the antibody concentration is in relative excess compared to antigen and if gel diffusion coefficients are equal, bands are formed close to the antigen-containing well; the opposite is observed in situations of antigen excess. The plate technique is simpler than the tube technique. It has, in particular, the advantage of allowing direct comparison of different antigen preparations. Various antigen preparations are placed into separate wells arranged in a circle, the center of which contains an antiserum-filled well. When the same antigen preparation is simultaneously placed into two adjacent wells, the two precipitation lines join and fuse if the wells are close together (Figs. 9.12 and 9.13); this phenomenon is a "reaction of identity." If two different antigenic solutions are placed into two adjacent wells, the precipitation lines intersect, producing a "nonidentity reaction." Finally, if the two antigenic solutions give rise to cross-reactions and if one of them has been used to produce antiserum, the bands will fuse, but beyond the point of fusion, a projection is noted that extends the precipitate line formed

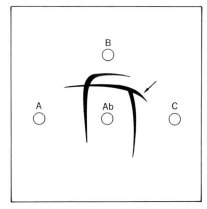

**Fig. 9.13** Analysis of cross-reactions by Outcherlony's technique. The antiserum, placed in the central well, has been prepared against antigen B, which precipitates it, giving two precipitation lines. It is also precipitated by antigens A and C. Antigen A possesses a determinant identical to that of antigen B, and the precipitate given by antigen A is a direct extention of one of the two precipitates given by B. It is a reaction of total identity (antigen B could also be contaminated by antigen A, which would explain why antigen A only possesses one of the two determinants presented by B). Antigen C possesses a determinant similar to that of B (partial identity reaction). The projection indicated by the arrow is located on the opposite side of the well that contains antigen B, against which the antiserum has been produced.

by the immunizing antigen, yielding a "partial identity, or cross-reaction" (Fig. 9.13). This projection, which is generally less dense than the main precipitate, represents antibodies that react with antigenic determinants not shared by the two antigens. This reaction generally corresponds to a smaller quantity of antibodies than does the main reaction, which explains why the projection is not very dense and tends to be seen closer to the central well, where antibody concentrations are greater. The incurvation of this projection is clearer when antigen diffusion is faster (e.g., because of low molecular weight). The precipitate is linear when the antigen and the antibody have approximately similar molecular weights; if the antigen is of higher molecular weight than is the antibody, the precipitate has a curve that is concave in the direction of the antigen (the converse is seen when the antigen has a lower molecular weight than does antibody). When there are determinants that give rise to cross-reactions between two antigens that were not used to prepare antisera, the projection is directed toward the antigen reacting less well with the antiserum, or there may be two distinct projections. These projections will have weak intensity and will be seen only if particularly careful inspection is carried out. As in tube immunodiffusion, plate immunodiffusion permits analysis of antigen-antibody mixtures; the number of precipitates represents the minimal number of precipitating systems.

### Radial Immunodiffusion (Mancini)

Agar into which a monospecific antiserum was previously incorporated is placed on a glass slide. The antigen solution deposited in a well diffuses into the agar, forming a blurred precipitate, the exterior diameter of which is proportional to the initial antigen concentration. This technique was developed by Mancini to quantify certain antigens. Monospecific antiserum is used, and the ring diameters of several known amounts of antigen are recorded. Mancini's technique is routinely used to measure Ig and complement.

The use of low antiserum concentrations makes the assay more sensitive but does not allow evaluation of high antigen concentrations that correspond to antigen excess, and therefore do not precipitate. For weak antigens (or low antigen concentrations), particularly IgD, it is possible to augment the precipitate by addition of a protein precipitating agent such as tannic acid. One may thereby detect amounts as minimal as 0.3 mg/100 ml of IgD. It is also possible to utilize radiolabeled antigens and quantify by autoradiography.

### Immunoelectrophoresis (Grabar and Williams)

Another simple and discriminative technique of immunodiffusion is immunoelectrophoresis. The technique consists of introducing an antigen mixture into a well cut in an agar plate and applying an electric field for 1 or 2 hr to separate antigen molecules according to their electrophoretic mobility. The electric field is then discontinued, and a polyspecific antiserum is added to a groove that parallels the direction of migration of the antigen preparation. Antibodies and antigens are allowed to diffuse freely toward one another, giving rise to precipitates analogous to those described in Outcherlony's technique, with similar standards for interpretation. Immunoelectrophoresis has been particularly rewarding in detecting the presence of more than 30 proteins in normal human serum.

### Radioimmunoelectrophoresis

The immunoelectrophoresis technique may be modified to study antibodies directed toward haptens (which do not give rise to visible precipitates) or to study small amounts of antibody. The antigens are placed into a well and fractionated by gel electrophoresis in the usual way. A groove is then prepared, and radioactive monospecific antiserum plus an anti-Ig antiserum are added. The antigen combines with the specific antibody, and the complexes are precipitated by the anti-Ig serum. The nonprecipitated proteins are eluted after washing and fixation, and the plates are read by autoradiography.

### Crossed Electrophoresis (Laurell's First Technique)

Laurell has proposed another variant of immunoelectrophoresis that allows quantitative analysis of antigens. The technique begins like classic electrophoresis. The various antigens present in the gel are separated linearly. A narrow strip of gel that contains the fractionated antigen is cut out. This gel band is placed onto a new gel plate into which weak antiserum concentrations were previously incorporated. The electric current is then reapplied perpendicular to the direction of the first electrophoresis. Precipitation zones develop at each antigen-antibody front. Precipitation lines are higher for more concentrated antigens. Analysis of the various precipitates is easier than in classic immunoelectrophoresis. In addition, for a given antibody concentration, the position of the peak is grossly proportional to antigen concentration.

### Rocket Immunoelectrophoresis (Laurell's Second Technique)

A simple modification of the preceding technique permits easy and rapid measurement of antigen concentrations. A monospecific antiserum is incorporated into a gel slide. Different dilutions of the antigen preparation being tested are placed into parallel wells. An electric current is then applied perpendicular to the line of wells. A rocket-like blurring ("trails") forms and extends as far as the antigen is in excess. The existence of a linear relationship between antigen concentrations in the holes and precipitate heights leads to precise and sensitive measurements of antigen concentration (Fig. 9.14).

### Counterimmunoelectrophoresis

This technique is very similar to the previous method in which the antiserum is placed into a row of wells that parallel wells that contain antigens. A current is then applied perpendicular to the lines of wells, and the maximal antigen dilution (or antibody dilution) that gives a precipitate is noted, by comparison to controls of known antigen (or antibody) concentrations. This technique is particularly useful for the detection of antibodies that precipitate the antigens that do not migrate well, if at all, in agarose gel unless an electric field is applied.

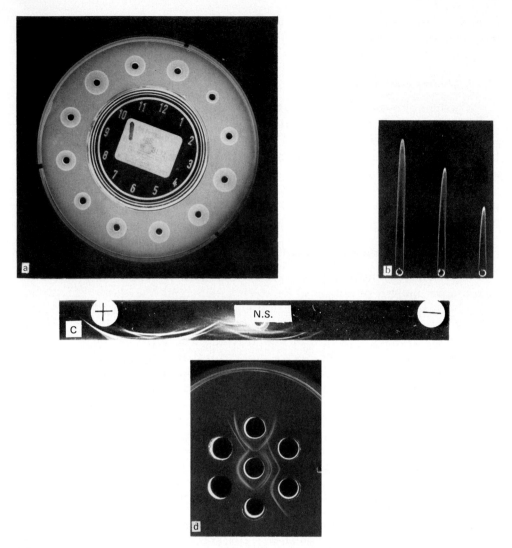

**Fig. 9.14** Applications of gel immunodiffusion. (a) radial immunodiffusion (Mancini); (b) rocket immunoelectrophoresis (Laurell); (c) immunoelectrophoresis (normal serum); (d) double immunodiffusion (Outcherlony).

### Nephelometry

The precipitation of antigen-antibody complexes involves an increase in the turbidity of the medium, which it is possible to measure directly by using different, very sensitive methods (particularly laser beams). After adding an antiserum directed against the particular protein under consideration (e.g., Ig or complement factors), the quantity of antigen present may be measured. The technique may be made more sensitive by the addition of polyethylene glycol.

This technical approach has been found to be extremely useful in laboratories dealing with a large number of samples because of its rapidity of execution.

# V. ANTIGEN-ANTIBODY REACTIONS USING CELLULAR OR PARTICULATE ANTIGENS

We have discussed in the preceding text various techniques for the study of reactions between antibodies and soluble antigens, including equilibrium dialysis, the Farr test, fluorescence quenching, and immunoprecipitation. It is also possible to study the reaction between antibodies and cellular or particulate antigens. These techniques, commonly used in serology, include agglutination reactions, neutralization reactions, and reactions that involve complement fixation (complement fixation, cytolysis, and opsonization).

## AGGLUTINATION REACTIONS

The agglutination reaction represents binding of agglutinating antibodies to cells. It is particularly applicable to bacteria and erythrocytes. Red blood cells can be directly studied or used to support soluble antigens bound to their surface (passive hemagglutination).

### Agglutination Mechanisms

Agglutinating antibodies agglutinate cells in a 0.15 M sodium chloride solution, as contrasted with nonagglutinating antibodies. This simplistic concept of agglutinating and nonagglutinating antibodies is only relative, however. The phenomenon depends on the molecular structure of the antibody (IgM or IgG), hence its valence, on the density of antigenic receptors on the cell surface, and on the medium employed (ionic strength). Generally speaking, agglutinating antibodies are IgM and nonagglutinating antibodies are IgG, but some IgG agglutinating antibodies exist. Nonagglutinating antibodies may be detected by artificial agglutination techniques (Coombs test, enzymatic red blood cell treatment, centrifugation, addition of macromolecular solutions).

Cell agglutination (e.g., of erythrocytes or bacteria) is not necessarily immunologic. Nonimmunologic agglutination may occur in the absence of antibodies by addition of polycations, macromolecular substances, protamine sulfate, or glucose. Phytohemagglutinin provokes agglutination of erythrocytes by binding to receptors present on their surface.

Agglutination requires a sufficient ionic strength (usually 0.15 M sodium chloride) to neutralize the negative charges normally present on the surface of bacteria or red blood cells so that the red blood cells may come into contact. Conversely, the addition of a solution of too high ionic strength may provoke agglutination in the absence of antibodies. Sera may not agglutinate at the usual molarity, but the reaction may occur in the presence of an albumin medium (see p. 605). For mixtures of several cell types (e.g., red blood cells and leukocytes), the two cell types separately agglutinate. This observation is compatible with the lattice theory of precipitation. Agglutination is the result of both a decrease in repulsive electrostatic forces between cells (the antibodies acting, then, directly through their positive charges) and of the creation of bridges between cells.

When a bacterium or any other cell is injected into a foreign host, it is lysed, and the immunogens present on the surface and inside the cells stimulate antibody production. However, only antibodies directed against the structures present on the membrane give rise to agglutination reactions. These antigens are called "agglutinogens." It is interesting to note that a given antigen is much more immunogenic as part of the cell surface, as compared to purified extracts, probably because the proximity of other structures on the cell membrane permits development of cooperation phenomena between various B- and T-lymphocyte populations.

Certain sera lose their ability to agglutinate at high concentrations and must be diluted 100- to 1000-fold to become agglutinating. This is analogous to the prozone phenomenon described earlier in immunoprecipitation. When high concentrations of fluorescein-labeled antibodies are incubated with cells, these cells appear to be coated with antibody but do not agglutinate. It is probable that in great antibody excess, simultaneous binding of both antibody sites (one Ig molecule) to two cells is minimized; therefore, agglutination does not occur. This explanation, however, is not entirely adequate, because the presence of nonagglutinating or blocking antibodies may also explain the prozone phenomenon.

### Coombs Test (or Antiglobulin Test)

In the 1940s, Coombs developed in ingenious method to detect nonagglutinating antibodies based on the antigenicity of Ig when it is bound to red blood cells by its Fab fragment. The Ig antigenic site (Fc fragments) can then be recognized by anti-Ig sera. The incubation of antibody-coated red blood cells with anti-Ig serum provokes agglutination (indirect Coombs test). A modification used to study hemolytic anemias is the direct Coombs test, which consists of incubating a patient's red blood cells coated in vivo with incomplete antibodies with the anti-Ig serum. A variant of the Coombs test is to use anticomplement antibodies that bind to complement molecules previously fixed onto antibody-coated red blood cells.

### Agglutination Applications in Serology

Hemagglutination techniques used in serology are semiquantitative procedures in which variable antiserum dilutions are mixed with a given cell or particle concentration, either in a tube or on a slide. The mixture is incubated at 4°C for variable times (5 to 60 min) and then agitated. Agglutination is read either visually (macroscopically) or under the microscope. Macroscopic reading detects, for red blood cells, the aspect of the sedimented pellet that is compact and has neat edges (negative reaction) or is more outstretched with irregular edges (positive reaction). The pellet may be resuspended by agitation and the amount of agglutinates noted in the medium. Numerous antibodies agglutinate only at 4°C (so-called cold agglutinins). The agglutination titer is defined as the highest dilution that gives agglutination. This titer is generally evaluated at one dilution and gives only a semiquantitative idea of the amount of antibodies present. A failure to note the presence or absence of agglutination in one tube (one dilution) represents a 100% error in evaluating the quantity of antibody. Titers are influenced not only by the amount of antibody present but also by their affinity and the number and distribution of antigenic determinants present on the indicator cells. This multiplicity of factors explains why agglutination gives only relative information, thus allowing recognition of positive antisera without quantification. More recently, the introduction of particle counters and autoanalyzers has permitted fairly precise definition of 50% of hemagglutinating doses ($HD_{50}$).

### Passive Hemagglutination

The agglutination target cell may be a red blood cell, a bacterium, or an inert particle (latex, bentonite). Passive agglutination involves precoating of red blood cells and inert particles by soluble antigen. This coupling onto the red blood cell may be accomplished by various means, which most classically consist of treating the red blood cells with tannic acid that makes them capable of reacting spontaneously with soluble antigens, like proteins or nucleic acids. Another method involves mixing red cells and antigens in the presence of chromium chloride or glutaraldehyde. It should be noted that some materials, namely, certain polysaccharides, spontaneously bind to red blood cells. The inhibition of passive hemagglutination by soluble antigen permits antigen quantification. A major application is in the measurement of plasma or urinary hormones, including urinary chorionic gonadotropins for the detection of pregnancy. Here, a standard antiserum is incubated with test urine; this incubation is followed by incubation with red blood cells or particles coated with the hormone under study. Agglutination does not occur (positive test) if the urine contained the hormone, because the hormone has previously neutralized the agglutinating antibodies in the antisera.

## NEUTRALIZATION REACTIONS

The preceding techniques are based on particulate conformation of certain antigens, which permits direct observation of macroscopic agglutination. Macromolecular or soluble cellular antigens may also be studied if endogenous (intrinsic) functions are lost (inhibited) after combination with antibody.

### Enzyme Neutralization

An antibody may inhibit the enzymatic activity of a protein if the enzymatic site is identical or close to the antigenic site. Antibody binding then masks the enzymatic site. Enzymatic and antigenic sites, however, may be relatively independent. For example, antiperoxidase antibodies do not inhibit the biologic activity of this enzyme. A common application of enzyme neutralization is in the field of bacteriology (detection of antistreptolysins, antistreptokinases, and antistaphylolysins).

### Toxin Neutralization

Antitoxin antibodies specifically neutralize the biologic effects of toxins. The lethal, inflammatory effects induced by toxins in animals may be neutralized by injecting an antitoxin serum. Toxin neutralization may also be observed in vivo. Thus, human subjects who possess antitoxin antibodies do not show the inflammatory reaction normally seen after intradermal injection of a small amount of toxin. This is the principle of Schick's (for diphtheria) and Dick's (for scarlet fever) reactions.

### Virus Neutralization

Antivirus antibodies decrease virus virulence, as expressed by cytopathogenicity. They also inhibit viral growth, and these activities may be used for purposes of quantification. Additionally, one may also examine the ability of antibody to inhibit viral hemagglutination, which normally occurs when virus is added to red blood cells. This phenomenon is used in Hirst's reaction for influenza.

### Phage Neutralization

Phages that infect bacteria have the property of provoking lysis. This characteristic property permits phage enumeration: bacteria are incubated with various phage dilutions, which are then placed into gelose-containing petri dishes. One then counts lysis plates, in which bacteria have been destroyed by phages. If the phage suspension is incubated with an antiphage antiserum before being added to bacteria, plaque (lysis) formation is inhibited. Study of various antiserum dilutions permits evaluation of the minimum quantity of antibody required to produce phage inactivation and thus the testing of antiserum in a sensitive and quantitative way. The technique may be applied to studies of other antigens by fixing them onto phages.

## REACTIONS USING COMPLEMENT

Numerous serologic reactions are based on the ability of Clq, and then of other complement components, to bind to immune complexes. Complement present in the initial serum is inactivated by heating at 56°C for 30 min, thus destroying Clq. Complement is obtained from a standardized source. Fixation of complement is quantified by measuring the amount of complement consumed (complement fixation) or by studying the biologic effects of complement activation (cytolysis, immunoadherence).

### Complement Fixation

An antigenic standard preparation is incubated with the test serum, which was previously heat inactivated. Complement, titrated by hemolytic dosage, is then added to these reagents, and the preparation is heated at 37°C for 30 min (or at 4°C for 16 hr). At the end of this fixation phase, sheep red blood cells and a standardized antisheep erythrocyte serum are added. The preparation is again incubated at 37°C for 15 to 30 min, and the amount of complement consumed in the latter reaction is determined. If the test serum contained complement-fixing antibodies directed against the antigen preparation, the complement activity will decrease during the fixation phase, and subsequent sheep red blood cell hemolysis will be proportionately decreased. One must initially verify that the serum in question does not by itself inactivate complement in the absence of antigen. This kind of anticomplementary property is present particularly in certain antisera that contain soluble immune complexes that bind Clq.

A seldom-used variant of complement fixation is conglutination. Conglutinin, present in normal ruminant serum, has the property of binding to the hidden determinants of the third component of complement after C3 fixation onto immune complexes. It is a euglobulin of molecular weight 750,000. Conglutinin agglutinates sensitized erythrocytes at subagglutinating antibody concentrations and infrahemolytic complement concentrations. Immunoconglutinin is an antibody that reacts similarly to conglutinin with hidden C3 determinants (perhaps also C4), somewhat analogous to rheumatoid factors (antibodies that react with IgG antigenic determinants; see chap. 28). Conglutinin or immunoconglutinin may be used in the complement fixation reaction by hemagglutination titration before and after incubation with a mixture of immune complexes and complement.

### Cytolysis

Antibodies directed against cellular structures may provoke lysis of the cells that bear these structures after binding the nine complement factors. Cellular lysis is easiest to evaluate for erythrocytes, because hemoglobin release is measured. With nucleated cells, the number of dead cells may be determined by uptake of stain (trypan blue) or by measuring the release of $^{51}Cr$ previously fixed onto the cells. In this procedure, one incubates cells with different antiserum and complement dilutions for 90 min at 37°C, followed immediately by estimation of cellular lysis. Prozone phenomena may be observed. Results are expressed as a hemolysis or cytotoxicity index:

$$\frac{\% \text{ of dead cells in the presence of } - \% \text{ of dead cells in the presence of antiserum + complement} \quad \text{complement alone}}{100\% - \text{ dead cells in the presence of complement alone}} \times 100.$$

This phenomenon also explains the treponema immobilization reaction. Treponema in the presence of antireponema antiserum and complement lose their mobility.

### Immunoadherence and Opsonization

Red blood cells and primate platelets, like many other cells, contain surface receptors for the third complement factor (C3). If one adds to particulate antigens (bacteria, viruses, leukocytes) their corresponding antibodies and complement, the particles are coated with C3. If admixture with red blood cells or platelets (considered here as "indicators") occurs, the particulate antigens, coated with C3, bind onto red blood cells and platelets and provoke agglutination. This immunoadherence reaction was initially described by Nelson.

Opsonization is closely similar to immunoadherence. Macrophages have surface receptors for the Fc fragment of IgG and for C3. The ability of macrophages to phagocytose bacteria is strongly augmented by prior incubation of bacteria with specific antibodies and complement. Macrophages may, for example, be obtained from the mouse peritoneal cavity. One may study, in a semiquantitative way, the ability of antibodies to enhance macrophage phagocytosis of bacteria.

## VI.  CONCLUSIONS

### COMPARATIVE SENSITIVITY OF SEROLOGIC REACTIONS: UNITARY HYPOTHESIS

Obviously, the methods discussed in the preceding pages do not show identical sensitivity (defined in terms of detection of minimum antibody amount). Precipitation is not very sensitive, whereas hemagglutination is much more sensitive; maximum sensitivity is achieved with phage neutralization. Table 9.5 lists the sensitivities of these serologic techniques, expressed in micrograms of

**Table 9.5  Comparison of the Sensitivity of Serologic Tests (Minimal Detectable Concentrations of Antibodies)**

| Test | Micrograms of antibody per milliliter (evaluated by nitrogen content) |
|---|---|
| Precipitation in liquid medium | 20 |
| Precipitation in gel | |
|    Simple diffusion (Oudin) | 10–100 |
|    Double diffusion (Outcherlony) | 3–20 |
|    Radial diffusion (Mancini) | 3–20 |
|    Immunoelectrophoresis | 50–200 |
| Bacterial agglutination | 0.01–0.01 |
| Direct hemagglutination | 0.5–1 |
| Passive hemagglutination | 0.001–0.01 |
| Hemolysis | 0.001–0.01 |
| Complement fixation | 0.1 |
| Toxin neutralization | 0.01 |
| Passive cutaneous anaphylaxis | 0.01 |
| Phage neutralization | 0.001 |
| Radioimmunoassay | 0.001 |

antibody per milliliter. Immunoprecipitation is seldom positive when antisera are diluted more than 10 to 50 times, whereas one commonly observes agglutination titers of 1 : 1000 to 1 : 10,000.

The multiplicity of serologic reactions poses important theoretical questions regarding antibody pluripotentiality. Is one given antibody responsible for the numerous biologic activities observed in an antiserum, or do multiple antibodies exist for each activity? Is, for example, the same anticholeric antibody responsible for protecting guinea pigs from lethal infection by *Vibrio cholerae*, the agglutination of *Vibrio* in vitro, the precipitation of filtrates obtained from the culture medium, and *Vibrio* phagocytosis by macrophages? It has been long believed that multiple antibody categories existed and variously represented agglutinins, precipitins, opsonins, and neutralizing antibodies. This view was abandoned when Heidelberger showed that antipneumococcal antibody precipitation by capsular polysaccharides simultaneously eliminates all biologic activities of antipneumococcal antisera and that these activities are recoverable after dissociation of precipitates. Subsequent to this observation, it was thought that each antibody molecule was capable of affecting, in adequate concentration, all biologic activities for antibodies of a given specificity—that was the unitary theory. In fact, it is now apparent that although one antibody may possess several biologic activities, antibodies are not totipotent. Thus, certain antibodies do not show precipitating activity (in particular, low-avidity antibodies). Others are not cytotoxic, because they do not fix complement. Generally speaking, biologic activities that distinguish antibodies are associated with differences in class, subclass, or avidity.

# BIBLIOGRAPHY

ARQUEMBOURG P. C. Immunoelectrophoresis. Theory, methods, identification, interpretation, ed. 2. Basel, 1975, Karger.

CHASE M. W. and KUHNS W. J. Specificity of serological reactions: Landsteiner centennial. Ann. N.Y. Acad. Sci., 1970, *169*.

CROWLE A. J. Immunodiffusion. New York, 1961, Academic Press.

EISEN H. N. Immunology. An introduction to molecular and cellular principles of the immune response, ed. 2. New York, 1974, Harper and Row.

EISEN N. and SISKIND G. W. Variations in affinities of antibody during the immune response. Biochemistry, 1968, *3*, 996.

GELL P. G. H., COOMBS R. R. A., and LACHMANN P. J. Clinical aspects of immunology, ed. 3. Oxford, 1975, Blackwell, 1754 p.

HOLBOROW E. J. Standardization of immunofluorescence. Oxford, 1970, Blackwell.

KABAT E. A. and MAYER M. Experimental immunochemistry. Springfield, Ill., 1975, Thomas.

KIRKHAM K. E. and HUNTER W. M. Radioimmunoassay methods. Edinburgh, 1971, Livingstone Churchill.

LANDSTEINER K. The specificity of serological reactions, ed. 2. 1945, Harvard Univ. Press; New York, 1962, Dover.

SONSKEN P. H. (Ed.) Radioimmunoassay and saturation analysis. Brit. Med. Bull., 1974, *30*.

WEIR D. M. (Ed.) Handbook of experimental immunology. Vol. I. Immunochemistry. Oxford, 1973, Blackwell.

# ORIGINAL ARTICLES

Avrameas S., Tandou B., and Chuilon J. Glutaraldehyde, cyanuric chloride and tetrazotized o-dianisidine, as coupling agents in the passive haemagglutination test. Immunochemistry, 1969, *6*, 67.

Coombs R. R. A., Mourant A. E., and Race R. R. A new test for the detection of weak and incomplete Rh agglutinins. Brit. J. Exp. Path., 1945, *26*, 255.

Fagraeus A., Epsmark J. A., and Jonsson J. Mixed haemadsorption; a mixed antiglobulin reaction applied to antigen on a glass surface. Immunology, 1965, *9*, 161.

Farr R. S. A quantitative immunochemical measure of the primary interaction between I BSA and antibody. J. Infect. Dis., 1958, *103*, 239.

Johnson M. M., Bremmer K., and Halle K. The use of a water-soluble carbodiimide as a coupling reagent in the passive haemagglutination test. J. Immunol., 1956, *97*, 791.

Sela M. and Haimovich J. Detection of protein with chemically modified bacteriophages. *In* H. Peters, Ed., Proteins of the biological fluids. New York, 1970, Pergamon Press, Elmsford.

**Part 3**

# THE PRINCIPAL TYPES OF IMMUNE RESPONSES

# Chapter 10

# PHYSIOLOGY OF ANTIBODY PRODUCTION

## Jean-François Bach

I. FATE AND LOCALIZATION OF ANTIGENS

II. HISTOLOGIC CHANGES IN LYMPHOID ORGANS

III. QUANTITATIVE VARIATIONS IN ANTIBODY
PRODUCTION

IV. QUALITATIVE VARIATIONS IN ANTIBODY
PRODUCTION

V. REGULATION OF ANTIBODY PRODUCTION
BY ANTIBODIES (FEEDBACK)

VI. ANTIGENIC COMPETITION

VII. SPECIFIC LOCAL IMMUNITY

In the preceding chapters, the elements of the immunologic machinery were described. We have discussed antibody-producing cells, the biochemical basis of immunoglobulin structure, and the antigens that elicit immunoglobulin production. We shall now describe the fate of antigens, the changes induced in lymphoid organs, and qualitative and quantitative variations in antibody production that follow antigen introduction, namely, the physiology of antibody production.

## I. FATE AND LOCALIZATION OF ANTIGENS

It was previously thought (instructionist theory) that antibody-forming cells incorporate the stimulating antigen. New selective theories of antibody formation (see p. 560) negate this theory, because only brief contact between antigen and membrane receptors is sufficient for immunocytic stimulation.

## TECHNIQUES

Numerous methods can be used to follow the in vivo fate of antigens. These methods fall into two categories: those that are directly based on antigenicity detection and those based on detection of labeled antigens. The latter methods are often more sensitive than the former but, at variance with them, are independent of the maintenance of immunogenicity.

In the first category, the methods largely consist of preparation of organ extracts, collected at various times after antigen administration, and testing of their immunogenicity in a new host. These methods are not very sensitive (1 mg for bovine serum albumin), although amounts as low as 1 μg of some bacterial antigens have been detected in this way. Immunofluorescence is informative because it allows histologic localization of antigens. It is also, however, a relatively insensitive technique, because antigen detected is of the order of 1 μg to 1 mg/g of tissue. One may also label antibodies with ferritin, which is electron dense and thus visible on electron microscopy, and apply the labeled antibodies on tissue sections from animals that have received antigens.

In the second category, the most widely used technique is isotopic labeling ($^{131}$I, $^{125}$I, $^{14}$C, $^{35}$S, $^{3}$H). Labeled antigens may be detected by the total counts in the organ or in extracts of the organ or by autoradiography with light or electron microscopy. The latter technique is especially applicable to tritium or $^{125}$I. It is also possible to examine the fate of antigen by electron microscopy when the antigen is a viral particle or heterologous ferritin.

## ANTIGEN LOCALIZATION IN ORGANS

Antigen distribution depends on numerous factors, including route of administration, immune status of the host, the particular structure and size of antigen, endogenous immunogenicity, and age of the recipient. Paradoxically, the dose of antigen, which has a marked influence on the quantity and quality of the antibodies produced, has little influence on antigen localization regardless of the time after antigen administration. Similarly, the delay following antigen localization has more influence on the absolute concentration of the antigen than its relative localization in each organ.

After intravenous injection, antigens are cleared from the blood more rapidly when their size is larger and when their immunogenicity is higher. Antigen aggregation considerably accelerates the clearance of soluble antigens. Particulate antigens, such as bacteria or heterologous erythrocytes, are eliminated by phagocytosis in a few hours. This phagocytosis is enhanced by opsonins.

Xenogeneic serum proteins persist in the blood for several days. Their elimination involves three phases: a relatively short period, that represents movement into extravascular spaces, a period of slow degradation, and a rapid elimination period linked to the appearance of antibodies and formation of phagocytosable immune complexes. The second phase is not observed in preimmunized animals.

The immune phase of antigen elimination merits additional comment. The antibodies that are produced initially form small soluble complexes with antigen.

The size of these complexes increases as more antibody is produced. Because complex elimination is more rapid when their size is large, the clearance rate of the antigen is augmented when antibody synthesis increases. Complement fixation by complexes further accelerates elimination. We will comment later on mechanisms of immune complex elimination. Irrespective of whether particulate or soluble antigens are examined, the major site of antigen localization is in the liver and then, in decreasing order (absolute amounts), the spleen (which contains the highest antigen concentrations), lungs, lymph nodes, and bone marrow. Preexistence of antibodies favors liver localization. Antigen persists in liver for long periods of time; it is possible that the antigen is progressively released from the liver, but this possibility has not been conclusively proven.

After subcutaneous administration, antigen remains close to the site of injection for some time, especially in regional lymph nodes, where it is present several minutes after administration. These lymph nodes undergo histologic alterations described on p. 332. After intravenous administration, the major portion of antigens is localized in the liver. However, the hepatic antigen concentration does not exceed that in the regional lymph nodes. Antigen retention by lymph nodes is related to immunogenicity and to the presence of antibodies. Aggregated antigens are especially prone to retention in the lymph nodes, at least initially.

Finally, irrespective of route of administration, a small proportion only of antigens localizes in lymphoid tissues, despite the fact that these tissues contain the highest antigen concentrations, and despite the fact that these organs are those in which the various phases of the immune response will occur. Antigen function in nonlymphoid tissues is unknown.

## LOCALIZATION OF ANTIGENS INSIDE LYMPHOID ORGANS

### Sinus Phagocytes

Particulate or soluble antigens are phagocytosed by cells of the reticuloendothelial system, particularly in peripheral and medullary sinuses of lymph nodes and in tissue between follicles. In the spleen, the antigens are phagocytosed by macrophages localized in the red pulp of the marginal zone, the white pulp, and periarteriolar zones. Antigens are present in the active immunocyte proliferative zones, confirmation of which has been shown by electron microscopy with ferritin used as the antigen. These studies localize the antigen within stellar phagocytic cells alongside medullary sinuses in direct contact with immunocytes. Phagocytic cells rapidly incorporate antigen, which is initially present throughout the cytoplasm, suggesting simple diffusion. Within a few hours, the antigen is found in vacuoles that rapidly fuse to form larger vacuoles, which persist for several weeks. The interdigitations observed between phagocytes and plasma cells (with plasma cells agglutinating around macrophages) are of considerable morphologic interest, but their significance is now only poorly understood. It must be emphasized (as demonstrated by Nossal, who performed the most significant studies with low antigen doses) that only phagocytes contain antigen.

*Follicles*

Immunofluorescence reveals significant localization of polysaccharidic an-tigens in follicles. Studies performed by Ada and Nossal with electron microscopy and autoradiography showed that flagellar antigens from purified *Salmonella* labeled with $^{125}$I also localize in follicles, even after administration of low antigen doses, of the order of 0.01 µg (which decreases "overload" risks).

These authors also noted that flagellin localization in primary folllicles was followed by the appearance of germinal centers at point of contact with the antigen. When the antigen penetrates the secondary follicle, it remains localized at the periphery of the germinal centers. There is a correlation between follicular antigen localization and immunogenicity.

Follicular antigen localization is enhanced by the presence of antibodies in the immunized animal or even by incubation of the antigen and the antibodies prior to injection. Conversely, follicular localization of flagellin is diminished in axenic rats. Thus, combination of antibodies and antigens is necessary for follicular localization, perhaps due to binding of the Fc-IgG fragment to follicular cells. Antigens bind to the surface of dendritic cells of germinal centers without true cell penetration. Dendritic cells, which contain few phag-ocytic vacuoles, have thin cellular prolongations onto which antigens bind. The role of antibodies in the follicular localization of antigen probably explains the absence of germinal centers in agammaglobulinemic states.

*Absence of Antigen Inside Lymphoid Cells*

In the 1960s, it was reported that tritiated haptens coupled to heterologous proteins (autoradiography) were present in plasma cells or lymphocytes in the spleen or lymph nodes. Similarly, injected ferritin has been observed within lymphocytes and plasma cells of mice. If some molecules of labeled antigen are indeed observed within lymphocytes of primary follicles and in plasma cells of medullary lymph nodes, their biologic significance is not clear. An artifact is possible, because antigen is present on the surface of dendritic cells or in phagocytes at the point of contact with monocytes. In more recent years, numerous negative results have been reported with very sensitive autoradiog-raphy techniques. One might therefore postulate, in conclusion, that antigens probably do not penetrate lymphoid cells but remain on the surface. It is obvious, however, that it is not possible to exclude antigen penetration of precursor antibody-forming cells, because there is no morphologic criterion for recognizing such precursors.

## II.  HISTOLOGIC CHANGES IN LYMPHOID ORGANS

The spleen is the main site of morphologic changes after intravenous injection of antigen. Large cells with basophilic or pyroninophilic cytoplasm appear as early as day 1 in the white pulp, in the periarteriolar zone. These cells proliferate into immunoblasts, plasmablasts, plasma cells, and intermediate cells. These cells are progressively replaced by small lymphocytes. Simultaneously, germinal centers develop in follicles. These germinal centers will persist for several weeks, but the white pulp and periarteriolar zones normalize as antibody production (high serum titers) continues. Analogous modifications are observed in regional lymph nodes after local (subcutaneous) antigen administration. Secondary reactions give rise to modifications similar to those described for primary reactions but at an accelerated rate. Immunohistochemical methods have shown antibody-containing cells, particularly numerous plasma cells, at the periphery of nodules and in medullary cords of the spleen, more rarely in nodules themselves. In secondary responses, the antibody-containing plasma cells are not numerous in nodules, but a high percentage of cells in the germinal centers (generally medium or large lymphocytes) show a diffuse and light cytoplasmic fluorescence.

The study of antibody-forming cells, by local hemolysis or by rosette techniques with dissociated cells (see p. 508), shows a rapid increase in the number of these cells on day 2 after antigen administration, with (plaque technique) peak values seen on the fourth day for primary responses and on the third day for secondary responses. We shall see later that each cell contains antibodies of one specificity and one class (usually IgM for the first 4 days and IgG thereafter). IgM production is less evident in secondary responses.

# III.  QUANTITATIVE VARIATIONS IN ANTIBODY PRODUCTION

Injection of one antigen leads to antibody production after a short lag period. The production is accelerated and particularly intense during the "secondary responses" observed after a second antigen injection. In the sera of normal animals, independently of all deliberate immunization, antibodies directed against numerous antigens are present (natural antibodies).

## NATURAL ANTIBODIES

Natural antibodies are found in the serum of animals that have not been deliberately immunized. Thus, adult mice have serum antibodies (and also antibody-forming cells detected by local hemolysis) directed toward sheep red blood cells, independently of immunization with sheep erythrocytes. In fact, adult animals have been repeatedly exposed to multiple antigenic stimulations, in particular to bacterial and viral antigens, either ingested with food or inhaled. Many of these microbial antigens give cross-reactions with sheep red blood cells. The question is posed whether these repeated immunizations explain natural antibody production. The use of axenic animals has provided a partial answer to this question.

Pigs delivered by cesarean section are bred in sterile rooms and fed antigen-free food made of protein hydrolysates. When adults, these animals have a serum immunoglobulin level lower than normal (but not true agammaglobuli-nemia). These antigen-free pigs do not produce natural antibodies, and no antibody-forming cells against sheep red blood cells are found in their lymphoid organs. They are, however, perfectly capable of producing antibodies after immunization with sheep red blood cells, and once introduced into conventional breeding, they produce natural antibodies. These observations, reported by Sterzl (Prague), corroborate the view that natural antibodies are the result of repeated immunization by undetected environmental antigens. In this hypothesis, the difference between "natural" and "immune" antibodies is essentially quantitative. It implies that the immune response observed in normal animals after a first injection of sheep red blood cells is not a true primary response.

There are also qualitative differences between natural and immune antibodies. The affinity of natural antibodies is generally much lower than that of immune antibodies. This difference might seem paradoxical, because immunizations that provoke their production are multiple and given in low dosage; these conditions favor the production of high-affinity antibodies. The weak affinity of natural antibodies is probably explained by the fact that these immunogens show determinants close to those of the antigens used to measure the antibodies but distinct from them, and also that many of their determinants are not found on the antigens used for antibody detection. Another difference between natural and immune antibodies relates to the depression of their production by passive administration of antibodies. Such injection depresses immune antibody production without affecting natural antibody production. This discrepancy is probably also explained by differences in affinity and specificity for the antigen. Natural antibodies are observed for numerous bacterial and viral antigens, heterologous erythrocytes, and some erythrocyte groups, particularly ABO groups in man.

## PRIMARY RESPONSE

One may distinguish between primary responses observed after the first injection of an antigen and secondary responses observed after second injection, taking into consideration the falsely "primary" nature of the primary responses, at least for natural antibodies. There are three separate phases within a primary response; a lag phase between antigen administration and appearance of detectable levels of serum antibody, a phase of increasing antibody titers, and a phase of decreasing titers.

### Lag Phase

The interval between the injection of the antigen and the appearance of the first antibody in the serum is variable and relates to the antigen involved: 20 hr for the $\phi \times 174$ bacteriophage, 3 to 4 days for sheep erythrocytes, 5 to 7 days for soluble proteins, 10 to 14 days for bacteria, and more than 3 weeks for diphtheria toxin. More specifically, the duration of the lag phase depends on dose of antigen, its form (the lag phase is shorter for particulate antigens), and the sensitivity threshold of the method used to detect antibodies. The utilization of very sensitive techniques for antibody detection in serum or on cells demonstrates that the lag phase may be as short as a few hours (3 to 4 hr according to Sercarz and Baker). Litt has observed lysis of heterologous erythrocytes in lymph nodes as early as 7 min after antigen administration; however, the immunologic basis for the hemolysis was not proven.

### Growth Phase

Serum concentration of antibodies increases exponentially at the end of the lag phase. Doubling time, defined as the time necessary for a twofold increase in antibody concentration, is about 6 hr for $\phi \times 174$ bacteriophase in the guinea pig and for poliovirus in the rabbit. The doubling time is longer after administration of low antigen doses. The peak response is obtained at variable times, also depending on the antigen studied: 4 to 5 days for heterologous erythrocytes, 9 to 10 days for soluble proteins, and as long as 3 months for diphtheria anatoxin. Antibody concentration may remain at this high plateau for several days but then decreases rapidly.

### Decreasing Phase

The level of serum antibody is dependent on the rates of synthesis and of degradation of antibodies. Degradation rate varies with the class of antibody (daily antibody degradation is about 7% for IgG, 25% for IgA, and 18% for IgM) and also with the total Ig concentration of the same class. Thus, the half-life of IgG (measured after perfusing trace amounts of labeled IgG) is 11, 23, or 70 days, depending on whether the IgG concentration is high, normal, or low (more detailed data on Ig metabolism are found on p. 224). When antibody production is less than antibody degradation, the serum level of antibodies decreases and becomes nil after a few days or, more rarely, after a few weeks. The factors responsible for rapid diminution of antibody production will be discussed further.

## SECONDARY RESPONSE

### Antibody Kinetics

A second injection of antigen causes a rapid increase in serum antibody to peak values higher than those seen in primary responses. This peak occurs earlier, and the lag phase is about half as long. The minimal antigen dose that gives a significant response is lower. The increase in antibody concentration is accelerated but remains exponential; the doubling time is about 7 hr for anti-$\phi \times 174$ phage antibodies. A third or fourth injection may further augment the antibody response (Fig. 10.1).

### Specificity

The specificity of the antigenic determinants that induce a secondary response is not different from that of determinants capable of provoking a primary reaction or of combining with antibodies. Alteration of the antigen molecule, which prevents combination with antibodies, also abolishes the ability to provoke secondary responses. An exaggerated secondary response is observed when the second antigen administered has determinants in common with the

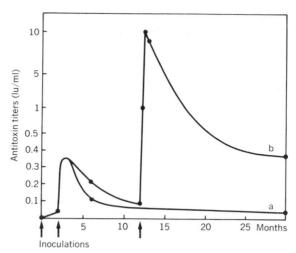

**Fig. 10.1** Primary and secondary responses of human subjects to tetanus anatoxin. (a) two injections; (b) three injections. (From D. G. Evans, Lancet, 1943, *2*, 316.)

first antigen. However, the response is less intense than that obtained when the same antigen is injected twice. Conversely, the immune response is of the primary type if the second antigen does not share determinants with the first antigen.

Immunization with antigens that give rise to cross-reactions with the first antigen administered may have unexpected effects. Thus, in man, when adults are vaccinated with influenza viruses, they may paradoxically produce less antibodies against the influenza type used for the vaccination than against strains encountered during childhood, which may have occurred 60 years earlier. This phenomenon is called "antigenic original sin": immunologic memory acquired by the subject after an initial contact with the antigen is as long-lasting as Adams's stain after his first contact with sin. This phenomenon has been the basis of retrospective epidemiologic studies that defined the serotype of viruses from past epidemics, for example, in influenza during the 1918 epidemics when the virus in question was unknown. The immunologic basis for the original antigenic sin phenomenon has been extensively studied by Fazekas de St. Groth. The first immunization leads to the generation of memory cells with multiple specificities. When the animal is subsequently stimulated by an antigen that gives rise to cross-reactions with the first antigen administered, the subpopulation of cells that recognize the common determinants is selectively stimulated. The antibodies produced are completely absorbed by the two antigens, although one occasionally observes antibodies against antigenic determinants present on the first, but not the second, antigen. Data recently obtained with respect to the carrier-hapten system provide new information on this phenomenon. One postulates that the second antigen shares with the first antigen carrier determinants that stimulate memory T cells; these T cells collaborate with memory B cells, the reactivation of which leads to production of antibodies against the first antigen. Thus, when guinea pigs are sensitized against the benzylpenicilloyl poly-L-lysine carrier-hapten conjugate or dinitrophenyl (DNP) poly-L-lysine, a second immunization with poly-L-lysine coupled simultaneously to the two haptens (benzylpenicilloyl and DNP) produces a primary response to the hapten against which the guinea pig had not been sensitized and a secondary response to the first hapten, closely analogous to "original antigenic sin." This hypothesis does not, however, explain why the second virus, or second antigen, may sometimes stimulate production of antibodies against determinants of the first virus, or antigen, that were not present on the second virus (antigen).

It is noteworthy that, in rare cases, false secondary responses, which are not antigen specific, can be observed. Thus, patients with rickettsial typhus may show increased antibody titers against bacteria to which they had been previously sensitized, even though there is no determinant shared between these bacteria and Rickettsia. It is possible that the nonspecific stimulation is linked to the release of soluble mediators by T cells, which then activate B cells by a mechanism similar to the allogeneic effect described on p. 538.

### Immunologic Memory

This phenomenon is the capacity of an animal or of cells to respond to an antigen by a secondary pattern, after a first exposure to the antigen. The response is maximal when the second stimulus is applied soon after the first one, but immunologic memory persists for a long time, several months in the mouse and several years in man, even when serum antibody concentrations have become very low or even nil (below the detection threshold). It should be noted that when the second injection is made very close in time to the first one, the secondary stimulus may be partially inoperative, because antigen is being eliminated by the antibodies still present in high serum concentrations. This effect of timing probably explains the apparent augmentation of immunologic memory within the first few months after the first antigenic stimulation especially when the latter was performed with high antigen doses. Generally speaking, antigen doses required to induce immunologic memory are lower than those needed to obtain antibody production. A particularly useful protocol for obtaining a secondary response consists of first injecting low antigen doses (priming doses), followed by high doses of antigens.

We have already noted the specificity of immunologic memory. Let us also mention that memory is carried both by B and T cells and that, schematically, T-cell memory is directed against carrier determinants, whereas B-cell memory is directed against haptenic determinants. Therefore, to elicit a secondary response, an antigen should have both carrier and haptenic determinants. In transfer experiments, one may obtain a secondary response by separate injections of T cells from animals sensitized to the carrier and of B cells from animals sensitized to the hapten (this is the classic Mitchison experiment discussed on p. 535).

## IV.  QUALITATIVE VARIATIONS IN ANTIBODY PRODUCTION

Antibodies produced during primary or secondary immune responses vary not only quantitatively with respect to time but also qualitatively with respect to class and affinity.

## CLASS VARIATIONS

IgM (19S) antibodies are produced before IgG (7S) antibodies. Mercaptoethanol treatment, which dissociates IgM into biologically inactive 7S subunits, destroys the biologic activity of sera obtained in the first few days after immunization. Mercaptoethanol does not, however, alter the activity of sera collected after the 10th day; sera, then, contain only IgG antibodies, the activity of which resists mercaptoethanol action (Fig. 10.2).

The presence of IgG antibodies is probably underestimated in the first few days after immunization, because pentavalent IgM molecules are much more avid, and therefore more efficient biologically, than IgG molecules (750 times more for hemagglutination). IgG production starts very early, on the second or third day, and the apparent increase on days 5 to 6 is partly due to cessation of IgM production, thereby unmasking the presence of IgG. The apparent transition from IgM to IgG antibody production directed against diphtheria toxoid in rabbits is, for example, much less abrupt when precise measurement of the absolute amount or active concentrations of IgM and IgG molecules is performed.

The IgM-IgG sequence is also observed at the cellular level by hemolysis plaque or rosette techniques (see p. 508). There is, however, controversy regarding the mechanism of the IgM-IgG switchover at the cellular level: some authors have described the simultaneous presence of the two classes inside a single antibody-forming cell, whereas others propose the existence of two distinct cell lines (cellular mechanisms involved in the cessation of IgM secretion will be discussed on p. 342 with the feedback effect of antibodies).

Thymus-independent antigens (defined on p. 158) mostly give rise to IgM antibody production. This is the case, for example, of antibodies directed against pneumococcal capsule polysaccharides in the horse and for antibodies against the lipopolysaccharides of Salmonella endotoxin or Forssman antigens of erythrocyte stroma in the rabbit.

Most antigens simultaneously provoke the formation of antibodies that contain either κ or λ light chains. One should mention, however, the sole

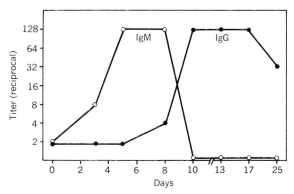

**Fig. 10.2**  Primary response to SRBC in the rabbit. IgM and IgG antibodies have been separated by ultracentrifugation on a sucrose gradient. (After Y. Borel.)

**Table 10.1   Augmentation of Affinity of Anti-DNP Antibody During Immunization: Role of Antigen Dose**

| Dose of antigen used for immunization (DNP-BGG) | Average intrinsic association constant* with ε-DNP-L-lysine at | | |
|---|---|---|---|
| | 2 Weeks | 5 Weeks | 8 Weeks |
| 5 mg | 0.86 | 14 | 120 |
| 250 mg | 0.18 | 0.13 | 0.15 |

\* Measured at 30°C and expressed in liters mole$^{-1}$ × 10$^{-6}$.

After H. N. Eisen and G. W. Siskind, Biochemistry, 1964, **3**, 996.

presence of Igs containing κ chains in certain antisera obtained after repeated immunization with DNP in the guinea pig or in some cold agglutinins in man.

## AFFINITY VARIATIONS

Antibody affinity increases during the immune response (by a factor of 10,000 for anti-DNP IgG in the rabbit). This increase, which is particularly clearcut for IgG antibodies, is most apparent after injection of low doses of antigen. (Table 10.1) The increased antibody affinity in immune responses is probably explained by a progressive decrease in the concentration of antigen in contact with immunocompetent cells. Its effects are more rapidly visible at lower antigen doses. If one postulates that antibodies produced by B cells have the same specificity and affinity as do recognition receptors of B cells that give rise to antibody-forming cells, it follows that at the low antigen concentrations that persist for a few days postimmunization, only B-cell clones with a high affinity for the antigen are still stimulated. The increase in affinity is also found at the cellular level: antigen concentrations necessary to inhibit hemolytic plaque formation decrease with immunization. Repeated administration of antigen delays the appearance of high-affinity antibodies.

In parallel to the augmentation of antibody affinity with time, one observes a paradoxical increase in the number of antibody specificities. The latter phenomenon is linked to the long lag period that precedes antibody production. The appearance of high-affinity antibodies against new determinants of the antigen molecule has two practical consequences: antigen-antibody complexes are less easily dissociated (i.e., the global avidity of the antiserum for the antigen increases more than expected on the basis of increased association constants for each antibody), and new cross-reactions may occur. These cross-reactions, linked to high-affinity antibodies, replace the cross-reactions due to low-affinity antibodies produced in the first days of the immune response.

## SECONDARY RESPONSES

Secondary responses are essentially associated with production of IgG of high affinity. (Table 10.2) It is of interest to note that thymus-independent antigens,

**Table 10.2   Augmentation of Anti-DNP Antibody Affinity in Secondary Responses**

| | *Average intrinsic association constant with 2,4-dinitrotoluene, a DNP analog (liters mole$^{-1}$ × $10^{-6}$)* |
|---|---|
| Primary response, studied 14 days after injection of 1 mg of DNP-hemocyanin in Freund's complete adjuvant (four rabbits) | 0.14, 0.03, 0.20, 0.15 |
| Secondary response, studied 7 months later, 8 days after injection of 1 mg of the same antigen (three rabbits) | 34, 84, >500 |

which essentially give rise to IgM antibody production after a first antigen dose, do not produce a secondary response after booster injections.

## V.  REGULATION OF ANTIBODY PRODUCTION BY ANTIBODIES (FEEDBACK)

We have already mentioned several factors involved in the regulation of antibody production that modify its kinetics. Let us mention also the role of Ig concentration, which modifies the catabolism of the immunoglobulins of the corresponding class and that of antigen concentrations related to the dose of administered antigen. Another critical factor is the antibody itself, which, through a feedback mechanism, depresses the synthesis of antibodies that have the same specificity. The concept of immunosuppressive antibodies is not new. At the end of the last century, it had been noticed that the simultaneous injection of toxin and antitoxin antibodies abolishes the toxin's biologic effects and also prevents immune responses of the animal against this toxin (however, without preventing the appearance of immunologic memory). Thus, secondary responses are not different from those observed in subjects who have received toxin alone. Before discussing the mechanisms of action of immunosuppressive antibodies on antibody synthesis, we will review the data obtained from experiments of passive antibody transfer.

### SUPPRESSION OF ANTIBODY PRODUCTION BY PASSIVE ANTIBODY TRANSFER

Passive administration of anti-sheep red blood cell (SRBC) antibody to mice simultaneously or within 5 days after administration of SRBC suppresses anti-SRBC antibody production. Suppression is strictly antigen specific, because only antibodies directed against the antigenic determinants present on the antigen molecule are immunosuppressive. Thus, in another system, incubation of

Proteus (bearing O and H antigens) with anti-O antibodies suppresses anti-O antibody production without altering anti-H antibodies. The intervention of the active antibody site is confirmed by the suppressive activity of Fab fragments, in contrast to the absence of effect of Fc fragments. The binding of antibody to antigen does not prevent the antigen molecule from localizing in lymphoid organs at the usual immunization sites, because antibodies selectively directed against part of the antigen molecule's determinants suppress only antibody development against these determinants. The intensity of antibody-induced immunosuppression depends on the time of antibody injection relative to antigenic administration and on the amount, class, and affinity of these injected antibodies.

### Kinetics

Suppressive antibodies may be injected before, simultaneously with, or after antigen. When administered before the antigen, antibodies are particularly active immunosuppressants for long periods of time when used at high doses and with a high ratio of IgG to IgM. When injected with the antigen, antibodies may either suppress or increase immune responses, depending on the ratio of antigen to antibody molecules. Exacerbation of the immune response is due to increased antigen localization at antigen-recognition sites, particularly lymph node follicles, and bears on all of the antigen molecule's determinants, not only on those to which the antibody is directed. For example, anti-SRBC antibodies incubated with DNP-coupled SRBC increase both anti-SRBC and anti-DNP antibody synthesis. Antibodies suppress immune responses when the antigen to antibody ratio is such that the majority of antigenic molecules are blocked by antibodies. However, in some cases, particularly for antigens that have a low catabolic rate (such as lipopolysaccharides), antibody synthesis may reappear long after complex (antigen and antibody) injection, probably at a time when the antibody has been degraded but antigen persists. When injected after the antigen, antibodies maintain their high suppressive activity, at least during the 24 to 48 hr after antigenic administration. This paradoxical fact is explained by the small amount of antigen that must then be neutralized, because a large proportion of antigen molecules has been phagocytosed in the preceding few hours. Antibody suppression is still effective when administered as late as 4 days after antigen injection. Secondary responses are much less suppressible than are primary responses.

### Role of the Class and Affinity of Injected Antibodies

IgG antibodies are better suppressors than are IgM antibodies at equal titers. When taking into account the much greater biologic activity of IgM at equal molarity, the question is raised as to whether IgM suppressive activity is linked to contamination by IgG antibodies. Some authors have reported that IgM antibodies may augment the immune response, a phenomenon never observed with IgG antibodies. In addition, high-affinity antibodies are much more suppressive than are low-affinity antibodies for a given class and for an equal titer. It seems, however, that in experimental systems that contain only IgM antibodies, IgM may, indeed, have a true suppressive action.

## ROLE OF ANTIBODIES IN THE REGULATION OF ANTIBODY PRODUCTION

The intervention of antibodies in the regulation of antibody synthesis, by a mechanism similar to that described above, is implied by cessation in exponential growth of antibody production at a time when high-affinity IgG antibodies appear, which are the most efficient suppressors of antibody production. A counterpart to antibody intervention is also suggested by the long-lasting antibody synthesis seen in lymphoid cells placed in a microenvironment deprived of antibodies. When one transfers spleen cells from SRBC-immunized mice into a syngeneic, irradiated, nonimmunized host (without anti-SRBC antibody) and then restimulates the host with SRBC, the number of anti-SRBC antibody-forming cells (detected by plaque formation) increases up to 1000-fold compared to the values seen after the initial application. This spectacular increase is prevented by prior passive administration of suppressive antibodies. Regulation of antibody synthesis by antibody probably also explains the cyclic production of IgM antibodies observed after immunization with *Escherichia coli* endotoxin. This slowly degradable antigen gives rise to a vigorous antibody production after a first stimulation, leading to neutralization of accessible determinants and cessation of increase in antibody production. When these antibodies have been degraded, the persisting antigen provokes a new increase in antibody response. Passive antibody administration prior to the onset of the serum antibody increase abolishes this response. Lastly, there is a probable intervention of IgG antibodies on IgE production in "hyposensitization" therapy in allergic states.

## ABSENCE OF EFFECTS ON IMMUNOLOGIC MEMORY

Whereas passive injections of antibodies almost completely suppress antibody production, no effect is evident on preexisting immunologic memory. Sensitized animals in which passive antibodies are administered several days before a booster antigen injection display a normal secondary response.

## MECHANISM OF ACTION OF IMMUNOSUPPRESSIVE ANTIBODIES

The simplest hypothesis to explain antibody-suppressive action is the masking of the antigen, which is, then, no longer recognized by immunocompetent lymphocytes and is rapidly eliminated. Antibody-forming cells, once differentiated, become insensitive in vitro to the suppressive action of antibodies. In addition, their life-span is apparently limited to a few days. The maintenance of antibody production, and even more so its increase, requires permanent recruitment of new antigen-sensitive cells. This recruitment proceeds from cells that themselves do not produce antibodies but that have surface recognition receptors for antigens. The number of these cells shows exponential augmentation during the immune response because of continuous recruitment by the antigen, which, in turn, increases the number of antibody-producing cells. High-affinity antibodies, either present at high concentration in the serum or passively injected, enter in competition with the receptors of antigen-sensitive cells and prevent their recruitment by the antigen. Thus, antibodies that are produced by clones with relatively weak-affinity IgM receptors are easier to suppress than IgG antibodies that are produced by clones with high-affinity IgG receptors and passive antibody injection preferentially suppresses low-affinity antibody production.

This simple and logical explanation for the mechanism of action of suppressive antibodies should, however, be accepted with caution, because many of the experimental data mentioned in preceding pages are still controversial, particularly those on the suppressive effect of Fab fragments and on the selective blocking of the action of antibodies directed against the determinants toward which injected antibodies are directed. The specificity of the immunosuppressive effect is not supported by observations on fetomaternal erythrocytic incompatibilities. Rhesus-negative mothers produce less antibodies against the Rh-positive antigens of their fetus when the Rh incompatibility is associated with an ABO incompatibility. In this system, natural ABO antibodies diminish, as a whole, the availability of fetal erythrocytic antigens in the mother. Similarly, immunization of guinea pigs with complexes of human $\gamma$ globulins and anti-Fc antibody in antibody excess prevents the production of antibodies, not only against Fc determinants but also against various determinants of the immunoglobulin molecules. The specificity of the immunosuppressive action of antibodies could, in fact, depend on the antigen to antibody concentration ratio and on the nature of the antibody: only small amounts of antibody would lead to specific suppression. The possibility of a central effect of suppressive antibodies is suggested by the experiments of Rowley and Fitch. Incubation of normal spleen cells with anti-SRBC antibodies prevents these cells from producing anti-SRBC antibodies after transfer into an irradiated host secondarily immunized with SRBC. Diener and Feldmann have additionally shown that a brief incubation of spleen cells with antigen-antibody complexes may suppress in vitro antibody production, perhaps by an action on receptors of antigen-sensitive cells.

The involvement of an antibody feedback mechanism in the regulation of antibody production must be distinguished from the hypothetical suppressive action of antiidiotypic antibodies produced against the idiotypes of the antibodies specific for the immunizing antigen as demonstrated, for example, for phosphorylcholine in mice (see p. 573).

# VI.  ANTIGENIC COMPETITION

Antigenic competition is defined as the transient and nonspecific suppression of one immune response by another immune response. Simultaneous or close injections of two unrelated antigens usually produce two distinct and independent responses. However, it has been observed that in certain conditions, antibody production or delayed hypersensitivity against one of the two antigens is less than the response obtained when each antigen is injected separately. The maximum depressive effect is observed when the second antigen is injected 2 to 4 days after the first one. Competition is even more evident when the second antigen is given after a booster injection of the first antigen. Mechanisms of antigenic competition are not known with certainty. There are numerous possible hypotheses, including (1) competition for a nutritive factor or, even more simply, spatial competition; the cells that react to the first antigen have insufficient space for the development of a cellular reaction against the second antigen; (2) a blocking of the reticuloendothelial system by macrophage overload, provoking an alteration in the capture or treatment of the second antigen by macrophages that have caught the first antigen or in their capacity to present the antigen to B or T cells; (3) T-cell paralysis (there is no antigenic competition in thymus-deprived mice); (4) release of soluble factors; (5) intervention of suppressor T cells; or (6) the existence of pluripotential cells.

## VII.  SPECIFIC LOCAL IMMUNITY

There is a first specific defense barrier against foreign antigens at the level of the respiratory system, gut, and genital mucosae. This defense barrier operates independently of serum antibodies or of the direct action of T cells. This immunity is linked to local production of IgA antibodies in tissues and plays a crucial role in defense against many infections. IgA is the predominant immunoglobulin in fluids, such as saliva, tears, milk, and gastrointestinal secretions, and in tissues in continuity with the external environment. Unlike serum IgA, which has a 7S sedimentation constant, a molecular weight of 165,000 daltons, and a rapid electrophoretic migration, secretory IgA has a molecular weight of 390,000. The molecular weight difference is due to a secretory piece of 60,000 daltons, which links two IgA molecules identical to those found in the serum. This secretory piece is a glycoprotein that contains 10% sugar. Its function may be to make IgA molecules less sensitive to proteolysis, but it may also play an important role in the transport of IgA molecules through mucosa cell membranes. IgA-bearing cells represent the majority of Ig-bearing cells in the gut, whereas they are a minority in the spleen and lymph nodes. This difference in location suggests that secretory IgA is essentially locally secreted and is not extracted from the circulation. IgA plasma cells in gut-associated lymphoid organs are found in reduced number in germ-free animals. However, another route has recently been described for the entry of IgA into the intestine. A large proportion of the blood IgA is passed into the bile by the hepatocytes but only in the dimeric or polymeric forms. IgA may therefore reach the intestinal contents by means of the bile.

   Local specific immunity provided by IgA appears to play an essential role in the defense against numerous local infections. Colostrum and milk IgA antibodies probably have a critical function in defending the newborn against gut infections. Interestingly, IgA does not appear during development until the eighth week of life, although the secretory component is already secreted in normal newborn saliva. In species other than man, gastrointestinal mucous membrane is permeable to IgA, which may then have a systemic effect. In fact, the secretory IgA system has as its most important function in the defense against inhaled or ingested bacteria and viruses. Secretory IgA with specificities against various microbes have been isolated. It has been proven that the cure of upper respiratory system infections is tightly linked to local IgA production in nasopharyngeal mucous membranes, whereas there is no relationship between cure and the serum antibody level. Similar observations have been made for gut infections, where good correlations have been demonstrated between the response (cure) to choleric infection in guinea pigs and "copro-antibody" titers (with no relationship to the serum antibody levels). These correlations probably explain the relative inefficiency of parenteral vaccination against cholera. Lastly, one may note the high frequency of respiratory infections in children with the ataxia-telangiectasia syndrome, who have no circulating or secretory IgA.

# BIBLIOGRAPHY

ADA G. L., PARISH C. R., NOSSAL G. J. V., and ABBOT A. The tissue localization, immunogenic and tolerance-inducing properties of antigens and antigenic fragments. *In* Antibodies. Cold Spring Harbor Symp. on Quantitative Biology. 1967, Vol. 32, p. 387.

BIENENSTOCK J. The physiology of the local immune response and the gastro-intestinal tract. *In* L. Brent and J. Holborow, Eds., Progress in Immunology. II. Vol. 4. Amsterdam, 1974, North Holland, p. 197.

HALL J. G. and ANDREW E. Biliglobulin: a new look at IgA. Immunology Today, 1980, 1, 100.

HEMMINGS W. A. Antigen absorption by the gut. Lancaster, 1978, MTP Press.

LIACOPOULOS P. and BEN-EPHRAIM S. Antigenic competition. Progr. Allergy, 1975, *18*, 97.

NOSSAL G. J. V. and ADA G. L. Antigens, lymphoid cells and the immune response. New York, 1971, Academic Press.

SISKIND G. W. Manipulation of the immune response. Pharmacol. Rev., 1973, *25*, 319.

STEINER L. A. and EISEN H. N. Variation in the immune response to a simple determinant. Bact. Rev., 1966, *30*, 383.

TOMASI T. B. The gamma A globulin. First line of defense. *In* R. A. Good and D. W. Fisher, Eds., Immunobiology. Stanford, Conn., 1971, Sinauer, p. 76.

WEISS L. The cells and tissues of the immune system. Structure, functions, interactions. Englewood Cliffs, N.J., 1972, Prentice-Hall, 252 p.

WERBLIN T. P. and SISKIND G. W. Effect of tolerance and immunity on antibody affinity. Transpl. Rev., 1972, *8*, 104.

WIGZELL H. Regulation of immunity at the cellular level. Quart. Rev. Biophys., 1969, *1*, 347.

## ORIGINAL ARTICLES

EISEN H. N. and SISKIND G. W. Variations in affinities during the immune response. Biochemistry, 1964, *3*, 966.

MÖLLER G. and WIGZELL H. Antibody synthesis at the cellular level. Antibody-induced suppression of 19S and 7S antibody response. J. Exp. Med., 1965, *121*, 969.

Chapter 11

# IMMEDIATE HYPERSENSITIVITY

**Jacques Benveniste**

I. INTRODUCTION

II. ANAPHYLAXIS

III. ANTIGENS

IV. ANTIBODIES

V. CELLS

VI. MEDIATORS

VII. MECHANISMS OF CELLULAR ACTIVATION
AND MEDIATOR RELEASE

VIII. CONCLUSIONS ON THE MECHANISMS
OF IMMEDIATE HYPERSENSITIVITY

IX. OTHER FORMS OF HYPERSENSITIVITY

## I. INTRODUCTION

The words "immediate hypersensitivity" (IH) and "allergy" merit precise definition. In fact, nowhere else in immunology are concepts so vague and limits so variable. The first observation by Magendie in 1837 and the subsequent pioneering studies of Richet and Portier at the beginning of this century had seemed mysterious and peripheral to classic immunity, even paradoxical, because hypersensitivity (anaphylaxis) was reported, rather than the usual protection afforded by immune reactions. The role of circulating antibodies in (cutaneous) anaphylaxis was demonstrated in 1921 by Prausnitz, who successively injected into himself the serum from a donor named Küstner who had been sensitized to fish, and then antigens extracted from fish and observed the appearance of a localized erythema. Thus passive cutaneous anaphylaxis, the Prausnitz-Küstner reaction, was discovered, but it was not until 1967, when an IgE myeloma was recognized by Johansson, and the molecules of IgE were isolated from serum by Ishizaka and his colleagues, that a firm immunochemical basis was given to the role of these antibodies. The demonstration of the role of basophils and mastocytes, and later the discovery of antigens (allergens) that provoked the production of IgE antibodies, permitted a more complete description of a coherent system that defines IH. The interaction between allergen and IgE, bound to the surface of basophils or mastocytes, at the level of a surface receptor for the Fc fragment of IgE leads to degranulation of these cells, with release of mediators that are responsible for the localized or systemic effects of IH. We shall limit our description of the mechanisms of immediate hypersensitivity to the phenomena that derive from the process just defined, specifically excluding events that relate to activation of the complement or kinin systems, since the latter probably plays an accessory or nil role. We note, however, that even though the IgE nature of the antibodies in question is well established, the participation of IgG antibodies in basophilic and mastocytic degranulation has not been formally excluded. Allergy may be defined according to its etymologic significance ("different state"), which has led some authors to use it as a synonym for immunity. Usually the term allergy is used to encompass all symptoms and diseases secondary to activation of IH mechanisms; however, because of potential ambiguities we prefer "immediate hypersensitivity" and will use this term in this chapter. After describing clinical manifestations of anaphylaxis, we will then discuss in order the various elements of IH reactions: antigens, antibodies, effector cells, and other mediators.

## II.   ANAPHYLAXIS

### ANAPHYLACTIC SHOCK (Table 11.1)

Injection of small amounts of horse serum (as low as 0.0001 ml) into guinea pigs may sensitize them against the proteins of that species. A second horse serum injection 15 days later may produce within a few minutes an intense reaction of anaphylactic shock including dyspnea due to the vigorous contraction of bronchiolar muscles and, possibly, suffocation and death. Lung autopsy reveals intense exudation and increased pulmonary volume. In other species, anaphylactic shock has different symptoms. In the rabbit, the most striking event is an intermittent constriction of the pulmonary arteries, leading to death due to acute right ventricular insufficiency. Deposition of immune complexes and leukocyte-platelet aggregates occurs in the pulmonary capillaries, followed by bronchiolar vasoconstriction. In the dog (used by Portier and Richet in their first experiments with sea anemone venom), the dominant event is a generalized vasodilatation of small blood vessels, particularly in the kidney, spleen, and liver, which leads to vascular collapse. The mouse is not very susceptible to anaphylaxis, except for a few strains. In man, anaphylactic shock is associated with dyspnea, which may lead to severe respiratory distress, followed by vascular collapse.

    Localization of the main symptoms in the respiratory tract is linked to binding of allergens in the lungs. However, anaphylaxis also provokes systemic

**Table 11.1  Anaphylaxis in Different Species**

| Species | Principal reaction site | Pharmacologic agents involved | Principal manifestations |
|---|---|---|---|
| Guinea pig | Lungs (bronchioles) | Histamine<br>SRS-A | Respiratory distress, bronchiolar constriction, emphysema |
| Rabbit | Heart<br>Pulmonary vessels | Histamine<br>Serotonin<br>SRS-A<br>PAF | Capillary obstruction with formation of pulmonary leukoplate-let thrombi, right ventricular insufficiency, hepatic and intestinal congestion |
| Rat | Intestine | Serotonin | Circulatory collapse, peristaltic augmentation, intestinal and pulmonary hemorrhages |
| Mouse | ? | Serotonin | Respiratory distress, emphysema, right ventricular insufficiency, intestinal hyperemia |
| Dog | Hepatic vessels | Histamine<br>Serotonin? | Hepatic congestion, abdominal and thoracic visceral hemorrhage? |
| Human | Lungs (bronchioles)<br>Larynx | Histamine<br>SRS-A<br>ECFA? | Dyspnea, hypotension, rash and pruritus; circulatory collapse; acute emphysema; laryngeal edema; secondary urticaria |

After K. F. Austen.

release of mediators, including, initially, histamine, the serum level of which becomes elevated during anaphylactic shock. Antihistamine injection prior to allergen injection prevents anaphylactic shock; a histamine injection into guinea pigs causes a syndrome similar to that seen in anaphylaxis, including bronchiolar constriction and vascular vasodilatation. As we shall see, histamine is contained in pulmonary mastocytic granules and is released after contact with the allergen. One should recognize, however, that the role of histamine is less clear-cut in species other than the guinea pig, where other mediators, such as serotonin and SRS-A, appear to have an important role. The relative contribution of each mediator may be due, at least partly, to its concentration at localized sites, which vary considerably from species to species. Thus, mastocytic histamine content is 7 to 16 ng in the dog but reaches 10 to 40 ng in the rat.

## PASSIVE (PCA) AND ACTIVE CUTANEOUS ANAPHYLAXIS

PCA, described by Z. Ovary, is a local form of IH. It is obtained by intradermal injection of an antiserum (eventually highly diluted). Twenty-four to 72 hr later, the corresponding antigen is injected intravenously simultaneously with, or just after, injection of Evans blue dye. The PCA reaction consists of an increase in local vascular permeability, which causes the appearance of Evans blue dye in the skin at the site of antiserum injection. Extravasation of Evans blue dye can then be measured. The PCA reaction is due to the binding of antibody to skin cells. The capacity to develop a PCA is transmitted by intravenous injections of antigen and is therefore a passive response. In man, the PCA reaction described by Prausnitz and Küstner is manifested as an erythematous area appearing at the common site of injection of antigen and antibody. In most species, the sensitizing antibodies are described as being homocytotropic, that is, they bind to cells, namely, cutaneous mast cells of the same species. However, the guinea pig, and to some degree the rat and the mouse, may be sensitized by IgG antibodies from man, rabbit, mouse, and rat, these antibodies being nonreaginic and heterocytotropic. In this latter case, the sensitization period is 2–3 hours.

It is possible to modify the protocol described above. Thus, in reverse passive cutaneous anaphylaxis (RPCA), the antigen, generally heterologous serum, is injected locally prior to antibody injection. The Ig contained in the heterologous serum binds to the injection point in the skin. Intravenous injection of an antiheterologous Ig serum produces a reaction similar to PCA. This experimental protocol is used to study the capacity of antibodies to bind to the skin.

Active cutaneous anaphylaxis may be demonstrated in actively immunized animals. In such cases the Evans blue is injected intravenously at the same time that the antigen is given locally. The diagnosis of allergic sensitization in man is based on this principle.

## III.  ANTIGENS

By definition, allergens are antigens capable of provoking an allergic reaction, for example, IH. All antigens do not cause IH and are therefore not allergens,

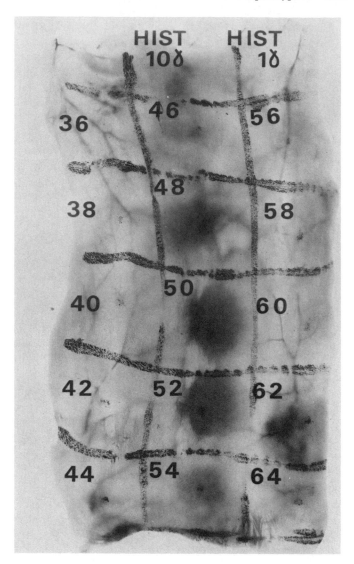

**Fig. 11.1**  Passive cutaneous anaphylaxis. Antiperoxidase rabbit serum has been fractionated on a DEAE-Sephadex column. The different fractions obtained were injected
under the skin of a rabbit, and, 72 hr later, peroxidase and Evans blue were injected
intravenously. The photograph was taken 10 min after such an injection. One observes
staining of the skin at the sites of injection of fractions 48–54, indicating an increase in
local vasopermeability. Fractions 38–44, which contain as much precipitating antibody
as does fraction 50, are, however, devoid of any anaphylactic activity.

even in allergic subjects. Allergens are pathogenic in certain indviduals but are
completely harmless in others, and some antigens may provoke an allergy in
animals but not in man. The reasons for these variations among species, between
individuals of the same species, and between antigens are not well known. One
should, however, note that some complex antigens are more frequently implicated in IH. One hopes that the recent progress in isolation and characterization

of antigenic constituents will permit a better understanding of the biochemical basis of their selective stimulating action on IgE production.

Numerous allergens have been described, and it would be tedious to list them all. We shall, instead, quickly describe the characteristics of the most important ones, categorized as either the inhaled antigens or the ingested antigens. In the first group, one must particularly mention pollen allergens, house dusts, hairs and danders from domestic or laboratory animals (horses, dogs, cats, guinea pigs, rabbits); among ingested allergens, the most frequently encountered are those derived from milk, eggs, and fish. In addition, numerous drugs, the number of which increases annually, may provoke an allergic reaction. Lastly, fungi, bacteria, and their products, and even vegetable fibers, are frequently allergenic.

The demonstration of allergenic activity of a given substance is difficult because of the frequent presence of contaminants in allergenic substances. For example, a person apparently allergic to products encountered at work may be, in fact, sensitized to fungi or bacteria that are contaminating these products.

## POLLEN ALLERGENS

The most common pollens are herbaceous: ragweed and barley in the United States, barley and the various common herbs in Europe. It has been calculated that 2.5 km$^2$ of ragweed may produce 16 tons of pollen during a season. Pollen consists of particles 10 to 100 μm in size. It is carried by winds and is deposited in nasopharyngeal, laryngeal, or tracheal mucosa. Pollen contains numerous constituents, but only a few are allergenic. Various fractionation methods have isolated two major allergens of ragweed, the E and K antigens, and two minor components. E and K antigens have a molecular weight of about 40,000 daltons. The E antigen is responsible for 90% of the allergenic activity of the total extract, although it represents only 6% of the protein content. Fractions (I and II) of comparable size and electrophoretic mobility have been isolated from ryegrass. More recently, two minor antigens have been described in ragweed; these components (called Ra$_3$ and Ra$_5$) differ from the other ragweed antigens by their small molecular weight (respectively, 11,000 and 5000). The isolation of these several antigens explains the heterogeneity of immune responses seen in allergic states. Some subjects are sensitive to all allergens, but others are only sensitive to some of the allergens. One should note, however, that most individuals allergic to pollen are sensitized to the major allergens, like ragweed E antigen and group I of ryegrass. We shall later see that variability in response has a genetic origin. Comparable immunochemical analyses have been performed to demonstrate the presence of distinct allergenic fractions in "Timothy pollen" and in most herbaceous pollens. Pollens from trees are much less allergenic than those of herbs. Some trees produce only small amounts of pollen and therefore do not cause much sensitization; other trees, like pines, may produce large amounts of pollen but are very rarely responsible for sensitization.

## HOUSE DUSTS

House dusts contain extremely heterogeneous allergens, including those contained in fungi, bacteria, vegetable debris, and human or animal epithelial fragments. It now seems that the most frequently encountered antigen is a substance from the acarian *Dermatophagoides pteronyssinus*: the existence of allergic symptoms has been directly correlated with infestation by these acarians. In support of this correlation, reactivity to house dust is often linked to the finding of positive cutaneous reactions to *Dermatophagoides* extracts. To date, purified extracts of acarian allergens have not been obtained, and opinions differ as to the origin of these allergens. Are they fragments of human epidermis infested by the arthropod, or are they true acarian constituents?

## INGESTED ALLERGENS

Among the numerous allergens capable of provoking digestive allergies (the diagnoses of which are made difficult by the nonspecificity of clinical manifestations), cow milk and eggs are most frequently involved. However, all hypersensitivity reactions to cow milk are not necessarily linked to the presence of IgE antibodies, and a role of non-IgE precipitating antibodies has been suggested. Further difficulties in diagnosis relate to the fact that antigens absorbed through the digestive tract are probably modified by acid hydrolysis during digestion. Despite all of these problems, allergenic activity has been found in the lactoglobulin fraction of milk and, more rarely, in $\alpha$ lactalbumin, casein, and bovine serum albumin, which are the other protein components of cow milk. The molecular weight of lactoglobulin is 36,000 daltons. An allergenic fraction, an ovomucoid of similar molecular weight (31,500), has been isolated from chicken eggs. An active allergenic faction has also been isolated from cod extracts. The latter is an acidic protein with an approximate molecular weight of 14,500. This fraction is still heterogeneous; it forms multiple precipitation lines against specific antisera.

## DRUG ALLERGENS

Numerous drugs are capable of causing allergic reactions, which may be clinically dramatic. All of these reactions do not necessarily represent IH, because other mechanisms may also be involved (including delayed hypersensitivity and immune complex pathology).

It is difficult to be precise when listing potentially allergenic drugs, because in practice it is often impossible to perform the diagnostic provocation tests. Some drugs do, however, appear to cause more frequent allergic reactions. The most allergenic, and also best studied, is penicillin. Other antibiotics, such as chloramphenicol, streptomycin, and tetracycline, are capable of provoking severe allergies. One should also mention sulfonamides, aspirin, and allopurinol. An important practical difficulty encountered in performing drug IH tests is that the drugs are generally only allergenic afer some degradation occurs, or simply following coupling to host proteins. Penicillin gives rise to several types of conjugates, two of which play a major role: the penicilloyl and the penicillamine antigens.

## CONCLUSIONS

The reason why some biologic or chemical agents have the selective property of provoking IgE antibody production is not well established. One may, however, note that most substances extracted from inhaled or ingested allergens have a molecular weight of about 30,000. Attempts by various authors to demonstrate structural analogies among these different allergens have not been conclusive. The possibility that a given antigen may provoke basophilic and mastocytic degranulation seems to be linked to their structure, which includes at least two subunits. Experiments performed with haptens of different valences have indicated that a minimum of two antigenic determinants are needed to produce binding between two adjacent IgE molecules fixed to basophilic membranes and to cause cell degranulation.

# IV.  ANTIBODIES

The antibodies (formerly called reagins) responsible for IH phenomena belong to the IgE class. Other antibodies may oppose the action of IgE; they are called blocking antibodies. Blocking antibodies may appear spontaneously or during or after desensitizing treatment with increasing allergen doses; they belong to the IgG class. The intervention of IgG reagins in IH reactions has been suggested by some authors, but they do not seem to play an important role in the onset of allergic manifestations in man. We shall see later that this is not so in certain animal species.

The existence of reaginic antibodies was known from the initial experiment of Prausnitz-Küstner. Subsequent workers initially associated serum reaginic activity with the presence of IgA and later with IgD antibodies. In 1967, Ishizaka showed that reaginic activity belonged to a new Ig class, IgE. Almost simultaneously, Johansson and Bennich isolated an atypical myelomatous protein called IgND, which was shown to be identical to Ishizaka's IgE. The discovery of this myeloma case, followed by two others in the United States, allowed recovery of large amounts of pure IgE for production of large quantities of anti-IgE sera necessary for the detection and measurement of serum IgE. IgE is heavier than IgG (molecular weight, 190,000; sedimentation constant, 8S); its carbohydrate content is relatively high. IgE migrates electrophoretically like IgG1 and is altered by heating (heating to 56°C, for 30 min to 2 hr, abolishes its capacity to bind to tissues). It may also be reduced by mercaptoethanol. IgE does not bind complement.

The most striking characteristic of IgE is its capacity to bind to tissue mastocytic surfaces, after injection into the skin. Whereas IgG disappears rapidly (within a few hours) after injection, IgE remains bound at the injection site for several days or, sometimes, several weeks. This long-lasting fixation is the basis for the classic methods for the detection of reaginic activity, passive cutaneous anaphylaxis and Prausnitz-Küstner's test. The binding involves structural characteristics of the Fc fragment that are lost by prior heating. The Fab extremity of this Ig bears antibody activity, as in other Ig classes. IgE binding to receptor sites and mastocytes occurs slowly. A lag time of 72 hr after serum injection is required before IgE can be detected in tissues by the passive anaphylaxis technique. IgE has been demonstrated in guinea pigs, mice, rats, rabbits, dogs, and monkeys. IgG1 reaginic antibodies, distinct from IgE, have been described in the guinea pig, mouse, and rat. These antibodies may be demonstrated 2 to 4 hr after subcutaneous injection and persist in the skin no longer than 1 to 2 days. They resist heating for 30 min at 56°C, and their sedimentation constant is 7S.

We have indicated previously that some investigators believe that there exist in certain individuals IgG class reaginic antibodies. One may, indeed, show the presence of antibodies capable of sensitizing the skin of human or primate recipients within a few hours, and this property is maintained, even after heating at 56°C for 2 hr. This passive sensitization is not inhibited by the injection of IgE antibodies. It is possible, therefore, that certain hyperimmunized individuals do have IgG with the property of binding to tissues (simulating rodent IgG1); nevertheless, these antibodies do not seem to play such a universal and biologically important role as does IgE.

It is important to recognize that serum IgE levels are very minimal in normal subjects; they range between 0.1 and 1 μg/ml. This low concentration indicates that IgE do not exert most of their function while in the circulation. Physiologic function relates to binding to receptor-bearing cells, followed by antigen fixation at the IgE antibody site; IgE then stimulates degranulation and release of mediators contained in the granules. Therefore, demonstration of IgE anaphylactic antibodies in the serum does not necessarily mean that they play a role in vivo in the degranulation of effector cells, and one must be cautious in interpreting elevations in serum IgE level or even specific IgE antibodies.

The examination of serum IgE levels is already in routine clinical use and does not seem to provide information superior to that produced by in vivo provocation tests. In certain cases, antigen-specific circulating IgE has been detected, even though the patient did not show IH directed toward this antigen (e.g., degranulation of basophils in the presence of the antigen).

## V.   CELLS

Basophils (Fig. 11.2) and mastocytes are the effector cells in IH. Eosinophilic polymorphs might also play a role, although concrete evidence is not yet available. Although of very different origin, basophils and mastocytes both contain numerous, highly osmophilic granules (densely stained with electron microscopy) that fix metachromatic stains, particularly toluidine blue, which makes them appear red. These granules contain heparin and proteins that act to support various IH mediators. This similarity between basophils and mastocytes is reminiscent of that (described in chap. 5) between monocytes and macrophages; however, there is no evidence that the two cells are derived from a common cell lineage. Mastocytes and basophils are capable of "degranulating" in several situations. Degranulation may have two aspects. Most often, mastocytes

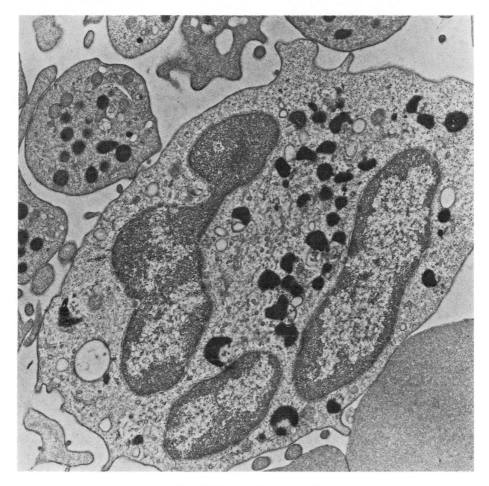

**Fig. 11.2**  Rabbit basophil.

degranulate by exocytosis; the granules open to the outside, dissolving as they release their mediators. This type of degranulation has been observed in human basophils by phase contrast microscopy. The second type of degranulation has been seen in the rabbit. It does not involve granular exocytosis but seems to occur by diffusion into the cytoplasm.

The list of stimuli capable of provoking degranulation of basophils and mastocytes is increasing. Numerous chemical agents, such as 48/80, octylamine, and polymyxin B, are capable of stimulating degranulation. C3a and C5a anaphylatoxins cause degranulation of mastocytes and, apparently, also of basophils. Certain drugs (in particular, basic molecules, such as Synacthen or polymyxin B) are able to directly cause basophilic degranulation without intervention of the IgE system. However, the main triggering factor remains the IgE system. It is significant in this respect that basophils and mastocytes are apparently the only cells of the organism capable of binding IgE to their membrane. The binding of antigen to the Fab part of previously fixed IgE molecules provokes within seconds cell degranulation and mediator release.

We have indicated that a role of eosinophils in allergy is suspected but has not yet been demonstrated. One should, however, note that mastocytes and basophils release an eosinophil chemotactic factor and that eosinophils are particularly rich in arylsulfatase, which is a potent inhibitor of slow-reacting substance of anaphylaxis (SRS-A), one of the mediators of allergic reactions.

## VI. MEDIATORS

If we limit ourselves to the IH definition given at the beginning of this chapter, that is the phenomena that result from the interaction of an antigen with an IgE molecule on the surface of a mastocyte or basophil, the number of known IH mediators is relatively small. Mediators include histamine, serotonin, SRS-A and other leukotrienes, the eosinophil chemotactic factor of anaphylaxis (ECF-A), and the platelet-activating factor (PAF-acether). Most of these mediators are not species specific and are active in all animal species studied; however, there are variations in sensitivity among species.

Histamine is probably the most important of the mediators of allergy. It is produced by basophils and mastocytes under the influence of a histidine decarboxylase and is stored in the granules, from which it is rapidly released during anaphylactic degranulation. Its low molecular weight (110 daltons) allows rapid diffusion through body tissues. Its action is twofold: edema with increased vasopermeability and contraction of smooth muscles (Fig. 11.4).

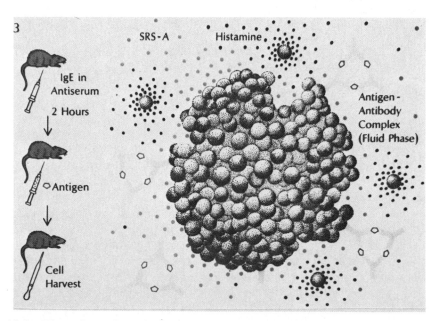

**Fig. 11.3** Histamine release in the peritoneal cavity by mastocytes in the rat sensitized in vivo with IgE after contact with antigen. (From R. P. Orange and K. F. Austen. *In* R. A. Good and D. W. Fisher, Eds., Immunobiology, ed. 5. Stamford, Conn., 1973, Sinauer, p. 115.)

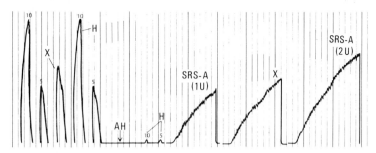

**Fig. 11.4** Utilization of guinea pig ileal contraction to dose some anaphylaxis mediators. Contraction given by the test sample (X) can be compared to that evoked by 5 and 10 ng of histamine (H), which is blocked by antihistamine (AH) and by one or two SRS-A units. (From R. P. Orange and Austen. *In* R. A. Good and D. W. Fisher, Eds., Immunobiology, ed. 5. Stamford, Conn., 1973, Sinauer, p. 115.)

Antihistamine administration nearly completely abolishes the passive cutaneous anaphylactic reaction in the rabbit. Serotonin has an effect comparable to that of histamine; its molecular weight is about 400 daltons. It is found in rat and mouse mastocytes and in platelets, particularly in man. SRS-A was described in 1938 by Feldberg and Kellaway. It causes a slow and prolonged contraction of guinea pig ileum, which is not blocked by antihistamines. SRS-A is released in anaphylactic reactions. It was shown to originate from mastocytes, macrophages and polymorphonuclear neutrophils. It is likely that SRS-A plays an important role in the pathogenesis of asthma, although its bronchoconstrictive effect in guinea-pig is blocked by aspirin (a cyclooxygenase blocker and thus an inhibitor of thromboxane and prostaglandin formation). A novel group of compounds, the leukotrienes (LT) have been recently discovered. Leukotrienes are arachidonic acid derivatives containing or not various sulfur side chains. The biologically active molecules (LTC, LTD, LTE, LTB) are released from several inflammatory cell types including murine macrophages, human polymorphonuclear cells and rabbit platelets. Some of these molecules (LTC, D, E) contribute to the SRS-A ileum contracting activity released from cells or specifically sentitized lungs. In addition LTC and LTD are bronchoconstrictors, LTD increases permeability of vasculature and LTB is a potent chemotactic agent. Leukotrienes might therefore be important mediators both in immediate hypersensitivity reactions and in inflammation. ECF-A has been found in alveolar fluid from human lungs that have just experienced anaphylactic reactions. ECF-A is defined by its chemotactic reactivity to eosinophils, which may explain the appearance of eosinophils at the site of an anaphylactic reaction. It was believed to be a small peptide. However recent reports indicate that most of the ECF-A activity is due to a lipid, the leukotriene B. PAF-acether was initially discovered in rabbit basophils. It is a mediator released by basophils that acts on platelets (which it is able to aggregate as well in the rabbit as in man) and also increases vascular permeability. It has been implicated in the vasopermeability changes associated with immune complex (IC) deposition in serum sickness. PAF-acether release is seen during anaphylactic reactions in the rabbit. It has recently been isolated from human and pig leukocyte preparations, macrophages, neutrophil polymorphs, platelets, and from rat kidney. Lastly, a lyso-2 compound derived from or precursor of PAF-acether released from the same cells as PAF-acether inactive on platelet aggregation, has been shown to induce chemokinesis and enzyme secretion from polymorphonuclear cells. In addition to these major anaphylactic mediators, other systems have been described, but their involvement in allergic reactions is not so clear-cut. Anaphylatoxins, two peptides of low molecular weight, are degradation products of the third and fifth complement factors that have a very important degranulating action on mastocytes. Bradykinin is capable of reproducing certain aspects of the anaphylactic reaction but whose involvement in the allergic reactions is difficult to establish. Lastly, it seems that during allergic reactions, phospholipids other than PAF-acether are released; the role of these phospholipids is completely unknown. They may have an action on vasopermeability.

The results obtained from recent studies suggest that the origin of the mediators of immediate hypersensitivity should be reconsidered. Although it appears that histamine and serotonin seem to be quite specific to basophils and mastocytes, SRS-A, PAF, and ECF-A also appear to be equally liberated by macrophages and neutrophils. These three mediators, therefore, arise from different cell types, and their liberation depends on the type of stimulus involved. One stimulus may involve IgE in the liberation of these substances from basophils and, in the case of SRS-A, from mast cells. Another stimulus, involving the intervention of IgG antibodies, or phagocyte stimulation, may provoke the liberation of these mediators from neutrophils and macrophages. Numerous possibilities for cell/mediator interaction may, therefore, exist, all of which result in local increases in vasopermeability and smooth muscle contraction. In turn, these actions encourage the diffusion of molecules, molecular aggregates, and cells from the intravascular compartment to the extravascular compartment. Finally, it has been recently shown that PAF has a bronchoconstrictor action by the intermediary of platelets. In the guinea pig, this action is independent of the arachidonic acid/prostaglandin pathway.

## VII.  MECHANISMS OF CELLULAR ACTIVATION AND MEDIATOR RELEASE

The interaction between the antigen and IgE on the mastocyte and basophil surface initiates a series of very complex intracellular events that have only now begun to be elucidated. The cyclic AMP-GMP system is implicated in the regulation of this response, which requires the presence of calcium ions and glucose and occurs only at 37°C (which demonstrates that mediator release is an active phenomenon and not simple lysis, as had been proposed earlier). The sequence of biochemical or intracellular events initiated by the interaction of antigen and cell-bound IgE includes several steps. The first phase involves calcium-dependent interaction of a membrane serine esterase sensitive to diisopropylfluorophosphate (DFP). The following phase is energetic: it requires glucose and is inhibited by deoxyglucose. A further step, again calcium dependent, implicates the cyclic AMP-GMP system and seems to terminate the

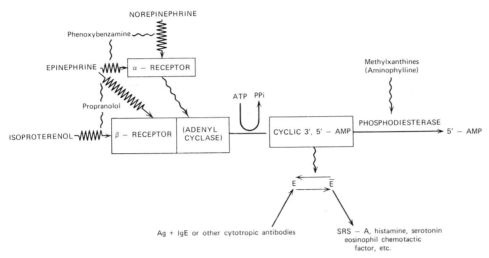

**Fig. 11.5** Modulatory effects of the cyclic AMP system on immunologic release of SRS-A and vasoactive amines. α-Receptor stimulation inhibits adenylcyclase activity, whereas that of β receptors enhances it. Mediator release would be under the control of a hypothetical enzyme (E), which would be activated (E′) and act in the presence of calcium. (From K. F. Austen, 1974.)

sequence. The exact order of the various metabolic phases is, however, not yet definitively established. In addition, differences are observed when the anaphylactic reaction is induced on previously sensitized tissues, such as lung, as compared to initiation of III on separated cells, such as rat peritoneal mastocytes.

The activity of the cyclic AMP system in the anaphylactic reaction is the inverse of that observed in secretory systems: a decrease in cyclic AMP level activates the system (Fig. 11.5). Histamine itself may exert a negative control action on mediator release. It has not been demonstrated that all mediators show this biochemical sequence.

## VIII.   CONCLUSIONS ON THE MECHANISMS OF IMMEDIATE HYPERSENSITIVITY

The last decade has seen considerable progress in understanding the mechanisms responsible for IH. This progress has had diagnostic and therapeutic consequences. Techniques for measuring IgE have appeared, although they have not yet significantly altered our diagnostic approach to allergic diseases. Thus, in drug allergy, we are still looking for a simple test that would permit direct evaluation of degranulation of effector cells to replace the use of skin tests. Demonstration of the presence of IgE is insufficient (even when specific IgE are involved), because the presence of IgE does not define allergy. IgE fixation on basophils and mastocytes and the response of these IgE-coated cells in the presence of antigen are extraordinarily variable among subjects (this

**Table 11.2  Anaphylactic Mediators**

| Mediator | Structure | Source | Properties Used for Identification |
|---|---|---|---|
| Histamine | | Mastocytes<br>Basophils<br>Platelets<br>Others | Contracts guinea pig ileum<br>Inhibited by antihistamine<br>Spectrofluorometry |
| Serotonin | | Enterochromaffin cells<br>Mastocytes<br>Platelets | Contracts guinea pig ileum and<br>rat uterus. Inhibited by lysergic<br>acid |
| PAF-acether | 1-O-Alkyl-2-acetyl-glyceryl<br>-3-phosphorylcholine | Basophils<br>Platelets<br>Macrophages<br>Neutrophils | Platelet aggregation in the<br>presence of cyclooxygenase<br>blockers and ADP scavengers<br>Increase in vasopermeability |
| SRS<br>(Leukotrienes) | | Mastocytes<br>Macrophages<br>Neutrophils | Contracts guinea pig ileum<br>Not inhibited by antihistamines or<br>destroyed by chymotrypsin |
| ECF | Val-Gly-Ser-Glu ?<br>Ala-Gly-Ser-Glu ?<br>Dihydroxy derivative of arachidonic acid<br>(LTB$_4$) ? | Mastocytes<br>Neutrophils | Chemotactic for eosinophils |
| Kinins<br>Bradykinin | Arg-Pro-Pro-Gly-Phe-Ser-Pro-Phe-Arg | Kininogen<br>Plasma α-globulin | Contracts rat uterus<br>Destroyed by chymotrypsin |
| Lysyl-bradykinin | Lys-Arg-Pro-Pro-Gly-Phe-Arg | Tissues | Contracts human bronchiola. No<br>effect on rat uterus |
| Methionyl-lysyl-<br>bradykinin | Met-Lys-Arg-Pro-Pro-Gly-Phe-Ser-Pro-Phe-<br>Arg | Tissues | Contracts guinea pig ileum |

variability is the basis for the definition of the allergic subject). From the therapeutic viewpoint, significant progress has been made with the introduction of sodium cromoglycate, which blocks mastocyte degranulation (by a mechanism not yet elucidated). This agent is effective in treating allergic asthma. Research is directed at finding methods for blocking IgE antibody production, preventing their binding to the mastocyte, preventing mastocyte degranulation, and inhibiting the action of other mediators than histamine.

## IX.   OTHER FORMS OF HYPERSENSITIVITY

IH, as described in the preceding pages, is linked to the action of anaphylactic antibodies (IgE in man and IgG1 in guinea pigs) and corresponds to the first category in Gell and Coombs' classification (chap. 1). Other mechanisms may also be responsible for hypersensitivity. Certain antibodies may bind complement, which then releases anaphylatoxins (class II of Gell and Coombs). These anaphylatoxins, which are degradation products of the third and fifth components of complement, may be released independent of the presence of antigen-antibody complexes after activation of the alternative pathway of the complement system. This hypothesis explains in vitro anaphylatoxin release after administration of polysaccharides and inulin. We have seen that anaphylatoxins induce the release of histamine, which causes symptoms that closely simulate the anaphylaxis described earlier.

Arthus' reaction is a semidelayed hypersensitivity reaction that features necrosis provoked by polymorphs, which are attracted to and activated by immune complexes. The reaction described by Arthus in 1903 may be seen in numerous species (rat, rabbit, mouse, guinea pig, and man) and belongs to class III of Gell and Coombs. The reaction consists of precipitation of an antigen injected under the skin by its antibody within cutaneous vessels in animals that produce precipitating antibodies. A passive Arthus' reaction is induced directly by injecting the antigen under the skin and injecting the antibody intravenously or indirectly by intravenous injection of antigen and cutaneous placement of the antibody.

Because the antibodies are precipitating, it is not surprising that after diffusion of antigen and antibody into the vessel walls, a precipitation occurs that is comparable to the gel precipitation reaction of Outcherlony. After the precipitation phase, rapid activation of the complement sequence occurs with release of C3a and C5a subfragments, which have a potent chemotactic action on polymorphs.

Within a few hours, polymorphs invade the injection site, and one may see numerous leukocytes phagocytosing ICs. Lysosomal proteolytic enzymes released during this process are responsible for both major clinical characteristics of Arthus' reaction, edema, and induration. Anatomically, the reaction is manifested by arteriolar lesions that show adherence and aggregation of leukocytes and platelets into the walls, thrombus formation, capillary wall hemorrhage, and necrosis. These abnormalities last a few hours and then completely disappear. Macroscopically, the reaction shows indurated erythema or a hemorrhagic tendency and even necrosis.

Although it is common to classify Arthus' reaction as an IH reaction, it is quite different from passive cutaneous anaphylaxis. Arthus' reaction does not require previous fixation of antibodies to tissues; it may be provoked by intravenous administration of antigen a few minutes after subcutaneous injection of antibody. Mastocytes are completely irrelevant to the reaction, which entirely depends on complement activation by ICs formed in situ and on the attraction of polymorphs. Antihistamine cannot inhibit Arthus' reaction, but it completely disappears if the animal is depleted of polymorphs or complement.

The passive anaphylactic reaction develops within a few minutes, whereas Arthus' reaction requires several hours. However, Maillard and Voisin have shown that the presence of anaphylactic antibodies at the site of the reaction facilitates the onset of Arthus' reaction initiated by precipitating IgG2 antibodies that were not anaphylactic.

A generalized Arthus reaction has been described in the guinea pig after administration of significant amounts of antigen in animals with circulating precipitating antibodies. These animals show delayed shock without true anaphylaxis, but hypotension, leukopenia, thrombocytopenia, and blood coagulation abnormalities are present, along with diminished serum levels of complement factors.

Arthus' reaction is the basis of certain incidents and accidents that occur after injection of serum and vaccines into subjects that possess circulating antigen or antibody. Arthus' reactions are responsible for some human diseases, including pigeon-breeder's disease. Certain pulmonary complications of measles have also been linked to an Arthus-type reaction. Gell and Coombs' classification gives an important place to delayed hypersensitivity reactions (type IV), which will be the subject of the following chapter.

**Table 11.3   Different Types of Allergic Reactions**

|  | *Anaphylaxis* | *Arthus' Reaction* | *Delayed Hypersensitivity* |
|---|---|---|---|
| Lag time in sensitized animals | 0–20 min | 30 min to 6 hr | 18 to 48 hr |
| Macroscopic aspect | Erythema, edema (urticaria) | Hemorrhagic necrosis, petechia | Erythema, indurated nodules |
| Histology | Edema, late eosinophils | Platelet thrombi, polymorphs, neutrophils | Mononucleated cells |
| Immunoflorescence | 0 | IgM, IgG, C3 | ? |
| Transfer | Serum IgE | Serum (IgM, IgG) | T lymphocytes |
| Antigenic specifity | Small determinants (minimum benzenic nucleus; maximum, hexapeptide, hexasaccharide) |  | Macromolecules (proteins, especially on cell surfaces) |
| General manifestations | Anaphylactic shock |  | Fever, tuberculinic shock |

Finally, another type of hypersensitivity is represented by Shwartzman's reaction, although, strictly speaking, this reaction is not one of immunologic hypersensitivity. Shwartzman's reaction is a hemorrhagic necrosis of certain organs observed after endotoxin injection into animals or humans presensitized by an earlier endotoxin injection, 6 to 48 hr before. The necrotic reaction is localized if the first endotoxin dose is injected intradermally and if the second dose is administered intravenously. The reaction is generalized (it features bilateral cortical necrosis of the kidneys) when both injections are intravenous. This reaction is not one of immunologic hypersensitivity, because the interval between the two injections is not sufficient to allow antibody production to develop and because the reaction is obtained when the two endotoxins have no antigenic relationship and may even be nonimmunogenic. In the local reaction, "preparative" endotoxin administration leads to granulocytic accumulation. Thus, it is of interest in this respect that immune complexes or tuberculin may be substituted for endotoxin in a subject sensitized to the former. The provoking agent induces release of lysosomal polymorph hydrolases that will produce lesions of small blood vessel walls and favor deposition of platelets, leukocytes, and fibrin aggregates. The generalized reaction seems to be due to different mechanisms that are less well understood. It does not seem to involve polymorph accumulation. Blocking of the reticuloendothelial system (RES) by endotoxins is suggested by the fact that it is possible to replace the preparative injection by administration of Thorotrast, which blocks the RES. The generalized reaction seems to include intravascular coagulation and fibrin deposition in vessels, both because of a poorly functioning RES and because of fibrinolysis blockade. In fact, this reaction touches on the subject of mechanisms of intravascular coagulation and their relationship to complement. (A discussion of this important problem is, of course, not within the scope of this immunology text.) It should be noted that Shwartzman's reactions may simulate certain immunologic reactions, particularly anaphylactic reactions, and that certain immunologic factors, such as immune complexes, may play the role of "preparators" or "provocators" in Shwartzman's phenomenon.

# BIBLIOGRAPHY

Austen K. F., Lewis R. A., Stichschulte D. J., Wasserman S. I., Leid R. W., and Goetzl E. J. Generation and release of chemical mediators of immediate hypersensitivity. *In* L. Brent and J. Holborow, Ed., Progress in immunology. II. Vol. 2. Amsterdam, 1974, North Holland, p. 61.

Becker E. L. Nature and classification of immediate-type allergic reactions. Adv. Immunol., 1971, *13*, 267.

Bennich H. and Johansson S. G. O. Structure and function of human IgE. Adv. Immunol., 1971, *13*, 1.

Brocklehurst W. E. Assay of mediators in hypersensitivity reactions. *In* D. M. Weir, Ed., Handbook of experimental immunology, ed. 2. Oxford, 1973, Blackwell, p. 43.1.12.

Goetzl E. J., Wasserman S. I., and Austen K. F. Modulation of the eosinophil chemotactic response in immediate hypersensitivity. *In* L. Brent and J. Holborow, Eds., Progress in immunology. II. Vol. 4. Amsterdam, 1974, North Holland, p. 41.

Gupta S. and Good R. A. Cellular, molecular and clinical aspects of allergic disorders. Comprehensive Immunology. Plenum Press, New York, London, 1979, 628 pp.

HOLGATE S. T., LEWIS R. A., and AUSTEN K. F. The role of cyclic nucleotides in mast cell activation and secretion. *In* Immunology 80 (M. Fougereau and J. Dausset eds.), Acad. Press, New York, 1980:846.

ISHIZAKA K. Regulation of the IgE response. *In* Immunology 80 (M. Fougereau and J. Dausset eds), Acad. Press. New York, 1980, 815.

ISHIZAKA K. The identification and significance of gamma E. *In* R. A. Good and D. W. Fisher, Eds., Immunobiology. Stamford, Conn., 1971, Sinauer, p. 84.

JOHANSSON S. G. O., BENNICH H., and BERG T. The clinical significance of IgE. *In* Progress in clinical immunology. Vol. I. New York, 1972, Grune & Stratton, p. 157.

KING T. P. Chemical and biological properties of some atopic allergens. Adv. Immunol. 1976, *23*, 77.

LICHTENSTEIN L. M. Anaphylactic reactions *In* Mechanisms of Immunopathology (S. Cohen, P. A. Ward, and R. T. McCluskey eds.), John Wiley & Sons, New York, 1979, 13.

LICHTENSTEIN L. M. Anaphylactic reactions *In* Mechanisms of Immunopathology (S. Cohen, P. A. Ward, and R. T. McCluskey eds.), John Wiley & Sons, New York, 1979, 13.

OVARY Z. *In* J. F. Acroyd, Ed., Immunological methods, CIOMS Symposium. Oxford 1961, Blackwell, p. 259.

PIPER P. D. Mediators of anaphylactic hypersensitivity. *In* L. Brent and J. Holborow, Ed., Progress in immunology. II. Vol. 4. Amsterdam, 1974, North Holland, p. 51.

STANWORTH D. R. Some thoughts on the mechanism of triggering of mast cells (and basophils) by cytophilic antibody-antigen interaction, of possible relevance to an understanding of other immunological release processes. *In* L. G. Sivestri, Ed., The immunological basis of connective tissue disorders. Amsterdam, 1975, North Holland, p. 73.

SULLIVAN T. J. and KULEZYCKI A. N. Immediate hypersensitivity responses. *In* Clinical Immunology (Parker C. W. ed.), Saunders, Philadelphia, 1980, 115.

WARD P. A. Mediators of inflammatory responses. *In* Mechanisms of Immunopathology (S. Cohen, P. A. Ward, and R. T. McCluskey eds.), John Wiley & Sons, New York, 1979, 1.

WARD P. A., DATA R. and TILL G. Regulatory control of complement-derived chemotactic and anaphylatoxin mediators. *In* L. Brent and J. Holborow, Ed., Progress in immunology. II. Vol. 1. Amsterdam, 1974, North Holland, p. 209.

## ORIGINAL ARTICLES

ISHIZAKA K. and ISHIZAKA T. Biologic function of IgE antibodies and mechanisms of reaginic hypersensitivity. Clin. Exp. Immunol., 1970, *6*, 25.

KAY A. B. and AUSTEN K. F. The IgE-mediated release of an eosinophil leucocyte chemotactic factor from human lung. J. Immunol., 1971, *107*, 889.

ORANGE R. P., AUSTEN W. G., and AUSTEN K. F. Immunological release of histamine and slow reacting substance of anaphylaxis from human lung. I. Modulation by agents influencing cellular levels of cyclic 3'5' adenosine monophosphate. J. Exp. Med., 1971, *134*, 136s.

Chapter 12

# DELAYED HYPERSENSITIVITY

## Jean-Pierre Revillard

I. INTRODUCTION: CONCEPT OF DELAYED HYPERSENSITIVITY AND OF CELL-MEDIATED IMMUNITY

II. INDUCTION AND EXPRESSION OF DELAYED HYPERSENSITIVITY

III. TRANSFER OF DELAYED HYPERSENSITIVITY

IV. EXPRESSION OF DELAYED HYPERSENSITIVITY IN VITRO

V. SUPPRESSION OF DELAYED HYPERSENSITIVITY

VI. INVESTIGATION OF DELAYED HYPERSENSITIVITY IN MAN

VII. CONCLUSIONS: DELAYED HYPERSENSITIVITY AND IMMUNITY

## I. INTRODUCTION: CONCEPT OF DELAYED HYPERSENSITIVITY AND OF CELL-MEDIATED IMMUNITY

Manifestations of delayed hypersensitivity (DH) were observed by Jenner, who in 1801, noticed the inflammatory reaction provoked by vaccine injected into the skin of subjects who had previously had chicken pox or vaccination. While studying experimental tuberculosis, in 1890, Robert Koch described hypersensitivity to tubercle bacillus. An initial bacillus inoculation into a guinea pig does not produce an immediate reaction, but 10 to 14 days later, a nodule appears at the inoculation site accompanied by regional adenopathy. During the next few weeks, the local lesion evolves slowly toward necrosis and ulceration and persists until death of the animal. If, after a few weeks, one inoculates a second dose of tubercle bacillus, the local induration appears early (24 hr), ulcerates, and then heals. The reaction to the second injection is "Koch's phenomenon." It represents both hypersensitivity, because the local reaction appears more rapidly than after the initial inoculation, and an increase in resistance to the bacillus, because the lesions go on to heal. Local reaction in the tuberculous guinea pig may also be produced by dead tubercle bacilli and be heated filtrates of the bacterial culture, for example, tuberculin. These preparations have no effect in nontuberculous controls.

Koch's phenomenon, tuberculin hypersensitivity, was used by Mantoux to detect subjects who presented with either evolving or cured tuberculous infection. Von Pirquet introduced (in 1906) the word "allergy" to describe this phenomenon, in which introduction of an infectious agent or a foreign substance (antigen) modifies the organisms's reactions to subsequent injection.

Strictly speaking, allergy is used to describe this state of protection and hypersensitivity. Today, however, allergy is used exclusively to describe hypersensitivity manifestations. In 1921, Zinsser described bacterial allergy, which he carefully separated from other hypersensitivity reactions, such as anaphylaxis, Arthus' reactions, and serum sickness disease.

The first criterion that permits differentiation is a 12 to 48 hr period during which the local reaction reaches its peak, thus the adjective "delayed" hypersensitivity, in contrast to immediate hypersensitivity (anaphylaxis) and semidelayed hypersensitivity (Arthus' phenomenon). Microscopy of the DH reaction has shown a predominance of mononucleated cells within the inflammatory perivascular infiltrate: this predominance of these cells is not seen in immediate hypersensitivity of in Arthus' phenomenon. Finally, attempts to passively transfer DH have regularly failed with serum from sensitized animals. Landsteiner and Chase later showed that DH could be transmitted by live lymphoid cells. These transfer experiments have been extended to other forms of hypersensitivity; and it is now appropriate to designate as cell-mediated hypersensitivity (or, more simply, cellular hypersensitivity) allergic reactions that may be transmitted by lymphoid cells and not by humoral antibodies. This property is seen in other forms of immune responses (Table 12.1), including resistance to numerous infectious agents (intracellular facultative parasites),

**Table 12.1   Reactions of Cell-Mediated Immunity**

| Antigen | Immune reaction |
|---|---|
| Bacteria, viruses | Delayed hypersensitivity |
| Yeast, protozoa, parasites | Acquired cellular resistance |
| Proteins with complete adjuvant | Delayed hypersensitivity |
| Proteins injected without complete adjuvant | Basophilic cutaneous hypersensitivity (Jones and Mote reaction) |
| Haptens (with autologous protein) | Contact dermatitis |
| Transplantation antigens | Allograft rejection Graft versus host reaction |
| Tumor antigens | Rejection of tumor |
| Tissue antigens | Certain experimental autoimmune diseases |

antitumor immunity, and allograft rejection due to cell-mediated immunity, as opposed to that mediated by humoral immunity.

Initially based on findings from transfer experiments, the traditional separation of humoral from cellular immunity has gained more substantiation, when the differences between thymus-dependent (T) and thymus-independent (B) systems were established. Humoral immunity has, as an effector cell, a B-type lymphocyte that has become (with or without T-cell cooperation) a plasma cell that secretes specific antibodies. In cell-mediated immunity, the antigen-sensitive cells and the effector cells are both thymus dependent. The effector cell is a circulating T lymphocyte capable of reacting specifically on contact with the antigen. The conditions and effects of these interactions are the essence of present-day studies of the DH mechanism.

Characteristics that permit differentiation between cell-mediated hypersensitivity and other forms of allergy (Table 11.3) cannot be studied in a single experimental system. The DH skin reaction that occurs after intradermal injection of antigen is distinctive in man and in the guinea pig but is more difficult to observe in the mouse, rat, or chicken, species in which the effects of neonatal thymectomy, bursectomy, or thoracic duct cannulation have been studied. Skin allograft rejection and resistance to facultative intracellular parasites are models of cell-mediated immunity better adapted to the latter animal species.

## II.  INDUCTION AND EXPRESSION OF DELAYED HYPERSENSITIVITY

## INDUCTION

### Bacterial, Viral, and Mycotic Infections

The experimental and clinical model of the DH reaction is tuberculin hypersensitivity. It may be induced by tuberculous infection, inoculation of bacilli with attenuated virulence [Bacillus Calmette-Guérin (BCG)], or injection of Freund's complete adjuvant. Skin reaction may be provoked by *Mycobacterium tuberculosis*, BCG (BCG test), tuberculin, or tuberculinic purified protein derivative (PPD). *M. tuberculosis* polysaccharidic antigens induce antibody formation without cellular response. Repeated PPD injections in man do not elicit DH.

Numerous bacterial antigens other than protein antigens of *Mycobacterium tuberculosis* may induce DH. These antigens include *Salmonella typhi*, *Brucella abortus* (melitin test), *Corynebacterium parvum*, streptococci (M protein, streptokinase/streptodornase), and the protein antigens (but not polysaccharides) of pneumococci. In all of these examples, it should be noted that only natural infection or inoculation of living bacteria leads to DH development. Injection of killed bacilli induces only a humoral response.

Most viral infections induce DH; the earliest discovered example was DH associated with antipox virus vaccination (vide supra). The DH reaction may be obtained by use of more or less purified preparations of measles, mumps, or herpes virus. Only natural infections and vaccinations with living virus give rise to DH; inoculation of killed virus induces only antibody production. All mycotic infections, including candidiasis, aspergillosis, cryptococcosis, blastomycosis, coccidioidomycosis, and histoplasmosis, induce DH. Among the protozoan infections, leishmaniosis and toxoplasmosis are known to produce DH. Intradermal tests are usually performed with crude extracts of these various pathogenic agents.

### Delayed Hypersensitivity After Protein Injection

The injection of a protein antigen dissolved in aqueous solution induces antibody formation but does not generally produce durable DH, unless the antigen is introduced in an emulsion of Freund's complete adjuvant. This adjuvant includes mineral oil, an emulsifying agent, and killed mycobacteria (e.g., *M. tuberculosis*, strain HR 37, 1 mg/ml). It can only be used in an animal. Dead bacilli may be replaced by BCG or by peptidoglycan purified from bacterial walls (see chap. 33). Complete Freund's adjuvant considerably increases antibody production. The dose of injected protein used is very important; low doses, of the order of 1 to 50 μg in the guinea pig and the rabbit, favor DH induction, whereas doses that approximate 1 mg preferentially provoke antibody formation. A vigorous humoral response probably plays an inhibitory role in induction and expression of manifestations of DH. Indeed, injection of emulsified antigen in incomplete adjuvant may prevent development of DH. However, it is possible to obtain DH by injecting protein antigen in the absence of complete adjuvant by administering multiple serial low-dose injections, of the order of 1 μg of purified protein, by injecting heat-denatured or chemically modified (by binding of haptenic groups) proteins, or by administering antigen-antibody complexes formed in antibody excess.

All of these injections must be intradermal. Other modes of antigen introduction may lead to antibody synthesis but not to DH. DH obtained by these procedures is called basophil cutaneous hypersensitivity, or Jones and Mote's reaction.

This type of hypersensitivity, which may be transmitted by lymphocytes but not by serum, differs from the prior examples in terms of weaker intensity, presence of basophil polymorphs (5 to 30%) in the cellular infiltrate, and a transient nature. It may occur 8 days after sensitization but disappears 1 to 4 weeks later, when the circulating antibody titer rises. This type of hypersensitivity probably corresponds to skin reactions observed after insect bites in man. Hypersensitivity reactions to mosquito bites (salivary antigens) are immunologically specific. The initial bites provoke no reaction; the next bites produce DH and, after a few weeks, immediate hypersensitivity. Repeated bites may lead to "desensitization," with loss of skin reaction.

### Hypersensitivity by Cutaneous Contact

Some low-molecular-weight molecules (less than 1000 daltons) are strongly electrophilic and are thus able to form covalent bonds with sulfhydryl or amino protein groups present in the skin. These substances sensitize a subject in such a way as to produce a DH reaction after a second contact, for example, "contact allergic dermatitis." Sensitizing substances most often used experimentally include picryl chloride, dinitrochlorobenzene (DNCB), dinitrofluorobenzene (DNFB), and oxazolone. These substances, which in themselves are irritants, are introduced percutaneously in the presence of Freund's complete adjuvant or in the form of haptens bound to cellular membranes. The test is then performed 15 days later by percutaneous application of a nonirritating allergen concentration. The immunogen is a conjugate of the chemical agent and the proteins of the surface epidermal cells, particularly the histocompatibility antigens of Langerhans cells. Contact dermatitides are very commonly seen in man: they may represent sensitization to cosmetics, medicines, or various chemical products (professional dermatosis).

### Transplantation and Tumoral Antigens

Allograft rejection is accompanied by a cell-mediated immunity reaction that may be demonstrated by a DH cutaneous reaction to the donor's transplantation antigens. Brent and Medawar have shown that if a guinea pig (A) is sensitized by a skin graft from a histoincompatible guinea pig (B), the subsequent injection of antigenic tissue extract from B into the skin of A provokes a DH tuberculin-type reaction (direct reaction). In addition, if lymph node cells from guinea pig A are injected into the skin of guinea pig B, they react to transplantation antigens and also induce a DH reaction (indirect reaction or local transfer of immune lymphocytes). Similar observations have been made with specific antigens from virus-induced tumors and less consistently with antigenic extracts prepared from chemical carcinogen-induced tumors.

## HISTOLOGIC AND CYTOLOGIC APPEARANCES OF DELAYED HYPERSENSITIVITY INDUCTION

When an antigen in an emulsion of Freund's complete adjuvant is injected, an inflammatory granuloma forms that consists of macrophages derived from circulating monocytes, T and B lymphocytes, and lymphoblasts. The intracytoplasmic vacuoles of the macrophages contain lipid droplets and mycobacteria. The arrangement of the granuloma ensures direct contact between lymphocytes and macrophages. When the antigen is applied cutaneously to induce a contact dermatitis, it binds to the surface of Langerhans' cells. These cells are distinguished from other epidermal cells, such as melanocytes and keratinocytes, by their lobulated nucleus, their clear cytoplasm containing typical granules, their intense ATP-ase activity, and their dendritic prolongations. They form a sort of tangential streak containing 460 to 1000 cells/mm$^3$. These cells, which are also found in the dermis, lymph nodes, and thymus, are of mesenchymatous origin. Although only slightly phagocytic, they possess some characteristics in common with macrophages—notably, the presence of Ia antigens in the mouse or HLA-DR antigens in man—and they have the capacity to stimulate allogeneic T lymphocytes in mixed culture. These cells leave the epidermis to reach the regional lymph nodes by means of the afferent lymphatic vessels.

Cellular changes associated with DH may be observed in lymph nodes draining the site of cutaneous antigen introduction (skin allograft or oxazolone application). The morphologic changes seen in the first days after antigen introduction include an increase in lymph node volume, due largely to lymph node retention of circulating lymphocytes. Later, hyperplasia of the deep cortex appears (the paracortical area; see p. 35). Until the fifth day, the enlarging paracortical area compresses the medulla, but after the sixth day, the superficial cortex and the medulla also undergo hypertrophy.

Cytologic study of the paracortical area shows large pyroninophilic cells or immunoblasts, which may constitute, by day 4, 10% of the total lymph node cell population. This peak immunoblast percentage precedes by 24 hr the appearance of generalized DH and the capability of lymph node cells to achieve DH transfer. The presence of "grains" in immunoblasts by autoradiography (prepared from lymph nodes of recently immunized animals injected with tritiated thymidine) indicates that these cells are rapidly dividing. Two to 3 days after thymidine injection, small lymphocytes are labeled. However, the number of grains per nucleus then progressively decreases, demonstrating evolution of the large pyroninophilic cells into small lymphocytes by successive divisions. After the sixth day, labeled lymphocytes exit from the lymph node and migrate to the spleen and other lymph nodes. Immunoblasts themselves derive from small lymphocytes, having undergone the lymphoblastic transformation phenomenon (see Fig. 12.3).

## EXPRESSION OF DELAYED HYPERSENSITIVITY

### Cutaneous Reaction

Intradermal injection of 0.1 μg of PPD tuberculin into a sensitized subject causes no reaction in the initial 10 hr. Thereafter, erythema and induration appear, with progressive augmentation in size, reaching a maximum at 24 to 70 hr, then followed by a very slow reduction in size of the lesion. The intensity of the cutaneous reaction may be quantified by measuring the diameter of the erythema and induration or the thickness of the affected skin. The evolution of central necrosis, sometimes accompanied by vesiculae and ulcerations, comprises a particularly intense DH. To avoid severe cutaneous reactions, it is recommended that these tests be performed with low antigen doses (1 tuberculin unit or 0.02 μg of PPD). If there is no reaction at low dose, higher doses (5, 10, or 50 tuberculin units) are selected. The 5-unit dose is recommended for epidemiologic studies. The 50-unit dose may be used initially if the clinical context suggests a DH deficiency. It is noteworthy that PPD doses necessary to obtain a local reaction in the guinea pig are 50 to 100 times greater than those required in man.

Antigen introduction may be performed by skin reaction, application of a ring, or percutaneously. These techniques are not as well suited for quantification as is intradermal application. Percutaneous application is used to study contact dermatitis (patch test). In the highly sensitized animal, corneal instillation of the sensitizing chemical substance or intracorneal injection of 10 to 50 μl of antigen provokes a delayed reaction that consists of redness, edema, and corneal opacification.

Local DH reactions must not be confused with Arthus reaction, which begins earlier, reaches peak intensity between 4 and 6 hr, and is not accompanied by induration (only erythema and edema occur). However, an intense Arthus's reaction that lasts more than 24 hr may be difficult to distinguish from a DH reaction, particularly because these two phenomena may occur closely in time.

Histologic aspects of DH reactions are distinctive. If a biopsy is performed during the first 12 hr, an increase in capillary permeability is observed, often with the presence of a few polymorphs. At 48 hr, the lesion consists of a mononucleated cell infiltrate (Fig. 12.1). The predominant cells are macrophages that originated from circulating monocytes that originally traversed the vascular wall at the reaction site (Fig. 12.2). In some tissues, where intense and prolonged DH is seen, the macrophages acquire a syncytial appearance. Other mononucleated cells include B and T lymphocytes and lymphoblasts that result from *in situ* transformation of small lymphocytes; it is not uncommon to later see occasional plasma cells. In contact dermatitis the epidermal Langerhans cells are surrounded by lymphoid cells after the third hour following antigen application. Subsequently, the number of Langerhans cells in the epidermis diminishes and correspondingly increases in the dermis. Those cells surrounded by lymphocytes undergo rupture of their cytoplasmic membranes, suggesting a cytotoxicity phenomenon.

### Systemic and Focal Manifestations

Intraperitoneal injection of high doses (about 5 mg) of tuberculin produce tuberculin shock in *M. tuberculosis*-sensitized guinea pigs. Three to 4 hr after

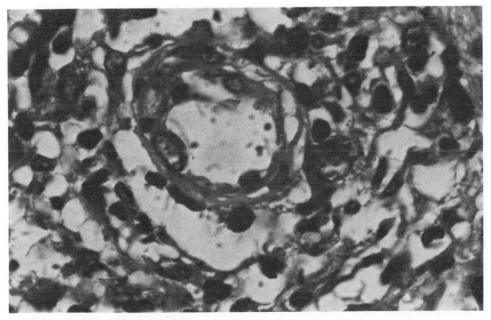

**Fig. 12.1** Delayed hypersensitivity skin reaction to tuberculin in man. Lymphocytic and macrophagic infiltration around the dermal venule. Note the modest edema and absence of polymorphs. (From S. Colon.)

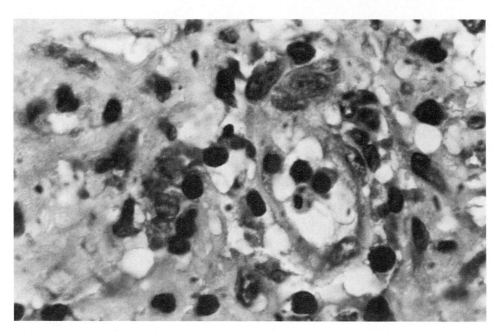

**Fig. 12.2**  Delayed hypersensitivity skin reaction to tuberculin in man. Accumulation of lymphocytes and macrophages around a dermal capillary. Note capillary wall changes, adherence and diapedesis of mononucleated cells, tight contact between lymphocytes and macrophages, and initiation of fusion of certain macrophages (first stage of giant-cell formation). × 500. (From S. Colon.)

injection, the animal is prostrated; body temperature decreases, and respiratory abnormalities develop, followed by vascular collapse and death within 48 hr. The antigenic specificity of this reaction is not proven, and contribution of a nonspecific hypersensitivity of the Sanarelli-Shwartzman type cannot be excluded.

In man, injection of high tuberculin doses in strongly sensitized individuals may be accompanied by a weak generalized reaction that features headache, malaise, and prostration.

Tuberculin fever constitutes the purest general manifestation of DH. Two to 4 hr after intravenous injection of a low tuberculin dose, fever (40° to 41°C) develops, which oscillates and then disappears within 48 hr. Arterial pressure is unaltered, and there is no vascular shock. The peripheral blood shows a rapid and significant decrease in number of monocytes, while polymorphs and platelets remain normal. Antihistamines are not preventive or curative. Histologic examination shows a distinct edema of vessel walls and a perivenous infiltrate of mononucleated cells, especially in the lungs.

The decrease in number of circulating monocytes may be induced by intravenous injection of a lymphokine-rich supernatant (migration-inhibitory factor) obtained by incubation of sensitized lymphocytes in the presence of antigen. The intraperitoneal injection of antigen into sensitized animals also induces the disappearance of macrophages from the peritoneal exudate (Nelson and Boyden's phenomenon).

Injection of antigen into subjects who present with DH may be associated with various focal reactions, including keratitis, conjunctival erythema, arthritis, adenitis, and inflammatory reactions in the lungs. These reactions are probably a consequence of the interaction of antigen with sensitized lymphocytes already present in the tissue where the antigen localizes. This is suggested by exacerbation of reactivity of prior intradermal reaction sites after a subsequent tuberculin test.

### Delayed Hypersensitivity-Antigenic Specificity

The antigenic-specific sites responsible for DH induction and manifestations are not identical to those that react with antibodies (see p. 156). When a guinea pig is immunized with 2,4-dinitrophenyl bovine serum albumin (DNP-BSA), a DH reaction occurs when the immunogen itself is reapplied: the reaction is weaker if the carrier protein (BSA) is used alone and nil if the hapten (DNP) is bound to another protein. The DH reaction is thus specific for the hapten-protein conjugate (Gell and Benacerraf). This property is common to all immunologic phenomena that result from direct interaction between antigen and T lymphocytes, such as humoral responses of the secondary type and tolerance induction.

# III. TRANSFER OF DELAYED HYPERSENSITIVITY

One of the chief characteristics of DH, common, by definition, to all cell-mediated immune reactions, is the inability to transfer this type of immunity by serum from sensitized donors, whereas transfer may be achieved by use of lymphoid cells from the same donors. Although this finding is generally accepted, papers regularly are published that claim DH transfer by use of serum. Acceptance of these observations requires that no antigen has been included in the serum used for transfer experiments.

## HISTORY

The first demonstration of transfer of tuberculin DH was performed by Helmoltz in 1909 (guinea pig) by use of defibrinated blood. One year later, Bail reported on a series of remarkably well-controlled experiments. A homogenate of spleen and of a noncaseous lymph node preparation from a tuberculous guinea pig was injected into healthy recipients; 24 hr later, application of a weak tuberculin dose induced lethal shock in the recipients. These results could not be obtained with a mixture of M. tuberculosis and lymphoid tissues from normal animals, thus excluding antigenic transfer, and not by a homogenate of tuberculous guinea pig liver, which demonstrated the role of the lymphoid system in this type of hypersensitivity. Serum from tuberculous guinea pigs could not produce the transfer, thus eliminating a role for circulating antibodies.

In 1942, Landsteiner and Chase established the basis of our present knowledge of the DH mechanism by achieving (in the guinea pig) transfer of picryl chloride contact sensitivity by use of living cells from peritoneal exudates taken from sensitized donors. The donor had been previously immunized by intraperitoneal injection of picrylated erythrocyte stromas mixed with paraffin oil and killed *M. tuberculosis*. The peritoneal exudate induced by paraffin oil consisted of approximately two-thirds macrophages and one-third polymorphs and lymphocytes. Neither the supernatant obtained after centrifugation of the exudate nor the peritoneal cells destroyed by freezing or heating at 48°C achieved the transfer.

## TRANSFER OF DELAYED HYPERSENSITIVITY IN AN ANIMAL WITH LIVING CELLS

### Syngeneic Transfer in the Guinea Pig

Transfer experiments of tuberculin DH and contact hypersensitivity to various haptens (picryl chloride, *o*-chlorobenzoyl chloride) performed by Bloom and Chase in the guinea pig have provided information on the mechanism of the transfer process. Success of transfer depends on the number of injected cells (Table 12.2) and the intensity of donor DH.

The integrity and viability of injected lymphoid cells are an absolute necessity; using eight to 10 times the number of cells sufficient under normal conditions, it has not been possible to obtain DH skin reactions in recipients when the donor cells were damaged (incubation in the presence of chloroform, heating at 48°C for 30 min, freezing and thawing, destruction by ultrasound, separation of subcellular fractions, treatment with actinomycin D or puromycin). In all cases, the supernatant obtained after centrifugation, deprived of living cells, is inactive, even when mixed with viable peritoneal cells from an unsensitized guinea pig. In vitro incubation of sensitized donor cells in the presence of specific antigen does not eliminate transfer capability, whereas the supernatant still remains inactive. These experiments exclude the existence of a preformed active substance in the transfer-producing cells. Interestingly, in vitro irradiation of lymphoid cells does not modify transfer ability.

### Histocompatibility and Duration of Adoptive Immunity

The DH reaction remains positive for several days after injection of cells into recipients that have received lymphoid cells from a sensitized donor. It

**Table 12.2  Number of Cells Obtained from Picryl Chloride-Sensitized Guinea Pigs After Injection of Picrylated Erythrocytic Stromas in the Presence of Freund's Complete Adjuvant, 35 to 60 Days Before the Experiment**

| Cell source | Number of cells obtained per animal | Minimum number of cells necessary for transfer |
|---|---|---|
| Peritoneal exudate | $1.5–2.5 \times 10^8$ | $1–1.5 \times 10^8$ |
| Lymph node | $4–6 \times 10^8$ | $6–9 \times 10^8$ |
| Spleen | $3.5–4 \times 10^8$ | $3–5 \times 10^8$ |

becomes negative after the 10th day, unless there is active immunization of the recipient by the antigen transmitted with donor cells. Transfer duration is much longer between mice of the same pure strain (adoptive transfer); it is shortened when the recipient has been presensitized against the donor transplantation antigens. These data may be explained by destruction of the lymphoid cells from the histoincompatible donor. The early experiments on transfer of DH were performed in guinea pigs selected from the same colony (Harley strain) but not selected for histocompatibility. When these experiments were reperformed in pure strains of mice or guinea pigs, it became apparent that the transfer of DH could only be regularly obtained among animals of the same strain. In the mouse, the donor and recipient must possess identical I-A genes on the H-2 region. These observations underline the importance of histocompatibility antigens in the cellular interactions that subserve the development of the DH reaction. Cell-mediated immunity may not be accomplished by cell transfer across a species barrier.

### Tranfer with Labeled Lymphoid Cells

One may assume from the preceding experiments that transferred lymphoid cells from the sensitized donor accumulate at the site of antigen injection in the recipient. By labeling donor lymphocytes with repeated injections of tritiated thymidine, it can be shown, in fact, that the cell infiltrate of the DH reaction actually contains less than 10% labeled cells. The remaining cells come from the nonsensitized recipient. There is no preferential attraction of donor cells by the antigen: it can be shown that the number of labeled cells is nearly the same for a nonspecific inflammatory reaction (turpentine) as compared to the DH reaction induced by an antigen against which the recipient, but not the donor, is sensitized. If in the same type of experiment, tritiated thymidine is injected into the recipient immediately before transfer, 70 to 90% of the infiltrating cells are labeled, which demonstrates that they are rapidly dividing endogenous cells.

### Nature of the Cell Responsible for the Transfer

Transfer experiments in the guinea pig have been performed in most cases with nonpurified suspensions of lymphoid cells that include a mixture of macrophages and various lymphocyte populations. Macrophage elimination based on adherence or phagocytosis does not diminish lymphocyte transfer capacity. (Transfer of graft immunity by thoracic duct lymphocytes confirms this observation.) In the mouse, treatment of the cellular suspension by an anti-θ serum and complement suppresses the adoptive transfer and thereby shows the critical role of T lymphocytes in transfer experiments. The participation of T-cell subpopulations has been more precisely delineated by the use of antisera directed against the Lyt 1,2, and 3 antigens. T cells that bring about the transfer of DH carry the Lyt 1 marker, just as the "helper cells" do in the antibody response. However, a second subpopulation of T cells carrying the Lyt 2 and 3 markers is necessary for the transfer of cell-mediated immunity (resistance to infection with *Listeria monocytogenes*).

Injection of purified T lymphocytes into lethally irradiated recipients does not allow development of a cell-mediated immunity hypersensitivity reaction, unless there is simultaneous administration (to the recipient) of rapidly dividing bone marrow cells that contain macrophage precursors that form the essential part of the skin infiltrate. These bone marrow cells may be obtained from either sensitized or unsensitized donors.

From all these data, one may imagine a sequence as follows: a small number of T lymphocytes capable of reacting specifically with the antigen makes contact with the tissue-bound antigen. This contact results in the accumulation of nonsensitized cells (lymphocytes and monocytes) that constitute the characteristic DH reaction infiltrate. The recruitment of nonsensitized cells by activated T lymphocytes requires certain humoral mediators, which we will discuss further (Fig. 12.3).

## TRANSFER OF DELAYED HYPERSENSITIVITY IN MAN

### Transfer with Living Cells

DH transfer experiments in man, initiated by H. S. Lawrence in 1949, involve many difficulties. Adult humans have been exposed to large numbers of bacterial antigens, which creates difficulty in selecting recipients for transfer experiments. Intradermal and subcutaneous leukocyte injections, followed by intradermal injection of 250 tuberculin units (at the same locus) induces at 24 hr a local reaction, which is followed by a delayed reaction after the sixth day. These findings have been duplicated with streptococcal antigens (intact streptococci, streptokinase, M protein). Attempts to transfer contact allergy to simple chemical substances have shown inconsistent but generally negative results.

Similar transfer experiments with living cells in man have yielded significantly different results when compared to DH transfer experiments in the guinea pig. The number of lymphoid cells required to achieve transfer in man (approximately equivalent to 100 ml of blood) is relatively less than that needed in the guinea pig. Second, DH reactions may persist in the recipient for several months or even several years after transfer, which represents a much longer duration than the leukocyte life-span in histoincompatible recipients. These observations led Lawrence to suggest that a factor contained in donor lymphocytes was transmitted to the recipient lymphoid cells, which rendered them capable of reacting specifically with antigen. The "tranfer factor" was demonstrated by DH transfer experiments with cellular extracts.

### Tranfer Factor

Transfer of DH to tuberculin and streptococcal M protein was achieved in man by Lawrence in 1954, by use of leukocytes destroyed by freezing and thawing, and later by a leukocyte dialysate treated by deoxyribonuclease. The dialysate (dialyzable transfer factor) retains its activity after ribonuclease and trypsin treatment. The precise chemical nature of the active principle is not known. Some studies suggest that it is a peptide coupled to a relatively small ribonucleic acid.

The biologic properties of the transfer factor are distinctive: transfer factor has no antibody properties: it is not neutralized by the antigen; and it induces

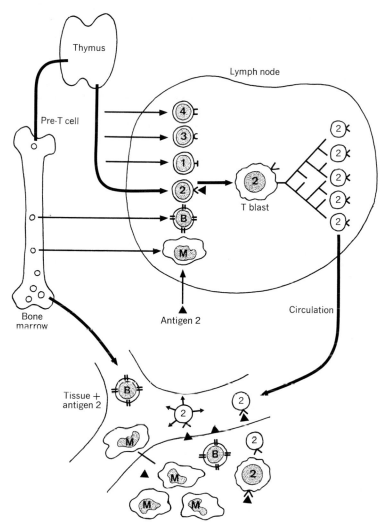

**Fig. 12.3** Schematic representation of the main phases of delayed hypersensitivity induction and expression. T cells recognize the antigen. Antigen 2 reactive clone proliferates and then leaves the lymph node. The active inflammatory reaction is associated with the release by sensitized T cells of mediators that act on lymphocytes, monocytes, and capillary permeability and have direct cytotoxic effects. As mentioned in the text, most of the scheme illustrated here is questionable. In particular, delayed hypersensitivity induction or interaction between antigen and clone 2 precursor cells probably occurs more at the tissue periphery than in the lymph node itself.

DH in the recipient but not antibody production against the corresponding antigen. Transfer factor exists preformed in mononucleated cells from sensitized subjects. In vitro, it can provoke both lymphoblastic transformation of the unsensitized recipient's lymphocytes in the presence of specific antigen and production of the macrophage migration-inhibitory factor. However, the immunologic specificity of these effects has not been demonstrated.

Transfer factor from leukocyte dialysates has been used therapeutically in numerous cases of cellular immunodeficiency. The results differ according to the type of deficiency. DH reactions usually remain negative in severe combined immunodeficiencies and in Hodgkin's disease. A local but nonsystemic transfer is usually observed in sarcoidosis. In immunodeficiencies of variable expression (ataxia telangiectasia, chronic granulomatous candidiasis, lepromatous leprosy, and various neoplasias), DH skin reactions usually become positive in the recipient. DH transfer is not always associated with a favorable therapeutic effect, although in some cases the response is spectacular. In 50% of children with Wiskott-Aldrich syndrome treated by transfer factor, a complete and prolonged remission of clinical symptoms occurs. Note, however, that negative skin reactions in DNCB sensitized children may become positive after injection of transfer factor.

## IV.  EXPRESSION OF DELAYED HYPERSENSITIVITY IN VITRO

### LYMPHOBLASTIC TRANSFORMATION

#### Description

When lymphocytes from a subject who exhibits DH to a specific antigen are cultured in vitro in the presence of the antigen, some lymphocytes transform into large blast cells. These lymphoblasts are defined by dimension (12 to 15 μm in diameter) and cytologic aspects, including nuclei with clear chromatin that contain two or three nucleoli, intensely basophilic cytoplasm with vacuoles, and a pale peripheral crescent. On electron microscopy, the nuclear chromatin is clear, and the cytoplasm is filled with ribosomes but is deficient in endoplasmic reticulum. On scanning microscopy, the cells are "spiky," with cytoplasmic ramifications. Various morphologic features intermediate between those of lymphocytes and blasts are also observed. May-Grünwald-Giemsa staining permits calculation of the percentage of transformed cells among surviving cells. This percentage is interpretable only if cells are viable, spreading is homogeneous, and when at least 2,000 cells are read.

Tranformed cells divide; cell proliferation may be measured either by counting the percentage of metaphases after exposure to colchicine or, more simply, by measuring incorporation into the cellular DNA of a radioactive precursor, such as tritiated thymidine. By autoradiography, cells that have nuclear grains appear to be lymphoblastoid morphologically. Therefore, the same cells that transform also proliferate.

#### Lymphoblastic Transformation and Delayed Hypersensitivity

At variance with transformation in mixed cultures of allogeneic lymphocytes (mixed lymphocyte reaction), transformation in the presence of antigen is obtained only with cells from an animal previously sensitized to the antigen. This phenomenon is specific, because only the immunizing antigen is capable of lymphoblastic transformation. The specificity is the same as that for skin tests in DH. Lymphoblastic transformation is obtained more easily from sensitized animals with predominant DH than in those that present with only humoral responses. In the latter animals, proliferation in the presence of antigen is observed with lymph node or spleen cells and more rarely with circulating blood lymphocytes. These differences are not absolute, because circulating lymphocytes from subjects with immediate allergic hypersensitivity mediated by reaginic antibodies may transform in vitro in the presence of the allergen.

### Kinetics

The appearance of the first lymphoblastic cells in cultures of human peripheral lymphocytes after 48 hr occurs at the same time as does increased tritiated thymidine incorporation. Thymidine incorporation increases exponentially at day 2 and is maximal between days 5 and 9. Observation of cells by microcinematography and phase-contrast microscopy shows that cell division occurs at a rate of one mitosis every 10 to 12 hr. The initial number of cells that react to an antigen has been estimated by extrapolation to be less than 1%.

After 48 hours, the proliferation is strictly clonal and all the lymphoblasts are derived from the division of other lymphoblasts. On the other hand, at the beginning of the culture, there is a recruitment of cells as a result of the action of humoral factors described below. The initial stages of the reaction have mainly been studied in cultures of lymphocytes stimulated by mitogens (see chap. 3), but the results obtained in these systems are wholly applicable to lymphocyte cultures stimulated by specific antigens. The only specific phenomenon that initiates the reaction is the interaction between T-lymphocyte receptors and the antigen present on the monocyte surface. In the absence of monocytes, soluble antigen is incapable of provoking T-lymphocyte transformation. During the first four hours after this activation, a redistribution of the cell-surface receptors has been described. This is accompanied by activation of Na-K-ATPase, penetration of calcium into and potassium out of the cell, modifications of lipid biosynthesis with increased cell-membrane fluidity and increased levels of cyclic GMP without any alteration of cyclic AMP. The intermediate stages of activation between the 4th and 24th hour include the development of cytotoxic activity and the liberation of humoral mediators, protein and ribosomal RNA synthesis, activation of RNA polymerase and ornithine decarboxylase, and synthesis of polyamines. It is only after 48 hours that the phenomenon of transformation into a lymphoblast takes place, followed immediately by DNA synthesis and cell division. Substances that interfere with the initial stages, acting on actin or tubulin (cytochalasin, colchicine, vincaleukoblastine) or on potassium transport (ouabain) inhibit lymphoblastoid transformation.

### Role of Monocytes and Macrophages

The elimination of adherent cells on nylon fibers, plastic surfaces or Sephadex G-10 beads, and to a lesser degree, the elimination of phagocytic cells suppresses the proliferative response in the presence of antigen. The interactions between monocytes and T cells therefore represent an essential stage in the initiation of transformation. These interactions have been studied by the demonstration of the agglutination of lymph node cells around peritoneal macrophages. The reaction is seen to occur in two stages. The first stage, observed after the first hour, is independent of the presence of antigen. It is reversible, calcium-dependent, and the integrity of macrophage metabolism is essential for its development. It is inhibited by the addition of cytochalasin B or by treatment of the macrophages with trypsin. B or T lymphocytes from allogeneic or syngeneic animals are equally agglutinated. The second stage, observed at 24 hours, is antigen dependent. Only T lymphocytes from an antigen-sensitized syngeneic animal are agglutinated. This is an irreversible reaction, which is not sensitive to cytochalasin B or mitomycin and requires the integrity of macrophage and lymphocyte metabolism. The addition of alloantibodies inhibits the phenomenon. The macrophage-lymphocyte interaction is accomplished by means of the intermediary of the histocompatibility antigens controlled by the I-region of the major histocompatibility complex. The addition of antisera directed against Ia antigens on the macrophages inhibits the transformation induced by the presence of antigen. In man, the addition of anti-HLA-DR antibodies suppresses the proliferative response.

Monocytes do not undergo transformation and do not interfere with the extent of the proliferative response. However, they play an essential role in the presentation of the antigen: monocytes incubated in the presence of the antigen, then washed, constitute an excellent stimulant for the lymphocytes of a sensitized donor. This stimulatory effect is seen equally well with monocytes from a nonsensitized subject as with monocytes from a subject who has been sensitized against the antigen in question. However, the stimulatory effect is only exerted on lymphocytes bearing the same histocompatibility antigens (Ia or HLA-DR) as the monocytes. The proliferative response induced by the antigen may, therefore, be considered as an autologous mixed lymphocyte reaction against "self" antigens (Ia or HLA-DR) associated with the specific antigen introduced into the culture. Furthermore, in addition to this direct interaction with T lymphocytes, macrophages have a regulatory effect on the proliferative response that is exerted by means of the intermediary of humoral factors. These may be amplifier (lymphocyte-activating factor) or suppressor (low-molecular-weight suppressor factor).

### Role of T and B Lymphocytes

T lymphocytes are indispensable for the initiation of the proliferative response. Their destruction by anti-T cell sera and complement inhibits the transformation. Most of the cells carry T-cell markers. However, as indicated above, purified T-lymphocyte populations do not transform in the presence of antigen. Similarly, it is not possible to demonstrate convincingly a direct binding of soluble antigens to receptors on the surface of T cells.

B lymphocytes are not essential for the proliferative response. However, some lymphoblasts observed at the peak of the response bear B-cell markers (especially the presence of membrane immunoglobulins). The transformation and proliferation of these lymphocytes are partly a result of the liberation of mitogenic or transforming factors by T lymphocytes activated by the antigen in the presence of adherent cells.

## CELL-MEDIATED CYTOTOXICITY

The mononuclear cells of an animal possessing cell-mediated hypersensitivity are capable of destroying, in vitro, target cells bearing on their surface the antigen utilized for sensitizing the donor. This phenomenon has been mainly analyzed in allograft models (chap. 13), but it may be observed in cell-mediated responses against haptens or viral antigens. Several cytotoxic mechanisms may be involved: direct action of cytotoxic T cells; cytotoxic action of antibodies in the presence of lymphocytes (K cells) or macrophages; release by lymphocytes of factors that are cytotoxic to certain target cells (lymphotoxin) or substances that provoke the activation of macrophages, which then become cytotoxic toward adjacent cells; or interferon synthesis, stimulating the production of cytotoxic cells against tumor cells (NK cells).

In fact, the main mechanism of the cell-mediated immune response is the cytotoxicity exerted by T lymphocytes. The mechanism of this cytotoxic reaction will be examined in the following chapter. It involves lysis following direct contact between the specific receptor on cytotoxic T cells and the antigen present on the surface of the target cell. This lysis is accomplished in the absence of antibody and complement. In the mouse, cytotoxic T lymphocytes belong to a subpopulation bearing the Lyt 2 and 3 antigens. The production of cytotoxic T lymphocytes necessitates cooperation between macrophages and T cells bearing the Lyt 1 marker. This production is under the control of suppressor T cells in such a manner that the cytotoxic response is more readily induced in vitro than in the intact animal.

The cytotoxic T-cell response obeys the phenomenon of syngeneic restriction (described on p. 87) according to which the cytotoxic T lymphocytes simultaneously recognize the "self" transplantation antigens, H2-D and H2-K, and the antigen against which the cellular response is directed (virus, hapten, etc.). There exists, therefore, at this level, a notable difference compared with the proliferative response previously examined, in that the macrophage-T lymphocyte interaction is accomplished by means of structures coded for by the I-region of the major histocompatibility complex.

## VIRAL REPLICATION TEST

Replication of numerous viruses (mumps, measles, poliomyelitis) occurs in T lymphocytes activated by an antigen or by a mitogen but not in quiescent T lymphocytes. It is thus possible to quantify the number of activated T lymphocytes by provoking lysis plaque formation on a cellular monolayer of indicator cells sensitive to the cytopathogenic effect of the virus (Bloom's test).

When lymph node cells from a guinea pig sensitized with BCG are incubated in the presence of tuberculin (24 hr), one of 1000 cells forms a lysis plaque. This number increases linearly with time, even after addition of an antimitotic substance (vinblastine) to the culture. The infected cells is therefore not the transformed cell (lymphoblast) whose exponential growth is limited in the presence of antimitotics. Lysis plaque formation is not seen after removal of adherent cells, thus suggesting a role for macrophages in this reaction. When the number of lymphoid cells in the culture is varied, the number of lysis plaques is proportional to the square of the number of lymphocytes; thus, formation of the lysis plaque requires two different cells.

## MACROPHAGE MIGRATION INHIBITION TEST

When spleen fragments are cultured on a glass surface, cells migrate to form a halo around the explant. In 1932, Rich and Lewis cultivated spleen fragments from tuberculous rabbits and observed that after tuberculin addition, cell migration was inhibited. Thirty years later, George and Vaughan designed a culture technique in capillary tubes inspired by the same phenomenon, which was later modified by David and Bloom.

### Migration of Peritoneal Cells in Capillary Tubes (Fig. 12.4)

Three days after intraperitoneal injection of oil in the guinea pig, the peritoneal exudate contains an average of 70% macrophages, 15% lymphocytes, and 15% polymorphs. These cells are washed and introduced into capillary tubes of 1.3- to 1.5-mm diameter. After centrifugation, the tubes are cut at the interface of the cell supernatant. They are placed horizontally on the transparent bottom of a migration chamber. After 16 to 24 hr of incubation at 37°C, the cells form a layer around the capillary orifice. An identical migration is obtained with cells from an animal sensitized to tuberculin. However, if the antigen is added to the migration chamber, a significant decrease in the migration surface occurs. The migration area is measured (planimetry) in the absence and

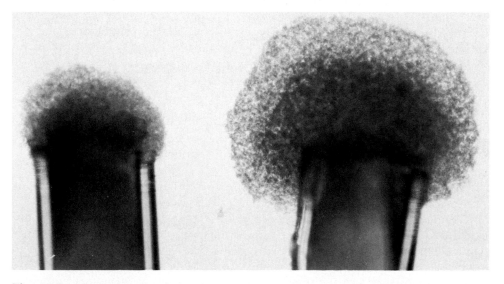

**Fig. 12.4** Migration of guinea pig peritoneal cells in a capillary tube. *Right*, normal migration; *left*, migration inhibited by the presence of semipurified human MIF. (From C. Vincent.)

presence of the antigen and is quantified by the migration index:

$$MI = \frac{(\text{average migration area with antigen})}{(\text{average migration area without antigen})} \times 100.$$

The inhibition index may also be defined:

$$\left(I - \frac{\text{migration area with antigen}}{\text{migration area without antigen}}\right) \times 100.$$

### Inhibition Specificity and Mechanism

Various characteristics of the inhibition phenomenon suggest that it is an in vitro phenomenon of DH. Inhibition is specific for the antigen used for sensitization because migration of peritoneal cells remains normal in the presence of a different antigen. Inhibition in the presence of antigen is obtained only with cells from animals immunized in the presence of Freund's complete adjuvant. Intravenous immunization with the same antigen induces antibody production but no migration inhibition of peritoneal cells in the presence of antigen. The addition of a small number of lymphoid (lymph node or peritoneal) cells from a sensitized animal to the peritoneal cells of a normal animal inhibits migration of the latter in the presence of antigen. Addition of serum from a sensitized animal to normal peritoneal cells does not prevent their migration in the presence of antigen. However, some antigen-antibody complexes may inhibit migration.

If cell populations from the peritoneal exudate of a sensitized animal are separated by fractionation, migration of purified macrophages or purified lymphocytes is not inhibited in the presence of the specific antigen. However, when small numbers of lymphocytes obtained from sensitized animal are added to purified macrophages from another animal (sensitized or nonsensitized), migration inhibition occurs in the presence of the specific antigen. If in similar experiments the sensitized lymphocytes are pretreated with a proteolytic enzyme (trypsin), their ability to induce migration inhibition in the presence of the specific antigen is lost. Their capability is again recovered spontaneously after 24 hr of culture. This finding suggests that lymphocytes of the sensitized animal react with antigen by means of a specific receptor, protein in nature, that is present on the cell membrane.

The observation that normal macrophages may serve as indicators in the reaction of lymphocytes sensitized to the antigen is the basis for a two-phase experimental system in which lymph node or peritoneal lymphocytes from tuberculin-sensitized guinea pigs are incubated in vitro with tuberculin. The culture supernatant is then collected and introduced into a migration chamber that contains normal macrophages. Their migration (in the absence of antigen) is inhibited relative to that of macrophages that migrate in a normal medium. The supernatant thus contains a factor called "migration-inhibitory factor" (MIF). If lymphocytes are incubated under the same conditions but in the absence of antigen, or if the antigen is added at the end of culture, migration is no longer inhibited.

## Biologic Effects of Activated Lymphocyte Supernatants

The biologic effects of activated lymphocyte supernatants are listed in Table 12.3. The effects have been classified according to the nature of the target cells on which these actions occur. A particular emphasis has been put recently on the so-called Interleukin 2 (IL 2) (see Table 12.3).

## Substances Responsible for These Effects

DH mediators are not immunoglobulins. Precipitation by 33% ammonium sulfate or passage on an anti-immunoglobulin immunoadsorbent column (specific for the species that produces the factor) does not reduce the biologic effects of the supernatant. These substances are not immune complexes. In some studies, it has been possible to eliminate from the supernatant the antigen that allowed production of the activation products. In this setting, the antigen-free supernatant maintains its biologic activity. Dumonde has proposed the term "lymphokine" for these substances.

Are lymphokines one or multiple? To answer this question, supernatants may be heated or exposed to various enzymes (trypsin, chymotrypsin, neuraminidase) to determine if various biologic activities are affected. These supernatants may also be fractionated (chromatography, electrophoresis, or ultracentrifugation) to see whether various biologic activities are separable. These techniques have shown several distinct factors, including a chemotactic factor, lymphotoxin, and macrophage migration-inhibitory factor (MIF) but the macrophage activating factor (MAF) and MIF have not yet been clearly chemically separated. All are glycoproteins of a lower molecular weight than albumin (Table 12.4). The biochemical characteristics of human lymphokines are slightly different from those of the guinea pig. Human MIF has a molecular weight of about 25,000 daltons and migrates with albumin on preparative electrophoresis. It resists the action of neuraminidase and may be separated from the factor that inhibits the migration of guinea-pig leukocytes. Human lymphotoxin has a molecular weight of the order of 90,000 daltons and migrates in the postalbumin position. These different factors have not yet been sufficiently purified to permit radioimmunoassay of the substance responsible for these different biologic effects.

## Humoral Mediators of Delayed Hypersensitivity

Intradermal injection of semipurified lymphokines produces a local inflammatory reaction characterized by increased capillary permeability and an accumulation of mononucleated cells with maximal infiltrate (volume) achieved at 6 and 12 hr. This reaction is identical to DH, except for more rapid kinetics. On this basis, it has been assumed that lymphokines are released in vivo by activated sensitized lymphocytes that are in contact with the tissue-bound antigen. Because lymphokines are produced in small amounts (less than 1 μg of MIF from $10^{10}$ lymph node cells cultured for 24 hr), they may act locally at the site of their production. Note that circulating lymphocytes do not usually produce lymphokines in patients with immunodeficiencies or in those subjected to immunosuppressive agents.

**Table 12.3  Biologic Effects of Lymphocytic Activation Products**

| Target cells | Factors | Effects observed |
|---|---|---|
| *Macrophages*: | Migration inhibitory factor (MIF) | Inhibits macrophage migration in vitro |
| | Macrophage activating factor (MAF) | Induces or increases the cytotoxic effect of macrophages against tumor cells, some normal cells and microorganisms |
| | | Increases macrophage adherence |
| | | Increases glucosamine incorporation, pinocytosis, production of plasminogen activator, prostaglandins (PGE2) and complement factors (C2), intracellular $Ca^{2+}$ influx and cyclic GMP level |
| | | Alters several enzymatic activities |
| | Macrophage chemotatic factor (MCF) | Provokes migration of macrophages or monocytes through membrane pores (Fig. 12.5) |
| | Macrophage mitogenic factor | Induces macrophage proliferation |
| | Macrophage agglutinating factor (MAgF) | Agglutinates macrophages in suspension |
| | Macrophage Ia$^+$ recruiting factor (MIRF) | Induces the appearance of a Ia$^+$ macrophage-rich exudate after intraperitoneal injection |
| *Polymorphs*: | | |
| All types | Leukocyte migration inhibitory factor (LIF) | Inhibits migration of polymorphs |
| Neutrophils | Neutrophil chemotactic factor (NCF) | Attracts neutrophils |
| | Neutrophil migration inhibitory factor (NIF) | Inhibits migration of neutrophils |
| Basophils (and mastocytes) | Basophil chemotactic factor (BCF) | Attracts basophils |
| | Histamine releasing factor (HRF) | Induces basophil degranulation |
| | Histamine producing cell stimulating factor (HCSF) | Induces histamine synthesis and mastocyte proliferation |
| | Basophilopoietin | Induces proliferation of basophils |
| Eosinophils | Eosinophil chemotactic factor (ECF) | Attracts eosinophils |
| | Eosinophil stimulation promoter (ESP) | Increases migration of eosinophils |
| *Lymphocytes*: | | |
| | Lymphocyte mitogenic factor (LMF) or blastogenic factor (BF) | Provokes lymphoblastic transformation and division of normal (B) lymphocytes |
| | Interleukin 2 (IL 2) formerly called: | Induces and maintains clonal growth of activated T cells |

**Table 12.3 Continued**

| Target cells | Factors | Effects observed |
|---|---|---|
| | · T cell growth factor (TCGF) | |
| | · Thymocyte mitogenic factor (TMF) | |
| | · Thymocyte stimulating factor (TSF) | |
| | · Co-stimulator | |
| | · Killer cell helper factor (KHF) | |
| | · Secondary cytotoxic T cell-inducing factor (SCIF) | |
| | Non antigen-specific helper factors, e.g.: | Stimulates the differentiation of antibody-producing B cells |
| | · T cell replacing factor (TRF) | |
| | · Non-specific mediator (NSM) | |
| | · Soluble enhancing factor (SEF) | |
| | Allogeneic effect factor (AEF) | Stimulates the differentiation of antigen-activated B and T cells. Induces an autologous cell-mediated response |
| | Non antigen-specific suppressor factors, e.g.: | Suppresses the differentiation of antigen-activated B and T cells |
| | · Soluble immune response suppressor (SIRS) | |
| | · Antibody inhibiting material (AIM) | |
| | · Immunoglobulin-binding factor (IBF) | |
| | Antigen-specific helper and suppressor factors (see p. 542) | |
| *Cell Lines*: | | |
| | Lymphotoxin (LT) | Exerts cytotoxic effect on certain cell lines (such as L cells) |
| | Proliferation-inhibitory factor (PIF) and cloning-inhibitory factor | Inhibit cellular proliferation and clone formation |
| | Interferon (type 2) | Diminishes the cytopathogenetic effect of viruses on cultured cells. Increases NK activity |
| | Collagen-producing factor | Induces collagen production |
| *Hemopoietic cells*: | Colony-stimulating factor (CSF) | Stimulates differentiation of bone marrow stem cells in myeloid or monocytic cells |
| *Osteoclasts*: | Osteoclast-activating factor (OAF) | Augments the osteoclastic activity measured by $^{45}$Ca release from embryonic bones in vitro |

388

**Table 12.3   Continued**

| Target cells | Factors | Effects observed |
|---|---|---|
| *In vivo effects*: | Skin-reactive factor (SRF) | Augments the capillary permeability measured by extravascular diffusion of labeled albumin. Contributes to the inflammatory reaction in guinea pig skin by infiltration with mononucleated cells. |
| | MIF, interferon, lymphotoxin | Diminish the level of circulating monocytes (given i.p.) and the number of peritoneal macrophages (given i.v.) |
| | Endogeneous pyrogen-activating factor (EPAF) | Stimulates macrophages to induce pyrexia |

# V.   SUPPRESSION OF DELAYED HYPERSENSITIVITY

There exist several methods for suppressing DH reactions. Various mechanisms of suppression are implied. In the tolerance mechanism, antigen introduction renders the animal incapable of producing antibodies and sensitized lymphocytes after second contact with the antigen. In the immune deviation mechanism, after a first contact with the antigen, production of certain antibody classes and/or suppressor lymphocytes prevent the development of DH following administration of the same antigen in emulsion with complete Freund's adjuvant. In desensitization, injection of specific antigen may temporarily suppress preexisting DH. Lastly, immunosuppressive and anti-inflammatory treatments suppress induction or expression of DH.

## TOLERANCE

In 1928, Frei described the phenomenon of specific tolerance in man. DH was induced by intradermal injection of neoarsphenamine into most normal adults, but DH did not occur in patients who had previously received intravenous neoarsphenamine (then used for treatment of syphilis). At about the same time, Sulzberger showed that intracardiac injection of this substance in the guinea pig prevented the development of contact hypersensitivity to this antigen.

Addition of picryl chloride or DNCB to food induces a specific tolerance to these substances in the guinea pig. After absorbing a total dose of 45 to 50 mg, this tolerance persists for 9 to 12 months. Intravenous injection of dinitrobenzene sulfonic acid (DNB-SO$_3$) prevents the development of contact hypersensitivity to DNCB. Tolerance is obtained when massive doses (200 mg) are injected at 15-day intervals into the peripheral vein or by an intracardiac route. However, two consecutive injections of 50 μg of picryl chloride into the mesenteric vein render most guinea pigs incapable of sensitization to this

**Table 12.5  Characteristics of Lymphokines and of Transfer Factor**

| | Migration-inhibitory factor | Chemotactic factor | Lymphotoxin | Blastogenic factor | Skin-reactive factor | Transfer factor |
|---|---|---|---|---|---|---|
| Chemical nature | Protein | Protein | Proetin | Protein | Protein | Ribonucleotide |
| Molecular weight | 23,000–55,000 | 35,000–55,000 | 35,000–55,000 | 25,000 | | 700–4000 (dialyzable) |
| Protease | Sensitive | | | | Sensitive | Resistant |
| DNase | Resistant | | Resistant | | Resistant | Resistant |
| RNase | Resistant | | Resistant | | Resistant | Resistant |
| Neuraminidase | Sensitive | Resistant | Resistant | | | Resistant |
| Heat (56°C) | Stable | Stable | Sensitive | | Sensitive | Stable |
| Other characteristics | Albumin mobility | Albumin mobility | Albumin mobility | | | Nonantigenic |

hapten. Lymphocytes from tolerant animals are not capable of transferring contact hypersensitivity to picryl chloride. Tolerance may be terminated by injecting lymphoid cells from a sensitized guinea pig. In the animal rendered tolerant by picryl chloride administration (diet), intraperitoneal injection of picrylated heterologous proteins in the presence of adjuvant induces antibody production with immediate hypersensitivity. The same guinea pigs remain refractory to DH induction by picryl chloride.

Tolerance specific to allografts follows neonatal injection of allogeneic cells and represents one of the best models of specific suppression of cellular immunity (see p. 586). In the guinea pig, in utero injection of tuberculin or killed BCG prevents induction of DH to tuberculin after subsequent injection of killed tubercle bacilli, but induction of DH to living BCG is unaffected. If living BCG is injected in utero, sensitization but not tolerance is produced.

## IMMUNE DEVIATION

Administration of solubilized antigen intravenously or antigen absorbed onto an alum gel for subcutaneous injection induces IgG-class antibody production in the guinea pig. If the same antigen mixed with Freund's complete adjuvant is subsequently injected, neither DH nor complement-fixing antibody results. The experimental model of immune deviation must be considered in conjunction with active facilitation experiments in allograft systems (see p. 586). In the latter, injection of solubilized transplantation antigen prevents rejection of tumor allografts. These animals generate the so-called facilitating antibodies, which block either induction of a cellular response or its expression on tumor graft. Cellular responses to administration of specific antibodies cannot be schematized as easily. Depending on the antibody class and the nature of in vivo immune complexes, either a stimulation or reduction of the cellular response may be seen. Suppressor T cells may also contribute to immune deviation in some experimental models where lymph-node and spleen cells from animals immunized with antigen in complete Freund's adjuvant were shown to transfer the "deviation," preventing recipients from developing a DH response.

## DESENSITIZATION

Desensitization consists of injecting specific antigen into a previously immunized (DH) subject. Partial desensitization follows simple intradermal antigen injection. Desensitization is enhanced if higher antigen concentrations or greater numbers of injection sites are used. This desensitization is short-lived. The proposed mechanism is the inactivation of limited numbers of T lymphocytes that are capable of specific reaction with antigen. Intravenous injection of hapten (dinitrobenzene sulfonic acid, 500 mg) or of protein antigen into guinea pigs with DH to these substances specifically suppresses the DH reaction during the next 24 to 48 hr. Desensitization is usually associated with generalized erythema, followed by localized desquamation. Mechanisms similar to desensitization probably explain the absence of DH seen in some anergic forms of tuberculosis

The DNCB test consists of inducing contact dermatitis by applying an acetone DNCB solution onto the skin. Two to 4 weeks later, sensitization is determined by performing a percutaneous test with DNCB diluted 1:100 times the sensitizing concentration. Most normal subjects are sensitized by the initial application. Absence of sensitization may indicate a deficiency of T cells capable of reacting with the antigen, activation of suppressive phenomena by T cells or B cells, or a nonspecific deficiency in the inflammatory response.

The PHA test consists of an intradermal injection of 0.1 ml of a PHA solution. This mitogen provokes a DH response whose maximum intensity occurs between 24 and 48 hours after the injection. This test examines, in vivo, the production of inflammatory mediators by T lymphocytes.

Investigation of the nonspecific inflammatory response induced by an injection of cantharidin or lauryl sulphate is recommended each time one finds a DH deficiency in vivo. These tests examine the nonspecific component of the response. The simultaneous use of these three categories of test (DNCB, PHA, inflammatory reaction) permits the in vivo investigation of one of the possible mechanisms involved in an apparent DH deficiency.

## INVESTIGATION IN VITRO

### Lymphoblastic Transformation Test

Lymphoblastic transformation is a clinical investigation tool in current use. DH is usually associated with "transformation" of lymphocytes that have been cultured in the presence of the specific antigen, shown not to be toxic to the cultured cells. Conversely, observation of a blastic transformation in vitro does not necessarily imply the existence of DH to the tested substance, because this transformation may represent a nonspecific mitogenic effect on lymphocytes from unsensitized subjects (e.g., cord blood lymphocytes) or may be a correlate of a humoral type of hypersensitivity rather than DH.

If a DH deficiency exists in vivo and a proliferative response is observed in vitro on culture of the patient's lymphocytes in the presence of the antigen, this leads to the search either for a deficiency in lymphokine production (MIF or chemotactic factor) or an inhibitory effect of the patient's serum. This may be demonstrated on the patient's lymphocytes or on the cells of a normal subject cultured in the presence of the patient's serum. The list of inhibitory factors of lymphoblastic transformation is now quite long. The demonstration of these factors in vitro does not, however, always lead to conclusions concerning their eventual role in the intact animal.

### Leukocyte Migration Test

Human macrophages cannot be used as an indicator of the migration reaction. Therefore, techniques must be derived from the test described above in the guinea pig.

TWO-PHASE TECHNIQUE

Sensitized blood lymphocytes are cultured along with specific antigen in serum-free medium. The concentrated supernatant (five- to 10-fold) is then applied to guinea pig peritoneal cells. The cellular migration area is compared to that obtained with supernatant in which the antigen has been added at the end of the culture.

ONE-PHASE TECHNIQUE

Lymphocytes from the test subject are mixed with guinea pig peritoneal cells or horse monocytes (one human lymphocyte for every four to five monocytes or macrophages). The MIF produced by lymphocytes in contact with the antigen acts directly on heterologous monocytes or macrophages, which serve as the indicators of migration.

Human leukocyte migration may be studied directly in capillary tubes (Søborg and Bendixen). Leukocytes are centrifuged in capillary or microcapillary tubes and after 4 to 6 hr at 37°C in the presence of foal serum, the migration area is measured. Sensitized lymphocytes in contact with the antigen release a factor that inhibits polymorph migration. Leukocyte migration can also be studied in gel (Clausen). Wells are prepared in a petri dish that contains humidified gelose, and leukocytes, previously incubated with the antigen, are introduced. Polymorphs migrate at the interface of the petri dish and the gelose, and the diameter of the resultant cellular disk is measured.

The correlation between peritoneal cell migration inhibition and DH is

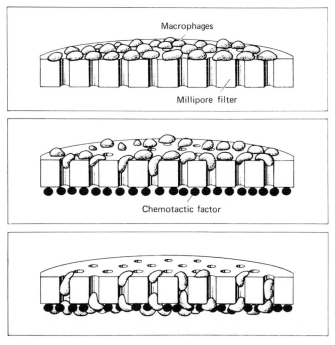

**Fig. 12.5** Demonstration of chemotactic factor in a Boyden chamber, Guinea pig macrophages are placed on the upper face of a Millipore filter, and the supernatant of sensitized lymphocytes cultivated in the presence of the specific antigen is placed in the lower compartment. Macrophage movement through the filter indicates the presence of chemotactic factor in the supernatant. (From J. R. David. In R. A. Good and D. W. Fisher, Eds., Immunobiology, ed. 5. Stamford, Conn., 1973, Sinauer, p. 151.)

well established in the guinea pig. This correlation is not firm for leukocyte migration tests in man, however. When an antigen causes migration inhibition after addition to a patient's cells, as compared to normal migration with cells from a healthy donor, a state of sensitization is presumed, but one does not know the immunologic mechanism and its relationship to disease.

### Lymphokine Study

Lymphocyte activation products are not generally studied clinically. These products may, however, be useful in studying certain immunodeficiencies, in recognizing the presence of inflammatory factors (skin-reactive factor), or in detecting chemotactic factor (Fig. 12.5) or interferon production by a patient's lymphocytes in the presence of a mitogen or the specific antigen.

## VII.  CONCLUSIONS: DELAYED HYPERSENSITIVITY AND IMMUNITY

The inflammatory reaction that is a consequence of cellular hypersensitivity is essential to the production of clinical manifestations and tissue lesions that characterize numerous bacterial, viral, or mycotic infections and may also play an important role in recovery from these infections. Severe clinical pictures are seen in anergic tuberculosis, lepromatous leprosy, chronic mucocutaneous candidiasis, and in unusually common and severe viral infections which develop in deficiencies of cell-mediated immunity. These clinical observations imply a close association between hypersensitivity and immunity. Experimental studies of DH and acquired cell resistance reveal mechanisms that are common to these two types of cellular immune responses.

DH and cellular immunity deficiencies may have several causes. In addition to hereditary immunodeficiencies, many conditions, including malformations (thymus aplasia, intestinal lymphangiectasia), iatrogenic factors (irradiation, chemotherapy), metabolic deficiencies (renal failure, malnutrition), and chronic or repetitive infections, may induce nonspecific decreases or even total suppression of the DH reaction (rubella, measles, hepatitis, malaria, leishmaniosis, infectious mononucleosis). Malignancies of the lymphoid system are also associated with an important, although probably secondary, deficiency of cellular immunity.

## BIBLIOGRAPHY

ASKENASE P. W. Effector cells in late and delayed hypersensitivity reactions that are dependent on antibodies or T cells. In: Immunology 80 (M. Fougereau and J. Dausset eds.). Acad. Press, New York, 1980:829.

ASHER M. S., GOTTLIEB A. A., and KIRKPATRICK C. H. Transfer factor: Basic properties and clinical applications. Academic Press, New-York, 1976.

BLOOM B. R. In vitro approaches to the mechanisms of cell-mediated immune reactions. Adv. Immunol., 1971, 13, 101.

BLOOM B. R. and DAVID J. R. In vitro methods in cell-mediated and tumor immunity. New York, 1976, Academic Press.

COHEN S. Lymphokines in delayed hypersensitivity. In: Immunology 80 (M. Fougereau and J. Dausset eds.) Acad. Press, New York, 1980, 860.

COHEN S. and YOSHIDA T. Lymphokine mediated reactions. In: Mechanisms of Immunopathology (S. Cohen, P. A. Ward, and R. T. McCluskey [eds]). John Wiley & Sons, New York, 1979, 49.

CROWLE A. J. Delayed hypersensitivity in the mouse. Adv. Immunol., 1975, 20, 197.

DAVID J. R. Lymphocytic factors in cellular hypersensitivity. In R. A. Good and D. W. Fisher, Eds., Immunobiology. Stamford, Conn., 1971, Sinauer, p. 146.

DEWECK A. L., KRISTENSEN F., and LANDY M. Biochemical characterization of lymphokines. Acad. Press, New York, 1980, p. 622.

GOWANS J. L. Lymphocytes. Harvey lectures, 1970, 64, 87.

LAWRENCE H. S. Transfer factor. Adv. Immunol., 1969, 11, 195.

LAWRENCE, H. S. Cellular immunity in clinical immunobiology. In F. H. Bach and R. A. Good, Eds., Clinical immunobiology. New York, 1972, Academic Press, p. 47.

MILLER J. F. A. P. MHC restrictions in cellular cooperation. In: Immunology 80 (M. Fougereau and J. Dausset eds.). Acad. Press, New York, 1980:359.

MOLLER G. [ed.]. Accessory cells in the immune response. Immunol. Rev., 1980, 53, p. 232.

REMOLD H. G. Purification and characterization of lymphocyte medidators in cellular immunity. Transpl. Rev., 1972, 10, 152.

REVILLARD J. P. Ed. Cell-mediated immunity. In vitro correlates. Basel, 1971, Karger.

TURK J. L. Delayed hypersensitivity, 3rd ed. Amsterdam, 1980, North Holland.

VALENTINE F. T. and LAWRENCE H. S. Cell-mediated immunity. Adv. Intern. Med., 1971, 17, 51.

WAKSMAN B. H. Atlas of experimental immunobiology and immunopathology. New Haven, 1970, Yale University Press.

# ORIGINAL ARTICLES

ASHERSON G. L., ZEMBALA M., MAYHEW B., and GOLDSTEIN A. Adult thymectomy prevention of the appearance of suppressor T cells which depress contact sensitivity to picryl chloride and reversal of adult thymectomy effect by thymus extract. Eur. J. Immunol., 1976, 6, 699.

ASHERSON G. L., ZEMBALA M., PERERA M. A. C. C., MAYHEW B., and THOMAS W. R. Production of immunity and unresponsiveness in the mouse by feeding contact sensitizing agents and the role of suppressor cells in the Peyer's patches, mesenteric lymph nodes and other lymphoid tissues. Cell. Immunol., 1977, 33, 145.

CHESS L., MACDERMOTT R. P., SONDEL P. M., and SCHLOSSMANN S. F. Isolation and characterization of cells involved in human cellular hypersensitivity. In L. Brent and J. Holborow, Eds., Progress in immunology. II. Vol. 3. Amsterdam, 1974, North Holland, p. 125.

CLARK R. A. F., DVORAK H. F., and COLVIN R. B. Fibronectin in delayed-type hypersensitivity skin reactions: Associations with vessel permeability and endothelial cell activation. J. Immunol., 1981, 126, 787–793.

COHEN S., PICK E., and OPPENHEIM J. J. Biology of the lymphokines Med. Press., 1979, 626.

DVORAK H. F., DVORAK A. M., SIMPSON B. A., RICHERSON H. B., LESKOWITZ S., and KARNOFSKY M. J. Cutaneous basophil hypersensitivity: a light and electron microscopic description. J. Exp. Med., 1970, 132, 558.

GEHA R. S., JONSEN M. E., AULT B H., YUNIS E., and BROFF M. D. Macrophage T cell interaction in man: Binding of antigen-specific human proliferating and helper T cells to antigen-pulsed macrophages. J. Immunol., 1981, 126, 781–786.

GRISCELLI C., REVILLARD J. P., BETUEL H., et al. Transfer factor therapy in immunodeficiencies. Biomed., 1973, 18, 220–227.

LAWRENCE H. S. Transfer factor and cellular immunodeficiency disease. New Engl. J. Med., 1970, *283*, 411.

LAWRENCE H. S. Selective immunotherapy with transfer factor. Clin. Immunobiol., 1974, *2*, 115.

McCLUSKEY R. T., BENACERAFF B., and McCLUSKEY J. W. Studies on the specificity of the cellular infiltrate in delayed hypersensitivity reactions. J. Immunol., 1963, *90*, 466.

REMOLD H. G. The interaction of MIF with macrophages and macrophage activation. *In* L. Brent and J. Holborow, Eds., Progress in Immunology. II. Vol. 3. Amsterdam, 1974, North Holland, p. 145.

SMITH K. A., LACHMAN L. B., OPPENHEIM J. J., and FAVATA M. F. The functional relationship of the interleukins. J. Exp. Med., 1980, 151.

STINGL G., KATZ S. I., SHEVACH E. M., ROSENTHAL A. S., and GREEN I. Analogous functions of macrophages and Langerhans cells in the initiation of the immune response. J. Invest. Derm., 1978, *71*, 59.

# Chapter 13

# TRANSPLANTATION IMMUNITY AND CYTOTOXICITY PHENOMENA

## Jean-François Bach

I. INTRODUCTION

II. A FEW DEFINITIONS

III. NATURAL HISTORY OF A GRAFT

IV. IN VITRO ALLOGRAFT REACTION: CYTOTOXICITY PHENOMENA

V. MECHANISMS OF GRAFT REJECTION

VI. GRAFT-VERSUS-HOST REACTION

VII. THE FETUS CONSIDERED AS AN ALLOGRAFT

# I. INTRODUCTION

The fate of a graft to a large extent depends on histocompatibility differences between donor and recipient. When donor and recipient are not genetically identical, the graft is irreversibly rejected. Rejection essentially involves immunologic phenomena. These various and complex phenomena include both cell-mediated and humorally mediated immunity. They define "transplantation immunity." In vivo and in vitro reactions caused by T cells that react with alloantigens (proliferation in mixed lymphocyte reactions and lymphocytotoxicity tests) will also be discussed in this chapter, even though their significance goes far beyond simple graft immunity. Leukocyte groups and histocompatibility concepts will be discussed in a subsequent section (chap. 23).

## II.   A FEW DEFINITIONS

There are many possible graft combinations between donor and recipient. When the graft is obtained from the same individual in whom it is later placed, the term used is "autograft." When the donor is a genetically identical brother or sister (homozygous twins) or an animal of the same strain, the graft is syngeneic. Allograft refers to a situation in which the donor is genetically different from the recipient but is of the same species. This type of graft, of course, is most common between nonhomozygous persons. When donor and recipient are not of the same species, the graft is a xenograft. These definitions have replaced the old terminology, which included isograft, homograft, and heterograft (Table 13.1). "Isologous" was a particularly inapt terminology, because it was used differently in transplantation (syngeneic) and transfusion (both syngeneic and allogeneic) work. "Graft" refers to transplantation of tissue or cells (e.g., bone marrow grafts and graft-versus-host reactions), whereas "transplantation" refers to grafts that involve vascular anastomosis, for example, organ grafts.

First-set (primary) rejections are observed when the recipients have never previously received a graft from the same donor. Second-set (secondary) rejections are those that occur in recipients who previously received a graft from the same donor. We shall see, however, that first-set grafts may be rejected in secondary fashion if antigens in previous grafts from different individuals contained antigens common to the new graft donor.

## III.   NATURAL HISTORY OF A GRAFT

Before envisaging mechanisms of graft rejection, the natural history of a graft in terms of function, morphology, and, in particular, immunologic aspects will be examined. We shall discuss first- and second-set rejections and skin and organ grafts which are associated in some degree with different rejection mechanisms.

## MORPHOLOGIC AND FUNCTIONAL ASPECTS

### Skin Grafts

Skin autografts (syngeneic grafts) are rapidly vascularized (2 to 3 days) and look nearly normal under the microscope on day 4 and 5. Skin architecture is normal, and there is no cellular infiltrate. Only scattered cells may be present, due either to inflammation or to surgical trauma. The epidermal cells may show intense mitotic activity.

The primary allograft initially behaves like an autograft (thus its application to cutaneous burn patients when autografts are not available). Vascularization is normal. In a few more days, the allograft is infiltrated with lymphocytes, lymphoblasts, plasma cells, and macrophages localized especially in perivascular areas. By day 7, the graft thickens, and necrosis begins. At about day 10 (in a

**Table 13.1  Terminology Utilized in Transplantation**

| Old name | Old adjective | New name | New adjective | Definition |
|---|---|---|---|---|
| Autograft | Autologous | — | — | Donor and recipient are the same individual |
| Isograft | Isologous | Syngraft (nonutilized) | Syngeneic | Genetically identical donor and recipient |
| Homograft | Homologous | Allograft | Allogeneic | Donor and recipient of the same species are genetically different |
| Heterograft | Heterologous | Xenograft | Xenogeneic | Donor and recipient from different species |

situation of strong incompatibility), blood flow to the graft ceases, arterioles obstruct, and the graft becomes completely necrotic. A few days later, the graft is eliminated and the underlying tissue rapidly becomes repleted by granulation tissue. When weak histocompatibility differences are present, the above process is delayed occasionally for as long as several months. Rarely does a graft persist indefinitely despite chronic rejection, as shown by histologic examination (biopsy).

Secondary allografts (performed several weeks to a few months after the first graft) are rejected in an accelerated fashion. In the very first days (up to day 3 or 4), the morphologic appearance of secondary allografts is nearly identical to that of first-set grafts, except in cases in which the graft has not been vascularized (white graft). However, as soon as the graft vascularizes, the process accelerates, and the graft is completely rejected by day 7, with the infiltrating cells concentrated around vessels. It is important to recognize that the second-set rejection is specific for the first donor (i.e., a second graft from a donor not genetically related to the first donor will not undergo accelerated rejection unless there are antigens common between the two donors).

### Organ Grafts

The fate of allogeneic organ grafts is fundamentally identical to that of skin grafts, because both eventually slough and die, but the rejection processes involved are slightly different. The initial difference lies in the intensity of rejection; skin grafts reject faster than do organ grafts.

Morphologic rejection of organ grafts begins when the transplant is infiltrated by mononucleated cells, which include transformed lymphoid cells that contain polyribosomes (Fig. 13.1) (we do not know with certainty whether these cells are of the B, T, or K lineage) and macrophages. Numerous arterioles and glomeruli (in kidney grafts) undergo necrosis, and the organ is rejected. In cases of presensitization (by prior graft, pregnancy, or transfusion), this cellular infiltration is less marked and may even be absent. Platelets aggregate in capillaries and, sometimes, in arterioles, followed by the arrival of polymorphs and fibrin, leading to thrombus formation. In chronic rejection, which occurs during immunosuppression, the predominant lesions are seen in arterioles, with endarteritis narrowing the arterial lumen. In the glomerulus, the basement membranes thicken, and there is a relatively modest cellular proliferation.

The rejection of organ grafts may be recognized early because of depressed function of the grafted organ. Considerable effort has been made in man to detect early rejection phenomena. For kidney grafts, rejection results in renal failure recognized by a reduction in clearance and an elevation in serum creatinine and urea concentrations concomitant to decreased renal blood flow. For cardiac grafts, modifications of the electrocardiogram and decreased cardiac output occur. In liver transplants, bilirubinemia increases, and transaminase titers elevate; pancreatic grafts show hyperglycemia; decreased oxygen saturation and hemoglobin concentrations are seen in lung grafts. These rejection signs may occur without further biological or clinical manifestations, especially in cases of chronic rejection associated with weak histocompatibility differences or on therapeutic immunosuppression. They are also observed in so-called

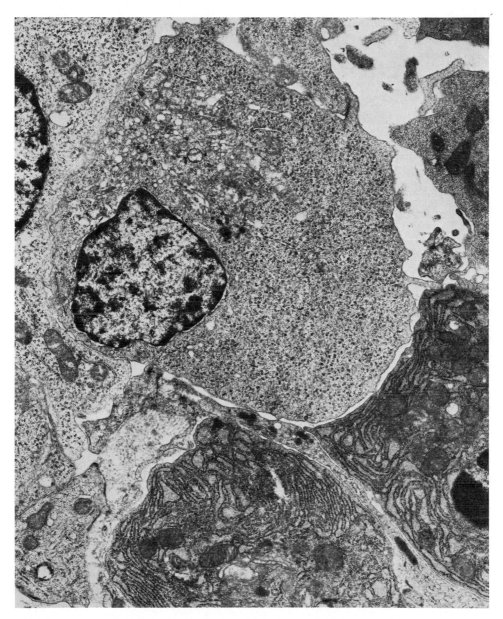

**Fig. 13.1** Cells infiltrating the parenchyma of a transplanted human kidney. The middle immunoblast, the cytoplasm of which is filled with polyribosomes, contains very little endoplasmic reticulum and few mitochondria. Below this cell is a fragment of cytoplasm from a plasma cell, characterized by the presence of very numerous ergastoplasmic lamellae ×15,000. (From B. Nabarra.)

*rejection crises,* in association with heavy infiltrates of mononucleated cells. Such crises probably represent rejection reactions that are reversible under the influence of steroid treatment or sometimes spontaneously.

Second-set organ rejections are accelerated or even hyperacute, producing renal cortical necrosis at the time of operation or in the first few days after transplantation.

### Special Situations

#### LARGE SIZE SKIN GRAFTS

Large grafts survive slightly longer than do small ones.

#### PRIVILEGED SITES

Some sites, such as the anterior eye chamber, cerebral tissue, and the jugal pouch of hamsters, permit prolonged survival of incompatible allografts, probably because of the absence of lymphatic drainage. At these sites, a barrier seems to prevent transplantation antigens from leaving the organ and, especially, to prevent the entry of lymphoid cells. A sialomucin barrier further augments isolation of the hamster's jugal pouch, which may even accept xenografts. The placenta also represents a cellular barrier that probably contributes to protection of the allografted fetus (see p. 426).

#### PRIVILEGED TISSUES

Some nonvascularized tissues are particularly resistant to rejection. Cartilage coated with sialomucin is not rejected after grafting into allogeneic hosts. However, cartilage xenografts (probably subjected to the action of antibodies) are rejected.

#### XENOGRAFTS

The fate of xenografts depends on the extent of differences between donor and recipient species. Nonetheless, in general, skin and organ xenografts are rejected rapidly. If the recipient has cirulating antidonor antibodies (which may be represented by natural antibodies in many species), there will be no graft vascularization and "white graft" rejection will occur. If there are no preexisting antibodies, a cellular infiltrate is followed by necrosis of the grafted organ, similar to the situation that occurs after allografting. Second-set xenograft rejections are always acute and are associated with the presence of antigraft antibodies.

## IMMUNOLOGIC ASPECTS

Graft rejection is considered to be exclusively immunologic. Before studying the facts that form the basis for this assertion (see p. 416), let us first review the major immunologic reactions seen during allograft rejection (without prejudging their contribution to rejection).

### Reactions of Lymphoid Organs

Regional graft lymph nodes (skin or organ) rapidly increase in size. The paracortical zones (see p. 35) enlarge, and numerous lymphoblasts are observed as early as the second or third day. Simultaneously, the rate of flow from efferent graft lymphatics increases. This increased flow may be directly studied in organ grafts. Numerous transformed cells are also observed in lymphatic ducts that drain regional lymph nodes. These same lymphoblasts are seen in circulating blood, in such a number that they have been claimed to be an early sign of rejection (in fact, this increase in number is to a large extent nonspecific).

### Cellular Reaction

The cellular reaction relates to cell-mediated immunity and is essentially performed by T cells. It is the first reaction to occur, as assessed by in vitro tests. Recipient lymphocytes from blood or regional lymph nodes destroy donor cells in vitro. We shall later examine the various lymphocytotoxicity tests and discuss their respective significance. Such lymphocytotoxicity is donor specific and the peak cytotoxicity is observed slightly before or at the time of rejection (Fig. 13.2). In the presence of the donor antigens (either as soluble spleen cell extracts or as integral cells), recipient leukocytes show inhibited migration outside of capillary tubes, thus indicating the existence of delayed hypersensitivity, at least in guinea pigs. In the rat or mouse, in which red blood cells bear transplantation antigens, the recipient lymphocytes and donor red blood cells form rosettes. The origin of these rosette-forming cells (RFC) is ambiguous; they may be either of B or T lineage (see p. 512). One should note also that an increased number of recipient lymphocytes have the capacity to transform and proliferate in the presence of mitomycin C-treated or irradiated donor cells (in mixed lymphocyte culture), although this increase is very transient and of little clinical value.

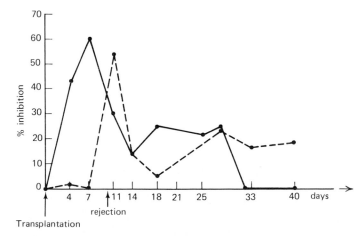

**Fig. 13.2**  Kinetics of cytotoxic activity of lymph node lymphocytes (——) and serum (–––) of Lewis rats after allografting skin from (Lewis × August) $F_1$ rats. Cytotoxicity is evaluated by inhibition of growth of August rat fibroblasts. (From M. Debray-Sachs and J. Hamburger, J. Immunol. 1973, *110*, 661.)

*Humoral Reaction*

Numerous antibodies are produced in allograft recipients. Cytotoxic antibodies detected by lysis of donor cells in the presence of complement are seen rather late, generally after graft rejection, irrespective of whether the target cells are leukocytes, fibroblasts, or donor renal cells. Agglutinating antibodies (leukoagglutinins, hemagglutinins) may also be detected using red blood cell sensitized by polyvinylpyrrolidone or proteolytic enzymes. Blocking antibodies can also be demonstrated by virtue of their effects on lymphocytotoxicity, on mixed lymphocyte reactions, or on leukocyte migration inhibition. These blocking antibodies, which may, in fact, circulate in the form of immune complexes, are often found, unlike cytotoxic antibodies, in well-tolerated grafts. Recently, IgG-class antibodies that cause unsensitized mononucleated cells to lyse donor cells sensitized with the recipient's serum have been detected. These antibodies are called lymphocyte dependent antibodies (LDA) (see p. 413).

*Search for an Immunologic Rejection Test*

The richness and diversity of recipient immunologic reactions toward donor antigens observed in the animal have prompted numerous studies of their relationship to early detection of rejection in transplanted patients. This problem is crucial, because earlier rejection diagnosis might permit more efficient immunosuppressive treatment. Provocative findings have been obtained with leukocyte migration inhibition and lymphocytotoxicity tests. Unfortunately, application is complicated because of probable contributions by blocking factors, which oppose rejection (imperfectly quantified by in vitro models that detect blocking antibodies), and by immunosuppressive treatment, which nonspecifically alters lymphocyte populations (see chap. 33). The complexity of this situation may explain why such slow progress is being made in this field.

# IV.  IN VITRO ALLOGRAFT REACTION: CYTOTOXICITY PHENOMENA

## MIXED LYMPHOCYTE REACTION

When lymphocytes from two genetically different individuals are mixed together and cultured in vitro, they transform into lymphoblasts and proliferate. This proliferation is evaluated in the mixed lymphocyte reaction (MLR) by enumerating the transformed cells or, better yet, by measuring tritiated thymidine incorporation into DNA.

### Description

Changes in lymphocytes that occur in MLR represent the blast transformation described in chapter 3. The response is weaker than that observed with phytohemagglutinin (PHA) and develops more slowly. Thus, MLR tests are evaluated later than are PHA transformation tests, around 6 or 7 days in man and at 3 to 5 days in the mouse (Fig. 13.3).

Unidirectional reactions may be produced by inactivation of one of the two populations by irradiation or mitomycin treatment. Such inactivation prevents proliferation but does not, however, always prevent production of blastogenic factor, which may, in some cases, induce transformation of nonirradiated lymphocytes that would not normally transform on a genetic basis (histocompatibility of the irradiated lymphocytes) or due to immunologic reasons (immunodeficiency). In animals, one-way reactions may also be obtained by mixing cells from a pure strain with cells from a hybrid of that and a second strain.

MLR is essentially a primary reaction. Donor sensitization by prior injection of allogeneic cells or skin grafting produces only transient and slight modification of the reaction, with accelerated kinetics and a slightly increased trans-

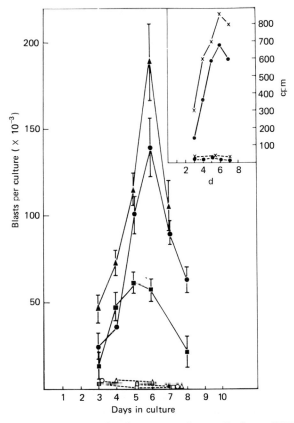

**Fig. 13.3** Mixed-lymphocyte reaction between spleen cells from C3H (H-2$^k$) and DBA/ 2 (H-2$^d$) mice. ▲, 1.5 × 10$^6$ C3 H + 3 × 10$^6$ DBA/2 (m); ●, 1.5 × 10$^6$ DBA/2 + 3 × 10$^6$ C3H (m); ■, 0.75 × 10$^6$ DBA/2 + 1.5 × 10$^6$ C3H (m). Cells were treated in vitro by mitomycin (m) and evaluated in terms of blasts per culture; open symbols correspond to one-way cultures (with a single-cell population). The inset shows evaluation by incorporation of tritiated thymidine (×) or tritiated uridine (●) in the C3H + DBA/2 (m) culture. (From P. Hayry et al., Transplant. Rev. 1972, *12*, 91.)

formation rate. One should note the very good MLR proliferative response of lymphocytes taken from the umbilical cord, which are not supposed to have been exposed to antigens other than those of the mother. Unexpectedly, the MLR is not stronger toward lymphocytes from other species as compared to a mixture of lymphocytes from the same species. MLR is not limited to proliferation. During MLR, MIF secretion may occur, as does generation of cytotoxic cells that react specifically to the sensitizing population. This phenomenon is known as the cell-mediated lympholysis test (CML). In vitro sensitization is also associated with the appearance of "memory" at the origin of secondary MLR or CML in the case of new stimulation.

## Implicated Cells

### RESPONDING CELLS

These cells are essentially T lymphocytes, as already mentioned (see p. 73). This conclusion has been reached from evidence of the presence of θ antigen on activated cells and of the T6 marker when responding cells are obtained from chimeric mice that possess T cells that bear that marker; evidence of the absence of MLR in T cell-deprived animals (after neonatal thymectomy or ALS treatment) or in children with a thymic immunodeficiency, as contrasted with the normal response of neonatally bursectomized chicken or agammaglobulinemic patients; and from evidence of inhibition of the MLR by treatment with anti-θ serum. In addition, some studies, which have not yet been confirmed, have demonstrated B-cell proliferation (by use of chromosomal markers). This proliferation may be due to secondary recruitment because of secretion of blastogenic factors by T cells. Finally, macrophages (or monocytes) are a prerequisite for the reaction to begin; it has been claimed that the supernatant of macrophage cultures may be substituted for macrophages. The lymphocytes that proliferate in MLR belong to the subpopulation that bear the Lyt 1 antigen in the mouse.

### STIMULATING CELLS

Stimulating cells are lymphocytes but transformation may also be induced by allogeneic monocytes, fibroblasts, or skin cells; however, the latter observation is controversial. Among the lymphocytes, various investigations have suggested that B lymphocytes are better stimulators than are T lymphocytes. These results are disputed, and it seems that either B or T cells may stimulate MLR. One should note the unusual finding (for immunology) that only living cells stimulate; dead cells or cellular extracts do not give rise to any detectable response. Moreover, transplantation antigens that stimulate MLR are different from those that induce transplantation antibody production. (This critical difference will be discussed again in chap. 23.) Sero-defined (SD) antigens give rise to antibody production, whereas lymphocyte-defined (LD) antigens stimulate MLR (Fig. 13.4).

## Percentage of Reactive Cells

By cellular dilution techniques, 1 to 3% of circulating lymphocytes have been shown to react in an MLR. This number is of the same order as that seen

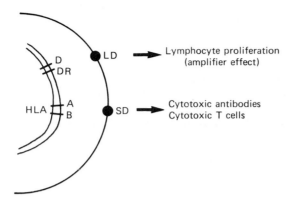

**Fig. 13.4** SD antigens (serologically defined) and LD antigens (defined by mixed lymphocyte reaction). It should be noted that the DR antigens (D-related) are serologically defined. Their identity with the D antigens and their role in the allograft response are still a matter of some controversy.

in graft versus host reactions (GvH) (see p. 422). It is a much higher percentage involvement than that of antigen-reactive cells that give rise to antibody production (0.1%). This high proportion of alloantigen-reactive cells, corroborated by the high number of cells binding antibodies directed at anti-allogeneic antibody associated idiotypes raises important theoretical considerations (which will be discussed later; see p. 572).

Reactive cells represent clones specific for antigens of the stimulating cells, because initial culture treatment with heavily tritiated thymidine (which destroys the first proliferating cells) induces a selective incapacity of the cells to thereafter respond to the initial stimulating cells but without diminishing their ability to respond to nonrelated cells.

## LYMPHOCYTOTOXICITY PHENOMENA

### Introduction

During rejection, lymphocytes from skin allograft-bearing mice are capable of destroying target cells obtained from the donor after minimal (short time) exposure in vitro. The nature of cytotoxic cells and the mechanisms of cytotoxicity have been extensively studied during recent years and will be reviewed in the following pages. From these observations, and from the fact that neonatal thymectomy prevents both the appearance of cytotoxic cells and graft rejection, the thymus was believed to play an essential and perhaps exclusive role in the maturation of cytotoxic lymphocytes. It has since been recognized that it is possible to observe cytotoxicity in the absence of T cells, for example, in nude mice. Non-T cells (called "killer" K cells) can destroy target cells coated with IgG antibodies, independently of presensitization. In addition, it has been shown that macrophages, previously armed by T cell-produced mediators and a still ill-defined population of "natural killer" cells, can be cytotoxic, suggesting yet other mechanisms of cellular cytotoxicity.

## Cytotoxic T Lymphocytes

DESCRIPTION OF THE TECHNIQUE

Cytotoxic cells may be produced in vivo after injection of allogeneic cells or grafting of allogeneic skin or tumor. In the first few days after alloimmunization, spleen cells are isolated and incubated with target cells that bear donor alloantigens. A target often used, especially in Brunner's technique, because of the high sensitivity to lymphocyte cytolytic action, is the transplantable P-815 mastocytoma cell (H-$2^d$). Cell lysis is obtained in the absence of complement. Lysis may be precisely measured if target cells have been previously labeled with $^{51}$Cr. By incubating cells with $^{51}$CrO$_4$Na$_2$, which binds to all of the membrane or cytoplasm, labeling of live cells is achieved. Chromium is released on cell death. Its valence is now altered, and, in principle, no further incorporation into new cells occurs.

Another technique, microcytotoxicity, originally described by Takasugi and E. Klein, consists of measuring inhibition of tumor cell or fibroblast growth (by cell count or evaluation of chromium, thymidine or proline release by detached cells) in the presence of cytotoxic cells. However, the significance of these techniques is less clear-cut than that of chromium release after short-term incubation, especially regarding the T-cell nature of cytotoxic cells, because some non-T cells appear to be involved. Takasugi and Klein's technique is primarily used for detecting weak cytotoxic reactions.

Recently, it has been possible to establish and maintain clones of cytotoxic T cells in the presence of T-cell growth factor, now called Interleukin 2 (produced by PHA and Con A-activated or MLR stimulated T cells). These T-cell clones carry the Lyt-2 and 3 antigens and show the same fine H-2 specificity as the cytotoxic T cells from which they are derived. One may predict that the use of such clones will lead to major progress in the knowledge of the nature and the mode of action of cytotoxic T lymphocytes.

KINETICS OF CYTOTOXIC CELLS

Cytotoxic lymphocytes are detected as early as the sixth day after allogeneic skin or tumor grafting, with peak numbers observed between days 9 and 16. Secondary responses observed after a secondary antigenic stimulation give rise to an accelerated course (peak on day 6) and a more intense response. Cytotoxic cells, highly similar to those that appear in vivo after skin grafting, may also be generated in vitro in an MLR (cell-mediated lympholysis; see Fig. 13.5 and Table 13.2).

T-CELL NATURE OF CYTOTOXIC CELLS

In vitro elimination of T cells in the mouse by incubation with anti-θ serum in the presence of complement abolishes cytotoxicity, whether cytotoxic cells have been generated in vivo or in vitro. T cells act separately, without need of other cell populations, since purified T-cells obtained, for example, by passage on nylon fibers or on columns coated with anti-Ig antibodies, show increased cytotoxicity compared with that of the original cells. Addition of macrophages

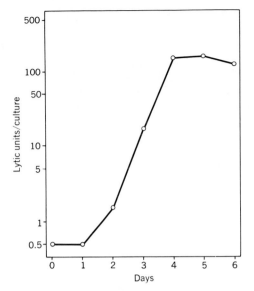

**Fig. 13.5** Cell-mediated lympholysis. Kinetics of cytotoxic cells generated during a mixed-lymphocyte reaction (C57BL/6 cells sensitized to DBA/2 cells). (From J. C. Cerottini, H. O. Engers, F. R. McDonald, and K. T. Brunner, J. Exp. Med. 1974, 140, 708.)

does not augment cytotoxicity. Lastly, when parental thymic cells are injected into irradiated $F_1$ mice, the recipient spleen cells become capable of specifically lysing cells that bear the other parental antigens, even after elimination of B lymphocytes and macrophages. B lymphocytes are eliminated by passage on columns coated with anti-Ig antibodies, and macrophages are eliminated by incubation of the cells on plastic in the presence of carbonyl iron and application

**Table 13.2  Cytotoxic Activity of Lymphocytes on the Fifth Day of a Mixed-Lymphocyte Culture**

| Responder cells (H-2) | Stimulating cells (H-2) | Target cells (H-2) | Percentage of $^{51}$Cr release (for different ratios of responder/target cells) | | | | |
|---|---|---|---|---|---|---|---|
| | | | *0.3:1* | *1:1* | *3:1* | *10:1* | *30:1* |
| C57BI/6 (b) | DBA/2 (d) | P-815 (d) | 12 | 32 | 71 | 98 | 95 |
| | | L-1210 (d) | 16 | 34 | 79 | 92 | 96 |
| | | EL4 (b) | 0 | 0 | 0 | 1 | 4 |
| | | GIL4 (b) | 0 | 1 | 2 | 2 | 1 |
| BALB/c (d) | C57BI/6 (b) | EL4 (b) | 8 | 21 | 44 | 72 | 92 |
| | | L-1210 (d) | 0 | 1 | 3 | 5 | 8 |
| DBA/2 (d) | C57BI/6 (b) | EL4 (b) | 7 | 16 | 27 | 55 | 76 |
| | | P-815 (d) | 0 | 1 | 2 | 4 | 8 |

After J. C. Cerottini, M. O. Engers, H. R. McDonald, and K. T. Brunner, J. Exp. Med. 1974, **140**, 703.

of magnetic field. It should also be noted that the cells of the thymus itself may be sensitized in vitro in the CML system.

Among the T cells, the cytotoxic lymphocytes belong to the subpopulation defined by the Lyt 23 antigens. It is not impossible, however, that the Lyt 123$^+$ cells may play the role of cytotoxic-cell precursors, under certain conditions, to the same extent as Lyt 23$^+$ cells. In addition, we shall see that Lyt 1$^+$ cells seem to play an important amplifier role in the differentiation of Lyt 23$^+$ cytotoxic lymphocytes.

A second addition of mitomycin-treated stimulatory cells to the mixed culture, after the first peak, stimulates the appearance of a new wave of cytotoxic T cells, which arise from memory cells, sensitized by the first stimulation. This reinduction may also be obtained in vitro several weeks after an in vivo stimulation. It is an interesting fact that certain polyclonal activators, such as pokeweed mitogen and, to a lesser degree, Con A, may also reinduce the appearance of cytotoxic T cells.

CYTOTOXICITY MECHANISMS

Cytotoxicity consists of three phases: establishment of contact between cytotoxic cells and target cells, development of cytotoxic activity, and death of the target cell.

*Contact Establishment.*   Cytotoxic cells are antigen specific inasmuch as they may kill only cells that bear the alloantigens that originated the sensitization. However, specificity essentially relates to target recognition by specific receptors, and cytotoxicity itself is probably nonspecific. The existence of specific receptors has been directly demonstrated in absorption experiments: immune lymphocytes are incubated on monolayers of macrophages or fibroblasts syngeneic to the immunizing cells. Nonadsorbed cells do not show any cytotoxicity when exposed to a new monolayer of target cells identical to the previous ones. It is even possible to demonstrate, conversely, that elution of cells bound to the mono layer provides a cytotoxic cell-enriched suspension. Similar results have been reported in unimmunized animals but, essentially, in xenogeneic combinations. Specific binding may still be obtained after glutaraldehyde treatment of fibroblast monolayers, implying a passive nature of target cell involvement. Conversely, recognition of target cell antigens by lymphocytes is probably an active phenomenon, because such recognition is abolished by metabolic inhibitors and because no adsorption of cytotoxic cells occurs on fibroblast monolayers at 4°C. Recognition is not inhibited by anti-Ig serum.

*Development of Cytotoxic Activity.*   Contact between aggressor and target cells causes, still ill-defined, metabolic changes in cytotoxic cells that may be associated with secretory activity. Intracellular levels of cyclic adenosine monophosphate (AMP) and guanosine monophosphate (GMP) may play an important role, because an increased cyclic GMP level augments lymphocytotoxicity, whereas increased cyclic AMP levels have the opposite effect.

The development of the cytotoxic action also depends on the presence of calcium and glucose. It is blocked by deoxyglucose, by numerous metabolic inhibitors, and by cytochalasin B.

It is interesting to note that the continual presence of functional effector cells throughout the cytotoxicity test is not obligatory. In fact, the effector cells may be functionally inactivated some minutes after the establishment of contact, before significant chromium liberation has occurred, without any subsequent diminution of the ultimate amount of isotope released. It therefore seems that a short intermediate phase exists after the recognition phase that still requires the presence of functional T cells. During this phase the irreversible cellular lesion (lethal hit) of the target cell is induced. The origins of the mechanisms that produce this lesion are still hypothetical. The lesion may be secondary to the direct contact established between the membranes of the effector and the target cells, for example, by means of the intermediary of an enzyme located on the membrane of the effector cell. The cytotoxic activity of membranes isolated from sensitized T cells supports this contention, but the specificity of the cytotoxicity exerted by membranes remains to be confirmed. Alternatively, the effector cell may release substances that are secondarily toxic to the target cell. The cytotoxic activity of certain cytotoxic-cell culture supernatants would be compatible with this hypothesis. However, foreign cells that do not share common antigens with the specific target are not destroyed when added to the culture, suggesting that cytotoxic lymphocytes must be in direct contact with their target. Cytotoxicity is polarized: a cytotoxic cell is capable of sequentially lysing several target cells and therefore is not destroyed by the cytolytic process (although remaining sensitive to the action of another cytotoxic cell directed against it). Finally, one should also mention an intermediate hypothesis in which the recognition phase initiates a series of metabolic steps involving the unmasking or activation of cytotoxic molecules on the effector-cell surface. These molecules may then directly attack the membrane of the target cell.

*Target-Cell Death.* Microcinematographic studies show that killer cells leave the target after exerting their "killer" action. The target cell then undergoes a series of still poorly understood modifications, eventually leading to death.

### K Cells

Mononucleated cells obtained from nonimmunized subjects are capable of destroying target cells coated with antibodies in the absence of complement. This phenomenon is called "antibody-dependent cell-mediated cytotoxicity" (ADCC). Mononucleated cells from normal human blood destroy chicken red blood cells coated with antichicken red blood cell antibody or liver cells coated with the corresponding antibody within a few hours (Fig. 13.6). More recently, ADCC has been observed with respect to transplantation antigens, by use of anti-HLA antibodies obtained after pregnancy, transfusion, or kidney grafting.

NATURE OF THE LYMPHOCYTE DEPENDENT ANTIBODY (LDA)

Antibodies that give rise to ADCC are essentially of the IgG class. Very low antibody concentrations suffice, for example, antichicken red blood cell serum diluted $10^6$ times in the human lymphocyte-chicken red blood cell system, conditions under which no lysis occurs if complement rather than K cells is added. The reaction is inhibited by aggregated IgG or immune complexes. Cytotoxicity occurs when the antibody is preincubated with the target cells but not when lymphocytes are added, indicating that LDA antibody is not cytophilic

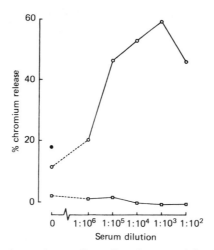

**Fig. 13.6**   The antibody-dependent cell-mediated cytotoxicity (ADCC) phenomenon of mononucleated cells from normal human peripheral blood toward liver tumor cells (Chang) coated with anti-Chang rabbit IgG antibodies at several dilutions (shown on the abscissa). Cytotoxicity is measured after 20 hr of incubation by evaluation of release of $^{51}$Cr previously fixed on Chang cells. (From G. Holm and P. Perlmann, Antibiot. Chemother. 1969, *15*, 295.)

for lymphocytes. Lastly if K cells are non T cells, LDA antibody production, nonetheless, seems to depend on T cells, as does that of other IgG antibodies.

K-CELL NATURE

The ADCC phenomenon is seen in neonatally thymectomized rats or mice, nude mice, and in children with thymic immunodeficiency. It is also observed in agammaglobulinemia with B-cell absence. Furthermore, elimination of circulating B lymphocytes and mature monocytes by nylon filtration or of T lymphocytes by sheep red blood cell rosette elimination in man (see Table 4.7, p. 69), or by in vitro treatment with anti-θ serum in the mouse, proportionally increases cytotoxic activity. K cells are present in considerable numbers in blood and spleen but, conversely, are few in number in lymph nodes and are absent in the thymus. These data suggest therefore that they are not T or B cells (as defined by the presence of membrane Ig or complement receptors). And they are probably not monocytes, because K cells do not adhere to nylon and do not have monocyte morphology. K cells could represent either a new lymphocyte population or be atypical or immature B cells or monocytes. In addition, it appears that T cells, monocytes, or macrophages exert K-cell activity in certain experimental conditions.

CYTOTOXICITY MECHANISMS

Like monocytes and B cells, K cells have receptors for the IgG Fc fragment; thus, one may observe a decrease of ADCC after depletion of rosettes formed with antibody-coated erythrocytes (EA) and successive eliminations of B and T lymphocytes. Binding of K cells to immune complexes present on the target cell is a prerequisite, because nonsensitized cells are not destroyed when added simultaneously with sensitized cells. The exact mechanism of the reaction is as yet poorly defined. The reaction occurs only at 37°C and rapidly progresses, with significant lysis apparent as early as the second hour.

SIGNIFICANCE

It is difficult to extrapolate these in vitro data to in vivo situations. Of considerable interest are the potential applications of ADCC to antitumor immunity, antigraft immunity, and immunopathology. For example, one can conceive of weak concentrations of IgG antibodies, incapable of producing cytotoxicity in the presence of complement, that might produce lysis of tumor cells. Another type of cytotoxicity that is produced by nonimmunized lympho- cytes may be similar to the ADCC phenomenon: after PHA stimulation, normal human T lymphocytes acquire the ability to destroy certain target cells, such as heterologous red blood cells in the presence of PHA. Such cytotoxic phenomena must be distinguished from the polyspecific cytotoxic activation of lymphoid cells that have been treated by polyclonal activators such as concanavalin A (such cytotoxicity is expressed in the absence of the activator).

## Macrophage Cytotoxicity

Monocytes have receptors for the Fc fragment of IgG molecules and seem capable of ADCC. Additionally, macrophages may be armed by mediators released by sensitized T cells in the presence of the antigen. This arming, which has been demonstrated for lysis of allogeneic tumor cells, has been seen to occur in vivo and in vitro. The factor produced by T cells [macrophage-arming factor (MAF)] had initially been claimed to be graft or tumor antigen specific,

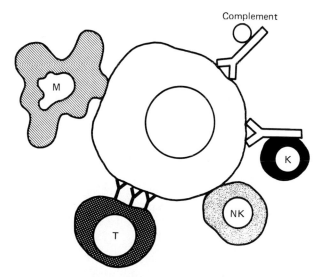

**Fig. 13.7**  The principal effector mechanisms in allograft rejection: antibody-plus complement, K cells, NK cells, T cells, and macrophages.

but this hypothesis has not been substantiated. It seems clear that macrophages have a cytotoxic action that is essentially nonspecific.

### Natural Killer Cells

There exist, in the absence of any known sensitization, a population of mononuclear cells capable of lysing certain virus-transformed lymphoblastoid cell lines. These natural killer cells (NK cells) do not appear to be B cells, T cells (although again their relationship to immature T cells has been suggested by some data), monocytes, macrophages, or K cells. Unlike the latter, they can act without the presence of antibody. Their level of activity in a given strain of mouse seems to be linked to the major histocompatibility complex and can be correlated with resistance to tumors induced by the virus infecting the cell lines that serve as their in vitro target. The role of NK cells in graft rejection is hypothetical but must be taken into consideration, particularly in bone marrow grafts.

# V.  MECHANISMS OF GRAFT REJECTION

Graft rejection involves the intervention of numerous effector agents, both cellular and humoral. The MLR and CML reactions have provided a great deal of information concerning the cytotoxic effects of T lymphocytes in the rejection of allografts differing at the MHC and their central position in this role is not in doubt. Nevertheless, it is still true that numerous other effector mechanisms may be involved and that important regulatory mechanisms exist, which modify the rejection response either in a positive (amplifier) manner or, on the contrary, by acting as a brake.

## IMMUNOLOGIC NATURE OF GRAFT REJECTION

The intervention of lymphocytes is essential and is found at several levels: in the cellular infiltrate at the moment of rejection, in the transfer of graft immunity by purified lymphocytes, in the involvement of lymphocytes in the mixed lymphocyte reaction and in cytotoxicity phenomena, and in the prolongation of graft survival by immunosuppressants, such as ALS. The demonstration of various immunologic reactions consequent to grafting is also suggestive of the immunologic nature of rejection. Lastly, specificity of the rejection reaction, as evidenced by the study of accelerated rejection following a second graft, indicates that it is an immune response.

## RESPECTIVE ROLES OF CELLULAR AND HUMORAL IMMUNITY

Primary rejection of allografts involves cell-mediated immunity effected by T cells. From this fact, which is fairly well documented, arises the generalization that all types of allograft rejection are due exclusively to T cells. We shall see, in fact, that the situation is more complex in hyperacute rejections (as observed in preimmunized individuals) and in chronic rejection (as seen in cases with a weak histocompatibility difference or under immunosuppression). Here, antibodies play a more important role.

### Intervention of Cell-Mediated Immunity

Some of the arguments that suggest intervention of T cells in graft rejection are indirect, including the presence of numerous lymphoid cells in the graft, persistence of anti-H-2 antibody production in mice in which rejection of skin allografts is prevented by ALS treatment, and the absence of allograft rejection in neonatally thymectomized or nude mice. One may also mention the exclusive role of T cells in initiating the mixed lymphocyte reaction, lymphocytotoxicity, and the GvH reaction, all of which are presumed models of allograft reaction. In fact, the most decisive arguments arise from transfer experiments. While it is practically impossible to transfer graft immunity by serum from presensitized animals (except in very high dose), transfer is obtained by use of lymphocyte preparations without simultaneous antibody transfer. Similarly, a local inflammatory reaction (analogous to a cutaneous delayed hypersensitivity reaction) results when sensitized lymphocytes are transferred into the skin of animals that bear alloantigens responsible for sensitization, whereas no reaction occurs after transfer of serum from sensitized animals, except in very high dose. Lymphocytes from nonsensitized animals also give a significant reaction (the normal lymphocyte transfer test described by Brent and Medawar).

### Intervention of Humoral Immunity

Various antibodies are regularly found in the serum of animals that reject skin or organ grafts. Some of these antibodies are IgG, give rise to ADCC in vitro, and may thus be the cause of lymphocytotoxicity through the intermediary of K cells. Cytotoxic antibodies are responsible for the onset of hyperacute rejection. In addition, in the chronic rejection that occurs with immunosuppression, Ig deposits in the graft are visible by immunofluorescence. These data suggest a possible role of antibodies, particularly in hyperacute or chronic rejection. One should, however, also mention blocking or facilitating antibodies seen in some presumably tolerant animals (obtained, for example, by neonatal injection of allogeneic cells; see chap. 20). These antibodies, under certain circumstances, particularly in chronic rejection, may oppose rejection. A particular role for anti-Ia antibodies (see chap. 23) in facilitation has been recently suggested but still remains to be evaluated.

### Conclusions

A survey of the data summarized above makes a definitive judgment difficult. It is likely that rejection is most often initiated by several factors, which are sometimes synergistic and at other times antagonistic (e.g., blocking factors); however, it is not possible in a particular case to say what is predominant. Overall, cytotoxic antibodies appear to be incriminated in hyperacute rejection in preimmunized subjects (and in xenografts, whether primary or not), while cytotoxic T cells are implicated in primary allograft rejection that involves strong histocompatibility differences with no immunosuppression. The special case of organ grafts in man is particularly difficult to interpret, because grafts with weak histocompatibility differences (resulting from donor selection) and immunosuppression are usually involved. These factors attenuate humoral and T-cell cytotoxic reactions, thus producing the potential for introduction of other parameters of the allograft immune response, including LDA antibodies, blocking antibodies, and armed macrophages. For any particular rejection case, it seems impossible to decide which mechanism is responsible if, indeed, there is a predominant one.

## PRESUMED SEQUENCE OF EVENTS

The sequence of immunologic events consists of several phases.

### Recognition of Transplantation Antigens

SD or LD transplantation antigens are localized in the graft; some fraction of these antigens leaves the graft by a vein or lymphatics. Circulation, better called "recirculation," of numerous T lymphocytes favors the influx of a considerable number of such cells into the graft, but circulating B lymphocytes also enter the graft. Once in the graft, T lymphocytes directly contact SD and LD antigens through specific receptors whose immunoglobulin-related nature is probable on the basis of the presence of idiotypic determinants, but not proven. Approximately 1 to 6% of T lymphocytes that enter the graft carry receptors for graft antigens. Possibly two different T-cell populations recognize SD and LD antigens.

### Lymphocyte Proliferation and Differentiation

Lymphocytes that recognize LD antigens transform and proliferate. These lymphocytes will help other lymphocytes to recognize specific SD antigens and differentiate into cytotoxic cells. At the same time, other cells differentiate into transplantation antibody-producing cells.

### Movements of Sensitized Lymphocytes

We have seen that lymphocytes seem to recognize transplantation antigens present in the graft. However, many of these lymphocytes then leave the graft, as is shown by the numerous lymphocytes and lymphoblasts present in efferent lymphatics and regional lymph nodes. These lymphocytes, followed by isotopic labeling, later return to the graft, where they are probably retained by specific receptors. It appears that lymphocytes from graft efferent lymphatics, and *a fortiori* lymph node lymphocytes, have already acquired lymphocytotoxic properties.

### Effector Mechanisms

Graft destruction is largely achieved by cells that infiltrate the graft (at least in acute rejections without immunosuppression). These cells include T lymphocytes, cytotoxic macrophages, K cells coated with LDA transplantation antibodies, and plasma cells that produce local cytotoxic antibodies. Mechanisms of destruction are largely unknown. For hyperacute rejection and, contrarily, chronic rejection, humoral antibodies secreted in distant lymph nodes seem to play an essential role.

# REGULATION OF GRAFT REJECTION

When incompatibility exists at the level of the major histocompatibility loci, the effector mechanisms described above usually result in rapid rejection of the whole graft, even before the regulatory mechanisms have become effective. In the opposite situation of minor histocompatibility or even in cases of strong histoincompatibility in recipients undergoing therapeutic immunosuppression, graft rejection is retarded or even prevented altogether. This attenuation of the rejection involves several mechanisms whose respective roles remain to be elucidated.

## Facilitating Antibodies

We have seen above that besides cytotoxic antibodies, certain antibodies seem to be capable of restraining graft rejection, in particular, it seems, anti-Ia antibodies. The role of these antibodies, acting either in the free form or as complexes with antigens, is probable but as yet not definitively established. The in vitro models that permit their demonstration (specific inhibition of MLR or cytotoxicity phenomena) are somewhat deceptive since their presence correlates poorly with the outcome of the graft. In particular, blocking antibodies are often absent from the serum of subjects whose grafts have progressed favorably despite a major histoincompatibility with the donor. We should mention, however, controversial results that suggest a favorable role in graft survival for cold lymphocytotoxins directed against B lymphocyte antigens. Moreover, it has been observed that the administration of blood transfusions before grafting seems, in general, to exert a beneficial effect on graft outcome (except in those cases that develop cytotoxic antibodies detected on a direct cross match immediately before transplantation). This beneficial effect does not appear to be explicable simply on the basis that transfusion results in the exclusion of "good responders" that develop antibodies detected before transplantation and would have rapidly rejected the graft. The possible intervention of blocking or facilitating antibodies developed in response to the transfusions must also be taken into consideration.

## Suppressor T Cells

Suppressor T cells specific for the antigens present on the stimulator cells may be demonstrated in the first few days of an MLR. These suppressor T cells also seem to occur in vivo because pretreatment with small doses of cyclophosphamide (Cytoxan), which is known to relatively selectively eliminate suppressor T cells, has been readily shown to augment the in vivo generation of cytotoxic T cells after immunization with allogeneic cells. Cell transfer experiments have confirmed that it is possible to delay graft rejection by the injection of purified

T cells from skin-graft bearing animals in whom rejection has been prevented by injections of antilymphocyte serum and donor bone marrow cells (Brent). All these studies result in the conclusion that specific suppressor T cells are active in the regulation of the effector mechanisms for graft rejection. This suppression, which is antigen-specific, must be distinguished from the nonspecific suppression of the MLR observed after stimulation of suppressor cells by mitogens such as concanavalin A.

### Amplifier T Cells

The concept of amplification of the effector mechanisms involved in graft rejection arises from results obtained in several experimental systems. The most supportive results have been obtained in the CML system described above. It has been demonstrated that the Lyt 1$^+$ cells that respond to LD alloantigens by proliferating, help the Lyt 23$^+$ cells to differentiate into cytotoxic T cells. The intervention of soluble factors (T-cell growth factor or interleukin 2) in this amplifier effect has been recently demonstrated by several authors.

This mechanism could explain the rejection, apparently initiated by T-cell stimulation, by a variety of antigens (often viral) that are unrelated to the transplantation antigens of the graft donor.

Finally, T cells may also act by stimulating cytotoxic activity in macrophages by means of the intermediary of the lymphokines they produce (in particular MAF).

### Idiotypic Suppression

We have seen that the alloantigen recognition receptors on B and T cells carry the idiotypes of antibodies that recognize the same transplantation antigens (see p. 86). It has been shown that allograft-bearing rats produce, after the tenth day, antibodies directed against the idiotypes of antibodies synthesized against the alloantigens of the graft. The activity of these anti-idiotypic antibodies in the regulation of graft rejection has been suggested by the suppression of rejection obtained after autoimmunization of rats with antibodies directed against the graft antigens. The antibodies are polymerized by glutaraldehyde treatment and injected in the presence of complete Freund's adjuvant (Binz and Wigzell). It is possible that T cells with anti-idiotypic specificity intervene conjointly with anti-idiotypic antibodies.

## GENETIC CONTROL OF GRAFT REJECTION

As has been seen, the fate of a graft is directly dependent on genetically determined histocompatibility differences that exist between the donor and the recipient. In addition to this principal genetic control, which will be discussed in further detail in chapter 23, it should be mentioned that the genetic control of the allograft response may also exist at other levels. In man, it appears that high and low responders exist, and this occurs as much at the cellular level as at the humoral level. In particular, antibody production after repeated transfusions is very variable and depends on the subject. The immunologic mecha-

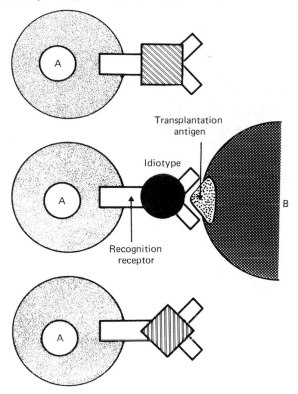

**Fig. 13.8**  T-cell recognition receptors for alloantigens. The clone of cells from subject A specifically recognizes the transplantation antigens carried by the cells of subject B by idiotype-bearing receptors that are shared with antiallogeneic A anti-B antibodies.

nism at the base of these reponder differences is at present poorly understood. Preliminary results suggest that cytotoxic responses are, like antibody production, under the control of Ir genes. In contrast, however, in the mice selected by Biozzi, both high and low responders, in terms of antibody production, reject grafts normally (see p. 700).

## PREVENTION OF GRAFT REJECTION: TOLERANCE AND FACILITATION

Considerable efforts have been applied in attempts to prevent immunologic rejection with the goal of maintaining prolonged survival of organ grafts. Immunosuppression may be antigen specific or nonspecific.

### Nonspecific Immunosuppression

Graft rejection in the animal is delayed by antimetabolites (6-mercapto-purine, azathioprine, methotrexate), alkylating agents (cyclophosphamide), methylhydrazine, and antilymphocyte serum (ALS). The latter makes possible a potentially indefinite graft survival. In man, prolonged survival of kidney grafts has been obtained by use of whole body irradiation and, in particular, azathioprine along with corticosteroids. We shall later discuss these immuno-suppressive methods (see chap. 33).

### Specific Immunosuppression

A specific tolerance to skin allografts may be obtained experimentally by injecting donor bone marrow cells along with ALS to a skin graft recipient or by injecting allogeneic cells into a newborn. Considerable controversy exists with respect to the mechanism of this specific immunosuppression (the animals respond normally to other grafts). Is this phenomenon true tolerance, in other words, inactivation or elimination of clones that respond to the antigens, or is it blocking, by suppressor T cells, antibodies, or antigen-antibody complexes, of the normal rejection mechanisms that are normally expressed? We shall look at this important problem again (see p. 586).

# VI.   GRAFT-VERSUS-HOST REACTION

The graft-versus-host reaction (GvH) in one sense represents the opposite of the graft rejection reaction just described. In GvH, the recipient is attacked by immunocompetent cells that have been injected into a host unable to reject them.

## CONDITIONS FOR OCCURRENCE

The GvH reaction is seen when grafted cells, essentially T lymphocytes, are fully immunocompetent, and the host is unable to reject grafted cells because of immunologic or genetic peculiarities. The aggressor cells may be splenic, lymph node, or peripheral in origin. The host may be immunoincompetent for genetic reasons, for example, when parental cells are injected into an $F_1$ hybrid [e.g., CBA to $F_1$ (C57B1/6 × CBA) mice].

The host may also be rendered immunoincompetent by immunosuppressive methods, such as irradiation of administration of cyclophosphamide, or be spontaneously immunodeficient, as is the case for newborn animals. One should mention also GvH reactions seen in parabiosis, where reciprocal transfusion of considerable amounts of lymphocytes may lead to a GvH reaction in the absence of overt immunosuppression.

## DESCRIPTION

The clinical picture of the GvH reaction is one of rapid progression to lethal cachexia. The most frequent symptoms are diarrhea, emaciation, growth retardation, splenomegaly, hepatomegaly, and hemolytic anemia. A particularly intense proliferative reaction occurs in the spleen, peaking at 8 to 10 days, followed by splenic atrophy. Microscopy reveals the presence of numerous blast cells and a few pyroninophilic plasma cells, plus destruction of malphigian follicles. Alternatively, progressive reconstitution of the splenic architecture may be observed when GvH is less intense. Conversely, in more severe forms, complete splenic atrophy occurs during the last few days before death, secondary to necrosis, fibrosis, and infarction. Lymph node atrophy is also observed, similarly preceded by a period of hypertrophy. The reaction is also associated with increased phagocytic activity, which may be evaluated by clearance of intravenous colloidal carbon or gold.

The GvH reaction may be quantified by various means. Mortality rate, date of death, and growth retardation are useful parameters because they assess the toxicity of GvH. A more sensitive and precise assay (and therefore more often utilized) consists of measuring splenomegaly, for example, the splenic index:

$$\frac{\text{spleen weight/body weight of injected mouse}}{\text{spleen weight/body weight of control mice}}$$

Alternatively, colloidal gold clearance, which is augmented in the GvH reaction, may be measured.

It is possible to induce a chronic GvH reaction and thus create a true chronic allogeneic disease, by repeated injections (over several weeks) of small doses of allogeneic cells. In addition to these systemic manifestations of GvH, immunosuppression may be observed (as assessed by decreased antibody production and the appearance of tumors) and glomerulonephritis may occur, linked to immune complex deposition, especially of anti-H-2 antibodies and H-2 antigens.

Let us lastly mention *local GvH reactions* which are often used as simple assays for T-cell competence. One may thus study the increase in popliteal lymph node weight after injection of allogeneic cells in the hind foot-pad.

## MECHANISMS

The immunologic nature of the GvH reaction seems well established, at least during the initiation phase. The ability to induce a GvH reaction may be suppressed by immunosuppression of the donor; the exclusive role of lymphocytes is demonstrated by the effect of purified lymphocytes. One may demonstrate, at least in combinations that involve weak histocompatibility differences (non-H-2 in the mouse), an immunization factor. The GvH reaction is more intense when the donor has been previously sensitized by the corresponding antigens. The immunization factor clearly indicates the reaction specificity. The absence of GvH reactions against certain alloantigens in animals rendered tolerant to these alloantigens at birth confirms this specificity (see p. 588). The exclusive intervention of T cells in the initiation of the reaction is also well established. No GvH reaction is obtained with cells from neonatally thymectomized mice or nude mice. Treatment in vitro with anti-θ serum or in vivo with ALS (given to the donor or to the recipient), selectively eliminate T cells also suppresses the GvH reaction.

The proliferative phase of the GvH reaction causes splenomegaly. This phase corresponds to the blast transformation observed in vitro when allogeneic

rejection cannot simply be explained by the absence of a maternal immune reaction. There are potentially "protective factors." A barrier between mother and fetus has been envisaged. This barrier may be the uterus itself, representing a privileged site, or the placenta. The nongravid uterus is not a privileged site, because various antigens, particularly transplantation antigens or allogeneic tissue placed into the normal uterine lumen, induce both humoral and cellular rejection reactions. However, the gravid uterus with decidual cells has been reported to be a privileged site for grafts of tumors or allogeneic cells independent of the trophoblast.

The trophoblast itself may also be a barrier. Trophoblast cells carry transplantation antigens, as shown by cytotoxicity tests performed after trypsinization. However, fetal histocompatibility antigens seem to be coated with inert fibrinoid material or sialomucin, which protects them from the action of maternal lymphocytes or antibodies. In addition the HLA-A and B antigens are only found (with β-2 microglobulin) in small quantities (5% of the quantity found on splenocytes) on trophoblasts. ABO antigens are either absent or weakly expressed on the trophoblast. The existence of trophoblast-specific antigens has been reported but remains to be corroborated. The presence of a trophoblastic barrier is thus uncertain; anyhow, this barrier is only partial, because a few fetal cells are found in the mother, and vice versa.

It is also possible that hormonal abnormalities during gestation may modify immune responses. The immunosuppression of high-dose corticosteroids is well known (see chap. 33). In fact, pregnant females have nearly normal immunocompetence. Skin allografts are normally rejected by pregnant women or mice, and delayed hypersensitivity skin reactions to tuberculin are normal, except immediately before parturition. One cannot exclude a role for very high local concentrations of placental hormones (steroids or gonadotropins). Thus, gonadotropins depress the normal in vitro lymphocyte response to PHA and mixed lymphocyte reactions. Other nonspecific factors may also have an immunosuppressive action as has been suggested; for example, for α-fetoprotein.

A final hypothesis is specific blocking of the fetomaternal immune response by humoral or cellular mechanisms. Observation that skin allografts of the same genotype as the fetus are more slowly rejected than are grafts with equal incompatibility, especially at the end of gestation and immediately postpartum, favors this hypothesis. However, the differences in graft survival are modest, and in man rejection of paternal grafts is sometimes accelerated. On the other hand, tumor grafts seem to be more easily accepted at the end of gestation. Gestation may partly diminish presensitization. The demonstration by the Hellströms of a specific blocking of lymphocytotoxicity reactions of mother to fetus by maternal serum favors a facilitation hypothesis. Blocking of the mixed lymphocyte reaction of the mother to the fetus by maternal serum seems to have the same significance as does discovery of Ig deposits in the placenta and elution (at acid pH) of maternal antibodies directed against fetal graft antigens. IgG3, which does not fix complement and easily crosses the placenta, could play a preferential role in this hypothesis. However, blocking specificity remains controversial, and the mode of action of blocking sera remains obscure. The Hellströms' results have been difficult to reproduce. The intervention of suppressor T cells has also been suggested, but this remains to be demonstrated.

**Table 13.3  Putative Mechanisms That Prevent Fetus Rejection**

Weak expression of alloantigens by the fetus

Mother's nonspecific immunosuppression due to placenta or other hormones or to other factors (e.g., $\alpha$-fetoprotein)

Absence of cell transfer from mother to fetus

Uterus as a privileged site, especially during pregnancy

Trophoblast as a barrier with weak expression of alloantigens (coated by sialomucin and polysaccharides)

Factors that block specifically the mother's immune response: humoral (blocking antibodies, antigen-antibody complexes) or cellular (suppressor T cells)

## CONCLUSIONS

None of the numerous mechanisms mentioned, which are summarized in Table 13.3, is in itself convincing. The role of the antigenically neutral barrier (probably represented by the placenta) is undoubtedly predominant. Blocking factors could also play an important role because of the weak antigenicity of trophoblast, without these factors being sufficient to inhibit skin allograft rejection.

## *BIBLIOGRAPHY*

BACH J. F. Cells involved in allograft rejection. Nature and characteristics of cells involved in recognition of transplantation antigens. *In* L. Brent and J. Holborow, Eds., Progress in immunology. II. Vol. 5. Amsterdam, 1974, North Holland, p. 115.

BACH J. F. The immunological follow-up of the kidney allograft recipient. *In* Proc. 5th Int. Congr. Nephrol. Mexico. Basel, 1974, Karger, Vol. 3, p. 40.

BACH F. H., BACH M. L., and SONDEL P. M. Differential function of major histocompatibility complex antigens in T lymphocytes activation. Nature, 1976, *259*, 273.

BEER A. E. and BILLINGHAM R. E. Immunoregulatory aspects of pregnancy. Fed. Proc., 1978, *37*, 2374.

BILLINGHAM R. and SIVERS W. K. The immunobiology of transplantation. Englewood Cliffs, N.J., 1971, Prentice-Hall.

BRENT L. Pathogenetic role of delayed hypersensitivity and antibody in allograft reactions. *In* Cell. Interactions in the Immune Response. Convoc. Immunol. Buffalo, New York. Basel, 1970, Karger, p. 250.

BRUNNER K. T. and CEROTTINI J. C. Cytotoxic lymphocytes as effector cells of cell mediated immunity. *In* B. Amos, Ed., Progress in immunology. New York. 1971, Academic Press, p. 385.

CALNE R. Y. (Ed.) Clinical organ transplantation. Oxford, 1972, Blackwell, 539 p.

CARPENTER C. B., D'APICE A. J., and ABBAS A. K. The role of antibodies in the rejection and enhancement of organ allografts. Adv. Immunol., 1976, *22*, 1.

CARPENTER C. B., and STROM T. B. Transplantation Immunology. In Clinical Immunology (Parker C. W. [ed]). Saunders. Philadelphia. 1980, 376.

CEROTTINI J. C. and BRUNNER K. T. Cell-mediated cytotoxicity. Allograft rejection and tumor immunity. Adv. Immunol., 1974, *18*, 67.

CEROTTINI J. C. and BRUNNER K. T. Mechanism of T and K cell-mediated cytolysis. *In* F. Loor and G. Roelants, Eds., B and T cells in immune recognition. Chichester, 1977, Wiley, p. 319.

CEROTTINI J. C. Clonal analysis of cytolytic T lymphocytes and their precursors. In: Immunology 80 (M. Fougereau and J. Dausset [ed]). Acad. Press New York, 1980, 622.

DUPONT B. and HANSEN J. A. Human mixed lymphocyte culture reaction: genetic, specificity and biological implications. Adv. Immunol., 1976, 23, 107.

EDWARDS R. G. and COOMBS R. R. A. Immunological interactions between mother and foetus. In P. G. H. Gell, R. R. A. Combs, and J. Lachmann, Eds., Clinical aspects of immunology, ed. 3. Oxford, 1975, Blackwell.

ENGERS H. D. and MacDONALD H. R. Generation of cytolytic T lymphocytes in vitro. Contemp. Top. Immunobiol., 1976, 5, 145.

FAULK W. P. Immunology of the maternofoetal relationship. In: Immunology 80 (M. Fougereau and J. Dausset [Eds]). Acad. Press, New York, 1980:1093.

GOLSTEIN P. and SMITH E. T. Mechanism of T cell-mediated cytolysis: the lethal hit stage. Contemp. Top. Immunobiol., 1977, 7, 273.

HAMBURGER J., CROSNIER J., KREIS H., and BACH J. F. Renal transplantation theory and practice. Baltimore, 1982, in press.

HAYRY P. Anamnestic response in mixed lymphocyte culture-induced cytolysis (MLC-CML) reaction. Immunogenetics, 1976, 3, 417.

HAYRY P., ANDERSSON L. C., NORDLING S., and VIROLAINEN M. Allograft response in vitro. Transpl. Rev., 1972, 12, 91.

HENNEY C. S. T cell-mediated cytolysis: An overview of some current issues. In: Contemp. Topics Immunobiology. Plenum N.Y., 1977, 245.

LINDQUIST R. Mechanisms of transplantation immunity. In: Mechanisms of Immunopathology. (S. Cohen, P. A. Ward, and R. T. McCluskey [eds]). John Wiley & Sons, New York, 1979, 323.

McKEARN T. J. A biological role for anti-idiotypic antibodies in transplantation immunity. In: Immunological tolerance and enhancement (F. P. Stuart and F. W. Fitch [eds]). MTP Press Ltd., Lancaster, U. K. 1979:61.

MÖLLER G. [Ed]. T cell stimulating growth factors. Immunol. Rev., 1980, 51.

MOLLER G. [Ed]. T cell clones, 1981, 54.

MÖLLER G. (Ed.) Liver transplantation. Transpl. Rev., 1969, 2.

MÖLLER G. (Ed.) Specificity of effector T lymphocytes. Transpl. Rev., 1976, 29.

NABHOLZ M. and MIGGIANO V. C. The biological significance of the mixed lymphocyte reaction. In F. Loor and G. Roelants, Eds., B and T cells in immune recognition. Chichester, 1977, Wiley, p. 261.

PERLMANN P. and HOLM G. Cytotoxic effects of lymphoid cells. Adv. Immunol. 1969, 11, 117.

RAPAPORT F. T. and DAUSSET J. Human Transplantation. New York, 1969, Grune & Stratton.

WAKSMAN B. H. The antiallograft response effector mechanisms. In L. Brent and J. Holborow, Eds., Progress in immunology. II. Vol. 5. Amsterdam, 1974, North Holland, p. 127.

WELSH R. M. Mouse natural killer cells: induction, specificity and function. J. Immunol., 1978, 121, 1631.

WILSON D. B., HOWARD J. C., and NOWELL P. C. Some biological aspects of lymphocyte reactive to strong histocompatibility cell antigens. Transpl. Rev., 1972, 12, 3.

## ORIGINAL ARTICLES

BAKER P. E., GILLIS S., FERM M. M., and SMITH K. A. The effect of T cell growth factor on the generation of cytolytic T cells. J. Immunol., 1978, 121, 2168.

BEER A. E. and BILLINGHAM R. E. Concerning the uterus as a graft site and the foetus as a natural parabiotic organism hemograft. In Ontogeny of acquired immunity. Ciba Foundation Symp. Amsterdam, 1972, Elsevier, North Holland, p. 149.

DENNERT G. Cytolytic and proliferative activity of a permanent T killer cell line. Nature, 1979, 277, 476.

FORMAN J. and MÖLLER G. The effector cell in antibody-induced cell-mediated immunity. Transpl. Rev., 1973, *17*, 108.

GREENBERG A. H. and WOLOSIN L. B. The nature of the K cell and the role of antibody-dependent cell mediated cytotoxicity (ADCC) in the rejection of tumours. Ann. Immunol. (Paris), 1977, *128c*, 485.

HENNEY C. S. On the mechanism of T-cell mediated cytolysis. Transpl. Rev. 1973, *17*, 37.

JEANNET M., PINA V. W., FLAX M. H., WINN J. H., and RUSSELL P. S. Humoral antibodies in renal allotransplantation in man. New Engl. J. Med., 1970, *282*, 111.

KIESSLING R., PETRANYI G., KARRE K., JONDAL M., TRACEY D., and WIGZELL H. Killer cells: a functional comparison between natural immune T cells and antibody-dependent in vitro systems. J. Exp. Med., 1976, *143*, 772.

LOHMANN-MATHES M. and FISCHER H. T-cell cytotoxicity and amplification of the cytotoxic reaction by macrophages. Transpl. Rev., 1973, *17*, 149.

MIYAJIMA T., HIGUCHI R., KASHIWABARA H., YOKOYAMA T., and FUJIMOTO S. Anti idiotypic antibodies in a patient with a functioning renal graft. Nature, 1980, 283, 306.

PEDERSEN N. C. and MORRIS B. The role of the lymphatic system in the rejection of homografts: a study of lymph from renal transplants. J. Exp. Med., 1970, *131*, 436.

ROEHM N. W., ALTER B. J., and BACH F. M. Lyt phenotype of alloreactive precursor and effector cytotoxic T lymphocyte. J. Immunol., 1981, 126, 353.

STIMPFLING J. H. The use of PVP as a developing agent in mouse haemagglutination tests. Transpl. Rev., 1961, *27*, 109.

TERASAKI P. I., KREISLER M., and MICKEY R. M. Presensitization and kidney transplant failures. Postgrad. Med., 1971, *47*, 89.

WAGNER H., ROLLINGHOF M., and NOSSAL G. J. V. T-cell mediated immune responses induced in vitro. A probe for allograft and tumor immunity. Transpl. Rev., 1973, *17*, 3.

WAGNER H., ROLLINGHOFF M., and SHORTMAN K. Evidence for T-T cell synergism during in vitro cytotoxic allograft responses. *In* L. Brent and J. Holborow, Eds., Progress in immunology. II. Vol. 3. Amsterdam, 1974, North Holland, p. 111.

Chapter 14

# ANTITUMOR IMMUNITY

**Jean-Paul Lévy**

I.   DEFINITION
II.  TUMOR ANTIGENS
III. ANTITUMOR IMMUNE REACTIONS
IV.  IMMUNOTHERAPY

## I.   DEFINITION

Tumor immunology deals with immunologic phenomena that develop in the host of a spontaneous or experimentally provoked tumor, whether these phenomena tend to inhibit or, alternatively, to enhance tumor development. It implies the existence of antigenic structures peculiar to malignant cells that are not present in normal cells of the same tissue in healthy animals at the same stage of development, and raises the possibility that these antigens may provoke an effective immunologic reaction that permits tumor rejection, analogous to that which occurs in an allogeneic graft. In many respects, problems of tumor immunology are reminiscent of those seen in transplantation immunology, but with the very special condition that the entire reaction occurs between the host and a product of its own tissues.

## II.   TUMOR ANTIGENS

### DEFINITION, INTEREST, AND NOMENCLATURE OF TUMOR ANTIGENS

Any malignant cell structure, absent in or on healthy cells of the same tissue at the same stage of development and capable of inducing immunologic reactions either in the host or by inoculation in a foreign host, may be considered a

430

tumor antigen. The interest in studying these antigens by immunologic methods is at least twofold.

The demonstration of antigens peculiar to malignant tissue is important in understanding the nature of malignancy; the expression of these antigens may directly or indirectly relate to the abnormality responsible for "malignant transformation." One may postulate, for example, that an abnormal membrane protein that modifies the relationship of the cell with the surrounding medium (thus an altered perception of regulatory signals) can possibly be the cause of the tumor and constitute an antigen. Immunology therefore provides a valuable method to study characteristics of malignant cells.

Tumor antigens are the theoretical target of the antitumor immunologic reaction by which the organism seems able to defend itself. It is essentially this aspect that defines tumor immunology as it will be examined in this chapter.

The term "neo-antigen" has been abandoned, because it is recognized that most tumor antigens are not "new" to the host or limited to the tumor cell. The term "tumor-specific antigen" (TSA) is used for the very rare antigens that are truly specific for the malignant cells; that is, never present in normal adult or embryonic tissue of the same species, even during virus infection.

TSA located on the cell surface are potentially able to cause cell rejection and are designated as tumor-specific transplantation antigens (TSTA). However, most antigens capable of provoking a rejection reaction (i.e., "transplantation antigens") are not specific for the malignant cell but may be found on embryonic cells or on cells infected by certain oncogenic viruses without being transformed by these viruses. These antigens are called tumor-associated transplantation antigens (TATA).

## LOCALIZATION OF TUMOR ANTIGENS

### Cell-Surface Antigens

Cell-surface antigens are important in tumor rejection because they are accessible to circulating antibodies and lymphoid cells. The tumor cell membrane is a complex antigenic mosaic that includes normal structures such as histocompatibility antigens, and tumor antigens. The latter may be capable of inducing immunologic rejection of the tumor (TSTA or TATA); however, numerous reactions directed against other surface tumor antigens do not lead to in vivo rejection. A particular problem is that of adsorption of antigenic substances on the malignant cell surface; these substances originate in the extracellular medium and may incorrectly be considered structural antigens of the membrane.

### Intracellular Antigens

Intracellular antigens are located in the nucleus or cytoplasm and are not implicated in cell rejection but do represent important markers of malignancy.

### Soluble Antigens

Membrane or intracellular antigens may be released into the medium during cell necrosis or by shedding from living cells. These soluble antigens are present either in the blood or in the culture medium. Their solubilization has several potential consequences. (1) Their detection in the blood at a distance from the tumor may reveal the presence or reappearance of the tumor after initial treatment (e.g., hepatoma and α-fetoprotein). (2) Solubilization may provoke or augment an immune reaction because it is an antigenic stimulus. (3) Conversely, circulating antigens may intervene to block immunologic reactions by combining with the antibody or with effector cells, which are specific for rejection phenomena.

## METHODS FOR STUDYING TUMOR ANTIGENS

### Immunization of Foreign Hosts

Antitumor antibodies may be produced by inoculating tumor homogenates or living tumor cells into animals of another strain or species. Because these inocula bear normal histocompatibility antigens, they will be recognized as a foreign graft by the host and will be rejected. Obviously, such antisera must first be absorbed to eliminate antibodies directed against antigens common to the tumor and healthy tissues. By this means, carcinoembryonic antigens of human colonic tumors and hepatoma-produced α-fetoprotein were discovered and, more recently, antigens associated with human leukemias. However, since tumor-cell antigenicity is generally weak and present in conjunction with strong antigens of normal cells, nonspecific absorption may occur, thus causing loss of antitumor activity. Additionally, it is sometimes difficult to be sure that a given reaction is directed against tumor antigens and not normal minor antigens. For this reason, "tumor antigens" have been described that were in part histocompatibility antigens. Quantitative variations in the expression of tumor antigens according to the stage of cell differentiation may also obscure the problem. It is sometimes impossible to obtain adequate pure controls (normal tissues of the same organ). One simple example is human leukemia: circulating blood cells or normal bone marrow cells may not represent a good control because of wide differences in the distribution of cell types in these two populations and in leukemic cell suspensions. The ideal control in this case is a suspension of pure normal hematopoietic stem cells, which at the present time cannot be identified or isolated. Thus, the nature of a leukemic cell antigen described by heterologous immunization is problematic. Is this antigen a tumor antigen, or is it a normal antigen that corresponds to an individual specificity of the patient? Alternatively, is it an antigen present on all cells at this particular stage of differentiation, whether or not malignant? The recent demonstration that all the antigens described in human leukemias—using antisera raised in other species—belong to this last category (they were once considered as probably being specific to leukemic cells), underlines the importance of this problem. Due to the considerable antigenic diversity of normal membranes, these questions are particularly important when cell membrane antigens are being studied.

### Immunization of the Natural Host

The reactions of the natural host can be theoretically directed only against antigens that the host normally does not possess. Thus, antibodies or lymphoid cells from tumor-bearing animals may react against tumor antigens. The serum of tumor bearers is especially interesting for study of reactions directed towards autologous malignant cells. If the patients were not previously transfused, grafted, or multiparous, one may utilize their serum against the tumor cells of another subject. The most ideal condition is that provided by autologous reactions. Similar results can, however, be obtained by testing antibodies or lymphoid cells of one individual against tumor cells of another individual, provided they are identical twins or, in experimental systems, that they belong to the same inbred strain.

## NATURE OF TUMOR ANTIGENS

There are four main categories of tumor antigens: viral antigens, individual antigens peculiar to certain tumors, carcinoembryonic antigens, and differentiation antigens.

### Viral Antigens

Viral antigens are found on tumors induced by DNA or RNA oncogenic viruses. In the DNA virus group, polyoma virus, SV 40, human adenovirus, and oncogenic viruses of the herpes group (herpes virus Saimiri, Lücke's virus, Marek's virus) have been most extensively studied. A human herpes virus associated with Burkitt's lymphomas and nasopharyngeal carcinoma, the Epstein-Barr virus, belongs to this group. RNA oncogenic viruses are present in many vertebrate species as widely disparate as fish, chickens, mice, cats, and monkeys. These viruses induce leukemias, various hematopoietic tumors, connective tissue tumors, and, in some species, mammary tumors. The possibility that such viruses exist in man is likely, but to date no virus has been isolated in humans; they may exist in an incompletely expressed form. In man, as in many other species, these viruses do not necessarily result in tumor-induction; oncogenic mutants seem to be the exceptions among the viruses of this group.

Antigens that correspond to virus-induced tumors seem to be entirely dependent on the viral genome and therefore are identical on different tumors when the same virus is etiologic in different animals within the same species or in different species. Some of these antigens are present inside cells, where they may be detected by immunofluorescence (on fixed cells) or by complement fixation by using cell homogenates. Other viral antigens, which are often complex, are located on the cell surface. An example of the latter is the membrane antigen (MA) in Burkitt's lymphoma. This antigen is a structural constituent of both the virion envelope and the host cell membrane. In tumors caused by RNA oncogenic viruses, all virus-producing cells contain a strong cell-surface antigenicity linked to the synthesis of several viral polypeptides, themselves secondarily included on the surface or inside the virion. These polypeptides may have variable specificities, common either to RNA viruses that parasitize one species or one vertebrate class or, conversely, peculiar to certain viruses. Viral antigens of the cell membrane, the total number of which has not been identified in experimental systems, are unknown in man, with the exception of the MA antigen of Burkitt's lymphoma. These antigens generally induce clear-cut immunologic reactions; several of them, sometimes present on the same cell, may play a TATA role. The existence of TSTA is less likely, because the same antigens may be present on virus-infected cells that have not been transformed (malignant). However, TSTA appear to exist in cells trans- formed by avian sarcoma virus. Experimentally, one may demonstrate viral antigens in vivo by rejection of the tumor graft by a sensitized syngeneic animal (TATA). Regardless of whether they are TATA, these antigens may also be identified in vitro by immunofluorescence (on living cells), by cytotoxicity in the presence of complement, or by electron microscopy with ferritin-conjugated antibodies. In addition they induce an intense cell-mediated immune response mediated by T cells.

### Individual Tumor Antigens

Individual tumor antigens are present, in particular, in experimental tumors induced by chemical carcinogens (methylcholanthrene- or dibenzan- thracene-induced sarcoma in the mouse, azo-dye-induced hepatoma in the rat). They are most often associated with solid tumors. Their existence in leukemia is likely but has not been well studied. Antigens of this type have not yet been identified in man for various technical reasons. They are specific for a given tumor in one individual and are not found in other tumors induced by the same carcinogen in the same species or in the same strain. If the initial tumor is transplanted into other animals of the same strain, the antigenicity is maintained. They are weakly immunogenic; however, in vivo rejection, and antibody production, or in vitro cell-mediated immunity reactions may be obtained in animals from which the tumor was removed or after hyperimmu- nization by inactivated cells (a requirement, because grafting of living cells leads to death of the host). There is, however, no cross-reaction between tumors, which differentiates these antigens from viral antigens. Their nature is not known.

### Carcinoembryonic Antigens

Carcinoembryonic antigens (CEA) are substances normally present in the embryo at some given stage in its development, and are absent in the adult or are present only in trace amounts. Their reappearance in association with tumors seems to be very common and is perhaps even universal. We do not know if CEA has a contributory role in malignancy or is simply a correlate of "dedifferentiation." Included among these antigens are the α-fetoprotein of hepatic primitive tumors, and CEA from colonic and other human tumors. However CEAs are sometimes detected in various other nonmalignant patho- logic states. Other human CEA are presently under study. It has recently been demonstrated that the cell surface of most experimental tumors is the site of numerous CEA, several of which are often present together. These antigens may co-exist with the two previous antigenic categories, but, apparently, there is no relationship between their presence and the etiology of the tumor. Their existence was only recently discovered and is almost undoubtedly the basis for some immunologic cross-reactions previously noted between different tumors. Generally, these antigens exhibit a weak immunogenicity that induces only

**Table 14.1   Experimental Tumors**

| Inducing agent | Example | Induced tumor |
|---|---|---|
| Physical or chemical agents | Methylcholanthrene | Sarcoma |
| | | Leukemia |
| | | Carcinoma |
| DNA virus | Polyoma, SV-40 | Heterogeneous tumors |
| | Adenovirus | (sarcoma, undifferentiated |
| | | sarcoma) |
| RNA virus | Avian type C | Myosarcomas, leukemias |
| | Murine type C | Fibrosarcomas, leukemias |
| | Feline type C | Fibrosarcomas, leukemias |
| | Bovine type C | Leukemias |
| | Simian type C | Mammary carcinomas |
| Spontaneous | | Variable |

minor reactions in the host. Thus, α-fetoprotein and colonic CEA can be demonstrated after immunization of heterologous hosts, but they do not appear to play a role in spontaneous tumor reactions. After immunization by normal embryonic tissues, a weak antitumor protection may be observed in certain animals; however, as a rule, CEA do not cause rejection reactions or are at best only weak TATA as compared to the two types of antigens previously described.

### Differentiation Antigens Associated with Tumors

The cell surface undergoes important changes during differentiation, in the embryo and also in all adult tissues. Membrane structures specific to certain stages of differentiation are antigenic and may be recognized by a foreign host. It is possible that, under certain conditions, the original host may also recognize these antigens if they are abnormally expressed. The precise nature of these antigens is unknown. Their existence has been demonstrated on certain tumors. They may intervene in in vitro reactions, but do not play the role of TATA in vivo. An example is the TL antigen present in certain mouse leukemias. This antigen is a thymic differentiation antigen (see chap. 4) that disappears from thymocytes leaving the thymus. It may be present on certain leukemia cells, even in TL-negative mice. Here, it is possible to induce a specific antibody reaction; however, this reaction has no effect on the outcome of the tumor, perhaps because of antigenic modulation (a property of the antigen that disappears from the cell surface in the presence of the specific antibody; see p. 83). It has recently been demonstrated that all the antigens demonstrated by means of xenoantisera on the surface of human leukemic cells and, probably, those responsible for cellular stimulation in in vitro mixed lymphocyte cultures are differentiation antigens that are characteristic of several hemopoietic stem cells and their precursors.

## CONCLUSIONS REGARDING TUMOR ANTIGENS

There is no doubt that most tumor cells bear tumor antigens, especially on their surface, and that these antigens constitute a complex antigenic mosaic.

They may include one or several TATA, possibly causing in vivo immunologic rejection. It is certain that strong antigenicity resulting in in vivo rejection is mainly a property of virally or chemically induced tumors. In other cases, notably in most tumors that arise spontaneously and that only possess embryonic or differentiation antigens, the responses are weak or absent. It is quite possible that this weak antigenicity is the most frequent situation in human tumors.

## III.  ANTITUMOR IMMUNE REACTIONS

### DEMONSTRATION OF AN EFFICIENT IMMUNOLOGIC CONTROL OF IN VIVO GROWTH OF SOME TUMORS

#### Effect of Immunosuppressive Agents

Host immunosuppression by irradiation, chemical immunosuppressants, or antilymphocyte sera may considerably enhance the development of tumors in experimental systems. By these means, a tumor may develop in animals from a naturally resistant strain. The high sensitivity of newborn animals to certain carcinogenic factors, especially viruses, is mainly due to the immaturity of their immune system. Also, early thymectomy significantly increases the sensitivity to numerous tumors.

In man, these observations have clinical analogues: malignant tumors appear at a very high rate in children with certain constitutional immune deficiencies, and patients exposed to prolonged immunosuppression, particularly after renal transplantation, develop malignant tumors, especially sarcoma of hematopoietic organs at rates considerably higher than that of the general population. Both of these observations suggest that an immunosurveillance mechanism that operates normally, regularly eliminates tumor clones; inhibition of this mechanism by means of immunosuppression could facilitate tumor development. However, it cannot be excluded in such observations that chronic stimulation of the precursors of immunocompetent cells results in an increased level of somatic mutation.

#### Preventive Antitumor Vaccination

Prophylactic antitumor vaccination is possible in several experimental systems, particularly in malignant virus-induced tumors (the animal is protected against any tumor induced by the same virus) and in chemical carcinogenesis (protection here strictly relates to the same transplanted tumor). In these systems, the grafting of irradiated or homogenized tumor cells or repeated resection of the tumor at the beginning of its development provides effective immunization. Vaccination can also be obtained by injecting living allogeneic cells that bear the same virus-induced tumor antigens and will be rejected because they bear normal histocompatibility antigens. These immunizations are the basis of the definitions of TATA and TSTA.

These observations are, however, limited in scope. (1) The immunity obtained requires repeated immunization and most often results only in weak protection against a limited number of tumor cells (in the order of $10^4$ to possibly $10^6$). Protective immunization against a large number of cells is observed only in cases of virus-induced and virus-producing tumors. (2) Cross-protection is possible only for viral tumors: a given oncogenic virus always induces the same antigens on cell surfaces. Unfortunately, within a given species, different oncogenic viruses exist that may have specific antigens for each virus subgroup. For example, immunization against a given leukemia protects only against the corresponding virus-induced leukemia. For chemically-induced tumors or spontaneous tumors, the protection only operates against the specific tumor; the only animals protected will be those of the same strain in which the tumor is grafted. Obviously, such a model has no corollary in man. However, these experiments may be applicable to immunotherapy in autologous conditions, for example, in individuals treated to prevent the recurrence of the initial tumor.

### Transfer of Antitumor Immunity

Immunologic control of tumors is suggested by the two types of experiments described above and has been corroborated by the transfer of protection against a tumor between animals. Antibody transfer is not very efficient except in very special circumstances related to experimental conditions difficult to achieve for spontaneous tumors. Adoptive transfer of immunity by use of histocompatible lymphocytes may, however, produce efficient protection against subsequent grafting of a tumor of the same antigenicity, which indicates a major role for cell-mediated immunity in antitumor immunity.

## NATURAL FORMATION OF ANTITUMOR ANTIBODIES

Antibodies present in the carrier of an autochtonous tumor or in an animal immunized with the tumor of another animal of the same strain are of great interest in the study of antitumor immunologic reactions.

In contrast, antibodies obtained by immunization of animals of other species do not necessarily prove that the natural host can produce antibodies of identical specificity.

### Experimental Tumors

Carriers of experimental tumors may exhibit circulating antibodies cytotoxic in the presence of complement, and one hypothesis has been that these antibodies are operative in vivo in destroying tumor cells. More commonly, however, noncomplement-fixing (noncytotoxic) antibodies are revealed. Here again, an in vivo role may be envisaged since these antibodies may have opsonin characteristics and permit the recognition of sensitized tumor cells by macrophages. Moreover, they may perhaps allow the recognition of tumor cells by non-T-killer cells (K cells, see below) but we do not know whether this mechanism operates in vivo. These antibodies may, instead, be deleterious to the host, since they may block all antigenic cellular sites, thus preventing the access of effector (cytotoxic) T-lymphoid cells. In fact, blocking of the immune reaction at the effector cell level is observed only in artifical systems in which malignant cells are previously incubated with specific high-activity sera (such as those obtained by hyperimmunization). It seems unlikely that such high-titer antibodies are present in vivo. In most cases, the usual characteristic of antitumor antibodies is their low titer.

### Antitumor Antibodies in Man

Human antitumor antibodies have been observed in association with numerous tumors. However, most of the older studies must be considered keeping in mind that no consideration was made with respect to histocompatibility differences, and that, in fact, these antibodies mainly recognized normal histocompatibility antigens on malignant cells. In a smaller number of cases, antitumor antibodies have been demonstrated under technically valid conditions but their significance is uncertain, with the exception of Epstein-Barr virus (EBV) linked tumors, such as Burkitt's lymphoma and nasopharyngeal carcinoma. Although the etiologic role of the virus remains unproven, its regular association with these two tumors confers them specific antigens. Carriers of these tumors have antibodies that are also present in the general population, but at much higher levels. Anti-EBV antibodies are of three types. (1) Numerous antibodies are directed against intracytoplasmic antigens that are constituents of the virion during synthesis, namely, viral capsid antigen (VCA) and early antigen (EA). These antibodies provide evidence of the past viral infection but not of malignancy or antitumor reaction. They are present worldwide and are seen in most adults. (2) Antibodies against Epstein-Barr nuclear antigen (EBNA) are more interesting because they recognize antigens located on chromosomes and present in malignant cells. However, because of their location, these antigens do not play a role in tumor rejection. (3) Antimembrane antigen (MA antibodies of different specificities, recognize antigens peculiar to the virion envelope and the malignant cell. Because they are directed against cell-surface antigens, they should play a role in rejection. It is noteworthy that the same antibodies are found in infectious mononucleosis, an early curable manifestation of the EBV infection.

Antibodies associated with other human tumors are less well defined. They occur in melanomas, numerous nervous system tumors, osteosarcomas, and uncommonly in malignant hematopoietic states. Most of them are directed against intracellular constituents and have unknown significance. In some cases, the antibody is directed against a cell membrane constituent, but here again, the differentiation between tumor antigen and histocompatibility antigen has not yet been well established. Conversely, well-defined human tumor antigens, such as $\alpha$-fetoprotein and CEA, are not clearly associated with the cell membrane and at most they are only weakly antigenic and, consequently, cause no detectable rejection.

### Role of Antibodies in Tumor Rejection

The role of antibodies in tumor rejection is difficult to assess. Experimentally, antibodies appear more often in resistant strains than in animals from strains sensitive to certain oncogenic agents. Very marked immune reactions against membrane antigens, probably TATA, are seen in numerous experimental systems, especially in virus-induced tumors, even as the tumor develops. Some tumors, particularly leukemia, may develop despite the immune response and show no evidence of inhibition. Very often, the tumor grows while antibody levels decline; such decline may permit tumor development or, on the other hand, the increased tumor mass may absorb noneffective circulating antibodies. Similarly, in Burkitt's lymphoma, patients with very long remissions sometimes show high titers of anti-MA antibodies over long periods of time, with decreasing titers occurring a few months before relapse. It seems that a soluble antigen of unknown significance (massive virus synthesis?) absorbs the circulating antibody, which may explain why there is no inhibitory effect of humoral immunity.

Finally, an antitumor antibody response is present in some experimental and human cases. With very few exceptions, it is a weak response. A correlation between antibody response and antitumor protection has been suggested in some systems but in most cases has not been demonstrated. In conclusion, the exact role of antibodies in tumor rejection remains hypothetical. Note that the transfer of antitumor protection by antibodies is not successful under the usual experimental conditions.

# NATURAL DEVELOPMENT OF CELL-MEDIATED ANTITUMOR REACTIONS

## Techniques

One series of techniques evaluates the preexisting sensitization to tumor cells as well as primary in vitro reactions. These techniques include in vitro lymphocyte transformation (tritiated thymidine incorporation) in the presence of isologous or autologous tumor cells and the macrophage migration inhibition test, in which the tumor antigen is presented by complete cells, tumor extracts, or soluble antigens. These techniques also include the study of skin reactions that occur after injection of inactivated tumor cells or homogenates. In all cases, however, the significance of the reaction observed is difficult to evaluate, and in particular, its relationship to tumor rejection cannot be established. Very often one cannot even be sure that these reactions are directed against tumor antigens or really involved in tumor rejection.

A second series of reactions supposedly evaluates the final phase of the effector immune response. These reactions explore the capacity of lymphoid cells to inhibit or to destroy tumor cells in vitro. The most popular of these techniques has initially been the microplaque cytotoxicity assay (i.e., microcytotoxicity assay, MA), which is analogous to older methods of inhibition of in vitro growth of tumor colonies. Other methods are based on the chromium release test (CRT) in which chromium-labeled tumor cells are incubated with immune lymphocytes whose activity is evaluated by the chromium release into the supernatant. The CRT phenomenon is purely cytolytic, whereas MA evaluates both cytolysis and cytostasis, and both specific and nonspecific reactions. Various other techniques differentiate between cytostasis and cytolysis.

### Demonstration of Sensitization of the Subject to His Tumor

Lymphocyte transformation in vitro after cocultivation with tumor cells and macrophage migration inhibition have not been extensively employed in experimental systems. They permitted, however, recognition of lymphoid cell reactions in the presence of autologous tumor cells. In man, these techniques have been extensively studied. It has thus been observed that leukemic patients in remission have lymphoid cells that transform in vitro in the presence of their own blasts, which were collected during the active leukemic phase (preserved in liquid nitrogen). Similar phenomena have been described for other tumors, in particular, melanomas. They probably represent a presensitization of lymphocytes after initial contact with the tumor. However, it has recently been shown that normal T cells may be stimulated in vitro by autologous B lymphocytes or by blasts carrying Ia-type antigens. Since identical antigens exist on numerous tissues, especially in the skin, the interpretation of experiments performed with mixed lymphocyte tumor reaction (MLTR) must be reviewed. At the present time, their significance in terms of antitumor responses appears to be in doubt. Positive skin tests have been noted with variable frequency, depending on tumor or author. It is, however, difficult to correlate the reactions with tumor status and to ascribe any prognostic significance to the results. In addition, these systems involve several technical uncertainties especially related to antigens.

### Presence of Cells Capable of Destroying Tumor Cells in Tumor Carriers

Application of the microcytotoxicity assay (MA), first studied in experimental systems and, subsequently, in human tumors, permitted the Hellströms (after 1969) to demonstrate cell-mediated immune reactions by means of in vitro inhibition of tumor cell growth by the subject's own lymphoid cells. In some cases, especially in experimental systems and more rarely in human tumors, it could be shown in vitro (by the CRT technique) that lymphocytes were cytotoxic for tumor cells. It was initially believed that MA and CRT represented the same unequivocal reactions. It has since been established that the cell-mediated immunity reaction is very complex and involves effector cells of multiple natures (Fig. 14.1).

Thymus-dependent cytolytic cells (CTLs), initially defined by CRT, are capable of directly destroying tumors cells. These cells are highly efficient in destroying tumor cells in vitro but perhaps have limited usefulness in vivo. They are found in experimental systems in which rejection of deep-seated tumors generally occurs. After tumor rejection, their activity persists, albeit at reduced levels. In man, antitumor cells of this type have not yet been definitively identified, but it is likely that they do exist in a few cases, in particular in Burkitt's tumors. Other cells, designated as K (killer) cells, act indirectly through the intermediary of antibodies (ADCC or antibody-dependent cell-mediated cytotoxicity). They do not show antitumor specificity and possess only surface receptors for the Fc fragment of IgG. By this means, they bind to circulating antigen-antibody complexes. If the antigen-antibody complexes correspond to antibodies directed against the tumor, K cells may be able to recognize tumor cells and exert a cytolytic or cytostatic action. Such activity develops only in

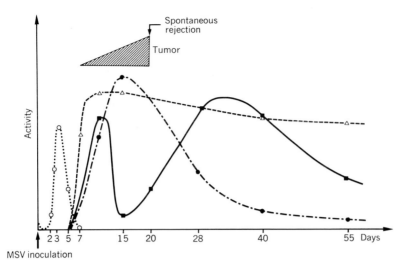

**Fig.14.1** Schematic representation of immunologic activity of mouse lymphoid cells against MSV virus-induced sarcoma, evaluated by four different methods: MLTR [mixed lymphocyte tumor reaction (stimulation index), ○], CA [cytostasis assay (tritiated thymidine incorporation), △], MA [microagglutination (semiquantitative scale), ■], CRT [chromium release test (percentage of specifically released chromium), ●]. (From J. C. Leclerc and J. P. Levy, 1974.)

antibody excess (as compared to antigen excess), because the existence of free antibody sites is required for K cells to recognize the tumor cells. If antigen is in excess and blocks these free sites, K-cell action is inhibited: circulating K cells may therefore be inhibited by soluble antigens derived from the tumor. Conversely, unarmed K cells should react easily with tumor cells sensitized by an IgG antibody. The nature of K cells is unclear. They may represent one particular lymphoid line that is neither T nor B ("null cells") or they may be similar to monocytes without complete macrophage differentiation. In particular, they are less adherent and less phagocytic than are macrophages. In fact, it is possible that any cell possessing surface Fc receptors may play the role of a K cell, including macrophages and even polymorphs. As far as macrophages are concerned, a nonimmunoglobulin arming factor, probably derived from T cells, has been described. The specific macrophage-arming factor (SMAF) may activate macrophages toward tumor cells. However, the existence and nature of SMAF are still not definitively established. In addition to this presumably specific role of macrophages, macrophages show predominantly nonspecific activities. It is known that macrophages "activated" by various stimulations, including bacteria, are capable of exerting in vitro a cytolytic action against most tumor cells. However, if macrophages play a very important, nonspecific role in the in vitro MA-type reaction, the in vivo significance of such reactions is uncertain. It is possible that within the tumor, activated macrophages contribute to the destruction of tumor cells. The fact that this action is not specific for rejection antigens suggests that its significance in vivo is probably minimal, except if it is triggered by a specific antitumor stimulus mediated by T cells.

# GENERAL SCHEME OF IN VIVO ANTITUMOR IMMUNITY PHENOMENA

A relatively simple general blueprint for tumor rejection was proposed by the Hellströms in 1969 from data obtained in MA experiments. In this proposal, lymphoid cells present in tumor carriers are capable of destroying tumor cells. A circulating blocking factor initially considered to be antibody, but now recognized to be an antigen-antibody complex, has the ability to inhibit the action of effector lymphoid cells. Today, however, it is known that the reactions observed in these experimental systems are due mostly to K-cell and macrophage activity, including nonspecific reactions. It is doubtful whether this contribution is essential for rejection in vivo. The role of blocking factors is particularly unclear, notably because they do not show much action on T-killer cells. Finally, the in vivo rejection mechanism is still not established, but the following points can be considered:

### Tumor Cell Recognition

In the initial phase of the antitumor reaction, T cells recognize antigenic tumor cells. At this stage, macrophages may possibly also destroy tumor cells nonspecifically; however, the existence of this phenomenon in vivo has not been demonstrated, exclusive of macrophage activation by concurrent inflammatory reactions. Such inflammation is usual in tumor transplants but can hardly be considered as a model for spontaneously arising tumors.

### Direct Cytolytic Action

Following tumor recognition and initiation of the immune response, cytolytic T cells analogous to those demonstrated by CRT might intervene by direct lytic action. These cells are easily detected in virus-induced experimental tumors. They are very similar to those found in transplantation immunity (directed against an allogeneic graft). They may play a major role in immunosurveillance; however, their activity is limited and may be overcome by rapidly growing tumors. Tumor prognosis is probably determined at this stage: strongly antigenic tumors are eliminated and are never or only rarely clinically detectable. Conversely, minimally antigenic or nonantigenic tumors pass through this stage without elimination by immunologic processes. Note that it is not clear if this kind of T-killer cell reaction exists against nonviral tumors, especially human tumors.

### Antibody Synthesis

T-cell induced cytolysis, when it exists, is followed by other reactions. Antibody synthesis probably plays an essential role. There are two possibilities. Antibodies may be relatively potent, providing further protection against the reappearance of the same malignant clone or a clone of the same antigenicity, if the initial T-cell reaction has been highly efficient. Antibodies may be relatively weak but may function through the intermediary of an ADCC mechanism (K cells or macrophages). However, K-cell reactions are difficult to interpret. In vivo, their importance in rejection is most certainly limited for at least two reasons: first, they are very easily blocked by the excess antigen released by tumor cells; second, an important portion of the reaction observed in vitro seems to be directed against embryonic differentiation antigens that have almost no role in in vivo rejection. These reactions may be satellite phenomena to the main reaction: they could represent immune reactions against tumor-released antigens but not necessarily involved in actual rejection. Most of the reactions reported in man may be due to K cells. Therefore their exact significance has not yet been established.

### Nonspecific Macrophage Reactions

Nonspecific macrophage reactions seem to accompany tumor development and contribute to cell necrosis and other inflammatory phenomena. Activated macrophages are frequently found in association with T cells inside tumors undergoing rejection. However, there is no relationship between this reaction and the antigens involved in rejection. Therefore the recognition in a given animal of a macrophage-mediated reaction is not a priori related to the ability of the animal to reject the tumor since this rejection is always a very antigen-specific phenomenon.

Finally, T-cell mediated immunosurveillance seems to be the determinant phase in the immunologic control of tumors. This phenomenon occurs very early, probably long before clinical discovery of the tumor. All of the other phenomena described above have uncertain significance and may not be related to rejection. At the present time, the data obtained in man are insufficient, and no definite conclusions can be reached. Additional study of human tumors under adequate experimental conditions is necessary before the significance of these reactions in tumor carriers is understood. Such a view is substantiated by the recent recognition that nonspecific antitumor reactions may be observed in many normal subjects. The cells of normal subjects are capable of destroying various tumor cells nonspecifically. Because of this, most of the previously described specific reactions were probably nonspecific. Two prerequisites are necessary to define significant antitumor immunologic reactions in man. The first is to determine precisely the effector cells involved. It is possible to demonstrate weak but significant T-killer-cell responses after non-T-cell elimination. To search for these T cells inside the tumor itself may be an especially valuable approach. The second is to define the antigenic specificity of the reaction mediated by the effector cells. Note also that the recently described "natural killer cells" (see p. 416) could play a determinant role in the so called "antitumor immune surveillance."

### Natural Antitumor Cytotoxic Activity (Natural Killer Cells)

NK activity appears to exist in normal subjects in all species studied, including man. NK activity appears to be attributable to lymphocytes of the "null" type (neither T nor B). Its mechanism is arguable. For some, it is identical with ADCC and therefore mediated by antibodies and K cells, whereas, for others, it is an entirely different phenomenon. The first hypothesis would be connected with the relationship of NK activity to circulating natural antibodies that might be capable of reacting with numerous tumor cells for unknown reasons. Some experimental studies have suggested a link between spontaneous

NK activity in certain mouse strains and their ability to reject tumor grafts. At present, no conclusions may be drawn as to the actual significance of this phenomenon in vivo. The apparent nonspecificity of NK reactions (for numerous syngeneic malignant cells, allogeneic malignant cells, and even xenogeneic cells) has placed in some doubt the fact that they play any role whatsoever. However, this nonspecificity may only be apparent because of the coexistence of multiple NK populations that recognize different antigens. It should also be noted that, at present, NK activity is a phenomenon that is mainly described in in vitro systems in which artifacts associated with the culture conditions may not always be excluded. Recently, it has been demonstrated that interferon can stimulate NK cell activity. NK cells might therefore, by this mechanism, play an efficient role in immunosurveillance against malignant cells and cells infected by viruses.

In conclusion, data concerning the NK phenomenon are still somewhat fragmentary. Its intervention in antitumor defence may be important, but it still remains to be established with certainty in both experimental systems and in man.

## GENETIC CONTROL OF THE IMMUNE RESPONSE

It is known that most immune responses are genetically controlled (see Chapter 24). Such genetic control has been observed for several antitumor immune responses. The genes that control the immune response to certain experimental leukemias have been identified in the mouse. At least one such gene is located in the major histocompatibility complex (H-2), more precisely the I region of the H-2 complex, alongside most other immune response genes (see p. 000). Their mode of action is not well understood; they may contribute to antibody synthesis, cell-mediated immunity, or both, or may even, in some cases, affect antigen expression. They appear to have a significant role in the onset of spontaneous mouse leukemias; however, control of this disease is polygenic, and regulatory mechanisms are not all immunologic. In mouse leukemias, the gene that controls the immune response is less important than are the genes that control relationships between host and virus at the cellular level. Recently, it has been shown in mice that the T-killer cells reacting with virus-induced tumor antigens of the tumor cell surface recognize, in fact, a complex antigen involving a viral product and a H-2 antigen. The determining antigen for cell-mediated reaction could be an "H-2 modified" specificity (see p. 87). Therefore the role of normal histocompatibility antigens could be decisive in immunosurveillance, their alteration by virus products allowing the recognition of the tumor cell and its elimination.

## TUMOR ESCAPE FROM IMMUNOLOGIC CONTROL

### Total Absence of Antigenicity

Most likely, the hypothesis implicating total absence of antigenicity is rarely applicable since most experimental tumors bear antigens whose role in rejection is probably weak but not necessarily nil. One might imagine that some animals possess a genetic formula that does not permit recognition of certain tumor antigens; thus, it is possible that some tumors have no immunogenicity for their host. Moreover, it is conceivable that no protective mechanism has been selected during evolution, for example, in the case of the antigens on chemically-induced tumors that are not found in the natural state. In contrast, total absence of antigenicity is apparently not exceptional for spontaneous tumors, differentiation antigens having no reason to be recognized by the autologus host.

### Antigenic Modulation

Antigenic modulation is observed with certain membrane antigens, such as TL antigen. These antigens disappear from the cell surface in the presence of specific antibody; thereafter, the cell resists the action of antibodies, and cell growth proceeds. This phenomenon is undoubtedly rare and cannot serve as the basis of a general model of tumor escape from immune reactions. It does, however, explain why some surface antigens are not TATA.

### Blocking of Immunologic Reactions

Blocking of immune reactions by circulating factors seems to be less important than was initially thought several years ago. Target cell blocking by antitumor antibody, which prevents access of effector cells to target cells, seems unlikely, because the antibody titer seen in vivo is always weak. Blocking of antitumor reactivity by antigen-antibody complexes is probably more significant, especially for K-cell reactions; but the significance of these reactions in vivo remains unclear. In addition, all studies of in vivo experimental systems that have attempted to recognize a role of blocking factors have shown disappointing results.

### Weak Tumor Antigens and Delayed Onset of Reaction

The two phenomena, weak tumor antigens and delayed onset of reaction, most often seem to be associated. If antigens are weak and consequently induce a slow and weak reaction or if antigens are strong but the reaction is delayed, the net result may be identical: by the time that rejection effector cells are present in sufficient quantity, the number of malignant cells will be too great for effective rejection. Several mechanisms may favor this escape from immunosurveillance: progressive immunoselection of less immunogenic cells during the regular elimination of malignant clones by means of immunosurveillance, transient or prolonged immunodepression of the host, localization of tumor cells at sites of poor accessibility (e.g., the thymus or bone marrow for hematopoietic cells), and intervention of a factor secreted by some cells of transplanted experimental tumors (e.g., trophoblastic cells) that may inhibit macrophage migration to the tumor focus, and possibly exert a toxic effect on macrophages. Such a factor might delay recognition of malignant cells by macrophages, thus delaying the onset of the immunologic reactions.

### Facilitation Reaction

A facilitation reaction is also possible. Some experiments seem to indicate that a very weak immune response may accelerate development of malignant cells. The mechanism of such facilitation is not well known, but its existence is likely.

On the whole, no conclusion can be drawn. However, one can say that (1) viral tumors are generally antigenic, and (perhaps for this reason) occur infrequently in man; (2) chemically induced tumors are sometimes but not always antigenic; and (3) spontaneous tumors are generally very weakly antigenic and probably easily escape immunologic control, if it exists.

# IV.  IMMUNOTHERAPY

## PASSIVE IMMUNOTHERAPY

Either antibodies or lymphoid cells sensitized to the tumor may be transferred to a tumor carrier.

Transfer of sensitized lymphoid cells between animals of the same pure strain may protect a previously immunosuppressed recipient against a tumor graft. However, rejection of a previously established and developing tumor is much more difficult. Immunotherapy of this type is limited in man by histocompatibility differences, and passive immunotherapy probably has no therapeutic usefulness. However, cell transfer between homozygous twins or bone marrow grafting is theoretically possible.

Passive antibody transfer in animals is not very efficient. In man, its usefulness is especially limited because of the existence of antibodies directed against the normal antigens of the recipient when the serum is prepared in another species. These limitations explain why passive immunotherapy has usually been abandoned in humans.

## ACTIVE IMMUNOTHERAPY

### Specific Active Immunotherapy

A subject may be immunized against his own tumor cells, which were previously homogenized or inactivated. The patient may also be immunized with tumor cells obtained from another subject. This technique presupposes that a common antigen on the tumor is able to trigger rejection. This hypothesis is unlikely for most human tumors but it can not always be excluded. Since the immune responses are probably at best very weak, the value of such therapy in subjects with developed tumors is unlikely; on the contrary, it may have an application for subjects who previously underwent surgical, x-ray, or chemical treatment that reduced the number of tumor cells. In experimental systems, documented protection is seen mainly in animals free of tumors (prophylaxis). Immunotherapy may, however, be logical in man as adjunctive treatment. In clinical practice, its application together with most conventional therapy seems illogical since the latter are immunosuppressive. This paradox raises ethical problems in deciding on maintenance chemotherapy, which may be effective in maintaining remissions, whereas the role of immunotherapy has not been established. Clinical trials have been performed by different groups after stopping conventional treatments but their results are still controversial.

### Nonspecific Active Immunotherapy

Enhancement of the level of host immune reactions should permit better antitumor control. Animals that receive adjuvants, such as BCG (Bacillus Calmette-Guérin) are often more resistant to tumor cell implantation. The role of these adjuvants in the rejection of established tumors is, however, difficult to assess. Antitumor protection and, conversely, growth facilitation have been observed accordingly, and the determining factor is still very much uncertain. In clinical practice, nonspecific BCG immunotherapy has been extensively applied to many malignant diseases. Its practical value is the subject of rather heated debate, which indicates that in light of our present knowledge, results are difficult to evaluate.

The association of specific and nonspecific immunotherapy is in theory the best means of stimulating antitumor immunity in patients and is presently most often utilized. Prolongation of remissions in malignant hematopoietic and solid tumors has been reported, but the overall significance of these results is as yet difficult to assess.

## THE PLACE OF IMMUNOTHERAPY IN TUMOR TREATMENT

Nonspecific preventive immunotherapy is not possible because it would necessitate the use of immunotherapeutic adjuvants applied for many years to thousands of individuals to provide statistically valid information. Specific preventive immunotherapy is thwarted by the multiplicity of antigens involved in both human and animal tumors. Nonspecific curative immunotherapy or the association of specific and nonspecific immunotherapy may provide an additional therapeutic weapon against certain human tumors in remission, but the real value of its contribution has not been established. Experiments in progress are necessarily performed in an empiric way. They must be executed under rigorous conditions so that future interpretation may be facilitated. At present, immunotherapy is still essentially experimental. The prognosis of malignant tumors has apparently not been drastically modified.

## BIBLIOGRAPHY

ALEXANDER P. Foetal antigens in cancer. Nature (Lond.), 1972, 235, 137.

BALDWIN R. W., BOWEN J. G., EMBLETON M. J., PRICE M. R., and ROBINS R. A. Cellular and humoral immune response to neoantigens associated with chemically-induced tumours. In L. Brent and J. Holborow, Eds., Progress in immunology. II. Vol. 3. Amsterdam, 1974, North Holland, p. 239.

BAUER B. Virion and tumor cell antigens of C type RNA tumor viruses. Adv. Cancer Res., 1974, 20, 275.

DORE J. F. and KOURILSKY F. M. Human leukemia associated antigens and immune reaction (a review). In Present problems in haematology. Amsterdam, 1974, Excerpta Medica, p. 59.

FAHEY J. L. and ZIGHELBOIM J. Tumor immunology. In: Clinical Immunology (Parker C. W. [ed]). Suanders. Philadelphia, 1980:445.

GOLD P. Embryonic origin of human tumor specific antigens. Progr. Exp. Tumor Res., 1971, *14*, 43.

HELLSTRÖM K. E. and HELLSTRÖM I. Cellular immunity against•tumor antigens. Adv. Cancer Res., 1969, *12*, 167.

HERBERMAN R. B. Cell-mediated immunity to tumor cells. Adv. Cancer Res., *19*, 207.

HERBERMAN R. B. Tests for tumor associated antigens and their clinical value. In: Clinical Immunology Update. Elsevier, New York, 1979, 23.

HERBERMAN R. B. [Ed]. Natural cell mediated immunity against tumors. Acad. Press, New York, 1980, 1360 p.

HERBERMAN R. B., TIMONEN T., ORTALDO J. R., BONNARD G. D., and GORELIK E. Natural cell-mediated cytotoxicity. In: Immunology 80 (M. Fougereau and J. Dausset [ed]). Acad. Press, New York, 1980, 691.

ITO Y. Immunology of DNA virus induced tumours. In: Immunology 80 (M. Fougereau and J, Dausset [eds]). Acad. Press, New York, 1980, 668.

KLEIN G. The Epstein-Barr virus. *In* A. S. Kaplan, Ed., The Herpes viruses. New York, London, 1973, Academic Press, p. 521.

KLEIN G. Tumor immunology. Transpl. Proc., 1973, *5*, 31.

KLEIN G. Immunological surveillance against neoplasia. Harvey lecture (N. Y., Academic Press), 1975, *59*, 71.

LAMON E. W. The immune response to virally determined tumor associated antigens. Biochem. Biophys. Acta, 1974, *355*, 149.

LENNOX E. S. The antigens of chemically induced tumours. In: Immunology 80 (M. Fougereau and J. Dausset [eds]). Acad. Press New York, 1980, 659.

LEVY J. P. Antigens associated with C type RNA virus induced tumors. *In* L. Brent and J. Holborow, Eds., Progress in immunology. II. Vol. 3. Amsterdam, 1974, North Holland, p. 249–259.

LEVY J. P. and LECLERC J. C. The murine sarcoma virus induced tumor: exception or general model in tumor immunology. Adv. Cancer Res., 1977, *24*, 1.

MARTZ E. Mechanism of specific tumor cell lysis by alloimmune T lymphocytes; resolution and characterization of discrete steps in the cellular interaction. In: Contemp. Topics Immunobiology. Plenum, N. Y. 1977:301.

MITCHISON N. A. and KINLEN L. J. Present concepts in immune surveillance. In: Immunology 80 (M. Fougereau and J. Dausset [eds]). Acad. Press, New York, 1980, 641.

MÖLLER G. (Ed.) Tumor associated embryonic antigens. Transpl. Rev., 1974, *20*.

MÖLLER G. (Ed) Experiments and the concept of immunological surveillance. Transpl. Rev., 1976, *26*.

MÖLLER G. (Ed) Natural killer cells. Immunol. Rev., 1979, 44.

PREHN R. T. Immunological surveillance: pro and con. Clin. Immunobiol., 1974, *2*, 191.

PREHN R. T. Immunomodulation of tumor growth. Amer. J. Pathol., 1974, *77*, 119.

RIETHMULLER G., WERNET P., and CUDKOWICZ G. Natural and induced cell mediated cytotoxicity. Acad. Press., New York, 1979, 242 p.

ROSENBERG S. A. [Ed]. Serologic analysis of human cancer antigens. Acad. Press, New York, 1979, 712 p.

SOUTHAM C. M. and FRIEDMAN H. (Eds.) International Conference on Immunotherapy of Cancer. Ann. N.Y. Acad. Sci., 1976, 277.

SPREAFICO F. and ARNON R. [Eds]. Tumor associated antigens and their specific immune responses. Acad. Press, New York, 1979, 359 p.

WESTON B. J. The thymus and immune surveillance. Contemp. Topics Immunobiol., 1973, *2*, 237.

# Chapter 15

# NONSPECIFIC IMMUNITY

## Robert M. Fauve

I. DEFINITION
II. FACTORS IMPLICATED IN NONSPECIFIC IMMUNITY
III. MODIFICATIONS OF NONSPECIFIC IMMUNITY

## I. DEFINITION

Immunity refers to the ability of an organism to repel certain pathogens (Littré). Immunity is considered nonspecific when it develops in the absence of prior contact with the antigen(s) specific for the pathogenic agent.

This "built-in" resistance provides the organism with the ability to resist most microorganisms with which it is in continuous contact. Unfortunately, nonspecific, sometimes called natural, resistance is not effective against some particularly virulent pathogens. The latter may only be eliminated if the organism develops specific immunity or increased levels of nonspecific immunity. Conversely, the virulence of certain pathogens may be enhanced when the level of specific or nonspecific immunity is decreased. Nonspecific immunity may be either decreased or enhanced after treatment with substances that have no common antigenic determinants with the pathogen against which immunity is directed.

We shall examine various factors responsible for nonspecific immunity. Most of this knowledge derives from studies of experimental bacterial infections. However, the same mechanisms are very often involved in the defense against viruses, bacteria, parasites, and even, occasionally, tumor cells.

## II. FACTORS IMPLICATED IN NONSPECIFIC IMMUNITY

To infect a living organism, a pathogenic agent crosses anatomic barriers that oppose penetration. Infection results in disease when the agent survives and multiplies despite various humoral and cellular defenses.

## ANATOMIC BARRIERS

Anatomic barriers are contained in skin and mucosae. The cutaneous and mucosal layers are continuously coated by secretion products of glandular cells. Thus, protection is both mechanical and chemical.

### Mechanical Protection

It is generally believed that because of intercellular juxtaposition, the skin is impermeable to infectious agents. In fact, certain viruses and bacteria are capable of passively crossing such barriers. In addition, some parasites (ankylostomes, furcocercariae) are capable of moving actively between skin cells. The mucosal cell barrier is coated by a film of mucus. The mucous film in the upper respiratory tract is propelled toward the digestive tract by motile filaments (cilia).

### Chemical Protection

In the skin, sweat is an important defense mechanism, due both to its acidity (lactic acid) and its high content of fatty acids, of which the bactericidal and parasiticidal role has been well demonstrated. A deficiency in certain fatty acids (oleic and undecylic acids) explains infection by *Microsporum audouini*; localization in the plantar aspect of the foot of certain mycoses is due to the paucity of sebaceous glands in this area. One should also note that the bactericidal effect of these fatty acids develops only if skin humidity is not excessive. The mucosae of the respiratory, digestive, and genital tracts are also replete with bactericidal and virulicidal activities linked to lysozyme, mucoprotein, and other substances.

Lysozyme is a basic protein that is a mucolytic enzyme. It acts by separating N-acetylglucosamine and N-acetylmuramic acid in mucopeptide complexes of the bacterial wall. In the presence of lysozyme, some bacteria are lysed, whereas others are killed without overt lysis. Lysozyme is also present in conjunctival, nasal, and salivary secretions and thus plays an important role in defending the organism against many saprophytic bacteria. However, there is only weak bactericidal activity against more virulent bacteria, even when IgA potentiates its action. The virulicidal action of mucoproteins occurs not only in mucus but also in plasma and urine. Their activity is very intense toward certain myxoviruses, particularly influenza. The viruses bind to cells after combination with a mucolytic enzyme or neuraminidase located on cellular mucopolysaccharidic receptors. Neuraminidase splits the link between the terminal group of N-acetylmuramic acid and internal constituents of the cell surface. Under these conditions, mucoproteins in the secretions of the infected host serve as a substrate for the viral enzyme, thus preventing virions from binding to normally sensitive receptors of the cells.

Gastric hydrochloric acid has a very important bactericidal effect. Patients who undergo gastrectomy or are achlorhydric are less resistant to bacterial intestinal infections. The anti-infectious role of urinary and vaginal mucosal acidity has long been known. In the latter organ, this acidity is due to lactic acid that originates from glycogen degradation caused by *Döderlein's bacillus*. The specific role of intestinal bacteria is not well established, but there seems to be a definite protective role. For example, massive ingestion by guinea pigs of *Shigella dysenteriae* usually has no consequence. Conversely, axenic guinea pigs (bacteriologically sterile) develop fatal infections. The protection is due to bacterial growth inhibition in the presence of other bacteria (by means of toxic substances, colicins, nutritional competition), but there is also a direct action of bacterial metabolites on the intestinal mucosa that protects the organism against invasion by intestinal bacteria. Interestingly, axenic animals present hypoplastic lymphoid organs, the role of which is essential in specific and nonspecific immunity. In this context, we shall recall the complications of moniliasis and staphylococcal enteritis that occur after the administration of broad-spectrum antibiotics. All mucous secretions contain serum constituents that have anti-infectious activity, despite their usual low concentration. These materials are also found in variable concentrations in extracellular spaces of all organs. Cells of most tissues are contained within a network of collagen and elastic fibers, which are embedded in a gel of hyaluronic acid-rich mucopolysacharide. This viscous gel impedes the mobility of infectious agents (hyaluronidase produced by certain bacteria or parasites has, therefore, a role in spreading infections). The low pH of these extracellular spaces is also protective, as is their low oxygen tension. High oxygen levels in the alveoli seem to relate to localization of tubercle bacilli. Conversely, a sudden decrease in oxygen content causes germination of anaerobic bacillary spores. A dramatic example of this phenomenon is the appearance of localized tetanus after reinjury to an old wound secondary to transient, local anaerobiosis.

## HUMORAL DEFENSES

Independent of disease, there are several substances in mammalian serum that play an important role in immunity. These substances include complement, lysozyme, and interferon, in addition to less well-defined substances, such as basic polypeptides, nonspecific opsonins, β-lysin and C-reactive protein.

### Complement

Complement consists of a set of cofactors present in normal serum that are necessary for expression of antibody activity. These cofactors (discussed in chap. 8) are by themselves inactive. However, when complement binds to antigen-antibody complexes, lysis of animal or bacterial cells may occur. Similarly, complement is implicated in the ingestion phase of phagocytosis, in anaphylactoxinic reactions, in polymorph chemotaxis, and in immunoadherence and conglutination reactions. Thus, complement plays an important role in many immune reactions. One might think that complement deficiencies would be associated with altered defense mechanisms against infections. It is surprising that animals with selective complement factor deficiencies survive normally and often show normal resistance to bacterial infection (see p. 279).

### Lysozyme

Lysozyme will be discussed in the next chapter. It should be mentioned that only very few pathogenic bacteria are sensitive to its action.

### *Interferon*

For many years, it has been known that a virus-infected animal is able to resist a subsequent infection by a second virus unrelated to the first one. This phenomenon represents viral interference. It was established that interference could be induced even when the first virus was made noninfectious by heating or ultraviolet rays. In 1957, Isaacs and Lindenmann demonstrated that chicken embryos exposed to inactivated influenza virus contain a cell-free extract that prevents viral multiplication in chorioallantoic membranes. This antiviral factor, "interferon," is a glycoprotein of variable molecular weight, depending on the conditions under which it is obtained. The entire antiviral activity is destroyed by proteolytic enzymes but is retained despite heating and acid treatment. Interferon has recently been obtained in its pure state (De Maeyer) and its amino-acids sequence has been determined after its gene has been cloned in bacteria.

Interferon is synthesized within cells soon after viral infection. In fact, metabolic inhibitors, such as actinomycin D, which blocks RNA synthesis, and puromycin, which blocks protein synthesis, prevent cellular synthesis of interferon. Interferon is species specific. Synthesis is very rapid; when a mouse is infected with influenza virus, interferon appears in the serum within a few hours, persists at high concentration for 3 days and disappears about the seventh day, at a time when antibody synthesis has become maximum. The amount of virus in the lungs begins to decrease when interferon synthesis is maximum. The preponderant role of interferon in primary viral infections is well illustrated by the findings that irradiated animals are capable of resisting certain viral infections despite depressed antibody synthesis. RNA viruses (arbovirus, myxovirus, paramyxovirus, picornavirus, and reovirus) are not the only in vivo and in vitro inducers of interferon. DNA viruses, such as those of the pox, herpes, papova and adeno groups, and, under certain conditions, gram-negative or positive bacteria, rickettsia, and certain parasites, may also induce interferon synthesis. Extracts of microorganisms that contain endotoxin, tuberculin, and some ribonucleotides may also induce its synthesis. Similarly, in the presence of certain antigens, sensitized T lymphocytes produce an interferon, described as type II interferon, which has a molecular weight different from that produced by virus-infected cells.* The mechanism of action of interferon has not yet been elucidated; however, immediately after penetration of interferon inside the cell, viral multiplication stops. Interferon does not protect chicken embryo cells from viral infections during the first third of embryonic life. If this is also true for mammals, it might explain the appearance of fetal malformations only during the first trimester of pregnancy. If protein synthesis is blocked, interferon action ceases. For this reason, it is proposed that interferon causes synthesis of a protein that in itself is antiviral: translation-inhibitory protein (TIP). TIP may prevent synthesis of various constituents of virions. Recently, the use of highly purified interferon preparations has shown that the spectrum of activity of interferon extends beyond resistance to viral infection. For example, when an

---

* According to a recent terminology, based on the autigenicity of the various types of interferon, type-I interferon is called Interferon α (IFN-α) or β (IFN-β) depending on its leukocyte or fibroblast origin, and type-II (immune) Interferon is called Interferon γ (IFN-γ).

animal is treated with large amounts of interferon, resistance to certain tumors is increased. In addition, it has recently been shown that interferon can influence immunologic reactions, such as graft immunity.

### Basic Proteins

β-lysin should be distinguished from other substances less well defined, including certain basic polypeptides. β-lysin is a cationic protein with a molecular weight of 6000 that is contained in platelets. It is thermostable and acts on gram-positive bacteria, as a cationic detergent, to lyse the cell membrane. Its action on many gram-positive bacteria is certain, but it has no action against many virulent bacteria, including *Listeria monocytogenes* and smooth pneumococci.

Independent of these essential factors, a bactericidal action of less well-defined substances has been reported. In certain inflammatory conditions or in response to nonspecific immunostimulation, other humoral factors may appear, the action of which has not yet been elucidated.

## CELLULAR DEFENSES

When an infectious agent crosses a mucocutaneous barrier and resists physicochemical conditions opposed to its survival, it next comes into contact with a certain number of cells (phagocytic cells) whose main function is its destruction. Phagocytic cells have already been more completely described in chapter 5. In this chapter, we will only briefly summarize their properties. Phagocytic cells are mainly polymorphs, monocytes, and macrophages. They derive from the bone marrow and penetrate, by diapedesis, into the extravascular spaces. Their main function is phagocytic, but they also metabolize numerous substances. Phagocytic cells adhere to inert or living particles and then ingest them. The particles may be digested but, on the other hand, some virulent infectious agents may multiply within phagocytes. In an apparently healthy mammal, no polymorphs and very few macrophages are present in extravascular spaces. Macrophages are found chiefly in spleen, liver, lymph nodes, lungs, bone marrow, and adrenal glands. However, if an organ is traumatized by introduction of a foreign body or infection, a series of reactions eventually results in the onset of an inflammatory reaction during which leukocytes congregate at the site of aggression. At the same time, the inflammatory reaction induces not only local changes in the whole organism but also alterations that lead to enhancement of nonspecific immune reactions. Independent of inflammation, other factors may change nonspecific immunity. These factors include sex, age, genetic makeup, and suppression or stimulation of the immune system.

## III.   MODIFICATIONS OF NONSPECIFIC IMMUNITY

## INFLAMMATION

Originally defined by this term because of the cardinal signs of erythema, edema, pain, and localized warmth, inflammation actually represents the organism's response to various insults through multiple neurologic, vascular, humoral, and cellular mechanisms. The complexity and interrelationships of these factors make it difficult to summarize the cascade of events that constitute the inflammatory reaction (Table 15.1). We will first schematically describe the inflammatory process and will then give details about certain aspects, particularly those that relate to immune responses.

Tissue injury by trauma, infectious agents, injected substances, increased temperature, and radiation initially induces vasodilatation, which is followed rapidly by increased vascular permeability. The latter effect is often associated with morphologic changes in capillary endothelial cells. These changes result in platelet adhesion and aggregation and in leukocytic adhesion at the site of cellular alteration. Platelet aggregation coincides with the onset of activation of various steps in blood coagulation that release mediators that participate in the inflammatory reaction. After adherence occurs, leukocytes pass through vessel walls into extravascular spaces (diapedesis). Leukocytes (especially polymorphs and, later, monocytes and lymphocytes) are directed to the attracted tissue or the irritant by chemotactic factors. Within the extravascular space, polymorphs release the by-products of their metabolism or their lysis, which, in turn, releases enzymes that induce mastocytic degranulation, with subsequent release of new mediators. Monocytes also leave the vessel to phagocytose cellular debris and to transform into macrophages. Products of macrophage metabolism or cell lysis thus reinforce the inflammatory reaction. Unlike polymorphs and monocytes, very few lymphocytes are found in inflammatory foci, except in peculiar situations. Paralleling leukocyte diapedesis, an exudation of plasma occurs that contributes to edema and brings various materials to the inflammation site, particularly coagulation factors and complement components, which both enhance inflammation. Accumulation at the site of the inflammatory focus of serum components, phagocytic cells, and certain mediators induces an alteration in the lymphoid system that permits entry into the circulation of substances that will act on antibody-forming organs and cells implicated in specific or nonspecific immune reactions. All these various events define the acute inflammatory reaction. Later, macrophages ingest the inflammatory agent and also eliminate cellular debris. The healing phase consists of fibroblast proliferation and collagen synthesis. If the causal agent is not easily resorbed, the role of macrophages is essential, but under certain conditions (infection by bacteria), lymphoid cells may also intervene. The transition from acute to chronic inflammation is most marked when inflammation is induced by foreign, poorly resorbed substances like adjuvants (used in immunization; see chap. 33). These substances include calcium or aluminum phosphates, mineral oil, and mixtures of mineral oil and mycobacteria (Freund's complete adjuvant). We shall now examine, in the order of their appearance, the various factors implicated in inflammation (see Table 15.1).

### Experimental Models

There are many models of experimental inflammation. In fact, any agent that alters tissue homeostasis induces an inflammatory reaction. The resultant inflammatory reaction may be directly observed in the living animal or by examining the tissue (biopsy) in which inflammation has been produced.

**Table 15.1 Inflammation Mechanisms**

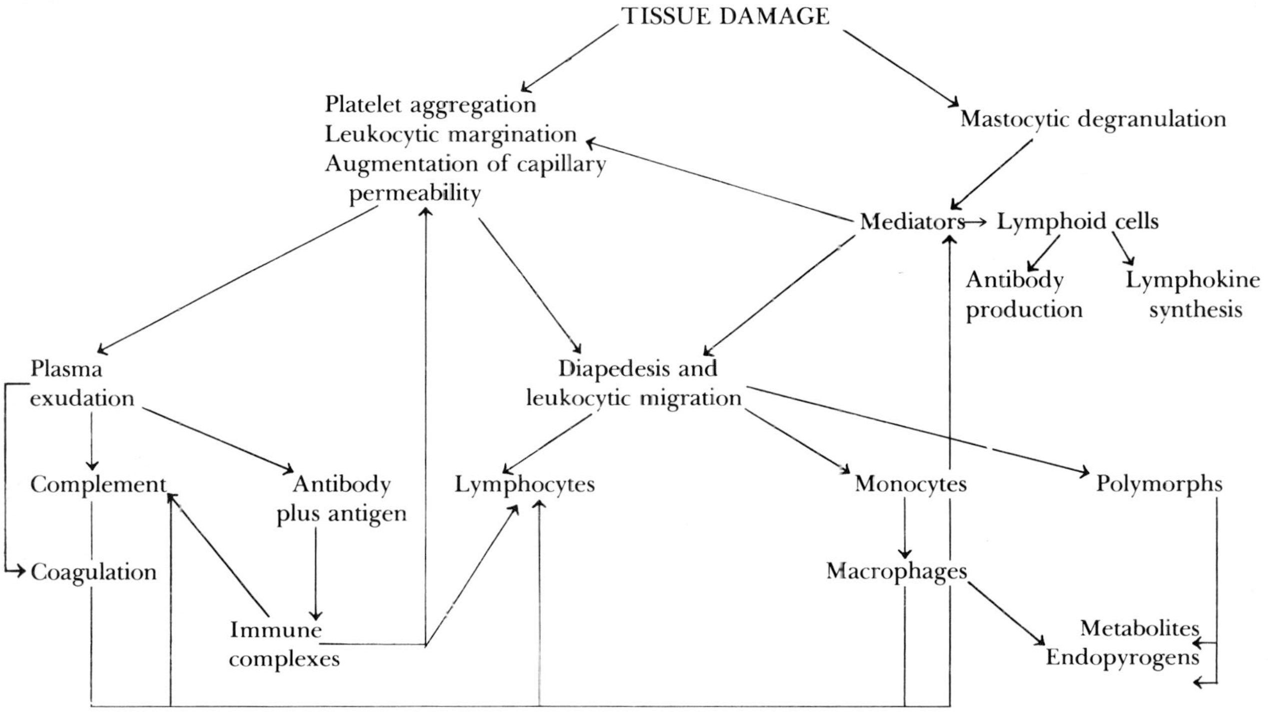

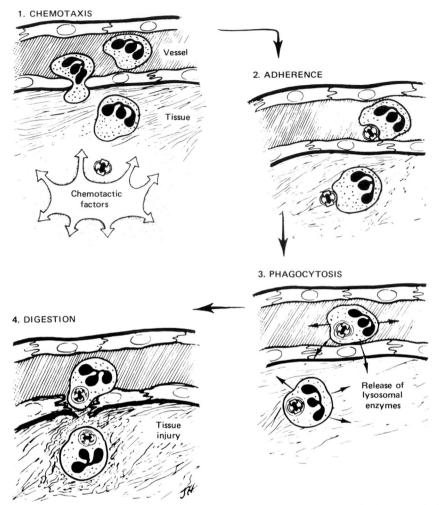

**Fig. 15.1**  Polymorph chemotaxis by an immune complex. Tissue lesions are induced by the release of lysosomal enzymes. (From J. A. Bellanti, Immunobiology, Philadelphia, 1971, Saunders, p. 233.)

In the living animal, the inflammatory reaction may be observed by use of a special apparatus like the Clark chamber. This chamber consists of two transparent plates fixed onto both sides of a perforation in a rabbit's ear. It is possible to observe, microscopically, changes in the connective tissue and vasculature. If the tissue under study is then altered, it is possible to follow the different phases of the inflammatory reaction and thus study the effect of various drugs. Algire's chamber, which is used in the mouse, is based on a similar principle. Other techniques allow evaluation of the intensity of edema and vascular permeability after induction of an inflammatory reaction (heat or injection of irritating substances) in mouse or rat paws by measuring the thickness of the paw as a function of time. It is also possible to quantitate plasma exudation into a skin inflammation by injecting certain stains that bind to albumin. During inflammation, stained albumin can be detected in the exudate, and the diameter of the inflammed area is an index of capillary permeability.

At necropsy, it is possible to collect tissue for histochemistry. One may also, in the mouse, measure the intensity of diapedesis by enumerating and examining the leukocytes that appear in the peritoneal cavity after injection of various inflammatory substances (peptone, glycogen, mineral oil). To study chronic inflammation, one may use nonabsorbable foreign bodies that are inserted subcutaneously and induce and inflammatory granuloma, which is then studied by use of histologic and biochemical techniques.

### Platelet Aggregation and Coagulation

Even minimal tissue alteration induces in nearby capillaries platelet adhesion to the capillary endothelium. This adhesion requires thrombin and divalent calcium ions. Adenosine diphosphate release by these platelets promotes adhesion of other platelets that aggregate and cause leukocyte adhesion. At this point in time, the platelets release serotonin. Platelet thrombus formation produces local coagulation. If thrombin is present, fibrinogen is transformed into fibrin. During these successive phases, some coagulation factors intervene in the inflammatory reaction. Thus, Hageman's factor, activated by blood contact with affected vessels, in turn, activates the kinin-forming system and increases leukocytic adhesion. Thrombin, a proteolytic enzyme with a molecular weight of 30,000, is also involved in particular at the platelet level, by stimulating mediator (serotonin) release. Fibrin has a chemotactic role. The plasminogen-plasmin fibrinolytic system acts (through plasmin) on $\alpha_2$-globulins to produce other mediators, especially kinins.

### Leukocyte Margination (Leukocyte Adhesion)

Soon after platelet aggregation, leukocytes adhere to vascular walls. Margination is enhanced in the presence of fibrin deposits. This phenomenon is not necessarily linked to increased capillary permeability. Once fixed onto endothelial cells, leukocytes (especially polymorphs) and, in lesser numbers, monocytes and lymphocytes may penetrate vessels if the inflammation is severe enough (diapedesis).

### Increase in Capillary Permeability

Capillaries are composed of endothelial cells tightly linked together by desmosomes. Capillary endothelial cells are surrounded by a basement membrane. Capillary permeability is increased by the contraction of endothelial cells caused by certain tissue factors, specific antigens, and, most importantly, mediators like bradykinin, histamine, and serotonin. The kinetics of increased capillary permeability vary according to species, site of activity (tissue), and type of inflammation. Increased vascular permeability induces (plasma) exudation, diapedesis, and extravascular migration of leukocytes.

EXUDATION

Plasma exudation causes the appearance of numerous substances within the extravascular space. These substances include antibodies, bactericidal substances, coagulation factors, and complement components, which also act to perpetuate the inflammatory reaction. Antibodies, in the presence of their corresponding antigen and complement, exert a chemotactic action on lymphocytes and, in addition, increase vascular permeability. Bactericidal substances lead to lysis and provoke phagocytic stimulation, with release of some bacterial products with probable chemotactic and vasodilatory actions. The importance of coagulation factors has already been emphasized. Complement components intervene at several levels. Complement activation may be induced by antigen-antibody complexes, by fixation of C-reactive protein (CRP) on a number of substrates or by a direct action of plasmin on the C3 component of complement. In the latter case, plasmin detaches a C3 fragment (C3a) that has anaphylatoxinic properties. The trimolecular complex (C5, C6, and C7) produced after the interaction of C1, C4, C2, and C3 has an important chemotactic effect on phagocytic cells.

LEUKOCYTE DIAPEDESIS AND MIGRATION

We have seen that at the beginning of inflammation, leukocytes adhere to vessels. Polymorphs, monocytes, and lymphocytes penetrate between endothelial cells to perforate the basement membrane and enter the extravascular space. The special nature of the extracellular space (collagen and elastic fibers plus mucopolysaccharides) favors cell movement. When leaving the vessels, leukocytes do not show any preferential migration. However, the presence of immune complexes, cellular debris, polymorphs, and monocytes appears to attract them. It is important to note that the relative proportions of neutrophils, basophils, eosinophils, monocytes, and lymphocytes vary according to the nature of the inflammatory agent. For example, some parasites induce a selective migration of eosinophilic polymorphs, which also appear in the inflammatory foci in the course of allergic reactions. As a consequence, numerous metabolites are produced, and variations in antigen and immune complex uptake and in endopyrogen and mediator release are seen. Metabolic products of leukocytes, especially phagocytic cells, cause a fall in local pH, largely due to the production of lactic acid by leukocytic glycolysis; antigen and immune complexes are preferentially taken up by certain polymorphs, especially eosinophils and macrophages. Macrophages originate from the monocyte transformation that occurs after diapedesis. Antigen uptake is particularly important for particulate antigens (cells, bacteria, parasites). Phagocytic cells degrade and extract antigenic determinants, which then directly stimulate antibody synthesis. During phagocytosis or lysis, polymorphs, monocytes, and macrophages may release endopyrogens. These substances, which have a molecular weight between $10^4$ and $2 \times 10^4$, are proteins. Very low concentrations are effective: levels of 30 to 50 ng exert intense pyrogenicity in the rabbit. These substances are not produced by lymphocytes. Leukocytes release other mediators, including vasoactive amines, proteases or migration-inhibitory factor, which we shall now examine.

### Inflammation Mediators

Inflammation mediators include vasoactive amines, polypeptides, and other substances.

### VASOACTIVE AMINES

Histamine is present in all tissues, with higher concentrations in tissues rich in mastocytes. Histamine is present in the granules of mastocytes, together with serotonin and heparin. Histamine release from mastocytic granules is provoked by proteolytic enzymes, macromolecular substances like dextran, basic compounds (48/80), denaturing agents, heat, decreased pH, and in the presence of antibody-antigen reactions. Histamine is a vasodilator and thus increases capillary permeability. In addition, histamine augments in vitro ingestion by phagocytic cells, particularly by neutrophil polymorphs.

Widely distributed in animals and vegetables, 5-hydroxytryptamine is found chiefly in mammalian mastocytes and platelets and is a strong vasodilator.

### PROTEASES

The inflammation mediator enzymes include plasmin, kallikrein, and a globulin permeability factor.

### POLYPEPTIDES

Two polypeptides are particularly important in inflammation: a nonapeptide, bradykinin, and a decapeptide, kallidin. These peptides originate from a plasma globulin (kininogen) that is degraded by a protease, kallikrein, and have very important vasodilating effects.

### OTHER SUBSTANCES

Adenosine and adenylic acid may be released in burned patients. They also have a vasodilator effect on arterioles.

Hyaluronidase is found in increased concentration in inflammatory states, even in the absence of infection. Its vasomotor role is unclear, but by impairing viscosity, hyaluronidase enhances leukocytic movement.

Lactic acid, produced by polymorphs and macrophages, provokes capillary vasodilatation.

Prostaglandins were initially isolated from seminal fluid. They derive from prostanoic acid (Fig. 15.2c), which itself derives from fatty acids. Several prostaglandin species have been identified, all derivatives of prostanoic acid. Prostaglandins are present in numerous tissues, especially in human platelets [prostaglandins $E_1$ and $E_2$ ($PGE_1$ and $PGE_2$)], which release them in response to thrombin deposition. $PGE_1$ and $PGE_2$ induce mastocytic degranulation and, therefore, histamine release. Possibly related to this action is evidence that intradermal injection of $PGE_1$ and $PGE_2$ augments capillary permeability by means of mediator release.

### FUNCTIONS OF MEDIATORS

Inflammation mediators exert focal and systemic actions.

It is well established that they produce localized vasodilation and increased capillary permeability. In addition to an effect on lymphatic vessels, they act directly on leukocytes. Thus, nucleotides may augment macrophage pinocytosis,

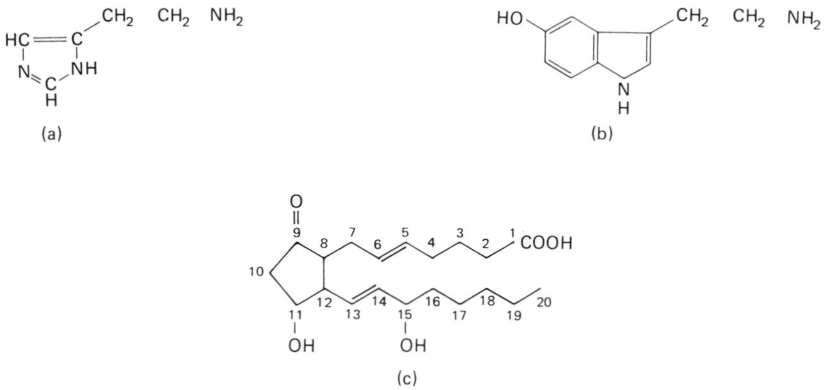

**Fig. 15.2**  Mediators of inflammation. (a) Histamine or β-iminazothylamine. (b) Serotonin or 5-hydroxytryptamine (5-HT). (c) Prostaglandins.

and certain concentrations of bradykinin increase the motility of polymorphs and especially, macrophages. Preliminary reports indicate that bradykinin may induce leukocyte division.

At a distance, mediators with pyrogenic action have an effect on bone marrow. It is known that the serum of a patient or animal undergoing an acute inflammatory reaction contains elevated levels of CSF (colony-stimulating factor), which is a substance capable of stimulating the growth of macrophage clones or polymorphonuclear clones in bone marrow. Finally, some of these mediators may act on the reticulohistiocytic system.

### Consequences of the Inflammatory Reaction

The consequences of the inflammatory reaction are obvious at the local level. They appear as a local increase in the concentrations of the humoral and cellular mediators of inflammation. At more distant sites, the effects are too numerous to detail here, and comments will be confined to the more important aspects.

Within hours of the induction of the inflammatory reaction an increase in the synthesis of several proteins of hepatic origin occurs, this being partly due to the effect of endopyrogens on the hypothalamic region. The proteins of the acute phase of the inflammatory reaction (acute-phase proteins) include orosomucoid, antitrypsin, ceruloplasmin, fibrinogen, haptoglobin, C3, and C-reactive protein (CRP). This latter protein, whose molecular weight varies between 115,000 and 145,000 (according to species), is of hepatic origin and consists of five subunits, whose sequence is known. Structure is similar to that of the P constituent of amyloid substance and Clt. Serum concentration may increase a thousandfold during inflammatory processes. CRP may induce the agglutination and precipitation of numerous substrates in a nonspecific manner and can stimulate phagocytosis. Similarly, it can activate complement by the classical pathway and may bind selectively to T lymphocytes and inhibit their function. Finally, CRP has been found to be capable of inhibiting the release of serotonin and β-glucuronidase from platelets by inhibiting platelet aggregation.

Recently, Fauve et al. investigated (in mice) the effects of a local inflammatory response provoked by nonbiodegradable, nonantigenic, nondiffusible irritants that were injected at a site distant from that of the introduction or multiplication of pathogenic agents. They found that mice so treated showed increased resistance toward *Salmonella typhimurium, Listeria monocytogenes, Yersinia pestis, Candida albicans, Schistosoma mansoni,* as well as against a very malignant mouse tumor, Lewis carcinoma. The same experimental observations were made in axenic mice and in thymus-deprived mice (nude). Considerable augmentation of the bactericidal activity of macrophages has been shown as well as a preferential differentiation of bone marrow stem cells toward leukocytes. It has also been possible to isolate from inflammatory granulomas a serum protein that, when injected into a mouse, totally protects it from a lethal inoculum of *L. monocytogenes.* In addition, it has been found that normal mouse macrophages become cytostatic for malignant cells when incubated in the presence of serum from a mouse undergoing an inflammatory response. These results prove that, at least in the mouse, following an inflammatory reaction, certain substances are released that show a significant stimulatory activity on the effectors of immune responses.

## AGE

Impaired defenses of the organism to infectious agents at the beginning of life are well established. Independent of the immaturity of acquired specific immunity, it is known that young animals show a lesser degree of inflammatory response than do adults. One such striking example is the negative Schick's reaction in young children. The reduced estrogen production may be responsible for the increased susceptibility of children to gonococcal vaginal infection. Estrogen lack explains the absence of glycogen in vaginal epithelial cells. Glycogen absence causes decreased lactic acid production and a consequent increase in vaginal pH, allowing proliferation of gonococci, which would not be possible at lower pH. Aged subjects also show less resistance to infection.

## SEX

It is usually stated that female animals exhibit more effective nonspecific immunity than do males, probably because of the stimulating effect of estrogens on reticulohistiocytic cells. However, sex differences are not so clear-cut in humans. Morbidity and mortality secondary to pertussis and infectious hepatitis are higher in women, whereas mortality from tuberculosis after 40 years of age is much greater in men. Similarly, syphilis is probably less severe in women.

## GENETIC FACTORS

By studying inbred mice and rats, it has been found that nonspecific resistance to infection is closely linked to genetic factors. It has even been possible to obtain selected rabbit and mouse strains that are either sensitive or resistant to tuberculosis or to murine typhoid fever. It has also been shown that in certain cases (toxoplasmosis, viral infections), resistance correlates with numbers of macrophages and with the ability of these cells to deal with infectious agents. The importance of genetic influences has been demonstrated in man. The relative resistance of white populations to tuberculosis is well known. Conversely, black people with sickle cell trait are much less sensitive to malarial infection than are whites. It is now known that falciform red blood cells contain an abnormal hemoglobin that is not suitable for parasites.

## NUTRITIONAL FACTORS

In animals, various nutritional deficiencies have unfavorable effects on inflammatory reactions and on phagocytic cells. These effects are best established for deficiency states that involve essential amino acids and vitamins B and C. In vitamin C deficiency, the bactericidal action of phagocytic cells is impaired. Guinea pigs similarly deficient show impaired inflammatory granuloma at the site of mycobacteria injection. There are numerous other examples. Particularly interesting is the contribution of folic acid, in the rat and monkey, to normal granulopoiesis.

## FACTORS THAT DECREASE NONSPECIFIC IMMUNITY

A rupture in anatomic barriers allows easier penetration of infectious agents. Such a rupture occurs, for example, after trauma. Irradiation, alters the intestinal mucosa and permits passage of massive numbers of intestinal bacteria into the blood. Similarly, the alterations of ciliated respiratory cells secondary to the administration of anesthetics increase the risk of infection. Also, increased bronchial secretions and stasis favor multiplication of infectious agents.

Diminished or inhibited inflammatory reactions lead to a considerable decrease in nonspecific immunity, as is seen after administration of various anti-inflammatory substances (such as cortisone) and immunosuppressive treatment (such as antimitotic substances or ionizing radiation). Independent of their local action, some of the above substances may decrease leukopoiesis. In addition, radiation and glucocorticoids depress the activity of phagocytic cells within the reticulohistocytic system (see chap. 33). Macrophages from treated animals show decreased motility and impaired bactericidal potency. A striking example is provided by the effect of corticosteroids on mouse pneumococcal infection. Mice may be protected against this infection following injection of sera from immunized animals. However, such seroprotection is totally ineffective in animals previously treated with corticosteroids, which decrease granulopoiesis and prevent afflux of polymorphs to the site of infection. Some diseases severely impair nonspecific resistance to infection. These diseases include diabetes, in which the low pH in the inflammatory focus follows the release of $\alpha$-ketoglutaric acid and $\beta$-hydroxybutyric acid, but not of lactic acid. The first two compounds are much less bactericidal than is lactic acid. During silicosis, alveolar macrophages are destroyed after phagocytosing silica particles, and the anti-infectious capability of the lung is diminished. Thus, a Bacillus Calmette-Guérin (BCG) injection normally well tolerated by guinea pigs causes death if the animal is silicotic. Important clinical examples are the impaired bactericidal abilities of phagocytic cells in the Chediak-Higashi syndrome and in chronic granulomatous disease.

## AUGMENTATION OF NONSPECIFIC IMMUNITY

It has been known for nearly 100 years that it is possible to enhance anti-infectious resistance with substances that have no antigenic relationship to the infectious agent. This phenomenon is known as nonspecific immunostimulation. As examples, we will consider bacteria, mycobacteria, anaerobic corynebacteria, and synthetic polynucleotides. (see p. 951).

## *BIBLIOGRAPHY*

BRAUN W. and UNGAR J. Non specific factors influencing host resistance: a reexamination. Basel, 1973, Karger.

COLVIN R. B., and DVORAK H. J. Role of granulocytes in cell mediated immunity. In: Mechanisms of Immunopathology (Cohen S., Ward P. A., and McCluskey R. T., [eds]). John Wiley and Sons, New York, 1979, 69.

DeMAYEER E. and DeMAYEER GUIGNARD J. Interferons. In: Comprehensive Virology (H. Fraenkel-Conrat and Wagner R. R. [eds.]). Plenum New York, 1979:205.

FAUVE R. M. Inflammation and natural immunity. In: Immunology 80 (M. Fougereau and J. Dausset [eds]). Acad. Press New York, 1980:737.

FLOREY H. W. (Ed.) General pathology, ed. 4. London, 1970, Lloyd-Luke.

Van FURTH R. (Ed.) Mononuclear phagocytes. Oxford, 1970, Blackwell.

GONTZEA I. Nutrition and anti-infectious defence. Basel, 1974, Karger.

GRESSER I. Interferon and the immune system. In: Immunology 80 (M. Fougereau and J. Dausset [eds]). Acad. Press, New York, 1980:710.

Haemopoietic stem cells. Ciba Found. Symp. 13. Amsterdam, 1973, Excerpta Medica.

Immunopotentiation. Ciba Found. Symp. 18. Amsterdam, 1974, Excerpta Medica.

KLEBANOFF S. J. Cytocidal mechanisms of phagocytic cells. In: Immunology 80 (M. Fougereau and J. Dausset [eds]). Acad. Press, New York, 1980, 720.

LEPOW I. H. and WARD P. A. Inflammation. Mechanisms and control. New York, 1972, Academic Press.

MINATO N., REID L., CANTOR H., LENGYEL P., and BLOOM B. R. Mode of regulation of natural killer activity by interferon. J. Exp. Med. 1980, 152, 124.

NELSON D. S. Macrophages and immunity. Amsterdam, 1969, North Holland.

ROCHAE SILVA M. and GARCIA LEME J. Chemical mediators of the acute inflammatory reaction. Oxford, 1972, Pergamon Press.

SMITH R. T. and LANDY M. (Eds.) Ecology and relative contribution of various lymphoreticular cells to tumor resistance. *In* Immunology of the tumor host relationship. New York, 1975, Academic Press.

STEWART W. E. The interferon system. Springer Verlag, New York, 1979, 421 p.

WAGNER W. H., HAHN H., and EVANS R. (Eds.) Activation of macrophages. Workshop conf. Hoechst. Vol. 2. Amsterdam, 1974, Excerpta Medica.

WILKINSON P. C. Chemotaxis and inflammation. Edinburgh, 1974, Churchill Livingstone.

WILLIAMS R. C. Jr and FUNDENBERG H. H. (Eds.) Phagocytic mechanisms in health and diseases. New York, 1972, Intercontinental Medical Book.

ZUCKERMAN A. and WEISS D. W. (Eds.) Dynamic aspects of host-parasite relationships. Vol. 1. New York, 1973, Academic Press.

ZWEIFACH B. W., GRANT L., and Mc CLUSKEY R. F. (Eds.) The inflammatory process, ed. 2. Vols. I, II, and III. New York, 1974, Academic Press.

## Chapter 16

# IMMUNE RESPONSES DIRECTED AGAINST INFECTIOUS AND PARASITIC AGENTS

**Philippe H. Lagrange and André Capron**

I.   INTRODUCTION
II.  BACTERIA
III. VIRUSES
IV.  PARASITES
V.   APPENDIX: VACCINATIONS AND SEROTHERAPY

## I. INTRODUCTION

The entry of an infectious agent into an organism initiates a series of reactions that terminate in anti-infectious immunity. This immunity confers to the individual specific protection against subsequent contact with the same pathogen. These reactions represent not only the principle of induced resistance but also include phenomena that alter the pathophysiology of the infectious disease and are capable of altering the response of the host to the infectious agent.

It has long been established that many patients who recover from a transmissible infection (acute disease) secondarily possess an acquired resistance to subsequent contact with the same infectious agent. Once isolation of specific microbes became possible, this fundamental observation was employed to provide preventive and even curative immunization against many transmissible diseases. Moreover, information regarding anti-infectious immunity enhanced our knowledge of biologic immune reactions toward foreign substances, thus providing an important stimulus to the general understanding of immunology.

The pathophysiology of clinical and biologic manifestations of infectious diseases served to clarify the relationships between the infectious agent and the infected host. The pathologic properties of a microorganism are not uniform.

Activities linked to exotoxin production (e.g., diphtheria, tetanus, or botulism) may be opposed to those that relate to the proliferation of microbes and to the action of their metabolic products. In fact, these two mechanisms may coexist during the course of an infectious disease (e.g., in *Clostridium perfringens* infection). Whatever the mechanism(s) involved, the response of the infected host confers on the infection additional characteristics. The infectious syndrome and its evolution represent the sum of the effect of the action of macroorganisms plus host reactions.

The analysis of anti-infectious immune responses include both innate and acquired immunity. The first response represents a spontaneous reaction to a specific pathogenic agent. This reaction involves various constitutional factors, including species, race, sex, heredity, and age, some of which are part of the nonspecific immunity discussed in chapter 15. Endogenous immunity also includes adaptation of an individual or a group of individuals to a pathogen after a prior contact with the infectious agent in which no overt manifestations were apparent. In fact, data from various experimental systems have led to a reexamination of this ancient concept, which, in turn, is leading to a revised classification of the various factors involved in anti-infectious defense mechanisms. This new approach involves two separate components: nonspecific defense mechanisms independent of the specific antigens of the infecting microorganism, and factors specific for the infecting agent. Nonspecific defense factors are those that oppose penetration, persistence, or multiplication of pathogenic agents within living organisms. Nonspecific defense mechanisms are the first to develop after infection is recognized and even represent a prerequisite for the next phase, specific defense. Specific defenses are, thus, time delayed. However, only specific immunity may be capable of limiting the infection and producing an eventual cure, which is followed by acquired resistance of variable duration. Moreover, evidence of humoral and cellular immune reactions may indirectly facilitate diagnosis of the disease.

In addition to these host-beneficial effects, the immune response to certain infections may cause secondary diseases entirely independent of persistent bacterial or viral infection. Although the data available are limited at present, postinfectious immunopathology will undoubtedly rapidly expand.

There are at least four processes by which anti-infectious specific immunity may exist in an individual. *Natural acquired immunity* can develop after infection by a pathogenic agent (penetration by a living microorganism), regardless of whether actual disease is induced. *Induced acquired immunity* represents the resistance acquired after vaccination by either living or dead microorganisms; alternatively, the vaccine may represent part of the bacterial product. *Natural passive immunity* refers to passive immunization of the fetus or newborn by maternal antibodies, by means of transplacental passage or colostrum or milk ingestion. *Passive induced immunity* is achieved by injecting recipients with serum, cells, or cellular extracts taken from an immune donor.

## II.   BACTERIA

A specific immune response induced by bacterial infections generally and simultaneously involves various elements of immunologic defense: antibodies,

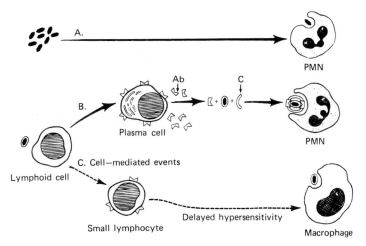

**Fig. 16.1** Schematic representation of the relative role of antibodies and cell-mediated immunity in bacterial phagocytosis. (A) Phagocytosis of a capsulated organism without intervention of specific immunity. (B) Phagocytosis facilitation by antibodies and complement. (C) Macrophage activation by T cells. (From J. A. Bellanti, Immunobiology. Philadelphia, 1971, Saunders, p. 265.)

macrophages, B and T lymphocytes, and complement proteins. Although in certain infections only one of these factors plays a predominant role, more often protection is the result of synergistic associations of the various specific and nonspecific factors discussed earlier. The systemic or localized humoral and cellular reactions observed in a particular case depend on the type of bacteria, its mode of entry, route of dissemination, and each bacterium's specific pathogenic effects. For example, the type of in vivo bacterial multiplication (extra- or intracellular) determines the mechanisms of specific host resistance. Bacteria that multiply extracellularly (streptococci, staphylococci) generally provoke defense reactions that involve production of specific antibodies. Bacteria that multiply intracellularly (mycobacteria, *Brucella*, *Listeria*) tend to induce cell-mediated defense reactions. In fact, the exact mechanisms by which such different defenses are induced have not yet been clearly defined. A first approach to study these mechanisms derives from clinical observations of immunodeficiencies (acquired and hereditary) that predispose an individual to certain infections. A second approach is that of animal experimentation. This approach involves studying the experimental pathogenic potency of a bacterial agent in various immune states in an attempt to reproduce in the animal conditions present in man during a given infection. Thus, by depleting certain cell populations and then replacing them by cell transfers, the role of each cell population in defending against a given infectious agent is examined. Selective depletions may be obtained in neonatally thymectomized or adult thymectomized animals, which are then exposed to sublethal irradiation and cellular reconstitution (bone marrow) or to corticosteroid treatment or immunosuppressive agents (cyclophosphamide or antilymphocytic serum). Another study technique involves transmitting adaptive immunity, specific for a given bacteria, by means of purified and selected cell preparations.

# ANTIBODIES

Antibodies are the essential factors of specific defense against bacteria that secrete exotoxin or that multiply extracellularly.

## *Production*

Antibody production varies according to the specific infectious agent, inoculation route, and stage of infection, both in quantitative and in qualitative terms. For example, bacterial infection of the respiratory or gastrointestinal tract causes secretory IgA levels to rise, without perturbation of the serum IgA level. Conversely, if the same bacteria are inoculated parenterally, circulating IgM and IgG are formed, but there is no secretory or serum IgA production. Again, infection by gram-negative bacteria (e.g., enterobacteria) merely induces IgM formation. The composition of the bacterial wall explains why antibody production is in part specific (directed against wall antigens) and, at the same time, nonspecific (linked to the presence of wall lipopolysaccharides), due to polyclonal antibody production. Lastly, each Ig class varies throughout the infection. Most often, primary responses are first associated with IgM production, which is followed by that of IgG; secondary responses usually show only IgG production. Thus, the Ig-class response may allow, in some cases, recognition of successive stages of infection. An example of this recognition occurs in *Salmonella* infections, in which detection of anti-H antibodies (antiflagella) versus anti-O antibodies (antisomatic) allows definition of the chronologic status of the infection. Note that, in parallel with class variations, the specificity and affinity of each Ig type varies during the chronologic course of the immune response (see p. 337).

## *Functions*

Specific antibody functions in anti-infectious defense were recognized very early (about the time of Pasteur), when it was shown that convalescent sera could be used prophylactically in antidiphtheria serotherapy.

The use of human γ-globulin in congenital immunodeficiencies (especially agammaglobulinemia) reduces the incidence and gravity of otherwise lethal infectious episodes. Similarly, suppression of maternal colostrum in newborn calves is followed by lethal septicemia due to *Escherichia coli*; the protecting element in colostrum is maternal Ig. Except for such special situations in which acquired or passive protection involves circulating or localized Ig, exclusive protection by antibodies is well established only in relation to bacterial exotoxin neutralization. Under other circumstances, specific Ig is only an adjuvant to nonspecific defense factors, acting by enhancement of bacterial phagocytosis or destruction.

### NEUTRALIZATION OF BACTERIAL EXOTOXIN

The predominant anti-infectious function of serum antibodies is neutralization of bacterial exotoxin. It is particularly apparent when clinical symptoms of the disease relate to toxin action and when intervention of cellular phago-cytosis is of little importance in defense. Such is the case for botulism, tetanus, and diphtheria. Toxin-antitoxin reactions hold a historical place in immunology. They represent one of the better models of the antigen-antibody reaction and have permitted the first applications of anti-infectious therapy by use of vaccination and preventive or curative serotherapy.

Circulating antitoxin antibodies may be demonstrated by at least two methods. The first technique consists of precipitating toxin by antitoxin and measuring the quantity of precipitate obtained or the speed of formation of the precipitate. Second, the neutralizing capacity of the serum may be quantified. The latter approach involves quantitative suppression of the toxin's properties by antiserum. For example, the dermonecrotic action of diphtheria toxin observed after localized injection of toxin is inhibited if the subject has circulating antitoxin antibodies; this phenomenon is known as the Schick reaction.

Similarly, one may measure the neutralizing action of serum when placed in contact with toxin in animals or in cell cultures. The action measured is expressed in units that relate to the noxious action of the toxin, such as lethal dose, hemolytic dose, or cytolytic or dermonecrotic dose. Serum preventive action is determined as a function of these harmful actions with reference to international toxin and antitoxin standards. These methods are both quantitative and qualitative and thus allow an examination of toxin specificity (e.g., toxi-notypy of botulism bacilli) and of antiserum potency, for example, for preventive therapy.

Neutralization of a toxin's effects reflects a direct action of antibodies without complement intervention. Titration of neutralizing power, compared to the dosages obtained by flocculation, reveals the importance of antibody avidity in neutralization. A serum neutralizes to a greater extent when its antibodies are more avid for the toxin. This point is of particular importance when specific antiserum is required, because hyperimmunization is possible only in donors with prior immunity. Only in such animals can hyperavid sera of high neutralizing potency be obtained.

Protective action of antibodies (exclusively of the IgG class) may be explained by neutralization of toxin subunits by steric blocking that prevents subsequent binding to synaptic receptors. With time, toxin transforms sponta-neously into toxoid, a protein molecule of the same antigenicity as toxin but not itself toxic. This transformation may be artifically reproduced by the simulta-neous action of heat and formaldehyde (Ramon's technique). The reaction is irreversible, and anatoxin is formed. Anatoxin is not toxic and is used for vaccination. Preventive vaccination by anatoxin provides nearly complete pro-tection, especially if booster injections are made at 10-year intervals. By this method, collective prophylaxis of the disease is achieved by diminishing its incidence; the disease can be completely eradicated if a large enough proportion of the population is vaccinated.

In perspective, it should be noted that whereas antibodies neutralize the noxious actions of bacteria exotoxins, specific sera offer no protection against the noxious effects of endotoxins originating, for example, in gram-negative bacilli.

ACTION ON PHAGOCYTOSIS

In addition to their direct role as antiexotoxins, antibodies play an indirectly protective role by enhancing cellular phagocytosis and phagocytic activity. Antibodies attract (recruit) phagocytic cells to sites of bacterial multiplication (chemotaxis) and facilitate preferential ingestion by bacteria (by opsonization) of pathogens that have obligatory extracellular multiplication. This effect is especially important when a capsule, or products of bacterial metabolism, retards phagocytosis. When there is a capsule, bacteria may remain free and extracellular, because no other defense system is operative until antibodies appear on the scene.

For example, pneumococcal virulence is apparently linked to the capsule that surrounds the pneumococcal wall. Whereas pneumococci are normally only slowly eliminated from the circulation after intravenous inoculation, injection of a small amount of antibody specific for the capsular mucopolysaccharide-type antigen (e.g., S III) causes very rapid elimination of encapsulated pneumococci of the same type. The effect of antibodies on pneumococcal phagocytosis (by neutrophil polymorphs) may be directly examined in vitro. The importance of the opsonizing activity of antibodies has also been demonstrated by experiments in mice rendered tolerant to pneumococci of the relevant type (these mice are totally deprived of type-specific antibodies). After an intravenous tolerogenic injection of 0.5 mg of type-III mucopolysaccharide, the injection of only one encapsulated type-III pneumococcus causes a lethal infection in these mice.

Antibodies that enhance phagocytosis can be observed for numerous microorganisms, including pneumococci, streptococci, some gram-negative bacteria of the enterobacteria family (in the smooth form), and meningococci of the A and C groups. Independent of the presence of a capsule that opposes phagocytosis, some bacteria (e.g., staphylococci) release products, before or after phagocytosis, that prevent the inflammatory reaction by means of inhibition of recruitment of new phagocytic cells.

Mechanisms of the adjunctive action of antibodies on phagocytosis may be due to chemotaxis or opsonization. Formation of specific (antigen-antibody) immune complexes, called cytotaxigens, may activate the complement system, whose components may also have a chemotactic effect. Only complement-binding Ig (i.e., IgM and certain IgG subclasses) exert chemotaxis. Opsonization is performed by the IgG classes (IgG1 and IgG3 in man) that contain intact Fc and Fab fragments. The bacteria-antibody complex initially binds to the macrophage by the Fc fragment. The whole complex is then actively ingested. Injection of antisera directed against phagocyte membranes decreases ingestion of opsonized bacteria; however, this effect varies, depending on the type of opsonization. One distinguishes between opsonization obtained with large amounts of antibodies and that achieved by use of very small amounts of antibodies, a distinction that implicates activation of the complement system (in particular, the first three factors, C1, C4, and C2, or the properdin system; both mechanisms lead to C3 activation).

A distinction must be made between opsonization and binding of certain bacteria to polymorphs without endocytosis. Some bacteria (like *Mycoplasma pneumoniae* on mouse peritoneal macrophages) adhere spontaneously to phag-ocytes but are ingested only if previously incubated with serum that contains specific antibodies.

ACTION ON BACTERIOLYSIS

Antibodies directed against antigens of certain gram-negative bacterial walls may induce bacterial lysis in the presence of fresh guinea pig serum. The conjoint action of antibodies and complement has been studied by electron microscopy. Fenestrations appear in *E. coli* walls similar to those produced by complement action on red blood cell membranes. In red blood cells, only one hole leads to complete lysis of the erythrocyte. However, for bacteria, comple-ment action must be followed by the lytic action of lysozyme on the mucopeptide wall. Lysis occurs only after an opening appears in the cytoplasmic membrane. This phenomenon has been observed with gram-negative bacteria (*Salmonella, Shigella, E. coli, Vibrio cholerae*), which are usually resistant to the dual action of antibodies and complement due to a lipid deficiency in the wall.

They lytic action of specific antibodies is mostly executed by IgM immu-noglobulins. A single IgM molecule can induce bacterial lysis after complement fixation. Complement-binding IgG may also cause lysis, but at least two molecules bound closely together are necessary to initiate complement activation and subsequent lysis. A bacteriolytic action of IgA secretory-type Ig has been suggested; however, IgA does not fix complement and lysis is probably associated with activation of the complement system by the alternative pathway.

### Conclusions

Neutralization of bacterial exotoxins, enhanced phagocytosis, and bacteri-olysis represent three major beneficial aspects of specific antibodies in antibac-terial protection. One should note, however, that other antibodies offer no protection and may in certain cases sensitize. We will discuss this point later under "Postinfectious Immunopathology."

## CELLS

Specific humoral reaction (favorable or not) represents only one of the reactions observed in bacterial infections. Bacteria that multiply intracellularly also provoke intense host cell responses. These bacteria induce recruitment and proliferation of T lymphocytes sensitized to specific bacterial antigens; these T lymphocytes then cause delayed hypersensitivity reactions (i.e., tuberculin type), release chemical mediators (lymphokines), activate macrophages, and produce specific antibodies after interaction with B cells by means of secondary reaction kinetics. The importance of cell-mediated immunity is underscored by the high incidence of some bacterial infections in immunodeficiencies bearing on T lymphocytes, as in thymic aplasia and immunosuppressive treatments.

Purely cell-mediated immune reactions are well recognized. A classic example is Koch's phenomenon, which includes two parallel reactions: delayed hypersensitivity to tubercle protein constitutents, which occurs 24-48 hr after injection of the infected guinea pig, and acquired immunity to the infecting *Mycobacterium tuberculosis* (premunition), which occurs only if the primary infection persists. Development of premunition immunity depends on the type, virulence, and quantity of mycobacteria in the initial lesion. Cell-mediated immunity plays an important role in defenses against microorganisms other than *M. tuberculosis,* which also have the property of persisting and multiplying inside phagocytic cells (especially monocytes and macrophages). As in Koch's phenomenon, these bacteria simultaneously induced delayed hypersensitivity and resistance.

Induction of delayed hypersensitivity to some antigens necessitates prior ingestion of the antigen by macrophages. In antibacterial cell-mediated resistance, bacteria may cause a nonspecific hyperactivation of the reticuloendothelial system immediately after the primary infection. This hyperactivity, of variable duration according to the type of bacteria involved, explains misinterpretations regarding the specificity of antibacterial cell-mediated immunity. During the secondary response (at the time of reinfection), antibacterial defense also includes macrophage activation. This activation requires T lymphocytes specifically sensitized during the first infection. Antigenic specificity is linked to T cells and not to activated macrophages, which are also activated against bacteria other than those that caused the original T-lymphocyte sensitization. A second contact of the antigen with T lymphocytes causes increased monocyte production and preferential migration of monocytes to the infection site, where the reaction takes place. In addition, T lymphocytes stimulate macrophage metabolism with significant elevations in bactericidal potency. These observations have been made for the rat and mouse infected by human or attenuated bovine mycobacteria (Bacillus Calmette-Guérin, BCG), *Listeria, Brucella,* and *Salmonella.*

We will now describe the experimental systems used to establish these conclusions and will then envisage the nature and function of the immunocompetent cells engaged in anti-infectious responses. Finally, we will describe the cellular interactions that lead to macrophage activation and formation of granulomatous lesions at the site of bacterial implantation.

### Description of Experimental Systems

Numerous experiments have examined the role of immune phagocytes in the development of resistance to tubercle bacilli, *Brucella, Salmonella, Listeria,* and toxoplasma. These observations are complicated in certain cases by simultaneous nonantigen specific activation of macrophages due to intracellular germs, concomitant with specific activation dependent on immune T lymphocytes. The latter activation is usually more important in vivo. The systematic study of mechanisms of specific macrophage activation in antibacterial immunity was performed by Mackaness. Because experimental tuberculous infections were difficult to produce and satisfactorily quantify, Mackaness studied *Listeria monocytogenes*, which is a gram-positive pathogenic bacterium. Following intravenous administration (mice), bacteria form inflammatory foci that contain polymorphs and macrophages in the liver and spleen. Their number is maximum on the second or third day, at which time macrophages become bactericidal and destroy surviving bacteria. This state of acquired resistance is controlled both by T lymphocytes, which release soluble chemical mediators that condition the influx of monocytes and macrophages, and by the functional activation of these cells by the scheme just mentioned.

### Nature of Immune Lymphocytes

The experimental studies mentioned above have permitted identification of the origin, production, and fate of immune lymphocytes specifically sensitized against bacteria.

ORIGIN

After introduction of living bacteria into a living organism, the antigenic stimulation thereby produced leads to lymphocyte accumulation within lymphoid tissues of the contiguous region, especially within thymus-dependent areas (paracortical lymph node areas and periarteriolar zones of the white pulp of the spleen). These cells, specifically sensitized to bacterial antigens, recirculate since they are long-lived T cells. They do not appear in neonatally thymectomized or antilymphocyte serum-treated mice. They are not seen in normal mice after injection of dead bacteria.

PROLIFERATION AND PRODUCTION

T cells recruited specifically to the infectious foci and the regional lymphoid tissue subsequently proliferate. The precocity, degree, and duration of proliferation depend on numerous factors, particularly the type of bacteria, dose, and virulence. Proliferation occurs in specifically sensitized cells, since, in transfer experiments, donor administration of antimitotic drugs suppresses the adoptive protection normally conferred to new recipients by injecting cells from the spleen or lymph node, peritoneal cavity, or peripheral blood from immune animals.

Protection is most often associated with transfer of delayed hypersensitivity and is maximal at the time of the proliferation peak. The duration of the transmitted protection varies according to the system studied; it is prolonged for mycobacteria and short for *Listeria* infections. It is always possible that transmitted protection is misinterpreted because of contamination of cells with bacteria.

CELLULAR MIGRATION

Specific immunocompetent cells or their descendents do not accumulate in thymus-dependent areas of the lymphoid tissue because they rapidly emigrate. They are found in the lymph node medulla, then in the efferent lymph, and finally thoracic duct and blood. These cells are responsible for anti-infectious immunity, as shown by studies in which cells obtained by thoracic duct transfer confer adoptive immunity to new recipients with the same time delay seen in delayed hypersensitivity. Because they originate from rapidly dividing precursors, they may be studied by radiolabeling their DNA (e.g., tritated thymidine). Specifically sensitized lymphocytes of the first generation do not recirculate (i.e., return to the peripheral lymphoid tissues and lymph after initial blood passage). Conversely, these lymphocytes enter the inflammatory exudates, especially within the peritoneal cavity. Limited cell multiplication may occur at this level. The passive protection conferred by cell transfer is short in duration for *Listeria* and of longer duration for *M. tuberculosis*. In fact, this apparent contradiction is due probably to a qualitative or quantitative difference in memory cells, particularly easily induced by mycobacteria infections. It may also be due to a persistence of bacterial antigen in the particulate form. The latter hypothesis is corroborated by the finding that only living mycobacteria are able to induce long-lasting and delayed hypersensitivity. Tuberculin itself is not protective, although it may induce a secondary response and induce delayed hypersensitivity.

### Functions of Sensitized Cells

Sensitized T lymphocytes confer delayed hypersensitivity and are capable of transferring passive protection. In the experimental systems examined above, neither serum from hyperimmune animals nor B-cell injections can be used to transfer delayed hypersensitivity or specific antibacterial protection. Adoptive immunity is transmitted only to virginal recipients by lymphoid cells, which in the mouse contain the θ antigen. Their role in anti-infectious resistance also requires mononucleated phagocytic cells for both delayed hypersensitivity and antibacterial protection. Once T lymphocytes recognize the antigen and begin to proliferate, they attract phagocytic mononucleated cells to the site of infection and stimulate phagocyte metabolic and bactericidal activities.

Recent observations in the *L. monocytogenes* system have shown the importance of the major histocompatibility complex in the specific recognition of antigen by T-dependent lymphocytes at the level of the macrophage membrane.

The necessity for concordance between the major histocompatibility complexes of the lymphocyte and macrophage appears to be linked to the obligatory expression of the specific bacterial antigen in contact with the phenotypic patterns governed by the I region of the major histocompatibility complex. This restriction has not only been demonstrated for helper lymphocytes but also for those responsible for delayed-type hypersensitivity.

#### ACCUMULATION OF PHAGOCYTIC CELLS

The accumulation of phagocytic cells represents the essential element of secondary responses in cell-mediated immunity, whether the specific antigen is reinjected as living or killed bacteria or as bacterial extracts. Only a small percentage of the total lymphocytes present in the lesion (4–7%) are specifically sensitized immune lymphocytes. The accumulating cells include monocytes and nonsensitized lymphocytes. The accumulation results from diffusion of soluble chemotactic factors, which differ from macrophage migration-inhibitory factor (see p. 387). Under certain circumstances, this accumulation leads to granuloma formation, characteristic of bacterial infections.

#### MACROPHAGE ACTIVATION

Macrophage activation is manifested by significant changes in morphology and metabolism, including an increased capacity to spread on glass and enhanced motility of the membranous veils. These changes relate also to an augmentation in energy metabolism, reflected in increased glucose and oxygen consumption. There is also an increase in lysosomal content and accelerated activity of the endoplasmic reticulum.

In vitro studies have shown that these changes are associated with increased bactericidal potency (Fig. 16.2), for example, more rapid and intense destruction of bacteria. However, in vitro at least, such bactericidal activation is not antigen specific: all bacterial species that show intracellular localization are more effectively destroyed, even though in vivo macrophage activation is more efficient for bacteria that originate the sensitization. However, only the specific bacteria are capable of reinducing cell-mediated immunity. Macrophage activation by species-specific T lymphocytes coincides with an increase in the specific humoral response. These specific antibodies may enhance phagocytic activity directed towards certain bacteria (*Salmonella* and *Brucella*).

### Conclusions

Cell-mediated antibacterial resistance consists of preferential macrophage recruitment to the site of infection and by increased bactericidal action induced by soluble mediators released by immune T lymphocytes in response to specific sensitization after contact with the bacterial antigen. These mediators are produced in response to certain bacteria that have as common characteristics the ability to survive and to multiply within cells. Immunity requires two populations of mononucleated cells: circulating blood monocytes that give rise to macrophages and recirculating T lymphocytes.

## POSTINFECTIOUS IMMUNOPATHOLOGY

Immune responses that occur after penetration of a bacterial agent into a living organism most often result in destruction of the pathogenic agent, cure of the

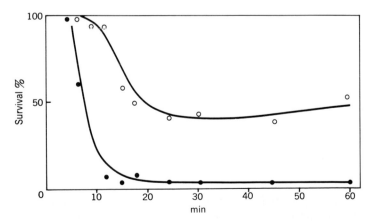

**Fig. 16.2** Macrophage activation. Increase of the bactericidal activity of macrophages toward *Salmonella* (*S. typhimurium*) coated with anti-*Salmonella* antibodies. O, Normal macrophages; ●, activated macrophages. (From G. B. Mackaness, Hosp. Pract. 1979, 73.)

infection, and a state of acquired resistance specific for the infecting microbe. In certain cases, however, these immune reactions are not limited to host-beneficial actions but may lead to delayed pathologic manifestations that may continue to evolve despite resolution of the infection. These manifestations were formerly described as "allergy" without prejudging the mechanism. The term "allergy" includes anaphylaxis, serum sickness disease, Arthus's reaction, delayed hypersensitivity reactions, and autoimmune diseases, all of which may be observed during bacterial infections.

## III.  VIRUSES

Immunity to viruses is based on the same principles as those discussed above for bacteria. We will therefore limit ourselves to a description of experimental models for the study of antiviral immunity and to a discussion of the mechanisms involved. There is, however, an essential difference between viruses and bacteria that must first be stressed, namely, that viral multiplication or replication occurs only inside living cells. This stipulation implicates the existence of specific membrane receptors on virus-sensitive cells and of a metabolic capacity of the host cell to induce the protein synthesis necessary for replication. This explains why all animal cells are not susceptible to every virus; some cells, such as neutrophil polymorphs, do not permit viral replication.

The study of antiviral immunity initially focused on resistance acquired after childhood infection (measles, varicella, mumps) or vaccination. The observation that some viral infections predominated in children with specific immunodeficiencies (Table 16.1) or in subjects submitted to therapeutic immunodepression has facilitated such studies. Ultimately, use of animal model systems permitted differentiation of the various mechanisms that control antiviral defense with some unique features that depend on the type of virus. In parallel, the concept of postinfectious immunopathology refers to immune reactions induced by these viruses.

Host-specific defense mechanisms differ according to the type of virus, mode of penetration, type of cell infected, and viral persistence within the cells. These various mechanisms include humoral and cellular factors in the form of local or systemic immunity and may follow each other chronologically. Local immunity often limits extension of the disease, whereas systemic immunity tends o restrict extension at a distance, in particular, movement of a virus to more susceptible cells or toward cells with a weak regeneration potential, including cells within the central nervous system.

### ANTIBODIES

Antibodies have long been considered the main element of antiviral resistance. This concept is incorrect, and today the preeminent role of T cells in virus elimination is definitely established. One observes the appearance of serum antibodies that neutralize virion infectivity during the course of infection. These antibodies may be detected in vivo in virus-sensitive animals or in vitro by cell

**Table 16.1   Viral Infections in Immune Deficiency**

| | |
|---|---|
| Hypogammaglobulinemia (normal cellular immunity) | Poliomyelitis |
| Selective deficiency of cellular immunity | Vaccinia |
| | Herpes |
| | Varicella |
| | Zoster |
| | Cytomegalovirus |
| | Measles |

culture. Serum absorption by means of specific viral antigens suppresses the protective effect of serum. These antibodies appear late in the circulation and are active only when injected soon after contact with the infecting agent. They are nearly always ineffective if injected after the onset of clinical symptoms. Thus, the role of antibodies seems limited to reinfection immunity. This apparent situation is, however, not a universal rule.

The role of antibodies in defense is corroborated by their effects on coxsackie viruses in mice pretreated by immunosuppressants. Coxsackie B3 infection regularly kills newborn mice but is not lethal for healthy adults. However, adult mice given cyclophosphamide develop lethal infections. This

**Table 16.2   Host Responses to Viruses**

| | *Response* | *Examples* |
|---|---|---|
| Acute infection: | Virus eliminated | Enteroviruses, rhinoviruses, myxoviruses |
| | Virus persists to produce: | |
| | Reactivation episodes | Herpes simplex, Varicella-zoster |
| | Chronic disease | Measles and subacute sclerosing panencephalitis (SSPE) |
| | No change | Adenoviruses |
| Chronic infection: | Progressive disease: | |
| | Inflammatory | Chronic active hepatitis and hepatitis B virus, progressive multifocal leukoencephalopathy and a polyoma virus |
| | Noninflammatory | The "spongiform" encephalopathies, Kuru and Jakob-Creutzfeldt syndromes |
| | Malignant change | Burkitt's lymphoma and Epstein-Barr virus; perhaps also nasopharyngeal carcinoma |
| | No disease | Cytomegalovirus, hepatitis B virus (Australia antigen) carriers, LCM and arenaviruses in normal (rodent) hosts |

After J. Nagington. *In* P. G. H. Gell, R. R. A. Coombs, and P. J. Lachmann, Eds. Clinical Aspects of Immunology. Oxford, 1975, Blackwell, p. 131.

lethal progression may be eliminated if the animal receives immune sera from healthy adult donors (Table 16.3). This phenomenon is not explained by interferon production, because mice treated by cyclophosphamide show serum interferon levels with kinetics highly similar to those of virions present in the circulation.

### Mechanisms of Action of Antibodies

The protection offered by antibodies may reflect neutralization of the infectivity of virions. Neutralization prevents viral penetration by obstructing virus fixation onto membrane receptors of recipient cells. Thus, bacteriophage-neutralizing sera prevent bacteriophage fixation onto receptors of recipient bacteria. This neutralizing action simulates that of bacterial antitoxin serum, which intervenes (e.g., in diphtheria) by preventing binding of toxin onto certain cell receptors.

Viral neutralization may also occur because of a combined action of antibody and complement, as in the case of herpes simplex virions in rabbits and with rubella. This neutralizing action may be due to (1) stabilization of antibody-virion complexes formed during the initial immunization with low-avidity antibodies; (2) lysis of the viral envelope, simulating hemolysis or bacteriolysis; (3) enhanced phagocytosis by polymorphs that does not allow viral multiplication and also suppresses infection of sensitive cells; or (4) cytolysis in the presence of complement, directed against virus-infected target cells that contain a viral antigen in their membrane.

The infectivity of certain viruses is not diminished by antibodies, even when in considerable excess. Immune complexes of virions and specific antibodies may develop. However, the host may produce antibodies directed against these complexes (i.e., antiglobulin factors) that may in themselves display a neutralizing activity. Antiglobulins explain why rheumatoid factors are detected during the course of many viral infections. Circulating immune complexes carrying antiglobulin are rapidly eliminated by phagocytic cells that have a receptor for the Fc fragment of IgG. However, some viruses, for example, herpes simplex, are not completely neutralized and, in fact, may multiply within phagocytic cells.

Protection against certain viruses, particularly enteroviruses and arboviruses, is largely linked to neutralization of the infectious potency of virions by

**Table 16.3   Mortality of Adult CBA Mice after Intraperitoneal Injection of Coxsackie B3 Virus, and Treatment by Cyclophosphamide; Protection by Passive Antibody**

| Treatment | Number of mice | Death (%) |
|---|---|---|
| No treatment | 16 | 0 |
| Cyclophosphamide (72 hr after virus) | 16 | 100 |
| Cyclophosphamide plus antibody (4 and 15 days after virus) | 14 | 0 |

After A. C. Allison.

circulating antibodies that prevent virion extension to highly susceptible cells (e.g., central nervous system, heart). This explains why agammaglobulinemic children are more prone to develop paralytic lesions after contact with wild viruses or vaccine strains of poliomyelitis virus. It is also possible that local IgA immunoglobulin secretion plays a protective role. In fact, the presence of specific serum IgG does not prevent virus implantation in the intestinal mucosa or dissemination into adjacent areas.

### Duration of Protection

Viral infectious diseases may be separated into two groups according to the duration of the protection conferred. The first group achieves a short-lived immunity. These diseases generally have a short incubation period and a localized infectious focus. They include myxovirus and paramyxovirus infections. Two factors may limit the possibility of immunization. The first factor relates to the short duration of antigenic presence and rapid regeneration of antigen-bearing cells, which do not allow sufficient time for recruitment of immunocompetent cells that might produce antibodies. This factor applies, however, more to serum antibodies than to localized antibody production. The second factor relates to variations in virus-specific antigens. The appearance of variants is particularly well known for group-A myxoviruses. Humoral immunity to one variant does not afford protection against a new variant. Only the prediction of the antigenic constitution of new variants permits preventive protection. The second group of viral infections features those that have long incubation periods and significant viral dissemination, and induce specific antibody production. Virus antigenic stability, a high incidence of inapparent infections, and minimal reinoculations may explain why immunity is induced by these viral infections.

### Harmful Effects of Antibodies

Paradoxically, specific antibodies that appear after viral infection may aggravate the cellular lesions produced by the virus. Antibodies may even produce lesions, under conditions in which viruses themselves have no cytopathogenicity. Certain complement-fixing antibodies may be cytotoxic for infected cells that express neoantigens on their surfaces. On the other hand, some noncomplement-fixing antibodies protect cells by inhibiting the activity of cytotoxic antibody by means of competition for the antigenic site. These mechanisms may explain the persistence of herpes virus despite the presence of antiherpes serum antibodies.

Another harmful effect of antibodies relates to circulating immune complexes. When infection is provoked by the murine virus of lymphochoriomeningitis (LCM), an immune complex disease is produced that features severe glomerulonephritis. A similar mechanism has been suggested to be operative in man to explain the pathogenesis of cases of polyarteritis nodosa associated with Australia antigen-containing immune complexes. Conversely, viral diseases transmitted vertically (in utero or at birth), such as adenovirus infections, show persistence without detectable clinical manifestations. They lead to formation of soluble immune complexes that inhibit T-lymphocyte function but that have no effect on B lymphocytes.

## CELLS

As we have seen, antibodies may represent an important source of protection against selected viruses, such as enteroviruses and arboviruses. Unfortunately, in other cases, injection of serum from immune donors has no preventive effect on the infectious disease: the course of infection is uncomplicated in agammaglobulinemic children. One must then incriminate cell-mediated immunity in antiviral defenses. This interpretation is corroborated by evidence that children with immunodeficiencies of Ig production alone show recurrent bacterial infections and may present with paralytic poliomyelitis, even though they react perfectly normally to smallpox vaccination and recover normally after viral hepatitis and measles. Conversely, systemic vaccinia has been described in subjects who present immunodeficiencies exclusively bearing on T cells in whom Ig production is normal. Similarly, children with the Wiskott-Aldrich syndrome, who possess an isolated cellular deficiency (see p. 897), are peculiarly susceptible to herpes simplex, measles viruses, and cytomegalovirus. Hodgkin's disease, which is associated with cell-mediated immunodeficiency, is more often complicated by severe herpes infections than are lymphosarcomas.

Lastly, the increase in certain viral infections, particularly those produced by herpes viruses (herpes simplex, cytomegalovirus, varicella, zoster), is well established in patients who receive therapeutic immunosuppressive treatment with azathioprine, which is known to affect primarily T cells (see p. 956).

The role of cell-mediated specific immunity in experimental antiviral immunity is well known. This role was suggested by the presence of delayed hypersensitivity against viral antigens (vaccinia, measles, mumps, herpes) after infection. In the guinea pig, viral antigens promote blast transformation of circulating lymphocytes and macrophage migration-inhibitory factor production. Additional evidence in the mouse is provided by the fact that experimental infections, such as lymphochoriomeningitis and ectromelia, are prevented by administration of purified immune T-cell injections. Ectromelia is an exclusively murine infection due to a pox virus but is very similar to human pox. After virus penetration through skin excoriations of the mouse paw, the virus multiplies locally and then disseminates through the lymphatics and blood to reach the spleen and liver. It is at this stage that the favorable or unfavorable outcome of the disease is determined. Cure occurs normally 4–6 days after infection because of circulating sensitized T lymphocytes. These cells recognize the specific viral antigen in the liver and promote hepatic lesion infiltration by monocytes. Circulating antibodies do not appear until day 7 or 8 and, in any case, do not seem to be responsible for the cure. The disease evolution is unfavorable in nude or T cell-depleted mice. T-cell injections restore immunity in irradiated mice, whereas sera from immune donors have no effect. Similar findings have been described for other viruses (Table 16.4).

**Table 16.4  Effects of Suppression of Cell-Mediated Immunity on the Outcome of Certain Viral Infections in Mice**

| Virus | Number of mice | Treatment | Mortality (%) |
|---|---|---|---|
| Herpes simplex | 25 | Normal rabbit serum | 0 |
| | 14 | Neonatal thymectomy | 71 |
| | 13 | Antilymphocyte serum | 100 |
| Yellow fever | 58 | No treatment | 16 |
| | 24 | Antilymphocyte serum | 96 |
| Coxsackie B3 | 25 | No treatment | 0 |
| | 22 | Neonatal thymectomy | 0 |
| Ectromelia | 26 | Normal serum | 20 |
| | 26 | Antilymphocyte serum | 100 |

After A. C. Allison.

## Mode of Action of T Lymphocytes

RECRUITMENT OF MONOCYTIC CELLS

This recruitment represents the major defensive function of T lymphocytes. In the absence of T cells, there is no monocytic invasion, and ectromelia viruses disseminate throughout the entire hepatic parenchyma. Monocytes also accumulate in the cerebrospinal fluid of immune mice inoculated intracerebrally with LCM viruses. Such localization permits both qualitative and quantitative studies. As described above for cutaneous delayed hypersensitivity reactions (see p. 374), monocytic recruitment is similarly achieved, even though only a small percentage of T cells is present in the lesions. By use of radioactive markers, specifically sensitized T lymphocytes constitute 4–7% of the infiltrating cells.

The mechanism of monocytic accumulation simulates that described for bacterial antigens. Recirculating immune T lymphocytes cross liver sinusoids to reach virus-infected cells and then release soluble chemotactic factors (directed toward monocytes). It is difficult, however, to know to what extent the accumulation of phagocytic cells, which does not allow viral replication, contributes to disease regression. It is not now known to what extent, or how, immune interferon (type II), which is secreted by both stimulated lymphocytes and macrophages, may intervene.

CYTOTOXICITY

Sensitized specific T cells may express toxicity toward infected cells expressing on their membrane the specific viral antigen. Cytotoxicity may be evaluated by means of the trypan blue dye test or by release of previously fixed $^{51}$Cr onto target cells. Studies have been performed for ectromelia, myxovirus infections, and lymphochoriomeningitis. In ectromelia, peak numbers of cytotoxic cells are seen on Day 6. Specificity is clear-cut despite the low number of these cells relative to the total spleen cell number (between 1 and 10%). It is difficult to know to what extent direct cytotoxicity detected in vitro contributes to protection in vivo. However, in some cases, the cure coincides with peak numbers of cytotoxic cells. Recently, Zinkernagel and Doherty showed that lymphocytic cytotoxicity in mice infected with lymphochoriomeningitis was expressed only toward infected cells bearing the same H-2 antigenic specificities as the sensitized mouse. Such a restriction has obvious implications for the specificity of T-cell receptors (see p. 87).

### INTERACTION WITH B CELLS

T cells may also intervene in host defense by collaborating with B cells that produce antibody. This possibility may apply particularly for tobacco mosaic virus, Japanese B-encephalitis, myxovirus, and herpes virus. When production of antibodies is delayed following a cure, T-cell function is limited to prevention of reinfections. Specificity differences between B and T cells, with respect to antigenic variants and long persistence of T-type memory, may explain the hypothesis of "original antigenic sin," according to which infection by a virus with antigenic determinants that cross-react with those of an earlier viral infection induces antibody production more effectively with respect to the former virus than to the second one, even when serial infections occur years later (see p. 336).

### INTERFERON PRODUCTION

Stimulation of immune lymphocytes by viral or other antigens or by a nonspecific mitogen causes type II interferon production by these lymphocytes. Type II interferon differs from type I interferon in several physicochemical and antigenic characteristics. Similarly, macrophage activation is associated with production of monocyte interferon. Interferon is a nonspecific anti-viral protein that protects other cells in its vicinity, not by opposing viral penetration but by preventing replication. The production of type II interferon is diminished or even absent in the course of such viral infections as varicella, herpes zoster and herpes simplex, seen in patients suffering from malignant lymphomas or undergoing immunosuppressive therapy. However, in healthy individuals, interferon production is only seen at the time of recovery and therefore seems to be a consequence of rather than a reason for recovery from the disease. Some viruses (e.g., herpes) are resistant to the action of type I interferon. Immune interferon may play an important role in host resistance to certain viral infections.

### VIRUS-INDUCED TUMORS

A final aspect of cell intervention in antiviral immunity concerns, at least in animals, defenses directed toward virus-induced malignant tumors. The most important example is polyoma virus. When injected into newborn mice, this virus may induce a high incidence of mammary and salivary carcinoma, osteosarcoma, and other tumors. The tumor cells are transplantable and produce intense immune responses in normal animals. If the virus is transferred by in vitro cultures, it retains its ability to induce malignant cell transformation.

When inoculated into normal adult mice, the virus multiplies within various organs, but tumors do not appear, which suggests that these mice, unlike newborns, have resistance mechanisms directed against the viral oncogenicity. It is of interest that adult thymectomized mice or antilymphocyte serum-treated mice develop tumors after polyoma virus injection. In this setting, injection of immune donor T cells produces protection. It is possible, however, that in experiments that involve antilymphocyte sera, the mice are deficient not only in T cells but also in K cells (see p. 413), which may be cytotoxic to infested cells that express viral antigens coated with the corresponding antibodies. In this respect, it should also be noted that production of lymphocytodependent antibodies (ADCC, see p. 413), may be thymus dependent. The differences in resistance between adult and newborn mice might represent T-cell immaturity of newborns. Conclusions drawn from study of the polyoma virus may apply to other viruses and may explain the peculiar susceptibility to oncogenic viruses that is observed at the beginning and at the end of life.

## CHRONIC VIRAL INFECTIONS

Despite diverse antiviral immune responses, viral infections may become chronic. Examples include congenital viral infections (vertical transmission), persistent infection due to slow viruses, and infections by viruses insensitive to antiviral defense mechanisms.

### Congenital Viral Infections

Congenital viral infections are transmitted vertically. Virions pass from mother to fetus or to newborn. The disease may be overt or latent, but virions are always present. An effective defense mechanism directed toward the infection never occurs, suggesting an acquired tolerance to the viral antigens. One of the best models of congenital viral infections is mouse lymphochorio-meningitis (LCM). The infection may be transmitted vertically or by injection of large doses of virus into the newborn (within 24 hr of birth). The virus does not in itself induce any clinically pathologic effect. Viruses multiply and spread throughout most tissues. Lesions of the central nervous system are universal but do not produce neurologic signs. After several weeks, immune complex deposition is associated with infiltrates of mononucleated cells, particularly within the renal glomeruli and in the choroid plexus. At variance with newborn mice, adult mice that receive high doses of virus develop a lethal disease characterized by central nervous system lesions. These lesions are not always due to the viral cytopathogenicity but may be caused by mononucleated cells (T-lymphocytes and monocytes under the influence of immune T cells). Death is prevented by neonatal thymectomy or antilymphocyte serum injection and does not occur in T cell-deprived mice (nude mice or thymectomized, irradiated, bone marrow-reconstituted mice). The T cell-depleted mice are chronic virus carriers. Transfer of immune T cells from normal adults to congenitally infected mice does not cause neurologic lesions but very clearly increases circulating antibody levels. Thus, congenital viral infection seems to induce tolerance in immune T cells (particularly in regard to cytotoxicity) without preventing B-cell production of antibodies. However, these antibodies may lead to formation of circulating immune complexes that may produce other pathologic effects, a situation we will discuss later.

### Persistent Viral Infections

Persistent viral diseases include those caused by slow viruses (scrapie, visna, maedi) or by infections that feature viral reactivation (zoster, varicella, herpes, subacute sclerosing panencephalitis). In these cases, the antiviral immune response does not prevent development of clinical signs. This ineffectiveness of the immune defense has at least three explanations, depending on the mechanism of viral dissemination. For viruses that spread between cells and pass through the *extracellular fluid* (vascular or extravascular), only the absence of immune responses explains the persistence of the infection. For viruses with *intracellular cytoplasmic extensions* (the virus travels along cytoplasmic axons or dendritic neurons, as in the case of herpesvirus), an abnormality of antigenic expression at the level of the membrane may explain the ineffectiveness of defense mechanisms. For viruses with *nuclear extensions* (characterized by genomic incorporation of a provirus in the host cell), the modified genome is transmitted from mother to daughter cell. The absence of any antigenic expression of the viral genome in the form of neosurface antigens may explain the absence of an immune response. We will now examine some examples that illustrate these three possibilities.

The absence of an immune response in the first hypothesis may be due to subthreshold concentrations of virus. This hypothesis may explain the absence of immune responses, both cellular and humoral, in scrapie (shaking scrapie of sheep).

Herpesvirus infections are associated with a highly effective immune response (including neutralizing antibodies and cellular reaction). Persistence of infection is explained by the presence of blocking serum factors, particularly immune complexes similar to those described in certain tumor states. Similar immune complexes have been demonstrated in patients with cytomegalovirus infection and subacute sclerosing panencephalitis. In the latter, blastic stimulation and macrophage migration-inhibitory factor production by lymphocytes are blocked by a factor present in the serum and cerebrospinal fluid.

In the second hypothesis, the absence of viral antigenic expression at the level of the infected cell membranes may either be extrinsic (when the antigenic pattern is masked by, for example, a noncomplement-binding antibody) or intrinsic (as with macrophage-ingested viruses that remain intact but do not replicate). The latter has been verified experimentally for viruses of LCM, lactodehydrogenase, and Aleutian mink disease. Reactivations might then be associated with metabolic changes in host cells instead of with a depression of the immune response.

A final hypothesis is that of viral genome integration in the host cell not associated with antigenic expression on the host cell surface. This hypothesis seems applicable to RNA viruses that contain RNA-dependent DNA polymerase.

Viral reactivation would then occur during blast cell transformation, which would nonspecifically depress the viral genome.

## VIRAL IMMUNOPATHOLOGY

As for bacteria, antiviral immune responses have a positive and favorable role in eliminating the infectious agent but also may initiate pathologic changes. Analysis of these various roles is complicated in viruses, because some viruses affect various immune responses of the host, including cell-mediated immunity (for cytomegalovirus), or, alternatively, the virus may cause inhibition of lymphocyte proliferation induced by phytohemagglutinin or a soluble antigen or may transiently modify various lymphocyte membrane receptors (in the case of Newcastle virus disease). Postviral immunopathology may relate to the action of antibodies, cytotoxic cells, or circulating immune complexes.

### Cytotoxic Antibodies

Cytotoxicity of antiviral antibodies toward host cells and their role in antiviral defense depend on the density of the viral antigen expressed at the level of membranes, on cellular susceptibility to lysis by complement, and on the nature and concentration of antiviral antibodies. Cytotoxicity may be inhibited by noncomplement-fixing antibodies. In some situations, antibody-dependent cell-mediated cytotoxicity (ADCC) may also play a role.

### Cytotoxic Cells

Lymphocytotoxicity of T cells has been described during LCM infections in adult mice. Such direct cytotoxicity may be controlled by genes present in the major histocompatibility complex (see chap. 24).

### Immune Complexes

Immune complexes have been demonstrated in various viral infections (LCM, lactodehydrogenase virus infections, Aleutian mink disease, murine leukemia, and equine infectious anemia). Australia antigen-containing immune complexes have been seen in some cases of polyarteritis nodosa and in immunoglobulin deposits in subjects dying of viral hepatitis. Another example is the infection produced by respiratory syncytial virus in subjects previously parenterally vaccinated; here, a second infectious contact induces an Arthus phenomenon in the lungs.

### Conclusions

Immune responses elicited by viral infections may be used for virus classification. The first group, which includes enteroviruses and arboviruses, provokes humoral immunity, either localized or systemic, depending on the route of viral introduction. The second group includes viruses that preferentially induce cell-mediated immunity; this group includes pox virus, herpes virus, certain myxoviruses, and paramyxoviruses. T lymphocytes are activated with secondary effects on monocytes. Interferon production is also stimulated. Also in this category are viruses that induce T-cell (and K-cell) immunity, for example, polyoma virus in the mouse. The third group includes arenoviruses, which are transmitted vertically, do not cause a clinical disease, and are transmitted but well tolerated by the infected host. However, adult infection produces a disease because of immune reactions to virus-infected cells.

# IV.  PARASITES

The interest of the study of immune response in parasitic infections may be considered at two levels. On one hand, parasitic infections are very common throughout the world (one of every three individuals carries parasites). Some very prevalent parasitic diseases (malaria, 600 million infested individuals; bilharziosis, 300 million; filariosis, 80 million) have an important impact on public health and affect the growth and development of the countries affected. There is at present no known effective immunologic control demonstrable for human parasitic diseases. On the other hand, the very chronic life-span of parasites in immune hosts provides a potential model for the study of numerous immunologic mechanisms (acquired host antigens, antigenic variation, immunosuppression, circulating antigens).

The great diversity of parasites and their complex biology make it difficult to apply general principles to all host-parasite systems. It is important, however, to review some characteristics of parasite biology that have an obvious effect on the immune response.

### Parasite Size

Diversity of size is considerable: several micrometers for *Leishmania* and several meters for *Taenia*.

### Migration and Localization in the Organism

The immunologic response to blood parasites (*Schistosoma, Trypanosoma, Plasmodium*) and tissue parasites (*Filaria*, for example) is very different from that to intestinal parasites. Complex patterns of migration within the body (liver fluke, *Ascaris, Schistosoma*), induce a diversity of immune responses during the migratory cycle.

### Multiplication Potential

Protozoa multiply within the host, whereas helminths do not. Morphogenesis of the helminths is associated with a characteristic moulting (nematodes) or structural or metabolic modifications (trematodes, cestodes).

### Parasitic Specificity

Numerous parasites are specific for certain hosts, only one in some cases. Adaptation of a given parasite to different hosts initiates varying pathogenic effects and immune responses. *Schistosoma*, for example, causes variations in response that range from perfect adaptation (man, hamster) to rejection of the parasitic population (rat). Parasitic specificity is emphasized by natural immunity patterns in certain hosts: of 8,000 species of parasitic protozoa, only 20 are found in man. The factors that cause sensitivity, on the one hand or natural resistance, on the other, are not known and do not necessarily depend on immunologic factors. For example, susceptibility versus resistance to infection by *Plasmodium* does not depend on serum factors but is related to the presence or absence of receptors specific for parasites on the surface of host red blood cells. Similarly, genetic mutations responsible for sickle cell anemia confer partial resistance to *Plasmodium falciparum* infection (in man). The incomplete review of these few factors underlines the complexity of immunologic pictures seen in parasitic diseases and the highly variable pattern of acquired immunity.

## EXPRESSION OF IMMUNITY IN PARASITIC DISEASES

It is often difficult, or even impossible, to show acquired immunity in various parasitic infections. For a long time, it was thought that parasites were weak immunogens. Three different profiles of immune responses were suggested.

### Apparent Absence of Acquired Immunity

This phenomenon is seen in infestation by African trypanosomiases (*Trypanosoma gambiense* or *rhodiense*), of American trypanosomia (*Trypanosoma cruci*), amoebic meningoencephalitis, visceral leishmaniosis, amoebiasis, and some nematode diseases (e.g., ankylostomosis). No evidence of acquired immunity is present. The parasites persist for very long periods, even for the life-span of the host.

### Nonsterilizing Immunity (Type I)

In several parasitic infections, an immune response that leads to acquired resistance to reinfection is induced that results in persistence of the parasite at controlled levels. Such a response is characteristic for numerous helminthic infections and has been described in schistosomiasis as concomitant immunity. For protozoa, the same phenomenon is called premunition. This phenomenon is seen in human and simian malaria, cattle infections by *Babesia* or *Theileria*, and in toxoplasmosis in the mouse and other animal species.

### Sterilizing Immunity (Type II)

In certain cases, immunity is associated with clinical recovery, including complete elimination of the parasite and subsequent long-lasting resistance to reinfection. This outcome is seen in human cutaneous leishmaniosis, rodent trypanosomiasis, and cattle pulmonary dictyocaulosis.

In most cases (type I or II), immunity is species specific or even disease stage specific (human malaria, african trypanosomiasis). With helminths, induction of an immune response or susceptibility to such a response varies considerably during the life cycle. Most often, immunity is altered during one particular stage of development, which defines stage-specific immunity. With most helminths, adult worms represent the major stimulus to immunity. Once immunity is well established, it acts against all invading forms. This is not, however, always true. Probably different immune mechanisms intervene at different stages of parasitic development.

The various aspects of immune response to parasites result from three components of the immune response: parasitic antigenicity, nature of the effector mechanisms, and parasite possible mechanisms of escape from such a response so as to allow survival of the parasite.

## PARASITIC ANTIGENICITY

The analysis of parasitic antigens shows that protozoa and helminths contain a very complex mosaic of antigens. Immunoelectrophoresis has identified a minimum of 25–30 components for each parasite. Bidimensional electrophoresis allows differentiation of as many as 60 different antigens. Within this mosaic, there are highly specific antigens that are good immunogens. They induce early production of antibodies detectable by common serologic techniques.

Antigenic analysis shows the existence of important shared antigenic relationships among various species of nematodes or cestodes, but marked disparity among different trematodes. In protozoa, cross-reacting intergeneric and interspecific reactivity is common and relates to the taxonomic status of these parasites. Within each species, stage-specific antigens may be identified. Each stage of schistosomal evolution shows antigens common to all stages and also stage-specific antigens.

This specificity is true also for protozoa, for example, trypanosomes. Here, antigens specific for the blood form, and clone-specific antigens may be demonstrated. Antigenic variations within a single strain have been demonstrated in trypanosomes and *Plasmodium*. These variations seem to result from phenotypic changes induced by antibodies. In trypanosomes, variant antigens are surface glycoproteins constituting the cell coat.

Most antigens that have been identified have characteristic enzymatic activities (hydrolases, hydratases). Modern affinity chromatography techniques that employ enzyme inhibitors or immunoadsorbents have now permitted purification of some parasitic antigens (hydatid, schistosomes).

At the functional level, somatic and metabolic antigens are differentiated. As a rule, most immunogenic antigens are metabolic. They represent either digestive excretory products or glandular secretions, especially for certain helminths (schistosomes), or surface antigens released by the permanent turnover of the external cytoplasmic membrane. Thus, in many parasitic infections (*Plasmodium, Babesia, Trypanosoma, Haemonchus, Trichinella, Schistosoma*), soluble antigens may be detected in the serum and/or urine of infested hosts. The existence of circulating immune complexes has, moreover, been demonstrated in malaria, trypanosomiasis, and schistosomiasis.

Numerous parasites, especially helminths, possess antigens that show cross-reactivity with the host (host antigen). These antigens may be synthesized by the parasite (glycoprotein antigens) or selectively incorporated within erythrocytic or cellular membranes (as for certain glycolipid antigens).

# NATURE OF EFFECTOR MECHANISMS

## Components of Immune Mechanisms

Parasitic infection by protozoa or helminths induces antibody production and, in certain cases, cell-mediated immunity. The distinction between these two types of response is not clear-cut. Transfer experiments with either serum or sensitized cells alone are generally unsuccessful.

### HUMORAL RESPONSE

Although many types of antibodies are found in most parasitic infections, these antibodies generally have little or no protective action.

*Production of Nonspecific Immunoglobulins.* Immunoglobulin synthesis is notably elevated in various parasitic diseases. In malaria, very high levels of IgG and IgM (up to seven times the normal level) are observed, but only 5% of IgG shows specific antibody activity against *Plasmodium*. Nonspecific Ig production probably explains the occurrence of autoantibodies, cold agglutinins or immunoconglutinins in these hyperglobulinemic subjects with chronic malaria.

The elevation of IgM in trypanosomiasis is so marked that it has diagnostic value. IgM contains specific agglutinating antibodies and also heterophile and antiglobulin antibodies. Some of the IgM is in the monomeric form (7S).

The production of high IgE levels along with reaginic antibodies is a striking immunologic characteristic of helminth infections (nematodes, cestodes, trematodes). This feature appears to be linked to the potentiation of the IgE response by certain helminthic products. The potentiation may involve a great variety of antigens, because IgE antibodies to the parasite represent no more than 5–6% of the total IgE. The significance of the IgE response in helminthiasis will be discussed later.

*Production of Specific Antibodies.* In all parasitic infections, the presence of specific antibodies may be demonstrated in vitro by serologic tests (complement fixation, agglutination, hemagglutination, immunofluorescence, immunodiffusion, immunoenzymologic techniques) or in vivo (intradermoreaction). All of these tests are of diagnostic interest for parasitic infections but do not correlate with host immunity. This fact suggests that the parasite-infested organism elaborates, in addition to nonspecific Ig, specific antibodies that have no protective action.

*Protective Antibodies.* The only convincing examples of these antibodies, demonstrated by passive transfer, have been found with protozoa: rodent trypanosomiasis (*Trypanosoma lewisi* and *musculi*), human and experimental malaria, and African trypanosomiasis. In all of these cases, however, large amounts of serum are necessary to transfer protection. In addition, neutralization tests in which parasites are preincubated in immune serum prior to experimental inoculation demonstrate protective antibodies in malaria, African trypanosomiasis, and certain nematode infections.

The exact mechanisms of protection are poorly understood. In human malaria, protective antibodies seem to belong to the IgG fraction. In the monkey, antibodies act on merozoites at the time of their release into the plasma, thus preventing erythrocytic reinvasion by blocking specific receptors of the erythrocytic membrane. This type of inhibition is species specific but does have an effect to a lesser degree on variants of the same strain or even on heterologous strains. In trypanosomiasis, passive immunization produces specific protection against the variant. The antibody is complement dependent and is species and strain specific. In rat infection by *T. lewisi*, immunity may be passively transferred by a trypanocidal antibody that is complement dependent. In addition, there is a substance called ablastin associated with IgG1, which inhibits parasite reproduction in vivo and in vitro without affecting variability or mobility.

### ROLE OF THE THYMUS AND OF CELL-MEDIATED IMMUNITY

The thymus and T lymphocytes are implicated in the induction of immunity towards many parasites and practically all helminths so far studied. Protective immunity against *Nippostrongylus brasiliensis, Trichinella spiralis,* or *Hymenolepis nana* is considerably reduced by neonatal thymectomy or treatment by antilymphocyte serum. Cattle with thymic abnormalities show increased sensitivity to infection by *Fasciola hepatica.*

There are numerous examples that suggest that immunity in helminthiasis requires T lymphocytes for induction. Several aspects of the immune response to helminths are, in fact, thymus dependent, including reaginic antibodies (production is reduced in thymectomized animals), eosiniphilia (a classic sign of helminthic infection), and tissue basophil infiltration.

Thymus-dependent immunity may express itself by various effector mechanisms, both humoral and/or cellular. In monkey and rodent malaria, protective immunity holds the infection to a very low level. T lymphocytes play an essential role in this response, probably by a "helper" effect on the synthesis by B lymphocytes of variant-specific antibodies. This "helper" action is responsible for a more rapid and efficient response to the successive variants. A similar phenomenon probably active in infection by African trypanosomes (*T. brucei* and *T. gambiense*). The intervention of cell-mediated immunity in protection mechanisms has been demonstrated in some parasitic systems. Thus numerous in vivo and in vitro studies have shown the presence of delayed hypersensitivity in helminths and protozoa.

The most striking example of cell-mediated immunity in parasitology is that of cutaneous leishmaniosis in the experimental model of *Leishmania enrietti* (guinea pig), which is closely analogous to the *Leishmania tropica* that affects man. Clinically, infection is associated with intense delayed hypersensitivity and long-term immunity against reinfection. Delayed hypersensitivity may be transmitted passively by cell transfer. *Leishmania* antigens inhibit macrophage migration. Reinfection immunity is considerably reduced after thymectomy. On this basis, it is thought that immunity in cutaneous leishmaniosis is cell mediated and that specific T-cell deficiency is the cause of diffuse cutaneous leishmaniosis and disseminated lupoid forms.

In helminths, the best evidence for an intervention of cell-mediated immunity is granuloma formation. Granulomas that develop around schistosoma eggs are correlates of cell-mediated immunity. They cause considerable histologic alterations but have no apparent relationship to protective immunity.

## Effector Mechanisms

Analysis of the various humoral and cellular factors in host reactions to parasites raises the question of the nature of immunity effector mechanisms in parasitosis. These mechanisms are, in most cases, unknown, and this lack of knowledge probably explains why no effective vaccination has been achieved in human parasitosis. Certain experimental models, however, are amenable to some synthetic approaches. We shall mention here those of *N. brasiliensis* in the rat and *S. mansoni* in rodents and monkeys.

The *N. brasiliensis*-rat system represents the best model of two-phase effector mechanisms in which antibodies and sensitized lymphocytes cooperate or are associated.

The first phase is represented by the action of antibodies on parasites. These antibodies (IgG1 in most cases) produce degenerative lesions in the digestive cell cytoplasm and alter enzymatic secretions. However, the action of these antibodies, which do not require complement, does not ensure parasite expulsion.

The second phase, which leads to parasite rejection, requires the action of sensitized lymphocytes. Transfer of sensitized lymphocytes to irradiated rats produces rapid expulsion of worms previously damaged by antibodies. Normal worms, not exposed to antibodies, are slowly rejected and only in small numbers. The cell population required for phase two, has not been formally identified, but macrophages do not seem to play an important role.

These experimental observations are reminiscent of two natural situations (newborn rats and suckling rats) in which the first phase, humorally mediated, is not affected but in which lymphocytic immaturity prevents parasite expulsion. Finally, immunity to *N. brasiliensis* in the rat represents a good example of a two-phase effector mechanism, whose existence in numerous parasitic systems is suggested.

In the rodent-monkey *S. mansoni* system, induction of immunity is conferred by adult worms, and effector mechanisms act on immature forms or schistosomules during reinfection. The development of in vitro culture techniques and the use of appropriate experimental models has recently led to the identification of effector mechanisms, the most important of which has been found to be antibody-dependent cell-mediated cytotoxicity (ADCC).

After the initial discovery, in several experimental models (man, monkey, rat), that cytotoxic antibodies of the IgG class could cause the destruction, in the presence of complement, of schistosomal larvae, an important series of observations focused attention on the importance, both in vivo and in vitro, of two particular mechanisms:

1. In man, the baboon, and the rat, it was demonstrated that in the presence of IgG produced during infection with *S. mansoni*, normal eosinophils gave marked cytotoxicity responses against schistosomules. This mechanism is not dependent on complement and is associated in the rat with IgG2a. In this model, the induction of cytotoxicity by eosinophils appears to depend on a double signal. One is dependent on mastocytic mediators released when mast cells are activated by IgG2a or IgE antibodies, whereas the other involves the binding of Fc fragments of antibodies onto the appropriate eosinophil receptor.

The administration of antieosinophilic serum in mice results in significant reduction of the immunity when reinfection occurs.

2. In man, the baboon, and the rat, normal monocytes or macrophages destroy schistosomules in the presence of IgE immune complexes. Correlative study of these two mechanisms with that of the evolution of acquired immunity in the rat reveals that joint participation of anaphylactic antibodies is essential in the reinfection immunity against schistosomes in rodents. The involvement of complement, of which both the classic and alternative pathways may be activated by parasitic membranes (hence the existence of C3b receptors on macrophages and eosinophils) may also be envisaged as one of the important mechanisms of defence concurrent with the amplification of the specific cytotoxic process.

These two examples, using particularly well-studied models, indicate the complexity of facts and interpretations. However, the existence of effector mechanisms in parasitic systems is well established on the basis of both epidemiologic and experimental data.

The effect of the immune response on parasites is extremely variable, ranging from growth inhibition to cytolysis, including the alteration of certain essential physiologic functions. Of these functions, egg laying is of particular interest, because its immunologic control would have clinical relevance. An example is seen in experimental filariasis, in which egg laying and microfilariae production by adult females seem to be controlled by a cell-mediated immunity phenomena (*Litomosoides carinii*-rat system) and antibodies (*Dipetalonema viteae*-hamster system).

The reasons for the relative ineffectiveness of the immune response induced by parasites, attested to by their long survival in immune hosts, have been the subject of considerable recent study, but the findings are so far inconclusive.

## MECHANISMS OF PARASITIC SURVIVAL

The role of immunity in parasitism raises unique questions for immunologists. Survival of parasites, as a species, depends on host survival; often, induction of the immune response in the host is essential for host survival and for the perenniality of the parasitic cycle. Thus, induction of antiparasitic immunity results from a balance between dimensions and functions of the parasitic population and the host.

Analysis of the adaptive mechanisms by which the parasite has or will escape from the immune response during its evolution is even more complex, because each parasite has its own methods of survival. Therefore, we will only briefly outline a few particularly important mechanisms.

### Host Antigens

It has been clearly established that parasites (either larval or adult) have antigens common to the host, both intermediate and definitive. Such an acquisition has at least two possible mechanisms. The antigen may be synthesized by the parasite itself or be produced by the host and secondarily selectively incorporated into the parasite. Some of these antigens are localized at the worm (*Schistosoma*) surface; their acquisition at the beginning of the larval phase makes the parasite insensitive from that point on to cytotoxic antibodies. The recent demonstration of the existence of murine major histocompatibility products (K and I) and receptors for the Fc portion of IgG on the surface of larval forms of schistosomes are additional indications of the complexity of the surface structure of some parasites' surfaces. Existence of such antigens on the schistosome surface after the fourth day is beneficial for the parasite, because it protects it from the host immune reaction. Concomitant immunity to schistosomiasis and some other parasites may thus be explained.

### Soluble Antigens

We have mentioned above that circulating soluble antigens are present in certain parasitic systems. They play multiple roles with regard to parasite survival: antigenic competition, tolerance induction, suppressor T-cell stimulation, neutralization of high-affinity antibodies, formation of circulating immune complexes, and immune deviation are current hypotheses.

### Antigenic Variation

Protozoan antigenic variation (*Trypanosoma, Plasmodium*) is linked to differences in cell wall glycoproteins. These proteins are eliminated and then replaced by antigenically distinct glycoproteins. By reference to other systems, complex formation between antibodies and coat antigens may lead to a capping phenomenon in which the antigenic structures of the membrane are eliminated and replaced by a layer of different specificity. Regardless of the mechanism, antigenic variation is an essential factor for parasitic survival in the immune host because the antibodies elicited are highly specific for the variant.

### Immunosuppression Mechanisms

The existence of immunosuppressive phenomena in the majority of parasitic infections has now become a well-established fact. In man, as well as in numerous experimental models, parasitic infections produce a susceptibility to tumorigencsis, delayed allograft rejection, and alteration of the response to diverse xenoantigens. In addition, the increased production of immunoglobulins and the frequency of autoantibody development demonstrate the polyclonal activation of B cells that takes place during such an infection.

A number of mechanisms have been suggested in an attempt to explain the different aspects of immunosuppression that have been observed, including antigenic competition, nonspecific T-cell suppression, acquired tolerance, blocking antibodies, and blockade by antigen and circulating immune complexes. Although it is unlikely that a sole mechanism is responsible for the immunosuppressive phenomena observed in all parasitic models, the production of immunoregulatory substances by the parasite itself has now been confirmed in a number of models (schistosomiasis, filiariasis, trichinosis, trypanosomiasis, malaria, etc.). Substances of low molecular weight that inhibit the proliferation of lymphocytes, both in vivo and in vitro, have now been described, particularly with schistosomes. Their action, independent of suppressor T-cell function, appears to be linked to a direct role at the level of the lymphocyte membrane.

The recognition of these various survival mechanisms demonstrates how much the expression of antiparasitic immunity results from the establishment of a permanent equilibrium between the development of effector mechanisms and their regulation, which often appears to be controlled by the parasite itself.

## CONCLUSIONS

Parasite immunology, like parasite biology, is complex and diversified in many subtle ways. This brief discussion has not attempted to closely define all of the important concepts that have resulted from immunologic study of parasitic systems. Our theoretical knowledge remains imperfect, and the prospects of effective vaccination for parasitosis seem remote. Nonetheless, at least two important goals have been reached in parasite immunology. First, knowledge of parasitic antigenicity has permitted the establishment of precise and specific diagnostic methods for parasitic infections. Second, parasites, on the basis of their peculiar biologic characteristics and of the diversity of immune responses that they induce have become privileged models for immunologic research.

# V. APPENDIX: VACCINATIONS AND SEROTHERAPY

Infectious diseases, whether bacterial, viral, or parasitic, induce immune responses and eventually cause a favorable host response, for example, naturally acquired immunization. The study of these active immunizations has permitted recognition of relevant humoral and cellular factors and has provided insight into the bases of prophylactic, and even curative, immunization if administered prior to or at the time of contact with the infectious agent. Induced immunization may be active; for example, it may involve the subject's own immune responses to the vaccinal antigen. This type of immunization is called vaccination. Or immunization may be passive, consisting of transfer to a virginal individual of specific resistance factors (either humoral or cellular) from an immune donor. This type of immunization is called serotherapy. It also includes treatment by transfer factors (see chap. 31 and p. 376).

## PASSIVE IMMUNIZATION

Induced passive immunization of a virginal or immunodeficient recipient consists of transfer of serum from a normal or immune donor (man or animal). Most passively induced immunizations involve injection of Ig in the form of antibodies specific for a given antigen. This type of immunization is called seroprophylaxis or serotherapy.

### *Indications*

Despite progress in vaccination, serotherapy has important applications when the anticipated incubation period is so short that active protection by vaccine cannot be achieved and curative therapy is unavailable; when the antigen is not borne by an infectious agent, as is the case with newborn hemolytic disease; when there is no effective vaccine available; in immune deficiency states; and in subjects with multiple infections.

### *Nature of Immunoglobulins*

SPECIFIC

The spectrum of indications described above requires a variety of treatment administrations. For the first two situations, sera that contain high levels of specific antibodies of high avidity from hyperimmunized or convalescent subjects are employed. This approach applies to antidiphtheria or antitetanus seroprophylaxis and prevention of measles in infants.

NONSPECIFIC

In other settings, the sera utilized are active against several specificities. It is then necessary to use a sufficient amount of serum and to verify the absence of serioustoxicity despite multiple serum injections.

### *Deficiencies of Serotherapy*

The positive effects of serotherapy last for only a short time. Heterologous immunoglobulins are foreign antigens and are eliminated increasingly rapidly during the course of treatment and may thereby lead to hypersensitivity reactions. Thus, the use of animal immunoglobulins is waning. Such therapy is also very costly. Serotherapy is today used only in cases in which there is no curative anti-infectious treatment or time-effective actively induced immunization.

## ACTIVE IMMUNIZATION

Actively induced immunization confers immunity specific for the vaccinal infectious antigen. It is linked to the appearance in the vaccinated subject of one or more natural factors of specific resistance. Considerable effort has been devoted to ensure optimal conditions for the most effective and durable immunity.

### *Efficiency*

Evaluation of the protection induced by the vaccine is made possible by controlling the immune responses of the vaccinated subjects to the vaccinal antigen, by evaluating the vaccine's effect at the onset of infection by epidemiologic studies, or, most rarely, by controlled infectious trials.

IMMUNOLOGIC TESTS

Immunologic studies evaluate qualitatively and quantitatively the effect of one or multiple vaccinating injections. They focus on the production of specific antibodies or on the development of delayed-type hypersensitivity, irrespective of whether the predominant mechanism implicated in the particular infectious disease is humoral or cellular. Such simple tests are sometimes valid (antidiphtheria and antitetanus vaccination) but are not adequate in evaluating the effects of many other vaccinations. Therefore tests that more closely measure cellular or humoral protection mechanisms are being developed, while tests that examine only associated responses are less often employed.

EPIDEMIOLOGIC TESTS

Epidemiologic tests allow a critical appreciation of vaccination efficiency. They are performed to evaluate whether a decreasing frequency of infections in an endemic population is occurring in response to vaccine administration versus the matched control (without vaccine) population. Statistical interpretation mainly concerning the choice of control subjects, the current or evolutive microbacterial ecology, and the socioeconomic level, is very important. The high cost of such trials explains why they are usually limited in scope and why only a few precise markers are studied.

CONTROLLED INFECTIOUS TRIALS

The study of small groups of vaccinated individuals subjected to deliberate and specific infection has numerous advantages. Evaluation of results is easy because the number of subjects is limited and the selection of parameters that have a low rate of variability can be better codified. These studies do, however, have at least two drawbacks. First, the results are dependent on the criteria chosen. Thus, if a high infecting dose is employed, a relatively inefficient vaccine may appear inadequate, even though it might have been useful in clinical practice where natural infecting doses were lower. Second, and more important, from the ethical point of view, this method is subject to considerable criticism (most of these studies have used prisoner or soldier subjects).

## Site of Administration

The technique of application must take into account the mechanisms of specific resistance. If circulating antibodies represent the major source of defense, as in tetanus, parenteral injection should be used (subcutaneous, intradermal, or intramuscular). If anti-infectious mechanisms involve only local defense, for example, with IgA secretory antibodies, immunization should be local (digestive, nasal, ocular, or bronchial tract). Both routes may be used if dual action is applicable, as with oral or parenteral antipoliomyelitis vaccine.

The route of administration may vary according to the individuals vaccinated. Absence of pain, ready application to mass vaccination, a refusal to undergo parenteral injections by certain populations, and the absence of side effects, of course, explain the popularity of oral vaccination.

**Table 16.5 Principal Vaccines**

| Disease | Antigen preparation | Indications | Immunization route | Result |
|---|---|---|---|---|
| Diphtheria | Formaldehyde-treated toxin | Children | Subcutaneous | Satisfactory |
| Tetanus | Formaldehyde-treated toxin | Children | Subcutaneous | Satisfactory |
| Botulism | Formaldehyde-treated toxin | On exposure | Subcutaneous | Needs improvement |
| Whooping cough | Killed bacteria | Children | Subcutaneous | Satisfactory |
| Typhoid | Killed bacteria | Endemia | Subcutaneous | Satisfactory |
| Cholera | Phenol-treated bacteria | Endemia | Subcutaneous | Needs improvement |
| Plague | Formalin-killed bacteria | On exposure | Subcutaneous | Needs improvement |
| Pneumonia | Bacterial extracts | Endemia | Subcutaneous | Needs improvement |
| Meningitis | Bacterial extracts | Endemia | Subcutaneous | Needs improvement |
| Tuberculosis | Attenuated organisms Bacillus Calmette-Guérin (BCG) | Children | Intradermal | Needs improvement |
| Poliomyelitis | Attenuated or inactivated virus | Children | Oral | Satisfactory |
| Measles | Attenuated virus | Children | Subcutaneous | Satisfactory |
| Mumps | Attenuated virus | Children | Subcutaneous | Satisfactory |
| Yellow fever | Attenuated virus | Endemia | Subcutaneous | Needs improvement |
| Smallpox | Attenuated virus | Children | Subcutaneous or intradermal | Satisfactory |
| Rubella | Attenuated virus | Children | Subcutaneous | Satisfactory |
| Influenza | Inactivated virus | High-risk group | Subcutaneous | Needs improvement |
| Rabies | Inactivated virus | On exposure | Subcutaneous | Needs improvement |
| Hepatitis B | HBs antigen | High-risk group | Subcutaneous | Satisfactory (to be confirmed) |
| Typhus | Killed rickettsies | On exposure | Subcutaneous | Satisfactory |

## Duration of Immunization

The duration of protection afforded by a vaccine relates to the quality of the vaccine and to the amount of antigen administered. Inactivated (dead) and living vaccines must be distinguished.

Dead or inactivated vaccines consist of microbial elements (viruses, parasites, or bacteria) destroyed chemically or physically or of microbial products (purified) of the pathogen. Examples are diphtheria and tetanus anatoxins, which are exotoxins in crystallized form, highly purified and modified by heat and formol. Anatoxins have no toxicity but maintain antigenicity. However, except for anatoxins, it is usually difficult to extract the specific vaccinal antigen while maintaining the protective capability.

Living vaccines are live microbial elements, either attenuated (rendered nonvirulent in normal subjects) or innocuous in certain hosts, that confer cross-immunity to the virulent infectious agent (an example is vaccinia). However, living vaccines are always more dangerous than killed vaccines, at least theoretically. In fact, only living vaccines are effective in infections in which specific defense mechanisms are cell mediated. Examples include tuberculosis (BCG, Bacillus Calmette-Guérin), measles, or poliomyelitis. Attenuated living vaccines must be evaluated in terms of standardized viable units, maintenance of attenuation, and risks of possible contamination.

## Amount of Vaccinal Antigen

Doses of antigen used in inactivated vaccines are always higher than those used in living vaccines. In the latter case, viral proliferation in vivo induces

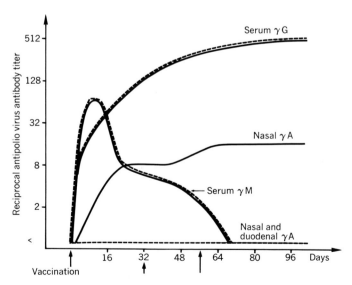

**Fig. 16.3**  Production of antibodies against poliomyelitis virus after administration of living (—) or killed (---) vaccine. (From A. J. Beale. *In* P. G. H. Cell, R. A. Coombs, and P. J. Lachmann, Clinical aspects of immunology, ed. 3. London, 1975, Blackwell, p. 1633.)

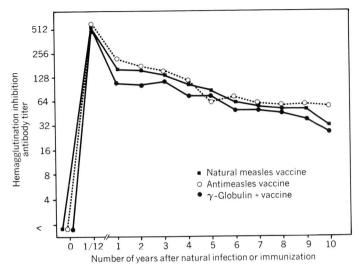

**Fig. 16.4**   Response of human subjects after natural measles or antimeasles vaccination. (From S. Krugman. *In* G. Edsall, in P. G. H. Gell, R. A. Coombs, and P. J. Lachmann. Clinical aspects of immunology, ed. 3. Oxford, 1975, Blackwell, 1605.)

optimal stimulation of specific resistance factors, which eliminate only pathogens when the dose of antigen produced is sufficient; with inactivated vaccine, it is necessary to administer the optimal quantity of antigen to induce a sufficient immune response. Several injections are usually necessary either to augment the intensity of the response or to increase the avidity of the antibodies produced. Only antigenic boosters ensure maintenance of a sufficient antibody level for 100% protection. In some cases, especially in certain antiviral vaccines in endemic countries, the immunity is subsequently reinforced by natural reinfections without detectable clinical signs. Boosters then become unnecessary.

The administration simultaneously of several vaccinal antigens (triple or quadruple vaccination) may increase the effectiveness of vaccinal antigens as compared to separate administrations. Potentialization seems to be due to the adjuvant action of some vaccinal preparations (see chap. 33). This effect is ascribed to lipopolysaccharides contained in the antityphic-paratyphic vaccine. In certain cases, the addition of inert adjuvants like calcium phosphate or aluminum hydroxide improves the immune response, especially antibody formation.

### Risks of Actively Induced Immunization

Some vaccines are perfectly innocuous and never are associated with side-effects, namely, antitetanus and antidiphtheria vaccines. Other vaccines, however, predispose one to severe complications, such as encephalitis associated with antivariola or antirabies vaccinations.

One must therefore take into account possible side-effects and the alternate risks of infection. Thus, in the United States, smallpox vaccination represents a risk probably greater than that of pox infection itself. Other less frequent complications of vaccination should be considered:

Certain antirubella vaccines (living attenuated vaccines) may cause placental lesions and fetal malformations when administered to pregnant women.

Certain oral attenuated living vaccines may induce dissemination of the vaccinal strain into the environment, with predictable effects on immunodeficient subjects who are unable to mount a normal response to the living organism.

Vaccination may lead to a hypersensitivity state with IgE production or delayed hypersensitivity. A subsequent infectious contact may then induce clinical hypersensitivity, sometimes more significant than the normal clinical infection (e.g., respiratory syncytial virus and measles virus).

When vaccination is very effective both in individual and whole populations, a decrease occurs in disease morbidity (e.g., diphtheria). This result may be followed by a tendency of large numbers of people to refuse vaccination. Collective susceptibility to infection increases, which may be harmful because certain infections are more severe in the adult than in children (e.g., poliomyelitis, measles).

Some bacterial or viral vaccinations alter collective immunity and may lead to the selection or appearance of genetic variants that are insensitive to acquired resistance factors (e.g., certain myxoviruses).

## BIBLIOGRAPHY

ALLISON A. C. Interactions of antibodies, complement components and various cell types in immunity against viruses and pyogenic bacteria. Transpl. Rev., 1974, *19*, 3.

BARON S. The biological significance of the interferon system. Arch. Intern. Med., 1970, *126*, 84.

BLANDEN R. V. T cell responses to viral and bacterial infections. Transpl. Rev., 1974, *19*, 56.

BLOOM B. R., TANOWITZ H., and WITTNER M. Game parasites play. *In*: Immune mechanisms and disease (D. B. Amos, R. S. Schwartz and B. W. Janicki [eds.]). Acad. Press, London, 1979, 69.

CAPRON A. R. G., CAPRON M., and DESSAINT J. P. ADCC as primary mechanisms of defense against metazoan parasites. *In*: Immunology 80 (M. Fougereau and J. Dausset [eds.]). Acad. Press, New York, 1980, 782.

COHEN S. Humoral responses to protozoal infections. *In*: Immunology 80 (M. Fougereau and J. Dausset [eds.]). Acad. Press, New York, 1980, 763.

COLLEY D. G. The immunopathology of schistosomiasis. *In* R. A. Thompson, Ed., Recent advances in clinical immunology. Edinburgh, 1977, Churchill-Livingstone, p. 101.

COOPER N. R. Humoral immunity to viruses. *In*: Comprehensive Virology (H. Fraenkel-Conrat and Wagner R. R. [eds.]). Plenum, New York, 1979, 123.

DEMAYEER E. and DEMAYEER-G. J. Interferons. *In*: Comprehensive Virology (H. Fraenkel-Conrat and Wagner R. R. [eds.]). Plenum, New York, 1979, 37.

DICK G. Immunological aspects of infectious diseases. MTP Lancaster U. K., 1979, 524 pp.

DOHERTY P. C. and ZINKERNAGEL R. M. T-cell mediated immunopathology in viral infections. Transpl. Rev., 1974, *19*, 89.

GLYNN A. A. Antibodies in infection. *In* L. Brent and J. Holborow, Eds., Progress in immunology. II. Vol. 4. Amsterdam, 1974, North Holland, p. 95.

Immunity in parasitic diseases. Colloque INSERM. Paris, 1978, INSERM.

JACKSON G. L., HERMAN R., and SINGER I. (Eds.) Immunity to parasitic animals. New York, 1970, Appleton-Century-Crofts.

MACKANESS G. B. Cell-mediated immunity to infection. *In* R. A. Good and D. W. Fisher, Eds., Immunobiology. Stamford, Conn., 1971, Sinauer, p. 45.

MITCHELL G. F. Responses to infection with metazoan and protozoan parasites in mice. Adv. Immunol., 1979, *28*, 451.

MITCHELL G. F. T cell dependent effects in parasitic infection and disease. *In*: Immunology 80 (M. Fougereau and J. Dausset [eds.]). Acad. Press, New York, 1980, 794.

NOTKINS A. L. Immunopathology of viral infections. *In* L. Brent and J. Holborow, Eds., Progress in immunology. II. Vol. 4. Amsterdam, 1974, North Holland, p. 141.

OGILVIE B. M. and JONES V. Immunity in the parasitic relationship between helminths and hosts. Progr. Allergy, 1973, *17*, 93.

OGILVIE B. M. and WILSON R. J. M. Evasion of the immune response by parasites. Brit. Med. Bull., 1976, *32*, 177.

OLDSTONE M. Immune responses, immune tolerance and viruses. *In*: Comprehensive Virology (H. Fraenkel-Conrat and Wagner R. R. [eds.]). Plenum, New York, 1979, 1.

OLDSTONE M. B. A., SISSONS J. G. P., and FUGINAMI R. S. Action of antibody and complement in regulating virus infection. *In*: Immunology 80 (M. Fougereau and J. Dausset [eds.]). Acad. Press, New York, 1980, 599.

PANDEL B. Interaction of viruses with neutralizing antibodies. *In*: Comprehensive Virology (H. Fraenkel-Conrat and Wagner R. R. [eds.]). Plenum, New York, 1979, 37.

Parasites in the immunized host: Mechanisms of survival. Ciba Foundation Symp. 25, Amsterdam, 1974, Elsevier North Holland.

SINCLAIR I. J. The relationship between circulating antibodies and immunity to helminthic infections. Adv. Parasit., 1970, *8*, 93.

SMITHERS S. R. and TERRY R. S. The immunology of schistosomiasis. Adv. Parasit., 1969, 7, 41.

STEWART W. E. The interferon system. Springer Verlag. New York, 1979, 421 pp.

SOULSBY E. J. L. Cell-mediated immunity in parasitic infections. J. Parasit., 1970, *56*, 534.

SOULSBY E. J. L. (Ed.) Immunity to animal parasites. New York, 1972, Academic Press.

STONER H. B. Specific and non-specific effects of bacterial infections of the host. Symp. Soc. Gen. Microbiol., 1972, *22*, 113.

VOLLER A. and FRIDMAN H. New trends and developments in vaccines. MTP Lancaster U. K., 1978, 323 pp.

ZINKERNAGEL R. M. H-2 restriction of cell-mediated virus-specific immunity and immunopathology: self recognition, altered self and auto-aggression. *In* N. Talal, Ed., autoimmunity, genetic, immunologic, virologic and clinical aspects. New-York, 1977, Academic Press, p. 363.

ZINKERNAGEL R. M. Cellular immune responses to viruses and the biological role of polymorphic major transplantation antigens. *In*: Comprehensive Virology (H. Fraenkel-Conrat and Wagner R. R. [eds.]). Plenum, New York, 1979, 171.

# ORIGINAL ARTICLES

GODAL T. The role of immune responses to Mycobacterium leprae in host defence and tissue damage in leprosy. *In* L. Brent and J. Holborow, Eds., Progress in immunology. II. Vol. 4. Amsterdam, 1974, North Holland, p. 161.

HIRSCH M. D., ZISMAN B., and ALLISON A. C. Macrophages and age-dependent resistance to herpes simplex virus in mice. J. Immunol., 1970, *104*, 1160.

LAGRANGE P. H., MACKANESS G. B., and MILLER T. E. Influence of dose and route of antigen injection on immunological induction of T-cells. J. Exp. Med., 1974, *139*, 528.

LAGRANGE P. H., MACKANESS G. B., and MILLER T. E. Potentiation of T-cell mediated immunity by selective suppression of antibody formation with cyclophosphamide. J. Exp. Med., 1974, *139*, 1529.

MACKANESS G. B. The influence of immunologically committed lymphoid cells in macrophage activity in vivo. J. Exp. Med., 1969, *129*, 973.

MAUEL J. Cell-mediated immune mechanisms in bacterial and protozoal infections. *In* L. Brent and J. Holborow, Eds., Progress in immunology. II. Vol. 4. Amsterdam, 1974, North Holland, p. 109.

SZMUNESS N., STEVENS C. E., HARLEY E. J., WILLIAM D. C., SALOVSKY R., MORRISON J. M., and KELLNER A. Hepatitis B vaccine: Demonstration of efficacy in a controlled trial in a high risk population in the United States. New Engl. J. Med., 1980, *303*, 833.

URQUHART G. M. Immunological unresponsiveness in parasitic infections. J. Parasit., 1970, *56*, 547.

ZINKERNAGEL R. M., ALTHAGE A., ADLER B., and BLANDEN R. V. H-2 restriction of cell-mediated immunity to an intracellular bacterium: effector T cells are specific to *Listeria* antigen in association with H-2I region-coded self-markers. J. Exp. Med., 1977, *145*, 1353.

## Part 4

## CELLULAR BASES OF
## ANTIBODY FORMATION

Chapter 17

# ANTIBODY FORMATION AT THE CELLULAR LEVEL

**Stratis Avrameas, Jean-François Bach, and Jean-Louis Preud'homme**

I.   INTRODUCTION
II.  ENUMERATION OF ANTIBODY-PRODUCING CELLS
III. CYTOLOGIC ASPECTS OF ANTIBODY FORMATION
IV.  BIOCHEMICAL ASPECTS OF CELLULAR IMMUNOGLOB-
     ULIN SYNTHESIS

## I.   INTRODUCTION

Antibody formation by lymphoid cells may be studied at various functional levels. The methods employed to study this phenomenon include quantifying the number of antibody-producing cells by hemolytic plaque and rosette techniques; localization of antibodies in cells by light or electron microscopy by various techniques, including determination of the immunochemical content of antibody-producing cells by use of antibodies labeled with ferritin or an easily detectable antigen like peroxidase; and examination of various biochemical aspects of cellular synthesis of immunoglobulins.

## II.   ENUMERATION OF ANTIBODY-PRODUCING CELLS*

The general principle of techniques used to count antibody-forming cells (AFC) consists of studying macroscopically or by light microscopy a visible phenomenon

---

* J.-F. Bach.

that relates to the biologic activity of antibodies secreted by the AFC. The visible phenomenon is hemolysis when the hemolytic plaque technique is used, and agglutination when the rosette technique is employed. The latter in fact detects antigen-binding cells, which may also be studied by means of autoradiography or fluorescence methods (fluorescent antigen). We shall see later that techniques based on simple binding of antigen to cellular receptors detect not only AFC but also antigen-sensitive cells, which do not secrete antibodies. The latter probably include T cells.

## HEMOLYTIC PLAQUE TECHNIQUE

### *Principle*

STANDARD TECHNIQUE

The hemolytic plaque technique, first described independently by Jerne and by Ingraham and Bussard in 1963 is similar in principle to the plaque technique, which was previously developed for bacteriophage counting. It consists of detecting minimal amounts of hemolytic antibodies localized around the AFC. Lymphoid cells are simultaneously incorporated with heterologous erythrocytes in a gel medium, either an agar slide layered in a petri dish or agar deposited on a microscope slide. Some lymphoid cells release diffusible hemolytic antibodies that lyse red blood cells in the immediate vicinity to form a lytic plaque (plaque-forming cells, PFC) after the addition of complement. Plaques are macroscopically visible and may be accurately counted by use of a simple magnifying lens.

VARIATIONS IN TECHNIQUE

Media other than agar may be used, for example, carboxymethyl cellulose (CMC), which additionally provides a nutritive medium for cell culture. Cell counts may be augmented by prior (to complement) addition of a serum directed against minimally hemolytic Ig (such as IgG and IgA). These anti-Ig antibody molecules bind to antibody molecules fixed on the red blood cell surface during the initial incubation. The resultant antibody complexes, in turn, bind complement factors, which then cause red blood cell lysis. This indirect technique may be performed with either polyvalent anti-Ig sera or Ig class-specific sera. The direct technique described first detects mostly IgM-PFC; the indirect technique reveals IgG-PFC in addition to IgM-PFC. Similarly, antiallotypic sera detect PFC formation by antibodies of a given allotype.

The plaque technique can be used to study antibody production against soluble antigens, polysaccharides, proteins, or haptens by prior fixation onto indicator red blood cells. The sensitivity of these techniques is increased when a liquid medium is used and when plaques are counted by light microscopy (Cunningham). Nossal and Bussard proposed another technique in 1970 that utilizes ultrathin preparations of carboxymethyl cellulose in oil, which provides even greater sensitivity and permits micromanipulation of PFC. By 1965, Berglund had proposed the use of ultrathin agar preparations (on microscope slides), which gave access to PFC and also permitted autoradiography and immunofluorescence modifications.

### Significance of PFC

A PFC background is present in nonimmunized animals (160–400 antisheep PFC per spleen, or approximately one to four PFC per $10^6$ cells). Most of these PFC are plasma cells, and they show the same properties as those of PFC after immunization. Sterzl showed the absence of PFC background in axenic pigs; thus, one may assume that PFC are natural antibody-producing cells.

PFC after immunization are antibody-producing cells that continue their secretion of antibodies in vitro. Secretion seems to occur approximately 20 min after synthesis (see p. 526). Plaque formation represents active secretion of antibodies by living cells (fixed cells do not form plaques). Plaque formation is blocked by potassium cyanide (0.1 M), puromycin, and cycloheximide. However when cycloheximide is added to the system, the cell may continue for several hours to secrete the antibodies synthesized prior to incubation with inhibitor. Treatment with actinomycin D has little effect on plaque formation, which suggests that messenger RNA, which is responsible for antibody synthesis, has a long life-span.

Direct plaques (as defined above) are formed mostly by IgM-secreting cells. However, cells that produce large amounts of IgG antibodies, as in secondary responses, may also form direct plaques prior to addition of anti-IgG serum. Furthermore, certain IgM PFC are not detected by direct techniques.

### Applications of the Technique

The hemolytic plaque technique has numerous applications, which will be discussed elsewhere in this chapter. These applications include cytologic studies by use of light or electron microscopy, micromanipulation of antibody-forming cells, and study of the nature of antibodies produced in single cells. At this point, we will examine postimmunization PFC kinetics as measured in vivo and in vitro by use of sheep red blood cells and will comment on the nature of antibodies secreted by PFC.

IN VIVO IMMUNIZATION KINETICS

The number of PFC increases rapidly in the spleen of mice immunized with sheep red blood cells (SRBC). Increased numbers are detected as early as the sixth hour. Peak response is seen on the fourth day: this peak averages approximately 50,000 direct PFC and 20,000 indirect PFC per spleen after intravenous immunization with $2 \times 10^8$ SRBC. The number of PFC decreases rapidly during subsequent days (Fig. 17.1).

After the same intravenous immunization, PFC are also found in lymph nodes and transiently in the circulating blood but in smaller numbers than in the spleen. PFC are not found in the thymus. In secondary responses, the increase in PFC occurs more rapidly, and PFC counts are higher.

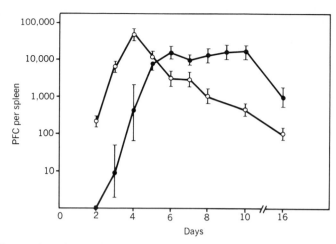

**Fig. 17.1**  Plaque-forming cell kinetics in spleens of mice subjected to primary immunization with SRBC. ●, Indirect plaques (IgG); ○, direct plaques (IgM).

IN VITRO IMMUNIZATION KINETICS

Mishell and Dutton have developed a culture technique that employs mouse spleen cells and that permits an in vitro primary response after addition of SRBC. PFC numbers increase as early as day 2, reaching maximum numbers by days 4–6 ($10^3$ PFC/$10^6$ cells).

ANTIBODY TYPE SECRETED BY PFC

PFC usually contain antibodies of only one specificity, one class, and one allotype. At the beginning of the primary response, the antibodies are IgM and later become IgG. IgG predominates even early in the secondary response. During a short time interval (days 3 and 4 of the primary response), PFC may produce both IgM and IgG (which probably represents the IgM-IgG switch) and may even produce double-specificity antibodies when two antigens are simultaneously injected. These data have obviously important implications but have not yet been fully confirmed.

## ROSETTE TEST

Several techniques are used to study antigen-binding cells under the microscope. The initial technique employed bacterial adherence. The rosette test, described independently by Biozzi and Zaalberg in 1964, is technically the easiest to perform.

Heterologous red blood cells and lymphoid cells from animals previously sensitized with the same red blood cells are incubated together. Simple contact of the two types of cells suffices to produce agglutination of red blood cells around certain "immunocytes" to form a typical rosette. A rosette is defined as adherence of at least four red blood cells around one lymphoid cell.

The rosette technique has added considerably to basic concepts of immunology: AFC and cells that bear immunologic memory form rosettes. The technique has been applied to clinical immunology for evaluating immunosuppressive agents and for diagnostic studies based on antigen binding.

### Description of the Test

Lymphoid cells of any origin and from any species may be used to form rosettes. In man, SRBC rosettes have particular significance, because they represent a nonspecific T-cell marker (discussed on p. 69).

In the initial step of the procedure, lymphocytes are isolated and purified. Lymphocytes and red blood cells are then combined in one of two ways by simple centrifugation at 200$g$ for 5 min or overnight incubation at 4°C. Resuspension is then performed to dissociate nonspecific agglutinates, but the procedure must not be so excessive as to dissociate rosettes, especially indirect rosettes formed with soluble antigen-coated red blood cells. An overly vigorous resuspension explains the negative results reported by some authors studying T cells. The cell suspension (e.g., $6 \times 10^6$ lymphocytes plus $25 \times 10^6$ red blood cells in a total volume of 1 ml of Hanks's medium) is inserted into a hematocytometer for rosette counting. The number of rosettes in relation to the number of lymphocytes is reported. Recognition of rosettes is relatively simple. The characteristic finding of a complete rosette includes a highly visible lymphocyte in the center; in the incomplete rosette, only a fraction of the circumference is coated with red blood cells; a morula may be seen in which the lymphocyte is not visible because it is hidden under a cluster of red blood cells (Figs. 17.2, 17.3).

All lymphocytes from an animal previously immunized with SRBC do not form rosettes. At peak immunization (on day 6), only 10–15 per 1,000 lymphocytes form rosettes. Rosettes are specific for one antigen; when the animal is immunized with two different red blood cell species, the great majority of rosettes contain only one red blood cell species.

### Table 17.1  Different Types of Rosettes

Rosettes due to antigen-specific receptors
    Xenogeneic erythrocytes (in the mouse and the rat)
    Erythrocytes coated with soluble antigens (B and T lymphocytes, macrophages)
    Allogeneic erythrocytes (in the mouse and the rat)
Autologous rosettes
    Markers of immature T cells(?)
Rosettes not due to antigen-specific receptors
    E rosettes formed with sheep red blood cells (in man), marker of T lymphocytes.
    EA rosettes formed by cells that have receptors for the Fc fragment of IgG (see p. 76)
    EAC rosettes formed by cells that have receptors for complement (see p. 75)
    Hybrid rosettes formed with erythrocytes coated with hybrid antibodies, two chains of which have antisheep red blood cell specificity and two others a specificity for receptors present on the surface of rosette-forming cells (for example, immunoglobulins)

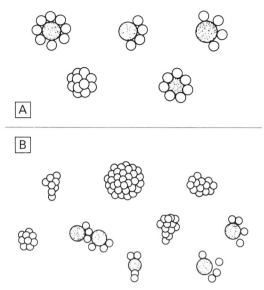

**Fig. 17.2** Rosettes. One easily distinguishes by light microscopy true rosettes (A) from nonspecific aggregates (B). Note that the scale is smaller in (B).

Similar results are obtained when erythrocytes are coated with soluble antigen (Fig. 17.4). Coupling of erythrocyte and antigen is performed by techniques used routinely for passive hemagglutination. The technique that employs chromium chloride is preferred because of the simplicity of its execution.

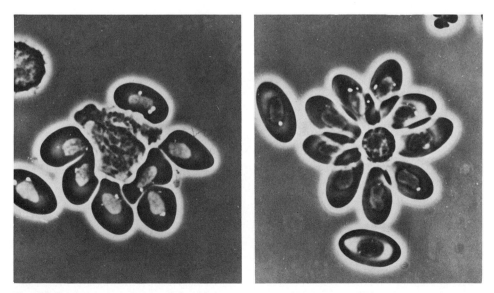

**Fig. 17.3** Rosettes observed by phase-contrast microscopy. *Right*, mouse spleen lymphocyte and chicken red blood cells; *left*, spleen macrophage and SRBC. (From F. Reyes and J. F. Bach, Cell. Immunol. 1971, *2*, 182.)

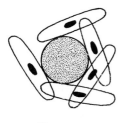

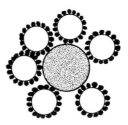

Direct test
(erythrocyte antigens;
e.g. pigeon erythrocytes)

Indirect test
(soluble antigen;
e.g., bovine serum albumin)

**Fig. 17.4**   Direct and indirect rosette tests.

### Significance of Rosette-Forming Cells (RFC) in the Mouse

The rosette test detects several categories of immunocompetent cells: antibody-producing cells, antigen-sensitive cells (not necessarily producing antibody), B and T cells, memory cells, and macrophages. This multiple screening has advantages, but extreme caution must be employed in its interpretation. It is necessary in each specific case to recognize or consider the nature of the cell involved. Possibilities include T cells susceptible to destruction by anti-θ serum, B cells, which resist anti-θ serum but are eliminated by passage on anti-Ig-coated columns, and macrophages, which adhere to glass (explaining their disappearance from the preparation after a 24-hr incubation at 4°C; this interesting variant is, in fact, the means by which macrophage-formed rosettes can be readily eliminated).

ANTIBODY-PRODUCING CELLS

Rosette-forming cells synthesize the receptors responsible for rosette formation as assessed after macrophage elimination by the absence or very low numbers of bispecific rosettes following double immunization. In addition, if each footpad of a mouse is injected with red blood cells from a different species, RFC formed in the respective regional lymph nodes are specific for the species injected into the corresponding paw. Conversely, when rosettes are due to cytophilic antibody passive fixation (on macrophages), rosettes of double specificity are observed, which are easily recognizable by employing pigeon and sheep RBC (the former cells are nucleated). It is important to recognize that passive rosette formation is not seen if spleen cells (depleted of macrophages) are incubated with anti-SRBC hyperimmune serum.

RFC contain significant numbers of plasma cells, which implies that antibody-producing cells may form rosettes. It has been directly shown by combining hemolytic plaque and rosette techniques that a high percentage of PFC forms rosettes.

ANTIGEN-SENSITIVE CELLS

RFC elimination from a spleen cell population results in a (transient) state of tolerance to the red blood cells used for rosette formation. Tolerance can be demonstrated by cell transfer into an irradiated recipient. RFC can be eliminated by initial rosette formation and subsequent application of the cell suspension on a Ficoll gradient. Red blood cells and rosettes (hence RFC) cross the gradient, while lymphocytes that do not form rosettes remain behind. Because the presence of RFC is required for development of the immune response and for the presence of specific receptors for the antigen, RFC are assumed to include antigen-sensitive cells in both the normal and the sensitized mouse.

### B AND T CELLS

The existence of B-RFC is shown by the presence of plasma cells and PFC in the center of numerous rosettes, by surface Ig on a high percentage of RFC, by retention of numerous RFC on anti-Ig-coated columns, and by the presence of RFC in T cell-deprived or nude mice. The existence of T-RFC is also supported by numerous data. These observations include the presence of $\theta$ antigen and heterospecific T-cell markers on a high percentage of RFC, the T-cell nature of numerous RFC in chimeric mice that have received T cells recognizable by alloantigenic or chromosomal markers, the finding of RFC among "educated" T cells (see definition p. 537), and the presence of RFC after filtration on anti-Ig-coated columns. The existence of T rosettes has been a controversial point, probably because of the marked fragility of T rosettes (due to small numbers of erythrocytes and high susceptibility to disruption by vigorous resuspension). In addition, the absence of rosettes in the neonatally bursectomized chicken deprived of B cells has raised the possibility that T rosettes may be due to red blood cell cytophilic antibodies. However, this hypothesis has not been confirmed in mice.

The RFC background in normal mice (Fig. 17.5) also contains, in addition to natural antibody-producing cells, macrophages and B and T antigen-sensitive cells. Spontaneous RFC of thymic origin observed in nonimmunized mice have been used as markers for detecting circulating thymic hormone (see p. 97).

### MACROPHAGES

Macrophages form rosettes after passive binding of cytophilic antibodies in vivo or in vitro. Such RFC are not antigen specific, because a given macrophage forms double-specificity rosettes after fixation of antibodies of two specificities.

### *Applications of the Rosette Technique*

The applications of the rosette test are numerous and correspond to the multiple cell categories detected by the test. We will discuss two particularly interesting ones.

### KINETICS OF ANTIGEN-BINDING CELLS AFTER IMMUNIZATION IN THE MOUSE

Prior to immunization, there exist 50,000–70,000 spontaneous anti-SRBC RFC per spleen. After red blood cell injection RFC numbers increase rapidly at an exponential rate with a doubling time that approximates 13 hr. The RFC

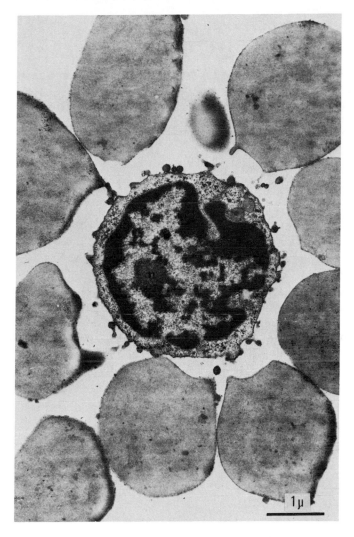

**Fig. 17.5** Rosette observed by electron microscopy. Small lymphocyte of unimmunized mouse spleen and SRBC. (From F. Reyes and J. F. Bach, Cell. Immunol. 1971, *2*, 182.)

number is about $1.6 \times 10^6$ per spleen at peak response (fifth, or sixth day). Doubling time decreases to about 7 hr in the secondary response (Fig. 17.6).

T- AND B-CELL RECEPTORS

Anti-Ig sera inhibit B-cell rosette formation. By means of rosette inhibition when antisera specific for Ig heavy chains are used, it has been shown that B-RFC possess IgM on their surface in the early primary response, and then IgG. The T-RFC receptors have been reported to be inhibited by antilight- but not by antiheavy-chain sera, except for questionable inhibition by anti-$\mu$ sera but these results are controversial.

## OTHER TECHNIQUES

### *Antibody-Forming Cells (AFC)*

Techniques other than use of the local hemolysis plaque may be employed to study AFC. These techniques include immunofluorescence studies of Ig-containing cells, bacteriophage neutralization with enumeration of antiphage antibody-producing cells (Zipp assay), bacterial immobilization by use of microdroplets that contain only one lymphoid cell, and bacterial colony inhibition tests that detect antiflagellin AFC.

### *Antigen-Binding Cells*

Techniques other than the rosette test permit study of antigen-binding cells, such as bacterial adherence, first described in 1950, which consists of replacing red blood cells with bacteria, and autoradiography with labeled antigens. The latter technique detects mostly B cells. It has, however, produced results very similar to those obtained with the rosette technique, when using heavily labeled antigens with which it has been possible to demonstrate the presence of antigen-binding T cells. As in RFC, the cells detected by autoradiography include antigen-sensitive B and T cells, since incubation of lymphoid cells with heavily labeled antigen leads to specific tolerance towards this antigen. The number of radiolabeled antigen-binding cells increases at higher antigen concentration, probably because of recruitment of cells that contain low-affinity receptors. Another technique (immunofluorescence) utilizes fluorescein-conjugated antigens or, even better, β-galactosidase (detected by its enzymatic activity by use of a substrate that releases fluorescing degradation products after hydrolysis). The latter technique is particularly sensitive and detects both T and B cells.

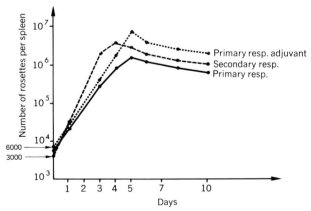

**Fig. 17.6**   Rosette-forming cell kinetics in mouse spleen. The RFC doubling time is 13 hr for the primary response and 7 hr for the secondary response. The duration of the exponential phase is 104 hr for the primary response and 79 hr for the secondary response. (From G. Biozzi.)

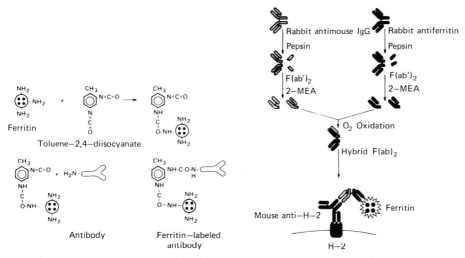

**Fig. 17.7** Principle of the ferritin-labeled antibody technique. *Left*, direct technique; *right*, technique that employs hybrid antibodies. (From J. Klein, Biology of the mouse histocompatibility-2 complex. Principles of immunogenetics applied to a single system. New York, 1975, Springer, p. 340.)

# III. CYTOLOGIC ASPECTS OF ANTIBODY FORMATION*

## METHODOLOGY

Immunocytologic methods associate cytologic principles and the specificity of immunologic reactions. They permit quantitation of AFC by use of light microscopy and provide a view of the ultrastructure of the site of antibody synthesis within the cell. The common feature of all immunocytologic techniques is the use of labeled antigen or antibody visible by light or electron microscopy. Antigens and antibodies may be labeled with proteins, such as ferritin (Fig. 17.7) and peroxidase, which are easily detectable.

To detect cell antibodies, the cellular preparations are initially fixed prior to incubation with labeled antigen. The excess antigen is then eliminated by washing, and the labeled antigen attached to the cellular antibody is detected by light or electron microscopy. Detection of cell antibodies may also be performed indirectly: the cells are first incubated with nonlabeled antigen and then washed and incubated with a labeled antibody specific for the antigen. Cellular preparations are then washed again and examined under the microscope.

Labels used for antigens and antibodies are fluorescent or radioactive substances, ferritin, and enzymes. The proteins labeled with fluorochromes are used to detect antibody-forming cells by light microscopy, whereas ferritin is used only for electron microscopy. Proteins labeled with radioactive elements,

* S. Avrameas.

or with enzymes, may be detected by either light or electron microscopy. We have already discussed the biochemical methods used for such labeling (see p. 136).

Fluorochromes illuminated by short-wave radiation emit a light wave that is visible by fluorescence microscopy. Ferritin is a protein molecule of large size (molecular weight 700,000) that contains 23% iron and is therefore electron dense and visible by electron microscopy. Enzymes are localized by light and electron microscopy or by cytochemical staining. Horseradish peroxidase is most often used in this type of labeling; it is detected by addition of diamino-benzidine and hydrogen peroxide. Proteins labeled with radioactive substances, preferentially $^{125}$I, require autoradiography in order to be detected by light or electron microscopy.

## LIGHT MICROSCOPY

The kinetics of antibody-forming cells obtained with immunocytologic methods are similar to those obtained using gel hemolysis, but kinetics obtained by both of these techniques differ somewhat from those obtained with the rosette test. Compared with the gel hemolysis techniques, immunocytologic methods detect two to four times more antibody-producing cells. However, this comparison is only relative because the gel hemolysis method can detect antibody-synthesizing cells that do not contain intracytoplasmic immunoglobulin, these not being detectable by immunocytologic methods (and vice versa).

Experiments performed with immunocytologic techniques show that after a single injection of antigen and before the appearance of antibody-producing cells, immunoglobulin-producing cells appear whose antibody possesses no antibody function directed against the sensitizing antigen. Recent studies demonstrate that direct relationships exist between immunoglobulin-producing cells and antibody-producing cells. The hypothesis proposed, and partially confirmed by micromanipulation experiments, is that the antibody-producing cells are derived from immunoglobulin-producing cells, at least in part.

Immunocytologic methods permit, as already discussed with rosettes and plaque-forming cells, to examine the type of antibody contained within a cell. In addition, they enable a study to be made of antibody contained in immunocytes. Nevertheless, immunocytologic methods are more complicated to perform and require more time and effort than do rosette or plaque techniques.

## ELECTRON MICROSCOPY (Figs. 17.8 to 17.11)

Ultrastructural studies of antibody synthesis have been performed with ferritin and, especially, peroxidase as antigens. When animals are immunized with a single antigen injection, the antibodies first appear in ergastoplasmic cisternae or in the Golgi apparatus of highly differentiated plasma cells. Two to 3 days after a booster injection, the antibodies first appear in the perinuclear space of

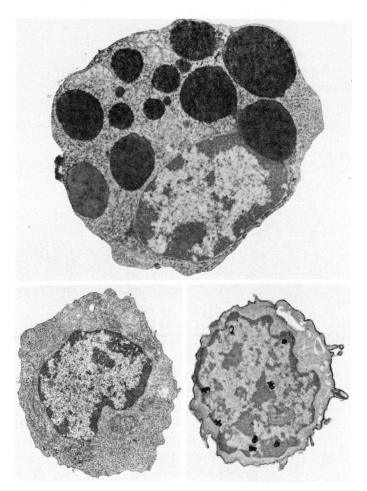

**Fig. 17.8** Cells secreting antiperoxidase-antibodies taken from the middle of a lysis plaque by macromanipulation, fixed, stained, and treated for intracellular detection of antiperoxidase antibody. *Top*, Mott cell in which antibody has accumulated in extremely dilated ergastoplasmic cisternae; *bottom left*, blast cell that contains antibody at the level of polyribosomes; *bottom right*, small lymphocyte with no detectable intracellular antibody stain but with antibodies present at the membrane level. (From D. Zagury and S. Avrameas.)

blast cells. Three to 4 days later, the cells contain a large number of ergasto-plasmic cisternae filled with antibodies, while the perinuclear spaces still contain some antibodies. In addition, at this stage, there is evidence of antibody in lamellae and vesicles of the Golgi apparatus. Four days after boosting, the antibodies are found in numerous ergastoplasmic cisternae of mature plasma cells. The Golgi apparatus does not contain antibodies. Five days after antigen injection, one observes virtually only mature plasma cells in which the antibodies are absent from the perinuclear space. The ergastoplasmic cisternae that contain

the antibody are now in close apposition to the plasma membrane, and their
limits cannot be well defined. At this stage, mature plasma cells may contain
diffuse antibody within the entire cytoplasm or antibody grouped in large
granules. Similar data are obtained at the level of PFC or RFC studied after
micromanipulation.

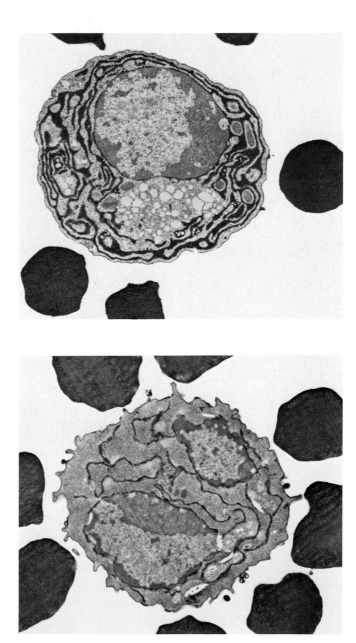

**Fig. 17.9** Cells forming rosettes with peroxidase-coated red blood cells (treated for
intracellular detection of antiperoxidase antibody). *Top*, mature plasma cell; *bottom*,
plasmablast. (From D. Zagury and S. Avrameas.)

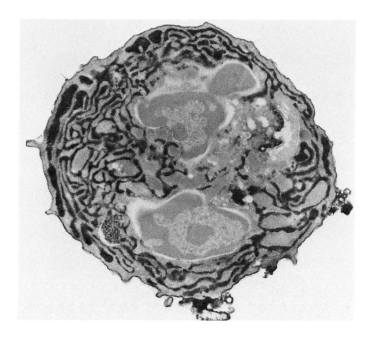

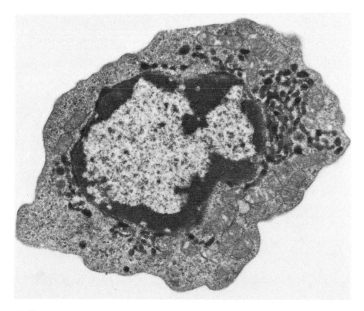

Fig. 17.10 Cells secreting antiperoxidase antibodies taken from the middle of a lysis plaque by micromanipulation. *Top*, mature plasmacell; *bottom*, plasmablast. (From D. Zagury and S. Avrameas.)

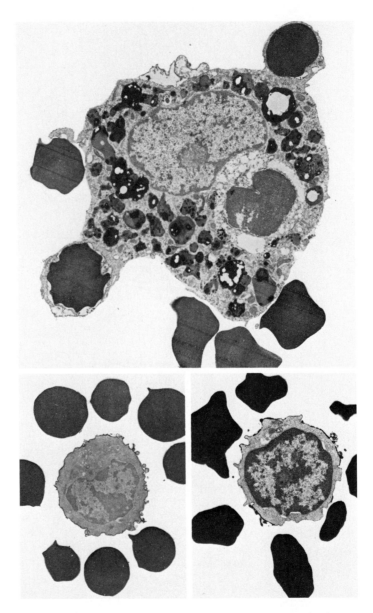

**Fig. 17.11** Cells forming rosettes with peroxidase-coated red blood cells in mice immunized with peroxidase. *Top*, macrophage; *bottom right*, small B lymphocyte revealed by rabbit antimouse immunoglobulin serum coupled with peroxidase; *bottom left*, small T lymphocyte revealed by anti-θ serum coupled with peroxidase. (From D. Zagury and S. Avrameas.)

# IV.  BIOCHEMICAL ASPECTS OF CELLULAR IMMUNOGLOBULIN SYNTHESIS*

Significant contributions have been made in the last decade toward an understanding of the mechanisms of immunoglobulins synthesis, assembly, and secretion. Our knowledge of these mechanisms is, however, still limited, and numerous questions remain unanswered. These studies have focused on synthesis by plasma cells of immunoglobulins (most studied materials are murine plasmacytomas). Only rare and limited studies of the biosynthesis of surface Ig located on lymphocytes are available; however, the mechanisms of synthesis, assembly, and intracellular transport of surface Ig seem basically the same as those applicable to plasma cells. Before envisaging biochemical mechanisms of Ig chain synthesis, it is necessary to recall basic concepts of structural genes of Ig, which are described in more detail in chapters 7 and 19.

## GENETIC ASPECTS

Several concepts of Ig structural genes and their expression are now well established.

### Locus

At variance with the earlier axiom of protein synthesis ("one gene corresponds to one protein"), there exist at least two genes that code for each heavy or light Ig chain. There are numerous arguments suggesting that one gene codes for the variable part (V gene) and one gene codes for the constant part (C gene) of Ig polypeptide chains. The mechanisms by which the two genes integrate to synthesize one single polypeptide chain which takes place at the DNA level have been discussed on p. 232.

Genetic and aminoacid sequencing studies have shown that there is a gene family for the λ light chains, another for the κ light chains, and a third for the various classes of heavy chains. The three loci are unlinked and the κ and H chains loci of the mouse have been found to reside on chromosomes 6 and 12. Preliminary data indicate that the genes coding for H chains in man are located on chromosome 2.

### Gene Expression

A fundamental concept is the extreme specialization of plasma cell in Ig synthesis. In fact, a given plasma cell generally synthesizes one antibody of a single specificity, one Ig with a single heavy chain class and subclass, and a single λ or κ light chain. In individuals heterozygous for Ig allotypes, a molecule synthesized by a given plasma cell contains only the allotypes that correspond to one of the two chromosomes (allelic exlusion). In the rabbit, in which allotypes are known on variable and constant regions, it has been demonstrated

---

* J.-L. Preud'homme.

that the Ig chain synthesized by one cell expresses the determinants linked in the *cis* configuration on the chromosome.

A few exceptions to these rules of immunocyte specialization must be mentioned. Lymphoblastoid lines in culture contain cells eventually capable of simultaneously synthesizing several light or heavy chains. Obviously, it is difficult to extrapolate from these lymphoid cells in culture to physiologic conditions. In normal subjects, there are very small numbers of double producing cells simultaneously secreting distinct heavy chains. Also, in a very few cases of double serum monoclonal Ig, both monoclonal Ig appear to be synthesized by the same cells (note that in the majority of cases, there are two distinct clones). These two exceptions probably relate to the existence of a physiologic "switch" from IgM to IgG or IgA synthesis at the level of a single cell or clone during the immune response. The genetic basis of this switch is discussed on p. 237. Indeed, one given cell or clone may synthesize serially an IgM and then an IgG molecule that contains the same light chain and the same variable part (hence, the same antibody activity). It is possible that during the switch, the cells may simultaneously express $C_\gamma$ and $C_\mu$ genes. On the other hand, cells producing two different antibodies have been found very transiently and in small number after immunization by two unrelated antigens. The mechanism responsible for this high degree of specialization of Ig synthesis by immunocytes remains unknown. Recent data tend to exclude a gene amplification process.

Gene expression in relation to the level of Ig synthesis has been studied as a function of the cell cycle by use of synchronous cells (i.e., cells whose cycle is in phase). These experiments show that secretory Ig is mainly synthesized at the end of the G1 phase and at the beginning of the S phase of the cell cycle. The mechanism of this time-preferential synthesis is unknown. Conversely, surface Ig are produced throughout the cell cycle.

## SYNTHESIS OF IMMUNOGLOBULIN POLYPEPTIDE CHAINS

Ig synthesis follows the general rules of protein synthesis. Transcription of information contained in structural genes occurs in messenger RNA and at the ribosomal level, with reading of the messenger by transfer RNA.

### Messenger RNA

The existence of two genes, one V and the other C, for each Ig polypeptide chain raises the question of what number of messenger RNA molecules is required for synthesis of each Ig chain. The study of nascent Ig chains by insertion of radiolabeled precursors has provided strong evidence that there is only one messenger RNA molecule for each single heavy or light chain, as opposed to two RNAs, one for the variable and the other for the constant part of the chain. Recent studies of Ig messenger RNA have confirmed these findings. In fact, since relatively pure preparations of Ig messenger RNA are now obtainable, Ig synthesis induced by messenger RNA can be studied in cell-free systems (preparations that contain ribosomes along with enzymes and metabolites necessary for protein synthesis) and in heterologous systems in which messenger RNA is introduced into cells that normally do not synthesize Ig but do synthesize protein (rabbit reticulocytes, certain cultured cells, eggs of selected amphibian species). These experiments have shown that synthesis of an entire Ig chain can be induced by a simple (one) homogeneous population of messenger RNA molecules. The exact structure of the Ig messenger RNA sequence is now known. It has been possible to isolate from a single light-chain messenger RNA molecule oligonucleotides whose sequence showed that some of them coded for the variable part, some for the constant part of the light chain, and others for the junction of constant and variable parts. The definite evidence for a single mRNA molecule for each Ig chain has recently been obtained by cell-hybridization experiments. The fusion of plasma cells producing two distinct Ig molecules resulted in hybrid cells that synthesized, in addition to parent Ig, hybrid molecules with all possible associations between heavy and light chains from each parent cell. In contrast, hybrid chains (i.e., chains with the variable part from one parent and the constant part from the other) were never found. Incidently, it is worth mentioning that fusion of certain myeloma cells adapted in culture with normal antibody-producing cells may result in hybrid lines that synthesize the antibody and no longer express the myeloma Ig chains. Implications of the availability of established lines producing pre-defined antibodies are obvious.

Studies in cell-free or heterologous systems, along with structural data, have permitted identification of certain characteristics of Ig messenger RNA. It has recently been shown that nuclear RNA contains a precursor messenger RNA (pre mRNA) of very high molecular weight (about 5,000 bases for heavy chain m-RNA) that separates at the level of the nucleus to give rise to a smaller (2,000 bases) messenger RNA, which reaches the cytoplasm. In addition, messenger RNA obtained from the cytoplasm of plasma cells synthesizing light chains is capable, in certain systems, of inducing synthesis of light chains larger than those normally produced by these plasma cells. Light chains appear to be initially synthesized as a precursor that contains approximately 20 additional amino acids at the amino terminal end. A further cleavage of these additional amino terminal residues gives rise to slightly shorter final light chains. The supplementary amino-terminal section is very hydrophobic and may play a crucial role in the linkage of the nascent chains at the ergastoplasmic membranes. The sequences of the supplementary sections vary from one subgroup to another but are closely analogous for light chains of the same subgroup. Therefore it is possible that the supplementary pieces are coded for by the V genes themselves, although certain results suggest the existence of a third independent group of genes that code for these pieces. The same type of hydrophobic amino-terminal supplementary sequence is now also known to exist for heavy chains. It has been estimated that the messenger RNA for a heavy chain contains about 1,250 bases, that of poly-A consisting of about 200 bases. Because the number of bases needed to code for the precursor of the light chain is approximately 690, the light-chain messenger RNA appears to have an excess of 350 bases that is not translated and has no known function. Heavy-chain mRNA contains about 2,000 bases and only 1,350 appear to be translated.

### Synthesis of Heavy and Light Chains on Different Polysomes

Identification of nascent Ig chains on polysomes after subcellular fraction-ation has shown that heavy and light chains are synthesized on distinct polysomes (polysomes of about 300S for heavy chains and 200S for light chains). These (not recent) findings, already confirmed by electron microscopy, had already shown that there are different messenger RNA molecules for heavy versus light chains.

### Free Versus Bound Polysomes

Plasma cells contain two varieties of polysomes; some are free in cytoplasm and others are linked to the endoplasmic reticulum. At least in hepatocytes, molecules that will be secreted (e.g., albumin) are synthesized by polysomes bound to the endoplasmic reticulum. Conversely, molecules that remain intra-cellular (e.g., ferritin) are synthesized on free polysomes. Ig synthesis on free versus bound polysomes has been studied after fractionation of the two polysome varieties. To date, rather contradictory data have been obtained, probably because of the inherent methodologic problems. The largest portion of Ig appears to be synthesized in ribosomes bound to ergastoplasmic mem-branes. Ribosomes connect to the ergastoplasmic membrane by their 60S unit and nascent chains develop within the cisternal lumen. Nevertheless, the possibility that significant synthesis of secretory Ig occurs in free ribosomes is still a matter of controversy.

## ASSEMBLY

After ribosomal synthesis of heavy (H) and light (L) chains, they are assembled into Ig molecules. The first phase of assembly is the formation of 7S $H_2 L_2$ molecules (final stage for monomeric IgG, IgA, IgD, and IgE). This phase may be followed by a second stage of polymerization of the monomers (polymeric IgM and IgA).

### Assembly of $H_2L_2$ Monomers

SITE OF ASSEMBLY

Within plasma cells, there exists a significant pool of free light chains with few free heavy chains. Relatively old experiments had shown the presence of light chains on heavy-chain polysomes; the two types of chains appeared to be linked by disulfide bridges. These data had suggested the hypothesis that free light chains bind to heavy chains while the latter are still bound to the polysomes and favor their release from the ribosomes. However, this hypothesis of disconnection of heavy chains by light chains is probably incorrect. Recent studies show that the findings of light chains on heavy-chain ribosomes is largely artifactual, that virtually no covalent bond exists between H and L chains at the level of ribosomes, and that the apparent absence of free heavy chains seems to relate to the relative insolubility of free H chains and their tendency to adhere to ribosomes. It would seem that most noncovalent assembly and all of the covalent bond assembly occur in ergastoplasmic cisternae.

INTERMEDIATES

Assembly of a monomeric Ig molecule from H and L chains follows two main pathways. In the first model, two H chains form an $H_2$ dimer. The addition of light chains successively results in an $H_2L$ then an $H_2L_2$ molecule. In the second model, an H and an L chain initially form an HL half molecule, through which the formation of inter-H bridges produces $H_2L_2$ molecules. Within one given species and one given Ig subclass, assembly corresponds to one given pattern. The Ig of a given subclass are preferentially assembled following one of the two models. It is possible that the $H_2$ or HL nature of the main intermediate is related to the number of inter-H disulfide bridges. One must emphasize that this is, in fact, a preferential but not exclusive mechanism. For example, with the $H_2$ dimer used as the main assembly pathway, a mouse IgG1 also uses HL as an intermediate to a lesser degree. In addition, in certain subclasses, like mouse IgG2b, all intermediates are used to an equal extent.

### Polymeric Immunoglobulins

The assembly of 11S dimeric IgA (i.e., secretory IgA) and IgM raises more complex patterns. In most cases, plasma cell cytoplasm contains only monomeric $H_2L_2$ molecules (the main intermediate for their assembly being the $H_2$ dimer for IgA and the half-molecule HL for IgM), whereas in very rare cases, polymeric molecules are also observed. Since Ig is released from the cell in polymeric form, polymerization and binding of the J piece (also synthesized by plasma cells) must occur at the moment of Ig secretion. The role of the J piece in polymer assembly is controversial. Some experiments have shown that the inability of intracellular monomeric subunits to form polymeric molecules is linked to the fact that sulfhydryl radicals necessary for polymerization are blocked within cells. In fact, three conditions seem necessary for polymerization: reduction of blocked residues, presence of the J piece, and presence of a particular enzyme. Other experiments have given conflicting results; thus, we are presently unable to say whether the J piece is really necessary for polymerization.

A peculiar problem is posed by secretory IgA (which includes dimeric IgA, the J piece, and the secretory piece). The secretory piece is synthesized by epithelial cells and is found in free form in these cells at the level of the Golgi apparatus and of the plasma membrane. It is possible that these surface-bound molecules of the secretory piece represent epithelial-cell receptors for IgA molecules that are secreted by plasma cells in the form of dimers that contain a J piece. IgA would hence attach to the membrane-bound secretory piece; the complex would then be incorporated by epithelial cells and transported in their cytoplasm to be later secreted into the intestinal lumen. It should be noted that synthesis of the J piece appears at a late stage in B-cell maturation, close to the plasmacyte stage, and is not limited to those cells that produce polymeric immunoglobulins. These latter bind the J piece to the immunoglobulin, which is then secreted, whereas, in a higher percentage of plasmocytes that secrete monomeric immunoglobulins (e.g., IgG), the J piece is degraded and not secreted. Recent data suggest that the J piece may play a role in the formation of inter-HL bridge.

## INTRACELLULAR TRANSPORT AND ADDITION OF CARBOHYDRATE RESIDUES

Heavy- and light-chain synthesis on respective polysomes is very rapid. It has been calculated that synthesis of light chain takes only 30 sec and that about 60 sec are required for formation of a heavy chain. Nonetheless, Ig are secreted only after a fairly long lag time of about 20 min for normal plasma cells and sometimes much longer for myeloma cells. This lag period corresponds to the time required for intracellular transport of Ig molecules, during which time carbohydrate binding to the polypeptide chain occurs. Mechanisms of intracellular transport of Ig are not very well documented. However, most of this transport seems to be performed within membrane structures. It is probable that secretory vesicles are ejected from the ergastroplasmic cisternae and then enter the Golgi apparatus, where vesicles of Golgian origin then leave the concavity of the Golgi apparatus and are propelled by cytoplasmic currents into the plasma membrane.

Binding of carbohydrates occurs sequentially, with glucosamine being the first carbohydrate residue to bind to Ig chains. In opposition to what was earlier suggested, glucosamine does not seem to bind to the polypeptide chain when it is still located on the polysome but only after it is released into the ergastoplasmic cisternae. Other carbohydrates bind sequentially later. Mannose is bound within the ergastoplasmic cisternae and Golgi apparatus. Glucose and galactose addition occurs much later, probably at the level of the Golgi apparatus and partly in Golgi vesicles. Sialic acid is the last sugar added, and this step occurs very close to secretion.

## SECRETION

Mechanisms of Ig secretion are relatively poorly documented. Some processes, including cell lysis, clasmatosis (separation of a cytoplasm fragment), and excretion of nuclear vacuoles, would seem inefficient and might cause important losses of cellular material. These mechanisms occur only under certain pathologic circumstances. As a rule, secretory granules seem to be incorporated into the plasma membrane; they secrete their contents outside of the cell by reverse pinocytosis. Some studies have suggested that carbohydrate addition plays an essential role in Ig secretion. However, recent studies appear to exclude this hypothesis; the role of carbohydrates in cellular mechanisms of Ig synthesis, transportation, and secretion is probably null.

## CONTROL OF IMMUNOGLOBULIN BIOSYNTHESIS

The mechanisms that control Ig biosynthesis are also very poorly understood. Binding of ribosomes to ergastoplasmic membranes may be essential for induction of synthesis. Moreover, recent studies suggest that intracellular $H_2L_2$ molecules may play a regulatory role.

Heavy chains could bind through their Fc region to an untranslated region of heavy chain messenger RNA and could block the sites of attachment of

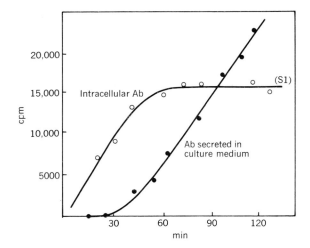

**Fig. 17.12**  Kinetics of cellular antibody production. Labeled amino acids are added at time 0 to a suspension of bone marrow cells from an immunized rabbit. Appearance of labeled antibodies is followed in cells and the supernatant. (From E. Helmreich et al., J. Biol. Chem. 1961, *236*, 464.)

messenger RNA to ribosomes therefore repressing heavy-chain synthesis. However, recent work has failed to confirm this appealing hypothesis.

The control of Ig secretion occurs under obscure mechanisms. The mechanisms by which Ig, which represent only 10% to 40% of the proteins synthesized by plasma cells, virtually constituting the totality of the secreted products, remain mysterious. Under certain conditions normal plasma cells may synthesize free light chains in excess (e.g., hyperimmune lymph nodes). However within physiological conditions, heavy- and light-chain synthesis is balanced (i.e., equimolar synthesis of light and heavy chains without synthesis of free light chains in excess). Conversely, in pathological conditions (myeloma), a very large excess of light chains may be synthesized by plasma cells. The cellular mechanisms leading to the balanced synthesis of light and heavy chains also remain unsolved. Heavy- and light-chain synthesis appears to be under independent control. It is worth noting that mutations in Ig production by plasmacytoma cells occurs with very high incidence. These events may affect production of heavy or light chains or both. In some lines, the cells spontaneously convert from IgG producers to light-chain producers, and then from light-chain producers to nonproducers. In other lines, a direct conversion from IgG producers to nonproducers is observed. The incidence of each of these events is high ($10^{-3}$ to $10^{-4}$ per cell per generation) and is increased by mutagenic agents (including drugs used in the treatment of plasma-cell dyscrasias in man). Mutagenesis also increases the frequency of the occurrence of primary structure variants. Such variants produce Ig chains which may show either deletions (often in the C3 domain of the heavy chain) or alterations in the heavy chain that lead to the appearance of serological, chemical, and assembly characteristics of a different subclass. An important recent observation has shown that the frequency of mutations affecting the variable regions, particularly the antibody site of immunoglobulins produced by a plasmacytoma, is even more elevated than the frequency of mutations affecting the production of chains or constant parts. As yet, it is too early to extrapolate this still-isolated observation to the normal immune response, but the possible implications of this for the problem of the origin of antibody diversity are obvious.

# BIBLIOGRAPHY

BACH J. F. Antigen-binding cells. In J. P. Revillard, Ed., Cell-mediated immunity. In vitro correlates. Basel, 1971, Karger, p. 51.

BAUMAL R. and SCHARFF M. D. Synthesis, assembly and secretion of mouse immunoglobulins. Transpl. Rev., 1973, 14, 163.

BUXBAUM J. The biosynthesis, assembly and secretion of immunoglobulins. Semin. Hemat., 1973, 10, 33.

JERNE N. K., HENRY C., NORDIN A. A., FUJI H., KOROS A. M. C., and LEFKOVITS I. Plaque-forming cells: methodology and theory. Transpl. Rev. 1974, 18, 130.

MISHELL R. I. and DUTTON R. W. Immunization of dissociated spleen cell cultures from normal mice. J. Exp. Med., 1967, 126, 423.

PARKHOUSE R. M. E. Assembly and secretion of immunoglobulin M (IgM) by plasma cells and lymphocytes. Transpl. Rev., 1973, 14, 131.

SCHARFF M. D. and LASKOV R. Synthesis and assembly of immunoglobulin polypeptide chains. Progr. Allergy, 1970, 14, 37.

SIGAL N. H. and KLINMAN N. B. The B cell clonotype repertoire. Adv. Immunol., 1978, 26, 255.

VITETTA E. S. and UHR J. W. Synthesis, transport, dynamics and fate of cell surface Ig and alloantigens in murine lymphocytes. Transpl. Rev., 1973, 14, 50.

WILLIAMSON A R. Biosynthesis of antibodies. Nature (London), 1971, 231, 359.

# ORIGINAL ARTICLES

ANTOINE J. C., BLEUX C., AVRAMEAS S., and LIACOPOULOS P. Specific antibody-secreting cells generated from cells producing immunoglobulins without antibody formation. Nature (London), 1978.

AVRAMEAS S., ANTOINE J. C., TERNYNCK T., and PETIT C. Development of immunoglobulin and antibody-forming cells in different stages of the immune response. Ann. Immunol. (Paris), 1976, 1270, 551.

BACH J. F., MULLER J. Y., and DARDENNE M. In vivo specific antigen recognition by rosette forming cells. Nature (London) 1970, 227, 1251.

BIOZZI G., STIFFEL C., MOUTON D., BOUTHILLIER Y., and DECREUSEFOND C. A kinetic study of antibody producing cells in the spleen of mice immunized intravenously with sheep erythrocytes. Immunology, 1968, 14, 7.

CHARREIRE J., DARDENNE M., and BACH J. F. Antigen recognition by T-lymphocytes. IV. Differences in antigen binding characteristics of T and B-RFC. A cause for variations in the evaluation of T-RFC. Cell. Immunol., 1973, 9, 32.

COOK W. D. and SCHARFF M. D. Antigen-binding mutants of mouse myeloma cells. Proc. Natl. Acad. Sci. USA, 1977, 74, 5687.

CUNNINGHAM A. J. and SZENBERG A. Further improvements in the plaque technique for detecting single antibody forming cells. Immunology, 1968, 14, 599.

DRESSER D. W. and WORTIS H. H. Use of an antiglobulin serum to detect cells producing antibody with low haemolytic efficiency. Nature (London), 1965, 208, 859.

Dwyer J. M. and McKay I. R. Antigen binding lymphocytes in human blood. Lancet, 1970, *1*, 164.

Ingraham J. S. and Bussard A. Application of a localized haemolysin reaction for specific detection of individual antibody producing cells. J. Exp. Med., 1964, *119*, 667.

Leduc E. H., Scott G. B., and Avrameas S. Ultrastructural localization of intracellular immuno-globulin in plasma cells and lymphoblasts by enzyme labelled antibodies. J. Histochem. Cytochem., 1969, *17*, 211.

Sterzl J. and Riha K. Detection of cells producing 7S antibodies by the plaque technique. Nature (London), 1965, *208*, 858.

Ternynck T., Rodrigot M., and Avrameas S. Kinetics of antibody and immunoglobulin-producing cells appearing in popliteal lymph nodes of mice stimulated with horse radish peroxidase. J. Immunol., 1977, *119*, 1321.

## Chapter 18

# CELLULAR INTERACTIONS IN IMMUNE RESPONSES

## Jean-François Bach

I.   INTERACTIONS BETWEEN MACROPHAGES AND LYMPHOCYTES

II.  COOPERATION BETWEEN B AND T LYMPHOCYTES IN ANTIBODY PRODUCTION

III. COOPERATION BETWEEN T LYMPHOCYTES

IV.  SUPPRESSOR T CELLS

Antibodies are secreted by plasma cells, more generally by B cells, while cell-mediated immunity is achieved by T lymphocytes. The generation of antigen-specific B- and T-effector cells relates not only to simple differentiation of precursor cells but also involves complex interactions between various cell types. These interactions, especially those between macrophages and lymphocytes and those of B and T lymphocytes, will now be examined.

## I. INTERACTIONS BETWEEN MACROPHAGES AND LYMPHOCYTES

The term "macrophage" was defined previously (see chap. 5). Note that the definition of macrophages is at best imprecise and that the interpretation of much of experimental data that claim macrophage participation must be viewed with caution.

### MACROPHAGES AND ANTIBODY PRODUCTION

Most of the studies regarding functional interactions between lymphocytes and macrophages deal with antibody production. Although there is no doubt that macrophages incorporate antigens and modify them by enzymatic digestion, a critical question remains as to whether macrophages are required for development of an immune response or, alternatively, whether they simply modify the development of immune responses. Arguments that favor macrophage intervention in antibody production have as their bases morphologic observations that show close contact between lymphocytes and macrophages and especially data that result from macrophage depletion or enrichment in relation to the integrity of lymphocyte suspensions.

### Morphologic Data

Adherence of lymphocytes to macrophages has long been observed on tissue sections or in vitro in lymphocyte cultures. Similarly, morphologic studies using isotope or ferritin-labeled antigens have shown that selective antigen binding to the surface of dendritic cells in germinal centers occurs just prior to cellular ingestion. The importance of the in vitro interaction between macrophages and either blast cells (activated by antigen) or plasma cells was corroborated by the finding that antibody-forming cells are generated within aggregates of macrophages and lymphoid cells.

### Effects of Macrophage Elimination

Macrophages are removed from lymphocyte suspensions by adherence to glass or plastic, by adding iron to the suspension, followed by passage through a magnetic field, or after treatment by antimacrophage serum (previously absorbed by lymphocytes to remove antilymphocytic activity; see p. 959). Such elimination of macrophages suppresses antibody production in response to numerous antigens in in vitro cultures and in vivo after cell transfer into lethally irradiated hosts. This immunosuppression is particularly marked when soluble or weak immunogens are studied. Immunocompetence of treated cells is restored by addition of adherent cells (even those obtained from nonimmunized animals) or, sometimes, by addition of the supernatant from macrophage cultures. Thus, in vitro, macrophages seem to have a role that at least suggests that they are nonantigen-specific auxiliary cells. At this point, it should be mentioned that macrophage-depleted cell preparations may regain their function after the addition of 2-mercaptoethanol (2ME). 2ME seems to act by stimulating the few remaining macrophages rather than replacing them, as it has no activity on a population that is completely deprived of macrophages.

### Intervention of Macrophages and Thymus Dependency

A correlation exists between the degree of thymus dependency of a given antigen (defined on p. 158) and the role of macrophages in producing antibodies to the same antigen. Thus, macrophages and T cells are both necessary for production of antibodies to sheep red blood cells (SRBC) and monomeric flagellin; however, the response to erythrocytes destroyed by ultrasound and the response to polymerized flagellin are independent of both macrophages and T cells. Similarly, those synthetic antigens that are more thymus dependent are also more easily digested by macrophages. Possibly, this phenomenon is linked to the mechanism of cellular collaboration between B and T cells, first described by Feldmann, in which T cells supposedly release specific factors that bind to macrophages and then present the antigen to B cells.

Macrophages probably also intervene by presenting the antigen to T cells. Recent data indicate that this interaction takes place, at least in secondary responses, only when macrophages and T cells share the same Ia antigens (see p. 689), or when macrophages presenting the antigen on the first and second challenge share the same Ia antigens, eventually different from those of T cells. It has thus been suggested that, as in other systems discussed on p. 87, T-cell receptors recognize a complex of the antigen and Ia molecules (here present on macrophage membranes). The intervention of macrophages in T-B cell cooperation is made still more complex by the description of macrophage released soluble factors (bearing Ia antigens?) whose role is still obscure.

Recent data have shown that in the complete absence of adherent cells, lymphocytes can no longer produce antibodies against thymus-independent antigens. Therefore, macrophages seem to act in the production of antibodies against thymus-independent antigens, although the number of adherent cells necessary for an optimal response appears to be much lower than that observed for thymus-dependent antigens.

### Antigenic or Informational Transfer

Purified macrophages that phagocytose an antigen (in vivo or in vitro) are capable of transmitting this antigen to a nonsensitized animal. Numerous antigens can be transferred more or less efficiently. Depending on the particular antigen, macrophages either depress or enhance immunogenicity. The mechanism of macrophage intervention during the initial phases of the immune response has been a matter of controversy ever since Fishman's pioneering studies. Fishman showed that peritoneal macrophage extracts obtained 30 min after ingestion of T2 phage were highly immunogenic; for example, these extracts permitted antigenic stimulation to occur in macrophage-depleted lymphocyte preparations. In addition, Fishman showed that the relevant molecules contained low-molecular-weight RNA (destroyed by ribonuclease). It was even demonstrated that when macrophage and lymphocyte donors had different allotypes, the antibodies produced by lymphoid cells contained the macrophage allotype. The ultimate demonstration by Askonas that these RNA preparations contained antigen, however, decreased the significance of these experiments, because it seemed possible that after macrophage treatment, the antigen was more easily bound to RNA. Immunogenicity would, then, be explained by the presence of a "super antigen." Allotype experiments could be explained less readily by this hypothesis; however, if the initial macrophage preparation was actually contaminated by lymphocytes, antibodies might be produced by the donor lymphoid cells.

Conversely, macrophages are sometimes able to prevent induction of immune tolerance (see chap. 20). Some antigens persist in the circulation for a few days after immunization. Such antigen that has escaped phagocytosis is often more tolerogenic when injected into a second host. Administration of aggregated antigen, followed by rapid phagocytosis, or the use of adjuvants to stimulate macrophages, favor immunity rather than tolerance. These data are the basis for the hypothesis according to which thymus-dependent antigens in direct contact with lymphocytic receptors induce tolerance, while antigens that are transferred to lymphocytes by macrophages may induce an immune response.

### Mode of Action of Macrophages: Arguments that Favor Direct Contact with Lymphocytes

Macrophages may digest antigens and release a super or modified antigen, which then enters into contact with lymphocyte surface receptors, without a requirement for direct contact between lymphocytes and macrophages. However, because lymphocyte and macrophage aggregates have been observed, it is possible that direct contact has a function. Feldmann has suggested that antigen-specific T-cell factors or complexes of these factors with antigen bind onto macrophages and then present the antigen to B lymphocytes, thus implicating direct physical contact.

It has been shown that a significant amount of the antigen in macrophages, whose immunogenicity is maintained despite digestion, is not localized in the cytoplasm but, instead, on the cell surface. A role for antigens on macrophage surfaces is also suggested by the disappearance of macrophage capacity to transfer antigens after trypsin treatment or addition of antibodies directed against the antigen in question. In addition, because they possess a receptor for the IgG Fc fragment, macrophages bind antigen-antibody complexes before contact with the lymphocytes. One should recall here the recent report, mentioned above, that macrophages secrete soluble factors, possibly contributing to the initiation of the immune response. In particular, a nonantigen-specific factor, a genetically controlled factor complexed with antigen (genetically related factor [GRF]), and an activating factor for B cells that acts like a polyclonal activator (B-cell activating factor [BAF]) have been described. It may also be recalled that such factors may be capable of replacing macrophages in certain in vitro systems. It appears that several of these factors such as BAF, and mitogenic factors are in fact a single entity recently given the name of lymphocyte activating factor (LAF) or Interleukin 1 (IL1), which nonspecifically stimulates several T-cell functions. All these factors secreted by monocytes and macrophages are occasionally collectively termed monokines. It should also be noted that under certain circumstances, macrophages appear to acquire suppressive properties—for example, after treatment with adjuvants of LPS, in tumor or parasite-bearing animals, or during graft-versus-host responses.

## MACROPHAGES AND CELL-MEDIATED IMMUNITY

Macrophages are involved in antigen recognition in cell-mediated immunity (probably in ways similar to that just described for antibody production), but much less is known about this activity. The information at hand includes antigenic transfer by purified macrophages that produce delayed hypersensitivity in a new recipient and the need for macrophages to obtain blast transformation in vitro in response to antigen in delayed hypersensitivity states.

In addition, macrophages seem able to intervene in the effector phase of cell-mediated immunity. Once "armed" by a T cell-secreted mediator (see p. 415), they become cytotoxic to tumor or allogeneic cells. Macrophages and sensitized T lymphocytes are probably both required for allograft rejection. This hypothesis is consistent with morphologic evidence of numerous macrophages within the cellular infiltrates of grafts during rejection.

# II. COOPERATION BETWEEN B AND T LYMPHOCYTES IN ANTIBODY PRODUCTION

B and T lymphocytes are implicated in the two main categories of immune responses (humoral and cell mediated), but this dichotomy is not absolute. We have already seen that neonatal thymectomy prevents antibody production to the so-called thymus-dependent antigens. This contribution of T lymphocytes to antibody production has led to the hypothesis of cellular cooperation of B and T lymphocytes.

## DIRECT DEMONSTRATION OF B- AND T-CELL COOPERATION

In 1966, Claman showed that irradiated mice were able to produce anti-SRBC antibodies after simultaneous injection of thymus and bone marrow cells; injection of only one of these two cell populations did not restore this capability (Fig. 18.1). This important study was confirmed by other workers with such antigens as bovine serum albumin or human γ-globulin in the mouse. More recently, the introduction of in vitro primary response techniques has permitted more analytical study of B and T cell collaboration. One should note that bicellular cooperation is also observed in secondary responses, in vitro and in vivo, and that cooperation develops only in principle when strict histocompatibility between B and T cells exists.

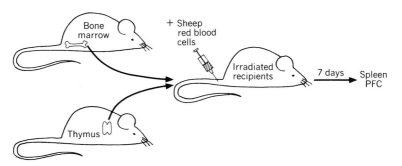

**Fig. 18.1** Principle of Claman's experiment that demonstrates cooperation between thymus and bone marrow cells.

## PRODUCTION OF ANTIBODIES BY B CELLS

The fact that production of antibodies to certain antigens (the so-called thymus-independent ones) may be obtained in the absence of T cells already indicates that B cells are capable of producing antibodies. One may thus assume that B cells produce antibodies to thymus-dependent antigens, with the help of T cells. Three different experimental designs have verified this important hypothesis.

The first experiment (by Davies) consisted of testing adult thymectomized mice, irradiated and repopulated by syngeneic bone marrow cells, and then grafted with a thymus obtained from an allogeneic donor (with, however, H-2 compatibility). When spleen cells from these mice (stimulated by SRBC) are transferred into a third strain of mice previously immunized to alloantigens of the bone marrow donor, the recipient mice do not produce antibodies; however, injection of the same spleen cells into hosts immunized against the thymus donor does not prevent antibody production. This experiment showed that antibodies are produced by bone marrow-derived cells.

These results were confirmed by Miller, who studied neonatally thymectomized mice. These mice recover their ability to produce anti-SRBC antibodies after injection of thymus or thoracic duct semiallogeneic cells. Miller showed that antibody-producing cells (which form hemolytic plaques) in these reconstituted mice are destroyed in vitro after addition of antialloantisera directed against the recipient antigens (i.e., B cells) but not by addition of antisera to the antigens of the T-cell donor.

The third experiment (performed by Nossal) provided direct proof of the B nature of antibody-producing cells. He used irradiated CBA mice that were restored to immunocompetence by addition of CBA spleen cells and bone marrow cells from CBA T6-T6 mice bearing a chromosomal translocation (T6 chromosome) easily recognizable in mitotic cells. It was demonstrated that the few mitotic cells that form hemolytic plaques all bore the T6 chromosome and were therefore B cells.

## CARRIER EFFECT AND CELLULAR COOPERATION

We have indicated earlier that haptens must be coupled to a carrier to induce antibody production. It was initially thought that the carrier effect related to the molecular environment conferred on the hapten molecule by the carrier. This hypothesis became less attractive when it was shown that introduction of inert determinants between carrier and hapten did not diminish the carrier effect, and that the binding energy of the antihapten antibody hapten-carrier complex was found mostly to be due to the hapten molecule alone. Mitchison suggested a much more satisfactory explanation for the carrier effect. Mice were immunized with the hapten-carrier conjugate NIP-OA (NIP is a hapten, 4-hydroxy-3-iodo-5-nitrophenylacetic acid, and OA is chicken ovalbumin). When cells from such mice were transferred into irradiated syngeneic hosts, the recipients produced antibodies only if injected with NIP coupled to the same carrier (NIP-OA). No antibody developed after injecting NIP bound to

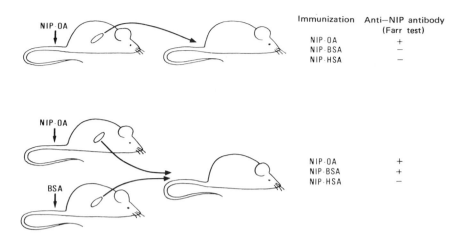

**Fig. 18.2** Mitchison's experiment that demonstrates cooperation between carrier- and hapten-specific cells in the carrier-hapten NIP-OA system.

another carrier, like bovine serum albumin (NIP-BSA). It was, however, possible to obtain anti-NIP antibody production after injection of NIP-BSA if at the same time cells from NIP-OA-immunized mice and spleen cells from mice immunized to BSA alone (not coupled to NIP) were administered (Fig. 18.2). Anti-BSA antibodies could not be substituted for BSA-sensitized cells. By use of an allotypic marker, it was shown that anti-NIP antibodies were secreted by the cells that originated in the NIP-OA immunized donor. The conclusions are that different cells respond to carrier and to hapten and that T cells respond to the carrier and assist B cells to produce antihapten antibodies. The latter conclusion was confirmed by transfer experiments in which anti-θ serum was used to selectively destroy carrier-specific cells and by the selective depletion of carrier-specific cells after administration of antilymphocyte serum in vivo.

The carrier effect is not restricted to hapten-protein conjugates. It may be demonstrated for protein molecule subunits, or even between erythrocyte antigenic determinants. Thus, T cells probably recognize some determinants of the antigen molecule, and they facilitate antibody production by B cells to other determinants. The nature of the determinants that result in stimulation of "helper" T cells and B cells has been discussed on p. 160.

## B- AND T-CELL SPECIFICITY

### B Cells

B cells produce antibodies of only one specificity, as assessed by the fact that antibody-forming cells are specific for the antigen used in immunization. On their surface, they have receptors specific for the same antigen (see p. 83). Although there is little doubt about B-cell specificity, the identity of recognition receptors and antibodies released into the serum is probable but not yet definitively demonstrated. We have noted that a hapten should be coupled to a carrier to achieve B-cell stimulation despite strong association of antibodies with haptens (see p. 286). In fact, B-cell receptors may also bind directly to haptens: B-cell incubation with a hapten inhibits the ability of these cells to cooperate with T cells in response to hapten-carrier conjugates. Similarly, experiments in which lymphoid cells are made specifically unresponsive after filtration on hapten-coated columns confirm the high specificity of B cells for haptens (independently of conjugation with a carrier). Finally, no arguments exist to suggest that the receptors on B cells and the antibodies they secrete have different specificities. However, it should be appreciated that the binding of antigen to surface receptors does not alone represent a sufficient stimulus to initiate B-cell differentiation.

### T Cells

T cells could possibly intervene by nonantigen-specific stimulation of B lymphocytes. In fact, although nonspecific stimulation probably occurs, it is probably not really exclusive. There are indeed numerous findings that suggest specificity of T-cell intervention in antibody production as in cell-mediated immunity.

Specificity for the carrier effect is nearly absolute, and this data, of course, favors the specificity of T-cell intervention. Double-transfer experiments also support the notion of this specificity. Irradiated mice receive thymus cells and SRBC. Their spleen cells are then injected into a second series of irradiated mice that also receive bone marrow cells and a second dose of SRBC. Five days later, anti-SRBC antibodies are produced. These antibodies do not develop, however, if SRBC injection of the first recipient is omitted, a finding that demonstrates the specificity of "educated" T cells previously exposed to the antigen injection. T-cell action is, indeed, specific, because injection of horse red blood cells into the first recipient does not allow the second recipient (stimulated by SRBC) to produce antibodies to SRBC.

These data have been recently directly confirmed by using helper T-cell clones, established and manufactured in the presence of T-cell growth factor (TCGF) or Interleukin 2 (IL2). Interestingly, these helper T-cell clones carry the Lyt 1 antigen, are Ia-restricted (see p. 690) and are blocked by anti-idiotypic antibodies.

Another argument that favors T-cell specificity in cellular cooperation is the existence of immunologic tolerance at a T-cell level. When inducing tolerance to a soluble protein (e.g., to human γ-globulin in the mouse), it is possible to show by transfer experiments that both B and T cells are tolerant, and, by definition, tolerance implies specificity.

### Comparison of B- and T-Cell Specificity

The above distinction between B-cell specificity for the hapten and T-cell specificity for the carrier does not necessarily apply to cell receptors. The techniques available at present do not provide a complete understanding of the respective specificities of B- and T-cell receptors. Indirect evidence favors the existence of different specificities for B and T cells. When guinea pigs are stimulated with native or reduced lysozyme, antibodies (thus B cells) are produced that are specific for one or the other lysozyme form, whereas T cells (detected by DNA synthesis in the presence of antigen or rosette formation with red blood cells coated with one or the other antigen) react simultaneously with both lysozyme forms. Similarly, sheep and pigeon red blood cells produce specific antibodies with a minimal cross reaction, but strong cross reaction is found at the T-cell level. It is possible that T cells have a receptor repertoire partially different from that of B cells. On the other hand, B- and T-lymphocyte receptors to a given antigen seem to share the same idiotypic determinants (see p. 86), which suggests that B- and T-cell receptor specificities are not fundamentally different. One important difference may bear on the apparent need for T cells of simultaneous recognition of conventional antigens and of antigenic products of the major histocompatibility complex (Ia antigens in the case of helper T cells in T-B cell cooperation) (see p. 692).

## ALLOGENEIC EFFECT

We have examined evidence that animals immunized with a hapten-carrier conjugate [e.g., 2,4-dinitrophenyl-keyhole limpet hemocyanin (DNP-KLH) conjugate] produce antibodies of an anamnestic type when again stimulated by the same DNP-KLH complex. The anamnestic response is not seen if the second injection uses a different carrier [e.g., DNP-bovine γ-globulin (DNP-BGG)]. Similarly, Katz and Benacerraf observed that guniea pigs sensitized to DNP-KLH do not show a secondary-type response to DNP after DNP-BGG injection. However, if, a few days before the DNP-BGG injection, the guinea pigs are given allogeneic lymphoid cells from an animal not sensitized to BGG, a more intense response results. A strong response, greater even than that obtained with cells sensitized to the carrier, has also been observed by use of various other antigen and hapten systems in the mouse and guinea pig. This phenomenon is called the "allogeneic effect," as it refers to the allogeneic reaction required for its development (Fig. 18.3).

Recent studies show that injection of allogeneic cells alone increases the level of anti-DNP and anti-KLH antibodies without further antigen injections. However, a contribution by weak antigens persisting after the first immunization cannot be excluded. The allogeneic effect is obtained as early as 24 hr after antigen administration, but there is no effect if the allogeneic cell injection precedes the first antigen dose. This finding suggests that B cells must be stimulated before becoming sensitive to the allogeneic effect. The allogeneic effect confers immunogenicity to products normally not immunogenic, such as the copolymer of glutamic acid and D-lysine (D-GL), normally a tolerogen. Similarly, the allogeneic effect allows mice that do not respond to certain synthetic antigens (see p. 688) to produce 7S antibodies to these antigens.

Finally, it is of interest that the allogeneic effect augments immunologic memory and antibody affinity (even in the absence of a second antigenic stimulation).

A graft-versus-host reaction (GvHR) is probably essential for the development of the allogeneic effect, because cells from irradiated allogeneic donors or $F_1$ hybrids of the recipient that are incapable of reacting against the recipient do not show any allogeneic effect. Conversely, the allogeneic effect is produced

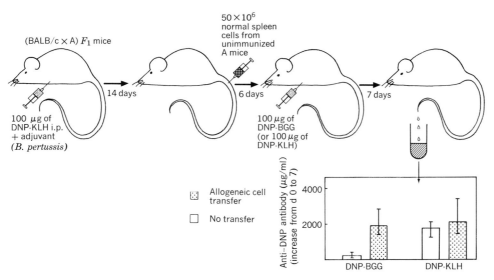

**Fig. 18.3**  Allogeneic effect. (From D. P. Osborne and D. H. Katz, J. Exp. Med. 1972, *136*, 439.)

by parental cells administered intravenously to $F_1$ hybrids. This finding suggests that the donor T cells, stimulated by the GvHR, enhance recipient B-lymphocyte function. Elimination of the recipient's T cells does not diminish the allogeneic effect. Finally the allogeneic effect may substitute for carrier-specific T cells. Note that in certain settings it may also act on helper T-cells themselves and augment their contribution to cellular cooperation.

The mechanisms of the allogeneic effect remain unknown. In vitro experiments suggest an action of soluble mediators and not a direct contact between activated T cells and allogeneic-effect sensitive cells. The fact that donor cells rather than recipient cells are involved may be explained by the short distance of action of mediators, which are secreted only when contact with the recipient's B lymphocytes is made. Note also that allogeneic reactions do not always stimulate but may sometimes be depressive. Such nonantigen-specific T-cell suppression of immune responses must be distinguished from antigen-specific T-cell induced suppression, which we shall discuss further in this chapter.

The allogeneic effect may be obtained in vitro (Schimpl and Wecker). The supernatant from mixed lymphocyte reactions added to a culture of nude mouse spleen cells permits the cells to respond to SRBC in vitro (Table 18.1). The factor involved seems to act on B-cell differentiation and not on proliferation. Cultures separated by a cell-impermeable membrane (two chambers) show that lymphocytes stimulated by Concanavalin A or an antigen may reveal the same effect. The biochemistry of the factors involved in the allogeneic effect is unknown. Preliminary studies indicate that these factors may be proteins with a molecular weight of 20,000–60,000 daltons. The presence of Ia antigens (see p. 690) on these factors has been reported but remains controversial. Of importance is the fact that the Schimpl's T-cell replacing factor (TRF) is distinct from T-cell growth factor (or Interleukin 2) described on p. 386.

**Table 18.1   Stimulation of the In Vitro Immune Response of Spleen Cells from Nude Mice by Supernatants of Mixed Lymphocyte Culture Between CBA and C57BL/6 Strains**

| Supernatant origin | PFC on Day 4 |
|---|---|
| O | 175 |
| CBA | 220 |
| C57BL/6 | 157 |
| CBA + C57BL/6 | 1680 |

After A. Schimpl and E. Wecker, Nature (London) 1972 *237*, 15.

## THYMUS-INDEPENDENT RESPONSES

We have already seen that T cells are not necessary for the production of all antibodies. Neonatally thymectomized mice produce significant amounts of antibodies (IgM type) after stimulation by so-called thymus-independent antigens, such as pneumococcal polysaccharides, *Escherichia coli* lipopolysaccharide, and polymerized flagellin. The latter antigen, unlike the others, stimulates T cells, even though T cells are unnecessary for the production of antiflagellin antibodies, except for IgG antibodies. Other thymus-independent antigens do not give rise to IgG antibodies, even in the presence of T cells. IgM antibodies to thymus-dependent antigens may be produced in neonatally thymectomized mice immunized with high antigen doses. Generally speaking, production of IgG, IgA, and IgE is more thymus dependent than is IgM production. However, it should be noted that IgM production against thymus-dependent antigens is depressed in neonatally thymectomized animals.

Thymus-independent antigens are biochemically essentially different from thymus-dependent antigens. The former are generally large polymeric molecules with high-density repetitive identical determinants. It is possible that the spatial distribution and not the biochemical nature of the antigens conditions thymus independence. However, all molecules with repetitive determinants are not necessarily thymus-independent antigens. Thus, L-amino acid copolymers are thymus dependent, whereas D-amino acid copolymers are not.

Macrophages have little effect on the response to thymus-independent antigens, and T cells, as discussed, are minimally, if at all, stimulated (when they are stimulated, their intervention does not modify the response). This absence of stimulation is unexplained. Most thymus-independent antigens are degraded very slowly and thus persist for a very long time, which may contribute to their thymus independence.

## MECHANISMS OF CELLULAR COOPERATION

The exact mechanisms of B- and T-cell cooperation in antibody production are unknown. The experimental data presented above suggest several hypotheses and exclude others. Two main mechanisms that are not mutually exclusive may be envisaged: direct interaction between B and T cells, perhaps through the intermediary of macrophages, and release of soluble mediators that act locally or at a distance.

### Direct Interaction Between B and T Lymphocytes: Antigenic Bridge Theory

This hypothesis was the first one proposed by Mitchison, following experiments on the carrier effect. As schematized in Fig. 18.4, the T-cell surface binds the antigenic molecule by its carrier determinant and presents it to the B cell by its haptenic determinant. The antigen is therefore a bridge between the B and T cells. In fact, this theory has apparently been invalidated by in vitro cooperation experiments. It has been shown that it is possible to obtain B- and T-cell cooperation when both cell populations are separated by a cell-impermeable membrane (Feldmann). Moreover, it would be difficult spatially, among all the lymphocytes circulating, for a few B and T lymphocytes specific for the same antigen to make contact. On the other hand, the apparent (and still controversial) need for histocompatibility of B and T cells has led to the hypothesis of complementary receptors on B- and T-cell surfaces linked to histocompatibility antigens, or at least to structures controlled by the major histocompatibility complex (e.g., Ia antigens; see p. 690). Receptors on B cells could, then, combine specifically with the corresponding receptors on T cells. Finally, it is difficult to conclude on the need for direct contact between B and T cells, as one may not easily extrapolate from in vitro to in vivo systems.

### Interaction Between Macrophages Coated with Antigen-Specific T-Cell Factor and B Lymphocytes

A theory first proposed by Lachmann, and later by Feldmann, modifies the antigenic bridge theory in relation to more recent findings. The T cell

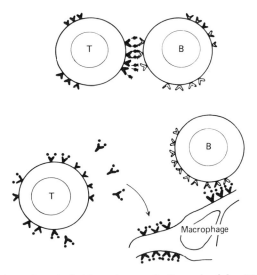

**Fig. 18.4** Mitchison's antigenic bridge theory (*top*), revised by M. Feldmann (*bottom*). (From M. Feldmann, Transplant. Proc. 1973, *5*, 45.)

**Table 18.2  Factors Involved in Cellular Cooperation**

| | Origin | Target | Response affected | M.W. | Presence of Ia antigens | Genetic restriction |
|---|---|---|---|---|---|---|
| *Antigen-specific factors* | | | | | | |
| *Helper factors* | | | | | | |
| Munro and Taussig's factor | Educated T cells (s) | B cells | Primary IgM | 50,000 | I-A | — |
| Feldmann's factor | Lyt 1$^+$ cells (s) | B cells + macrophages | Primary and secondary IgM & IgG | 50,000 | I-A | — |
| Tada's amplifier factor | Lyt 1$^+$ cells (e) | Sensitized T cells | Secondary IgG | | I-A | |
| *Suppressor factors* | | | | | | |
| Tada's factor | Lyt 23$^+$ cells (e) | Sensitized T cells | Secondary IgG | 40–50,000 | I-J | + (I-A) |
| Kapp, Thèze, and Benacerraf's factor | T cells from nonresponder mice (e) | T cells | Primary IgG | 40–50,000 | I-J | (Nonresponding recipient) |
| Feldmann's factor | Lyt 23$^+$ T cells (s) | Helper T cells | Primary, secondary IgM and IgG | 40,000 | I-J | — |
| *Nonantigen specific factors* | | | | | | |
| Allogeneic factor (Katz) | T cells (s) | B cells | Antibody production | 30–40,000 | I-A and β-2 microglobulin | + |
| T-cell replacing factor (TRF) (Schimpl and Wecker) | T cells (s) | B cells | Antibody production | 25–35,000 | | — |
| "Soluble immune response suppressor" (SIRS) | T cells incubated for 48 hr with Con A (s) | Macrophages, B cells, T cells (MLR) | Antibody production MLR | 48–67,000 | | |
| MLR suppressor factor | T cells stimulated in vivo by alloantigens (s) | ? | MLR | ? | ? | + (I-C) |

(e) = extract; (s) = supernatant.

542

produces a soluble antigen-specific factor, once called IgT because it was initially thought to be a monomeric 7S IgM. This molecule, complexing with antigen, binds to the macrophage's surface and, in turn, presents the antigen to B cells. T cells, preimmunized in vivo against a carrier, may thus interact specifically with B cells preimmunized in vivo to a hapten. The required presence of macrophages in the B cell-containing chamber (in two-chamber system) and hypothetical IgT cytophilia for macrophages favor this hypothesis, which still remains unproven.

### *Mediators Released by T Cells Without Direct Contact Between B and T Cells or Macrophages*

SPECIFIC MEDIATORS (Fig. 18.5)

Antigen recognition receptors on T cells might also intervene without intermediary macrophages to form complexes with the antigen that would then bind to B-lymphocyte antigen-binding receptors. Antigen-specific mediators of this type have been demonstrated (in the mouse) for (T,G)-A- -L response by Munro and Taussig. T cells educated to (T,G)-A- -L are prepared in irradiated mice that have been previously restored to immunocompetence by thymocyte injection and have been injected with (T,G)-A- -L. These (splenic) T cells are incubated in vitro with antigen, and supernatant (collected after 24 hr) is injected simultaneously with bone marrow cells into irradiated recipients that can then respond to (T,G)-A- -L antigen only. The antigen-specific factor that binds the antigen in vitro has a molecular weight of about 50,000. It does not bear Ig antigenicity but would bear Ia antigens encoded by the I-A subregion

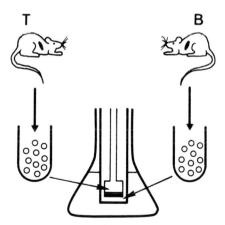

**Fig. 18.5** Experimental protocol employed by M. Feldmann to demonstrate the possibility of T- and B-cell cooperation without direct contact in the production of anti-DNP antibodies after the addition of DNP-KLH conjugate. The T cells (educated against KLH) are placed in the upper compartment. B cells (spleen cells from mice immunized with DNP-flagellin conjugate and treated with anti-θ serum) are placed in the lower compartment, which also contains macrophages. The two compartments are separated by a nucleopore membrane that is impermeable to cells but permits macromolecular exchange.

of the H-2 complex. In addition, B cells would bear acceptor sites for the factor that could also bear Ia antigens. Interestingly, however, the specific factor maintains its action on B cells, which do not have the same H-2 complex as that of the T cells. These data are very attractive, particularly because of their relationships with the genetic control of immune responses, but they are still insufficiently documented and merit further experimental confirmation.

Whatever the significance of Munro and Taussig's work, questioned by some, the production of soluble cooperation factors, which are antigen-specific, has been confirmed in several other systems, such as that of Feldmann (in vitro anti-DNP-flagellin response) and also that of Tada (in vivo response to DNP-KLH). These factors have been partially characterized (see p. 542). Like the factor described by Munro and Taussig, they carry Ia antigens, although it has not been demonstrated that such Ia antigens are identical to those present on B-lymphocyte surfaces.

NONSPECIFIC MEDIATORS

T cells might also act by the intermediary of nonantigen-specific mediators. This possibility is suggested by the allogeneic effect observed in vivo (GvH experiments) or in vitro (mixed-lymphocyte reaction). One must also note that in in vitro primary stimulation cultures (two chambers), activated T cells secrete both antigen-specific and nonantigen-specific factors.

### Other B-cell Activation Factors

B-cell activation is enhanced by various T cell-independent factors. Thymus-independent antigens, which are generally (but not always) B-cell mitogens, may play a nonantigen-specific role. Thus, Möller has proposed that the Ig receptor does not provide a direct signal for B-lymphocyte stimulation but that it may only serve to bind on the lymphocyte surface the antigen, which, in turn, would trigger the relevant B-lymphocyte clone through various possible mechanisms. In other words, the Ig receptors would essentially have a focusing function, which permits selective binding of the antigen to the specific cells, and thus be responsible for the characteristic specificity of the immune response. This is the one nonspecific signal hypothesis in which B-cell triggering is not performed by the antigenic determinants of the antigen molecule but rather by some polyclonal activator sites of the antigen, by T-cell factors, or by other factors. More generally, polyclonal B-cell activators, such as lipopolysaccharides, can reveal the genetic potentials of the B lymphocyte. The activation may take different aspects according to the state of differentiation of the B cell, including in particular antibody synthesis and/or DNA synthesis (hence the frequent but inconstant correlation between antigen thymus independency and mitogenicity).

The third complement factor could also possibly contribute to B-cell activation. C3 depletion has been reported to depress antibody production to thymus-dependent antigens. This observation suggests that C3 bound to antigen-receptor complexes may be a binding structure between immune complex, macrophage, and B cell (both cells have C3 receptors). C3 might also stimulate B cells. Stimulation does occur in the presence of products known to activate

C3, including trypsin, polyvinylpyrrolidone, *E. coli* lipopolysaccharide, and most thymus-independent antigens.

### Conclusions

It is difficult to choose among hypotheses, which, of course, are not mutually exclusive. Conclusions are difficult to make, because the individual experiments on which they are based are performed in very different systems (in vitro and in vivo) and are sometimes difficult to confirm. The contribution of T cells might represent presentation of antigen to B cells in a peculiarly immunogenic form. This presentation is perhaps repetitive, based on the structure of thymus-independent antigens. T cells would favor B-cell activation by direct membrane interaction (to be defined) or by release of antigen-specific or -nonspecific factors.

# III. COOPERATION BETWEEN T LYMPHOCYTES

Interactions between T lymphocytes in antibody production have been mentioned in relation to the allogeneic effect, in which T cells activated by a GvHR may stimulate T cell-mediated anticarrier function in addition to its direct effect on B cells. Additionally interactions between T lymphocytes have been described in cell-mediated immunity.

## SYNERGY BETWEEN T LYMPHOCYTES

Thymus and lymph node cells induce a GvHR when injected in a sufficient dose to newborn allogeneic $F_1$ hybrid recipients. A mixture of thymus and lymph node cells, in lower dose than that which produces a GvHR for each component, induces a significant GvHR. Synergy is also observed when thymus cells are replaced by spleen cells, and when blood cells are substituted for lymph node cells. It has been shown that the lymph node population recirculates and is long-lived; it is eliminated by short term antilymphocyte serum treatment. Conversely, the thymic population does not recirculate, has a short life-span, and is relatively resistant to antilymphocyte serum action (Cantor and Asofsky). Analogous experiments performed in vitro have shown a synergy between thymic and lymph node cells in the mixed-lymphocyte reaction and in the cell-mediated lymphocytotoxicity reaction (see p. 412). These observations recall the finding that θ-positive rosette-forming cells (RFC) in the thymus and spleen, on the one hand, and lymph node and blood RFC, on the other, oppose each other. The former cells are eliminated by adult thymectomy, and the second are removed by low doses of antilymphocyte serum.

These experiments indicate the existence of several T-cell subsets recently shown to bear different Ly antigens (see p. 65). It is, however, difficult to determine with certainty in some of these systems which are effector and which are helper cells. Mechanisms of the interaction are still unknown (secretion of soluble mediators, direct interaction, recruitment of cells from one population to another?).

ALLOGENEIC EFFECT AND CELL-MEDIATED IMMUNITY

The allogeneic effect, first described in relation to antibody production, may also be applicable to cell-mediated immunity. Guinea pigs undergoing a GvHR reject lymphoblastic leukemia cells, while they are not able to do so in the absence of the GvHR. This rejection represents an exclusively T-cell reaction. The allogeneic effect also may increase delayed hypersensitivity reactions.

# IV.   SUPPRESSOR T CELLS

As seen above, T cells have the ability to help B cells to produce antibodies. Some T cells may also act synergistically with other T cells. However, at variance with these amplifying actions, it is now known that T cells have a inhibitory action on B and T cells, thus suggesting a fine regulatory function. Experimental data with respect to suppressor T cells are derived from very different models, and these cells are not necessarily a unique cell type. Most likely, several categories of suppressor T cells exist. We shall examine successively several of these models.

## INCREASED RESPONSES BY T-CELL ELIMINATION

Antilymphocyte serum that inactivates T cells (see chap. 33), and adult thymectomy increase the response to thymus-independent antigens [e.g., pneumococcal polysaccharide (SIII), *E. coli* lipopolysaccharide, or polyvinylpyrrolidone (PVP); Table 18.3]. The response is normalized by thymocyte injections. Similarly, IgE production in the rat in response to immunization with a DNP-*Ascaris* conjugate (thymus dependent) is augmented and markedly prolonged after adult thymectomy. This elevated response is suppressed by administration of syngeneic thymocytes hyperimmunized to *Ascaris* or to the DNP-*Ascaris* conjugate; thymocytes immunized against DNP-BSA are without effect, which suggests that in this particular system, suppressor T cells are carrier specific. Taken together, these experiments suggest the existence of suppressor T cells, which are antigen specific at least in carrier-hapten systems and short-lived (they disappear after adult thymectomy). Such suppressor T cells, when injected

**Table 18.3   Effects of Antilymphocyte Serum (ALS) on Antibody Production Against SIII Pneumococcal Polysaccharide, Evaluated by the Local Hemolysis Plaque Technique**

| SIII | ALS | Cells (10^7) | PFC per spleen |
|:---:|:---:|:---:|:---:|
| + | − | — | 16,200 |
| + | + | — | 160,000 |
| + | + | Thymus | 52,000 |
| + | + | Spleen | 160,000 |
| + | + | Blood | 315,000 |

After P. J. Baker, J. Immunol. 1972, *105*, 158.

Table 18.4 Suppression of Anti-DNP Antibody Production in BALB/c Mice Preimmunized with DNP-KLH Conjugate and Treated with Thymus and Spleen Extracts

| Extract injected | Indirect PFC (IgG) |
|---|---|
| — | 11,100 ± 115 |
| Thymus from mouse immunized with KLH | 929 ± 291 |
| Thymus from mouse immunized with BGG* | 11,100 ± 193 |
| Spleen from mouse immunized with KLH | 2,930 ± 145 |
| Spleen from mouse immunized with BGG* | 13,600 ± 196 |

* BGG = bovine gammaglobulin.

After T. Tahemori and T. Tada, J. Exp. Med., 1975, *142*, 1241.

into normal recipients, depress antibody production in these animals. It should be noted, however, that athymic nude mice make a near-normal response to SIII and treatment of these mice by antilymphocyte serum does not augment this response. These unexpected data indicate that nude mice lack both suppressor T cells and a population of amplifier T cells (Baker).

## ANTIGEN-SPECIFIC T-CELL SUPPRESSION

We have seen above that rats immunized against DNP-*Ascaris* conjugates developed *Ascaris*-specific suppressor T cells. It has been shown ultimately that this suppression was achieved by a humoral mediator extracted from T cells. Tada has extended the observation of the antigen specific T-cell factor of the IgE system in the rat to the study of factors involved in the suppression of the IgG antibody response to keyhole limpet hemocyanin (KLH) in antigen-primed mice. Mice immunized with soluble KLH were shown to have T cells with suppressor activity, primarily for IgG antibody responses. Supernatants obtained from such cells by sonication and ultracentrifugation were shown to have carrier-specific suppressor activity for IgG, both in in vivo and in vitro responses. In vivo studies suggested that the T-cell factor may be under genetic control, since the suppressive effect could only be demonstrated in syngeneic but not in H-2 incompatible recipients. More precisely, it was shown that identity was required in a region now called I-J, located on the 17th chromosome between I-B and I-C subregions. Using an in vitro secondary antibody response system, the primary target of the antigen-specific suppressor factor was demonstrated to be the carrier-primed helper T cell rather than the hapten-primed cell. It was also shown, using alloantisera directed towards major histocompatibility complex products, that the factor was coded for by genes present in the I-J region. In addition, it was shown that the factor was retained on columns coated with the specific antigen but not on anti-Ig immunoadsorbents, which suggests that the factor is probably a non-Ig protein with antigen binding sites bearing Ia antigens. Its molecular weight has been evaluated around 50,000 daltons. Analogy with the antigen specific T-cell factor of Munro and Taussig (see p. 543) is obvious but not yet well worked out. It is hoped that the recent development of hybridomas or suppressor T-cell clones which secrete the suppressor factor, will expedite the characterization of these factors. Similar data have been obtained in the response to the terpolymer of L-glutamic acid, L-alanine, and L-lysine (GAT) in which the absence of response is probably explained by the generation of GAT-specific suppressor T cells. The nonresponding strains will respond to GAT coupled with methyl-BSA (MBSA). However, if they are preimmunized with GAT alone, they no longer respond to GAT-MBSA. The involvement of suppressor T cells in the failure to respond to GAT is also indicated by the ability of nonresponders to produce antibodies against GAT after pretreatment with low-dose cyclophosphamide (known to selectively eliminate suppressor T cells). Suppression in the GAT system is, as in Tada's system, mediated by a soluble factor that can be extracted from suppressor T cells. This factor, whose properties are summarized in Table 18.2, is only active in nonresponder recipients. Recent data show that it shares idiotypic determinants with anti-GAT antibodies. Finally, recent studies have shown for both the anti-DNP-KLH and anti-SRBC responses that, although Lyt $23^+$ cells have the fundamental role in suppression, the presence of adherent Lyt $123^+$ cells very significantly augment the suppression. However, opinions differ on their mode of action. Is the Lyt $123^+$ cell the effector agent (nonspecific) for suppression after specific induction by the Lyt $23^+$ cell and its suppressor factor? Alternatively, does the Lyt $123^+$ cell activate the Lyt $23^+$ cell, possibly after having been activated itself by a Lyt $1^+$Qa $1^+$ cell (feedback circuit of Cantor and Gershon)?

## NZB AND B/W MICE

NZB and (NZB $\times$ NZW)$F_1$ (B/W) mice are spontaneously autoimmune mice that present very early signs of thymic deficiency (difficulty in making thymus cells tolerant, cessation of thymic hormone secretion; see p. 712). These mice show exaggerated production of antibodies to thymus-independent antigens, such as pneumococcal polysaccharide or PVP, and even to thymus-dependent antigens early in life. In addition, their thymus cells, injected into irradiated allogeneic recipients, undergo exaggerated proliferation, suggesting that the regulatory cell population that controls proliferation is deficient. Both of these abnormalities are corrected by treatment with thymic hormone.

The implication of such a deficiency (in suppressor T cells) to the pathogenesis of autoimmunity are being studied extensively. Prevention of the onset of hemolytic anemia and other autoimmune manifestations by bimonthly injections of thymocytes or of supernatants of Con A-activated T cells favors such a role. It should also be noted that neonatally thymectomized and nude mice present early manifestations of auto immunity. Further arguments in favor of the depression or suppression of T cells in the onset of autoimmune diseases will be presented in chapter 25.

## ALLOTYPIC AND IDIOTYPIC SUPPRESSION

Injection into newborn rabbits of antiallotype sera directed against their own Ig depresses production of Ig of the corresponding allotype, and this inhibition may last for several weeks or months. Similarly, when a female rabbit is immunized with male rabbit Ig, the offsprings of the two rabbits show a deficiency in production of paternal allotypes. Allotypic suppression may also be obtained by injecting nonimmunized mothers with antibodies to paternal allotypes. Analogous results have been obtained in the mouse. In this species, the suppression obtained from maternal immunization is often transient (a few weeks), except for a few strains in which it is nearly permanent. An example of the latter occurs after immunization of BALB/c females (ultimately mated with SJL/J males) with SJL/J immunoglobulin. One should note that SJL/J mice display certain immunologic abnormalities, including reticulosarcoma at the age of one year or more, and gammopathies with abnormalities in certain Ig classes.

The presence of an active phenomenon in allotypic suppression is suggested by the fact that lethally irradiated "suppressed" mice do not recover Ig production of the suppressed allotype despite injection of spleen cells from normal syngeneic donors. Similarly, mixed spleen cells from suppressed SJL/J × BALB/c and from normal SJL/J × BALB/c donors do not restore the secretion of Ig that bears the suppressed allotype, when they are injected into lethally irradiated, nonsuppressed BALB/c recipients (whereas injection of normal donor cells does effect such reconstitution; Fig. 18.7). Suppressed donor cells injected into normal nonirradiated recipients cause suppression. A role for T cells is suggested by the elimination of the cells responsible for suppression after treatment with anti-θ serum in the presence of complement. Suppressor T cells are found in the spleen, thymus, lymph nodes, and bone marrow. Their mode of action remains obscure; helper T cells rather than antibody-producing B cells seem to be the target of this suppression (Herzenberg).

Eichmann has described a system of idiotypic suppression in the response

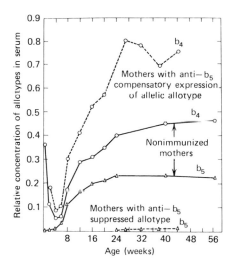

**Fig. 18.6**  Allotypic suppression in the rabbit. Example of Ab5 allotypic suppression. Ordinates are relative concentrations of Ab4 and Ab5 allotypes in sera of heterozygous rabbits, descendents of a homozygous Ab5 father and a homozygous Ab4 mother. Anti-Ab5 antibodies from anti-Ab5 immunized mothers (———) have caused a nearly complete and durable suppression of the Ab5 allotype and a compensatory increase in Ab4 concentration. (From S. Dray, Nature (London), 1962, *195*, 677.)

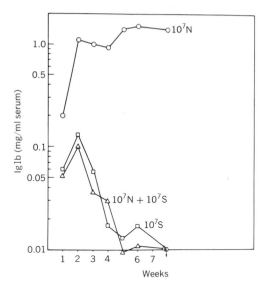

**Fig. 18.7** Spleen cell transfer from normal mice (N) or mice submitted to chronic suppression (S) into irradiated mice. Normal cell transfer restores production of the allotype, but the simultaneous injection of suppressed mouse cells prevents such restoration. (From L. A. Herzenberg and L. A. Herzenberg, Contemp. Topics Immunobiol. 1974, *3*, 41.)

to streptococcal A polysaccharides, perpetuated by a suppressor T cell, that may be analogous to the allotype suppression described above. The synthesis of antibody with certain idiotypic specificities may be depressed by treatment of mice by anti-idiotypic antibodies. High doses of antiidiotypic antibody cause immediate but transient suppression, whereas a low dose results in a delayed but chronic suppression. Such chronic suppression can be adoptively transferred to irradiated mice with spleen cells shown to be T cells. These suppressor T cells, which can recognize an idiotype expressed on the surface of B cells or even other T cells, may be of critical importance in the regulation of the immune response.

## SUPPRESSION BY POLYCLONAL ACTIVATION

In addition to activation of helper cells, the T-cell polyclonal activator Concanavalin A (Con A) can also activate a separate suppressor T-cell system. Con A-activated T cells can suppress the generation of cytotoxic lymphocytes to allogeneic cells in mixed lymphocyte reaction, mitogen-induced blast transformation, pokeweed mitogen-driven Ig secretion, and antibody production to thymus-dependent or thymus-independent antigens. Mouse spleen or lymph node cells incubated with Con A in vitro for 24 to 48 hr can be activated to become suppressor cells, as assessed by addition to cultures of normal spleen cells and antigen or to pokeweed mitogen-stimulated Ig-secreting cells. Con A-activated T cells release into supernatants a soluble immune response suppressor (SIRS) factor that also suppresses plaque-forming cell responses to antigens and Ig production in response to pokeweed mitogen (Rich and Pierce). SIRS, which is a glycoprotein with a molecular weight of from 48,000 to 67,000, is produced by Lyt 23$^+$ cells and possesses physicochemical properties similar to those of MIF. It seems to act upon macrophages.

## SUPPRESSOR T CELLS ASSOCIATED WITH HUMORAL IMMUNODEFICIENCY

The majority of patients with common variable hypogammaglobulinemia (see p. 898) have significant numbers of B cells (as assessed by membrane Ig), but they do not produce antibody in vivo and thus appear to have a defect in the terminal differentiation of B lymphocytes into mature Ig-synthesizing and Ig-secreting plasma cells. Most of these patients are not able to synthesize and secrete significant quantities of IgG, IgA, or IgM in vitro after pokeweed mitogen stimulation as normal lymphocytes do. That this defect is due to an excess of suppressor T cells is indicated by the fact that lymphocytes of some of these patients, cocultured with lymphocytes from normal individuals reduce IgG, IgA, and IgM synthesis by the latter lymphocytes by a factor of 85% to 100% (Waldmann). Similar results have been obtained with lymphocytes from patients with hypogammaglobulinemia of late onset, associated with a benign thymoma, in some patients with X-linked agammaglobulinemia and in selective IgA deficiency. It is not known, however, in all these clinical conditions if the excess of suppressor T cells is primary and possibly the cause of the agammaglobulinemia, or if it is secondary to it. The latter hypothesis is suggested by the transfer of agammaglobulinemia into normal chickens by grafts of thymus or spleen cells from adult agammaglobulinemic birds, neonatally bursectomized and irradiated.

## OTHER SYSTEMS

The existence of suppressor T cells is shown in several other experimental systems. These systems include tolerance states to soluble antigens (see p. 583) or to allografts (see p. 586); an absence of antigenic competition in thymus deprived mice; production of suppressor T cells (and suppressive antigen specific factor) in nonresponder mice to certain polypeptides (see p. 689); suppression of delayed hypersensitivity, assessed after sensitization by oxazolone or contact with picryl chloride (lymph node cells of mice rendered unresponsive by the injection of picryl sulfonic acid depress the passive transfer of contact sensitivity), in the immunologic enhancement of tumor growth and in the anergy observed in certain patients with fungal infections. Nonantigen specific factors, liberated during the course of the MLR, should also be mentioned in addition to the Ig-binding factor (IBF) produced by activated T cells that nonspecifically suppresses antibody responses in vitro.

## SERUM SUPPRESSOR FACTORS NOT PRODUCED BY LYMPHOCYTES

The manifold mechanisms of suppression discussed are mediated by T cells that either act directly or, as is more often the case, by means of the intermediary of antigen-specific or nonantigen-specific soluble factors. Certain immune responses may also be suppressed by antibodies (by means of the feedback mechanism described on p. 340 or by facilitation described on p. 586).

Other molecules that are nonantigen-specific and produced by cells other than lymphocytes may suppress immune responses. Their role in the physiological regulation of these immune responses is difficult to evaluate, but they probably do have such a role in certain situations (pregnancy, inflammation, etc.). Among the better documented of these factors one may mention: (1) the immunoregulatory α-globulins, (2) the α-globulin suppressor factors present in the sera of some cancer-bearing patients, (3) amylose-inhibiting α-globulin, (4) a lipoprotein that inhibits formation of E rosettes in hepatitis, (5) α-fetoprotein and other proteins associated with pregnancy, (6) C-reactive protein, (7) interferon. The prostaglandins, corticosteroids, estrogens, and cyclic nucleotides should also be mentioned.

## CONCLUSIONS

There is now accumulating evidence showing that T cells may suppress the function or the differentiation of B cells and other T cells (involved in B-cell help or in cell-mediated immunity). Such suppression probably has important implications in the physiologic regulation of immune responses as well as in the control of autoimmunity and in graft or tumor rejection.

It is likely, however, that various concepts of suppressor T cells are associated with different phenomena. Although information on this subject is still insufficient, it must be recognized that antigen-specific and nonspecific suppression should be distinguished. There is antigen-specific suppression (Tada's system) in the response to the DNP-*Ascaris* conjugate to KLH or to GAT. Conversely, antigen specificity is absent or not conclusively demonstrated in T-cell suppression of antibody responses to thymus-independent antigens or in Con A-induced suppression. The target cell of suppressor T cells is generally not well established and one may discuss in each system whether helper T cells or B cells are preferentially hit.

Lastly, the nature of the suppressor T cell is generally obscure. It has been claimed that the cells secreting the antigen-specific suppressor factor were mature Lyt 23[+] cells in the response to DNP-KLH or GAT, but recent data show that in these systems and others, Lyt 123[+] cells might also intervene. The role of the latter cells would explain the finding of large amounts of suppressor T cells in the thymus, their depletion after adult thymectomy, and their dependence on thymic hormone secretion. One should also mention here that not all cell-mediated suppression systems are T-cell dependent since macrophages and certain nonantigen-specific serum proteins not apparently produced by T cells may also suppress immune responses.

## *BIBLIOGRAPHY*

Asherson G. L. and Zembala M. Suppressor T cells in cell-mediated immunity. Brit. Med. Bulletin, 1976, *32*, 158.

BASTEN A. and HOWARD J. G. Thymus independence. Contemp. Topics Immunobiol., 1973, 2, 165.

CALDERON J. and UNANUE E. R. An evaluation of the role of macrophages in immune induction. Fed. Proc., 1975, 34, 1737.

CANTOR H. and BOYSE E. A. Regulation of cellular and humoral immune response by T cell subclasses. Cold Spring Harbor Symp. Quant. Biol., 1977, Cold Spring Harbor Laboratory, Vol. 41, p. 23.

CANTOR H. Control of the immune system by inhibitor and inducer T lymphocytes. Ann. Rev. Med., 1979, 30, 269.

COUTINHO A., GRONOWICZ E., MÖLLER G., and LEMKE H. Polyclonal B cell activators (PBA). In Mitogens in immunobiology (J. J. Oppenheim, D. L. Rosen, and Vreich L. [eds.]). New York, 1976, Academic Press, p. 173.

DIENER E. and LEE K. C. The role of macrophages and their soluble products in immune regulation. In T. E. Mandel, C. Cheers, C. S. Hosking, I. F. C. Mc Kenzie, and G. J. V. Nossal, Eds., Progress in immunology. III. Proc. 3rd Int. Congr. Immunol., Sydney. Amsterdam, 1977, North Holland.

GERSHON R. K. T-cell control of antibody production. Contemp. Topics Immunobiol., 1974, 3, 1.

GERSHON R. K. Suppressor T cell dysfunction as a possible cause for autoimmunity. In N. Talal, Ed., Autoimmunity: genetic, immunologic, virologic and clinical aspects, New York, 1977, Academic Press, p. 171.

GERSHON R. K. Suppressor T cells: miniposition paper celebrating a new decade. In: Immunology 80 (M. Fougereau and J. Dausset [eds.]). Acad. Press, New York, 1980:375.

GREAVES M. F., OWEN J. J. T., and RAFF M. C. T and B lymphocytes. Origins, properties and role in immune responses. Amsterdam, 1973, Elsevier North Holland.

HERZENBERG L. A. and HERZENBERG L. A. Short-term and chronic allotype suppression in mice. Contemp. Topics Immunobiol., 1974, 3, 41.

KAPP J. A., PIERCE C. W., THEZE J., and BENACERRAF B. Modulation of immune response by suppressor T cells. Fed. Proc., 1978, 37, 2361.

KATZ D. H. The allogeneic effect on immune responses: model for regulatory influences of T-lymphocytes on the immune system. Transpl. Rev., 1972, 12, 141.

KATZ D. H. Lymphocyte differentiation, recognition and regulation. New York, 1977, Academic Press, p. 749.

MAKELA O. The diversity and specialization of immunocytes. Progr. Allergy, 1970, 14, 154.

MILLER J. F. A. P. MHC restrictions in cellular cooperation. In: Immunology 80 (M. Fougereau and J. Dausset [eds.]). Acad. Press, New York, 1980, 359.

MÖLLER G. Ed. Antigen-sensitive cells. Transpl. Rev., 1969, 1.

MÖLLER G. Ed. Suppressor T lymphocytes. Transpl. Rev. 1975, 26.

MÖLLER G. Ed. Antigen receptors on lymphocytes. Transpl. Rev., 1970, 5.

MÖLLER G. Ed. Concepts of B lymphocyte activation. Transpl. Rev., 1975, 23.

MÖLLER G. Ed. Antibody suppression of gene products. Transpl. Rev., 1975, 27.

MÖLLER G., COUTINHO A., GRONOWICZ E., HHAMMERSTROM L., and SMITH E. Role of mitogenic components of thymus-independent antigens. In Mitogens in immunobiology (J. J. Oppenheim, D. L. Rosen, and Vreich L. [eds.]). New York, 1976, Academic Press, p. 291.

SCHIMPL A., HUBNER L., WONG C., and WECKER E. Nonantigen specific T-cell factors. In: Immunology 80 (M. Fougereau and J. Dausset [eds.]). Acad. Press, New York, 1980, 403.

SCHWARTZ R. S., RYDER R. J. W., and GOTTLIEB A. A. Macrophages and antibody synthesis. Progr. Allergy, 1970, 14, 81.

SINGHAL S. D. and SINCLAIR N. R. St. C. (Ed.) Suppressor cells in immunity. International Symposium London. University of Western Ontario, Canada, 1975.

TADA T. and OKUMURA K. The role of antigen specific T-cell factors in the immune response. Adv. Immunol., 1979, 1:28.

TADA T. and HAYAKAWA K. Antigen-specific helper and suppressor factors. In: Immunology 80 (M. Fougereau and J. Dausset [eds.]). Acad. Press, New York, 1980, 389.

Taussig M. J. and Munro A. J. Antigen specific T-cell factor in cell cooperation and genetic control of the immune response. Fed. Proc., 1976, 35, 2061.

Unanue E. R. The regulatory role of the macrophage. Adv. Immunol., 1972, 15, 95.

Unanue E. R. Cooperation between mononuclear phagocytes and lymphocytes in immunity. New Engl. J. Med., 1980, 303, 977.

Wigzell H. Specific fractionation of immunocompetent cells. Transpl. Rev., 1970, 5, 76.

# ORIGINAL ARTICLES

Askonas B. A. and Rhodes J. M. Immunogenicity of antigen-containing RNA preparations from macrophages. Nature (London), 1965, 205, 470.

Claman N. H., Chaperon E. A., and Triplett R. F. Thymus-marrow cell combination. Synergism in antibody production. Proc. Soc. Exp. Biol. (N.Y.), 1966, 122, 1167.

Coutinho A. and Möller G. Thymus-independent B cells induction and paralysis. Adv. Immunol., 1975, 21, 113.

Davies A. J. S., Leuchars E., Wallis V., Marchant R., and Elliott E. V. The failure of thymus-derived cells to make antibody. Transplantation, 1967, 5, 222.

Eardley D. D., Kemp J., Shen F. W., Cantor H., and Gershon R. K. Immunoregulatory circuits among T cell sets: Effect of mode of immunization on determining which Ly 1 T cell sets will be activated. J. Immunol., 1979, 122, 1663.

Eichmann K. Idiotype suppression. II. Amplification of a suppressor T cell with antiidiotypic activity. Eur. J. Immunol., 1975, 5, 511.

Feldmann M. and Basten A. Specific collaboration between T and B lymphocytes across a cell-impermeable membrane in vitro. Nature (New Biol.), 1972, 237, 13.

Fishman M. and Adler F. L. The role of macrophage RNA in the immune response. Cold Spring Harbor Symp. Quant. Biol., 1967, 32, 343.

Katz D. H., Hamaoka T., Dorf M. E., and Benacerraf B. Cell interaction between histoincompatible T and B lymphocytes. III. Demonstration that H-2 gene complex determines successful physiologic lymphocyte interaction. Proc. Nat. Acad. Sci. (Wash.), 1973, 70, 2624.

Mitchison N. A. The carrier effect in the secondary response to hapten-protein conjugates. II. Cellular cooperation. Eur. J. Immunol., 1971, 1, 18.

Nossal G. J. V., Cunningham A., Mitchell G. F., and Miller J. F. A. P. Cell to cell interaction in the immune response. III. Chromosomal marker analysis of single antibody-forming cells in reconstituted, irradiated or thymectomized mice, J. Exp. Med., 1968, 128, 839.

Pepys M. B. Role of complement in induction of antibody production in vivo. Effect of cobra factor and other C3 reactive agents on thymus-dependent and thymus-independent antibody responses. J. Exp. Med., 1974, 140, 126.

Pierce C. W., Kapp J. A., and Benacerraf B. Regulation by the H-2 gene complex of macrophage lymphoid cell interactions in secondary antibody responses in vitro. J. Exp. Med., 1976, 144, 371.

Rajewsky K., Schirrmacher V., Nass S., and Jerne N. K. The requirement of more than one antigenic determinant for immunogenicity. J. Exp. Med., 1969, 129, 1131.

Rich R. R. and Pierce C. W. Biological expressions of lymphocyte activation. III. Suppression of plaque forming cell responses in vitro by supernatant fluid of Concanavalin activated spleen cell cultures. J. Immunol., 1974, 112, 1360.

Schimpl A. and Wecker E. Replacement of T-cell function by a T-cell product. Nature (New Biol.), 1972, 237, 15.

Tada T., Taniguchi M., and David C. Properties of the antigen-specific suppressor T cell factor in the regulation of antibody response in the mouse. IV. Special subregion assignment of the gene(s) that code for the suppressive T cell factor in the H-2 histocompatibility complex. J. Exp. Med., 1976, 144, 713.

TADA T., TANIGUCHI M., and OKUMURA K. Regulation of antibody response by antigen-specific T cell factors bearing I region determinants. *In* T. E. Mandel, C. Cheers, C. S. Hosking, I. F. C. Mc Kenzie, and G. J. V. Nossal, Eds., Progress in immunology III, Proc. 3rd Int. Congr. Immunol., Sydney. Amsterdam, 1977, North Holland.

TANIGUCHI M., SAITO T., and TADA T. Antigen-specific suppressive factor produced by a transplantable I-J bearing T cell hybridoma. Nature, 1979, *278*, 555.

TAUSSIG M. J. T-cell factor which can replace T-cells in vivo. Nature (London)., 1974, *248*, 234.

TAYLOR R. B. and WORTIS H. H. Thymus dependence of antibody response. Variation with dose of antigen and class of antibody. Nature (London), 1968, *220*, 927.

Chapter 19

# ORIGIN OF ANTIBODY DIVERSITY

Jean-François Bach

I. INTRODUCTION

II. EXPERIMENTAL FINDINGS RELATIVE TO THE CLONAL
SELECTION THEORY

III. GENETIC BASIS OF SELECTIVE THEORIES

## I.  INTRODUCTION

### POSING THE PROBLEM

Antibody diversity is considerable. An individual is capable of synthesizing an estimated $10^5-10^7$ separate antibodies. The origin of this diversity has been the subject of speculation by immunologists since the beginning of the century. Recognition that the primary protein structure is totally under exclusive genetic control has shed new light on the problem. Is the number of genes specialized in Ig structure the same as the number of immunologic specificities? Are all of these multiple genes present in the germinal cell or do they appear randomly from mutations or recombination during immunocytic differentiation? Alternatively, can the antigen induce de novo synthesis of an antibody protein? We will try to answer these central questions in this chapter.

### IMMUNOLOGIC BASIS

The data on which the various theories are based are limited in number and can be summarized as follows: (1) antibodies are specific for the antigen that induces their formation; (2) an animal may respond simultaneously to many antigens administered simultaneously; (3) an antibody-producing cell synthesizes, as a rule, antibodies of the same specificity, isotype, allotype, and idiotype;

556

(4) the specific information corresponding to immunologic memory is borne by lymphocytes; (5) self-tolerance persists throughout life; (6) specific nonresponsiveness (tolerance) to foreign antigens can be induced; (7) the ability to produce antibodies of a given specificity is genetically controlled; (8) administration of some antigens may block the antibody response to other antigens; (9) prolonged stimulation by an antigen is associated with increased antibody affinity; (10) the antibody sites of immunoglobulins are determined by the sequence of amino acids in the variable part of their heavy and light chains; (11) antigens are not detected inside antibody-forming cells; (12) autoantibodies may be produced under certain circumstances; (13) the number of antibody-producing cells initially stimulated by an antigen is limited.

## THE PROBLEM RECONSIDERED

Antibody diversity is represented structurally by diverse amino acid sequences in the variable part of immunoglobulin light and heavy chains. The existence of constant and variable parts is in itself unusual (for proteins), the more so since, as earlier mentioned, the variable part presents extremely variable segments that exist alongside relatively constant segments. The genetic control of immunoglobulin chain synthesis must therefore include hypotheses super imposed on the general scheme of protein synthesis.

The simplest hypothesis proposes that each antibody corresponds to a separate gene (selective theories). On a Darwinian basis, variability, then, results from selection during evolution: the germinal selection hypothesis states that all genes that code for immunoglobulins are present in germinal cells. An opposite hypothesis proposes that variability appears randomly, from mutations or recombinations, during immunocytic differentiation in the fetus or in extrauterine life. This is the selective theory of somatic mutations or recombinations. The latter hypothesis has at least two alternative possibilities: totally random somatic mutations with nonfunctional clones either being spontaneously destroyed or eliminated under the influence of selective pressure, or somatic recombinations between a small number of cistrons present in the germinal cell.

In another hypothesis the antigen is said to induce de novo antibody synthesis (instructive theory). Here we must include a new mechanism that is not a priori compatible with the general genetic scheme of protein synthesis. However, the recent demonstration of a reverse transcriptional mechanism by RNA-dependent DNA polymerase in oncogenic viruses and in mammal cells might permit theoretically a restatement of instructive theories on a more plausible basis.

## HISTORICAL SURVEY

### Early Theories

The very first theory of immunity was probably that of Pasteur, who, in 1880, extrapolated from data observed in vitro (bacterial cell cultures) to in vivo defense mechanisms against infectious agents. Bacteria cultured in an appropriate medium stop growing after a time because they have exhausted a critical nutrient. Pasteur proposed, by analogy, that the growth of microorganisms in vivo exhausted the host organism of certain specific constituents that were necessary for germ growth. This hypothesis was abandoned when it was shown, a few years later, that sheep resistant to anthrax bacilli were, nonetheless, sensitive to the injection of large quantities of the same bacteria.

The first modern immune theory was proposed by Ehrlich in 1900. In a now classic article, Ehrlich proposed that antibodies are identical to preformed "lateral chains" (later called receptors) bound to cells (Fig. 19.1). Some of these

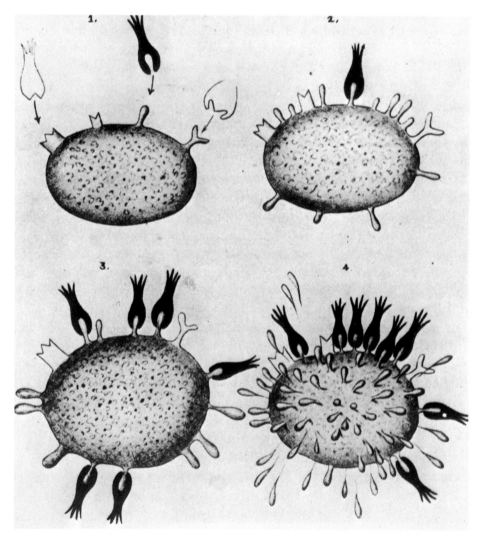

**Fig. 19.1** Ehrlich's theory. Contact between immunocompetent cells and antigen leads to multiplication and then release of cellular receptors. (From P. Ehrlich, Proc. Roy. Soc. [London], Ser. B. 1900, *66*, 424.)

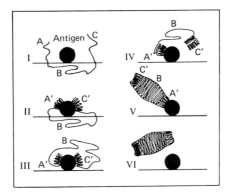

**Fig. 19.2**  Instructive theory. The antigen reacts with the antibody molecule and causes formation of a complementary structure. (From L. Pauling, J. Amer. Chem. Soc., 1940, *62*, 2643.)

receptors have structures complementary to those of specific antigens: when antigens bind to these receptors, synthesis of molecules identical to the receptors is stimulated. Some of these molecules appear in the serum as circulating antibodies. Two obvious merits of this theory were that it proposed a chemical basis for the antigen-antibody interaction, and that it implied that there exist preformed receptors to antigens. The "lateral chain" theory of Ehrlich was, nonetheless, vigorously attacked and in effect abandoned when Landsteiner showed that antibodies to artificial antigens, such as proteins coupled with dinitrobenzene or sulfanilic acid, could be formed. It seemed difficult to explain preformed receptors to an undefinite number of specificities, including artificial antigens.

### Instructive Theories

Theories that disputed the validity of Ehrlich's hypothesis were not proposed until 1930. At that time instructive theories were proposed by Breinl and Haurowitz and, subsequently, by Alexander and Mudd. These hypotheses state that the antibody molecule makes contact with the antigen molecule, with the latter serving as a template. Such contact modifies the antibody molecule, making it complementary to the antigen (Fig. 19.2). These theories obviously can explain the formation of thousands of different antibodies produced in response to synthetic antigens. Instructive theories were reevaluated and refined by Linus Pauling in 1940. Pauling postulated that all antibody molecules contain the same amino acid sequence and that the antibody molecule acquires specificity directly after contact with antigen. Karush stated that the structure that dictates specificity of antibody molecules was located at the level of disulfide bridges that connect cysteine residues in the polypeptide chain. He later postulated that antibodies initially consisted of reduced polypeptide chains that were secondarily folded in multiple ways. In the presence of antigen, the polypeptide precursor acquires a configuration complementary to the antigen. This configuration is stabilized by formation of disulfide bridges, and the antibody molecule then dissociates from antigen. Karush's model was the first to consider actual antibody molecular structure.

Instructive theories remain attractive to immunologists because they represent the simplest explanation for immunologic specificity. They do, however, represent no more than a working hypothesis. They are not satisfactory, for they fail to explain such concepts as immunologic memory and tolerance. Instructive theories do not take into account cellular aspects of antibody synthesis, especially the specificity of antibody-producing cells. Moreover, they contradict current concepts of protein synthesis, which state that proteins do not transmit the structural information they have received.

Burnet and Fenner proposed, in 1941, an interesting modification of instructive theories. They postulated that in penetrating cells, antigens induce changes in replicable enzymes responsible for antibody synthesis. This hypothesis had the advantage of providing an explanation for immunologic memory and the exponential increase in antibody titer after antigenic stimulation. Later, Burnet modified this theory to give DNA rather than enzymes the control function in antigen-modulated antibody synthesis. Nonetheless, all indirect instructive theories and related theories that implied, for example, RNA changes have the same major deficiency. They do not explain the molecular mechanisms by which an antigen may modify an enzyme or a nucleic acid.

### Selective Theories

The first selective theory, a modern form of Ehrlich's hypothesis, was proposed in 1955. Niels Jerne was the first to postulate natural selection. Jerne proposed that approximately one million different antibody molecules are formed during embryonic life (perhaps in the thymus). These molecules, then, may serve as models for antibody-producing cells, which synthesize identical molecules. The Ig molecule is considered a replicable unit (an hypothesis difficult to understand at a molecular level). Ig molecules that react with autoantigens are eliminated following combination with autoantigens that are met during fetal life, before the appearance of antibody-forming cells. The occasional reappearance of these autoantibodies reflects "copy mistakes." Antigens experienced after birth combine selectively with certain γ-globulins (preformed antibodies) that have a complementary configuration. Complexes thus formed are phagocytosed by specialized cells. The intracellular penetration of these selected globulins signals the synthesis of identical or only slightly modified molecules. This latter hypothesis explains the progressive improvement of the antibody complementary to antigens through a continuous process of selection. When the antigen is injected a second time, it encounters a specific globulin population; this fact explains the rapidity and intensity of secondary responses. When the antigen is eliminated, antibody synthesis decreases, and the level of specific γ-globulin decreases. This theory thus proposes the existence of antibody synthesis both before and after antigen injection. Jerne attributed the existence of preformed antibodies to a random production of a large variety of γ-globulins with cross-reactivities. The major objection to Jerne's theory is the experimental demonstration that immunologic memory is localized in cells and not in serum (see p. 537). The clonal selection theory proposed by Burnet and Talmage eliminated this objection by localizing selection to the cells, while maintaining other elements of Jerne's theory. Thus, clonal selection explained anamnestic responses, affinity increases during the course of immunization, the existence of natural antibodies, and the tolerance phenomenon.

In 1967, MacFarlane Burnet proposed the theory of clonal selection of acquired immunity. This hypothesis proposes that a family (clone) of cells reacts specifically to each individual antigen. The cells capable of producing antibodies to autoantigens are "forbidden;" they are eliminated during fetal life. Each cell from the clone has on its surface either the specific immunoglobulin or other molecules that have the same specificity for the antigen. The role of the antigen is to provoke, by interaction with these cellular receptors, proliferation and differentiation of immunocytes. Once stimulated, antigen-sensitive cells may give rise to plasma cells that produce large amounts of antibodies, to cells responsible for delayed hypersensitivity phenomena, or to memory cells. Burnet thought that the origin of diversity of antibody specificities is somatic mutations, which are particularly common during fetal life. The "forbidden" clones are eliminated during fetal life after contact with autoantigen.

This historical survey serves to remind us that beginning with Ehrlich's selective theory, and after a long period of time during which instructive theories prevailed, current opinion is once again oriented towards selective theories. We will not now reiterate findings that tend to refute instructive theories, but we will discuss experimental findings that support the clonal selection theory and then will analyze certain aspects of this theory that remain unproven or are obscure. We will finally envisage the genetic basis of selective theories, already discussed in chapter 7.

## II.  EXPERIMENTAL FINDINGS RELATIVE TO THE CLONAL SELECTION THEORY

### EVIDENCE THAT FAVORS A SELECTIVE THEORY

#### Absence of Antigen in Immunocompetent Cells

As discussed earlier (p. 332), antibody-forming cells, especially plasma cells, do not contain any antigen detectable by autoradiography or immunofluorescence techniques. One cannot, however, absolutely exclude the presence of antigens inside precursor cells on the basis of current methodology.

#### Biochemical Data Regarding Immunoglobulin Structure

##### DENATURATION-RENATURATION EXPERIMENTS

The reduction of IgG or its Fab fragment (disulfide bridges) in the presence of guanidine at high concentration destroys all organized spatial structure. However, if guanidine is removed by dialysis and the unfolded molecules are reoxidized, the immunoglobulin molecule will reassociate and present its original antibody site. This finding is incompatible with instructive theories, which imply the presence of antigen for formation of antibody-specific sites. The data rather suggest that the information present in the primary sequence of amino acids permits the tertiary structure to reform by folding. These facts are reminiscent of the case of ribonuclease, which after dissociation may spontaneously reassociate and regain its original enzymatic activity (see p. 144).

AMINO ACID SEQUENCE OF IMMUNOGLOBULINS

The sequence of several purified myeloma antibodies has been determined (see chap. 7). These sequences vary in their N-terminal portion of heavy and light chains. The differences express varying DNA nucleotide sequences and are inconsistent with an instructive theory.

### Genetic Control of Immune Responses

The immune response to certain antigens is controlled by immune response genes located close to genes that code for transplantation antigens (see chap. 24). The concept of discrete and separate genes for each antigenic determinant is not very compatible with instructive theories, according to which all information originates from the antigen.

## EVIDENCE THAT FAVORS CLONAL SELECTION

The above evidence favors a selective theory. In addition, numerous facts suggest that the selection operates at the level of antigen-recognizing cells.

### Existence of Surface Antigen Receptors on Immunocompetent Cells

B and T cells have on their surface antigen-specific receptors that are detectable by autoradiography or by the rosette test; 1–2/1000 lymphocytes of nonimmunized animals bind such antigens as bovine serum albumin or sheep red blood cells. The immunoglobulin nature of these receptors has been demonstrated for B cells and is suspected for T cells at least for the variable region (see chap. 4).

Cocapping experiments with membrane immunoglobulin and antigen receptors indicate that all B-lymphocyte membrane immunoglobulins are indeed antigen receptors. Recall also that individual B cells have surface immunoglobulin of a single class, allotype, and idiotype. The number of cells that bind the antigen increases during immunization and may decrease when tolerance is induced.

### Specificity of Antibody-Producing Cells (One Cell, One Antibody)

Antibody-producing cells, identified by hemolysis plaque and rosette techniques, are antigen specific and produce antibodies of a single class and allotype (see chap. 17). The simultaneous (and transient) presence of IgM and IgG molecules inside the same cell concurrent with the IgM-IgG switch observed in serum during immunization does not argue against the clonal theory, because variable parts of these antibodies are the same. The same remark applies to myeloma cells, which produce both IgM and IgG with the same idiotypes (see p. 522).

Note also the homogeneity of myeloma Ig, allelic exclusion (according to which a given Ig molecule from a heterozygous individual who is the progeny of homozygous parents bears only one allotype, either paternal or maternal in origin), and the evidence that an antibody-producing cell and its descendants express the same idiotypic specificities.

There now also exist numerous data to indicate that the descendants of a given B lymphocyte continue to produce the same antibody in a stable and durable manner. This has been shown particularly for Ig produced by murine plasmacytomas after multiple transfers. Similarly, B cells, either cultured in vitro or injected in infraoptimal quantities into irradiated animals (or even a single cell), produce antibodies that are perfectly homogenous in their allotypes, ability to bind antigen and even in their migration characteristics in isoelectric focusing.

### Existence of Antigen-Sensitive Clones

Antigen-binding cell clones may be separated by various techniques: passage of cells down glass-bead columns coated with the relevant antigen (Wigzell); incubation with a highly radiolabeled antigen, which leads to "suicide" of the antigen-binding cells (Ada); elimination of cells that form rosettes with sheep red blood cells by centrifugation on a Ficoll gradient that is crossed not only by red blood cells but also selectively by the erythrocyte-coated lymphocytes (Bach). In all three experiments, performed in normal and immunized mice, the elimination of antigen-binding cells suppresses the ability of the remaining cells to confer immunity to the antigen in irradiated animals. This absence of immunologic reactivity is antigen specific. The use of the fluorescent cell separator (described on p. 80) has enabled the even more direct demonstration that cells enriched in DNP-binding lymphocytes have an increased capacity to respond to DNP. Furthermore, the affinity of antibodies produced by such cells is correlated with the avidity of cells for DNP.

Antigen-binding and in vitro antibody production by B cells are inhibited in all these systems by incubation with anti-Ig sera and anti-idiotypic antisera corresponding to the antibody specificity under consideration. This latter crucial point has been particularly well demonstrated for phosphorylcholine and the carbohydrate antigens of *Streptococcus A*. Similar, although less conclusive, results have been reported for T cells.

### Conditions of High-Affinity Antibody Production: Antibody Feedback

Antibody affinity increases during the course of the immune response, paralleling a progressive decrease in antigen concentration. The injection of small antigen doses selectively stimulates production of high-affinity antibodies. Both observations may be explained by selective stimulation of high-affinity clones by low antigen concentrations. The antibodies produced have the same affinity as that of recognition receptors. The feedback phenomenon observed after passive antibody injection may be explained by competition of these antibodies with receptors on antigen-sensitive cells.

### Inhibition of Antibody Synthesis by in Vitro Treatment by Hapten

If lymphoid cells from mice immunized by a hapten-carrier complex are incubated in vitro with an excess of free hapten and are then transferred to irradiated recipients, there is no secondary response in the recipient when the same hapten-carrier complex is injected. Inhibition by free hapten is explained by binding of the hapten to lymphocyte receptors, which leads to neutralization of these receptors. The absence of direct immunocytic stimulation by the hapten might be explained by a requirement for a multivalent stimulation, which would involve interactions with both T lymphocytes and macrophages.

### Effect of Antigen Charge

One may separate rabbit IgG antibodies by ion-exchange chromatography into two portions with different charges. The negatively charged antigens selectively stimulate synthesis of positively charged antibodies and vice versa. These facts are compatible with the preferential binding of antigens to cells that possess surface receptors of opposite charge.

### Immunologic Tolerance

The decrease in the number of cells that bind the antigen sometimes observed in tolerance states suggests the possibility of clone deletion as the cause of certain tolerance states.

## EVALUATION OF CLONOTYPE NUMBER AND SIZE

An essential question in any discussion of antibody diversity is the evaluation of the number of antibodies that any individual is capable of producing and, consequently, in the selective theory hypothesis, the frequency of antibody-producing cell precursors against a given antigenic determinant in the lymphoid population.

A clonotype, that is, the antibody molecule produced by a B-lymphocyte clone, may be studied and defined in different ways: (1) by examination of the binding specificity with antigen, studied with strict comparison between the binding characteristics of the initial antigen and those of related molecules; (2) by charge—charge differences, as demonstrated by isoelectric focusing (usually in polyacrylamide gel), are a manifestation of the disparity in amino acid sequences of the variable or constant parts; (3) by idiotypic determinants—although two clones of different types may share the same idiotypes; (4) although it is rarely available for nonmyelomatous antibodies induced by immunization, determination of amino acid sequences of the variable part.

The number of clonotypes, that is, the repertoire of B-lymphocyte specificities, may be determined by analysis of the frequency of the cells specific for a given antigen associated with the identification of the number of clonotypes reactive toward that antigen.

The frequency of cells specific for a given antigen may be estimated by evaluating the number of cells that bind single antigens by rosette techniques, immunoenzymology, or autoradiography. The values obtained vary, according to the antigens studied, between 0.01 and 10 antigen-binding cells per $10^3$ cells. Kennedy's technique which consists of injecting a small number of cells at the same time as the antigen into an irradiated mouse and then counting PFC foci in the spleen, gives a value for sheep red cells of precursor frequencies of the order of $10^{-5}$.

Experiments that employ limiting dilutions are based on the same principle. Increasing numbers of cells are injected into irradiated recipients and the antibody response (all or nothing) is evaluated in the spleen by the hemolytic plaque technique. The results obtained, which follow Poisson's law, allow a theoretical evaluation of precursor numbers. The technique may be refined by injecting purified B-cell preparations in the presence of T-cell excess. Such techniques give estimations for phosphorylcholine on the order of 1 precursor cell per 40,000 to 50,000 cells.

The splenic foci and limiting dilution techniques have both been applied in vitro with resulting estimations of 1 per $10^5$ cells for sheep red cells, 1 per $5 \times 10^4$ cells for phosphorylcholine, and $1.5 \times 10^3$ to $10^4$ for NIP. By refining the technique and not taking into account the antibodies that possess a given idiotype, a figure of 1 precursor per $4-5 \times 10^6$ B cells is obtained. Conversely, higher figures are obtained when the techniques are performed using polyclonal activators that activate cells that produce weak affinity antibodies.

The determination of the number of clonotypes that exist for a given antibody is far from easy. Williamson has attempted such an evaluation for NIP, using isoelectric focusing analysis of the clonotypes present in an irradiated mouse that had received a limited number of cells from an NIP-BGG immunized mouse and is then immunized by the antigen. This technique has resulted in an estimate of about 10,000 anti-NIP clonotypes. A similar approach has led to a minimum estimate of 16,000 clonotypes for anti-DNP. Using an approximation of the figures for B-cell precursors of B cells producing anti-NIP antibodies (1 per 7,000–15,000) and those producing anti-DNP antibodies (1 per 500) and extrapolating these figures to other specificities, it may be concluded (Klinman) that the total number of possible clonotypes is about 5,000 (number of clonotypes per hapten) multiplied by 5,000–10,000 (frequency of different precursors corresponding to these different determinants)—in other words, it is of the order of 2.5 to $7.5 \times 10^7$ clonotypes.

Assuming an estimated number of total B cells of around 2 to $3 \times 10^8$ per mouse, it may thus be deduced that approximately 3 to 12 B cells are present in each mouse clonotype. Kohler has obtained a similar estimate for β-galactosidase.

These data and others derived from similar experiments have shown that (1) the maximal frequency of clonotypes in a nonimmune individual is about 1 precursor per $1-2 \times 10^6$ B cells, (2) the clones are of variable size (100,000 cells for β-galactosidase), and (3) consequently, in a given strain, the total number of specificities is on the order of $5 \times 10^7$.

suggests the same conclusions (especially with respect to the RNA messenger of the MOPC 21 murine L chain; see p. 232). (6) Lastly and most importantly direct DNA sequence analysis has confirmed the colinearity of V and C genes (with intervening non translated introns). Such studies have also shown the importance of J and D segments at the V-C junction (see p. 234).

The observed association of V and C segments has, nonetheless, important restrictions. There are three groups of translocation: $V_\kappa$, $V_\lambda$, and $V_H$. The $V_H$ sequences are always associated with $C_H$ sequences, and light-chain V genes are always associated with C genes of the corresponding chain. However, the fact that there is a pool of $V_H$ genes capable of associating with different $C_H$ genes and, in man, that $V_\lambda$ genes are capable of associating with three different $C_\lambda$ genes favors V and C gene independence. This hypothesis also explains the existence, mentioned above, of myeloma cells that produce two Ig molecules with the same idiotypes and the IgM-IgG intracellular switch that occurs during the immune response.

C and V genes belong to the same chromosome but are clearly distinct. Crossing-over places $V_H$ and $C_H$ genes of the same translocation group into proximity. Such crossing-over might be facilitated by mutual recognition of nucleotide sequences of terminal extremities that associate. It has been observed that the N-terminal extremities of $C_H$ fragments have the same sequence (for the three or four first amino acids) in each class ($\alpha$, $\mu$, or $\gamma$). This sequence could correspond, at the DNA level, to a palindromic structure that is a good candidate for the signal of V-C junction (see Fig. 7.40 p. 235).

## GERMLINE HYPOTHESES

### Description of the Germline Hypotheses

This hypothesis postulates that each Ig polypeptide chain is synthesized from a cistron present in the germinal line. All antibody diversity is thus inscribed in the genome of the individual and is hereditary, thus the analogy to other protein systems like hemoglobin. This hypothesis has the advantage of a genetic basis in common with other protein synthesis (with the same general limitations posed in other systems by lack of information about the molecular genetics of eukaryotes). The major problem (discussed on p. 244), is the large number of cistrons that would be necessary to explain production of all antibody specificities.

### Arguments in Favor of the Germline Hypothesis

All V chains do not present anarchic variability (or diversity). In some cases, one finds, in fact, a phylogenetic affiliation of variability subgroups from a common ancestor (see p. 207). Note, however, that this ancestral tree is based only on the comparison of subgroup-specific regions. A tree may be formed with all complete sequences, but obviously homologies are, then, less numerous.

Recall also that there probably exist antibody-producing cells of two specificities along with production of nonspecific Ig, both of which facts are poorly compatible with theories of recombination or somatic mutation.

Finally, it is important to note that Ig have the same limitations as do other coevolutionary proteins: the relative consistency of length, presence of certain positions that contain extremely variable amino acids while other positions contain amino acids of relatively constant composition, and the possibility that most mutations involve a single base substitution. In addition, the data now available on the DNA sequences for V genes (see p. 234) indicate the simultaneous existence, in the genome of a given cell, of several V genes both in the embryo and the adult.

In favor of the germline hypothesis, it is also worthwhile mentioning the programmed sequential appearance, in the course of ontogenesis in a given strain, of diverse antibody specificities in different species as well as the identity of spectrotypes observed in isogenetic xenopes obtained by hybridization after DNP stimulation.

### Evidence Against the Germline Hypothesis

Briefly, the main arguments are the large number of cistrons required, the existence of phylogenetically associated residues, and the presence of a-series allotypes on the variable parts of rabbit Ig. Still another question that must be answered by those who favor germline hypothesis concerns the evolutionary mechanisms that were responsible for the appearance and maintenance in genomes of cistrons that code for antibodies directed against rare and, in particular, synthetic antigens. Those who uphold the germline theory imply that there exists a vast pool of V cistrons that contains cumulative germline mutations and recombinations. This pool has to be sufficiently large to permit various organisms to face modifications in their environment. It is hard to say whether antigenic stimuli constitute in themselves a sufficient selective pressure. Perhaps such an assumption is possible for commonly encountered antigens, but certainly it is much less likely for exceptional antigens.

## SOMATIC RECOMBINATION HYPOTHESES

These hypotheses differ from the preceding ones in that they postulate the existence of a limited number of V cistrons in the germinal line. They are, nonetheless, compatible with the notion of coevolutionary genes and the existence of species-specific residues and allotypic specificities in variable parts (these points have been cited as objections to germline theories).

Variability is created by somatic recombinations between a limited number of germline cistrons. Hypotheses include extreme theories, totally somatic, with only two or three V cistrons in which variability is nearly all of somatic origin, and mixed theories (like those of Edelman and Gally), which involve between 10 and 100 V cistrons per translocation group. In the latter, variability is in part inscribed in the germinal line but then increases by somatic recombination within translocational groups (the latter theories are described and discussed on p. 246).

One must realize that the variability induced by such a model is considerable. Edelman and Gally postulated that the number of cistrons per translocation group is about 10. Thus, a variability on the order of $10^6$ would be expected.

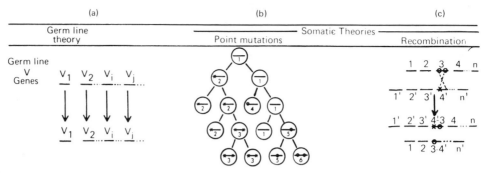

**Fig. 19.3** Selective theories of antibody diversity. (a) Germline theory. Each antibody is coded for by inherited genes not modified during somatic development. Genes are produced by mutations that occurred during evolution of the species. (b) Somatic mutation theory. A small number of inherited germline V genes become greatly diversified in somatic cells through successive point mutations, which are selected by prevalent antigens, self- or other. (c) Recombination theory. Inherited germline V genes become greatly diversified during somatic cell division by recombinations of sets of V genes. Recombinants are selected by prevalent antigens, self- or other. (From H. N. Eisen, Immunology. An introduction to molecular and cellular principles of the immune responses, ed. 2, New York, 1974, Harper & Row, p. 438.)

In addition, Edelman and Gally proposed that inside of the same immunocyte, a previously formed functional CV cistron might translocate onto another $C_H$ cistron. This complementary hypothesis would then explain the IgM-IgG switch inside of one immunocyte (the $V_H$ episome being successively translocated onto the $C\gamma$ instead of the $C\mu$ cistron), Oudin's observation of the same idiotypes on identical specificity antibodies that have different heavy chains, and the abnormally short heavy chains in heavy-chain disease (discussed earlier). Edelman and Gally's theory is a composite of germline and somatic theories and thus avoids many of the criticisms directed against the individual theories. Note, however, that additional hypotheses are implied (e.g., hypothetical enzymes, arbitrary estimation of the number of cistrons). It should be noted that recently obtained data on V gene DNA sequences demonstrate homologies in the nontranslated regions, which may further clarify these hypotheses, notably by simplifying the enzymatic hypotheses that have been necessary to explain intragenic recombinations.

Studies on V gene DNA sequences have recently brought direct argument for somatic recombinations both within the $V_H$ segment (particularly for $V_\lambda$ region in the mouse for which very few genes are present and at the V-J junction (see p. 234). In fact a major source of diversity of light chain arises from somatic recombination events that join one of several hundred V region sequences to one of J region segments. In addition to various combinations inherent in this process, the cross-over point of recombination can itself vary and thereby generate additional diversity. Heavy chain diversity is similarly generated but appears to involve the incorporation of a third region between V and J sequences.

# SOMATIC MUTATION HYPOTHESES

The underlying observation that supports hypotheses of somatic mutations is the large variety of stimuli to which any animal responds by producing specific antibodies. It is indeed difficult to explain how these stimuli would have represented sufficient selective pressure to select a gene and then maintain it in the germinal line throughout evolution. Somaticians distinguish between how populations and individuals react to new stimuli. Germline evolution would apply at the population level, and favorable mutations would accumulate in the germinal line. Somatic evolution would be a characteristic of individuals. Three categories of somatic mutations may be differentiated on the basis of origin of mutations.

### Spontaneous Mutations

Between 1959 and 1967, several models of somatic hypermutation were proposed. In 1959, Lederberg suggested a random hypermutation mechanism bearing on the entire germinal cistron. This hypothesis was abandoned when it was shown that all immunoglobulin chains contained the same constant region. Brenner and Milstein responded to this problem in 1966 by suggesting a cleavage enzyme that cleaves one of the two DNA chains at a recognition site. Such cleavage would release the V region extremity from which an exonuclease would then destroy a DNA fragment, leaving the C region intact. A DNA polymerase would then readily repair the DNA fragment. Errors might occur during repair, thus creating new V cistrons. In this hypothesis, mutations should be more numerous in the C adjacent part. However, this assumption has not been confirmed by sequence studies.

Lennox and Cohn then modified Brenner and Milstein's hypothesis by extending variability to the whole V cistron. The starting signal for enzymes, the generator of diversity, is no longer located only at the C-V junction but may be present anywhere on the V segment. The mutations, which occur randomly, can generate only a few functional structures in view of the strict constraints shown by subsequent sequential analysis. To answer this objection, somatic hypotheses were modified to include a hypothetical "somatic selection pressure" mutations, occurring randomly, are selected when they are located at points of functional advantage.

### Antigen-Induced Mutations

Cohn has proposed that the antigen is responsible for positive selection of the clone that produces the corresponding antibody. Somatic mutations would produce great antibody diversity and some of the specificities thus created would produce antibodies of high affinity for the specific antigenic determinant. The antigen selects the best adapted receptors, and this selection leads to proliferation of the corresponding clone. Such proliferation is the basis of mutations that generate and select the most specific receptors (and, hence, antibodies). The shortcoming of this hypothesis is that an important variety of antigens must make contact with the immune system and persist throughout all of development.

### Mutations Induced by Histocompatibility Autoantigens

In opposition to the theory of positive selection by the antigen, Jerne has proposed a theory of negative selection in which nonmutants are destroyed by histocompatibility antigens. According to this theory, the diversity of antibodies is the consequence of self-recognition. V cistrons present in the germinal line code for antibodies directed against histocompatibility antigens, including autoantigens. Lymphocytes that express receptors for alloantigens are maintained and are present in high percentage after birth. Lymphocytes that express receptors for histocompatibility autoantigens are heavily stimulated during fetal life by autoantigens. This cellular proliferation is associated with V cistron mutations in such a way that antibodies no longer are directed against histocompatibility antigens but, instead, against foreign antigens. Nonmutated cells are eliminated. A suggested site of mutation is the thymus, because cell proliferation is particularly intense in this organ. Recent studies by Zinkernagel (see p. 692) have confidently shown the role of the thymic epithelium in the acquisition of the repertoire of specificities recognized by T cells (see p. 87). Note that Jerne's theory is compatible with Ig allelic exclusion on the lymphocyte surface: for two immunoglobulins per cell to be expressed, two simultaneous mutations are necessary. This occurrence appears to be unlikely statistically.

Conversely, functional haploidy is not required, according to Jerne's theory, for lymphocytes that recognize alloantigens because they did not undergo mutation. Simonsen's experiments that show development of a graft versus host reaction in the chicken by only 50–100 lymphocytes corroborates Jerne's theory since they indicate that alloantigen-sensitive clones are large (1% to 2% of lymphocytes per specificity). Similar or even higher figures (5% to 6%) have been found using cell-dilution experiments in mixed-lymphocyte reactions (Wilson) and T-cell labeling with anti-idiotypic antibodies (Binz and Wigzell).

## CONCLUSIONS

All of the above selective hypotheses, both germline and somatic, are at least partly contradictory, and it is not possible to definitively accept any one of them. It fact, most recent data on DNA sequences indicate that all three hypotheses (germline, somatic mutations, and recombinations) intervene to some extent. Further studies will determine the precise number of V genes in each cluster. Latest evaluations indicate figures of $100–600V_K$ genes and $70–400V_H$ genes in the mouse.

## IV.   NETWORK THEORY

Jerne has recently proposed yet another theory in which the immune system is conceived to be a network of idiotypes and anti-idiotypic antibodies. If an antibody (Ab-1) is directed against a given exogeneous antigen, the individual has the capacity to produce Ab-2 antibodies with anti-idiotypic specificity for the Ab-1 antibody. Similarly, there will also be Ab-3 antibody with specificity against the Ab-2 antibody idiotypes, and so on. In addition, the Ab-1 antibody that recognizes the initial antigen (or epitope) can also simultaneously possess anti-idiotypic cross-reactivity toward an Ab-X antibody. This latter is considered by Jerne to be the internal image of the epitope. When antigen is administered, this network dissociates and antibody production results. Specifically, the antigen would inactivate its corresponding natural Ab-1 antibodies, thus transiently increasing production of the internal image Ab-X and, therefore, secondarily leading to production of the immune Ab-1 antibody (anti-Ab-X). Such a model could explain many immunologic phenomena that are otherwise difficult to understand. For example, tolerance to low antigen dose could be explained because Ab-1 antibody causes formation of large amounts of Ab-2, which suppresses Ab-1 antibody production by the mechanisms of idiotypic suppression (described on p. 215). Production of Ab-2 antibodies may, however, lead to the formation of Ab-3 antibodies, which may suppress formation of Ab-2 antibodies and, therefore, eliminate the suppression exerted by these antibodies on Ab-1 antibody production. The recent demonstration of the same idiotypic specificities on B and T lymphocytes (see p. 86) which would imply that both B and T cells participate to the network has enhanced interest in the hypothesis. More precise experimental demonstration of its theoretical bases is needed. However, one should already note that many of the elements required for the network have been shown to exist: (1) T- and B-lymphocyte reactions to idiotypes present on the animal's own Ig molecule have been demonstrated. (2) Antiidiotypic antibodies administered exogenously or produced endogenously suppress or stimulate T and/or B lymphocytes presenting with the relevant idiotypes. (3) Antiidiotype reacting T cells have been shown to suppress the production of antibodies carrying the idiotype. (4) The antibody response to phosphorylchlorine in BALB/c mice is followed by the production of antiidiotypic antibodies. Similarly, anti-idiotypic autoantibodies appear after allogeneic stimulation. (5) A given idiotypic determinant may be associated with several antibody sites (which do not necessarily bind the same antigen) and, conversely, the combination sites corresponding to a given antigen may be associated with several idiotypes.

# BIBLIOGRAPHY

COHN M. Selection under a somatic model. Cell. Immunol., 1970, *1*, 461.

COHN M. The take-home lesson. Ann. N. Y. Acad. Sci., 1971, *190*, 529.

EICHMANN K. Expression and function of idiotypes on lymphocytes. Adv. Immunol., 1978, *26*, 1.

GALLY J. A. and EDELMAN G. M. The genetic control of immunoglobulin synthesis. Ann. Rev. Genet., 1972, *6*, 1.

HOOD L. and PRAHEL J. The immune system. A model for differentiation in higher organisms. Adv. Immunol., 1971, *14*, 291.

HOOD L., WATERFIELD M. D., MORRIS J., and TODD C. W. Light chain structure and theory of antibody diversity. Ann. N. Y. Acad. Sci., 1971, *190*, 26.

MILSTEIN C. and MUNRO A. J. The genetic basis of antibody diversity. Annu. Rev. Microbiol., 1970, *24*, 335.

SEIDMAN J. G., LEDER A., NAU M., NORMAN B., and LEDER P. Antibody diversity. The structure of cloned immunoglobulin genes suggests a mechanism for generating new sequences. Science, 1978, *202*, 11.

SIGAL N. H. and KLINMAN N. B. The B cell clonotype repertoire. Adv. Immunol., 1978, *26*, 255.

SMITH G., HOOD, and FITCH W. Antibody diversity. Annu. Rev. Biochem., 1971, *40*, 969.

URBAIN J., CAZENAVE P. A., WIKLER M., FRANSSEN J. D., MARIAME B., and LEO O. Idiotypic induction and immune networks. In: Immunology 80 (M. Fougereau and J. Dausset [eds]). Acad. Press, New York, 1980:81.

VON BOEHMER H. Expression of receptor diversity in T Lymphocytes. In: Immunology 80, (M. Fougereau and J. Dasset [eds]). Acad. Press, New York, 1980:113.

## ORIGINAL ARTICLES

AVRAMEAS S., ANTOINE J. C., TERNYNCK T., and PETIT C. Development of immunoglobulin and antibody-forming cells in different stages of the immune response. Ann. Immunol. (Paris), 1976, *127c*, 551.

COHN M., LAGMAN R., and GECKELER W. Diversity 1980. In: Immunology 80 (M. Fougereau and J. Dausset [eds]). Acad. Press, New York, 1980:153.

EDELMAN G. M. and GALLY J. A. Somatic recombination of duplicated genes: an hypothesis on the origin of antibody diversity. Proc. Nat. Acad. Sci. (Wash.), 1967, *57*, 353.

GALLY, J. A. and EDELMAN G. M. Somatic translocation of antibody genes. Nature (London), 1970, *227*, 341.

JERNE N. K. The somatic generation of immunological reaction. Eur. J. Immunol., 1971, *1*, 1.

JERNE N. K. Towards a network theory of the immune system. Ann. Immunol., 1974, *125c*, 373.

# Chapter 20

# IMMUNOLOGIC TOLERANCE

## Jean-François Bach

I.   HISTORICAL SURVEY
II.  CONDITIONS FOR PRODUCING TOLERANCE
III. CELLULAR BASES OF TOLERANCE
IV.  IN VITRO TOLERANCE INDUCTION
V.   MECHANISMS OF TOLERANCE TO SOLUBLE ANTIGENS
VI.  TOLERANCE TO ALLOGRAFTS AND TUMORS

Immunologic tolerance may be defined as specific inhibition at the central level of immune responses to an antigen after previous contact with the same antigen. Under certain conditions, the organsim may not develop an immune response, either humoral or cellular, but may, instead, show a "paralytic" state that is antigen specific. Repeated administration of the antigen does not result in an immune response; however, the immune response remains normal to antigens that do not cross-react with the aforementioned antigen. This state of antigen-specific paralysis is called "tolerance." The term "immune paralysis," which is preferred by some, has the same meaning.

## I. HISTORICAL SURVEY

The first demonstration of tolerance was made in 1945 by Owen, who showed that, occasionally, both calves of a twining had circulating erythrocytes from both twins. Owen proposed that during embryonic life, the calves exchanged hematopoietic cells through placental vascular anastomoses. Cells that penetrated the partner colonized it, proliferated, and persisted (even though they would have been rejected in adults). Several years later, Billingham, Brent, and Medawar created an analogous chimera in the mouse: spleen cells from adult

A mice injected into newborn B mice render the latter tolerant to A donor skin grafts. One year later, Hasek reproduced the same phenomenon in the chicken by embryonic parabiosis: at the time of hatching, both chickens were mutually tolerant to skin grafts.

The universality of the tolerance phenomenon was demonstrated by use of soluble antigens, such as bovine or human serum albumin, after neonatal injection of these proteins into rabbits. Tolerance (to a soluble antigen) can also be induced in adult animals by administering high doses of antigen along with immunosuppressive treatment.

We will now describe tolerance to conventional antigens and then we will discuss tolerance in transplantation systems. Tolerance to autoantigens, which explains the usual absence of autoimmunity in normal animals, will be discussed in detail in chapter 25.

# II.   CONDITIONS FOR PRODUCING TOLERANCE

Numerous factors are involved in the initiation of tolerance, namely, form of the antigen, immunization method, level of immunocompetence, and species. Tolerance can be produced for both cell-mediated and humoral immunity systems. However, under certain circumstances, it dissociates. Such "split-tolerance," or immunodeviation, may suppress delayed hypersensitivity, although antibody production remains normal (for example, after dinitrophenyl-bovine γ-globulin injection in the guinea pig). Conversely, antibody production may be prevented, whereas delayed hypersensitivity is induced (an example is the immune response to acetoacetylated flagellin antigen) or tolerance may affect only a specific antibody class (IgG2 but not IgG1) in guinea pigs made tolerant to heterologous proteins.

## HOST IMMUNOCOMPETENCE

Tolerance can develop in most species. There are, however, several host factors that affect the ease with which tolerance is induced. Certain mouse strains are more easily made tolerant than are others: 10 mg of human deaggregated γ-globulin are required for BALB/c mice to develop tolerance, whereas 1 mg suffices for A/J mice, and 0.1 mg is effective for C57BL/6/J mice. Even more important is the level of immunocompetence (or immunologic maturity) of the host: the greater the individual's immunocompetence, the more difficult it is to induce tolerance. Animals with immunodeficiency are more easily rendered tolerant than are normal animals, regardless of whether immunodeficiency is spontaneous (linked to immaturity of the immune system in the fetus or newborn) or provoked (by various immunosuppressive agents).

### Fetus and Newborn

The capacity for antibody production and development of cell-mediated immunity does not appear until 8–15 days of age in the mouse and in newborn rabbits. Paralleling this immunologic immaturity, fetuses and newborns are particularly sensitive to induction of tolerance. Parenteral (intravenous) injection of human γ-globulin to newborn mice produces durable tolerance to this antigen, which persists several weeks or months if more injections follow (additional immunosuppression is unnecessary).

### Immunosuppressive Agents

It is possible to create tolerance by administration of high doses of soluble antigens in nonimmunosuppressed adult animals; however, nonspecific depression of immunocompetence considerably facilitates the creation of tolerance. Immunodepression may be achieved by total sublethal irradiation, administration of antimetabolites, alkylating agents, methylhydrazine, or antilymphocyte serum (see chap. 33), and by thoracic duct cannulation. For example, rabbits given 6-mercaptopurine several days prior to antigen injection develop tolerance specific for bovine serum albumin. Immunosuppressants permit tolerance to develop even in previously sensitized animals.

## NATURE OF THE ANTIGEN

Tolerance to many types of antigens has been induced.

### Immunogens and Tolerogens

Some antigens have two forms, "immunogenic" and "tolerogenic." Injection of the tolerogenic form induces tolerance to subsequent injections of the immunogenic form. The classic example of a substance that is both an immunogen and a tolerogen is γ-globulin, which is immunogenic in aggregates but is tolerogenic if the protein is present in soluble form. Commercial γ-globulin preparations are immunogenic because they are contaminated with very small amounts of aggregated γ-globulins. This immunogenicity is augmented by heating, which increases the amount of aggregates. Conversely, γ-globulins may be rendered tolerogenic by ultracentrifugation (e.g., for 90 min at 120,000g), because this procedure eliminates aggregates, leaving behind pure monomers. It is also possible to produce tolerogenic γ-globulin after deaggregation by in vivo filtration. Heterologous γ-globulins are injected into normal mice, and serum is collected several hours later. Aggregates are apparently removed from the circulation by the reticuloendothelial system. Other data suggest that macrophages may prevent tolerance induction. A correlation exists between the ease with which an antigen is phagocytosed and its ability to produce tolerance. In addition, reticuloendothelial blockade by, for example, carbon particles or mineral oil, will prevent tolerance induction. Finally, it should be noted that the sensitivity to tolerance induction towards BGG is 100 times greater in DBA/2 mice than in BALB/c mice and that this is due to adherent radioresistant cells, as shown in cell transfer experiments.

### Main Tolerogens

Many categories of antigens may be used to create tolerance, namely, heterologous proteins, bacterial and viral antigens, haptens, and synthetic polypeptides.

PROTEINS

As already mentioned, heterologous proteins are relatively easy to use for achieving tolerance, especially when aggregates are removed.

BACTERIAL OR VIRAL ANTIGENS

These (generally) particulate antigens are rapidly eliminated from the circulation. Such rapid elimination may explain why tolerance is difficult to induce, because only a low concentration may be expected to make contact with immunocompetent cells. One exception to this rule is pneumococcal polysaccharide, which persists for several months at high serum concentrations (probably because specific depolymerases are absent). This material is highly tolerogenic. Injection of as little as 250 μg of polysaccharide induces an almost completely tolerant state, without detectable circulating antibody, despite the fact that antibody-forming cells are detectable by the hemolysis plaque technique. This phenomenon is not true systemic inactivation; the "pseudotolerance" may, for example, result from antibody neutralization by persisting antigen (treadmill principle).

In high doses, however, polysaccharides may induce a true tolerance characterized by a lack of discernible antibody-forming cells (Fig. 20.1). Analogous results have been reported for detoxified *Escherichia coli* endotoxin (a lipopolysaccharide).

It is also possible to induce tolerance by use of monomeric subunits of

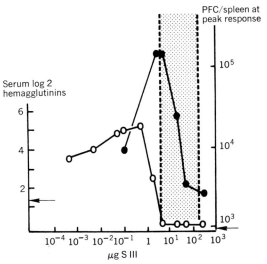

**Fig. 20.1**   Tolerance and pseudotolerance to S III pneumococcal polysaccharide. Note the discordant results for S III doses between 10 and 100 μg (dotted zone) between the absence of antibody (○) and the presence of hemolysis plaque-forming cells toward S III-coated red blood cells (●). Antibodies are absorbed by the antigen, persisting as they are produced. It is only at S III doses higher than 100 μg that PFC and antibodies are no longer observed. [From J. G. Howard et al., Proc. Roy. Soc. (London), Ser. B, 1971, *178*, 417.]

flagellin (*Salmonella* antigen) after acetoacetylation. Flagellin, which has a molecular weight of approximately 40,000 daltons, is cleaved by cyanogen bromide into four fragments, the largest (A fragment) of which is tolerogenic.

Tolerance states to viral antigens have not been well studied. Repeated injections of influenza virus, beginning at birth, produce a specific hyporeactivity. Neonatal injection of lymphochoriomeningitis virus induces a partial tolerance to this virus; however, tolerance is accompanied by antibody production and formation of immune complexes, which deposit along glomerular basement membranes to produce glomerulonephritis (see chap. 29).

### HAPTENS AND SYNTHETIC POLYPEPTIDES

Intravenous injection of large amounts of hapten (e.g., dinitrophenyl) into adult guinea pigs may produce tolerance, particularly towards antibody production and contact hypersensitivity. Such tolerance is generally considered to follow conjugation of the hapten to autologous proteins (the conjugate produced is usually more tolerogenic than immunogenic). Neonatal tolerance that involves delayed hypersensitivity can only be achieved through use of immunogenic conjugates, such as poly(Tyr)-ABA(polytyrosine-azobenzene arsonate). Neonatal tolerance to haptens conjugated to heterologous proteins like trinitrophenyl-bovine serum albumin can be induced in the rabbit. Such conjugates may also induce tolerance in adults after multiple injections in normal or cyclophosphamide-treated animals.

### OTHER ANTIGENS

Other antigens may induce tolerance, including heterologous red blood cells in newborns or adults (after injection of immunosuppressive agents such as cyclophosphamide). However, tolerance to these particulate antigens is very difficult to achieve, perhaps because they are too rapidly eliminated.

## ANTIGEN DOSE

The antigen dose is one of the most critical factors involved in the induction of tolerance.

### Tolerance at High Dose of Antigen

Generally speaking, tolerance is more easily induced and lasts longer when the antigen dose is large. For the same cumulative dosage, repeated administrations of smaller antigen doses are more effective than is a single large dose. It should be recalled, however, that once neonatal tolerance is induced, serial administration of low-dose antigen permits maintenance of tolerance throughout adult life.

### Tolerance at Low Dose of Antigen

Mitchison, in 1964, demonstrated that repeated injection of low doses (below the immunogenic dose) of bovine serum albumin (BSA) into adult mice induced tolerance. Similar results have been obtained with human serum albumin (HSA) in the rabbit. A tolerance to very low doses of antigen has also been obtained with flagellin in the mouse (doses of approximately $10^{-3}$ pg/g of body weight, injected serially, induced tolerance; Fig. 20.2). Unfortunately, these results have not been confirmed in the rat. In addition, tolerance to the administration of small doses has not been observed with other antigens, including RNase, lysozyme, ovalbumin, and diphtheria toxoid.

In conclusion, low-dose tolerance seems to be real but rare. It is only observed in certain species with antigens presenting both immunogenic and tolerogenic forms (very strong tolerogens like deaggregated BSA cannot be used to induce low-dose tolerance). The actual mechanisms remain obscure, but a major role is probably played by T cells.

## ROUTE OF ANTIGEN ADMINISTRATION

The route of administration of antigen influences induction of tolerance, especially in adults and for particulate antigens with limited diffusion. The converse holds for soluble proteins, which rapidly equilibrate between intra- and extravascular spaces, irrespective of the injection site. The intravenous route is generally more effective in inducing tolerance to particulate antigens.

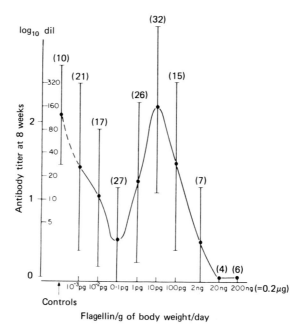

**Fig. 20.2**   The two antigen dose ranges that induce immune tolerance in newborn rats. *Abscissa,* different amounts of antigen (monomeric flagellin of *Salmonella adelaide*) injected; *ordinate,* serum agglutination titers, figures in parentheses indicate numbers of animals per group. (From R. G. Shellam and G. J. V. Nossal, Immunology, 1968, *14,* 273.)

In addition, some antigens may induce tolerance when injected by unusual routes. Thus, some haptens (e.g., picryl chloride in the guinea pig), injected intradermally bind to free amino groups of tissue lysines and give rise to antibody production and delayed hypersensitivity. Free hapten administered orally or in high intravenous doses inhibits subsequent attempts to sensitize by the intradermal route. These observations, which relate to the route of administration, may be explained by the binding of hapten to autologous proteins and by variations of its distribution volume in the organism according to the route of administration.

Of some interest is the fate of bovine γ-globulin (BGG), which, when injected into the mesenteric vein, deaggregates (probably in the liver) to become tolerogenic. Direct BGG injection into the thymus may also induce tolerance, which suggests thymic participation in the development of certain tolerance states.

# III. CELLULAR BASES OF TOLERANCE

## TRANSFER EXPERIMENTS

### Transfer from Tolerant to Irradiated Animals

After transfer, lymphocytes from tolerant animals confer tolerance to syngeneic irradiated recipients. The capacity to produce antibodies directed against pneumococcal polysaccharides is restored in lethally irradiated mice by injection of lymph node and spleen cells from normal animals. However, this restoration does not occur after administration of spleen cells obtained from mice made tolerant following polysaccharide injection 9 days earlier. Similar results have been reported for delayed hypersensitivity in the guinea pig (particularly for 2,4-dinitro-1-chlorobenzene). Tolerance follows when cells are collected during the first few days after induction of tolerance or after a longer period of time (e.g., up to 30 days for mice that receive deaggregated HGG). However, after 120 days, spleen cells do not transfer tolerance, even though the donor is still tolerant. This paradox has not been explained. It could involve antigenic persistence in a supertolerogenic form within certain privileged sites.

### Transfer from Normal to Tolerant Animals

While it is relatively easy, as has been said, to transfer tolerance to irradiated animals, the opposite phenomenon, which involves restoration, in a tolerant animal, of the immune response by transfer of normal cells, is much more difficult, if not impossible to obtain. No definitive explanation for this paradox has been proposed. It is possible that tolerance is associated with the presence of T cells suppressing B cell function (see p. 583). Perhaps persistence of the tolerogen renders the injected lymphocytes immediately tolerant. Circulating factors (especially antibodies) may also play a role.

## CELLULAR COOPERATION EXPERIMENTS

### Indirect Data

Both T and B cells are implicated in immunologic tolerance. Thymectomy in the mouse and bursectomy in the chicken perpetuate BSA tolerance. It has been observed that immunocompetence of thymectomized, irradiated, and bone marrow-reconstituted rats can be restored by administering normal thymic cells but not thymic cells from tolerant donors. This finding suggests that T cells play a central role in tolerance. These experiments have recently been reexamined systematically by various authors, particularly Weigle.

### Transfer Experiments into Irradiated Recipients

The design of these transfer experiments involves restoration of immunocompetence in irradiated mice by using mixtures of B and T cells obtained from normal or tolerant donors. Competence is assessed by serial measurements of antibody formation in recipient mice after stimulation by test and control antigens. Experiments with tolerant cells obtained from cyclophosphamide-treated mice have yielded inconclusive data (see p. 957). Some authors have reported that tolerance is transmitted by thymic cells, while others believe that bone marrow cells are crucial (especially in NZB mice that show T-cell abnormalities). Still others have reported that neither thymic nor bone marrow cells but only peripheral T cells in the spleen or thoracic duct confer tolerance. These conflicting findings were clarified by Weigle, who studied donor adult mice made tolerant to HGG by injection of deaggregated HGG and used syngeneic irradiated mice as the recipient of thymus and marrow cell inoculum.

Tolerance was found to be associated with both thymic and bone marrow cells (Table 20.1). When either T or B cells from tolerant mice are supplied, reconstituted mice also become tolerant. This experimental system has permitted precise definition of the kinetics of cellular tolerance. Tolerance studied at the level of spleen cells begins as early as 4 hr after tolerogen administration and is maximal by day 4. Tolerance kinetics at the level of B and T cells were also

**Table 20.1   Simultaneous Tolerance of B and T cells in Irradiated Mice Given Tolerogenic Human γ-Globulin***

| Cellular combinations | Indirect plaque-forming cells per spleen | |
|---|---|---|
| | TGG | HGG |
| nT + nBM | 9824 | 2508 |
| tT + nBM | 23,296 | 0 |
| nT + tBM | 22,425 | 0 |
| tT + tBM | 9797 | 0 |

* Abbreviations: n, normal donor; t, donor treated by tolerogen; T, thymus; BM, bone marrow; TGG, turkey γ-globulin; HGG, human γ-globulin.
After J. M. Chiller, G. S. Habicht, and W. O. Weigle, Proc. Nat. Acad. Sci. USA 1970, 65, 551.

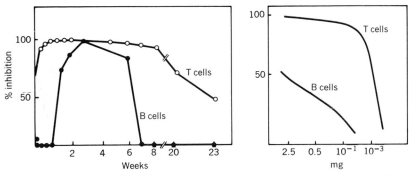

**Fig. 20.3**  B- and T-cell tolerance in mice rendered tolerant to deaggregated human γ-globulin (see text). Tolerance at the T-cell level occurs earlier, is more durable, and is obtained at lower tolerogen doses than is B-cell tolerance. (From J. M. Chiller et al., Science, 1971, *171*, 813.)

studied. Tolerance was induced by giving bone marrow or thymic cells from mice rendered tolerant for various lengths of time prior to cell collection. Still using HGG in the mouse, it was demonstrated that tolerance is rapidly induced in T cells (by the second day), persists for 120–130 days and begins to decrease after 150 days (Fig. 20.3). Tolerance induction in bone marrow cells takes longer to develop and is relatively short-lived (Fig. 20.3), even when high doses of tolerogen are employed.

Suppressor T cells were first demonstrated in tolerant mice by Basten and Miller; Weigle later showed that these cells are present during the first few weeks after induction of tolerance. Transfer of spleen cells from HGG-tolerant mice along with cells from mice immunized by aggregated HGG and with cells from mice immunized by the DNP-flagellin conjugate to irradiated recipients prevents the normal antibody formation in these mice that occurs after stimulation by the DNP-HGG conjugate. The suppressive action of tolerant mouse cells, which is HGG specific, is due to T cells, because it can be eliminated by pretreatment of (transferable) spleen cells with anti-θ serum. A role for these cells in induction or maintenance of tolerance seems plausible even if suppressor T cells are only transiently detectable, whereas tolerance persists. Suppressor T cells are apparently particularly important in low-dose tolerance, which seems to preferentially require T-cell participation (Fig. 20.3).

All of these data could explain the difficulties mentioned earlier involved in reconstituting immunocompetence in tolerant mice by giving normal or immune cells, the possibility of transferring specific tolerance by simple injection of tolerant cells, and the fact that it is impossible to induce tolerance to sheep erythrocytes in thymectomized, irradiated, and bone marrow reconstituted mice, unless they also receive thymic cells (reported by Gershon). Note that induction of tolerance in bone marrow B cells occurs later than in splenic B cells (which may become transiently tolerant after 3 days).

Antibodies secreted by B cells apparently play a minor role in tolerance: no HGG antibody-forming cell can be demonstrated in recipients made tolerant by injection of deaggregated HGG. The role of macrophages in tolerance induction is at present unclear. Like deaggregated HGG, tolerogens are incorporated in much smaller amounts by macrophages than are immunogens, such as aggregated HGG.

### Tolerance Breakdown

Tolerance to soluble antigens is not permanent. If no further tolerogen is administered, tolerance progressively disappears. When tolerance ceases, it is followed by the transient production of weak affinity antibodies, even in the absence of new antigenic stimulation. Administration of a new antigen dose may now produce a secondary-type response. All of these data are compatible with the hypothesis (mentioned earlier) of long-lived tolerance where T cells rather than B cells are implicated.

One may abrogate tolerance by injecting molecules that cross-react with the tolerogen (either the initial modified protein or a heterologous protein from another species). Thus, rabbits made tolerant at birth (by injection of 500 mg of BSA) produce anti-BSA antibodies when stimulated, as adults, with albumin from other species (e.g., HSA). The antibodies thus produced react with BSA and HSA shared determinants and are completely absorbed by both proteins. Subsequent BSA injection induces, in the same animal, a new tolerance state.

Interpretation of these facts is based on the concepts discussed above regarding tolerance at B- and T-cell levels. Indeed, if there is essentially a T-cell type of tolerance to BSA, in this example, HSA will stimulate, by its determinants not shared with BSA, exclusively anti-HSA T cells, and, by determinants common to BSA, BSA-specific B-cell precursors, which are not tolerant.

By analogy to carrier-hapten systems (discussed in chap. 18), it is possible that HSA stimulates T cells via its own "carrier" determinants and that it stimulates B cells by use of its "hapten" determinants that it shares in common with BSA (hence, production of anti-BSA antibodies). Another possibility to abrogate tolerance consists of inducing a graft-versus-host reaction, which leads to an allogeneic effect that substitutes for carrier-specific T cells, which are tolerant (see p. 538). Similarly, administration of the antigen in the presence of Freund's complete adjuvant (the latter stimulates T cells; see p. 946) may produce identical effects. These observations and hypotheses concerning tolerance abrogation are essential for the understanding of autoimmunity mechanisms because autoimmune manifestations may actually represent a loss of tolerance to autoantigens (see p. 722).

## IV.   IN VITRO TOLERANCE INDUCTION

It is possible to induce tolerance, in lymphoid cell cultures in vitro especially to thymus-independent antigens. Thus, by adding normal spleen cells to polymeric antigens with repetitive determinants, such as *E. coli* lipopolysaccharide, polymerized flagellin (POL), and highly substituted conjugates of POL (DNP-POL), tolerance is induced in these cells. One can also induce, in vitro, tolerance to normally nontolerogenic antigens, like the A fragment of flagellin, if the antigen is previously incubated with low concentrations of the antibody. Apparently, the antibody acts by aggregating monomeric determinants. It seems that repetitive determinants are required for in vitro tolerance to be induced; however, in vivo, the situation is quite different, in that protein monomers are tolerogenic, whereas aggregates of the same proteins are immunogenic. In vitro induction of tolerance to heterologous proteins (which are thymus-dependent antigens) is most difficult to achieve.

# V.  MECHANISMS OF TOLERANCE TO SOLUBLE ANTIGENS

We have reviewed the major factors of tolerance induction, defined precise transfer conditions, and described the major cellular events that accompany tolerance induction. Some conclusions regarding mechanisms can be derived from this information. Cell transfer experiments indicate that tolerance is localized in lymphoid cells. Because spleen cells from tolerant donors may transfer antigen-specific immunity to irradiated animals several weeks after tolerance induction, tolerogen localization in privileged sites may play an important role. Since tolerance is usually not reversed by normal cells, intervention of humoral or cellular factors in maintenance of tolerance induction is suggested. Antibody might act in various ways: by feedback mechanisms (see p. 340), by idiotypic suppression (see p. 215), or by modifying antigenic presentation (as in in vitro tolerance experiments). However, such a role for antibodies does not seem to be essential, because few, if any, hemolytic plaque-forming cells are present in tolerant animals. An intervening role for suppressor T cells, on the other hand, seems very plausible. Suppressor T cells specifically sensitized to the antigen might, indeed, cause specific immune paralysis. Their mode of action is uncertain, but it probably involves both B and T cells as target cells (see p. 546).

It is likely, by analogy to induction of immune responses by immunogens, that tolerance induction involves physical contact between the tolerogen and B- and T-lymphocyte receptors. The way the antigen presents itself is important, as can be seen when comparing tolerance induction in vivo (deaggregated proteins) or in vitro (repetitive determinants). Possibly, especially for HGG, polymeric aggregates stimulate T lymphocytes, whereas monomers block receptors and fail to activate cells. If one admits that T cells play a role in presenting thymus-dependent antigens to B cells, T-cell inactivation adequately explains tolerance to these antigens.

Another very important question still to be resolved is whether the clone of tolerogen-sensitive cells is destroyed or inactivated or is simply influenced by suppressor factors (antibodies or suppressor T cells). The effect of tolerance on the number of antigen-binding cells (autoradiography or rosette test) has produced contradictory findings. Absolutely normal, increased, and decreased (antigen-binding) numbers of cells have been reported. These discordant results may be explained by proposing that the number of antigen-binding cells is decreased only during the short time period of B-cell tolerance, because autoradiography essentially detects B cells. In fact, no solid data are yet available regarding antigen-binding T cells in tolerance. The presence of cells that bind antigen would exclude the hypothesis of elimination of a clone that reacts with the antigen; on the other hand, a decrease in or the absence of antigen-binding cells during tolerance induction does not necessarily indicate that the cells in question have been eliminated. Receptors may be masked by the tolerogen, subject to redistribution (analogous to the phenomenon of capping, described p. 82), or no longer synthesized.

# VI.  TOLERANCE TO ALLOGRAFTS AND TUMORS

Tolerance to allografts and tumors probably has the same mechanisms as does tolerance to soluble antigens. Tolerance induction to allografts may be obtained by neonatal injection of allogeneic cells (followed by ultimate regular similar injections), or by injection of allogeneic cells or cellular extracts directly into adult animals that are receiving high-dose immunosuppression [e.g., antilymphocyte serum (ALS) or methylhydrazine]. Such tolerance is difficult to achieve if major H-2 histocompatibility differences exist. Tolerance-induction to allografts requires a systematic search for the best protocol for sequential administration of graft, immunosuppressant, and tolerogenic lymphoid cells. To obtain tolerance with ALS, the tolerogenic cells must be administered early enough after ALS treatment so that immunosuppression exists at the time of cell administration (injection) but not so early that ALS in high concentration destroys the injected cells. Adult thymectomy considerably enhances tolerance induction. The persistence of tolerogenic cells (chimera) and their proliferation, observed in some settings, may also be important.

A role for antibodies in tolerance is unproven (it even seems unlikely) for soluble antigens, but represents an attractive possibility for transplantation tolerance. It remains a matter of considerable debate. A "central" theory proposes inactivation or elimination of cytotoxic T cells, and a "peripheral," or facilitation, theory suggests, instead, that blocking factors (facilitating or anti-idiotypic antibodies, suppressor T cells) oppose the action of T lymphocytes.

## SUPPRESSION

It is possible to increase skin, organ, or tumor graft survival by administering facilitating antisera. This possibility was shown by Kaliss (in 1958) for tumors and by Voisin (in 1965) for skin grafts. Facilitating sera are obtained by injecting allogeneic cells or tumors into normal recipients. The relevant antibodies are essentially noncomplement fixing and of the $\gamma_1$ class in the guinea pig. Facilitating antisera specifically block in vitro activities of sensitized lymphocytes, particularly lymphocytotoxicity and mixed-lymphocyte reactions.

The Hellströms and others have reported that animals apparently tolerant to an allograft or a tumor carry lymphocytes cytotoxic to the foreign cells. Furthermore, some of these animals possess serum factors that block the lymphocytotoxic reaction of Takasugi and Klein (tumor cell or fibroblast growth

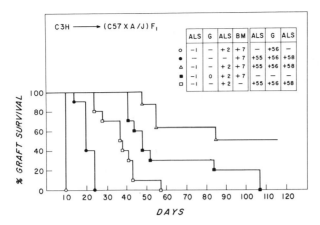

**Fig. 20.4** Effects of previous administration of bone marrow and antilymphocyte serum (ALS) on skin allograft survival from C3H mice to (C57BL/6 × A/J) $F_1$ mice. Some mice receive 0.5 ml of ALS on days −1 and +2 and 25 × 10⁶ bone marrow cells from C3H mice on day +7. Some mice in this group (△) do not receive skin grafts on day 0 but, instead, on day 56 and a new ALS treatment (days 56 and 58). Another group (■) receives a skin graft on day 0 but no ALS treatment. Control groups (□, ●, and ○) are submitted to the same protocol as the △ group, omitting either the bone marrow injection (□), or ALS on days −1 and +2 (●), or ALS on days 56 and 58 (○). Day 0 on the abscissa refers to the day of the second skin allograft (56 days after the first one). Differences in survival between △ and □ demonstrate the tolerogenic effect of bone marrow cell injection. (From A. P. Monaco et al., *in* Actualités néphrologiques Hôpital Necker, Paris, 1974, Flammarion, p. 39.)

inhibition; Table 20.2). These blocking factors may be antibodies or antigen-antibody complexes. Their action could be peripheral (at the level of the graft), in which case transplantation antigens would be masked, or central, perhaps representing immune complex neutralization of T-cell antigenic receptors. Anti-H-2 antibodies (demonstrable by hemagglutination) have been observed in mice made tolerant at birth (by injections of allogeneic cells). Lastly, tetraparental mice (see p. 688) have circulating lymphocytes capable of reacting against the cells of each parent, but they also possess a serum factor capable of

**Table 20.2  Blocking of Lymphocytotoxicity by Lymph Node Cells from W/Fu Rats Rendered "Tolerant" to BN Bone Marrow Cells at Birth by Their Serum**

| Target cells (fibroblasts) | Donor lymph node cells | Serum donor | Cytotoxicity (%) | Blocking (%) |
|---|---|---|---|---|
| BN | W/Fu "tolerant" to BN | W/Fu "tolerant" to BN | 0 | ≥100 |
|  |  | W/Fu normal | 36.8 | 0 |
| W/Fu | W/Fu "tolerant" to BN | W/Fu "tolerant" to BN | 0 | — |
|  |  | W/Fu normal | 0 | — |

After L. W. Wright et al., *Transplantation* 1974, *18*, 49.

blocking these reactions. The antigenic specificities of the facilitating antibodies are still unknown, but recent data indicate a particular role for anti-Ia antibodies.

Other blocking factors might intervene in the creation of allograft tolerance. Anti-idiotypic antibodies may bind to T cells and inhibit their immune functions. Their presence in allograft recipients is well demonstrated and they could play a role in active tolerance. Similarly, suppressor T cells could be involved in tolerance onset or maintenance. Such suppressor cells have been demonstrated in in vitro systems (MLC, CML) and in in vivo transfer experiments. Their specificity is probably essentially directed at donor alloantigens but also, possibly, at antidonor antibody and receptor idiotypes.

## CENTRAL INACTIVATION

There is, however, some evidence in opposition to a role for blocking factors in relation to mechanisms of complete tolerance. It is possible to terminate allograft tolerance by injecting competent cells (especially those from a specifically sensitized animal). In addition, spleen cells from mice rendered completely tolerant to H-2 alloantigens do not develop a graft-versus-host reaction when they are administered to an irradiated host that possesses these alloantigens, nor is a mixed-lymphocytic reaction or in vitro cytotoxicity toward donor lymphocytes ever seen. The observations mentioned above, which demonstrate cellular reactivity of the recipients toward the host, would only be seen in partial tolerance. Absence of a primary role for blocking antibodies in complete tolerance is also implied by an absence of detectable antibody in completely tolerant animals, and especially because induction of allograft tolerance is possible in neonatally bursectomized chickens, which produce no antibodies. These experiments do not, however, exclude the possible role of blocking suppressor T cells; these cells would play a role similar to that envisaged in tolerance to soluble antigens.

## CONCLUSIONS

On the basis of these data, one may assume that complete tolerance is due to elimination, or "central" inactivation, of clones reactive towards specific alloantigens, whereas partial tolerance may be due to blocking factors, either cellular (suppressor-T lymphocytes) or humoral (facilitating or anti-idiotypic antibodies, immune complexes). These conclusions might also apply to certain states of tumor growth, but these data are still more limited than are those for allograft tolerance.

## *BIBLIOGRAPHY*

ADA G. L. Antigen-binding cells in tolerance and immunity. Transpl. Rev., 1970, 5, 105.

ALLISON A. C. Immunologic tolerance. In F. H. Bach and R. A. Good, Eds., Clinical immunobiology. Vol. I. New York, 1972, Academic Press, p. 113.

BRENT L. Tolerance and enhancement in organ transplantation. Transpl. Proc., 1972, 4, 363.

Diener E. Cellular and subcellular aspects of tolerance induction. *In* L. Brent and J. Holborow, Eds., Progress in Immunology. Vol. 3. Amsterdam, 1974, North Holland, p. 217.

Doyle M. V., Parks D. E., Romball C. G., and Weigle W. O. Immunoregulation in tolerance and autoimmunity. In: Mechanisms of Immunopathology (S. Cohn, P.A. Ward, and R. T. McCluskey [eds]). John Wiley & Sons New York, 1979:107.

Dresser D. W. Immunological tolerance. Brit. Med. Bulletin, 1976, *32*.

Dresser D. W. and Mitchison N. A. The mechanism of immunological paralysis. Adv. Immunol., 1968, *8*, 129.

Feldman J. Immunological enhancement: a study of blocking antibodies. Adv. Immunol., 1972, *15*, 167.

Howard J. G. Cellular events in the induction and loss of tolerance to pneumococcal polysaccharides. Transpl. Rev., 1972, *8*, 50.

Katz D. H. and Benacerraf B. (Ed.) Immunological tolerance. New York, 1975, Academic Press.

McKearn T. J. A biological role for for anti-idiotypic antibodies in transplantation immunity. In: Immunological tolerance and enhancement (F. P. Stuart and F. W. Fitch [eds]). MTP Press Ltd. Lancaster U. K., 1979, 61.

Miller R. G. The role of accessory cells in specific immunological unresponsiveness. *In* L. Brent and J. Holborow, Eds., Progress in immunology. Vol. 3. Amsterdam, 1974, North Holland, p. 229.

Möller G. [Ed]. Mechanisms of B lymphocyte tolerance. Immunol. Rev., 1979, Vol. 43.

Möller G. [Ed]. Transplantation tolerance. Immunol. Rev., 1979. Vol. 49.

Möller G. [Ed]. Regulation of the immune response by antibodies against the immunogen. Immunol. Rev., 1980, Vol. 49.

Möller G. (Ed.) Suppressor T lymphocytes. Transpl. Rev., 1975, *26*.

Nisbet N. A. and Elves M. W. Immunological tolerance to tissue antigens. Orthopaedic Hospital, Oswestry, 1973, England.

Nossal G. J. V. The cellular and molecular basis of immunological tolerance. *In* Essays in Fundamental Immunology. Vol. I. London, 1973, Blackwell, p. 28.

Nossal G. J. V. and Schraeder J. W. B-lymphocyte-antigen interaction in the initiation of tolerance or immunity. Transpl. Rev., 1975, *23*, 138.

Stuart F. P. and Fitch F. W. Immunological tolerance and enhancement MTP Press Ltd. Lancaster U. K., 1979, 196.

Voisin G. A. Immunity and tolerance: a unified concept. Cell. Immunol., 1971, *2*, 670.

Weigle W. O. Immunological unresponsiveness. Adv. Immunol., 1973, *16*, 61.

Weigle W. O. and Skidmore B. J. Mechanism of activation and tolerance induction in B lymphocytes. Transpl. Rev., 1975, *23*, 250.

# ORIGINAL ARTICLES

Diener E. and Feldmann M. Antibody mediated suppression of the immune response in vitro. II. A new approach to the phenomenon of immunological tolerance. J. Exp. Med., 1970, *132*, 31.

Diener E. and Feldmann M. Mechanisms at the cellular level during induction of high zone tolerance in vitro. Cell. Immunol., 1972, *5*, 130.

Hellström I. and Hellström K. E. Cell-mediated immunity and blocking antibodies to renal allografts. Transpl. Proc., 1972, *4*, 369.

Hellström K. E., Hellström I., and Allison A. C. Neonatally induced allograft tolerance may be mediated by serum-borne factors. Nature (London), 1971, *230*, 49.

Mitchison N. A. Induction of immunological paralysis in two zones of dosages. Proc. Roy. Soc. Med., 1964, *161*, 275.

Möller E. and Sjoberg O. Antigen-binding cells in immune and tolerant animals. Transpl. Rev., 1972, *8*, 26.

# Part 5

# IMMUNOGENETICS

# Chapter 21

# INTRODUCTION TO IMMUNOGENETICS

**Charles Salmon**

   I.   HISTORICAL INTRODUCTION
   II.  GENETIC BASES
   III. IMMUNOLOGIC BASES
   IV.  APPLICATION OF BLOOD GROUPS AND POLYMORPH-
        ISM TO HUMAN GENETICS

## I. HISTORICAL INTRODUCTION

### MAIN BLOOD GROUPS

In 1900, Landsteiner discovered that serum from some individuals agglutinates other subjects erythrocytes. Thus, the first alloantigens, called A and B, were identified. The genetic transmission of these antigens was demonstrated in 1910 by Von Dungern and Hirszfeld. This discovery was a most important one, because it demonstrated for the first time human polymorphism and permitted transfusion therapy. Landsteiner and Wiener introduced experimental heteroimmunization. Antibodies were produced in animals, species-specific antibodies being eliminated by absorption. By this means, three other human blood group systems, MN, P, and, of special interest, LW (detected by immunizing rabbits with *Macacus rhesus* blood) were identified. Further progress was accomplished in 1939 by Levine, who discovered alloimmunization—a woman who had just delivered a child with a yet mysterious disease called erythroblastosis fetalis presented a circulating antibody that recognized the father's erythrocytes and those of the icteric child. The antigen identified was the Rhesus (Rh) antigen, similar but not identical to the LW antigen of Landsteiner and Wiener. Levine recognized that the fetal disease represented alloimmunization of the Rh-negative mother to the Rh antigen that the fetus had inherited from its father. Unlike the apparently spontaneous antibody formation of Landsteiner's

ABO system, this represented the classic reaction of an organism without a genetic marker to introduction of such a marker.

Because of the existence of several blood groups systems, it was thought that polytransfused patients and multiparous women might possess antibodies to multiple unknown antigens. Many laboratories worldwide began to investigate such sera, aided considerably by various technologic breakthroughs that had followed the Rh discovery, particularly Coombs' reaction. At the Lister Institute in London (Race and Sanger), a large number of new antigens was subsequently recognized.

## OTHER MARKERS

In 1958, Dausset first identified leukocytic and platelet antigens, soon to be called the HLA (A, B and C) antigens. Interhuman alloimmunization quickly focused on the developing field of organ transplantation. Utilization of cellular reactions, such as mixed-lymphocyte cultures, showed that biologic (individual) uniqueness could also be defined in terms of cellular recognition systems (HLA-D antigens). HLA antigens found numerous applications in transplantation and, more recently, in studies of association with certain diseases (see p. 695).

Furthermore, Grubb (in man) and Oudin (in animals, 1956) recognized in serum immunoglobulins a genetic variation similar to that described for red cells (allotypy).

## HUMAN IMMUNOGENETICS AND IMMUNOHEMATOLOGY

Coincidentally, immunologists became interested in globulins present on red blood cell surfaces of subjects with acquired hemolytic anemia. Wiener was the first to show that these globulins were antibodies, usually directed against blood group antigens that occur in high frequency, such as Hr antigens for IgG and I antigen for IgM antibodies. Due to precise analysis of antierythrocytic autoantibody specificity, autoimmune hemolytic anemia soon became a reference model for immunopathologists. Thus, immunogenetics and immunohematology developed together, both concerned with the fundamental problems of immunology represented by the existence of natural antibodies, allo- and autoantibody formation, and the definition of recognition systems.

Immunogenetics attempts to analyze immunologic phenomena by genetic methods or, conversely, to apply laws of formal or physiologic genetics to various immunologic problems. Matters of particular interest include polymorphism markers and the regulation of immune responses.

Immunohematology is the study of aspects of hematology that concern immune phenomena or employ immunologic methods. It is an integral part of immunogenetics.

## II.   GENETIC BASES

The genetic material, DNA, has three remarkable properties: replication, production of proteins, and mutation. The first of these properties involves formal genetics, and the second deals with physiologic genetics. These two properties of DNA, along with photosynthesis of vegetal chloroplasts, are the basis for life itself. The third property introduces genetic polymorphism and population genetics.

## CLASSIC (FORMAL) GENETICS

Mitosis, which terminates in DNA replication and thereby gene repetition, is the phenomenon that transmits characteristics of mother to daughter cells and thus determines somatic differentiation. Meiosis produces gene segregation and permits, by means of chromatic reduction, a compensatory mechanism, the actual transmission of self-identity from one generation to another. Classic Mendelian genetics refers to phenotypes. Its best-known application is in the transmission of immunogenetic characters, such as blood groups. We will now review some elementary applications of formal genetics that apply to blood groups.

### Gamete Purity

An AB blood group subject mated to an O group subject may only produce either A or B children. During meiosis, these characteristics (A and B) exclude each other; they are alleles.

### Independent Character Segregation

The descendants of a double heterozygote (e.g., AB MN) and a double homozygote (e.g., O NN) exhibit phenotypes in which gametes from heterozygotes (AM, AN, BM, BN) are represented in equal proportions. This proves that transmission of the A and B alleles is independent of that of M or N. Each of these groups is an allele couple, and the two are called "independent" blood group systems.

### Genetic Linkage

However, it appears that characters of both systems more often are transmitted together than would be expected on the basis of a total independence. Thus, these two characters are "linked," as in the case of Lutheran and ABH secretion systems, or for ABO and AK systems, or PGM and Rh systems.

Linkage is recognized by identifying the percentage of recombinants that issue from parental gametes. The closer together are the characters, the greater is the linkage.

In extreme cases genes that are very close to one another, are termed pseudoalleles. They are very rarely dissociated (by crossing-over during meiosis). The M or N and the S or s genes are pseudoalleles. Haplotypes represent the characteristics transmitted by one gene complex or closely linked genes (for example, MS, or DCe in the Rh system).

Several linkage groups may be present on one chromosome. This possibility has been demonstrated in man by cell hybridization experiments between human and mouse fibroblasts. Knowledge of those linkage groups has resulted in enormous progress in mapping the human chromosomes. Transmission of sexual X chromosomes is subjected to peculiar rules directly related to the male (XY) and female (XX) genetic constituents. Transmission of the $Xg^a$ blood group is such an example.

### Linkage Disequilibrium

Genetic linkage may be suspected when linkage disequilibrium is seen. In haplotypes, the genes are more often associated than might be expected if they were independent. Thus, the frequency of the Ms haplotype, which in the absence of linkage would equal the product of gene frequency multiplied by the frequency of the s gene, is in fact quite different. The difference between the observed frequency and the frequency that might be expected according to the independence hypothesis, indicates the extent of the linkage disequilibrium. This disequilibrium is even more significant if the linkage is direct. Thus, in the MNSs, Rh, Lutheran, and HLA systems, obvious linkage disequilibrium is seen, but this is not observed in looser linkages, such as in the Lewis system and the secretory system. Here there is no disequilibrium and the haplotypes are seen with a frequency that is in keeping with that of the genes of the Lele and Sese systems.

### Dominant and Recessive Characters

The terms "dominant" and "recessive" in classic genetics refer to characters, that is, phenotypes, not genes. A characteristic is dominant when it is expressed in the heterozygote and is called recessive when it is not expressed in the heterozygote. Thus, the $A_1A_2$ genotype is expressed as $A_1$, which indicates that $A_1$ is dominant and that $A_2$ is recessive. However, recently it has been possible to detect $A_2$ enzyme in an $A_1A_2$ genotype; therefore, for this gene product, the literal use of the term "recessive character" is somewhat inappropriate.

## PHYSIOLOGIC GENETICS OR THE PROTEIN FACTORY

Only proteins are primary products of genes. Blood group antigens, whose specificities are borne by carbohydrate molecules, are thus not direct gene products, as are protein genetic markers (for example, immunoglobulins).

**Table 21.1   Linkage Disequilibrium: The Example of MNSs**

| | |
|---|---|
| Frequency of M allele | 0.55 |
| Frequency of s allele | 0.66 |
| Expected frequency of Ms haplotype in the absence of linkage | 0.36 |
| Observed frequency of Ms haplotype | 0.28 |
| Difference between expected and observed frequency | 0.08 |

## POPULATION GENETICS AND POLYMORPHISM

Certain characters are identical in all individuals of a given species (isotypy). However, DNA mutations are responsible for differences in individuals of one species for a given monofactorial characteristic (produced by a single locus). This phenomenon is allotypy. The word was initially coined by Oudin to delineate antigenic differences in immunoglobulins present within the rabbit species. Allotypy now refers to any system of immunogenetic variation within species. Some authors, for example, Ropartz, propose its use even for nonantigenic characters. When the frequency of genetic mutation is very low, a monomorphic system is identified. Under these conditions, most genes are identical in the species. Such is the case for the two alleles ($Ve^a$ and $Ve^b$) of the Vel system; the former has a high frequency, whereas the latter occurs rarely. On the other hand, in some subjects, two genes may be seen at similar frequencies; the system here is called dimorphic (e.g., $Hp_1$, $Hp_2$). When a series of alleles coexists with relative stability within a population, the phenomenon represented is called equilibrated polymorphism. Most human genetic systems, in man, like blood groups and HLA antigens, correspond to this model.

Hardy-Weinberg's law states that gene frequencies do not appreciably change from one generation to another in a well-equilibrated system, at least for autosomal chromosomes. Some consanguinous subjects do have, to some degree, identical genes at a given locus. Thus, in a consanguinous population, the incidence of homozygotes increases. Another case of loss of balance represents genetic drift associated with loss of certain genes. Hardy-Weinberg's law implies that selection and mutation do not occur.

## ENZYMES AND ANTIGENS

Certain blood group antigens, such as those of the Rh system, are proteins and are direct gene products manufactured by erythroblasts. On the other hand, other blood group antigens possess a glycolipid or glycoprotein structure. In these cases, the antigenic specificity is carried by the carbohydrate fraction. Such is the situation for the antigens of the ABO, Hh, and Lewis systems (although the latter originate in the plasma and are secondarily absorbed onto the red cell surface); therefore, it can be seen that these specificities, whose gene-product character has, however, been perfectly demonstrated, are not primary products of the ABO, H, or Lewis genes, but must logically result from the specific transport activity of specialized enzymes, the glycosyl transferases.

All the current analyses show that this concept is the correct one; it has resulted in the successful identification of each enzyme predicted on the basis of the genomes of all individuals in the ABO, Hh, and Lewis systems. Thus, the biosynthesis of the ABH and Lewis blood group substances is now clearly understood. The genes of the A or B, H, and Lewis blood groups produce enzymes that, one after the other, build carbohydrate chains on a protein or lipid base, thus constituting the membrane glycoproteins and glycolipids of the corresponding blood groups.

# III.  IMMUNOLOGIC BASES

## ANTIGENS

Blood groups provide good examples for clinical and experimental definitions of general immunologic principles applicable to the understanding of human immunogenetics. The concepts of xeno-, allo-, and autoantigens approached in chapter 6 (p. 133) will now be presented in relation to blood groups.

### Xenoantigens

Some human blood group antigens, such as ABO, are widely distributed in nature, especially in bacteria (including intestinal saprophytes), plants, and animals. These antigens are known as xenoantigens. The peculiar environment of these various species probably explains the origin of unrecognized immunization responsible for "natural" antibody production. Furthermore, antigens present on the human red blood cell surface, although less prevalent, are not peculiar to erythrocytes or to humans. For example, red blood cells of certain pigs possess AP antigen, which is also present on human erythrocytes of the $A_1$ group. Similarly, rabbit, guinea pig, and opossum erythrocytes contain an antigen common to human red blood cells of the B group. The Forssman antigen, present on $A_1$ and $A_2$ human red cells, or sheep erythrocytes and guinea pig kidney cells, represents another example of a "ubiquitous" antigen. It is not present on ox erythrocytes, hence the clinical application of the Paul-Bunnell-Davidsohn's reaction.

### Alloantigens

Alloantigens, which represent various cell or plasma groups, reflect genetic variation within one given species. The antigens of interest to immunogenetics are products of nucleated cell genes (i.e., erythroblast for blood groups, mucous cells for secretion groups, lymphocytes or megakaryocytes for tissue groups, and lymphocytes for immunoglobulin groups). These cells synthesize antigens directly, if they are proteins, or by means of enzymes, for carbohydrate antigens, such as ABO blood groups. In some cases, it is impossible to identify directly the antigen and to demonstrate experimentally the corresponding antibody production. Here, we must be satisfied with considering as an antigen any substance to which an antibody binds. The antibody is then called "natural" (anti-A and -B, anti-Lewis, anti-Gm, anti-Inv).

Alloantigens, of which an ever-increasing number is being identified, are grouped together according to classic genetic analysis into marker systems, the best known of which are various blood, tissue, and immunoglobulin groups. Any new antigen must be examined by segregation analysis and compared to those already identified. Genetic independence is one of the bases for definition of group systems. An immunologic relationship between two antigens does not mean however, that the antigens belong to the same system. For example, ABO and H or Rh and LW antigens are phenotypically associated, even though they are produced by independent genetic units.

Some antigens are not included in well-defined groups because they have been recognized in only very few individuals. Although genetic transmission may yet be proven, genetic studies have not determined whether these antigens belong to already recognized systems or to new systems. For this reason, they are called "private" antigens. In addition, some antigens may be rare, or even absent, in certain races and are present at higher frequency in other races. Thus, Diego antigen is limited to the yellow race and Sutter antigen to blacks.

The immunogenic potency of the various human alloantigens is quantifiable. In humans, cell membrane antigens (HLA and blood groups antigens, especially Rh and Kell) are very immunogenic, whereas immunoglobulin alloantigens are less immunogenic.

### Autoantigens

Erythrocytes that bear Hr antigens (Rh systems) or I antigens (I system) may bind autoantibodies. Examples are hemolytic anemia of the IgG type, in which anti-Hr antibodies are found, and of the IgM type, in which anti-I antibodies are present. Similarly, P antigen of the P system may be the target of IgG autoantibodies or of the biphasic hemolysin of Donath and Landsteiner. Mechanisms of production of autoantibodies remain unknown (see chap. 25 and 27).

### Antigenic Specificity and Topochemistry

Many antigens are polyspecific. Thus, a large-sized antigenic molecule may have several specific sites. The term "partial antigen" refers to one of the molecular sites; the term "site," or "factor," has the same meaning. Blood groups provide numerous examples of partial antigens. $A_1$ antigen possesses several specific sites, including $A_1$, A, Ap, and Forssman. The "standard" Rh antigen is actually an antigenic mosaic.

Two closely reactive sites, both of which react with the specific antibody, may associate in space to create a new structure ("compound antigen"), which may then be recognized by a third antibody. The $Le^a$ and H structures, both of which are the target of a specific antibody (anti-$Le^a$ and anti-H), show a new combined spatial specificity that is recognized by another antibody (anti-$Le^b$). This specificity is a purely immunologic concept, because there is no $Le^b$ gene. Both Le and H genes, produce enzymes that transfer their own specific sugar, namely, fucose; the two fucoses create a new "immunogenetic" conformation in a broad sense of the term. There are, however, compound antigens that result from genetic associations, such as the Ce and ce antigens of the Rh system, which are only produced when both contiguous sites of genetic activity are in *cis* and not in the *trans* position. In other words, in some human sera, there may be an antibody that recognizes a complex antigenic structure that appears as the product of two contiguous genes. These two genes must belong to the same cistron, because subunits do not complement in the *trans* position.

We will see later (chap. 22) that the structure of erythrocytic surface antigens involves relatively complicated topochemical relationships. Many structures of the erythrocytic membrane show an analogy to the $Le^b$ antigen described above. These mixed antigens that result from structural associations of materials produced by independent genetic units are the cause of cross-reactions. Thus, erythrocytic membrane topochemistry poses a problem similar to that seen in salmonella polyosidic structures.

### Other Antigen Forms

#### HIDDEN ANTIGENS

Neuraminidase removes sialic acid from red blood cell membranes to uncover the T antigen, which is recognized by an antibody present in most human sera. Other examples of hidden antigens will be examined in chapter 22 (Rhesus system).

#### ADSORBED ANTIGENS

Some antigens are not synthesized by the cell that bears them but are, instead, adsorbed onto the cell surface in vivo by an incompletely understood mechanism. Such is the case of the Lewis antigen of human erythrocytes, which therefore reflects genetic properties of cells not yet identified.

#### FALSE ANTIGENS

From a genetic viewpoint, acquired B antigens are false antigens. During certain bacterial infections that occur in $A_1$ subjects, a B antigenicity appears on their erythrocytes. This phenomenon is, in fact, a somatic modification that relates to the action of a bacterial enzyme. Transformation of $A_1$- to B-reactive red blood cells (which appear as the phenocopy of $A_1B$ erythrocytes) can be produced in vitro. Bacteria able to induce this transformation synthesize a deacetylase that severs the $N$-acetyl radical of $N$-acetylgalactosamine to create galactosamine. The modified $A_1$ structure is very similar to the B structure.

#### PATHOLOGIC MODIFICATIONS

Pathologic alterations that occur in erythrocytic membrane antigens during some myeloproliferative diseases raise special and complicated issues. These alterations do not seem to be merely surface phenomena but, rather, represent an immunogenetic abnormality that directly involves gene function. The primary gene product, specific transferase, is abnormal, indicating that the molecular lesion is present at this early stage.

## ANTIBODIES

Antibodies to blood group antigens are most often alloantibodies; they may also be heteroantibodies or even autoantibodies. Some appear spontaneously, for example, anti-A, anti-B, or anti-Le$^a$ antibodies, and are therefore called "natural antibodies." Others, however, are classically "immune." Examples of the latter include anti-Rh and anti-Kell antibodies. Some blood group antibodies are IgM, whereas others are IgG or even IgA.

### Natural Antibodies

These antibodies seem to exist even before stimulation. When they consistently occur in all subjects without the presence of the specific antigen, they are called *regular natural antibodies*. The best examples are anti-A and anti-B allohemagglutinins. Conversely, they may occasionally be present in some subjects who do not possess the specific antigen; they are then termed *irregular natural antibodies*. An example is the anti-Le$^a$ antibody, which is present in some Le(a−) subjects.

REGULAR NATURAL ANTIBODIES

Mechanisms responsible for production of natural antibodies have already been discussed (p. 333). The appearance of natural anti-A or anti-B IgM antibodies in man may represent "hidden" stimulation, either bacterial or viral, because ABH group substances are omnipresent in the environment. In the chicken, anti-B antibody formation is linked to selected colibacilli; chicken bred in a germ-free environment develop few of these antibodies, whereas chicken infected by *Escherichia coli* O$^{86}$ show precocious generation of large amounts of antibody. Springer and Horton have shown in man that the introduction of *E. coli* O$^{86}$ (through the digestive tract or by inhalation) may induce production of anti-B allohemagglutinins in certain newborns.

One should recall, however, that the clonal theory supposes the existence of natural antibodies. In this respect, it is of considerable interest that rare subjects (of Bombay phenotype) who have no ABO or Hh blood group antigens (e.g., A, B, and H), not only produce anti-A and anti-B, but also anti-H antibodies. It looks as if the clones capable of producing anti-H antibodies had proliferated because they had not met the specific antigen. Thermodynamic study of anti-A and anti-B allohemagglutinins in man (by Wurmser et al.) indicates that the structure of antibodies that have the same specificity differs according to endogenous (native) blood group. Thus, anti-B antibody from an O subject possesses a structure different from that from an A subject. Natural antibodies are, like all other proteins, under genetic control. Thus, there is no contradiction between their genetic determinism and a contributary role of the environment, which may considerably increase their production. A final argument that militates against an exclusive role of the environment in antibody production is that anti-A$_1$ antibodies are present in A$_2$B group subjects, all of whom are exposed to similar environment. Other regular natural antibodies are seen in man. For example, subjects without P$_1$ or P antigens, nonetheless, produce an anti-P + P$_1$ + P$^k$ (anti-Tj$^a$) antibody. Recall also that Rh-null subjects possess an apparently natural anti-Rh$^{29}$ antibody.

IRREGULAR NATURAL ANTIBODIES

There are irregular natural antibodies in the Lewis system; anti-Le$^a$, anti-Le$^x$, and anti-Le$^b$ are present in subjects with the Le(a−b−) phenotype. The most common (highest incidence) antibody is P$_1$ present in P$_2$ subjects. Rare natural alloantibodies that correspond to antigens with very low frequency are seen in acquired hemolytic anemia or rheumatoid arthritis. A genetic basis for formation of irregular natural antibodies has been suggested by studies of certain families; however, the causes of their highly variable level are only poorly understood. Increased age, racial factors, presence of certain diseases (e.g., hepatic cirrhosis), and pregnancy seem to influence the formation of irregular natural antibodies.

### Immune Antibodies

Immune antibodies appear only after stimulation. Numerous blood group antibodies are immune. They appear after antigen introduction during transfusion or pregnancy (e.g., anti-Rh, anti-Kell), vaccination or injection of various substances (immune anti-A). Antibodies to leukocytic or platelet antigens appear more often than do antibodies directed against erythrocytic antigens. Among them, anti-Rh and anti-Kell antibodies are the easiest to produce. Some subjects show an enhanced capability of immunization against certain alloantigens by producing antileukocytic and antierythrocytic antibodies. Some of the factors controlling this predisposition are now known; production of alloantibodies is higher in females and during certain diseases, for example, hepatic cirrhosis.

### Autoantibodies

Blood group autoantibodies are generally undifferentiated structures of high frequency such as Hr, I, Sp$^1$, or P. For IgG autoantibodies, IgGl or IgG3 sensitizes the red blood cells that are recognized and phagocytosed by splenic reticuloendothelial cells after opsonization. For IgM autoantibodies, complement is adsorbed to the red blood cell surface, which is, in turn, phagocytosed by several tissues, especially Kupffer hepatic cells. Only rarely do autoantibodies directly cause intravascular hemolysis.

## ANTIGEN-ANTIBODY REACTIONS

### Reversibility and Equilibrium State

Reactions of antibody with group-specific antigens are controlled by the same rules described previously (chap. 9) for other antigen-antibody reactions. Because antigens are often cell borne, the techniques usually employed in hapten-antihapten systems (e.g., equilibrium dialysis) could not be utilized to study these reactions. Other methods have been developed and have provided considerable and important knowledge about the physicochemical characteristics of this reaction.

The antigen-antibody reaction is reversible. If Rh-positive A-group erythrocytes sensitized by standard anti-Rh antibody are incubated with nonsensitized Rh-positive B-group erythrocytes, and then separated by anti-A and anti-B sera, the antiglobulin reaction occurs in both A and B red blood cell populations. It appears, therefore, that anti-Rh antibody passes from one (A) to another (B) type of red blood cell. As with other antigen-antibody reaction types, links are not covalent but include weak intermolecular bonds (hydrogen bond type, ionic attraction, and Van der Waals forces), which are very efficient at short distances. Specificity of immunologic reactions is thus based on a high degree of complementary antigen and antibody reactive sites.

The antigen-antibody reaction is a reversible equilibrium phenomenon subjected to the general mass action law. The blood group antibody and its antigen are bound together in dynamic equilibrium, with a similar number of formed and disrupted linkages. Such an equilibrium is defined by the association constant ($K_a$) of the system. As in hapten-antihapten/antibody reactions, association constants and Scatchard's or Sips' (see p. 288) equations can be used.

An example of this quantitation is the protocol used by Hughes Jones to measure the equilibrium constant of the anti-D-D antigen combination. Variable amounts of erythrocytes are added to a single anti-D antibody dilution. When equilibrium is reached, the amount of antibodies bound to erythrocytes is measured by use of an $^{125}$I-labeled antiglobulin. Results are then expressed graphically, and the Sip's equation is used to determine the equilibrium constant.

Scatchard's and Sips' formulations permit measurement of immunoglobulin valence, the serum antibody concentration, and the number of antigenic sites on the erythrocytic surface. The number of antigenic sites ranges from 500,000 to 1,000,000 for normal A and B erythrocytes. Much lower numbers of Rh sites, from 5000 to 30,000, are seen for some phenotypes. For Kell antigen, the number of sites ranges from 2000 to 5000; for Lewis antigen (Le$^a$), 4000–8000 sites is the usual range. Variations in site numbers may depend on whether the subject is homozygous or heterozygous but this notion is not a general one, particularly for the ABO system. Measurement of numbers of antigenic sites of poorly agglutinable A erythrocytes (weak A phenotypes) has shown a distinct relationship between agglutinability and antigenic site number; in certain phenotypes, genetically transmitted erythrocytic heterogeneity has been observed by Cartron. The latter, rather unexpected, finding has not yet been explained.

### Thermodynamic Approach

The study of equilibrium constants as a function of temperature permits determination of the change, or variation, in free energy, $\Delta F^\circ$, and in enthalpy, $\Delta H$, (heat of reaction). This information has important applications to the study of blood groups.

A strongly positive enthalpy variation indicates a very exothermic reaction. More simply expressed, the mole to mole combination of an antibody to its antigen releases a large quantity of heat. In this case, binding of antibody to antigen is maximal at very low temperatures (i.e., 4°C) and is much weaker at 25°C and often null at 37°C. This property defines cold agglutinins. As an example, combination of anti-I antibody to its antigen releases 30,000–40,000 cal/mol. Natural allohemagglutinins of the ABO system are exothermic. They give —$\Delta H$ values that range from 2000 cal/mol for anti-B antibodies of O subjects to 20,000 cal/mol for anti-A antibodies of B subjects. Conversely, anti-Rh antibodies (practically always IgG) give a rather low-heat reaction and therefore are known as "warm" antibodies. In this case, agglutination is best obtained at 37°C.

### WURMSER'S METHOD

The thermodynamic study of combination of allohemagglutinins to their antigens was introduced to immunogenetics by René Wurmser and colleagues. Antibody concentration is measured by an original technique that is more precise than previous classic methods (double dilution titration); the technique involves counting maximal numbers of red blood cells that agglutinate in serum at 4°C ($N_4$). Under standard conditions, the number is proportional to antibody concentration. This method may be used to characterize an antibody if the same antigen is always used (Filitti-Wurmser) or to characterize an antigen when the same serum (Salmon) is always employed.

*Antibody Study.* Wurmser has been able to differentiate antibodies from $A_1$, $A_2$, and O subjects on the basis of the relationship between the blood group of the subject and the physicochemical properties of the antibodies produced. This relationship has led to the hypothesis that the nature of the antigen present on the erythrocytic membrane surface influences the structure and class of the allohemagglutinin.

*Antigen Study.* One may use a single antibody to study the reactivity of several types of antigen. Different thermodynamic properties may thus be demonstrated for antigen-antibody reactions involving anti-B antibodies between different families, whereas antigens in the same family give identical values. This finding indicates that a genetic variation in the ABO locus represents a familial mutant.

Wurmser's methods have thus significantly added to our understanding of blood group antigens. These methods are, nonetheless, limited from a physicochemical point of view: (1) The methods explore a narrow range of antigen concentrations at equilibrium in contrast with isotopic techniques that permit exploration of wider zones. (2) The method has been applied as yet to total sera, not to purified antibodies. The results observed may thus relate to variable concentrations of IgG, and IgM anti-B antibodies in serum. On the other hand, the use of minimally diluted serum in the presence of high antigen concentrations does not favor selection of higher affinity antibodies, which is often the case when purified antibodies are utilized.

### RADIOIMMUNOLOGIC METHODS

Isotopic methods of studying the binding of labeled purified antibodies to erythrocytes have permitted important progress in allowing measurement of equilibrium constants. These methods offer the possibility of exploring a much wider range of relative antibody and antigen concentrations. However, because they are hyperimmune, these antibodies are often more heterogeneous than are natural antibodies. Cartron's studies of weak A antigens illustrate the interest of such methods. The same anti-A IgG antibody preparation labeled with $^{125}I$ has been studied in the presence of various types of normal A cells of weak phenotype $A_3$, Ax, Aend, Am, and Ael. At variance with what has been observed for the B variation by use of Wurmser's method, no single heat-reactive group has been identified: all measurements varied between $-5$ and $-12$ kcal/mol.

Finally, thermodynamic analysis of blood group variants has not yet been completed. Wurmser's method permits only differentiation of products of various familial mutants. The radioimmunologic method employs antibodies of more heterogeneous affinity and rather analyzes common structures. One should await with interest the result of the studies now in progress concerning respective roles of IgM and IgG molecules according to Wurmser's methodology.

### Agglutination Reaction Applied to Blood Groups

Specificity and reversibility, which are the major characteristics of antigen-antibody reactions, also apply to immunohematologic techniques. However, most immunohematologic reactions are not concerned with the antigen-antibody reaction itself but, rather, with its nonspecific secondary manifestations, such as agglutination. Reversibility permits verification at any time that the phenomenon is one of antibody fixation. Dissociation of the complex may be obtained by heating at 56°C, by modifying pH (usually by acidification), by adding alkaline metal chlorides or ethylenediamine tetra-acetate, or by more drastic means, in the case of cell membrane or stroma, such as ether or alcohol treatment. Highly exothermic IgM generally elute better by heating, whereas IgG and anti-Rh elute better by use of ether or acidification.

When red blood cells are suspended in saline, they remain dissociated but, under certain conditions, may adhere to each other to form aggregates, which defines agglutination. Agglutination may follow fixation of an antibody to a specific antigen, but it is also possible to obtain agglutination independently of the antibody, by use of certain metallic ions, such as trivalent chromium, tannic acid, or colloidal silica, or even by use of simple changes in physicochemical characteristics of the medium or red blood cell surface. Antibody binding to the red blood cell surface is therefore only one of the possible causes of physicochemical changes that leads to loss of red blood cell stability in suspension. An antibody is agglutinating when it is capable of producing erythrocytic agglutination in 0.9% saline. Conversely, an antibody is nonagglutinating when its binding to erythrocytic surfaces is not sufficient to agglutinate erythrocytes in 0.9% saline suspension, even though it is possible to show (by elution) that the binding has occurred and even when "artifical agglutination" is obtained by various other means.

Agglutination depends on several factors, particularly the nature of the red blood cell surface, the type of antibody, and the medium characteristics.

#### AGGLUTINATION FACTORS

*Erythrocytic Surface.*   The most important factor is undoubtedly the number of specific receptor sites. Agglutination requires a minimal number of antigenic sites per red blood cell (see p. 606). Thus, standard Rh antibodies do not normally agglutinate normal Rh erythrocytes but do agglutinate $D^{--}$ red blood cells that contain a very high number of D receptor sites. In fact, agglutination may occur when a very small number of antigenic sites combines with antibodies. For example, at 4°C, as few as five anti-I antibody molecules per red blood cell surface induce agglutination.

The localization of the sites on the surface or deep within the erythrocyte are also of fundamental importance. As we have discussed, T antigen is accessible only to antibodies after neuraminidase treatment. More generally, membrane integrity is a very important factor. Red blood cells whose surface is altered (made rigid) by osmic acid or formol or red blood cells from patients with sickle cell anemia are not agglutinable, even though they have retained a good capacity of antibody binding. Conversely, in some phenotypes, in which amounts of sialic acid on the erythrocytic surface are considerably diminished, red blood cells can be agglutinated by certain normally nonagglutinating antibodies because of the diminished electric charge.

*Antibody.* Most agglutinating antibodies are IgM, whereas the majority of nonagglutinating antibodies are IgG. This distinction is explained by the smaller number of IgM molecules required on the red blood cell surface to induce agglutination. Thus, in the A-anti-A system, 25 molecules of IgM anti-A antibody on the red blood cell surface are sufficient for agglutination, whereas 20,000 molecules of the IgG class are required. Such a small number of IgM molecules does not seem very compatible with the hypothesis according to which agglutination is ascribed to formation of intercellular bridges. It is, in fact, possible for one IgM molecule to bind to two adjacent sites on the red blood cell surface. This possibility depends on the density of antigenic receptor sites and on the homogeneity of distribution. If, as a theoretical example, the sites are distributed uniformly (homogeneously), the mean distance between two Rh sites is of 70–75 nm (for an erythrocytic surface area of 163 $\mu m^2$, with a total density of 20,000–30,000 Rh sites per red blood cell). This distance exceeds the average IgM diameter (35 nm). These theoretical calculations favor the concept of a nonhomogeneous distribution of reactive sites, especially in relation to binding of five IgM subunits to the same red blood cell.

*Medium.* The agglutinability of an erythrocyte suspension depends on the dielectric constant and ionic strength of the medium, pH, and temperature. The role of temperature is multifaceted. Antibodies generally bind better at low temperatures because of the inherent exothermicity of immunologic reactions (described above). However, the speed of agglutination depends on antibody nature: IgG agglutinates more rapidly at 37°C, while the reaction for IgM is more rapid at 4°C.

PHYSICOCHEMICAL MECHANISMS OF AGGLUTINATION: ZETA POTENTIAL

Agglutination used to be explained by the lattice theory, discussed earlier (p. 307) with respect to immunoprecipitation. It is now believed that agglutination results from physicochemical phenomena that follow antibody binding to red blood cells. A stable erythrocyte suspension is subjected to two types of forces: repulsion forces secondary to red blood cell electrostatic charges and cohesion forces that relate to interfacial tensions between erythrocytes. Agglutination does not occur if red blood cells are not close enough to one another. Even in the lattice hypothesis, which concerns intercellular bridge formation, red blood cells sensitized by an IgG-type antibody must be close enough together (20–25 nm) for formation of intercellular bridges to occur.

In an electrolytic solution, erythrocytes are surrounded by a cloud of ions of opposed charges; their density decreases with distance from the erythrocyte, thus creating a potential difference between the cloud of cations (surrounding red blood cells) and the environment. This zeta potential can be measured by the electrophoretic migration speed of the red blood cell. The repulsion force between two red blood cells depends on the value of the zeta potential, below which the suspension remains stable and above which it becomes unstable. Artificial agglutination methods either decrease the zeta potential of red blood cells prior to the addition of nonagglutinating antibodies or increase the critical zeta potential at the time of sensitization. The zeta potential of a saline suspension of erythrocytes is $-16$ mV; sensitization by antibodies of red blood cells alters this potential. Nonsensitized red blood cells in saline suspension (0.15 M) agglutinate spontaneously when the zeta potential is less than $-7$ mV. Sensitized red blood cells agglutinate if the zeta potential is lower than $-18$ mV ($-18$ to $-23$ mV), when IgM antibodies are used, and when the zeta potential is about $-10$ mV ($-8$ to $-10$ mV) for IgG. In light of the normal value of the zeta potential, one may explain why IgM spontaneously agglutinates, whereas IgG does not agglutinate without a prior decrease in the zeta potential. According to Pollack, the zeta value ($\zeta$) relates to the red blood cell's electric charge ($\sigma$), the dielectric constant of the medium ($D$), and to the ionic strength of the medium ($\mu$), with the following relationship:

$$\zeta = f\left(\sigma, \frac{1}{D}, \frac{1}{\sqrt{\mu}}\right).$$

Thus, the zeta potential decreases when the surface electrostatic charge decreases, when the dielectric constant of the medium increases or when the ionic strength, that is, salt concentration, is increased. These three modifications are employed in artificial agglutination studies by addition of enzymes or macromolecules to the medium to increase the dielectric constant.

## IV.  APPLICATION OF BLOOD GROUPS AND POLYMORPHISM TO HUMAN GENETICS

The use of polymorphism markers in man has made possible an extremely precise definition of genetic individuality. About 30 systems are now available to define the individual biologically. Independent genetic markers that express the polymorphism of the human species have also been found in systems other than blood groups. Similar genetic systems are, in fact, present not only in red blood cells but also in other cells.

Within the erythrocyte, various enzyme groups are known: acid phosphatase, phosphoglucomutase, adenylate kinase, 6-phosphoglucose deaminase, glucose 6-phosphate dehydrogenase, adenosine deaminase, and hemoglobin itself expresses an individual variation.

In other blood cells, one must mention leukocyte and platelet groups and, in particular, the HLA system, with its high degree of polymorphism (numerous alleles are identified in the same locus).

In certain tissues, such as the digestive tract (especially salivary glands), Sese and Lewis systems have been demonstrated.

A considerable number of genetic systems exists for serum proteins: haptoglobins, lipoproteins, Gc proteins ($\alpha_2$-macroglobulin), immunoglobulins, which include four systems (Gm, Inv, ISf, Am), and the third component of complement (C3).

Thus, a detailed genetic formulation may be obtained for an individual; an example that utilizes 29 marker systems follows:

Blood groups: B  M  SS  $P_1$  ccddee  K−k+  Kp(a−b+)  Fy(a+b−)  Jk(a−b+)
     Lu(a−b+)  Do(a+)  Xg(a+)  Yt(a+b−)  Au(a−)
Secretion groups: Sec BH, sec $Le^a$ $Le^b$
Erythrocytic enzyme groups: PAc B AK 2.1 $PGM_1$ 1.1 $PGM_2$ 1.1 ADA 1.1 6PGD
       1.1 SGPT 2.1 Est D 1.1
Leukocyte groups: HLA-A9A28-B5B8-DW2-DR2
Serum groups: Gm(—1,—2,4,5,10,14) Inv(—1) Hp 2.2 Gc 2.1 C3 2.1

Such an approach may be used with reliability in problems of parentage and identity, for the more diversified and balanced the genetic polymorphism is, the more efficient the system.

## PATERNITY EXCLUSION

This application, often required legally, has become extremely accurate since one can use several polymorphic systems including ABO, Rh, MNS, Gm, and HLA. At present, the probability of excluding the paternity of a given child approximates 99%. Furthermore, a single irregular paternity that occurs within a family group cannot escape notice anymore if a sufficient number of marker systems is employed. The paternity exclusion will appear in one or the other system, and generally in several of them.

## TWIN BLOOD GROUPS

A major application of blood groups in identity problems is the analysis of genetic characters in twins. It is most often possible to recognize dizygous twins and, in other cases, to calculate the probability of monozygosity. Two recent remarkable discoveries in this context are respresented by chimerism in dizygous twins and heterokaryotic monozygotes.

### Diagnosis of Dizygotism and Chimeras

Recognition that twins are dizygous follows the discovery of differences in their phenotype. However, dizygous twins that include a boy and a girl, for example, may present the juxtaposition of both blood cell populations, probably due to exchange of blood cells during fetal life analogous to some twin pregnancies in cattle (see p. 586). Chorionic anastomoses permit exchange between twins of stem cells that will form the blood tissue. The cells are tolerated in the same way as are grafts in embryos. The genotype of the recipient twin may be deduced from specificities of saliva substances. An example is a brother genetically A who received an O graft. His sister was genetically O and received an A graft. It is interesting to note that she did not produce anti-A antibodies, despite prior contact with the A antigen, because of embryonic tolerance.

### Heterokaryotic Monozygotism

When the phenotype and genotype of mother and father are known, it is possible to establish the probability of twins having the same phenotypes if they are dizygotes. Conversely, apparently identical monozygous twins may not have the same karyotype: one is XO and the other is XX. These twins differ only by karyotype; the first has Turner's syndrome. The genetic analysis shows with certainty that the abnormality occurred after fertilization. This example depicts heterokaryotic monozygotism now known to have occurred in several dozen families worldwide. Systemic examination of karyotypes in various body tissues has shown that heterokaryotic monozygous couples are, indeed, mosaics. It is therefore likely that exchanges between twins, which occur rarely in dizygotism (then to be expressed by a chimera), are probably common in monozygotism.

## DOUBLE FERTILIZATION

Precise analysis of phenotypes lead to the even more striking discovery of mosaicism in nontwins. Analysis of both parent's contribution shows that the father provides different contributions to each of two cell populations. The observed mosaic results either from double fertilization, or of spermatocytic fertilization, or of fusion of the two zygotes. Thus, for each of these three hypotheses a new and unexpected phenomenon is demonstrated by means of precise phenotypic analysis.

## BLOOD GROUPS AND ABNORMALITIES IN SEX CHROMOSOMES

The discovery (in 1961) of a blood group system localized on the X chromosome opened up new possibilities for analysis of aneuploidies of sex chromosomes in the human species, achieved through study of the gene frequency in populations and by analysis of genetic transmission of the Xg(a) character. Generally speaking, immunogenetics has added considerable knowledge to our understanding of human chromosome mapping, especially for the Duffy and Rhesus systems, localized on the first autosome, and Xg system on the X chromosome.

## *BIBLIOGRAPHY*

Race R. R. and Sanger R. Blood groups in man, ed. 6. Oxford, 1975, Blackwell.

Rochna E. and Hugues-Jones N. C. The use of purified [125]I-labelled antiglobulin in the determination of the number of D antigen sites on red cells of different phenotypes. Vox Sang., Basel, 1965, *10*, 675.

WURMSER R. and FILITTI-WURMSER S. Thermodynamic study of the isohaemagglutinins. Progr. Biophys., 1957, *7*, 88.


## ORIGINAL ARTICLES

BODMER N. F. Evolutionary significance of the HL-A system. Nature (London), 1972, *237*, 139.

CARTRON J. P., GERBAL A., HUGHES-JONES N. C., and SALMON Ch. Weak A phenotypes: relationship between red cell agglutinability and antigen site density. Immunology, 1974, *27*, 723.

DAUSSET J. Iso-leuco-anticorps. Acta Haemat. (Basel), 1958, *20*, 156.

GRUBB R. Agglutination of erythrocytes coated with incomplete anti-Rh by certain rheumatoid arthritis sera and some other sera. The existence of human serum groups. Acta Path. Microbiol. Scand., 1956, *39*, 290.

HUGUES-JONES N. C. GARDNER B., and LINCOLN P. J. Observations of the number of available c, D and E antigen sites on red cells. Vox Sang. (Basel), 1971, *21*, 210.

LANDSTEINER K. and WIENER A. S. An agglutinable factor in human blood recognized by immune sera for rhesus blood. Proc. Soc. Exp. Biol. (N.Y.), 1940, *43*, 223.

LOPEZ M., BOUGUERRA A., LEMEUD J., BADET J., and SALMON C. Quantitative kinetics and thermodynamic analysis of weak $B_{60}$ erythrocyte phenotypes. Vox Sang. (Basel), 1974, *27*, 243.

## Chapter 22

# BLOOD GROUPS

**Charles Salmon**

I.   INTRODUCTION
II.  THE ABO AND ASSOCIATED SYSTEMS
III. RH SYSTEM
IV.  OTHER BLOOD GROUP SYSTEMS
V.   SERUM PROTEIN GROUPS
VI.  APPENDIX: ERYTHROCYTE GROUPING

## I.  INTRODUCTION

Blood group substances are produced in the erythroblast, which is a nucleated cell, and are detected on the surface of the mature erythrocytic membrane. They are genetically induced and independent membrane alloantigens.

They are genetic products that express gene activity either directly or through an enzyme intermediate, such as ABO-group glycosyl transferases. These products differ between subjects and are categorized into group systems that correspond to different genetic units.

The genetic units are transmitted independently of each other during meiosis, in conformity with Mendel's second law. Two given genetic units are located on different chromosomes or are separated very far from each other on the same chromosome.

These substances are antigens and are thus immunogenic, that is, capable of stimulating antibody formation. This property is the basis for interhuman alloimmunization following pregnancy or transfusion.

## II.  THE ABO AND ASSOCIATED SYSTEMS

Two main cell lines produce ABO substances: the erythroblast, in which synthesis of erythrocytic blood group antigens occurs, and mucous cells of the

**Table 22.1   Discovery of the Main Blood Groups**

| ABO | 1900 | Lewis | 1946 |
|---|---|---|---|
| MN | 1927 | Duffy | 1950 |
| R | 1927 | Kidd | 1951 |
| Rh | 1939 | Yt | 1956 |
| Lutheran | 1945 | Xg | 1962 |
| Kell | 1946 | | |

digestive tract, which, in 80% of humans, the so-called secretors, are the site of synthesis of an ABH-group substance in hydrosoluble form. A and B antigens are the end product of a long series of metabolic transformations in which several independent genetic systems collaborate. These systems are not necessarily identical in a given subject's erythroblasts and salivary cells.

There are three antigen systems in the erythroblast and two others in the mucous cell, which show numerous interactions. The three erythroblast systems are the classic Landsteiner *ABO system*, which controls the presence of A and B antigens on the erythrocyte, the *Hh system*, distinct from the ABO system, which was discovered after recognition of the Bombay phenotype, which determines the presence of the H substance (the H substance of O-group erythrocytes is an acceptor necessary for elaboration of A or B specificities; it is produced by the Hh system, not the ABO system), and the recently discovered I *antigen*. The role of the latter is discussed here because of the existence of complex HI, AI, and BI antigens. I specificity is probably in part an acceptor of H, A, and B substances.

The two systems unique to mucous cells are the *ABH secretion system*, Sese, which controls the presence of A, B, or H antigen in saliva (the Se gene appears to be a regulator of H-gene activity), and the *Lewis system*, which controls the presence of Le$^a$ substance in saliva (according to present theories, Lewis antigens on erythrocytic surfaces are not produced by erythroblasts but come from the plasma and secondarily adhere to erythrocytes).

## ERYTHROBLASTS

### *ABO System*

#### A AND B ANTIGENS AND ANTI-A AND ANTI-B ANTIBODIES OF ABO BLOOD GROUPS

In 1900, Landsteiner discovered that the serum of certain subjects agglutinated red blood cells from other subjects. He thus identified two antigens, A and B, and labeled "O" any erythrocytes not agglutinated by either of these antibodies. Subjects whose erythrocytes bear the A antigen have an anti-B agglutinin in their serum. Conversely, subjects with B antigen-bearing erythrocytes possess serum anti-A agglutinin. Subjects whose erythrocytes have no A or B antigen possess anti-A and anti-B agglutinins in their serum (Table 22.2). Two years later, a fourth group was discovered, subjects whose erythrocytes contained both A and B antigens and whose serum contained no anti-A and anti-B agglutinin. The scheme of "natural" anti-A and anti-B human

**Table 22.2   Four Classic ABO Groups**

|           | Antigen           | Antibody          | Frequency in caucasians (%) |
|-----------|-------------------|-------------------|------------------------------|
| A group   | A                 | Anti-B            | 45                           |
| B group   | B                 | Anti-A            | 9                            |
| AB group  | A and B           | None              | 3                            |
| O group   | Neither A nor B   | Anti-A and Anti-B | 43                           |

agglutinins was thus already perfectly clear; by convention, the four classic blood groups are defined in terms of erythrocytic antigen(s): A, B, AB, and O. In fact, the O group is recognized by negative reactions to anti-A and anti-B antibodies and not by direct identification of the specific antigen.

By 1910, Von Dungern and Hirzfeld demonstrated that A and B characters were genetically controlled; Bernstein showed in 1924 that transmission was Mendelian, with erythrocytic blood groups depending on the presence of two out of three A, B, or O alleles (or R according to Bernstein) on two loci of the corresponding erythroblast chromosome.

PHENOTYPE AND GENOTYPE

Serologically defined groups characterize phenotypes. The phenotype may differ from the genotype for the A and B groups. Indeed, if erythrocytes from an individual are agglutinated only by anti-A antibodies, they are said to belong to the A group, but this classification does not indicate whether the corresponding chromosome of their erythroblast nucleus contains two A genes or only one A gene associated with one O gene. Thus, the individual genotype of A phenotype may be AA or AO. Only family study permits in some cases differentiation of these two possibilities.

This distinction does not apply to AB and O groups, for which serologic study permits identification of not only the phenotype but also the genotype. In fact, both alleles are here recognized either directly (AB group) or indirectly

**Table 22.3   Frequency of ABO Groups in Various Ethnic Groups**

| Population       | Phenotype (%) |     |     |      |
|------------------|---------------|-----|-----|------|
|                  | O             | A   | B   | AB   |
| France           | 44            | 45  | 8   | 3    |
| Scotland         | 50            | 32  | 15  | 3    |
| Sweden           | 37            | 48  | 10  | 6    |
| Switzerland      | 40            | 47  | 9   | 4    |
| Pakistan         | 25            | 33  | 36  | 5    |
| India            | 32            | 29  | 28  | 11   |
| American Indians | 88            | 12  | 0   | 0    |
| Eskimos          | 54            | 43  | 1.5 | 1.5  |

After A. E. Mourant.

(O group). In the latter case, the absence of A and B antigens implies O-gene homozygosity.

Serum from B subjects contains an anti-A antibody absorbed by certain types of A ($A_2$) erythrocytes that agglutinates red blood cells of 80% of group-A subjects that are called $A_1$. Serum from B subjects, in fact, contains two distinct anti-A antibodies: anti-$A_1$ is active only against $A_1$ erythrocytes, while anti-A reacts with both $A_1$ and $A_2$ red blood cells. The same applies to serum anti-A antibodies in O subjects, in whom anti-B antibody is also present. Thus, a specific anti-$A_1$ antibody can be obtained by absorbing B subject serum onto $A_2$ red blood cells.

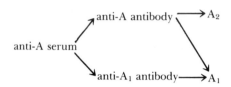

There are still other A and B group variants, the weak A and B antigens (see p. 637).

ABO blood group antigens are glycolipids. For each group, the immuno-dominant sugar that is responsible for immunologic specificity has been identified. This sugar is $N$-acetylgalactosamine for the A group and galactose for the B group. It is obvious that these blood group sugars are not primary ABO gene products. A and B gene products are, in fact, specific transferases, respectively, $N$-acetylgalactosaminyl transferase and galactosyl transferase, that transfer $N$-acetylgalactosamine or galactose to an "acceptor," the H substance. The latter substance (with fucose as the dominant sugar) is itself coded for by an H gene located in the Hh genetic unit independent of ABO genes.

## Hh System

Erythrocytes from O-group subjects, which possess neither A nor B antigen, contain an antigen related to the ABO system, the H antigen. This antigen is, in fact, the precursor of A and B antigens, in other words the basic material on which A and B gene products act. The H antigen is recognized by a specific antibody present in some $A_1$ or $A_1B$ subjects. O subjects who have neither the A nor B gene cannot transform the H precursor substance into A or B substance. Thus, all individuals, irrespective of ABO group, contain the H gene, which enables them to produce H substance. There is, however, one exception to this rule. It was discovered in Bombay, in the 1950s, that rare individuals, apparently of the O group, had no H substance on their erythrocytes and produced not only anti-A and anti-B antibodies (like the usual O individual) but also anti-H antibody. Their serum agglutinated all red blood cells, except their own. Family studies of these subjects have shown that the Bombay phenotype in the homozygous state represents a nonfunctional gene at the H locus. These subjects have normal genes of the ABO system because they are able to transmit those genes to their children. In the example shown (Fig. 22.1), the Bombay proposita transmitted to her first daughter a B gene obviously obtained from her mother. This interpretation was corroborated by demonstrating the presence of the corresponding galactosyl transferase enzyme. This enzyme has no H substrate to transform, and the B antigen is therefore not produced. Study of the Bombay phenotype is additional proof that the H substance is, indeed, the acceptor for A and B substances. It also shows that the H substrate is produced by a locus independent of ABO loci; the Bombay proposita whose family is represented in Fig. 22.1 had consanguinous parents and thus the hh genotype. At the same time, genetic analysis demonstrated that she was BO, that is, heterozygous at the ABO locus. This discordance between heterozygosity in one system and homozygosity in the other proves the genetic independence of the two systems. Indeed, in a subject homozygous for a rare gene, born of consanguinous parents, the chromosomal pair that carries the rare gene is a copy of the original chromosomal segment that originated in the common ancestor. The same reasoning demonstrated the independence of Hh and Sese loci (the latter is responsible for ABH secretion). For the sake of completeness, let us mention also that the enzyme that carries the specific fucose for the H substance is a fucosyl transferase.

### Erythroblast I Antigen

The H substrate probably overlays the I antigen, which is also produced by an ABO-independent locus. At variance with H, I specificity is, however, not absolutely necessary for A and B antigen formation because rare subjects without I antigen express H and ABO specificities. Interestingly, I reactivity of Bombay subjects and of H-deficient subjects is much greater than that of normal subjects.

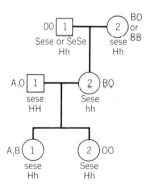

**Fig. 22.1** Family pedigree of a subject who carries the Bombay genotype. The Bombay proposita (no. 2 of the second generation) transmits the B gene to her daughter, although she is apparently of the O group.

### Other Systems

The analysis of reactive structures on the erythrocyte surface is not yet complete. Several genetic observations suggest that other systems, independent of ABO, H, and I, may also exist (Y, Z).

## MUCOUS CELLS

Mucous cells, especially those of salivary glands, are capable of extracting and then secreting in hydrosoluble form certain blood group antigens. Here again, three genetic systems are involved: Lewis (Lele), secretion (Sese), and Hh, which has already been described.

### Genetic Aspects (Fig. 22.2)

Only subjects with the Le gene produce the Lewis substance. Genetic analysis shows that this substance is a mendelian system that is independent of the systems mentioned earlier. The same is true for the Sese secretor system,

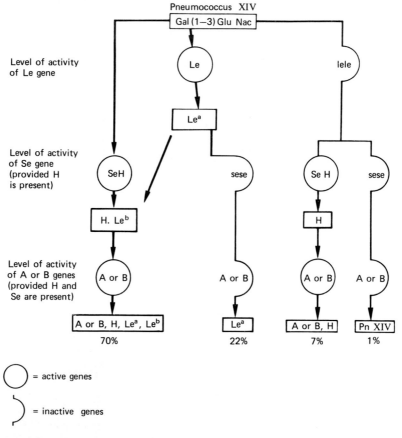

**Fig. 22.2** The synthetic pathways for Lewis, H and A, or B antigens in the four categories of salivary phenotypes.

**Table 22.4   Genes and Substances of Salivary Mucous Cells**

| Gene | Substance | | |
|------|-----------|---|---|
| Le Se | Le$^a$ | H | Le$^b$ |
| Le sese | Le$^a$ | — | |
| Lele Se | — | H | |
| Sese lele | — | — | |

whose genes control secretion of ABH substances. We have already discussed an argument that favors independence of these systems from ABO and Hh (see p. 615). The Hh system is present in salivary cells. Subjects who carry Se and H genes secrete H substance in their saliva, whereas subjects without Se gene, for example, sese homozygotes, do not secrete it. In addition, it is obvious that the newly formed H substance is immediately converted into an A or B substance by the ABO system enzymes coded for by the genes present in the genome.

The salivary secretions may appear as four different phenotypes, shown in Table 22.4. It is interesting to note that the quantity of Lewis substance is much greater in type-2 subjects than in type-1 subjects and that only type-2 subjects have the Lewis substance on their erythrocytes, because the Lewis soluble substance circulating in great quantity in the plasma may adsorb onto the red blood cell surface. As in the case of the erythroblast, new genetic systems are appearing. Thus, in some subjects, called $OH_m$, the H substance is present in the saliva but not on the erythroblast.

### Biochemical Aspects

Biochemical studies have permitted definition of the relationships among the Lewis, H, and ABO systems. Unexpectedly, group-specific substances, when purified and isolated, reveal multiple specificities. For example, A and B specificities are found on the same molecule in AB subjects. Salivary blood group-specific substances are glycoproteins that contain a central protein backbone on which oligosaccharide chains are attached laterally. Their immunologic specificty has been verified by enzymatic hydrolysis; proteolytic enzymes do not destroy immunologic specificity, whereas glucidolytic enzymes, which detach terminal sugars from lateral oligosaccharide chains, cause disappearance of specificity. It thus appears that group antigens relate to lateral chain sugars, and not to proteins, which indicates that the antigens are not primary gene products but result from activity of specific (gene-produced) enzymes.

If one adds to the soluble substance from an A-group subject (who secretes ABH and Le$^a$ substances encoded by AH, Le, and Se genes), the N-acetylgalactosaminidase enzyme (Fig. 22.3) N-acetylgalactosamine is removed and, at the same time, A specificity disappears. H specificity is then observed. Similarly, if fucosidase is added, only Lewis specificity remains. This specificity may, in turn, be removed by addition of another fucosidase, which splits fucose from C-4 in N-acetylglucosamine; a residual specificity of pneumococcus XIV now appears (due to the disaccharide galactose-N-acetylglucosamine) (Table 22.5).

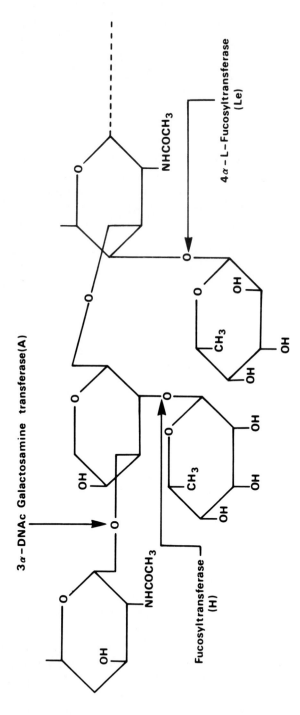

**Fig. 22.3** Biosynthesis of A, B, H, and Le specificities.

**Table 22.5   Successive Stages in the Degradation of Substance A, B, or AB by Different Glucosidases**

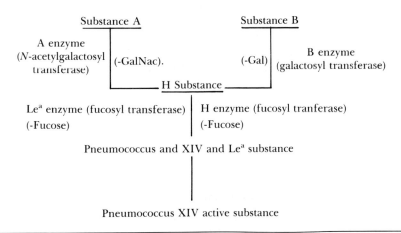

The disappearance of A and B gives rise to substance H, then Lewis substance, and then pneumococcal-XIV-type substance. The order in which these subjacent specificities appear has led to the concept that the synthesis occurs in the reverse order within the cell.

This disaccharide, present in all subjects, either in the form of 1,3-glucosamine or 1,4-glucosamine, could be called an isotype. If the order of antigen construction in living cells is the reverse of that seen in in vitro destruction of antigens, one deduces the existence of a basic galactose-glucosamine disaccharide on which a Lewis gene binds a fucose to C-4 of glucosamine; at the same time, an H gene binds another fucose to C−2 of galactose, if the Se gene is present. Finally, an A or B gene binds either an $N$-acetylgalactosamine or a galactose to the C-3 of the terminal galactose (Fig. 22.3).

This hypothesis implies that there are specific enzymes for each gene: 4α-L-fucosyl transferase for Lewis, 2α-L-fucosyl transferase for H, 3α-D-$N$-acetylgalactosaminyl transferase for A, and 3α-D-galactose transferase for B. This hypothesis has been entirely confirmed in recent years by direct demonstration of these enzymes. The principle of this demonstration is the following: $N$-acetylgalactosamine labeled with $^{14}$C is incubated with the serum in which the enzyme is being searched for. The acceptor onto which the enzyme is capable of transferring the sugar is then added. This substrate may be found in O erythrocytes or in extracts of human breast milk in the form of fucosyl-lactose. If the enzymes are present, the erythrocytes acquire A antigenicity or a radioactive tetrasaccharide is formed, depending on whether the substrate is a red blood cell or fucosyl-lactose.

Similarly, by incubating mucous gland extract from subjects with Lewis genes or, simply, serum of these subjects with the galactose-1,3-$N$-acetylglucosamine acceptor, α-L-fucose is transferred onto C-4 of glucosamine, indicating that subjects who possess the Lewis gene do have a 4α-L-fucosyl transferase that allows in vitro conversion of the base XIV substance into Le$^a$ specificity substance. It is also possible to obtain in vitro (by use of extracts or serum from

O-secretors) conversion of the base XIV disaccharide into H substance whether the disaccharide is formed by either 1,3 or 1,4 binding, which demonstrates that the H gene codes for another fucosyltransferase, a 2α-L-fucosyltransferase. When using an extract or serum from a subject with both H and Le genes, transfer of both 1,4-fucose and 1,2-fucose is obtained at least for the disaccharide substrate with 1,3 binding. Here, both H and Le[a] transformations occur.

An extract or serum from an A subject converts the H substrate into A substance; an extract or serum from a B subject transforms H substance into B substance. In the first case, the presence of 3α-D-N-acetylgalactosamine transferase is demonstrated; in the second case, 3α-D-galactose transferase is detected. Thus, one finds A enzyme in A subjects and B enzyme in B subjects, A and B enzymes in AB subjects, and no enzyme in O subjects. Nonsecreting subjects have enzymes of their ABO genes but do not contain (in their mucous cells) the fucosyl transferase that is present in their serum. Bombay subjects have no fucosyl transferase but have the enzymes that correspond to their ABO genome. Thus, the existence of a logical masterplan of synergistic functioning of independent genetic units is shown, as is a precise description of biochemical mechanisms associated with cell differentiation. Se and Le genes contribute within mucous cells to the production of these antigens within the erythroblast. For the same final product, for example, the A group, two different genetic pathways may be used by two differentiated somatic cells.

## ANTI-ABH ANTIBODIES

We have seen that in the ABO system, a given subject always possesses antibodies that correspond to the antigen(s) not present in his erythrocytes. This rule has no exception. These antibodies are consistently found in normal individuals. They are called "natural" because they seem to be present prior to any known stimulation. If a new A or B specific antigen is introduced into an organism that does not carry it, specific anti-A or -B antibodies appear, as if the antigen had determined the appearance of new molecules with an apparent identical specificty but different behavior. These antibodies, superimposed on the already present natural antibodies, are observed only after stimulation and are called "immune" antibodies.

The distinction between natural and immune antibodies is of great theoretical importance and has generated considerable thought. However, this differentiation is not absolute. Sera from subjects without any known prior stimulation may sometimes contain antibodies with some immune antibody properties, such as hemolytic ability. In addition, the determinism of the formation of the two types of antibody is not necessarily different. Detailed study of these two antibody categories is important due to their unique serologic and physicochemical differences.

### Natural Antibodies

Natural (or normal) antibodies include anti-A in B subjects, anti-B in A subjects, anti-A and anti-B in O subjects, and anti-H in the Bombay phenotype. These antibodies are always observed in subjects who lack the corresponding

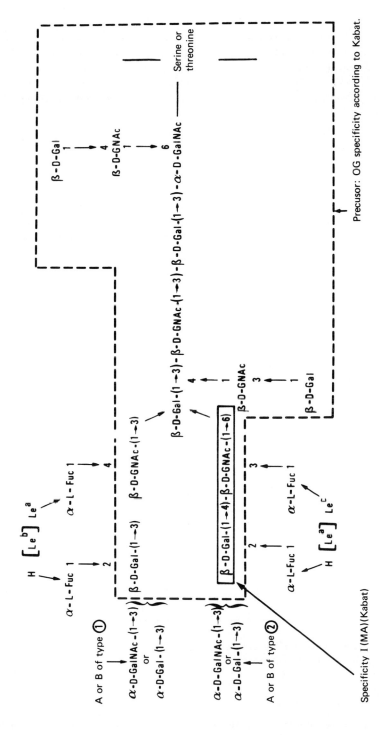

**Fig. 22.4** Structure of the carbohydrate part of the glycoproteins of A, B, H, and Lewis specificities. This figure represents the group of blood group specificities carried by a macroglycoprotein with the OG, I, H, Le[a], Le[b], H, Le[c], Le[d] specificities and the terminal specificities A or B or type 1 or 2. The A, B, H, Le[b], Le[a] specificities are classical. The Le[c] specificity (Gunson), Le[d] (Potapov), I and OG (Kabat et al.) specificities are all of recent definition.

antigen. Less commonly occurring antibodies that do not follow any known stimulation, include anti-$A_1$, anti-A of "weak A" subjects, and anti-H in some $A_1$ or $A_1B$ subjects (aside from the Bombay phenotype).

Natural anti-A and -B antibodies have some characteristics different from those of immune anti-A and -B: permanence, spontaneous agglutination, no hemolyzing ability, maximum activity at 4°C, neutralization by soluble substances, thermolability at 70°C, relatively homogeneous association constant for the homologous antigen (Wurmser). They are mostly IgM, which never cross the placenta.

### Immune Antibodies

Immune antibodies are only found after stimulation. Even if the environment is the source of unknown stimuli responsible for natural antibody formation, these antibodies (IgM class) are called "primary-response" antibodies, whereas immune antibodies (IgG class) are "secondary-response" antibodies. The role of the environment in natural and immune antibody production is well established (soluble blood group substances are found in animals and in vegetables) but is not exclusive.

Anti-A and -B immune antibodies differ from natural antibodies by the following criteria: their appearance is inconstant, they do not agglutinate spontaneously; they can hemolyze; their activity is maximal at 37°C; they are difficult to neutralize with soluble substances; they are thermostable at 70°C; their affinity for homologous antigen is very heterogeneous (Wurmser); and they are mostly IgG antibodies, which cross the placenta.

Anti-A immunization may appear under numerous and not always known circumstances:

Vaccination by diphtheria or tetanus toxoids: the toxoid antigenicity relates to the presence in the culture medium of hog stomach extracts rich in A substance.

Antitetanus or antidiphtheria serotherapy: until recently, most antisera were purified by pepsin enzymatic digestion. Sera thus treated are very rich in A substance.

Injection of certain pharmacologic preparations of animal origin that contain the A substance: examples are dealbuminated hog stomach extracts used in the treatment of gastroduodenal ulcers or pernicious anemias.

**Table 22.6   Average Concentration of Anti-B Allohemagglutinins in Various Pathologic Situations**

| | | |
|---|---|---|
| Alcoholic cirrhosis | 12 | $N_4^* \times 10^6$ |
| Autoimmune "complement-type" hemolytic anemia | 6.5 | $N_4 \times 10^6$ |
| Autoimmune "IgG-type" hemolytic anemia | 3.5 | $N_4 \times 10^6$ |
| Acute leukemia | 2.5 | $N_4 \times 10^6$ |
| Healthy subjects | 2.5 | $N_4 \times 10^6$ |
| Chronic lymphocytic leukemia | 0.5 | $N_4 \times 10^6$ |

* $N_4$ is the maximal number of erythrocytes agglutinated at 4°C by a given serum. This number is proportional to the concentration of specific ABO antibodies.

Injection of antigenic substances related to A antigen: an example is the Forssman antigen, which is present in paratyphic B bacilli (TAB vaccine).

Pregnancy: when the fetus is A or B and the mother is O.

Immunization duration is highly variable. Regular follow-up of donors known to be immunized against the A antigen have shown the disappearance of the immune antibody within a few weeks to a few months, occasionally as long as 20 months after immunization. Note that the possibility to artificially induce the formation of high titer immune antibody enables to obtain anti-A or -B test sera, notably by injection of small amounts of A or Bsoluble substances.

## ANTI-I AND ANTI-LEWIS ANTIBODIES

### I-System Antibodies

Antibodies that correspond to the I system are IgM autoantibodies. These generally exothermic antibodies are responsible for cold agglutinin disease (see p. 774).

### Lewis-System Antibodies

Anti-Lewis antibodies (anti-Le$^a$, anti-Le$^b$, anti-Le$^x$) are not infrequent and may be considered natural antibodies in man. Their appearance in relation to the erythrocytic and salivary phenotypes of the subjects who produce them is not completely understood. The classic anti-Le$^a$ antibody appears in all Le(a−b−) subjects of the A, B, or AB group who secrete ABH substances (Se, lele); anti-Le$^b$ appears in Le(a−b−) subjects who do not secrete ABH substances (sese, lele).

Anti-Lewis antibodies are generally agglutinating but may also be detected by Coombs' test, in the presence of complement. In certain cases, they may show hemolyzing ability, especially if test erythrocytes have been treated with trypsin. Anti-Lewis antibodies are IgM and do not cross the placenta. Because of this property and the fact that fetal erythrocytic phenotypes are usually Le(a−b−), they have no role in immunologic fetomaternal disease. Their existence must, however, be considered in cases of transfusion, because anti-Le$^a$ or -Le$^b$ hemolyzing antibodies may cause hemolytic accidents.

# III.  Rh SYSTEM

The classic Rh system had to be modified in 1961 when the differences between Rh and LW groups were clarified. They are in fact two genetically independent systems although they are phenotypically associated.

In the serum of most women having had a newborn with hemolytic disease, an alloantibody is present that recognizes 85% of the erythrocytes of white subjects (Rh positive). This alloantibody is anti-Rh. This type of antibody was first identified by Levine in 1939. Conversely, if a rabbit or guinea pig is immunized with human or *Macacus rhesus* monkey red blood cells the animal elaborates xenoantibodies that agglutinate not only *M. Rhesus* red blood cells but also all human red blood cells, with very few exceptions. This antibody is anti-LW antibody, first detected by Landsteiner and Wiener in 1940. After adequate dilution and absorption of species-specific satellite xenoantibodies, anti-LW xenoantibodies recognize the red blood cells of only 85% of white subjects, those defined above as Rh+. Rh+ subjects have, in fact, larger amounts of LW antigens than do Rh− subjects, and it is this fact that caused the confusion between Rh and LW. The very rare subjects who are not recognized by the nondiluted reagent are called LW⁻. They may produce an anti-LW alloantibody.

The clinically important antigen is the antigen recognized by the immune alloantibody in fetomaternal alloimmunization. The use of the term "Rhesus" is therefore improper, but because of long precedence, Levine has proposed that the antigen common to the *M. rhesus* monkey and man, identified by the xenoantibody or by the exceptional human alloantibody, be labeled LW antigen in honor of Landsteiner and Wiener. The name, anti-Rh, has been retained for the alloantibody responsible for the hemolytic disease of the newborn.

## IMMUNOLOGIC ASPECTS

Subjects whose erythrocytes are agglutinated by anti-Rh alloantibody (85%) are said to have the Rh+ or D+ phenotype. The 15% of the subjects who are negative are Rh− or D−. Techniques that permit artificial agglutination, developed between 1940 and 1945, especially Coombs' test, allow recognition of other antigens of the Rh system. These antigens include C, present in 70% of white subjects, E (30%), c(80%), and e antigens (98%). Rhesus-negative subjects who possess the C antigen are termed rh', and those with E antigen are known as rh''. It has been noted that these antibodies form couples and give antithetic reactions. Because anti-C and anti-c and anti-E and anti-e are antithetic, their specific antigens are presumed to be produced by alleles.

### *Phenogroups with Three Variation Units*

The recognition of these antithetic reactions led Fisher to postulate the existence of three closely linked locus pairs, or pseudoalleles (D(d), Cc, Ee). Blocked transmission of various haplotypes has been really observed. Major common haplotypes are shown in Table 22.7.

However, each series of antigens produced by the three genetic units shows many variations. The D standard Rh antigen itself is concerned and there are numerous varieties of weak antigens (D$^u$) that have considerable practical importance. Thus, D reactivity presents a quantitative variability with a gaussian distribution; the tail of the curve represents a population of very weak reactivity. Weak D antigens are the classic D$^u$, only detected by certain techniques and reagents. Thus, for standard Rh, as for many other blood group antigens, there are weak variants that are genetically transmitted.

Weakly reactive D antigens are seen in two other situations: some partial

**Table 22.7    Definition of the Main Haplotypes of the Rhesus System**

| Three-unit haplotypes (Fisher) | Current names (Wiener) | Approximate frequency |
|---|---|---|
| Haplotypes that possess the standard Rh gene (D) | | |
| DCe | $R_1$ | 0.40 |
| DcE | $R_2$ | 0.15 |
| Dce | $R_0$ | 0.02 |
| DCE | Rr | 0.00 |
| DC$^w$e | $R^w_1$ | 0.01 |
| Haplotypes that do not possess the standard Rh gene (D) | | |
| dce | r | 0.39 |
| dCe | r$'$ | 0.01 |
| dcE | r$''$ | 0.01 |
| dCE | $r_y$ | 0.00 |

Rh antigens, which are genetically transmitted, and depressed Rh antigen, due to a positional abnormality caused by allelic interaction. $D^u$ antigens are of clinical importance because they may cause immunization in a Rh− subject. Sensitive techniques are used to detect them to avoid alloimmunization of an Rh− recipient who would otherwise be transfused with "weak" D blood. Conversely, it is wise to avoid needless injections of anti-D immunoglobulins into $D^u$ women.

### Phenogroups with Five Variation Units

It was soon discovered that these three variation units did not explain all reactivities. The phenogroup produced by various Rh haplotypes also includes two other antigenic types: compound antigens and G antigen.

Compound antigens are produced only by haplotypes that possess two contiguous genetic markers. For example, Ce, ce, cE, and ce$^s$ antigens are produced only when the corresponding variants of Cc or Ee are in the *cis* position in the same haplotype.

The G antigen is defined by a reactivity present in all subjects who have either C antigen, D antigen, or both C and D and only very rarely in subjects who lack C and D antigens. Phenogroups thus include five variation units: C or c, G or non-G, D or non-D, compound antigens, and E or e.

### Polarized Antigen Production

DEPRESSED ANTIGENS

Certain phenogroups have only weakly expressed Ee reactivities or, usually, weak expression of both Cc and Ee. To date, any such phenogroup, including weak C or c and normal E or e reactivities has not been observed. The main haplotypes known presently, which are transmitted as a block, are the D(C)(e), D(c)(E), —(c)(e) complexes.

SILENT ANTIGENS: "DASH" PHENOGROUP

The "dash" phenogroup is a silent phenotype, either for the Ee antigens (Dc−) or for the Cc and Ee antigens (D− −). Antigenic D reactivity is then in excess. These individuals are very readily immunized, because they produce antibodies to naturally absent antigens, which appear as antigens produced by the Cc or Ee zone, the incidence of which is very high. They also are targets for autoantibodies of the IgG type, especially Hr, nl, Ee, or Rh 18.

Rh-NULL PHENOTYPE

The Rh-null phenotype defines subjects who lack all of the known Rh antigens. Two types are known: one is extremely rare (silent type) and results from the existence of two entirely silent haplotypes. The other phenotype (regulator type) is less exceptional. It seems to result from interactions with another genetic system by substrate inhibition or defect. In fact, within the ABO group, the O gene at the ABO locus is also silent; it resembles the first mentioned Rh−null phenotype. The second is reminiscent of the Bombay phenotype, in which A and B genes cannot express themselves due to lack of a substrate, although the corresponding enzymes are synthesized.

### Associated LW Antigen

The anti-LW antibody produced by guinea pigs immunized with *M. rhesus* erythrocytes or by the very rare LW− human erythrocytes reacts weakly with D− red blood cells and more strongly with Rh+ red blood cells. This difference caused the early confusion between the Rh and LW systems. Rh-null erythrocytes, which possess no DCE antigens, do not contain the LW antigen either, and this is probably not a coincidence.

### Rh Antigens and the Membrane

Rh antigens are most likely a part of the lipoprotein structures responsible for integrity of the erythrocytic membrane. D-reactive sites are much less numerous than those of the ABO system. Their number varies from 10,000 to 30,000 for normal phenotypes, with a maximum of 100,000 for the exceptional D− − phenotypes. The larger site number of D− − erythrocytes explains why they are readily agglutinated by anti-D antibodies (which are normally nonagglutinating). In addition, both with the regulator and the silent-type Rh-null, there is nearly constantly an abnormal fragility of Rh-null red blood cells in vivo. Levine has postulated that lipoprotein Rh antigens are functional membrane components, unlike glycolipid ABH antigens. Fragile Rh-null red blood cells and intact Bombay erythrocytes are thus explained, according to Levine, by the fact that ABH sites are more superficially imbedded within the membrane than are Rh sites.

ROSENFIELD'S NOMENCLATURE (Table 22.8)

In view of the complexity of Rh-reactive structures and the difficulty involved in their genetic interpretation, Rosenfield has proposed a practical

**Table 22.8    Rosenfield's Numerical Nomenclature and Wiener's Classification**

| DCE | Numerical | Rh-Hr | DCE | Numerical | Rh-Hr |
|---|---|---|---|---|---|
| D | Rh 1 | $Rh_0$ | — | Rh 17 | $Hr_0$ |
| C | Rh 2 | rh′ | — | Rh 18 | Hr |
| E | Rh 3 | rh″ | — | Rh 19 | $hr^s$ |
| c | Rh 4 | hr′ | vs or e′ | Rh 20 | — |
| e | Rh 5 | hr″ | $C^G$ | Rh 21 | — |
| ce | Rh 6 | hr | CE | Rh 22 | — |
| Ce | Rh 7 | $rh_1$ | $D^w$ | Rh 23 | — |
| $C^w$ | Rh 8 | $rh^w$ | $E^t$ | Rh 24 | — |
| $C^x$ | Rh 9 | $rh^x$ | LW | Rh 25 | — |
| V or $ce^s$ | Rh 10 | $hr^v$ | (c-like) | Rh 26 | — |
| $E^w$ | Rh 11 | $rh^{w2}$ | cE | Rh 27 | — |
| G | Rh 12 | $rh^G$ | — | Rh 28 | $hr^H$ |
| — | Rh 13 | $Rh^A$ | — | Rh 29 | — |
| — | Rh 14 | $Rh^B$ | $D^C_{or}$ | Rh 30 | — |
| — | Rh 15 | $Rh^C$ | — | Rh 31 | $hr^B$ |
| — | Rh 16 | $Rh^D$ | — | Rh 32 | — |
| | | | — | Rh 34 | — |
| | | | — | Rh 35 | — |

nomenclature that attempts to more precisely classify the antigens studied. Each defined test serum is given a number that corresponds to the Rh determinant that it recognizes. Thus, factors 1, 2, 3, 4, and 5 correspond to D, C, E, c, and e. A given phenotype is expressed by the test serum utilized for its characterization; a number is preceded by a minus sign if the reaction is negative. For example, a Rh negative phenotype may be written: $-1, -2, -3, 4, 5$ (ddccee). Such a nomenclature has obvious advantages for computer use but may be difficult to introduce into clinical practice.

## GENETIC ASPECTS

Fisher and Race's classic scheme introduced the concept of pseudoalleles. The existence of three pairs of genes is considered: Dd, Cc, and Ee. The antigen that corresponds to d has not yet been found. In addition, there are probably more than three antigenic variations and the analysis of compound antigens leads us to consider that C and E belong to the same cistron and do not complement in the *trans* position. Two genetic units are proposed: the D zone, which produces the D antigen or not, and the Cc Ee zone, which produces a large series of proper antigens. Any overview of the genetic nature of the Rh system must also explain three more phenomena:

That formation of specificities of the Rh gene complex is polarized. None of the compound antigens so far discovered associates D to E, but, conversely, all of them associate C with E. In addition, the fact that the D− − haplotype shows D excess suggests a failure of a basic substance conversion, as if there were polarity from D to C and then to E. But so far, no complex of − −E or

− −e has been detected. Such polarity might be explained by sequential action of one or several operons.

Several independent genetic systems are involved in the manifestations of a coordinated genetic activity. It has been demonstrated by segregation analysis that Rh and LW are independent. In addition, a Rh-null subject (of regulatory type) may transmit a normal Rh gene, just as a Bombay subject may transmit a normal A or B gene. However, the imaginary basic substance cannot be LW because some LW subjects have normal Rh antigens. Nevertheless, all Rh-null subjects are LW−. Therefore, the initiating substance must be a substrate for both Rh and LW.

Silent-type Rh-null subjects are also LW−. These subjects do not lack a priori the substrate produced by the $X_1r$ gene. Jouvenceaux and Gibblett imaginatively proposed a sequential activity, involving, alternatively, Rh, then LW, and, again, Rh. The first cistron involved is D, the second is LW, and the third is CE. If one notes that LW suppression is observed only when the Rh complex is totally silent but not when the complex is partially silent (D − − or Dc−), one must agree with Jouvenceaux that LW expression requires an active Dd segment. The antigenic relationship between D and LW would then be explained by the fact that D type permits formation of a greater quantity of LW than does d type. The Dd segment would therefore transform the substance produced by $X_1r$ into substance 2 (Rh 29), onto which independent LW and CE units would then act.

### Rosenfield's Hypothesis

Rosenfield, Allen, and Rubinstein have recently proposed a genetic basis for Rh antigen production that takes into account the polarization mentioned above. The operator $R^{29}$ gene first permits elaboration of the Rh 29 basic substance and then acts on operator genes $R^1$, $R^{17}$, and $R^{18}$. This genetic model explains a certain number of complex findings, but it must be admitted that the genetic function that leads to formation of Rh and LW antigens is still uncertain.

## Rh-SYSTEM ANTIBODIES

These antibodies are the most important of the immune antibodies in immu-nohematology. The D antigen itself is the most immunogenic antigen of all blood group systems. It is the main antigen responsible for fetomaternal alloimmunization. However, anti-E and -c antibodies are also frequently observed in polytransfused subjects and in women immunized by pregnancy, unlike anti-e, which is very rare. Thus, the Rh system is the second most important red blood cell group system, after ABO. Even in primary responses, anti-Rh antibodies are IgG antibodies. They usually do not agglutinate Rh+ red cells, and one must resort to artificial techniques of agglutination in searching for them in serum and in Rh grouping. Note also that some high-frequency antigens, (Rh17 and Rh18 in Rosenfield's nomenclature), are partic-ularly common targets of IgG autoantibodies in autoimmune hemolytic anemias (see p. 772).

# IV.   OTHER BLOOD GROUP SYSTEMS

The erythrocytic membrane has numerous other antigenic markers that express genetic "allotypic" variations within our species. It is possible to distinguish highly immunogenic antigens, such as the Rhesus system, which are responsible for most alloimmunizations in our species (Kell, Duffy, Kidd, and Bg systems), and those that are conversely poorly immunogenic but may, in certain cases, lead to the formation of irregular natural antibodies (MNS, P, and Lutheran systems). Finally, the $Xg^a$ antigen merits particular attention, because it is produced by a genetic unit localized on the X chromosome, hence the interest it has in human genetics.

About 15 genetically independent blood group systems have been identified. They are not, as is sometimes claimed, "subgroups," because each expresses the activity of an autonomous genetic unit. Some of them are highly polymorphic and equilibrated, for example, the MNS system. Others have a great hemotypologic value. They include $Di^a$ antigen of the Diego system, which has been found only in mongoloids, and the $Js^a$ antigen of the Kell system, which is peculiar to blacks.

More and more complex relationships between reactive structures of the erythrocytic membrane appear as various blood group systems are being uncovered. Independent of the classic relations between A and B or between H, I, or i antigens, there is coupling between Rh and Duffy, Lutheran and Auberger, and i and $P_1$. The significance of these relationships may either be genetic or phenotypic and is presently under study.

## IMMUNOGENIC SYSTEMS

### Kell System

The Kell antigen is present in about 8% of white subjects and is one of the most immunogenic antigens, frequently responsible for antibody formation in polytransfused subjects.

The Kell system is relatively complex. It includes a series of haplotypes, the most current of which produces the Cellano, $Kp^b$, and $Js^b$ antigens, with several variants. Mutant haplotypes may produce the Kell antigen (more common in whites than in blacks), the $Kp^a$ antigen in whites, and the $Js^a$ antigen in blacks. In fact, here again, synergistic activity is suggested between the basic system Kx, which may be produced by an X-linked gene, and the Kell gene complex itself. The Kx antigen may be present on normal leukocytes. It would be lacking in children with a X-linked disease called septic granulomatosis, in which polymorphs are unable to destroy previously phagocytosed bacteria. Anti-Kell antibody is an example of immune antibodies that may appear after transfusion or fetomaternal stimulation. It is usually revealed by Coombs' test (IgG type) but may also be detected directly when red blood cells are suspended in human serum. Its clinical importance has already been mentioned.

## Duffy System

The Fy$^a$ antigen of the Duffy system, present in 65% of white subjects, is more immunogenic than the Fy$^b$ antigen. Both antigens represent the product of two Fy$^a$ and Fy$^b$ alleles, but in black populations, subjects are not infrequently deprived of one or the other and thus exhibit the Fy(a−b−) phenotype. The anti-Fy$^a$ antibody is the most commonly occurring antibody. It may be responsible for transfusional hemolytic accidents. It has also been incriminated in fetomaternal alloimmunization accidents. It is generally detectable by the indirect Coombs' test by use of anti-IgG antibodies.

## Kidd System

This system has two alleles (Jk$^a$ and Jk$^b$). Here again, the Jk$^a$ antigen, present in 80% of white subjects, is the most immunogenic. Very rare subjects have neither Jk$^a$ nor Jk$^b$ and may produce an anti-Jk$^a$ Jk$^b$ antibody. Recently, it was demonstrated that this antibody recognizes all leukocytes from Jk(a+) or Jk(b+) subjects but not leukocytes from Jk(a−b−) subjects. Paradoxically, neither isolated anti-Jk$^a$ nor anti-Jk$^b$ reacts with normal leukocytes. It has been suggested that the antigen recognized by anti-Jk$^a$ Jk$^b$ antibody may be a Jk$^a$ and Jk$^b$ precursor present on leukocytes, similar to the Kx antigen of the Kell system.

The anti-Jk$^a$ antibody is relatively common in polytransfused subjects, and its identification is technically difficult. Nonetheless, it may cause hemolytic blood accidents and hemolytic disease of the newborn if it is an IgG antibody. The best technique for detection is a Coombs' test that employs trypsin-treated red blood cells in the presence of complement and of anticomplement serum. The anti-Jk$^b$ antibody is rarer but may also cause transfusion accidents and hemolytic disease of the newborn.

## Bg Antigens

There are on human erythrocytes antigens that correspond to selected HLA antigens (SD) of leukocytes and platelets. The Bg$^a$ antigen is identical to HLA-B7, Bg$^b$ to HLA-BW17, and Bg$^c$ to HLA-A28. Antibodies that correspond to these antigens are frequently observed in polytransfused subjects, especially in subjects who possess complex mixtures of immune alloantibodies, which greatly increases the difficulty of analyzing the specificities of antibodies present in these sera.

## Conclusion

Anti-Rh, D, C, E, e anti-Kell, anti-Fy$^a$, and anti-Jk$^a$ represent more than 98% of the antibodies found in transfusional immunization. They always appear first. The corresponding systems (Rh, Kell, Duffy, and Kidd) must therefore be considered first when transfusion is indicated.

# WEAKLY IMMUNOGENIC SYSTEMS

### MNS System

This system includes two series of pseudoalleles, M and N and S and s, organized in four haplotypes of decreasing frequency, Ns, Ms, MS, and NS. The fact that the frequencies are well equilibrated account for the polymorphism of the MNS system and for its contribution to segregation analysis. In fact, this system is further complicated by the existence of rare alleles in which the antigen is defined by a specific antibody (e.g., Mg antigen) and by the presence of alleles whose antigens are revealed by discrepancies that depend on which reagent is used, whether of human or animal origin. Their link with the MNS system is demonstrated by segregation analysis, e.g., for the $Mi^a$ antigen.

Considerable biochemical breakthroughs have been made in recent years. M and N specificities are linked to the presence of sialic acid [$N$-acetylneuraminic acid (NANA)]. They are carried by complex glycoprotein molecules, where oligosaccharidic lateral chains are linked to the amino acids of the protein chain (Pro, Lys, Arg) by O-glycosidic bonds. M and N specificities might result from specific sialyl transferase activities, which transfer two NANA units to different points of a basic disaccharide that bears T and Tn specificities that characterize hidden antigens. This hypothesis explains the polyagglutinability of neuraminidase-treated red blood cells.

### P System

The P system is a relatively complex one that has two main phenotypes: $P_1$ which carries $P_1$ and P specificities, $P_2$, which has only P specificity, and very rare phenotypes, which apparently represent nonconverted substrates [$P^k$, which lacks P, and Tj(a−), which lacks $P_1$, P, and $P^k$]. $P_2$ subjects sometimes produce an irregular natural anti-$P_1$ antibody; Tj(a) sera contain anti-P + $P_1$ + $P^k$ antibody, for example. These sera recognize antigens of all other subjects, except the Tj(a−) ones. $P^k$ subjects produce an anti-P antibody that recognizes antigens of all other subjects, except $P^k$ and Tj(a−).

At variance with M and N specificities (T and Tn, $Pr_1$ and $Pr_2$), which are glycoprotein in nature, $P^k$, P, and $P_1$ specificities are glycolipid in nature, just like ABH specificities of the erythrocyte. Lactosyl ceramide is the basic disaccharide structure onto which specific α-galactosaminyl transferases successively bind $P^k$ and P specificities. So formed, lacto-$N$-neotetraose ceramide is the basic tetrasaccharide structure, very similar to ABH specificities, onto which an α-galactosyl transferase adds the $P_1$ specificity. The $P_2$ phenotype, that is, the nonconverted P, could be due to the absence of the transferase.

### Lutheran System

This system is characterized by the existence of two alleles, $Lu^a$ and $Lu^b$, which give phenotypes Lu(a+b−) (0.2%), Lu(a+b+) (5.8%), and Lu(a−b+) (94%) in whites. Here again, there is a very rare silent phenotype, Lu(a−b−), of two types, one recessive and the other dominant.

# V.  SERUM PROTEIN GROUPS

We have seen (in chap. 7) that immunoglobulins have a genetic polymorphism, called allotypy, to be compared in many respects to those mentioned on the preceding pages for erythrocytes. Numerous other serum proteins present a similar polymorphism, and some authors have decided to designate them also under the term "allotypy." We will briefly review the major human serum protein allotypes.

## IMMUNOGLOBULIN ALLOTYPES

Four Ig allotype systems are recognized in man: Inv, Gm, Isf, and Am systems. The first one distinguishes the light chains of every Ig, the second and the third (Gm and Isf) determine heavy chains of certain IgG, and the Am system determines heavy chains of certain less IgA subclasses.

### Methodology

The allotypic character of human Ig is recognized by hemagglutination inhibition techniques. A specific antibody recognizes the allotype borne by Ig that is bound to erythrocytes, and this recognition induces red blood cell agglutination. For example, an anti-Rh specific antibody that bears a Gm (1) marker on its Fc fragment may bind to Rh+ erythrocytes. When the sensitized erythrocytes are incubated together with specific anti-Gm (1) antibody, the marker on the heavy chains of the bound antibody is recognized and causes agglutination of red blood cells. Some human sera inhibit such agglutination. One may deduce that these sera possess Gm (1) specificity on their own immunoglobulins.

The intial source of anti-Gm sera was subjects with rheumatoid arthritis [rheumatoid arthritis γ-globulin (Ragg)], and, in fact, in this setting, Grubb first discovered anti-Gm antibody. Unfortunately, these sera are often polyspecific and thus difficult to use despite their generally high titer. Recognition of antiallotypes of low titer but of restricted specificity in normal subjects [sera normal agglutinators (SNagg)] represented significant technical progress, which led to the discovery of the Inv system. The immune nature of SNagg has been demonstrated in certain situations, such as fetomaternal immunization and injection of blood or blood derivatives. However, anti-Gm post-transfusion immunization is fairly rare.

#### INV SYSTEM

This system includes three specificities, Inv(1), Inv(2), and Inv(3), with five phenotypes, Inv(1, 2, −3), Inv(−1, −2, 3), Inv(1, −2, −3), Inv(1, 2, 3), and Inv (1, −2, 3). In this nomenclature, the specificity is indicated by the number, and the absence of any specificity is denoted by a minus sign. The three allotypes are formed by a series of polyallelic genes: $Inv^{1,2}$, $Inv^1$, $Inv^3$, and $Inv^-$. The latter is a silent gene, which explains the sixth silent phenotype,

Inv($-1$, $-2$, $-3$), when it exists in a double dose. The biochemical basis of the Inv system is described elsewhere (p. 000).

GM SYSTEM

Allotypic specificities within the Gm system are now very numerous, Gm(1) to Gm(25) by the international nomenclature most generally used. Each specificity is transmitted like a mendelian character, but segregation analysis has shown that some allotypes are transmitted as a block. Studies that involve formal genetics combined with population analysis have permitted recognition of the most frequent haplotypes within the human races:

White race: Gm 1, 17, 21; Gm 1, 2, 17, 21; Gm 3, 5, 8, 10, 13, 14
Black race: Gm 1, 5, 13, 14, 17; Gm 1, 5, 14, 17; Gm 1, 5, 6, 14, 17
Mongoloid race: Gm 1, 17, 21; Gm 1, 2, 17, 12; Gm 1, 13, 17; Gm 1, 3, 5, 13, 14

It should be noticed that Gm(1) and (5) allotypes are never present in the same haplotype in whites, whereas coexistence is always the case in blacks, which means that black individuals are always of the Gm(1,5) phenotype. Similarly, all mongoloid people are Gm(1) because all haplotypes of mongoloid races include the Gm1 gene. Conversely, Gm(6) specificity is found only in black people. This specific polymorphism has made the Gm system particularly important in studying cross-breeding and evolution in primates. It has thus permitted dating the appearance of certain mutations during evolution. The mechanism by which such polymorphism is maintained is, however, unknown.

The various Gm specificities are borne by different molecules within each individual's serum. They represent the subject's phenotype. By use of methods similar to those previously described for Inv, it was recognized that Gm specificities are borne by IgG and that most markers are located on the Fc of the heavy chains. Only Gm(4) and Gm(17) specificities are located on the Fc fragment and need for their expression the quaternary structure of the IgG molecule. Interestingly, each marker is borne by a different IgG molecule.

### Relationships Between Allotypy and Isotypy

The Gm system provides an example of the very close relationship between allotypy and isotypy. Table 22.9 demonstrates, by use of four antisera [anti-Gm(1), anti-Gm(4), anti-Gm(5), and anti-Gm(21) along with anti-non-a and anti-non-g sera], how it is possible to define the isotypic class of a myelomatous protein or a purified antibody.

As can be seen, IgG1 does not bear the same markers as IgG3: the first contains Gm(1, 17) or Gm(3,4), and the second contains Gm(5) or Gm(21). This means that in subjects whose genome bears the haplotype "1, 17, 21," 1 and 17 markers are present in differentiated cells that synthesize IgG1, whereas the 21 marker is found in differentiating cells that synthesize IgG3. It must be admitted, then, that the two contiguous zones are not activated within the same differentiated cell.

Table 22.9    Relationships Between Allotypy and Isotypy of Human Immunoglobulins

| Isotypy | Allotypy | | | | Isotypy | |
|---|---|---|---|---|---|---|
| | Anti-Gm (1) | Anti-Gm (4) | Anti-Gm (5) | Anti-Gm (21) | Anti-"non-a" | Anti-"non-g" |
| IgG1 | + | − | − | − | − | − |
| | − | + | + | − | + | − |
| IgG3 | − | − | + | − | + | + |
| | − | − | − | + | + | − |
| IgG2 | − | − | − | − | + | + |
| IgG4 | − | − | − | − | − | − |

Such an analysis has been profitably put to use in studying modifications of genetic markers that occur during certain myeloproliferative diseases. By this means, it has been shown that in some cases, the changes bear on the characteristics of only one of two haplotypes, which argues in favor of genetic determinism of the abnormality. Note that when one determines the Gm phenotype of a subject, one is, in fact, grouping the precursor stem cells from which Ig-forming lymphocytes are made.

### Biochemical Basis of Specificities

The biochemical basis for Gm specificities of IgG heavy chains has already been discussed (p. 222). Note that the Fc fragment of Gm(1) IgG1 differs from that of Gm(−1) IgG1 by two noncontiguous amino acids of a pentapeptide located toward the middle of the Fc fragment. IgG2 and IgG3 chains, but not IgG4, have a peptide analogous to the Gm(−1) peptide of IgG1 chains. This peptide explains "non-a" specificity (see Table 22.9). In other words, the "non-a" peptide represents an immunologic specificity defined by an antibody that recognizes Gm(−1) IgG1, IgG2, and IgG3, as though it were an allotypic specificity for IgG1 and an isotypic one for the other two. Such specificities are presently called isoallotypic.

### Applications to the Study of Genetic Function

FUNCTIONAL HAPLOIDY

In the heterozygous state, no molecule is marked simultaneously by both alleles. For example, in a 1, 5 subject, no single protein has both markers.

Either Gm(1) or Gm(5) is present but not Gm(1, 5). An analogous phenomenon has never been observed in AB subjects, in whom all erythrocytes are both A and B. This means that only one of the chromosomes is involved in antibody synthesis.

ALLOTYPE PRODUCTION IN LYMPHOCYTE CULTURES

It has been shown by Ropartz that homozygous Gm(4, 5) lymphocytes placed in culture can produce Ig of Gm(1) and Gm(17) allotypes. Analogous results have been obtained after phytohemagglutinin stimulation or in mixed-lymphocyte cultures.

This finding has suggested that all subjects have a genetic potential that enables them to synthesize any Ig that carries the various allotypes. Gm system genes could therefore be regulatory genes transmitted by mendelian inheritance that repress structural genes. Artificial culture conditions would then modify the action of the regulatory genes and derepress structural genes.

### ISF SYSTEM

The third system of Ig allotypic markers is the ISf system, presently represented by only one allotype, ISf(1), whose specificity is borne by the Fc fragment of IgG1 molecules. It is interesting to note that in several myelomatous proteins, a Gm and an Isf factor have been found to occur simultaneously, which indicates that the heavy chains relate to at least two independent genetic systems. Another unexpected finding was the discovery that frequency of the Isf(1) marker increases with age.

### AM SYSTEM

This marker is specific for certain IgA2 immunoglobulins. It is borne by $\alpha_2$ heavy chains. The character identified in serum is also present in saliva. Two Am specificities are presently known, Am(1) and Am(2), but their relationships have not yet been clearly determined. Familial studies indicate that there is a relationship between the Am(2) and the Gm locus.

## $\alpha_2$-GLOBULIN ALLOTYPES (Gc GLOBULINS)

The Gc polymorphism ("group-specific component") relates to $\alpha_2$-globulins. In animals, antisera have been described that react with certain types of $\alpha_2$-globulins that differ between individuals. On immunoelectrophoresis, there may be one precipitation arc, either a rapidly migrating or a slow migrating protein, or two arcs that react with two protein types. A genetic system is thus defined, in which two alleles, $Gc_1$ and $Gc_2$, determine three phenotypes. In addition, there exists a silent allele of very rare frequency and numerous rare variants of $Gc_1$ and $Gc_2$.

## β-LIPOPROTEIN GROUPS

Two "allotypic" genetic β-lipoprotein systems have been identified, Ag ("antigen") and Lp ("lipoprotein").

### Ag System

In performing simple gel immunodiffusion with antibodies against human serum in polytransfused subjects, Allison and Blumberg (in 1961) observed that one of the sera was capable of precipitating 50% of normal human sera and that this trait was a dominant mendelian genetic character with autosomal transmission. They called this substance $Ag^a$ antigen. Other factors were soon recognized: $Ag^x$, $Ag^y$, $Ag^z$, and $Ag^t$. Genetic analyses showed that the $Ag^x$ and $Ag^y$ systems are probably alleles and that the Ag system is at least as complex as Rh, Kell, and Gm, Ag and $Ag^y$ characters are observed in heterozygotes; there is no functional haploidy, as in the Gm system.

### Lp System

This allotype is transmitted as a dominant and autosomal mendelian character. Two antigens are known, $Lp^a$ and $Lp^x$, associated with three phenotypes, $a+x-$, $a+x+$, $a-x-$. This genetic system is independent of the Ag system and of most other marker systems. Berg, who discovered this system, has shown that only part of the circulating β-lipoproteins of $Lp(a+)$ sera have the character and that antigens of the Lp and Ag systems are borne by entirely separate lipoprotein molecules. Thus, when an $Lp(1+)$ or an $Ag(a+)$ serum is treated with an anti-$Lp^a$ antibody to remove (by precipitation) all $Lp(a+)$ molecules, the supernatant still reacts with anti-$Ag^a$ serum.

## VI.   APPENDIX: ERYTHROCYTE GROUPING

Erythrocyte grouping is a prerequisite to any transfusion. The routine is to study the standard ABO and Rh groups. We will only discuss the main methods of grouping in detail but stress that in some circumstances, especially multiple transfusions, it is necessary to determine the entire Rh group (C, c, E, e) along with the Kell, Duffy, Kidd, and Lewis groups.

### ABO GROUPING AND ITS DIFFICULTIES

ABO grouping is performed by two complementary tests on both erythrocytes and serum.

The red cell test incubates known anti-B, anti-A, and anti-A plus anti-B sera with the erythrocytes to be tested. The erythrocytic antigen(s) define(s) blood group A, B, AB, or O.

The serum test consists of incubating the serum to be tested with known $A_1$, $A_2$, and B erythrocytes. Every individual has in his serum the antibody(ies) that corresponds to the absent erythrocytic antigen(s) (Table 22.10).

If red blood cells are agglutinated by anti-A and anti-A plus anti-B but not by anti-B, they bear only the A antigen. The subject may be tentatively considered to belong to the A group. His serum does not agglutinate A red blood cells ($A_1$ and $A_2$) but does agglutinate B red blood cells. He therefore possesses an anti-B antibody, which confirms the fact that he belongs to the A group. Concordance of findings in red blood cell and serum tests is required. If there is a discrepancy, no ABO group conclusion can be reached. The order of reagent examinations (anti-B, anti-A, anti-A + B) is unimportant but, once chosen, must not be changed.

**Table 22.10    Red Cell and Serum Tests of ABO Grouping**

| Anti-B | Anti-A | Anti-A+B | $A_1$ | $A_2$ | B | Groups and frequency in France (%) |
|---|---|---|---|---|---|---|
| − | +++ | +++ | − | − | +++ | A, 45 |
| − | − | − | +++ | +++ | +++ | O, 44 |
| +++ | − | +++ | +++ | +++ | − | B, 8 |
| +++ | +++ | +++ | − | − | − | AB, 3 |

The two most widely used techniques of agglutination are performed in Kahn tubes or on opalin slides. Although currently studied in certain laboratories, $A_1$ and $A_2$ subgroup determination is of no consequence in transfusion. Note that $A_1$ red blood cells are agglutinated by anti-$A_1$ reagents but not by anti-H reagents, while the reverse is true for $A_2$ red blood cells.

ABO group determination is generally uncomplicated. Any discrepancy between red blood cell and serum tests requires three additional controls, following preliminary washing of test erythrocytes:

"Auto control" involves patient's serum plus patient's own red blood cells. If the results are negative, this control eliminates spontaneous erythrocytic agglutination.

"AB control" involves AB serum plus erythrocytes to be tested. When negative, this control excludes erythrocytic polyagglutination and verifies the red cell test.

"Allo control" involves the patient's serum plus compatible O erythrocytes. This is, in fact, a simple agglutinin detection. This control, when negative, verifies the serum test.

If there is a discrepancy between erythrocyte and serum tests, with negative controls, the cause is usually a rare but normal group; less often, hypogammaglobulinemia is responsible for negative serum tests. If one of the controls is positive, one must think of an associated immunologic disease.

### Discrepancies with Negative Controls

O SUBJECTS WITH HEMOLYSIN

The tested serum may react less with A than with B erythrocytes. This occurs rarely in O-group subjects and must never be accepted without further study. It may represent anti-A hemolysin in the O subject's serum. Serum inactivation (20 min at 56°C), which destroys complement, suffices to normalize the serum test. Less commonly there is an unknown $A_x$, but in this case, $A_2$ erythrocytes are not agglutinated in the serum test.

WEAK A GROUPS

There are three main weak A groups (all very rare): $A_3$, $A_x$, and $A_m$.

$A_3$ is detected by anti-A and anti-A+B. It gives a dual population pattern on slide grouping. $A_3$ is sometimes associated with serum anti-$A_1$. $A_x$ is detected by anti-A + B and sometimes also by anti-A. Agglutination is weak, and there is no dual-population pattern. A serum anti-A is always present. $A_m$ gives no agglutination with test sera. The fixation elution test, employing anti-A, is required to detect the antigen. Similar B-group varieties ($B_3$, $B_x$, $B_m$) are even rarer.

DUAL POPULATION

Double populations are recognized on opalin slides. Whereas agglutinates are normally seen on the white background of opalin, dual population agglutinates appear on a pink background made of nonagglutinated red blood cells. A dual population may be due to an $A_3$ leukemia or malignant hemopathy of the myeloproliferative type, previous transfusions with O blood, or a chimera or mosaic (very rare).

$A_2B$ SUBJECTS WITH ANTI-$A_1$

This phenotype presents the only real difficulty in ABO typing, because the A antigen may be considerably weakened, independent of any relevant clinical disorder. Its presence can therefore not be recognized, and, because there is an anti-$A_1$ in serum, one may erroneously conclude that it is a B group. This pitfall justifies the use of $A_2$ erythrocytes in the serum test. Similarly, it is wise to check the red blood cell test results of all B subjects by use of a strongly positive anti-A reagent.

LEUKEMIC MODIFICATIONS

Certain malignant hemopathies may induce a very important alteration in A- or B-antigen expression, either on a fraction of red blood cells (giving then a dual-population pattern and simulating $A_3$), or on all erythrocytes (thus simulating $A_x$ or $A_m$). But, there are no anti-A antibodies in the serum. The abnormality represents an acquired modification of blood group. It may normalize during clinical remissions.

ABSENCE OF AN EXPECTED ANTIBODY IN THE SERUM TEST

The natural antibody expected in the serum test in relation to data obtained in the red blood cell test, may be absent when the subject is unable to produce antibodies, either due to newborn immune immaturity (antibodies present being of maternal origin) or to congenital or acquired agammaglobulinemia, myeloma, or chronic lymphocytic leukemia.

### Discrepancies with Positive Controls

There exist three possibilities: the auto control is positive (presence of cold agglutinins or rouleau formation), only the AB control is positive (polyagglutinability), or the allo control alone is positive (because of an irregular agglutinin).

COLD AGGLUTININS

This is a most difficult situation in which all three controls are strongly positive (agglutination is already seen in the tube in which blood is collected). Agglutination is most often due to autoantibodies bound to the patient's erythrocytes and less commonly to free antibodies in the serum. The bound autoantibodies may be eluted by washing red blood cells at 37, 40, or 45°C; the free antibodies can be absorbed onto O-group erythrocytes (the grouping may also be performed at 37°C).

ROULEAUX

In macroglobulinemia, myeloma, and hyperfibrinemia, abnormal red blood cell sedimentation may simulate agglutination. However, the AB control performed prior to erythrocyte washing is positive, while mere red blood cell washing is followed by a normal red blood cell test. The serum test is performed by slightly diluting serum in saline (1/2, 1/3). The protein responsible for the effect is then insufficiently concentrated, and the rouleaux disappear. One should note, however, that anti-A and anti-B hemagglutinins have also been diluted and may sometimes be difficult to detect.

POLYAGGLUTINABILITY

The polyagglutinability phenomenon (recognized by an AB positive control) may be due to contamination of the blood sample (it then suffices to obtain another blood sample) or to certain infectious diseases. There are several types of polyagglutinability: T, Tn, and acquired B. Diagnosis is difficult and requires the experience of a specialized blood center.

### Contribution of ABO Grouping to Pathology

We have named several diseases whose diagnosis may be recognized by irregularity in ABO typing. Let us briefly review them.

An ABO dual population (or, possibly, Rh) may be due to acute leukemia, refractory anemia, or myeloproliferative diseases.

A double population in several group systems, for example, ABO, MNS, Rh, and Kidd, may represent a mosaic or chimera with possible hermaphroditism (XX-XY).

Large quantities of A or B substance in the plasma suggest the presence of a gastrointestinal carcinoma (e.g., stomach or pancreas). These substances inhibit agglutination in the red blood cell test.

The presence of an anti-$P_1$ antibody may indicate the existence of a hydatic cyst.

The absence of detectable antibody on serum testing should lead to a search for a primary or secondary immunodeficiency (e.g., chronic lymphocytic leukemia).

Massive autoagglutination usually denotes cold agglutinin hemolytic anemia. The rouleaux phenomenon suggests Waldenström's macroglobulinemia or myeloma.

## Rh GROUPING

Determination of the standard (D) Rh phenotype is always performed along with ABO typing and is, of course, recorded on the usual blood group card. Rh+ refers to any subject whose red blood cells contain the standard Rh antigen (85% in the white race), and Rh− denotes any subject who lacks this antigen. Unlike ABO grouping, there is no possible serum test, because Rh− subjects do not normally have anti-Rh antibody. Standard Rh grouping must be performed not only for all subjects to be transfused but also for pregnant women with possible fetomaternal alloimmunization (which could cause hemolytic disease of the newborn; see p. 752).

### *Technique Description*

The anti-Rh reagent is a mixture of bovine serum albumin and selected antisera obtained either from pregnancy-immunized women or from male volunteers previously immunized. The anti-Rh antibody is not capable alone of causing agglutination of Rh+ red blood cells. The addition of bovine serum albumin modifies the dielectric constant of the medium and leads to agglutination of sensitized erythrocytes.

The technical conditions of Rh grouping are different from those of ABO grouping. The reaction is performed at 40°C on a slide or at 37°C in microtubes. The utilization of proteolytic enzymes, such as papain, bromelin, or trypsin, considerably increases sensitivity and permits immediate recognition of weak Rh ($D^u$) antigens (see p. 319). Automatic techniques (Autoanalyzer or Groupamatic) generally include use of bromelin or Polybrene (a bicationic molecule).

The albumin control must always be performed. Erythrocytes sensitized by any IgG antibody generally agglutinate in bovine serum albumin, which explains why red blood cells from patients with hemolytic anemia due to IgG-type autoantibodies, already coated with antibody before contact with anti-Rh reagent, agglutinate in the presence of albumin even when they are Rh−. Rh grouping of these patients is difficult. Elution of autoantibodies by heating to 56°C is not possible because of risk of Rh antigen alteration. Ether, which readily elutes IgG, is even more traumatic to erythrocytes, reducing them to stromatous state. The only viable solution is to use the very rare anti-Rh antibodies that are capable of agglutinating Rh+ red blood cells in saline suspension.

Practically speaking, routine grouping consists of testing erythrocytes with two anti-D reagents. If both reactions are positive and the control is negative, the subject is said to be Rh+. When both reactions and the control are negative, the subject is said to be Rh− (Table 22.11). In the case of a patient awaiting transfusion, no further testing is necessary. Conversely, if the subject is a prospective blood donor, weak Rh ($D^u$) and the satellite antigens C and E must

**Table 22.11   Results of Rhesus Grouping**

| Anti-D (1) | Anti-D (2) | Anti-C | Anti-E | |
|:---:|:---:|:---:|:---:|:---|
| + | + | | | Rh+ |
| − | − | | | Rh− |
| + | − | | | D$^u$ (weak Rh+) |
| − | − | + | − | rh′ |
| − | − | − | + | rh″ |
| − | − | + | + | rh′rh″ |

be evaluated. Conflicting reactions may be observed. The red blood cells of the tested subject are recognized as positive by one reagent and negative by another, suggesting the possibility of D$^u$.

### D$^u$

All blood group antigens are heterogeneous. We have already discussed various A antigens, for example, $A_1$, $A_2$, and weak A antigens. The standard Rh antigen does not escape this rule, and the term D$^u$ refers to all weak Rh antigens that present as positive Rh, which are more or less recognized by a specific reagent or technique. Weak Rh antigens may also be due to a positional effect (e.g., a $R_1r′$ subject produces weak standard Rh) or to incomplete Rh antigens that lack some portion of the standard Rh antigen. Recent improvements in reagents and techniques have increased D$^u$ detection threshold (Fig. 22.5). The laboratories that utilize automated grouping methods, including the use of bromelin or polybrene, detect weak Rh (Rh + ), which would have previously been considered to be negative or D$^u$ by standard techniques.

In practice, if the results are negative on both test sera, the laboratory has no reason to proceed further, since the aim of the blood group card is to choose

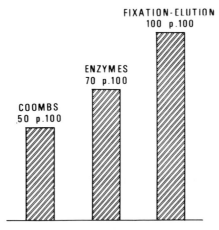

**Fig. 22.5** D$^u$ detection: proportion of positive results obtained according to the technique used.

# *BIBLIOGRAPHY*

Boorman and Dodd B. E. An introduction to blood group serology, ed. 4. London, 1970, Churchill.

Dodd B. E. and Lincoln P. Blood group topics. *In* Current Topics in immunology, London, Aronold, p. 141.

Dunsford I. and Bowrey C. C. Techniques in blood grouping. Edinburgh, London, 1967, Olivier and Boyd.

Goudemand M. and Salmon C. Immunohématologie et Immunogénétique. Flammarion, Paris, 1980, 592 p.

Kabat E. A. Blood group substances: their chemistry and immunochemistry, New York, 1956, Academic Press.

Mollison P. L. Blood transfusion in clinical medicine, ed. 5. Oxford, 1972, Blackwell.

Mourant A. E., Kopéc A. C., and Domaniewska-Sobczak O. The distrubtion of the human blood groups and other polymorphisms, ed. 2. 1 vol., 1050 p., London, 1976, Oxford Univ. Press.

Race R. R. and Sanger R. Blood groups in man. Oxford, 1968, Blackwell.

Rosenfield R. E., Allen F. H., Swisher S. N., and Kochwa S. A review of Rh serology and presentation of a new terminology. Transfusion (Phila.), 1962, *2*, 87.

Rosenfield R. F., Allen F. H., and Rubinstein P. Genetic model for the Rh blood group system. Proc. Nat. Acad. Sci. (Wash.), 1973, *70*, 1303.

Salmon C., Lopez M., Gerbal A., Bouguerra A., and Cartron J. P. Current genetic problems in the ABO blood group system. Biomed., 1973, *18*, 375.

Stratton F. and Renton P. H. Practical blood grouping, ed. 2. Oxford, 1967, Blackwell.

## ORIGINAL ARTICLES

Cartron J. P., Gerbal A., Badet J., Ropars C. and Salmon C. Assay of -N- acetylgalactosaminyl transferases in human sera. Vox Sang. (Basel), 1975, *28*, 347.

Landsteiner K. and Wiener A. S. An agglutinable factor in human blood recognized by immune sera for rhesus blood. Proc. Soc. Exp. Biol. (N.Y.), 1940, *43*.

Levine P., Celano M., Fenichel R., Pollack W., and Singher H. A « D like » antigen in rhesus monkeys, human Rh positive and human Rh negative red blood cells. J. Immunol., 1961, *87*, 747.

Wurmser-Filitti S., Jacquot-Armand Y., and Wurmser R. Sur les isohémagglutinines naturelles due systàeme ABO. Rev. Hémat., 1960, *15*, 201.

## Chapter 23

# TRANSPLANTATION IMMUNOGENETICS AND THE MAJOR HISTOCOMPATIBILITY COMPLEX

## Jean-François Bach

I.   INTRODUCTION

II.  SERO-DEFINED (SD) ANTIGENS

III. ANTIGENS INDUCING LYMPHOCYTE PROLIFERATION (LD ANTIGENS)

IV.  THE Ia AND DR ANTIGENS

V.   BIOCHEMISTRY OF THE MAJOR HISTOCOMPATIBILITY COMPLEX (MHC) PRODUCTS

VI.  IMMUNOGENETICS OF GRAFT REJECTION

## I.  INTRODUCTION

On the surface of nucleated cells, there are alloantigens responsible for allograft rejection, as there exist on erythrocytes alloantigens that provoke the production of hemolytic antibodies. Histocompatibility systems include all antigenic systems at the origin of rejection phenomena. Their study is of considerable interest from a theoretical viewpoint. Histocompatibility antigens represent a unique model of polymorphism for studying the complexity of systems that possess many alleles. They are practically ubiquitous, and genes that control them are codominant (each antigen is expressed when the allele is present in the genome). The demonstration of an association of immune response genes with genes that

The author thanks L. Degos for his critical appraisal of this chapter.

code for histocompatibility antigens has presented even wider prospects. Lastly, study of histocompatibility has found numerous clinical applications, particularly in selection of the best donor for an organ graft or, more recently, in the study of the genetic basis of some diseases.

Definition of histocompatibility antigens has long been essentially serologic. Thus, CBA mice immunized by C57BL/6 spleen cells produce antibodies directed against antigens of the C57BL/6 strain. These antibodies may be detected by various serologic techniques, such as hemagglutination, leukoagglutination, or lymphocytotoxicity. The former two techniques can also be used to study these antigens in man. Leukoagglutinins are produced after pregnancies, transfusions, allografts, or injections of allogeneic lymphocytes. In man, however, in contrast to rodents, transplantation (or histocompatibility) antigens are generally absent from mature red blood cells.

The serologic approach has permitted definition of the major histocompatibility systems, H-2 in the mouse and HLA in man. However, there are situations both in mouse and in man where an allogeneic reaction may develop in the absence of differences in loci that code for antigens that induce antibody production, which indicates the existence of antigens that stimulate selectively cellular responses. This phenomenon has led to the definition of structures that provoke cellular reactions: lymphocyte-defined (LD) antigens as opposed to serodefined (SD) antigens, recognized by their reaction with humoral antibodies. It should be noted, however, that the genes coding for the LD antigens, (Ia in the mouse and DR in man) that are only present on B lymphocytes, stimulate antibody production which diminishes the absolute character of the LD-SD dichotomy. In addition, SD and LD antigens appear to be controlled by neighboring genes on the same chromosome, in a region where immune response genes (Ir genes) are also located (see chap. 24). The possible relationships between SD and LD genes and functions of their products will be examined in the following pages.

**Table 23.1   Principal Functions Controlled by the Major Histocompatibility Complex**

1. Histocompatibility: graft rejection
2. Mixed lymphocyte reaction and cell-mediated lympholysis
3. Immune responses against defined antigens (Ir genes)
4. Cellular interactions between macrophages and T cells, T-T and B-T lymphocytes
5. Allogeneic restriction in the recognition of non-H-2 antigens by T lymphocytes
6. Allogeneic effect (see p. 538); chronic allogeneic disease (see p. 423)
7. Levels and polymorphism of some complement components
8. Hybrid resistance (Hh system) and allogeneic inhibition
9. Susceptibility to Friend or Gross virus-induced leukemias
10. Susceptibility to various autoimmune diseases (thyroiditis, encephalomyelitis)
11. Sensitivity to lymphocytic choriomeningitis

# II. SERO-DEFINED (SD) ANTIGENS (CLASS I)

## DETECTION AND QUANTIFICATION OF SD ANTIGENS

Numerous techniques may be used for serologic detection of histocompatibility antigens. These techniques must be sensitive, because alloantibodies are generally present at low concentrations. Historically, hemagglutination and leukoagglutination were first described in the mouse and in man, respectively, but while hemagglutination is still used in the mouse, the preferable techniques for use in humans are lymphocytotoxicity and complement fixation on platelets rather than leukoagglutination. Hemagglutination is only applicable to species that express histocompatibility antigens on red blood cells, such as the mouse and the rat but not man. Because of the low titer of antibodies present, it is often necessary to increase the sensitivity of the technique by treating red blood cells with polyvinylpyrrolidone (PVP), papain, or trypsin. Leukoagglutination is performed with lymphocytes isolated from the spleen (in the mouse and rat) or blood (in man). Cytotoxicity reactions are obtained by incubating spleen or blood lymphocytes with antiserum and complement (fresh guinea pig or rabbit serum) and evaluating the number of cells lysed relative to the total number of cells (percent) by incorporation of trypan blue (a stain that only penetrates dead cells) or by measurement of $^{51}$Cr release, a label previously bound to lymphocytes. Generally, this toxicity technique is used for cross-match performed before organ grafting to check for the absence of preformed antibodies to donor antigens. The complement fixation reaction on platelets is obtained by incubating antiserum with platelets in the presence of a standard amount of complement (fresh human serum) and measuring complement consumption by the reaction. Note, lastly, that determination of Ia-like human antigens is performed on B-cell enriched preparations (for example by E rosette depletion). This approach has permitted the definition of the DR antigens described on p. 663.

It is possible to quantify histocompatibility antigens of a given specificity in a cell suspension or a soluble antigen preparation by measuring the capacity of the preparation to absorb out the biologic activity of the specific antiserum. The cell suspension or the antigenic preparation is incubated with the antiserum and then titrated by one of the methods mentioned above.

## SOURCES OF ANTISERA: DISTRIBUTION OF TRANSPLANTATION ANTIGENS

Antibodies directed against histocompatibility antigens are normally formed after pregnancy or leukocyte injections (intradermal or intravenous leukocyte injections or transfusion of histoincompatible blood). They are also produced after skin or organ grafting. In man, the best serum sources are multiparous women or polytransfused subjects (such as hemodialyzed patients). Immunization of volunteers may also be used when antisera of a given specificity are desired. Generally, antisera are polyspecific, and their use as reagents for leukocyte grouping must be preceded by several absorptions with suspensions of cells that bear the antigens toward which unwanted antibodies are directed. It is now possible to obtain pure monoclonal antibodies directed at a single determinant by using the hybridoma technique. The existence of cross-reactions between the various antigenic groups produces further complications. Immunization with different tissues has shown that histocompatibility antigens are present in all tissues but at different concentrations. Unexpectedly, lymphoid cells contain the greater density of antigens, and the reason why is still not understood. Human red cells do not possess transplantation antigens excepts for certain well-defined antigens that are regarded as erythrocytic groups ($Bg^a$ = HLA-A7, $Bg^b$ = HLA-A17, $Bg^c$ = HLA-A23). In contrast, histocompatibility antigens are present on reticulocytes.

## MOUSE HISTOCOMPATIBILITY

Most of our knowledge of histocompatibility system genetics has been obtained since 1930, in the mouse, through the work of Gorer and Snell; the first H-2 "II" antigen was described by Gorer in 1936; Snell's laws, which define the mendelian inheritance of histocompatibility genes, are apparently applicable to all species.

### Snell's Laws

Following the results obtained during skin grafting studies in multiple combination between pure strains of mice, Snell has described five basic laws whose general validity (with several minor amendments) has largely been confirmed:
1.   Syngeneic grafts are not rejected.
2.   Allografts are rejected.
3.   Grafts from one parent (A or B) to an $F_1$ hybrid (A × B) are not rejected.
4.   Grafts from one parent (A) to an $F_2$ hybrid ($F_1$ mouse hybrids crossed with one another) or to mice resulting from a back-cross with the other parent ($F_1$ [A × B] and B) may be accepted, but only in a limited number of cases.
5.   Grafts from $F_2$ mice or from mice resulting from backcross mating to $F_1$ mice are not rejected.
These laws indicate that there exists a major histocompatibility system that controls graft rejection and whose genes are situated in the same chromosomal region. This region is the H-2 region in the mouse and, as will be seen later, the HLA region in man. The presence of such a "major" histocompatibility system does not exclude the existence of other antigen systems that may result in a subsequent, later, graft rejection in the absence of differences at the H-2 locus. These are the minor histocompatibility systems, for example, in the mouse the H-1, H-3, H-n systems.

### H-2 System

The H-2 system is controlled by two close loci, H-2K and H-2D, that seemingly derive from each other by duplication. "Crossing-over" frequency between the two loci is of the order of 0.5%. Genes of each locus control the production of separate molecules, as shown by biochemical studies that demonstrate the presence of two different molecules in lymphocytic membranes and by independent redistribution (or "capping") of antigens encoded by genes of H-2K and H-2D loci under the influence of the corresponding antisera. Migration of H-2K antigens by an anti-H-2K antiserum does not lead to redistribution of H-2D antigens and vice versa.

There are multiple alleles for each H-2 locus, hence the existence of numerous different H-2 molecules. Heredity is codominant: the antigen is expressed if the gene is present. The problem is complicated further by the fact that each H-2 molecule reacts with several alloantibodies; thus, the $H-2D^d$ molecule reacts with at least 12 known alloantibodies, if not more. It is still not known whether there is an independent antigenic determinant on the surface of the molecule for each antibody or if a relatively extended site controls the production of several antibodies; the true situation probably lies somewhere between these two extreme hypotheses. Recombinant analysis, that is, study of the crossing-overs that occur inside the H-2 region, also suggests, like the evidence obtained from the biochemical and capping studies mentioned above, grouping of specificities in two H-2D and H-2K loci. These specificities are defined by monospecific reactions obtained by use of a panel of antisera.

Basically about 50 specificities, classified 1-56, have been defined by serologic studies, and several frequently occurring groups (24 at present) associated with these specificities are designated by a superscript, $H-2^a \cdots H-2^1$. Some strains that possess minor modifications have been further distinguished by the use of a second letter ($H-2^{ba}$, $H-2^{bb}$) (Table 23.3). Thus, the AKR and CBA strains belong to the $H-2^k$ group , which possesses specificities 1, 5, 11, 23, 25, and 32. BALB/c and DBA/2 mice belong to the $H-2^d$ group, which has specificities 3, 4, 13, and 31. Specificity grouping in two loci has been established by analysis of recombinant mice, as the following example:

| Group | Specificities | |
|---|---|---|
| $H-2^d$ | 31 | 3, 4, 13 |
| $H-2^k$ | 11, 23, 25 | 1, 5, 32 |
| Recombinant | 31 | 1, 5, 32 |

In some rare cases, certain specificities are classified according to recombinants in one or another locus. This difficulty is explained by the fact that these specificities correspond to determinants that are common to two specificities and therefore give rise to a cross-reaction (this reaction was formerly interpreted as indicative of the existence of other loci).

Chromosomal localization of H-2D and H-2K loci has been achieved through use of several antigenic markers that are independent of histocompatibility systems. H-2 loci are localized at the ninth linkage group, that is, the 17th pair of chromosomes. The H-2K locus is nearest to the centromere, but, by convention and for historical reasons, the H-2K and H-2D loci are generally placed from left to right.

**Table 23.2  Genetic Nomenclature of the H-2 Complex**

| Complex | H-2 | | | | | | | | |
|---|---|---|---|---|---|---|---|---|---|
| Extremities | K | | | | D | | | | |
| Regions | K | I | | | | S | "X" | D | L |
| Subregions | H-K | IA | IB | (IJ)(IE) | IC | Ss | Lad | H-2D | H-2L |
| | H-K | Ir-Ia | Ir-Ib | | Ia | Ss | Lad | H-2D | H-2L |
| Loci | Lad | Ir-(T, G)-A-L<br>Ir-IgA<br>Ir-RE<br>Ir-OA<br>Ir-OM<br>Ir-BGG<br>H-2 I<br>Lad<br>Ia | Ir-LDH$_B$<br>Ir-Nase<br>Lad$_5$<br>Ia | | Lad<br>Ir-GLT$_5$ | Slp | H-2G | Lad | |

After J. Klein, Biology of the mouse histocompatibility-2 complex, New York, 1975, Springer, p. 14.

In addition, a new locus has recently been described (following analysis of recombinants by serology and capping). This lies close to, although independent of, the H-2D locus, and it is known as the H-2L locus. A further locus, the H-2G codes for antigens present on erythrocytes rather than lymphoid cells, but it is of uncertain significance.

One defines as "private" (H-2D or H-2K) specificities those that are observed in a single known haplotype (the haplotype is the set of H-2D, Ir, and II-2K alleles or genes). This definition is in contrast to that of "public" specificities, which are shared by two or more haplotypes. Further refinements consist of separating short public specificities, shared by two or three haplotypes (the most frequent), and long public specificities, shared by more than three haplotypes. Very few private specificities are known because of the limited number of ancestor laboratory mice, but these private specificities are probably very numerous, as indicated by studies of wild mice.

The level of antibody production and the biologic properties of anti-H-2 antibodies (class, cytotoxicity, and agglutinating potency) are quite variable, according to specificity and strain; private specificities often give rise to production of larger amounts of antibodies than do public specificities.

In conclusion, each haplotype bears an H-2K and an H-2D allele. Each allele is characterized by a particular antigenic specificity (private specificity) and/or by one or several public specificities, which may be found in other alleles. Studies performed in congenic mice (which differ by a single antigen; see p. 654) have shown that differences at both the D and the K extremities lead to skin graft rejection.

Two strains of mice, which are genetically identical except for a single locus, are described as being coisogenic. True coisogenicity is the result of point mutations in a pure strain. Partial coisogenicity may be obtained by a series of crossings that conserve the genetic material of one strain while retaining only a single gene of another strain (Fig. 23.1). Partially coisogenic strains, that is, strains that differ not only at the desired locus but also (probably) at the level of a chromosomal segment of indeterminate length adjacent to this locus, are described as congenic. Congenic strains that differ at a histocompatibility locus and consequently reject tissue grafts from the complementary strains are described as resistant congenic strains.

### Non-H-2 Systems

Mice from different strains but with the same H-2 specificities generally reject allografts, but only after a long delay, sometimes more than 100 days. Antigens responsible for this (delayed) rejection may be grouped into histocompatibility systems analogous to H-2. On the basis of the percentage of graft survival from parents to $F_1$ hybrids between partially purified strains, or between mice derived from multiple backcrosses—it has been estimated that in the mouse there are 15–30 minor histocompatibility systems, together including more than 500 genes. Isolation of these different systems has benefited greatly from the use of congenic mice, obtained by maintaining (by means of selected breeding) an exclusive difference at the level of one locus.

Thus, 10 non-H-2 loci have been described, and 16 others are under study.

**Table 23.3  D and K Series of H-2 Specifities**

| Haplotype H-2 | K-series antigens — Public | | | | | | | | | | | | | | | | | | | | Pri-vate | Main strains |
|---|---|---|---|---|---|---|---|---|---|---|---|---|---|---|---|---|---|---|---|---|---|---|
| | 1 | 3 | 5 | 7 | 8 | 11 | 25 | 27 | 28 | 29 | 34 | 35 | 36 | 37 | 38 | 39 | 42 | 45 | 46 | 47 | vate | |
| b | —* | — | 5 | — | — | — | — | 27 | 28 | 29 | — | 35 | 36 | — | — | 39 | — | — | 46 | — | 33 | A.BY, C57BL/6, C57BL/IO |
| d | — | 3 | — | — | 8 | — | — | 27† | 28 | 29 | 34 | — | — | — | — | — | — | — | 46 | 47 | 31 | BALB/c, DBA/2, NZB |
| j | 1? | — | ‡ | 7 | 8 | — | — | 27? | 28? | 29? | — | — | — | 37 | 38 | 39 | — | 45 | 46 | — | 15 | |
| k | 1 | 3 | 5 | — | 8 | 11 | 25 | ·§ | · | — | — | — | — | — | 38 | — | — | 45 | 46? | 47? | 23 | AKR, CBA, C3H |
| p | 1 | — | 5 | 7 | 8 | — | — | — | — | — | 34? | — | — | 37 | 38 | — | — | — | 46? | · | 16 | |
| q | 1 | 3 | 5 | — | — | 11 | — | — | 34 | — | — | — | — | — | — | — | — | 45 | — | 47 | 17 | DBA/1 |
| r | 1 | 3 | 5 | — | 8 | 11 | 25 | — | — | — | — | — | — | — | — | — | — | 45 | — | 47 | · | |
| s | 1 | — | 5 | 7 | — | — | — | · | — | — | — | 35 | 36 | — | — | — | 42 | 45 | · | — | 19 | SJL |
| u | c‡ | — | 5 | — | 8? | — | — | — | — | — | — | — | — | — | — | — | — | 45 | · | · | 20 | |
| v | 1 | 3 | 5 | — | — | — | — | · | · | — | — | — | — | — | — | — | — | 45? | — | · | 21 | |
| z | — | · | 5 | — | — | — | — | 27 | — | 29 | — | — | — | — | — | — | — | — | 46 | 47 | ? | |

## D-series antigens

| H-2 | 1 | 3 | 5 | 6 | 13 | 27 | 28 | 29 | 35 | 36 | 41 | 42 | 43 | 44 | 49 | Private | Main strains |
|-----|---|---|---|---|----|----|----|----|----|----|----|----|----|----|----|---------|--------------|
| b | — | — | — | 6 | — | 27 | 28 | 29 | — | — | — | — | — | — | — | 2 | A.BY, C57BL/6, C57BL/IO |
| d | — | 3 | — | 6 | 13 | 27 | 28 | 29 | 35 | 35 | 41 | 42 | 43 | 44 | 49 | 4 | BALB/c, DBA/2, NZB |
| j | — | · | — | 6 | — | 27 | ? | ? | — | — | — | — | — | 44 | — | 9 | |
| k | 1 | 3 | 5 | — | — | — | — | — | — | — | — | — | — | — | 49 | 32 | AKR, CBA, C3H |
| p | 1 | 3 | 5 | 6 | — | — | — | — | 35 | — | 41 | — | — | — | 49 | ? | |
| q | — | 3 | — | 6 | 13 | 27 | 28 | 29 | c‡ | c‡ | — | — | — | — | 49 | 30 | DBA/1 |
| r | 1 | · | 5 | 6 | — | — | — | — | — | — | — | — | — | — | 49 | 18? | |
| s | — | 3 | — | 6 | — | 27? | 28 | 29 | c‡ | 36 | — | 42 | 43 | — | 49 | 12 | SJL |
| u | — | 3 | — | · | 13? | 27? | 28 | 29 | — | — | 41 | 42 | 43 | — | 49 | 4 | |
| v | — | — | — | · | · | —? | 28? | · | — | — | — | — | 43 | — | 49 | 30 | |
| z | — | — | — | 6 | — | · | · | · | — | — | — | — | — | — | · | 30 | |

\* Absence of an antigen.
? Presence or absence of an antigen is uncertain.
‡ Some antisera give cross-reactions with the indicated H-2 haplotype.
§ Unknown.

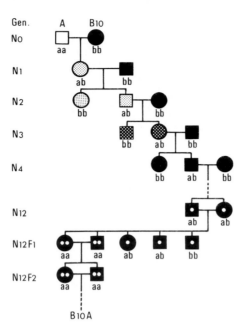

**Fig. 23.1** Production of congenic strains. A(aa) and B10(bb) mice are crossed and their descendants (ab) are back-crossed repeatedly with B10(bb) mice. At the twelfth generation, these descendants are crossed with one-another. The mice resulting from this crossing, being exclusively H-2ᵃ(aa), may then be considered as homozygotes and congenic (B10-A) to B10 mice from which they only differ by the chromosome segment corresponding to the a gene. (After J. Klein, Biology of the mouse histocompatibility-2 complex: principles of immunogenetics applied to a single system, New York, 1975, Springer, p. 32.)

H-1 and H-4 loci are located on the seventh chromosome, and H-3 and H-13 loci (weaker) are present on the second chromosome. H-5 and H-6 loci, also borne by the second chromosome, do not induce skin-graft rejection and are therefore not really histocompatibility loci (they are, rather, called Ea loci, because they are also found on erythrocytes and are, in fact, the analogs of human erythrocytic groups). Other loci are not localized (H-7 to H-30). In addition, there are histocompatibility genes on the X and Y chromosomes, which explains why, within one strain, grafts from males to females are rejected, whereas grafts from females to males are accepted. The development of male antigens depends on male hormones, because neonatal castration prevents their appearance. Administration of androgens does not induce their appearance in females.

The number of alleles per locus is variable and still rather hypothetical (12 for H-1, five for H-3, and four for H-7). The duration of graft survival between mice congenic at one non-H-2 locus varies considerably with the locus (20 days for H-4, 33 days for H-7, 37 days for H-8, 50 days for H-3, 71 days for H-10, 73 days for H-13, 164 days for H-11, and more than 250 days for H-1, H-9, and H-12). These values are only general estimates, because antigenic strength in a given system varies with the alleles present.

Slow rejection linked to non-H-2 systems permits study of factors not evident in the course of overwhelming H-2 graft rejections. It has thus been shown that large grafts sensitize more than small ones but are rejected less rapidly; that females respond better than do males; and that the weaker the system, the easier the induction of a nonresponse state (tolerance or facilitation). Non-H-2 antigens do not induce significant antibody production and are essentially detected by graft experiments. Non-H-2 differences often exhibit a cumulative effect and cooperate with H-2 differences.

### Hybrid Resistance

Applying the laws outlined by Snell, one would normally expect that a graft from a parent to an $F_1$ offspring would always be accepted. In fact, there exist a few exceptions to this rule when dissociated cellular suspensions are used. This "hybrid resistance" is controlled by the D extremity of the H-2 region. Cudkcowicz has shown that this phenomenon is probably explained by the presence of H-2-linked recessive genes. These genes in the homozygous parent code for the presence of antigens that are absent from the $F_1$ heterozygote. The locus in question has been called the "hybrid histocompatibility" or "hematopoietic" locus (Hh). This rejection system, which may have considerable significance after bone marrow grafting, surprisingly is radioresistant and not augmented by immunization. Hybrid resistance may be compared with the phenomenon of allogeneic inhibition whereby parental tumor cells or embryonic cells may be destroyed in vitro by $F_1$ cells. The causative cell is not a T cell but is derived from the bone marrow. It can be distinguished from precursors of antibody-forming cells. It has been termed the M cell. It has recently been suggested that it may be related to the NK cells with which it shares numerous similarities.

## HLA SYSTEM IN MAN

### HLA Antigens

In 1958, Dausset described the first human leukocyte group, the "Mac" group. It was soon shown that the histocompatibility system in man, called HLA (human leukocyte, locus A), was extremely complex. Several international workshops have classified more than 25 different groups. The HLA system is the equivalent of the H-2 system of the mouse and resembles it in many aspects. There are two major loci, HLA-A and HLA-B, with, respectively, about 13 and 19 alleles. There is also a third locus, HLA-C, localized between HLA-A and HLA-B (T1, T2, . . . antigens) and linked to the HLA-B locus. Each HLA allele controls the synthesis of an antigenic product borne by a particular molecule, but each of these molecules possesses several determinants, some of them specific to the HLA molecule (private specificities) and others shared with other HLA molecules, (public specificities). All of these private and public determinants probably occur on a single molecule, as suggested by simultaneous capping of private and public specificities.

Each individual possesses on each chromosome one allele per locus. These alleles are transmitted like codominant traits; that is, they are all expressed in the heterozygote. An example is given in Figure 23.2. Each parent transmits a haplotype. It is clear that every individual possesses one haplotype in common with each parent (haplo-identity) and that siblings may be identical (four identical antigens), haplo-identical (two antigens in common), or different (four different antigens). All HLA antigens are not yet known, and there are cases in which the four antigens cannot be determined (familial studies show that the absence of the antigen in question is not linked to homozygosity at one of the two loci). Recombinations between the two main loci are rare (of the order of

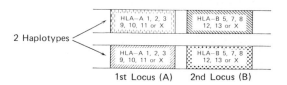

2 Haplotypes

1st Locus (A)          2nd Locus (B)

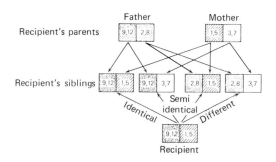

Fig. 23.2 Familial transmission of HLA antigens. Application to donor selection in organ transplantation. The father and mother always have one HLA haplotype in common with their children. A brother or sister may have 0, 1, or 2 haplotypes in common with each other.

0.5–1%, as in the mouse). It is, however, these recombinations that have made possible the demonstration of the presence of two distinct loci (Table 23.4).

When an individual is immunized with cells from a subject having the HLA antigens in common with him (e.g., HLA-A2, B5, and B12) and differing from him by one antigen (e.g., A3 in place of A9), the individual develops antibodies against the different antigen (anti-A3) and occasionally also develops antibodies against another antigen (for example, anti-A11). In the example cited, the donor cells absorb all the anti-A11 antibodies, even though they do not express the A11 phenotype. A number of cross-reactivities similar to the A3-A11 association have been demonstrated between antigens coded for by the same locus. Several antigenic determinants may be defined on each antigen molecule, the intensity of the cross-reaction depending on the number of common determinants. It is difficult to say whether or not these cross-reactions correspond to a similarity of private determinant structure or if several categories of antibody molecule exist, of which one recognizes a common public determinant. However, it is clear from data obtained from biochemical and capping studies that three HLA cistrons give rise to 3 distinct HLA-A, B, and C molecules and that only a single molecule exists per cistron (probably with 3 or 4 sites per molecule).

Because the number of alleles per locus is very high (Table 23.5), the number of possible haplotypes is considerable (more than 1700) and corresponds to a number of genotypes close to $10^6$. In the absence of association between the various alleles of the three SD loci, the frequency of each HLA haplotype should be a direct function of the frequency of each allele. However, such associations do exist in certain cases: A1 (first locus) and B8 (second locus) antigens are more frequently associated (6% cases) than would be expected from mere random association (1–2% cases). Similar findings have been reported for A3-B7 and A2-B12, which correspond to, in genetic terminology, "linkage disequilibrium," which results from a still obscure mechanism. It may involve selection or genetic derivation, or, more probably, it may be due to

**Table 23.4  Complete List of HLA Specificities (With New Terminology, as of January 1, 1977)**

| First SD(A) locus (formerly for some authors LA) | | Second SD(B) locus (formerly for some authors 4) | | Third SD(C) locus (formerly AJ) | | First LD(D) locus | |
|---|---|---|---|---|---|---|---|
| New terminology | Old terminology | New terminology | Old terminology | New terminology | Old terminology | New terminology | Old terminology |
| HLA-A1 | HL-A1 | HLA-B5 | HL-A5 | HLA-Cw1 | T1 | HLA-Dw1 | LD101 or W5a |
| HLA-A2 | HL-A2 | HLA-B7 | HL-A7 | HLA-Cw2 | T2 | HLA-Dw2 | LD102 or 7a |
| HLA-A3 | HL-A3 | HLA-B8 | HL-A8 | HLA-Cw3 | T3 | HLA-Dw3 | LD103 or 8a |
| HLA-A9 | HL-A9 | HLA-B12 | HL-A12 | HLA-Cw4 | T4 | HLA-Dw4 | LD104 or 12a |
| HLA-A10 | HL-A10 | HLA-B13 | HL-A13 | HLA-Cw5 | T5 | HLA-Dw5 | LD105 or 16a |
| HLA-A11 | HL-A11 | HLA-B14 | W14 | | | HLA-Dw6 | LD106 or 15a |
| HLA-A28 | W28 | HLA-B18 | W18 | | | HLA-Dw7 | LD107 |
| HLA-A29 | W29 | HLA-B27 | W27 | | | HLA-Dw8 | LD108 or Colin |
| HLA-Aw19 | Li$^e$ | HLA-Bw15 | W15 | | | | |
| HLA-Aw23 | W23 | HLA-Bw17 | W16 | | | | |
| HLA-Aw24 | W24 | HLA-Bw21 | W17 | | | | |
| HLA-Aw25 | W25 | HLA-Bw22 | W21 | | | | |
| HLA-Aw26 | W26 | HLA-Bw35 | W22 | | | | |
| HLA-Aw30 | W30 | HLA-Bw37 | W5 | | | | |
| HLA-A31 | W31 | | TY | | | | |
| HLA-Aw32 | W32 | HLA-Bw38 | W16.1 (Da31)  or | | | | |
| HLA-Aw33 | W19.6 | HLA-Bw39 | W16.2 (U18)  or | | | | |
| HLA-Aw34 | Malay 2 | HLA-Bw40 | W10 | | | | |
| HLA-Aw36 | Mo | HLA-Bw41 | Sabell (Da34)  or | | | | |
| HLA-Aw43 | BK | HLA-Bw42 | MWA | | | | |

**Table 23.5  Cross Reactions Between HLA Antigens**

| A locus | + + | A1, A3, A11 |
|---------|-----|-------------|
|         |     | A2, A28 |
|         | +   | A9, Aw29, A30, A32, A33, A31 |
| B locus | + + | B5, Bw31, Bw15, Bw21 |
|         |     | B7, Bw40, B27, Bw22 |
|         |     | B8, B14 |

population mixing, none of these hypotheses being mutually exclusive. The most frequently observed linkage disequilibria are the following: A1-B8-DW3, A2-B12 (particularly frequent in Great Britain), A3-B7, and A3-BW35. The linkage is even stronger for certain rare antigens—A29-B12 (frequent in Basques), A1-B17, A33-B14, A30-B13.

Important differences may exist in the frequencies of various alleles from one population to another. Thus, HLA-A1 and HLA-B8 alleles are particularly frequent in caucasians (including Europeans), whereas HLA-BW21 is essentially observed in the Mediterranean areas. A13 and BW22 antigens are especially frequent in Oceania. Conceivably, these facts may be of interest for retrospective studies of geographic migrations of populations.

## OTHER SPECIES

In the rat, the major histocompatibility locus is the Rt-1, H-1, or Ag-B locus (Table 23.7). There also are, as in the mouse, minor histocompatibility systems; these systems would explain, for example, the rapid rejection of skin grafts between Lewis and Fischer rats, which both have the Ag-B1 antigen. Major histocompatibility systems have also been described in the dog (DLA), *Macacus rhesus* (Rh LA), pig (PLA or SLA), rabbit (RLA), and even in the frog. In the chicken, the B-group locus is probably the major histocompatibility locus, but knowledge is less advanced in this species than in the others mentioned above. In some of these species, particularly the monkey and the pig, study of the LD antigens has already been initiated, and linkage between genes that control LD antigens and those that control SD antigens has been established.

## III.  ANTIGENS INDUCING LYMPHOCYTE PROLIFERATION (LD ANTIGENS) (CLASS II)

We have so far examined sero-defined (SD) antigens. There also exist, however, as mentioned above, structures (probably antigens) that selectively stimulate blast transformation in the mixed-lymphocyte reaction and probably in graft versus host reactions, the LD antigens. LD antigens are distinct from SD antigens. However, they are controlled by genes close to those that control SD antigens and are therefore also located in the major histocompatibility region. In addition, as will be seen further on, the LD genes are identical or at least

**Table 23.6  Frequency of the HLA-A, B, C, D and DR Genes and Antigens in the French Population**

| A Locus | | | B Locus | | |
|---|---|---|---|---|---|
| *Antigens* | *Antigen* | *Gene* | *Antigens* | *Antigen* | *Gene* |
| A1 | 25.1 | 13.4 | B5 | 15.2 | 7.9 |
| A2 | 44.8 | 25.7 | B7 | 18.2 | 9.5 |
| A3 | 22.6 | 12.0 | B8 | 16.7 | 8.7 |
| Aw23 } A9 | 4.3 | 2.2 | B12 | 32.5 | 17.8 |
| Aw24 } A9 | 18.2 | 9.5 | B13 | 5.4 | 2.7 |
| Aw25 } A10 | 3.9 | 1.9 | B14 | 8.8 | 4.5 |
| Aw26 } A10 | 8.3 | 4.2 | B18 | 11.3 | 5.8 |
| | | | | | |
| A11 | 11.8 | 6.0 | B27 | 7.8 | 4.0 |
| A28 | 9.8 | 5.0 | Bw35 (W5) | 15.2 | 7.9 |
| A29 | 10.3 | 5.3 | Bw40 (W10) | 13.7 | 7.1 |
| Aw30 | 2.4 | 1.2 | Bw15 | 12.3 | 6.3 |
| Aw31 | 6.8 | 3.5 | Bw39 } Bw16 | 0.9 | 0.4 |
| Aw32 | 9.8 | 5.0 | Bw38 } Bw16 | 2.4 | 1.2 |
| Aw33 | 1.9 | 0.9 | Bw17 | 5.9 | 3.0 |
| Others including | | 4.9 | Bw21 | 4.9 | 2.4 |
| Aw19, Aw23, | | | Bw22 | 7.1 | 3.7 |
| Aw24, A25, A26, | | | Bw37 | 2.9 | 1.4 |
| Aw34, Aw36 and | | | Bw41 | 4.9 | 2.4 |
| Aw43 | | | Others including | | 4.4 |
| | | | B15, Bw16, B17, | | |
| | | | B18, Bw21, Bw22, | | |
| | | | B37, Bw38, Bw39, | | |
| | | | Bw41, Bw63 | | |

| Locus C | | | Locus D | | |
|---|---|---|---|---|---|
| *Antigens* | *Antigen* | *Gene* | *Antigens* | *Antigen* | *Gene* |
| Cw1 | 10.0 | 5.0 | Dw1 | 19.3 | 10.2 |
| Cw2 | 14.9 | 8.0 | Dw2 | 15.2 | 7.8 |
| Cw3 | 26.0 | 14.6 | Dw3 | 16.4 | 8.5 |
| Cw4 | 19.7 | 11.1 | Dw4 | 15.6 | 8.2 |
| Cw5 | 14.0 | 7.4 | Dw5 | 14.6 | 7.5 |
| Others including | | 53.9 | Dw6 | 10.5 | 5.4 |
| Cw6, Cw7 and Cw8 | | | Others including | | 52.4 |
| | | | Dw7, Dw8, Dw9, | | |
| | | | Dw10, Dw11 and | | |
| | | | Dw12 | | |

| Locus DR | | | | | |
|---|---|---|---|---|---|
| *Antigens* | *Antigen* | *Gene* | *Antigens* | *Antigen* | *Gene* |
| DRw1 | 15.1 | 7.90 | DRw6 | 21.7 | 11.5 |
| DRw2 | 18.1 | 9.53 | DRw7 | 11.2 | 5.76 |
| DRw3 | 18.1 | 9.53 | DRw8 | 5.0 | 2.54 |
| DRw4 | 9.9 | 5.11 | Others including | 62.8 | 39.1 |
| DRw5 | 17.2 | 9 | DRw9 and DRw10 | | |

After G. Snell, J Dausset, and S Nathanson.

#### Table 23.7   Histocompatibility of Pure Rat Strains

| Rt-1 | H-1 | | Ag-B | | Main strain |
|------|-----|---|------|---|-------------|
| a | a | 4 | | | (DA) |
| b | b | 6 | | | Buffalo (BUF) |
| c | c | 5 | | | August (AUG) |
| d | d | 9 | | | BD V |
|   | e | 10 | | | BD VII |
| f | f | 10 | | | AS 2 |
| i | i | 1 | AS Fisher Lewis | | (FI) (LEW) |
| n | n | 3 | Brown-Norway | | (BN) |
| v | w | 2 | Wistar/Forth Yoshida | | (WF) (YO) |
| g | g | 7 | | | KGH |
| k | k | 8 | | | WKA |
| d | d | d | | | |

Examples: Ag-B$^4$, H-y$^a$, Rt-1$^a$.

very similar to the Ia or DR genes, giving rise to the population of anti-B-lymphocyte antibodies.

## MICE

Mixed-lymphocyte reactions between pure ordinary strains do not allow the demonstration of LD antigens, because most combinations with or without H-2 and non-H-2 differences give rise to positive reactions, without a correlation between the intensity of the response and antigenic strength evaluated serologically. The particular intensity of the response between strains that have differences only at the H-2 locus, however, indicates the essential role of the H-2 region in the control of the mixed-lymphocyte reaction (MLR).

Studies of recombinants have revealed that differences at the H-2K extremity are sufficient to provoke blast proliferation, whereas isolated differences at the H-2D extremity induce less stimulation. There is, in fact, an important LD locus close to, but distinct from, the H-2K extremity. In addition, there exists an LD locus close to, or identical with, the immune response gene loci (see chap. 24); recombinations that provoke differences in the I and Ss SIp regions without H-2D or H-2K difference give rise to a positive MLR, and, conversely, recombinations that involve H-2K locus differences but without I-region differences lead to little stimulation. In addition, recombinations that lack H-2K, I, or H-2D differences but that possess Ss SIp incompatibility result in little stimulation. There could be other LD loci in the H-2 region between the Ir, and Ss SIp loci and the Ss SIp region. In fact identification and classification of LD loci remains difficult, and some authors believe that the products of numerous H-2 region genes are capable of stimulating an MLR. In addition, another locus, M, which is independent of the H-2 complex, controls MLR independently of H-2 differences.

## MAN

Lymphocytes from HLA-identical siblings usually give rise to a negative MLR, whereas a strongly positive response is observed when HLA differences exist; the response is particularly clear-cut when the two haplotypes are different. These results suggests first that SD antigens control the MLR. Several recent observations, however, invalidate this simple hypothesis: the MLR is usually strongly positive in apparently nonrelated subjects who are identical at HLA-A and -B loci; a positive MLR is observed in 1% of cases between two HLA-A and -B identical siblings; and, in certain families, one observes the absence of stimulation despite the existence of differences at both HLA-A and -B loci. Systematic studies of recombinations between both A and B loci have shown that incompatibilities isolated on the first locus yield a weak or negative MLR, whereas incompatibilities at the second locus produce strong MLR.

Several explanations may be proposed:

It is possible that the MLR is controlled by private SD specificities not yet determined. It then becomes difficult, however, to explain the absence of stimulation in certain recombinations with known SD differences.

Non-HLA-SD differences could also intervene, and a cumulative effect of several of them could explain positive results without SD differences, by possible intervention of preimmunization. The degree of stimulation observed in the absence of SD differences does not favor this hypothesis, however.

The most satisfactory explanation, and the most commonly held, involves an LD locus different from HLA-A and -B loci that control SD antigens. This hypothesis is compatible with the observations mentioned above, particularly the absence of stimulation in certain pairs with an SD difference and the stimulation observed in the absence of SD differences, which are, in this hypothesis, explained by SD/LD recombinations.

Localization of the LD locus has not been definitively established. It seems, however, that there is, in contrast to what is observed in the mouse, a major LD locus located outside the SD locus, to the left of the second SD locus. The localization of a second LD locus, close to the HLA-A locus has been suggested.

One would normally expect from these data a high frequency of positive MLR in nonrelated SD-identical pairs, which probably are not LD identical. In fact, while there is, indeed, a majority of positive MLR between nonrelated SD-identical subjects, the frequency of negative MLR reaches 10% for certain SD haplotype combinations. This frequency indicates the existence of linkage disequilibrium between SD and LD loci, that is, an abnormal association of a few SD and LD alleles, especially with the HLA-A1-B8-DW3 haplotype.

Studies are in progress to define LD locus alleles and, more generally, the immunogenetics of LD antigens. Cells homozygous at the LD locus are used as stimulating cells. Absence of proliferation in response to one of these cells defines its LD group. One may also use "primed LD typing" (PLT). Cells are educated in a 10-day MLC to recognize certain MHC-controlled LD antigens. Such educated cells can be used to test whether the lymphocytes of any one individual carry the LD antigens that the PLT cells were taught to recognize. Eight LD groups have already been individualized, some of them linked to HLA-A and -B groups, such as HLA-B8 and -B7, because of the linkage disequilibrium mentioned above for A1-B8 and A3-B7 haplotypes. Cytotoxicity reactions with B lymphocytes used as target cells (after T-cell elimination) and to a lesser degree MLR inhibition by alloantisera without anti-HLA antibodies (obtained, in particular, from multiparous women or from lupus patients after absorption with platelets) will perhaps make possible a more direct serologic analysis of LD gene products.

In fact, the nature of alloantigens detected on B lymphocytes remains uncertain. Are they LD antigens, as would be suggested by the close or identical segregation of the genes that control some of these antigens and LD antigens, are they equivalent to mouse Ia antigens, which are also coded for by genes of the major histocompatibility region and essentially localized on B lymphocytes, or do they represent still another histocompatibility system?

## IV.  THE Ia AND DR ANTIGENS (CLASS II)

### Ia ANTIGENS

Another type of antigens has been defined following the results of studies on the genetic control of immune responses. These are the Ia antigens in the mouse and DR antigens in man, which appear to play a fundamental role in antigen recognition by T cells and in T- and B-cell interaction. They are related to the LD antigens described above. They are now grouped with these latter under the term class II antigens, which distinguishes them from class I antigens (H-2K and H-2D in the mouse and HLA-A, -B, and -C in man). This new classification appears to be more applicable than the classification into LD and SD antigens.

Independent of the S D antigens coded for by the H-2K and H-2D extremities of the H-2 region, there also exists a family of antigens coded for by the central I region genes and called Ia antigens. These antigens are defined by antibodies obtained by cross-immunization between recombinant mice that only differ from one another at the central portion of the H-2 complex. More than 20 specificities have now been described, but almost certainly many more remain to be discovered. Certain specificities are exclusive to a single haplotype and are therefore considered as private specificities, in contrast with public specificities common to several haplotypes. The public antigens that are controlled by different subregions possess specificities that are able to give rise to cross-reactions, as has been described for the H-2K and H-2D antigens. The majority of Ia specificities have been localized to the I-A subregion, the other specificities being situated in the I-C subregion. More recently, some specificities have been described in the I-E and I-J subregions, the latter coding for determinants present on suppressor T cells between I-B and I-C. No specificity has been described in the I-B subregion, whose existence is questionable anyway.

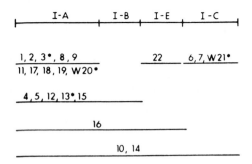

**Fig. 23.3**  Chromosomal location of Ia specificities.

The distribution of Ia antigens on the cell membrane has been studied by means of "capping" experiments that have also shown that the Ia specificities are carried by two different molecular structures and are, therefore, coded for by two different genes. The specificities coded by the I-A subregion migrate simultaneously and independently of those coded by the I-C subregion. This independence of molecules coded by different loci is reminiscent of the observations described for H-2K and H-2D molecules.

However, in contrast to the H-2D and H-2K antigens, Ia antigens are not ubiquitous. They have only been found on B lymphocytes and to a lesser extent on certain T cells (particularly on T cells stimulated by Con A), on macrophages, on spermatozoa, and on epidermal Langerhans' cells. The I subregion also contains the immune response genes, genes coding for determinants that activate lymphocytes in the MLR and cellular cooperation genes. The question arises as to the identity of these genes and those coding for the Ia antigens. Anti-Ia antibodies specifically block the MLR, which suggests that the molecules responsible for the lymphocyte stimulation may well include Ia antigens or products directly related to them. Moreover, several arguments suggest that the Ia antigens are products of the Ir genes, that is, they are in part or wholly responsible for their intervention in the regulation of immune responses. It should also be noted that soluble "helper" or suppressor factors produced by T cells, whether or not antigen-specific, also possess Ia specificity. Macrophages present antigens to T cells in association with Ia antigens. The activation of T cells as evaluated by in vitro proliferation induced by antigens may be blocked by anti-Ia antibodies. In the following chapter we will return to this discussion in further detail (see p. 000).

## DR ANTIGENS

The similarities observed between the H-2 and HLA complexes renders plausible the concept according to which equivalents of the Ia antigens of the mouse exist in man, that is, antigens present on B lymphocytes coded by the MHC and possibly linked to determinants that activate lymphocytes in the MLR and that are also implicated in the regulation of immune responses. The demonstration of a system of alloantigens on B lymphocytes, detected with the help of serum from multiparous women, has confirmed this idea. These antigens are controlled by a locus close to the HLA-D locus, hence their being denoted DR (D-related) antigens.

Sera from multiparous women, repeatedly absorbed with platelets to eliminate antibodies directed against HLA-A, -B, and -C specificities still contain antibodies that bind to allogeneic B cells, upon which they may be detected by indirect immunofluorescence. These "anti-B cell antibodies" are cytotoxic in the presence of complement, this being the basis of the test routinely used for their detection. In practice, peripheral blood lymphocytes are enriched in B cells before performing the cytotoxicity test. A more readily available source of B cells is provided by lymphoblastoid cell lines. Anti-DR antibodies present on lymphocyte membranes block Fc receptors by steric inhibition and inhibit the binding of radiolabeled immunoglobulin aggregates. Serologic methods permit the detection of DR antigens on cells other than B lymphocytes, such as macrophages, epidermal Langerhans' cells, and spermatozoa, this being a similar distribution to that of Ia antigens in the mouse.

Anti-DR antisera inhibit the mixed-lymphocyte reaction. This blockade appears to be exerted on the stimulating B lymphocytes by masking LHA-D determinants. Certain antisera, however, may also act on the responder cells, almost certainly due to the fact that currently employed anti-DR antisera are polyspecific. There is a good correlation between DR-typing by cytotoxicity or immunofluorescence and results of HLA-D typing, which suggests a direct association between the DR and HLA-D antigens. The study of DR antigens in families reveals a parallel distribution with that of the HLA-D specificities, which shows that the genes coding for DR antigens are included in the HLA complex. Several authors hold that the HLA-D and DR loci are confounded, but this contention remains controversial because of the apparent existence of recombinations between the two loci.

# V. BIOCHEMISTRY OF THE MAJOR HISTOCOMPATIBILITY COMPLEX (MHC) PRODUCTS

Considerable information on the biochemical nature of transplantation antigens has accrued over the past few years. The study of the peptide and sugar constituents of the different antigen classes has been made possible by their treatment with proteolytic enzymes (papain); ionic detergents, such as deoxycholate; or nonionic detergents, such as triton. Following this, the components are isolated by Sephadex chromatography, electrophoresis, or sucrose-gradient centrifugation. More recently, the amino acid sequences of a growing number of antigens have been obtained and this has enabled direct comparison of different types of antigens (H-2K or D, Ia or HLA-A, B, D, and DR) in different species.

The H-2K and H-2D antigens in the mouse and HLA-A and B antigens in man are glycoproteins of similar molecular weight (about 45,000) that are directly integrated within the cell membrane (Fig. 23.4). They are noncovalently linked to $\beta_2$-microglobulin, which is a molecule of about 100 amino acid residues of molecular weight 11,600 and showing a close homology with the C3 domain of IgG. The H-2 and HLA antigens contain four units, each being about 100 residues in length. The two central units are bound together by disulfide bridges, the complete assembly possessing a certain similarity with Ig suggesting the possibility of a common evolutionary origin. The carbohydrate moiety, which represents about 10% of the molecule, is constant for different antigens. In other words, it does not contribute to the antigenic specificity. The Ia antigens and HLA-D and DR antigens in man are less well characterized. These are also glycoproteins with, in general, two subunits, one being of molecular weight of about 35,000 ($\alpha$-chain), the other about 28,000 ($\beta$-chain). The two chains which are structurally distinct are tightly but not covalently associated. The molecule of the Ia antigen is not associated with $\beta_2$-microglobulin, unlike the TL and Qa-2 antigens (Fig. 23.5). Recent two-dimensional gel analyses have revealed a fluid polypeptide of molecular weight 31,000 whose significance is still ill-defined.

The partial identification of the amino acid sequences of H-2, Ia, and HLA antigens has revealed some interesting homologies. The K and D antigens are homologous and are probably derived from a common ancestral gene. In addition, the H-2K and D antigens possess considerable homologies with the HLA and B antigens. Simultaneously, homologies between the Ia and DR antigens have also been discerned (Table 23.8).

Both being associated with $\beta_2$-microglobulin, the K and D antigens present several analogies with immunoglobulin molecules, for example, extreme polymorphism, localization in the cell membrane, and implication in immune

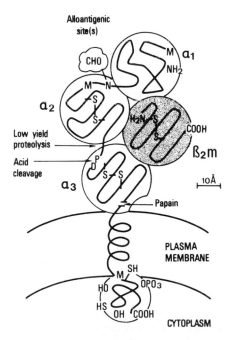

**Fig. 23.4**  Structure of H-2K and H-2D molecules.

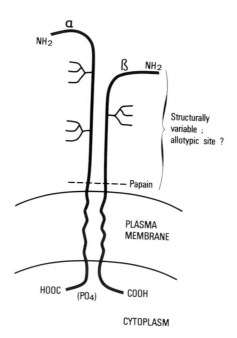

**Fig. 23.5**  Structure of Ia molecule.

responses. Furthermore, although only a marginal similarity exists between the N-terminal part of K and D antigens and that of IgG, one may find in transplantation antigens an internal fragment that has a strong homology with part of the V region of Ig. This homology suggests either that the transplantation antigens and Ig have a common ancestor (divergent evolution) or that the two regions in question acquired similar structures (convergent evolution).

At certain positions, the K and D antigens possess common amino acids that distinguish them from HLA-A and B (species-specific residues). This suggests, but does not prove, that the gene duplication that created the K and D genes occurred after the divergence of the species.

The H-2K$^k$ and H-2k$^b$ antigens differ from one another by 5 residues out of 17 (about 30%) and the H-2D antigens differ by 4 residues out of 14 (about 28%). This involves relatively numerous differences in alleles. The K and D antigens may therefore be regarded as complex allotypes. The partial identification of the sequences of the chains of Ia and DR antigens has also shown the existence of considerable homologies.

# VI.   THE MAJOR HISTOCOMPATIBILITY COMPLEX: IMMUNOGENETICS OF GRAFT REJECTION

## SPECIFICITY OF CYTOTOXIC CELLS

The specificity of allograft rejection may be analyzed by serum antibodies (which define SD antigens), by stimulation of blast transformation (which defines LD antigens), and by detection of effector cells in vitro cytotoxicity reactions (see p. 410). Most studies that have taken advantage of the latter property have been performed with the cell-mediated lympholysis technique (see p. 411), which explores the in vitro generation of cytotoxic cells in the MLR.

In the mouse, the target antigens for in vivo or in vitro sensitized cytotoxic lymphocytes are gene products encoded by the H-2D or H-2K regions of the H-2 complex. These antigenic structures are likely to be the same as the SD antigens, defined by serologic means. However, it has recently been shown that sensitization between two strains of mice differing only for the I-A-subregion generated cytotoxic lymphocytes with specific lytic activity directed against I-A gene products. The reverse situation, namely, that sensitization directed exclusively against SD antigens without LD antigenic participation does also lead to the generation of cytotoxic effector cells, has also been reported.

In man, the absence of a strict correlation between MLR and cytotoxic effects has also been observed; certain genetic combinations give rise to MLR without cytotoxicity or, more rarely, the reverse occurs. The study of recombinants has shown that, as in the mouse, the cytotoxic effect is directed against SD determinants. Cell-mediated lympholysis (CML) is, however, generally

**Table 23.8  N Terminal Amino Acid Sequences of H-2 Antigens, HLA Antigens and B₂-Microglobulin**

| | | Position | | | | | | | | | | | |
|---|---|---|---|---|---|---|---|---|---|---|---|---|---|
| | | 1 | 2 | 3 | 4 | 5 | 6 | 7 | 8 | 9 | 10 | 11 | 12 |
| H-2 antigens (mouse) | H-2Kᵇ | Met | Pro | His | · | Leu | Arg | Tyr | Phe | His | · | Ala | Val |
| | H-2Kᵇ | — | Pro | His | · | Leu | Arg | Tyr | Phe | Val | · | Ala | Val |
| | H-2Kᵈ | Met | — | His | · | — | Arg | Tyr | Phe | · | · | · | · |
| | H-2Dᵈ | Met | Pro? | His | · | Leu | Arg | Tyr | — | Val | · | Ala | Val |
| | H-2Dᵈ | — | Pro | — | · | — | — | Tyr | · | — | · | Ala | Val |
| HLA antigens | HLA-A₂ | Gly | Ser | · | Ser | Met | Arg | Tyr | Phe | Phe | Thr | Ser | Val |
| | HLA-B₇ | Gly | Ser | · | Ser | Met | Arg | Tyr | Phe | Tyr | Thr | Ser | Val |
| | HLA-B₁₂ | Gly | Ser | — | Ser | Met | Val | Tyr | Phe | Tyr | Thr | Ala | Val |
| β₂-microglobulin | Man | Ile | Gln | Arg | Thr | Pro | Lys | Ile | Gln | Val | Tyr | Ser | Arg |
| | Rat | Ile | Gln | Lys | Thr | Pro | Glx | Ile | Gln | Val | Tyr | Ser | Arg |
| | Mouse | | | Lys | | Pro | | | | Val | Tyr | | |

| Position | | | | | | | | | | | | | | |
|---|---|---|---|---|---|---|---|---|---|---|---|---|---|---|
| 13 | 14 | 15 | 16 | 17 | 18 | 19 | 20 | 21 | 22 | 23 | 24 | 25 | 26 | 27 |
| · | Ile | Pro | · | Leu | · | Lys | Pro | Phe | Ala | · | · | · | · | Tyr |
| · | Arg | Pro | · | Leu | · | — | — | Arg | Tyr | · | · | · | · | Tyr |
| · | · | · | · | · | · | · | · | · | · | · | · | · | · | · |
| · | · | Pro | · | — | · | — | Pro | · | Tyr | · | · | · | · | · |
| · | Arg | Pro | · | Leu | · | — | Pro | Arg | Tyr | · | · | · | · | · |
| Ser | · | · | Gly | · | Gly | Glu | · | · | Phe | Ile | · | Val | · | · |
| Ser | Arg? | Pro | Gly | · | Gly | Glu | · | · | Phe | Ile | · | Val | · | · |
| Ser | Arg? | Pro | Gly | · | Gly | Glu | · | · | Phe | Ile | · | Val | · | · |
| His | Pro | Ala | Glu | Asn | Gly | Lys | Ser | Asn | Phe | Leu | Asn | Lys | Try | Val |
| His | Pro | Pro | Glu | Asn | Gly | Lys | Pro | Asn | Phe | Leu | Asn | Lys | Tyr | Val |
| · | Pro | Pro | · | · | · | Lys | Pro | · | · | Leu | · | · | Tyr | Val |

associated with lymphocytic proliferation, which seems to have a potent helper effect. It is important to note that SD and LD antigens may not necessarily be present on the same cells because addition of lymphocytes that differ at the LD locus, but without SD differences to responder cells, permits the lymphocytes to generate a cytotoxic reaction against cells that differ only at the SD locus (and are LD identical).

Cytotoxic T lymphocytes can also be generated after sensitization against antigens which are not encoded by the MHC. This is in particular the case for viral antigens, haptenic alterations of syngeneic cells, or even minor histocompatibility antigens. Yet even under those circumstances, the cytotoxic phase is controlled by the MHC: educated T cells will recognize the sensitizing antigen most efficiently on syngeneic target cells. Initial observations were made by Zinkernagel and Doherty in mouse lymphochoriomeningitis (LCM). T cells from LCM-virus-infested mice are cytotoxic toward LCM-virus-infested lymphoid cells. However such cytotoxicity is restricted to virus-infested cells sharing the same H-2 complex with the killer cells.

This requirement for syngeneicity between killer and target cell is restricted to the K and/or D extremities of the MHC. Two kinds of explanations were proposed when this phenomenon was first described in the viral model of Doherty and Zingernagel and in a model of haptenic (TNP) modification of autologous spleen cells by Shearer. In the first hypothesis, cytotoxic T cells have two distinct receptors, one recognizing the sensitizing antigen and the other syngeneic H-2 antigens, the activation of both receptors being a requisite for triggering the cytotoxic process. In the second hypothesis, the antigen introduces a modification of H-2 antigens and it is this "altered self" which is recognized as a whole. Several experimental arguments argue in favor of the second hypothesis, such as (1) the absence of cytotoxic $F_1$ killer cells after sensitization against modified parental cells when testing against the other modified parent; (2) the absence of cytotoxicity inhibition when adding cold, unlabelled target cells, whether syngeneic unmodified or allogeneic modified; (3) the absence of cross-reactivity between wild and H-2 mutant target cells modified by the same virus; and (4) the absence of cytotoxicity against TNP-sensitized spleen cells when TNP is separated from spleen cell antigens by a tripeptide spacer. However, other lines of evidence suggest that T cells are endowed with two types of receptors, one type recognizing conventional antigens and the other being directed against determinants controlled by various segments of the MHC, in particular in T-cell cooperation with B cells or in T cell-mediated delayed hypersensitivity. The definitive explanation for restricted cytotoxicity remains to be established. It could be a compromise between both hypotheses, each T cell carrying two receptors encoded by two unrelated variable region genes but phenotypically associated in one single unit recognizing the antigen linked to products of MHC genes.

## GENETIC COMPOSITION OF THE MAJOR HISTOCOMPATIBILITY COMPLEX (CHROMOSOMAL CHART)

We have just alluded to the complexity of loci that control the production of histocompatibility antibodies, MLR, and generation of cytotoxic cells. In addi-

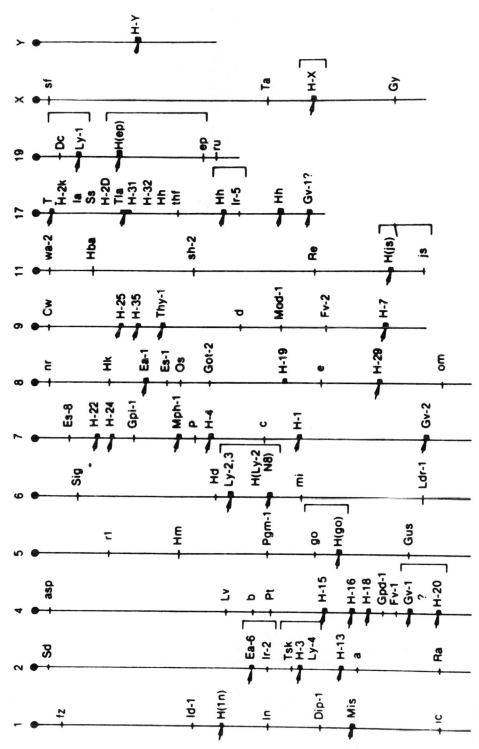

**Fig. 23.6** Chromosomal map of the mouse showing the chromosomes coding for membrane alloantigens (arrows). The other markers indicated are not involved in immune responses. (After G. D. Snell, J. Dausset, and S. Nathanson. Histocompatibility. New York, 1976, Academic Press, p. 28.)

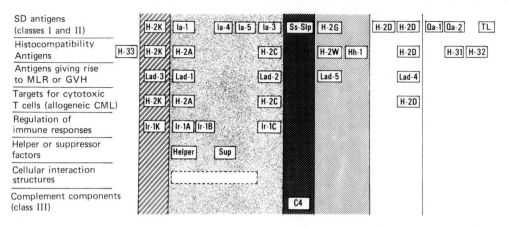

**Fig. 23.7** Functions controlled by different regions of the major histocompatibility complex. The presence of several genes in a given region does not necessarily imply that they belong to the same locus. (After J. Klein, Adv. Immunol. 1978, 26, 57.)

tion, we have seen that other genes are localized in the same region. We will now attempt to draw a chart of the major histocompatibility complex in the mouse and in man.

### H-2 Region

The serum level of the Ss protein (serum serologic), which is an $\alpha_2\beta$-globulin and probably the equivalent of the fourth component of complement in man, is present in the mouse at different levels (high or low) and is controlled by H-2 region genes. The same applies for another serum protein, "sex-limited" protein (Slp), observed in males, which is controlled by a gene identical to the Ss gene or very close to it. The Qa-1 and Qa-2 antigens are expressed on certain lymphocyte subpopulations. They are controlled by genes situated to the right of the H-2D locus. TL antigen, expressed on thymocytes and on certain leukemic cells (see p. 65), is controlled by the Tla region, close to the H-2D locus. Similarly, it seems that the θ antigen could be controlled by genes of the H-2 region, although it is not yet apparent whether regulation of the amount of θ antigen per cell or the number of θ⁺ cells is at issue. Some sexual characteristics linked to the serum level of testosterone and of its carrier protein are controlled by H-2K region genes, the Hom-1 genes (hormone metabolic). H-2 region genes control factors that inhibit the growth of allogeneic hemato-poietic cells (independently of classic SD or LD antigens); they are the Hh-1 factors. Lastly, H-2 region genes control RgV-1 factors and the susceptibility of mice to Gross leukemia virus and to other tumorigenic viruses. There does not appear to be any obvious relationship between these different markers and LD or SD genes (except perhaps for Hh-1 and RgV-1 genes, which are associated with immune responses). Such a relationship is, however, suspected for the immune response (Ir) genes (see chap. 24), also located in the H-2 region. The precise location of these genes in the H-2 region will be discussed in the next chapter.

In conclusion, it is still impossible to draw a definitive chart of the H-2 region, but the markers mentioned above, which permit precise analysis of recombinations inside the H-2 region, should make rapid progress possible. Figure 23.8 represents the map of the H-2 region according to present beliefs.

The identification of markers that are close to but outside the H-2 complex has been extremely useful. Thus, the T/t locus controls numerous embryonic abnormalities—malformation of the tail in heterozygotes (T/t), lethal malformation in homozygotes (T/T). This region has interesting possibilities since it appears to code for membrane molecules that are necessary for embryonic cellular interactions and could therefore represent the equivalent of the H-2 region, which, in the adult, controls cellular interactions in the immune response. Figure 23.8 represents the H-2 region with 12 known loci; K, Ia-1, Ia-4, Ia-3, Ss, Slp, G, D, L, Qa-1, Qa-2, and Tla.

### HLA Region

Markers in the HLA region are less numerous than in the H-2 region. Ir genes are only beginning to be studied, and it is obvious that knowledge will progress more slowly in man than in the mouse. Most data on SD and LD genes are obtained from family studies (Fig. 23.2). Nevertheless, it may be recalled that a link exists between certain components of the complement system and the HLA region (see p. 283). The polymorphism of factor B (Bf or C3PA) of C2 and of C4 is linked to HLA antigens and may be provisionally localized to the left of the HLA-D locus. In addition, it has recently been shown that the erythrocytic antigens, *Chido* and *Rodgers*, are in fact C4 components that have become secondarily attached to red cells. Other markers are known to lie close to the HLA region: erythrocytic glyco-oxalase (GLO) and the third enzyme of

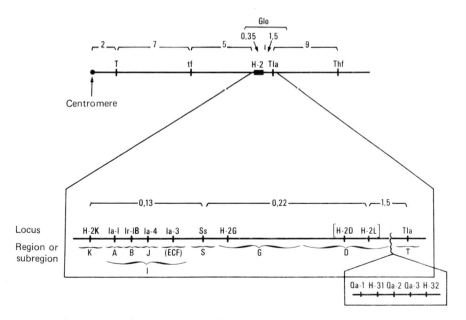

**Fig. 23.8**  The H-2 complex in the mouse (on the 17th chromosome).

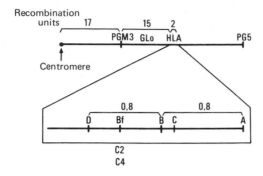

**Fig. 23.9**   The HLA complex in man (on the sixth chromosome).

phosphoglucomutase-3 (PGM-3). All these genes, like the HLA region, have been localized on the short arm of the 6th chromosome by means of cellular hybridization data and the study of families with pericentric inversion (Fig. 23.9).

## CONCLUSIONS: GENES AND ANTIGENS THAT INTERVENE IN GRAFT REJECTION

At this point, it appears useful to discuss what are, finally, the antigenic specificities responsible for skin or organ graft rejection.

In the mouse, the predominant role of the H-2 region is well established because skin grafts between congenic mice that differ only in the H-2 region are rapidly rejected. In addition, between ordinary mice of pure strains, H-2 differences regularly induce production of anti-H-2 antibodies, MLR, CML, and rapid graft rejection. Grafts between mice that differ at one of the two H-2K or H-2D loci are rejected, whereas grafts between recombinant mice that differ only at regions between the H-2K and H-2D extremities are not always rejected (even when differences include the S and I regions, sometimes with a positive MLR). However, graft rejections are observed when there are differences that bear on certain segments distinct from the H-2D extremities, particularly in the I-A and Tla regions, which suggests the existence of other histocompatibility loci. Even a fourth histocompatibility locus could exist in the region between the H-2D and Ir-1 loci. It is interesting to note, in this respect, that H-2K differences lead to more severe graft-versus-host reactions and more rapid rejection of allogeneic skin or tumor grafts than do H-2D differences. In addition, anti-H-2K antibodies are of higher titer than are anti-H-2D antibodies.

Whereas SD antigens may induce rejection even without an LD difference, induction of rejection by LD differences alone without SD differences, remains to be proven unequivocally. M locus differences, which induce the MLR, do not by themselves lead to graft rejection. The role of Ia antigens remains uncertain. Recent data (to be confirmed) give them a preferential role in the induction of tolerance (and facilitation?). With respect to the graft-versus-host reaction, it appears that the proliferation phase, the in vivo counterpart of the MLR, involves LD loci and that the cytotoxic phase involves SD loci. One must, however, point out that LD and SD loci are close together; the frequency of recombination between these loci is less than 1%.

Independent of these histocompatibility antigens, other organ antigen systems exist that may precipitate graft rejection. One example is the SK system, which controls the expression of alloantigens present on skin and brain. At this point, we might also mention the (ubiquitous) antigens present in males that may give rise to skin graft rejection in purely syngeneic combinations and that are therefore histocompatibility antigens. In man, much less data are available. HLA identity among siblings is associated with prolonged skin or kidney graft survival (Fig. 23.10), but skin grafts are still rejected within 20–25 days. Less clear-cut results, but still significant, have been reported between nonrelated subjects for skin grafts. Correlations between duration of kidney graft survival and HLA compatibility, the practical interest of which is obvious, have been the matter of considerable controversy. Whereas most authors do recognize the excellent correlation obtained when the donor is related to the recipient, this is not the case for grafts between nonrelated pairs. It is clear, however, that corroborative statistics obtained, particularly in France, England, the Netherlands, and Scandinavia, have revealed significant differences; the results are better in cases of good matches (HLA identity or one antigen mismatch) (Fig. 23.11). This justified the establishment of national and European organizations (France and Euro-Transplant) that enable transplant teams to select the best recipient when a cadaver kidney becomes available for grafting (with, of course, no ABO incompatibility and no preformed cytotoxic antibodies against the donor's lymphocytes, which might lead to hyperacute rejection). The longer survival of grafts between related (than between nonrelated) pairs for an equal number of HLA incompatibilities may be explained by the still insufficient

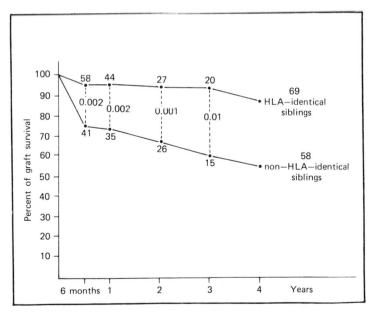

**Fig. 23.10** Actuarial curves of 127 renal transplantations between siblings (HLA genotype). (From J. Hors et al., in Cours international transplantation, Lyon 1973, Villeurbanne, 1973, Simep, p. 23.)

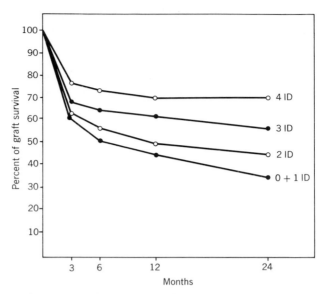

**Fig. 23.11** Actuarial curves of cadaver renal transplantations according to the number of identities (ID) at HLA-A and HLA-B loci. (From J. Dausset et al., N. Engl. J. Med. 1974, *290*, 980.)

quality of serologic techniques (unknown or badly determined groups have more influence in nonrelated pairs, generally incompatible in these groups, than in HLA-identical pairs who have inherited the same haplotypes and are most often compatible for these antigens) or by the existence of other loci (such as LD loci close to the HLA loci) for which related pairs will also be identical, whereas nonrelated pairs are not.

Correlations between the MLR and graft survival (independent of HLA antigens) have only been studied between related donors and recipients. Significant relationships have been observed, but these studies did not include sufficient number of recombinants (SD different and LD identical or SD identical and LD different) to determine the respective roles of LD and SD incompatibilities in rejection.

Recent results indicate that compatibility at the DR-locus is associated with better graft survival at identical levels of HLA-A and -B compatibility. It should also be noted that the ABO antigens play an important role, whereas the Rhesus antigens do not seem to intervene or only do so to a very slight degree (still contested). The role of incompatibility of Lewis erythrocyte antigens has recently been suggested. Conversely, "male" antigens do not seem to have any obvious role in graft rejection in male to female transplants. It may be noted that for the latter as for the minor antigens, it is probable that they do not intervene unless they are associated at the surface of the cell with HLA-A or -B antigens, which the donor and recipient have in common, as suggested by the studies of Zinkernagel. Thus, these minor antigens only have an effect in cases of partial HLA-A or -B identity.

In any case, it should be realized that a number of factors make it difficult to assess with certainty the value of HLA matching in cadaveric renal transplantation, notably:

1. the important effect of pregraft blood transfusions (see p. 419).
2. Host factors such as responder status. The intensity of immune responses varies from one individual to another independently of antigen strength. Some authors have reported that dialysis patients who failed to respond to a skin test with dinitrochlorobenzene had better subsequent graft survival than had patients who reacted positively.
3. Minor histocompatibility antigens, ABO blood groups and sex.
4. Centre variation.

Finally, the data available are insufficient to propose a definitive blueprint for these systems. Several hypotheses may be envisaged: the theory that involves cellular interactions between cells that react to LD antigens and cells reactive to SD antigens is the most attractive. It is reminiscent of interactions observed in the response to carrier-hapten conjugates (LD antigens could play the role of the carrier and SD antigens that of the hapten) or of cell interactions described between T-cell subsets (see p. 545).

# BIBLIOGRAPHY

BACH F. H., BACH M. L., SONDEL P. M., and SUNDHA RADAS G. Genetic control of mixed leucocyte culture reactivity. Transpl. Rev., 1972, *12*, 30.

BODMER W. F. (Ed.) Histocompatibility testing. Copenhagen, 1978, Munskgaard.

BENNETT D. The T locus of the mouse. Cell, 1975, *6*, 441.

DAUSSET J., DEGOS L., and HORS J. The association of the HL A antigens with disease. Clin. Immunol. Immunopathol. 1974, *3*, 127.

DEMANT P. H-2 gene complex and its role in alloimmune reactions. Transpl. Rev., 1973, *15*, 162.

FERRONE C. S., PELLEGRINO M. A., and REISFELD R. A. The major histocompatibility complex in man: biological and molecular approaches. Prog. All., 1976, *21*, 114.

FESTENSTEIN H. Immunogenetic and biological aspects of in vitro lymphocyte allotransformation (MLR) in the mouse. Transpl. Rev., 1973, *15*, 62.

GOTZE D. (Ed.) The major histocompatibility system in man and animals. Berlin, 1977, Springer Verlag, p. 404.

GRAFF R. J. and BAILEY D. W. The non-H-2 histocompatibility loci and their antigens. Transpl. Rev., 1973, *15*, 26.

HIRSCHBERG H., ALBRECHTSEN D., SOLHEIM B. G. and THORSBY E. Inhibition of human mixed lymphocyte culture. Stimulation by anti-HLA-D. Eur. J. Immunol., 1977, *7*, 26.

KISSMEYER-NIELSEN F., and THORSBY E. Human transplantation antigens. Transpl. Rev., 1970, *4*.

KLEIN J. Biology of the mouse histocompatibility-2 complex. New York, 1975, Springer.

KLEIN J. H-2 mutations: their genetics and effects on immune functions. Adv. Immunol., 1978, *26*, 56.

MÖLLER G. (Ed.) Strong and weak histocompatibility antigens. Transpl. Rev., 1970, *3*.

MÖLLER G. (Ed.) β2-microglobulin and HL-A antigens. Transpl. Rev., 1974, *21*, 3.

MÖLLER G. (Ed.) HL-A and disease. Transpl. Rev., 1975, *22*.

MÖLLER G. (Ed.) Specificity of effector T lymphocytes. Transpl. Rev., 1976, *20*.

MÖLLER G. (Ed.) Biochemistry and biology of Ia antigens. Transpl. Rev., 1976, *30*.

REISFELD R. A. and KAHAN B. D. Extraction and purification of soluble histocompatibility antigens. Transpl. Rev., 1971, *6*, 81.

SHEARER G. M., REHN T. G., and SCHMITT-VERHULST A. M. Role of the murine major histocompatibility complex in the specificity of in vitro T cell-mediated lympholysis against chemically-modified autologous lymphocytes. Transpl. Rev., 1976, 29, 233.

SHREFFLER D. C. Genetic and serological definition of the mouse major histocompatibility complex. In T. E. Mandel, C. Cheers, C. S. Hosking, I. F. C. Mc Kenzie, and G. J. V. Nossal, Eds., Progress in immunology III. Proc. 3rd Int. Congr. Immunol., Sydney. Amsterdam, 1977, North Holland, p. 311.

SCHREFFLER D. C. and DAVID C. S. The H-2 major histocompatibility complex and the I immune response region-genetic variation, function and organization. Adv. Immunol., 1975, 20, 125.

SNELL G. D., CHERRY M., and DEMANT P. H-2, its structure and similarity to HL-A. Transpl. Rev., 1973, 15, 3.

SNELL D., DAUSSET J., and NATHANSON S. Histocompatibility. New York, 1976, Academic Press, 401 p.

STROMINGER J. L. Structure of products of the major histocompatibility complex in man and mouse. In: Immunology 80 (M. Fougereau and J. Dausset [eds]). Acad. Press, New York, 1980:530.

TANIGAKI N. and PRESSMAN D. The basic structure and the antigenic characteristics of HL-A antigens. Transpl. Rev., 1974, 21, 15.

THORSBY E. The human major histocompatibility system. Transpl. Rev., 1974, 18, 51.

TING, A. The effect of HLA matching on Kidney-graft survival. Immunology Today. 1981, 2, 25.

VAN HOOF J. P. HLA and other important factors in renal allograft survival. Behring Inst. Mitt., 1978, 62, 53.

VITTETTA E. S. and CAPRA J. D. The protein products of the murine 17th chromosome: genetics and structure. Adv. Immunol., 1978, 26, 148.

WINCHESTER R. J., FU S. M., WERNET P., KUNKEL H. G. DUPONT B., and JERSILD C. Recognition of pregnancy serum of non-HLA alloantigens selectively expressed on B lymphocytes. J. Exp. Med., 1975, 141, 924.

WINCHESTER R. J. and KUNKEL H. G. The human Ia System. Adv. Immunol. 1979, 28, 222.

ZINKERNAGEL R. and KLEIN J. H-2 association specificity of virus immune cytotoxic T-cells from H-2 mutant and wild mice. Immunogenetics, 1977, 4, 581.

## ORIGINAL ARTICLES

DAUSSET J., HORS J., BUSSON M., FESTENSTEIN H., OLIVER R. T. D., CAIR B., PARIS A. M. I., and SAEMS J. I. Serologically defined HL-A antigens and long-term survival of cadaver kidney transplants. A joint analysis of 918 cases performed by France-Transplant and the London Transplant Groupe. New Engl. J. Med., 1974, 290, 980.

DEGOS L. and DAUSSET J. Human migrations and linkage disequilibrium of HLA system. Immunogenetics, 1974, 3, 195.

MOEN T., ALBRECHTSEN D., FLATMARK A., JAKOBSEN A., JERNELL J., HALVORSEN S., SOLHEIM B. G. and THORSBY E. Importance of HLA-DR matching in cadaveric renal transplantation: a prospective one center study of 170 transplant. New Engl. J. Med., 1980, 303, 850.

SILVER J. and HOOD L. Preliminary amino-acid sequences of transplantation antigens: genetic and evolutionary implications. Contemp. Top. Mol. Immunol., 1976, 5, 35.

# Chapter 24

# GENETIC CONTROL OF IMMUNE RESPONSES

**Jean-François Bach**

I.  INTRODUCTION
II.  GENETIC REGULATION OF ANTIGEN RECOGNITION: IR GENES
III.  GENETIC CONTROL OF THE ANTIBODY PRODUCTION PHASE

## I.  INTRODUCTION

The concept according to which immune reactivity, susceptibility to toxins and infectious agents, and propensity to develop immunologic diseases are dependent on hereditary factors is not new. Familial differences in susceptibility to the lethal effect of diphtheria toxin were discovered at the beginning of the century. Also observed were variations in sensitivity of guinea pigs to tuberculosis and of mice to *Salmonella*, as were important differences among various mouse strains to produce antibodies to sheep red blood cells (SRBC), ovalbumin, or type-1 pneumococcal polysaccharides. The existence of genetic control mechanisms for immune responses was demonstrated in 1943 by Scheibel, who showed, by genetic selection, that there were both good and poor antibody producers to diphtheria toxoid. However, not until 1963 was important progress made, with Benacerraf's discovery of gene-specific control of the immune response to simple antigens, and the demonstration by Biozzi, in 1970, of a polygenic system that controls the antibody production phase. These two essential concepts of genetic control of immune responses will be discussed in this chapter. The genetic determinants of Ig structure, which obviously are linked to genetic control of immunity, have already been discussed in relation to Ig structure (chap. 7) and the origins of antibody diversity (see chaps. 7 and 19).

The author thanks G. Biozzi for his critical appraisal of this chapter.

## II.   GENETIC REGULATION OF ANTIGEN RECOGNITION: Ir GENES

Despite the complexity of immune phenomena and the large number of antigens to which specific responses may develop, genetic control of the formation of antibodies to specific antigens follows fairly simple rules.

### HYPOTHESIS OF IMMUNE RESPONSE (Ir) GENES

Several autosomal dominant genes govern the immune response to simple antigens. An animal that possesses one of these genes will respond vigorously to the corresponding antigen by both antibody production and by delayed hypersensitivity (DH). However, animals without this gene will not develop a cellular reaction and are completely or partially unable to produce antibody to that antigen. We will next describe the major experimental models that led to the discovery of these genes. Three types of antigens were utilized: synthetic polypeptides, including only a few L-amino acids, sometimes conjugated to simple haptens and thus forming conjugates of limited structural diversity; weak natural antigens that differ very little from host proteins; and strong natural antigens injected at low doses and then immunogenic for only a few individuals.

### GENES THAT CONTROL THE RESPONSE TO SYNTHETIC POLYPEPTIDES

#### Response of Guinea Pigs to Poly-L-Lysine (PLL)

Levine and Benacerraf reported in 1963 that only a few Hartley guinea pigs immunized by the conjugate of the haptenic group 2,4-dinitrophenyl and of the poly-L-lysine polymer (DNP-PLL) produced anti-DNP antibodies. Similar results were obtained with DNP-GL (DNP conjugated to the copolymer of glutamic acid and lysine) or GL alone. "Responder" animals immunized by DNP-PLL or DNP-GL produce significant amounts of anti-DNP antibodies and develop a DH reaction to the conjugate. Conversely, "nonresponder" animals produce little or no anti-DNP antibodies and do not develop DH. Cross-breeding experiments then showed that the capacity to respond to DNP-PLL antigen was a function of a dominant autosomal gene. All guinea pigs of strain 13 are nonresponders, whereas strain-2 guinea pigs and $(2 \times 13)F_1$ hybrids are responders. The immune-response gene present in strain 2 but absent in strain 13 is called the "PLL gene" (Table 24.2).

It was subsequently shown that nonresponder guinea pigs could synthesize large amounts of anti-DNP antibodies after immunization by a DNP-PLL conjugate coupled to heterologous albumins, such as bovine serum albumin (BSA) or ovalbumin (the negative charge of which opposes the positivity of DNP-PLL). In these complexes, DNP (linked to PLL) acts like a hapten, and albumin behaves like a carrier. No response is obtained if the carrier is autologous albumin. Similarly, if nonresponder guinea pigs are first made

**Table 24.1   Principal Synthetic Polypeptides Utilized in the Study of Genetic Regulation of Immune Responses**

| Polypeptide | Description |
| --- | --- |
| PLL | A linear polymer composed entirely of Poly-L-lysine |
| DNP-PLL | Poly-L-lysine substituted with dinitrophenyl groups on the ε-amino groups of lysine |
| GA | A linear polymer of glutamic acid and alanine |
| GL | A linear polymer of glutamic acid and lysine |
| DNP-GL | A linear copolymer of glutamic acid and lysine substituted with dinitrophenyl groups on the ε-amino groups of lysine |
| GT | A linear copolymer of glutamic acid and tyrosine |
| GAT$_{10}$ | A linear copolymer of glutamic acid, alanine, and tyrosine in which tyrosine makes up 10% of the amino acid residues |
| (T,G)-A--L | A branched, multichain copolymer of the general structure shown in Fig. 6.3 (see p. 131). The copolymer has the structural formula: poly-L-(tyrosine, glutamic acid)-poly-D,L-alanine—poly-L-lysine. The structural formula is written this way to indicate that the amino acids in parentheses are in random sequence, the dash indicates a long stretch of poly-D,L-alanine, and the double dash indicates a branch point where the alanine joins the ε-amino groups of lysine, which forms the backbone of the molecule. Thus, the synthetic polypeptide is built on a chain of poly-L-lysine, with each lysine being substituted in its ε-amino group by a long side chain of alanine, attached to the amino terminus of which is a short random sequence of tyrosine and glutamic acid |
| (H,G)-A--L | Poly-L(histidine, glutamic acid)-poly D,L alanine-poly-L-lysine. Structural analog of (T,G)-A--L, in which tyrosine is replaced by histidine |
| (Phe,G)-A--L | Poly-L-(phenylalanine, glutamic acid)-poly-D,L-alanine--poly-L-lysine. A structural analog of (T,G)-A--L, in which tyrosine is replaced by phenylalanine |
| (T,G)-Pro--L | Poly-L-(tyrosine, glutamic acid)poly-L-proline--poly-L-lysine. This synthetic polypeptide has the same general structure as (T,G)-A--L and its congeners, but in this case, the side chains of poly-D,L-alanine are replaced by poly-L-proline |
| (Phe,G)-Pro--L | Poly-L-(phenylalanine, glutamic acid)-poly-L-proline- -poly-L-lysine. A structural analog of (T,G)-Pro--L, in which tyrosine is replaced by phenylalanine |

After B. Benacerraf.

tolerant to BSA and then immunized by the DNP-PLL-BSA complex, production of anti-DNP antibodies remains weak or nil. Interestingly enough, after immunization of nonresponder guinea pigs by the DNP-PLL-BSA immunogenic complex, anti-DNP antibody is produced but DH to DNP-PLL is not observed. This finding indicates that DH to DNP-PLL requires the presence of the PLL gene.

We therefore conclude that the deficiency of nonresponders does not apply

**Table 24.2    Relationships Between Ir Genes and the Major Histocompatibility Locus in Guinea Pig Strains 2 and 13, (2 × 13)$F_1$, and Backcross Animals**

| Antigen | Strain 2 | 13 | (2 × 13) $F_1$ | (2 × 13) $F_1$ × 13 50% | 50% | (2 × 13) $F_1$ × 2 50% | 50% |
|---|---|---|---|---|---|---|---|
| DNP-PLL-GL | + | | + | + | − | | |
| GA | + | | + | + | − | | |
| GT | | + | + | | | + | − |
| BSA (0.1 μg) | + | − | + | + | − | | |
| HSA (1 μg) | + | − | + | | | | |
| DNP-BSA (1 μg) | + | − | + | + | − | | |
| DNP-GPA (1 μg) | − | + | + | | | + | − |
| Specificities at H locus | | | | | | | |
| Strain 2 | + | | + | + | − | | |
| Strain 13 | | + | + | | | + | − |

After I. Green and B. Benacerraf.

at the level of the production phase of specific anti-DNP antibodies, because synthesis of such antibodies is obtained after conjugation to another carrier. The action of the PLL gene apparently bears on the recognition of carrier determinants, a function possessed by T cells (see chap. 18). Involvement of the PLL gene at the level of T cells is corroborated by the absence of DH to DNP-PLL when the PLL gene is not present. Complementary studies have shown also that the PLL gene controls the response to poly-L-arginine (PLA) and to copolymers of L-glutamic acid and L-lysine (GL).

Another immune response gene has been identified in the guinea pig. The GA gene controls production of antibodies to the copolymer of L-glutamic acid and L-alanine (Glu-60, Ala-40). Both GA and PLL genes are present in strain 2 but absent in strain 13. Conversely, the GT gene, which controls the response to the linear copolymer of L-glutamic acid and L-tyrosine (Glu-50, Tyr-50), is present in strain 13 and absent in strain 2.

### Responses of Mice to (T,G)-A— —L (Ir-1 locus) and Other Synthetic Polypeptides

In 1969, MacDevitt and Sela reported that mouse production of antibodies against branched synthetic polypeptides that contain several chains is controlled by a dominant autosomal gene, now called the Ir-1 gene. The antigen initially used was (T,G)-A- -L, which consists of lateral chains of poly-DL-alanine bound onto ε-amino groups of a long PLL chain. Short tyrosine and glutamic acid sequences are randomly included in lateral alanine chains. Later, histidine and phenylalanine were substituted for tyrosine to give (H-G)-A- -L and (Phe, G)-A- -L. C57 mice immunized against (T,G)-A- -L are good responders, as are (C57 × CBA) $F_1$ hybrid mice, but CBA mice are poorly responsive (Fig. 24.1).

No correlation between the level of the response and serum immunoglobulin concentration, Ig class, or allotype has been shown. The response to (T-G)-A- -L can be transferred by injecting spleen cells from good-responder $F_1$ mice into nonresponder, lethally irradiated parental mice. Thus, the genetic control

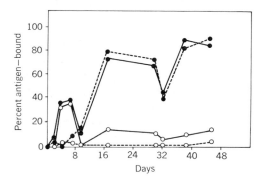

**Fig. 24.1** Primary and secondary responses of $C_3H$ and $C_3H$-SW mice to aqueous solution of (T, G)-A- -L. $C_3H$-SW mice (●) are good responders, whereas $C_3H$ mice (○) are bad responders. (—), total antibodies; (- - -), IgG antibodies. (From H. O. McDevitt, Hosp. Pract. 1973, *8*, 61.)

of immune responses is expressed directly at the level of immunocompetent cells and is not linked to humoral (in particular, endocrine) factors. The autosomal dominant genes that control the response to (T,G)-A- -L and (Phe, G)-A- -L belong to the same locus (Ir-1). The Ir-1 locus includes at least three tightly linked subloci with multiple alleles: Ir-1A, Ir-1B, and Ir-1C.

The genetic regulation of immune responses to other synthetic polypeptides has been similarly studied in the mouse. It has thus been shown that the response to the terpolymer that contains L-glutamic acid, L-alanine, and 10% L-tyrosine ($GAT_{10}$) is controlled by a dominant gene (not belonging to the Ir-1 locus). Specificity of Ir genes is emphasized by the fact that there is absolutely no response in nonresponders. Figure 24.2 lists the polypeptides that have been studied in the mouse by the above methods.

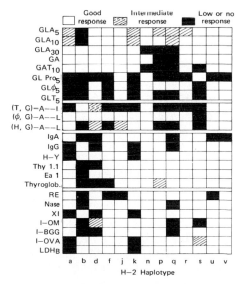

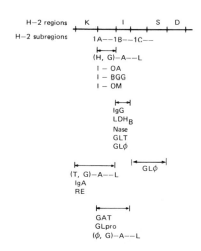

**Fig. 24.2** Ir genes in the mouse. *Left*: Immune responses controlled by Ir genes in mice representative of 13 haplotypes against four classes of thymus-dependent antigens: nonordered linear copolymers of L-amino acids, branched copolymers of L-amino acids, murine alloantigens, and foreign antigens. *Right*: Ir gene chart (Ir region of the H-2 complex). (From B. Benacerraf et al. In L. Brent and J. Holborow, Eds., Progress in immunology II. Vol. 2. Amsterdam, 1974, North-Holland, p. 182.)

## Gene Complementation

Certain crossing experiments have unexpectedly shown that descendents of nonresponder strains can occasionally produce a good response, clearly better than that of the two parental mice. Further study of several systems, particularly the response to the terpolymer Glu-Lys-Phe (GL$\phi$) has led to the interesting concept of "gene complementation" in the MHC. At least two genes are involved in the control of the response to GL$\phi$. One is situated in the I-C region ($\alpha$ gene), the other in the I-A region ($\beta$-gene). In fact, the situation is even more complex since strains possessing the $\alpha$-allele, which permits an anti-GL$\phi$ response, seem, in addition, to require two $\beta$-type I-A subregion alleles for the response to occur ($\beta$-$\beta$ complementation). These observations have been extended to other antigenic systems. Furthermore, similar observations have been made for suppressor T cells in the GT system. $F_1$ hybrids of H-$2^b$ and H-$2^a$ strains that do not produce suppressor T cells do, in fact, produce such suppressor T cells. Here, also, the situation seems to be complicated by the observation of restriction in the capacity of suppressor genes to complement one another when they are derived from different haplotypes (concept of "coupled complementation").

This gene complementation must not be confused with the observations (unconfirmed) of Munro and Taussig that have shown that recombinants of B10-M mice, a nonresponder to (T,G)-A- -L (because of the failure of their T cells to secrete antigen-specific factor), and B10-BR mice, also a nonresponder (because the sensitivity of their B cells to this factor is absent), are perfectly good responders.

## Response to Weak Alloantigens

Several dominant Ir genes, which control the response to weak alloantigens, have been identified in the mouse. The principal alloantigens studied include the Ea-1 antigen of wild mice erythrocytes, male antigens recognized by female mice, which are histocompatibility antigens controlled by the Y chromsome, $\theta$ antigen (Thy-1 in new terminology), transplantation antigens of H-2.2 and H-1.3 specificities, and allotypic determinants of IgA myeloma.

## Response to Suboptimal Doses of Strong Antigens

Suboptimal doses of bovine or human albumin in the guinea pig, bovine $\gamma$-globulin or chicken albumin in the mouse, and hapten-protein conjugates in both species lead to intense antibody production only in certain strains.

A response to low doses of BSA (0.1–1 $\mu$g in Freund's complete adjuvant) is seen in strain-2 but not in strain-13 guinea pigs. Such a difference in responses is not observed if 10–100 $\mu$g of BSA are used. (2 × 13) $F_1$ hybrid guinea pigs produce anti-BSA antibodies if 0.1 $\mu$g of BSA is given, as do 50% of the backcrossed animals from strain 13. The gene that controls this response is autosomal dominant (so-called BSA-1) and is linked to the PLL and GA genes.

These data show that immune response genes control the immune response to complex antigens administered in low dose. This may also be true for high antigen doses, but genetic regulation here is impossible to demonstrate because there exist on most complex antigens several carrier determinants; when the Ir gene for one or another carrier is absent, the carrier whose Ir gene is present substitutes for the nonrecognized carrier. However, at low antigen doses, only certain carriers are present in immunogenic concentrations, and genetic regulation may, then, be expressed.

## CHARACTERISTICS OF Ir GENES

### Specificity

It is possible that Ir genes that control immune responses of different specificities are always distinct or, alternatively, that a single gene may control the response to several nonrelated antigenic determinants. Data on the Ir-1 locus in the mouse and studies performed in the guinea pig show that a given Ir gene may be found in several pure strains and in wild animals, which show many differences in response to several antigens. These observations indicate that distinct Ir genes control the response to different polypeptides. For example, while PLL and GA genes are linked in strain-2 guinea pigs, many other guinea pig strains respond to only one or the other of these (PLL and GA) antigens.

This diversity of Ir genes obviously raises the question of the ultimate size of the Ir gene pool. A very considerable number of Ir genes has already been identified, within only a few years, on the basis of experiments using essentially simple synthetic antigens or complex antigens in suboptimal doses. Injection of high-dose antigens will probably involve more Ir genes. The number of Ir genes is however most likely lower than that of antibody specificities, because a single Ir gene controls production of antibodies of heterogeneous affinity and thus of heterogeneous specificity.

### Association Between Ir Genes and Genes That Code for Transplantation Antigens

DISCOVERY OF THE LINK BETWEEN Ir-1 AND H-2 LOCI

A large percentage of Ir genes in the mouse and guinea pig are tightly bound to genes that code for histocompatibility antigens, as first noted in studies on congenic mice.

No differences in response to (T, G)-A- -L can be demonstrated between the two strains of mice if there is no difference in their respective H-2 complexes. However, congenic mice, identical to nonresponder mice in all criteria except for a different H-2 complex, respond vigorously to (T, G)-A- -L. Thus, C3H mice (H-$2^k$) are not responsive to (T, G)-A- -L, whereas C3H-SW mice, which are congenic to C3H but differ in the H-2 complex, respond well. Conversely, C57BL/6 mice (H-$2^b$) are good responders, whereas B10BR mice, congenic to C57BL/6 mice except for the H-2 complex (they are H-$2^k$), are nonresponders. These observations led to systematic studies of relationships between the H-2 complex and Ir genes.

LOCALIZATION OF Ir GENES IN THE MOUSE

The Ir-IA locus controls the responses to (T, G)-A- -L, (H, G)-A- -L, and (Phe, G)-A- -L and is located inside the H-2 complex, on the 17th chromosome, to the left of the SsSlp locus (which controls the production of a serum β-globulin), and immediately to the right of the H-2K extremity (Fig. 24.3). Localization of this locus has been established by study of the immune responses of mice recombinant at the H-2 complex. Among the recombinations within the H-2 complex and its immediately adjacent structures, only recombinations located between the H-2D and H-2K extremities permitted dissociation of Ir genes and H-2 specificities. Recently, further study of recombinants has allowed separation of the original Ir-1 locus into three loci: Ir-1A, Ir-1B, and Ir-1C (Fig. 24.3).

The majority of the Ir genes have been localized in the I-A subregion: a few that require complementation are situated both in the I-A and I-C subregions. Only two genes have been localized to the I-B subregions (response against the antigenic determinants of an IgG myeloma of BALB/c mice and against staphylococcal nuclease).

At this point, it should be recalled that the Ia antigens expressed at the surface of B lymphocytes, macrophages, and certain activated T cells (see p. 662) have been localized in the I-A, I-C, and I-J subregions and also that helper and suppressor factors carry Ia antigens coded for by the I-A and I-J subregions respectively. This suggests that the Ia antigens on B lymphocytes are identical with those present on "helper" factors. The absence of specificities in the I-B subregion leads one to doubt the very existence of this subregion, whose

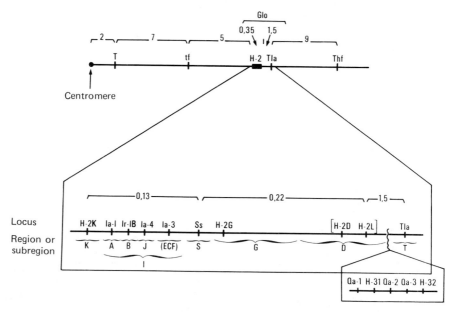

**Fig. 24.3** Major histocompatibility complex in the mouse (17th chromosome, linkage group IX).

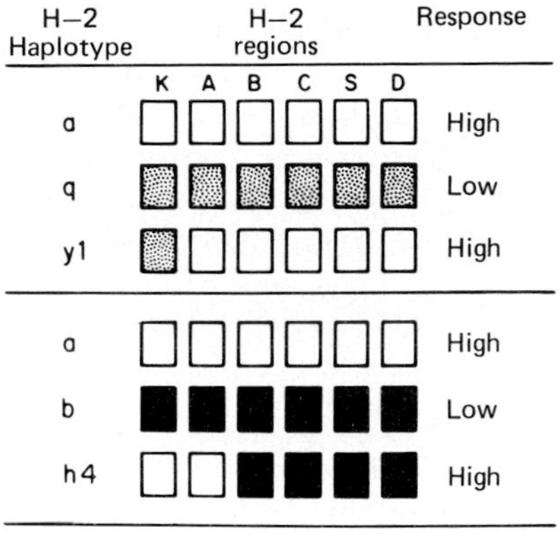

Fig. 24.4 — Principle of the localization of an immune response gene in the MHC.

| H−2 Haplotype | K | A | B | C | S | D | Response |
|---|---|---|---|---|---|---|---|
| a | □ | □ | □ | □ | □ | □ | High |
| q | ▨ | ▨ | ▨ | ▨ | ▨ | ▨ | Low |
| y1 | ▨ | □ | □ | □ | □ | □ | High |
| a | □ | □ | □ | □ | □ | □ | High |
| b | ■ | ■ | ■ | ■ | ■ | ■ | Low |
| h4 | □ | □ | ■ | ■ | ■ | ■ | High |

**Fig. 24.4** Principle of the localization of an immune response gene in the MHC. In the first experiment, the H-2$^a$ mice are good responders against (H,G)-A− −L, whereas H-2$^q$ mice are poor responders. The H-2$^{y1}$ recombinants, which only have the K-region in common with H-2$^q$ mice, are good responders, which suggests that the K-region is not implicated in the genetic control of the response to (H-G)-A− −L. In the second experiment the H-2$^a$ mice are good responders, whereas the H-2$^b$ mice are poor responders. The H-2$^{h4}$ recombinant obtained from these two strains, H-2$^a$ and H-2$^b$, by crossing over between the A and B regions, is a good responder, which leads to the conclusion that the response to (H,G)-A− −L is controlled by the A region. (After J. Klein Adv. Immunol. 1978, 26, 56.)

description is perhaps secondary to the existence, initially poorly understood, of complementation genes.

The H-2 region thus contains genes that code for both H-2 antigens and immune responses (Ir loci), genes that code for Ss and Slp proteins, TL antigen (see p. 670), a lymphocytic antigen induced by murine leukemogenic virus (MuLv), and G2-1-1 antigen, and genes that control mouse susceptibility to leukemia induced by Gross or Friend's virus. The H-2 complex also contains genes that code for antigens that stimulate mixed-lymphocyte reactions [lymphocyte-defined (LD) antigens (see p. 658)].

One should note, however, that genetic regulation of production of some antibodies may also be controlled by genes not located in the H-2 complex. This is particularly true for antibodies directed against lysozyme "loop peptide."

LOCALIZATION OF Ir GENES IN THE GUINEA PIG

Similar findings in the guinea pig show that PLL, GA, and BSA-1 genes are linked to the locus that codes for major histocompatibility antigens of strains 2 and 13. There is also a link between the GT gene and histocompatibility genes.

As mentioned earlier, strain-2 guinea pigs respond well to DNP-PLL, whereas strain-13 guinea pigs are nonresponders, but $F_1$ hybrids are good responders. This situation is explained by control of the DNP-PLL response by a single gene; thus, 50% of ($F_1 \times 13$) backcross animals are good responders. The regular presence of transplantation antigens of strain 2 in responsive ($F_1$

× 13) backcross guinea pigs has been demonstrated by Shevach and Green. Strain-13 guinea pigs are immunized by lymph node and spleen cells from strain-2 guinea pigs, in order to obtain a strain-13 antistrain-2 antiserum. This cytotoxic antiserum, in the presence of complement, kills cells from good-responder backcross $(F_1 \times 13)$ guinea pigs but has absolutely no effect on nonresponder cells. Thus, $(F_1 \times 13)$ backcross animals with the PLL gene have strain-2 antigens, but backcross animals without the PLL gene do not have them. In 94 outbred guinea pigs, it was impossible to dissociate the PLL gene from antigenic specificities of strain 2 (determined with specific 13-anti-2 sera; see Table 24.2).

More precisely, it has been demonstrated that in experiments involving the inhibition of blast transformation in response to antigen by diverse antisera against MHC products, the Ir genes are directly associated with the expression of Ia antigenic specificities.

OTHER SPECIES

Similar data have been reported in the rat, monkey, and man. For example, in the rat, there are Ir genes that control the response to (T, G)-A- -L and (H, G)-A- -L. These genes are linked to the major histocompatibility Ag-B locus. In man, the IgE response to ragweed has been reported to be linked to the HLA locus, but this observation has not yet been confirmed.

SIGNIFICANCE OF THE ASSOCIATION BETWEEN Ir AND HISTOCOMPATIBILITY
GENES

The relationship between Ir genes and genes that code for transplantation antigens raises the possibility that the apparent genetic control of antibody production discussed above is due to a cross-reaction between histocompatibility antigens and foreign antigens against which the antibodies are directed. Animals tolerant to their own histocompatibility antigens would, then, also be tolerant to foreign antigens that cross-react with the histocompatibility antigens. However, the "good response" of $F_1$ hybrids of responders and nonresponders, which possess the histocompatibility antigens of nonresponders, contradicts this hypothesis, unless these special histocompatibility antigens are recessive, which seems unlikely.

This possibility of "genetic tolerance" to foreign antigens is unlikely but its exclusion is essential to evaluate the biologic significance of Ir genes. Accumulating evidence against this hypothesis includes the following data:

Anti-H-$2^k$ sera do not react with (T, G)-A- -L, nor do anti-(T, G)-A- -L sera react with histocompatibility antigens of H-$2^k$ mouse cells (which are nonresponders to (T, G)-A- -L).

Injection of H-$2^k$ spleen or thymus cells into H-$2^b$ mice does not augment their immune response to (T, G)-A- -L.

Anti-(T, G)-A- -L antibodies are not absorbed by H-$2^k$ or H-$2^b$ cells.

Antibodies from mice that respond well to (T, G)-A- -L infused into nonimmunized H-$2^b$ or H-$2^k$ mice disappear from the serum of both strains with equal rapidity.

# NATURE OF CELLS THAT EXPRESS Ir GENES

We have seen above that in the two best-studied systems (antibody response to synthetic polypeptides controlled by the Ir-1 locus and guinea pig response to PLL), the immune reactivity of good-responder animals can be transferred to irradiated nonresponders by immunocompetent cells of animals that possess the relevant Ir genes. This transmission shows that Ir genes express themselves at the level of immunocompetent cells. We will now examine evidence concerning the particular B- or T-lymphocyte categories in which Ir genes are expressed.

## Evidence in Favor of Ir Gene Expression in T cells

### Ir GENES CONTROL CELL-MEDIATED IMMUNITY

We have seen that DH to synthetic polypeptides is Ir gene dependent. Ir genes are required for the development of such reactions in vivo (DH to PLL in the guinea pig) or in vitro [DNA synthesis in the presence of PLL or (T, G)-A- -L in mice immunized with these antigens]. Note also that stimulation of DNA synthesis in the presence of (T, G)-A- -L is essentially a T-cell function: it is suppressed by treatment with anti-θ serum and persists after elimination of B cells on nylon columns. Its regulation by Ir genes is strictly (T, G)-A- -L specific when tested against (H, G)-A- -L and (Phe, G)-A- -L, whereas these three antigens induce the production of cross-reacting antibodies. Lymphocyte blast transformation in the presence of antigen is inhibited by antisera raised against MHC gene products but not by anti-Ig sera.

### ANTIBODY PRODUCTION IS NO LONGER CONTROLLED BY Ir GENES IN THYMUS-DEPRIVED MICE

Good-responder mice, T-cell depleted by thymectomy and irradiation followed by bone marrow reconstitution, lose their ability to produce 7S antibodies to (T, G)-A- -L. In this setting, only 19S antibodies are produced, as is true also of nonresponder mice (whether thymectomized or not). Production of 19S antibodies in nonresponder mice shows that (B) precursors of antibody-forming cells are present in nonresponders and suggests that Ir genes may act at the IgM to IgG switch level, known to involve T cells. In fact, the primary IgM response that occurs after (T, G)-A- -L injection in aqueous solution, does not differ between good- and nonresponder mice. Furthermore Ir gene effects do not apply to thymus-independent responses of the IgM type, as is observed in responses to polyvinylpyrrolidone or lipopolysaccharides.

### THE ACTION OF Ir GENES APPLIES TO THE CARRIER

Production of antibody to a hapten conjugated to a synthetic polypeptide, used as a carrier, is dependent on the Ir gene that controls the response to the polypeptide. When this Ir gene is absent, antibody production to the hapten may still be induced by coupling the latter to another carrier for which the animal possesses the corresponding Ir gene. These observations show that Ir genes control the response with respect to the carrier determinant of a carrier-hapten conjugate.

In addition, suppressor T cells specific for the carrier may be produced by nonresponder mice in the absence of "helper" cells. Thus, immunization of H-$2^s$ mice with GAT, to which they are nonresponsive, prevents the immune response normally observed after immunization with GAT coupled to methylated BSA. Thus, a "nonresponse" could sometimes be linked to excessive production of suppressor T cells, thereby preventing antibody production, perhaps by means of soluble factors (see p. 547). Further experiments by Tada and Benacerraf's group have confirmed that the suppression could be linked to the production by T cells of a humoral mediator (see p. 548), bearing antigenic specificities encoded by the I region, at the level of a new "I-J" locus located between I-B and I-C (Tada).

### B CELLS FROM NONRESPONDER MICE MAY PRODUCE NORMAL AMOUNTS OF ANTIBODY UNDER SOME CIRCUMSTANCES

In some experimental systems, nonresponder mice may produce antibodies to antigens despite a lack of the corresponding Ir gene.

*Tetraparental Mice.*    Cells of two different H-2 specificities may coexist in the same host without a reciprocal graft-versus-host (GvH) reaction when they are grafted at a very early stage of embryonic development. Tetraparental, or "allophenic," mice, first described by Minz, are prepared by treating the eight-cell blastula with pronase to alter the pellucidal zone. Four cells of each line are then fused and grafted into pseudogestant females (mated with a vasectomized male). True chimeras are created, as demonstrated by study of the hemoglobin types or Ig allotypes. MacDevitt has produced tetraparental mice by fusing cells of good- and nonresponder mice differing also at the locus that controls immunoglobulin allotypes. The antibodies produced were identified by allotypes, thus revealing their origins from good- or nonresponder mice. These studies have shown that B cells from nonresponder mice can cooperate with T cells of good responders.

*Allogeneic Effect.*    If one considers two strains of congenic C3H mice, both nonresponders but of different H-2 composition (H-$2^k$ and H-$2^q$), their $F_1$ hybrids are also nonresponders. However, after injection of parental H-$2^k$ cells into these $F_1$ mice, they become good responders. Such an injection of parental cells to $F_1$ hybrid mice induces a GvH reaction, which causes an allogeneic effect (see p. 538). This allogeneic effect permits $F_1$ mice, which are normally nonresponders, to be responsive due to substitution of a "helper" effect that is not achievable by T cells alone, since they do not express the Ir gene.

### GOOD- AND NONRESPONDER MICE HAVE THE SAME NUMBER OF ANTIGEN-BINDING B CELLS

The binding of antigen to lymphoid cells may be studied by autoradiography (after incubation with radiolabeled antigens). By this technique, it can be shown that the number of cells that bind $^{125}$I-labeled DNP-GPA and GAT is not different between good- and nonresponder mice. This finding indicates that good- and nonresponder mice contain the same quantities of antigen-binding B cells because autoradiography essentially detects B cells (see p. 514). This observation is not, however, restricted to B cells because T cells may also be studied by autoradiography (using highly labeled antigens); antigen binding is also similar for T cells in good- and nonresponder mice, even before immunization, as shown by MacDevitt in the mouse with $^{125}$I-labeled (T, G)-A- -L. Only after immunization do differences between good- and nonresponder mice appear at both B- and T-cell levels.

CAN THE ACTION OF Ir GENES BE EXPLAINED BY THE PRESENCE OF SUPPRESSOR T CELLS?

The discovery of suppressor T cells raises the question of whether antigen-specific suppressor T cells might be controlled by the I region (Immuno suppression genes or Is gene), as is the case with T-helper cells, and thereby explain some of the results described above.

In the DNP-KLH system, Tada showed that the generation of a suppressor effect and the production of suppressor factors (described on p. 000) are under the strict control of a new locus situated in the I-J region between the I-A and I-C subregions. In addition, the suppressor factor bears antigens coded for by the I-J region. Benacerraf's group confirmed these results with synthetic polypeptides. Nonresponder mice to the copolymer $Glu^{60}$, $Ala^{30}$, $Tyr^{10}$ (GAT) produce antibodies against these antigens when it is coupled with a carrier, such as methylated bovine serum albumin (MBSA). It was shown that prior injection of GAT specifically suppressed the response to GAT-MBSA. Transfer experiments demonstrated that the suppression was attributable to Lyt $23^+$ suppressor T cells and could be induced by a soluble factor extracted from these cells. Analogous results were obtained with GT ($Glu^{50}$, $Tyr^{50}$ copolymer). Furthermore, it was demonstrated, with GT, that prior immunization with GT suppressed the response to GT-MBSA only in certain strains ($H-2^k$, $H-2^d$, and $H-2^s$; not $H-2^b$ or $H-2^a$). Use of congenic mice confirmed that the suppression was controlled by the MHC, more precisely by the I region. It was then not surprising that the pretreatment of nonresponder mice to GT with cyclophosphamide, which selectively inhibits suppressor T cells at low doses, allowed these mice to produce anti-GT antibodies. Although the suppressor T cells seem to explain numerous nonresponse states, their intervention does not, however, appear to be general since, for example, certain mice that do not respond to GT ($H-2^a$ and $H-2^b$) fail to produce suppressor T cells.

### The I Region and Macrophages

Rosenthal and Shevach have immunized $(2 \times 13)$ $F_1$ guinea pigs simultaneously with DNP-GL (to which strain 2 responds but not strain 13) and GT (to which strain 13 responds but not strain 2). They then studied the proliferative response of peritoneal lymphocytes in vitro in response to these antigens, presented either alone or within macrophages of strains 2, 13 and $(2 \times 13)$ $F_1$. The $(2 \times 13)$ $F_1$ peritoneal cells respond both to DNP-GL and to GT, whether presented alone or by $(2 \times 13)$ $F_1$ macrophages. Similarly, the lymphocytes of DNP-GL responders (strain 2) or GT responders (strain 13) respond to the antigen which they normally recognize when it is presented by syngeneic macrophages. Nevertheless, no response is observed when the DNP-GL is presented to $(2 \times 13)$ $F_1$ lymphocytes by strain-13 macrophages (nonresponder to DNP-GL) or when GT is presented by strain-2 macrophages (nonresponder to GT). Conversely, $(2 \times 13)$ $F_1$ lymphocytes respond, respectively to DNP-GL when presented by strain-2 macrophages and to GT when presented by strain-13 macrophages. These results, recently extended to the mouse and to in vivo systems, show that the macrophages that present antigens to T cells must share the same Ir genes as the T cells and therefore present the corresponding Ia antigens. Such findings, which extend the syngeneic H-2 restriction described for cytotoxic T cells to the interaction between macrophages and T cells, appear mainly to apply to secondary responses. In effect, it is possible to make macrophages and allogeneic T cells interact in primary reactions. It should also be noted that it is also possible to obtain a secondary response with macrophages that differ by their Ia antigens with T cells if the antigens are presented by the same macrophages as used in the course of the first stimulation. Only these macrophages are then able to initiate the secondary response. Note also that seemingly suppressor T cells do not show H-2 restriction in antigen recognition as helper or cytotoxic T cells.

### The I Region and Cooperation Factors

Cellular cooperation between B and T cells requires the intervention of several antigen-specific factors. It should be recalled that these factors, which appear after antigenic stimulation, are absorbed by the antigen (they bind the antigen and may act in the form of a complex with the antigen) and do not possess any antigenic determinants of Ig-heavy or Ig-light chains, have a molecular weight of about 40,000 daltons, and carry Ia determinants coded by the I-A region for "helper" factors and I-J region for "suppressor" factors. Some authors, such as Tada, have shown that the action of these factors requires I-region identity (I-A or I-J) between the factor-producing cell and the target cell. These results, however, have been questioned by other workers who report that the suppressor factors act on all the nonresponder strains without H-2 restriction, even in the total absence of restriction.

### Expression of Ir Genes in B Cells

Are Ir genes also expressed in antibody-forming cells and in their precursors? Evidence that there are no differences in specificities between antibodies produced by good responders and those produced by nonresponders does not favor the latter hypothesis. However, in certain systems, Ir genes do seem to control antibody specificity, perhaps by selecting highly thymus-dependent determinants.

The possibility of expression of Ir genes in B cells is suggested by cell dilution experiments (Shearer and Sela) that have sometimes shown exclusive Ir gene expression in B cells; in other situations, expression may occur in B and T cells, depending on the antigen and the mouse strain. Injection into an irradiated animal of syngeneic spleen cells in suboptimal amounts permits determination of the minimal number of cells necessary to restore immunocompetence (linked to that of precursors). For the lysozyme "loop peptide," for which Ir genes are present in SJL mice and absent in DBA/1 mice, the number of precursors is four times greater in SJL than in DBA/1 mice prior to immunization; this difference increases 25-fold after immunization. By injecting irradiated animals with an excess of thymus cells and a limited number of bone marrow cells or, conversely, with an excess of bone marrow cells and a small number of thymocytes, the good versus bad character of B- and T-cell precursors can be determined. The results differ depending on the antigen employed. Ir genes are expressed in B cells for (T, G)-Pro- -L and in both B and T cells for (Phe, G)-A- -L.

Munro and Taussig have shown that B cells from some nonresponder mice may be insensitive to the antigen-specific factor produced by T cells from responder mice. This finding indicates the possibility of two levels of Ir gene action, on T and B cells, respectively, possibly controlled by two different genes (see p. 543). In this scheme, effects on B cells would occur only at the level of interaction with T cells, which is still compatible with a selective action of Ir genes on thymus-dependent responses. This effect on B cells must be distinguished from the action on T cells that may alter production of the antigen-specific factor.

### Genetic Control of Cytotoxic T Cells (Zinkernagel and Doherty's Phenomenon)

Much less data is available on the effect of the MHC on the generation of cytotoxic T cells than on antibody production against thymus-dependent antigens. Nonetheless, it has been reported that H-2 mice immunized against TNP-modified syngeneic cells possess specific cytotoxic T cells for TNP conjugates with cells syngeneic at the H-2K end. This response is under the control of the H-2K region (and not the I region). Similar data show that, in addition, complementation genes exist for the cellular response to the male (Y) antigen.

Zinkernagel's experiments on the H-2 restriction of antigen recognition by cytotoxic T cells should also be recalled at this point (p. 87). We have seen that to kill a nucleated cell that bears on its surface virus-induced antigens, a minor histocompatibility antigen or a hapten, such as TNP, the T cells must recognize the antigens in question in association with H-2D and/or H-2K antigens. We have discussed two possible theories that may explain this fundamental observation: one involving a single receptor that recognizes a histocompatibility antigen-conventional antigen complex (altered "self"), the other involving two receptors, one for the histocompatibility antigen, the other for the conventional antigen*.

From the point of view of the ontogenesis of the recognition repertoire, the two-receptor hypothesis implies that the genes coding for the syngeneic H-2 recognition receptors (K and D for cytotoxic T precursors and I for the helper T-cell precursors) are selected or may be acquired independently of the genes coding for the conventional antigen. Conversely, the "altered self" hypothesis implies the selection of receptors that evolve by successive mutations from a prototype receptor directed against syngeneic determinants. Recent ontogenetic studies by Zinkernagel's group, on the one hand, and by Bevan

---

* The conventional antigen is the structure against which the immune response studied is directed (as opposed to histocompatibility antigens, which are the basis of the restriction).

studying minor histocompatibility antigens, on the other hand, tend to tip the balance in favor of the first hypothesis. In effect, these authors have shown that in a chimeric mouse of parental type A, reconstituted by $F_1$ (A × B) bone marrow, the cytotoxic T lymphocytes can only recognize the conventional antigen when it is present in association with the H-2 antigens of A, not when present in association with the H-2 antigens of B. Thus, in the course of the maturation of bone marrow T-cell precursors (which are A × B), a selective process (restriction) is operative in favor of T-cell clones recognizing self H-2A, independent of and before the recognition of the conventional antigen, which is introduced very much later. Of course, it might be supposed, according to Jerne's schema, that the A × B precursors in contact with A thymus begin to mutate away from A to escape the negative pressure exerted by the syngeneic A antigens. This leads us to the second model.

In addition, Zinkernagel has shown that the education or selection (in the case of $F_1$ marrow injected into a parental recipient) is operative at the level of the radioresistant part of the thymic epithelium. Thus, if (A × B) $F_1$ marrow is injected into a thymectomized irradiated syngeneic (A × B) $F_1$ recipient, who is then grafted with an irradiated parental (A or B) thymus, cytotoxic T cells are capable of recognizing semisyngeneic A or B (depending on the thymus grafted), whereas an irradiated $F_1$ thymus gives rise to T cells capable of recognizing either A or B equally well. It follows that if one grafts thymus-deprived individual A with a thymus B, the A marrow precursors will differentiate in the B thymus where, a priori, they will become educated against B antigens. These T lymphocytes, although mature, will be incapable of restoring the immunologic function of the host, A, since they will be confronted by antigens exposed in an H-2KA and H-2DA environment and will have to cooperate with B-lymphoid cells, derived from bone marrow, which present H-2IA antigens.

In fact, one of the great unanswered questions consists of knowing whether a T precursor can truly learn a new "self" in an allogeneic thymus or if the thymus merely acts as a selective and restraining influence on the diverse possible reactions against histocompatibility antigens expressed on precursor cells. This question arises particularly in the case of allogeneic (A marrow in B recipient) and semiallogeneic (A marrow in (A × B) $F_1$) chimeras. Are the A precursors educated against B antigens presented by the thymus? Opinions differ. Zinkernagel suggests that only syngeneic education is possible since A→B chimeras are immunologically incompetent and A to $F_1$ cannot be educated against B. Conversely, Matzinger, working with a minor histocompatibility system, has shown that A→B chimeras are competent and that cytotoxic T cells may be produced that are capable of killing cells bearing minor antigens in an H-2A and B context.

## NATURE OF THE Ir GENE PRODUCT: RELATIONSHIPS WITH HISTOCOMPATIBILITY ANTIGENS AND WITH FACTORS PRODUCED BY T CELLS

The Ir genes, which control specific responses to antigens, may, in theory, intervene by controlling the variable part of Ig. This hypothesis is unlikely

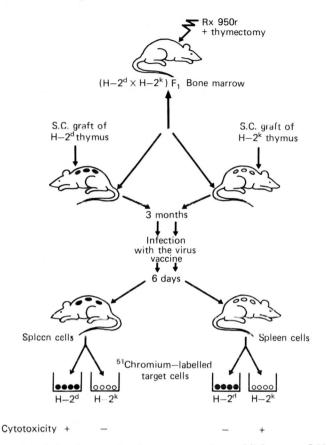

Rx 950r
+ thymectomy

$(H-2^d \times H-2^k)$ $F_1$ Bone marrow

S.C. graft of
$H-2^d$ thymus

S.C. graft of
$H-2^k$ thymus

3 months

Infection
with the virus
vaccine

6 days

Spleen cells

Spleen cells

$^{51}$Chromium—labelled
target cells

$H-2^d$   $H-2^k$

$H-2^d$   $H-2^k$

Cytotoxicity   +      —                          —      +

**Fig. 24.5**  The role of the thymus in the ontogenetic establishment of H-2 restriction. Adult $(H-2^d \times H-2^k)$ $F_1$ mice are thymectomized, lethally irradiated (950 R), and then reconstituted with an injection of $(H-2^d \times H-2^k)$ bone marrow, whose T cells are eliminated by anti-θ serum treatment. Thymus lobes from $H-2^d$ or $H-2^k$ mice are then grafted subcutaneously. Three months later, the chimeras thus obtained are infected with the virus vaccine, and the cytotoxic capacity of their spleen cells is assessed against virus-modified $H-2^d$ or $H-2^k$ target cells. Cytotoxicity is observed only when the target presents the same H-2 antigens as the grafted thymus.

because of the absence of any link between the Ir locus and the locus coding for the allotypes of immunoglobulin heavy chains in the mouse. Numerous other hypotheses have been envisaged, but, as yet, it is impossible to make a definitive choice among them.

In fact, two principal models may be proposed to explain the role and function of Ir genes.

In the first model, the function of the Ir genes is to code for Ia molecules on macrophages and B lymphocytes. The Ia molecules interact with thymus-dependent antigens in such a manner that the T cells (helper effect, delayed hypersensitivity, proliferation) differentiate with a specificity for each of two components (Ia and conventional antigen). This first model is, in fact, a variant of the schema described by Zinkernagel (see p. 87). In other words, when the Ia antigen, present on the macrophage surface is incapable of interacting with conventional antigen in such a way as to produce an immunogenic signal for T cells, the macrophage is incapable of stimulating the T cell and, thus, the animal is a nonresponder. Injection of antigen into this animal with operationally deficient macrophages may then result in the appearance of suppressor T cells (provided there is no deficiency of recognition at their level). This model assumes that the Ia antigen represents an Ir gene product. In some cases, the interaction of two Ia molecules on the macrophage is necessary, as is the case with GLφ.

Data concerning B cells are less clear. The model presumes that the same Ir genes are expressed on both B cells and macrophages. Ia molecules on B cells interact with antigen (bound to immunoglobulin receptors and representing a target for T cells specifically activated by the same complex of antigen and Ia molecule). Thus, one can explain the fact that T cells from (responder × nonresponder) $F_1$ mice cooperate only with the parental B cells (sensitized against the hapten) that possess the Ir gene in question. In such a situation, the Ia molecule of $F_1$ macrophages, associated with antigen, generate the production of memory T cells, and only B cells bearing the Ia molecules in question are recognized by T cells. This latter interpretation requires direct demonstration. It will also be important to determine whether macrophages must interact directly with T cells or by means of the intermediary of factors, such as "GRF" (see p. 533).

According to the second model, the Ir genes are first of all expressed at the level of the T cell, and they control the production of helper and suppressor factors. In this model, Ir genes would directly be involved in the expression of the T cell repertoire, perhaps at the level of the anti-self receptor. The presence of Ia antigens on helper and suppressor factors would be readily explained by such hypothesis.

It is difficult to choose between these two models. Perhaps they are both correct and reflect the control of specific immune responses by two distinct mechanisms, implying two classes of different molecules coded for by the I region.

## ROLE OF Ir GENES IN RELATION TO DEVELOPMENT OF INFECTIONS, NEOPLASIA, AND CERTAIN IMMUNOLOGIC DISEASES

Inasmuch as Ir genes in various species control numerous immune responses, including susceptibility to infections, neoplasia, and diseases that involve immunologic mechanisms, it seems likely that Ir genes contribute to the organism's suceptibility to various aggressions. In man, in whom Ir genes are ill-defined, correlations have been observed between the above-mentioned diseases and various histocompatibility antigens, which are coded for by genes that are probably physically close to Ir genes; however, this correlation is not necessarily due to direct association of disease and Ir genes.

### Experimental Animal Data

SENSITIVITY TO VIRUS-INDUCED LEUKEMIA

In the mouse, H-2 specificity and susceptibility to Friend's and Gross's leukemogenic viruses are related. Susceptibility to Friend's virus is dependent on two gene types, one independent of and the other dependent of H-2. These gene types determine the degree of splenomegaly that results from injection of high doses of virus; the disease is less marked in $H-2^b$ than in $H-2^d$ mice. Susceptibility to Gross's virus is apparently controlled by two genes. The Rgv-1 gene is linked to H-2 and determines resistance to the virus ($H-2^k$ mice are very susceptible). This is, in fact, a true Ir gene, because it confers to (BALB × B6) $F_1$ mice the capacity to respond to a new transplantion antigen induced by the leukemia (the GIX antigen). The two other genes, Rgv-2 and Rgv-3, are independent of H-2.

EXPERIMENTAL IMMUNOLOGIC DISEASES

Experimental allergic thyroiditis is linked to the H-2 complex in the mouse. Experimental allergic encephalomyelitis in the rat is linked to Ag-B antigens.

### Data Obtained in Man

Only preliminary data are available on the role of Ir genes in relation to the development of infection and disease in man, because Ir genes have not been very thoroughly explored in the human species. It has been reported that IgE production in response to ragweed, responsible for hay fever, seems to be correlated with the presence of HLA-B7 antigen, but this observation requires confirmation.

SUSCEPTIBILITY TO INFECTIONS

In certain settings, susceptibility to certain bacterial infections may be linked to HLA antigens. For example, patients with epiglottitis or meningitis caused by *Hemophilus influenzae* infections may have an abnormally high frequency of HLA-B14 and Bw15 antigens. Susceptibility to Australia antigen may also be genetically inherited; however, no correlation with HLA antigens has been formally demonstrated, except in hemodialyzed patients. In such patients, it has been found that those possessing the B8 antigen are particularly able to eliminate Australia (HBs) antigen.

HLA AND DISEASES

Considerable effort has been devoted in recent years in an attempt to correlate HLA groups with selected diseases of suspected immunologic origin. The highest correlation is found for ankylosing spondylitis and HLA-B27 antigen; this antigen is present in 80–90% of patients with the disease, as contrasted to a 10% occurrence in normal subjects (Table 24.3). Less spectacular correlations, which are, nonetheless, significant, have been found for other antigens and myasthenia gravis, gluten enteropathy, psoriasis, dermatitis herpetiformis, chronic active hepatitis, multiple sclerosis, diabetes mellitus, and Addison's disease.

It seems that the best correlations are observed with antigens HLA-B -D, and even -DR (Tables 24.3 and 24.4). In fact, apart from the rare disorders associated exclusively with HLA-B antigen (B5 and B27), the majority of diseases are mainly associated with the HLA-D and DR antigens. It is interesting to note that in the majority of cases, these disorders (mainly those associated with D and DR antigens) possess a common factor in that they are linked with more-or-less well-defined immunologic abnormalities and are more common in women.

The significance of correlations established between a given disease and HLA group must be subjected to rigorous statistical analysis. It must also be ensured that the patients and control-reference populations are obtained from comparable ethnic groups. The selection criteria for the patients must be strict and homogeneous. The study of the transmission of the illness and HLA phenotypes within a given family should be undertaken whenever possible.

Two types of association between an illness and its markers may be distinguished. In the first type, there is a simple genetic character, transmission being dominant. When the illness is transmitted, one always finds a certain allele in the immunogenetic system, which, in the family under consideration, represents a marker of the disease. This condition, however, is not absolute and depends on the degree of recombination between the gene of the illness and the gene of the immunogenetic system. Simultaneous transmission of the disease and the allele may occur within the family, but, when compared from one family to another, it is not always the same allele that is implicated. Congenital adrenal hyperplasia, due to 21-hydroxilase deficiency (HLA-linked); certain hereditary C-2 deficiencies (also HLA-linked), the nail-patella syndrome (linked to ABO groups); and elliptocytosis (Rh-antigen linked) are all examples of this.

More often, the diseases are not hereditary in the strict sense. A familial background may exist, but no genetic schema can account for some of these rare familial disorders.

**Table 24.3   Frequencies of Certain HLA Antigens in Normal Subjects and in Patients With Certain Diseases**

| Disease and HLA antigen | Patients (%) | Normal population (%) |
|---|---|---|
| Ankylosing spondylitis, B27 | 81 | 4 |
| Psoriasis, B17 | 22 | 4 |
| B13 | 13 | 4 |
| Juvenile diabetes B8 | 31 | 11 |
| Celiac disease, B8 | 45 | 11 |
| Hemochromatosis, A3 | 81 | 24 |
| Multiple sclerosis, Dw2 | 41 | 12 |

After J. Dausset.

**Table 24.4  HLA and Disease-Definite Associations**

| Condition | HLA | Frequency (%) Patients | Controls | Relative Risk* |
|---|---|---|---|---|
| Hodgkin's disease | A1 | 40 | 32.0 | 1.4 |
| Idiopathic hemochromatosis | A3 | 76 | 28.2 | 8.2 |
| | B14 | 16 | 3.8 | 4.7 |
| Behçet's disease | B5 | 41 | 10.1 | 6.3 |
| Congenital adrenal hyperplasia | B47 | 9 | .6 | 15.4 |
| Ankylosing spondylitis | B27 | 90 | 9.4 | 87.4 |
| Reiter's disease | B27 | 79 | 9.4 | 37.0 |
| Acute anterior uveitis | B27 | 52 | 9.4 | 10.4 |
| Subacute thyroiditis | B35 | 70 | 14.6 | 13.7 |
| Psoriasis vulgaris | Cw6 | 87 | 33.1 | 13.3 |
| Dermatitis herpetiformis | D/DR3 | 85 | 26.3 | 15.4 |
| Celiac disease | D/DR3 | 79 | 26.3 | 10.8 |
| | D/DR7 also increased | | | |
| Sjögren syndrome | D/DR3 | 78 | 26.3 | 9.7 |
| Idiopathic Addison's disease | D/DR3 | 69 | 26.3 | 6.3 |
| Graves' disease | D/DR3 | 57 | 26.3 | 3.7 |
| Insulin-dependent diabetes | D/DR3 | 56 | 28.2 | 3.3 |
| | D/DR4 | 75 | 32.2 | 6.4 |
| | D/DR2 | 10 | 30.5 | .2 |
| Myasthenia gravis | D/DR3 | 50 | 28.2 | 2.5 |
| | B8 | 47 | 24.6 | 2.7 |
| S.L.E. | D/DR3 | 70 | 28.2 | 5.8 |
| Idiopathic membraneous nephropathy | D/DR3 | 75 | 20.0 | 12.0 |
| Multiple sclerosis | D/DR2 | 59 | 25.8 | 4.1 |
| Optic neuritis | D/DR2 | 46 | 25.8 | 2.4 |
| C2 deficiency | D/DR2 | | | |
| | B18 | | | |
| Goodpasture's syndrome | D/DR2 | 88 | 32.0 | 15.9 |
| Rheumatoid arthritis | D/DR4 | 50 | 19.4 | 4.2 |
| Pemphigus (Jews) | D/DR4 | 87 | 32.1 | 14.4 |
| IgA nephropathy | D/DR4 | 49 | 19.5 | 4.0 |
| Hydralazine-induced SLE | D/DR4 | 73 | 32.7 | 5.6 |
| Hashimoto's thyroiditis | D/DR5 | 19 | 6.9 | 3.2 |
| Pernicious anemia | D/DR5 | 25 | 5.8 | 5.4 |
| Juvenile rheumatoid arthritis: | | | | |
|   pauciarticular | D/DR5 | 50 | 16.2 | 5.2 |
|   all cases | D/DRw8 | 23 | 7.5 | 3.6 |

* After A. Svejgaard. The relative risk expresses the increase in the risk of being afflicted with the disease when one possesses the antigen in question in comparison with the risk when one does not possess the antigen. Knowing the antigen frequency in patients (FP) and in controls (FC), the relative risk (R) is calculated according to the following formula:

$$R = \frac{FP\,(1 - FC)}{FC\,(1 - FP)}$$

NB: Other associations between HLA antigens and certain diseases have also been reported but require confirmation.

Doubtless the interpretation of these associations is not always the same. The most attractive hypothesis is that the disorder is linked to the presence of an Ir (or Is) gene in linkage disequilibrium with the HLA antigen. Different alleles at diverse Ir loci may explain an exaggerated or deficient response against certain antigens. It should, however, be noted that studies that tend to demonstrate the existence of Ir genes in man are still preliminary. In addition, the susceptibility to the disorder is generally dominant and the presence of an "unfavorable" gene should induce an abnormal immune response rather than an absent response since in the majority of cases (heterozygotes) a "nonpathogenic" allele exists.

The involvement of genes analogous to those described in good and bad antibody-producing mice (see p. 699) is barely probable, except, perhaps, for those diseases associated with HLA antigens A1, B8, and DR3, which seem to translate an overall immune hyperreactivity. Moreover, it should be noted that most the genes described by Biozzi are sited outside the MHC. The association with genes coding for complement factors or cellular interaction genes is also improbable, except, perhaps, for certain particular cases (abnormal function of variants of complement components).

A role for the HLA antigens themselves may also be evoked to explain a very strong association between HLA antigens and a disorder, such as HLA-B27, which is associated with ankylosing spondylitis in several ethnic groups, from European Caucasians to the Japanese. HLA antigens may have determinants in common with certain bacteria or viruses. This has, in particular, been suggested for Klebsiella (and HLA-B27) but has never really been demonstrated. The presence of elevated titers of anti-Gross virus natural antibody in mice susceptible to this virus is not wholly compatible with this hypothesis. Furthermore, homozygous subjects should be more sensitive to infection by the organism in question, and this has never been demonstrated. The HLA-antigen molecule may also play the role of receptor for a virus or hormone. Above all, the HLA-antigen molecule may associate with an antigen or a hapten and permit them to be recognized by receptors on T cells. Only certain HLA antigens could then give rise to immunogenic associations.

Finally, it should be recalled that even in the most evident cases (such as B27 and spondylitis) by far the majority of subjects bearing the antigen in question (10% of the normal population for B27) do not develop the disease, which clearly indicates that the phenomena associated with the presence of HLA antigens are not the only causative etiologic factors.

## III.  GENETIC CONTROL OF THE ANTIBODY PRODUCTION PHASE

Antibody titers present after immunization with a complex antigen [like sheep red blood cells (SRBC)] vary among strains, even in a given species. Antigenic complexity explains why it is difficult and even impossible to analyze Ir genes that correspond to each determinant. One may take advantage of this complexity to study the effect of genetic factors other than Ir genes, in hope that these effects may then be neutralized. By use of this approach, Biozzi has selected mice that vary in the ability to produce antibodies directed against SRBC. These antigens are very complex, probably representing a true mosaic of determinants. Biozzi has defined two mouse lines, high- and low-antibody producers.

## SELECTION OF HIGH- VERSUS LOW-RESPONDER MICE

The principle of the technique developed by Biozzi involves mating high- and low-anti SRBC agglutinin-producing mice (by measuring the peak response after injection of an optimal SRBC dose). Selection was studied in a group of 62 ordinary Swiss mice that were genetically unrelated (and included both sexes). A one-month interval is allowed to elapse between weaning and immunization to diminish the effect of maternal antibodies passively transferred to the newborn. Because the selection obtained for SRBC is also applicable to pigeon RBC, both kinds of red blood cells may be used alternatively in successive generations. After 15–20 generations, "good-producer" mice show titers of approximately 1/10,000, in contrast to a titer of 1/40 in bad producers (Fig. 24.6). Responses in both groups are quite homogeneous.

Most importantly, high producers respond well not only to SRBC but apparently to all antigens, for example, *Salmonella* antigens, bovine serum albumin, chicken egg albumin, hemocyanin, SIII pneumococcal polysaccharide, (thymus-independent) and DNP-BSA (Table 24.5). Similarly, low-SRBC responders are also unable to produce large amounts of antibody to any of these antigens. Selection bears on various antibody classes (IgG and IgM), anaphylactic

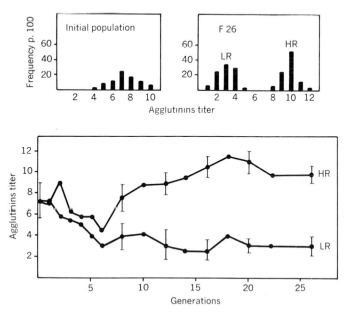

**Fig. 24.6** Separation of high- and low-responder mice during selective breeding, assessed by the production of antisheep red blood cell antibodies. (From G. Biozzi et al., Ann. Inst. Pasteur, 1974, *125c*, 119.)

McDevitt H. O. The role of H-2 I region genes in regulation of the immune responses. In: Immunology 80 (M. Fougereau and J. Dausset [eds.]). Acad Press, New York, 1980, 503.

MacDevitt H. O., Oldstone M. B. A., and Pincus T. Histocompatibility-linked genetic control of specific immune responses to viral infection. Transpl. Rev., 1974, 19, 209.

MacDevitt H. O. Regulation of the immune response by the major histocompatibility system. New Engl. J. Med., 1980, 303, 1514.

Möller G. (Ed.) HL-A and disease. Transpl. Rev., 1975, 22.

Möller G. (Ed.) Specificity of effector T lymphocytes. Transpl. Rev., 1976, 20.

Möller G. (Ed.) Acquisition of the T cell repertoire. Immunol. Rev., 1978, 42.

Mozes and Shearer G. M. Genetic control of the immune response. In Current Topics in Microbiology. Vol. 59. Berlin, 1972, Springer.

Mozes E. Expression of immune response (Ir) genes in T and B cells. Immunogenet., 1975, 2, 397.

Rosenthal A. S. Thomas J. W., Schroer J., and Blake J. T. The role of macrophages in genetic control of the immune response. In: Immunology 80 (M. Fougereau and J. Dausset [eds.]). Acad. Press, New York, 1980, 458.

Rude E. and Gunther E. Genetic control of the immune response to synthetic polypeptides in rats in mice. In L. Brent and J. Holborow, Eds., Progress in immunology. II. Vol. 2. Amsterdam, 1974, North Holland, p. 223.

Sachs D. H. and Dickler A. B. The possible role of I region determined cell surface molecules in the regulation of immune responses. Transpl. Rev., 1975, 23, 159.

Schreffler D. C and David C. S. The H-2 major histocompatibility complex and the I immune response region. Genetic variation, function and organization. Adv. Immunol., 1975, 20, 125.

Schwartz B. D., and Shreffler D. C. Genetic influences on the immune responses. In: Clinical Immunology (Parker C. W. [ed.]). Saunders, Philadelphia, 1980, 49.

Shearer G. M., Rehn T. G., and Schmitt-Verhulst A. M. Role of the murine major histocompatibility complex in the specificity of in vitro T-cell mediated lympholysis against chemically-modified autologous lymphocytes. Transpl. Rev., 1976, 29, 222.

Shearer G. M. and Schmitt-Verhulst A. M. Major histocompatibility complex restricted cell-mediated immunity. Adv. Immunol., 1978, 25.

Shearer G. M., Schmitt Verhulst A. M., and Rehn T. G. Significance of the major histocompatibility complex as assessed by T cell mediated lympholysis involving syngeneic stimulating cells. In: Contemp. Topics in Immunobiology. Plenum Press, New York, 1977, 221.

Stiffel C., Mouton D., Bouthillier Y., Heumann A. M., Decreusefonc C., Mevel J. C., and Biozzi G. Polygenic regulation of general antibody synthesis in the mouse. In L. Brent and J. Holborow, Eds., Progress in immunology. II. Vol. 2. Amsterdam, 1974, North Holland, p. 203.

Svejgaard A., Morling N., Platz P., Ryder L. P., and Thomsen M., HLA and disease. In Immunology 80 (M. Fougereau and J. Dausset [eds.]). Acad. Press, New York, 1980, 530.

Zinkernagel R. M. and Doherty P. C. MHC restricted cytotoxic T cells: studies on the biological role of polymorphic major transplantation antigens determining T cell restriction. Specificity, functions and responsiveness. Adv. Immunol., 1979, 27, 52.

# ORIGINAL ARTICLES

Engleman E. G. (Ed). Genetic control of the human immune response. J. Exp. Med., 1980, 152.

MacDevitt H. O., Deak B. D., Shreffler D. C., Klein J., Stimpfling J. H., and Snell G. D. Genetic control of the immune response. Mapping of Ir locus. J. Exp. Med., 1972, 135, 1259.

Matzinger P. and Waterfield J. D. Is self tolerance H-2 restricted? Nature, 1980, 285, 492.

Munro A. J., Taussig M. J., Campbell R., Williams H., and Lawson Y. Antigen-specific T-cell factor in cell cooperation: physical properties and mapping in the left-hand (K) half of H-2. J. Exp. Med., 1974, 140, 157.

TADA T., TANIGUCHI M., and DAVID C. S. Properties of the antigen-specific T cell factor in the regulation of antibody response in the mouse. IV. Special sub-region assignment of the gene(s) that code for the suppressive T cell factor in the H-2 histocompatibility complex. J. Exp. Med., 1976, *144*, 713.

ZINKERNAGEL R. F. Major transplantation antigens in T cell-mediated immunity: a comparison of the transplantation reaction with anti-viral immunity. Fed. Proc., 1978, *37*, 2379.

**Part 6**

# IMMUNOPATHOLOGY

# Chapter 25

# PRINCIPLES OF IMMUNOPATHOLOGY

**Jean-François Bach**

I.   INTRODUCTION
II.  AUTOIMMUNIZATION
III. EXPERIMENTAL IMMUNOLOGIC DISEASES
IV.  ETIOLOGY AND PATHOGENESIS OF AUTOIMMUNITY
V.   EXPERIMENTAL PATHOLOGY OF IMMUNE COMPLEXES

## I.  INTRODUCTION

The immune system is orientated toward rejecting foreign substances, particularly infectious agents, tumors and grafts. Most of these reactions generally have an ultimately favorable effect for the individual (except sometimes graft rejection), and normally the immune system does not react against its own constituents (Ehrlich's "horror autotoxicus").

However, there are several circumstances when abnormal stimulation of the normally reactive immune system or primary dysfunction of the lymphoid organs (hypo- or hyperfunction) may have unfavorable clinical consequences. These immunopathologic manifestations may be classified into five main categories: autoimmune diseases, immune complex diseases, immunoproliferative disorders (neoplasias of the lymphoid system), immunodeficiencies, and hypersensitivity reactions, including atopy.

This classification is, however, imperfect. Thus, for example, systemic lupus erythematosus (SLE) is associated with production of autoantibodies and immune complexes. Moreover, as we shall see, SLE and some other autoimmune diseases are probably linked to certain types of immunodeficiencies and may be rarely associated with lymphomas. This classification is, however, a practical one because it allows the grouping of most human immunologic diseases.

Additionally, it is in agreement with most immunopathologic experimental models that we will review in this chapter.

## II.  AUTOIMMUNIZATION

### DEFINITION

Autoimmunization is the immunization of an individual against his own constituents. Autoantibodies are antibodies produced by an individual against structures present within himself. Antigens toward which autoantibodies are directed are called autoantigens. They may be tissue antigens, or free molecules as immunoglobulins or coagulation factors. The concept of autoantibodies is based on the hypothesis of "self" and, as such, is difficult to define. It is often, in particular, hard to differentiate between autoantibodies and alloantibodies. Thus, anticolon antibodies were long considered to be true autoantibodies, but actually they are usually alloantibodies directed against digestive group substances. Similarly, SLE may be associated with true autoantilymphocytic antibodies (active against one's own leukocytes) and with alloantibodies directed against transplantation antigens (whether or not HLA), which are not borne by the patient's own lymphocytes.

### AUTOANTIBODY SPECIFICITY: THE CONCEPT OF ORGAN SPECIFICITY

Some autoantibodies are directed against organ-specific determinants (e.g., glomerular basement membrane, heart, or adrenals). In some cases, autoantibodies are not organ specific but are directed against determinants present in numerous or all organs, like antinuclear antibodies (Table 25.2). This distinction is not just theoretical but is clinically important, as we shall see later.

Table 25.1 lists the principal autoantibodies observed in human diseases, along with the techniques used for their detection. One should immediately note that more than one autoantibody is usually present in a given patient. Note also the imprecise definition of most of these autoantibodies. The technique most often utilized for detection is immunofluorescence, which does not allow precise biochemical definition of antigens. Cross-reactions between various autoantibodies are poorly defined, although they are often observed; for example, antiglomerular basement membrane antibodies in Goodpasture's syndrome react with alveolar basement membrane antigens. Little information is available on the specificity and affinity of autoantibodies, again because of the imprecise autoantigen definition. There are often difficulties in borderline cases on deciding whether an antibody titer is significant, especially for immunofluorescence reactions, which are only semiquantitative. All these difficulties explain why techniques that utilize purified antigen preparations are preferred, for example, in measuring anti-DNA antibodies by the Farr test by use of $^{14}$C-labeled DNA.

**Table 25.1  Main Autoantibodies**

| | Technique* | Diseases |
|---|---|---|
| Thyroglobulin | P, PH, IF | Thyroiditis, Graves' disease |
| Thyroid microsomes | IF | Thyroiditis |
| Receptors for TSH | Cyclic AMP synthesis | Graves' disease |
| Intrinsic factor | Blocking of fixation of vitamin $B_{12}$ on intrinsic factor | Pernicious anemia |
| Gastric parietal cells | IF, CF | Pernicious anemia |
| Adrenal gland cells | IF, CF | Addison's disease |
| Islets of Langerhans | IF | Diabetes mellitus |
| Epidermal cells | IF | Pemphigus |
| Cutaneous basement membranes | | Pemphigoid |
| Lens | Cutaneous reactions | Sympathetic ophthalmia |
| Glomerular and pulmonary basement membranes | IF, PH, radioimmunoassay | Goodpasture's syndrome |
| Erythrocytes | Coombs' test | Autoimmune hemolytic anema |
| Platelets | Thromboagglutination, CF, platelet survival | Some thrombocytopenic purpuras |
| Striated muscle (skeletal and cardiac) | IF | Myasthenia gravis, rheumatic fever |
| Smooth muscle | IF | Acute chronic hepatitis Biliary cirrhosis |
| Thymus | IF | Myasthenia gravis |
| Lymphocytes | Cytotoxicity | Numerous autoimmune diseases |
| Brain | Cytotoxicity | Multiple sclerosis |
| Spermatozoa | Agglutination | Some male sterilities |
| Ovarian cells (steroid secreting) | IF | Some female sterilities |
| Mitochondria (liver) | IF | Primary biliary cirrhosis |
| Salivary and lacrimal glands | IF | Sjögren's syndrome |
| Fc fragments of IgC | Rose-Waaler reaction Latex text | Rheumatoid arthritis, SLE |
| Nuclear antigens | IF, Le cells, Farr test | SLE, rheumatoid arthritis |

* P, precipitation; PH, passive hemagglutination; IF, immunoflourescence; CF, complement fixation.

## AUTOANTIBODY PATHOGENICITY

The interrelationship between organ-specific autoantibodies and clinical manifestations of organ dysfunction may be unclear. It is often difficult to decide whether autoantibodies are the cause of the clinical manifestations, an associated phenomenon (while another immunologic mechanism, such as cell-mediated immunity, might be causal), or are only the consequence of disease. Thus, antierythrocytic antibodies are responsible for the anemia observed in autoimmune hemolytic anemia, while antiheart antibodies are secondary to the tissue necrosis of myocardial infarction. It is likely that rheumatoid factor is associated with rheumatoid arthritis, without being either its cause or consequence. This difficulty probably explains the often unrewarding nature of the search for autoantibodies in many presumptive autoimmune diseases. Moreover, the usual absence of good animal models excludes experimental studies.

The best approach remains the search for a correlation between the presence of autoantibodies and the existence of defined clinical symptoms. It is, however, unusual for an autoantibody to be exclusively associated with one given disease or syndrome, with perhaps the exception of antinative DNA antibodies, which are found essentially in SLE (except for a few subjects with high titers and no clinical lupus signs). It is possible that the poor correlations seen may be explained in some cases by binding of antibodies to their target which reduces their serum concentration. It should also be remembered that certain antibodies may be produced in situ in the target organ, this possibly being the case in thyroiditis and multiple sclerosis.

We shall later examine the mechanisms of the pathogenic action of autoantibodies. One should, however, note now that the main mechanisms are cytolysis, opsonization, deposition in organs in the form of immune complexes, and induction of cytotoxicity by "K" cells against autoantibody-coated target cells (see p. 413). Antibodies also appear to intervene by stimulating the function of certain organs, for example, LATS in Graves' disease, which has a thyroid-stimulating hormone-like action.

## POSSIBLE ROLE OF CELL-MEDIATED IMMUNITY

Experimental autoimmune diseases are often associated with the existence of delayed hypersensitivity toward autoantigens that occurs concomitantly with autoantibodies. It is in fact a general feature of most immune responses to associate antibodies and cell-mediated immunity. The existence of cell-mediated immunity in autoimmune diseases is suggested by the positivity of certain in

**Table 25.2   Autoimmune Diseases**

| | |
|---|---|
| Organ nonspecific | |
|   Systemic lupus erythematosus | |
|   Rheumatoid arthritis | |
|   Sjogren's syndrome | |
|   Hemolytic anemia, leukopenia and thrombocytopenia of immunologic origin | |
| Organ specific | |
|   Endocrine glands | Thyroiditis, Graves' disease, Addison's disease, hypoparathyroidism |
|   Gastrointestinal tract | Pernicious anemia, Crohn's disease?,* ulcerative colitis |
|   Kidney | Goodpasture's syndrome |
|   Muscle | Myasthenia gravis, rheumatic fever? |
|   Eye | Sympathetic ophthalmia |
|   Skin | Pemphigus |
|   Spermatozoa | Some sterilities? |

* Question marks indicate the uncertain nature of autoimmune etiology.

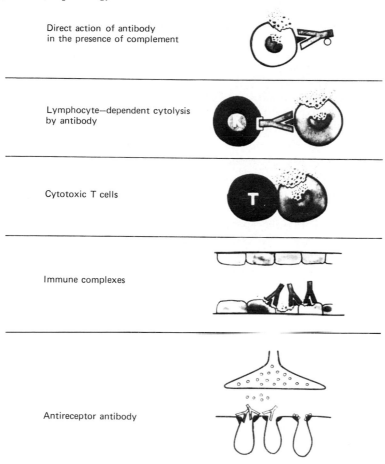

Direct action of antibody
in the presence of complement

Lymphocyte—dependent cytolysis
by antibody

Cytotoxic T cells

Immune complexes

Antireceptor antibody

**Fig. 25.1** Effector mechanisms in immunopathology.

vitro tests that are considered to be correlated with delayed hypersensitivity (lymphocyte transformation or leukocyte migration inhibition), but the contribution of antibodies in these tests is always difficult to eliminate. Additionally, we are confronted with the same problem discussed for autoantibodies, namely, to determine whether delayed hypersensitivity assessed in vitro is the cause or a consequence of the disease. In fact, as we shall see, most experimental autoimmune diseases seem to be associated with the action of antibodies, apart from experimental allergic encephalomyelitis, where cell-mediated immunity apparently plays the principal role.

# III.  EXPERIMENTAL IMMUNOLOGIC DISEASES

## SPONTANEOUS DISEASES

Several models of spontaneous autoimmune diseases have been described, particularly in the mouse.

### Immune Complex Disease of New Zealand Black (NZB) Mice

NZB mice were originally obtained in New Zealand from a radiation-induced mutation. These mice present multiple autoimmune manifestations, including, as early as 6 months of age, Coombs' positive autoimmune hemolytic anemia, antinuclear antibodies, and glomerulonephritis (GN) with Ig (Fig. 25.2) and DNA glomerular deposits (detected by immunofluorescence). These autoimmune manifestations are associated with other immunologic abnormalities, which may even precede them. As early as the first month of life, thymus cells become resistant to tolerance induction toward thymus-dependent antigens, such as sheep red blood cells (SRBC) or bovine serum albumin (see p. 582). Atrophy of the thymic epithelium is associated with premature cessation of thymic hormone secretion (Fig. 25.3). At 3 months of age, there is loss of the suppressor T-cell function, which probably explains the increased antibody responses, particularly observed against thymus-independent antigens (Fig. 25.4). The production of SIRS (defined on p. 550) is diminished together with the number of Lyt 123$^+$ cells. At 6 months of age, a progressive decline in all T-cell functions is noted, involving mitogen responsiveness, reactivity in the mixed-lymphocyte reaction, graft-versus-host reaction, and tumor rejection. It is only after 12–14 months that the number of θ-positive cells declines. At the same time, significant modifications of the lymphoid organs occur, with an initial lymphoid hyperplasia (pseudolymphoma) followed by a true lymphoma (type B) associated with a monoclonal macroglobulinemia.

It might be suggested that all these abnormalities are linked with a premature involution of the thymus, more precisely of the thymic epithelium, whatever its etiology (genetically controlled premature aging, viral infection, etc.). The correction of many of these abnormalities by thymus grafts or injections of thymic factor supports this hypothesis. An intrinsic deficiency of

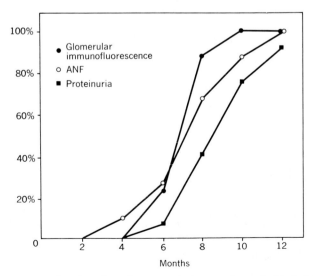

**Fig. 25.2** Appearance of antinuclear factor and glomerulonephritis in NZB mice. (After J. B. Howie.)

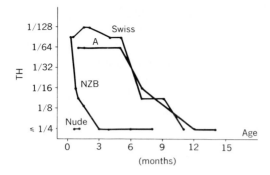

**Fig. 25.3** Serum level of thymic hormone in Swiss, A, NZB, and nude mice as a function of age. (After J. F. Bach and M. Dardenne, 1972.)

prothymocytes (i.e., pre-T cells) might also be envisaged, but the fact that epithelial cell grafts from NZB mice are (compared with those of other strains) incapable of restoring T-cell function in nude mice is in favor of the former hypothesis. It could also be postulated that the T-cell abnormalities are secondary to the action of circulating inhibitory factors, notably immune complexes and lymphocytotoxic antibodies. These antibodies seem to be preferentially directed against certain T-cell subpopulations, particularly suppressor T cells. The inconstant appearance of these antilymphocytic antibodies and the favorable effect of thymus grafts do not favor a role for these antibodies in the development of the disease, but they may contribute to the progressive decline in T-cell function observed during the life of the NZB mouse.

The links uniting the T-cell deficiency and pathogenesis of autoimmunity are very likely, but have not yet been definitely demonstrated. It is possible that the very early diminution in the suppressor T-cell population in these mice explains the secondary appearance of autoimmune manifestations. In this regard, it is significant that NZB mouse disease is transmitted by spleen cells

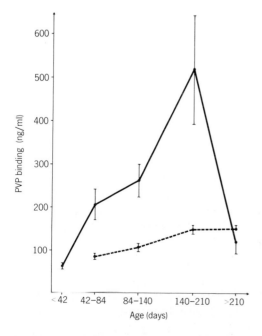

**Fig. 25.4** Augmentation of the production of antipolyvinylpyrrolidone (anti-PVP) antibodies in NZB mice (—) as compared to C57BL/6 mice (– – –) as a function of age. The level of anti-PVP antibodies is assessed by the Farr test. (After M. A. Bach, 1975.)

from aged animals to younger ones (which supposedly still have suppressor T cells) only when the recipients are treated with antilymphocytic serum to inactivate their own T cells and that neonatal thymectomy aggravates NZB mouse disease, whereas, as we have seen, thymus grafts or injections of thymic factors have the opposite effect. Reduction of the number of Lyt $123^+$ cells may play an important role in the loss of suppressor T-cell function. In fact, it seems that the phenomena are more complex than was initially thought. NZB mice appear to be capable of generating suppressor T cells, but these cells appear to be ineffective, perhaps because of a fault at the stage represented by the Lyt $123^+$ cells (see p. 548).

Several recent experimental pieces of evidence argue in favor of the presence of intrinsic B-cell hyperactivity in NZB and B/W mice. Spontaneous polyclonal activation is detectable very early in the life of these mice, even before birth. Other signs of polyclonal B-cell activation are found before thymic failure onset. Such a B-cell abnormality, however, does not appear to be absolute since the autoimmunity may be prevented by thymus grafts or injections of SIRS (see p. 550). These considerations may, in the near future, lead to new therapeutic approaches in systemic lupus erythematosus (in particular by stimulation of T cells with thymic factors). Preliminary results have been promising, but the early experiments have also shown that it is still difficult to control the effects of these treatments on diverse T-cell populations, particularly in controlling the action on helper T cells, which may be the source of the exacerbation of certain autoimmune manifestations. This may notably be the case when these products are administered late in the disease when suppressor T-cell precursors have doubtless disappeared.

Nevertheless, the T-cell deficit only represents one of the many factors favoring the development of autoimmune manifestations, beside viruses (see below), sex hormones (male hormones retard the evolution of the disease, p. 810), genetic factors, and environmental factors (nutrition, UV rays, etc.).

NZB mouse cells carry endogenous xenotropic type-C RNA viruses, which only infect the cells of other species in vitro but replicate in NZB mouse cells (as opposed to ecotropic viruses, which replicate in the cells of the same species).

Type C viral antigens are found on T- and B-lymphocyte surfaces and on the membranes of B/W mouse B lymphoma, in particular, the glycoprotein of the viral envelope (gp70) and the core protein (p30). Their role, possibly linked to H-2 antigens with which they seem to be tightly associated, remains to be defined. The preferential localization of the virus in lymphocytes may explain the incidence of antilymphocytic antibodies. The virus could also play a role of a nonspecific adjuvant for immune responses or might be the cause of a premature degeneration of the thymic epithelium. It has been reported that NZB mouse disease can be transferred to other mouse strains by cell free extracts of NZB mouse spleen, but these experiments do not appear to be reproducible. The isolation of a virus specific to NZB mice has also been described but has not been further confirmed.

### Other Mouse Spontaneous Diseases

Other strains of spontaneously autoimmune mice exist, such as certain mice of A strain or Swan mice (Swiss antinuclear), obtained by genetic selection based on the spontaneous presence of antinuclear antibodies in aged Swiss mice (Monier). After three or four generations, mice thus selected present autoimmune manifestations and glomerulonephritis analogous to those described above for NZB mice. Other strains of autoimmune mice have recently been described, particularly the MRL/1, MRN/n, and BXSB strains, which, like NZB mice, develop multiple autoantibodies (notably antinuclear) with deposits containing type C viral glycoproteins (gp70), elevated levels of Ig, lowered serum levels of complement factors, and thymic cortical atrophy. However, these mice present a profile of autoantibodies slightly different from those of B/W mice, a more rapid and severe evolution, with a greater degree of lymphoid hyperplasia, a greater frequency of arteritis (in MRL/1) and in BXSB mice a male predominance (MRL/1 males and females having a comparable evolution). These differences could relate to a different pattern of the Ir genes controlling autoantigen recognition but also to different nature of T- and B-cell imbalance (e.g. excess of helper T-cell functions). Finally, the early appearance of glomerular deposits of Ig and antinuclear antibodies in the nude mouse should be noted, as should the presence of antinuclear antibodies in SJL mice (concomitantly with a dysproteinemia with monoclonal Ig and lymphoid tumors).

### Obese Chicken Thyroiditis

A chicken strain derived from the white leghorn strain develops spontaneous autoimmune thyroiditis. These chickens have subcutaneous fat deposits, which predominate in the abdomen, simultaneously with bone and integumental abnormalities, plus an abnormal sensitivity to cold. The disease aggravates with age, leading to premature death. All of these abnormalities are due to thyroid insufficiency, as shown by serum hormone levels. The thyroid is infiltrated by lymphoid cells and germinal centers. By electron microscopy, numerous cells show a well-developed endoplasmic reticulum, suggesting local antibody synthesis. The disease is genetically determined: more than 90% of animals are affected after eight-generation selection, the trait being polygenic. The genetic control, linked to the B locus of the major histocompatibility complex, affects both the immune response and the target cells (the thyroid gland of obese chickens possesses before the appearance of the disease, certain functional abnormalities).

The obese chicken disease resembles in many respects Hashimoto's thyroiditis. It displays numerous immunologic abnormalities also found in Hashimoto's human thyroiditis. There are serum antibodies against thyroid antigens, in particular, thyroglobulin. These antibodies are detected by passive hemagglutination, immunoprecipitation, or immunofluorescence techniques and reach maximal titers at 17 weeks. Antithyroxin antibodies, which may contribute to the clinical hypothyroidism, are also found.

It is fortunately easy in the chicken to study the respective contribution of B and T cells to the autoimmune response after thymectomy and bursectomy. Thyroiditis is completely prevented by neonatal bursectomy and, conversely, is aggravated by neonatal thymectomy. The latter is reminiscent of similar observations made in NZB mice. These facts suggest that, as in NZB mice, a suppressor T-cell failure is operative, with obvious effects on the production of antithyroid antibodies but also more generalized effects, as suggested by the appearance of autoantibodies directed against other organs. At variance with NZB mice, no viral particle has yet been found, and transfer experiments with cell-free homogenates have been completely negative. A spontaneous thyroiditis has also been observed in BUF rats.

### Aleutian Mink Disease

A lethal disease, which affects the liver and kidneys, in particular, was seen in an Aleutian mink farm in 1941, following a mutation initially detected by change in fur color. The liver and kidneys are infiltrated with numerous plasma cells, which initially suggested a myeloma-like disease. In fact, the disease may be transmitted by tissue extracts obtained from sick minks, which contain viral particles. Renal disease is an immune complex-induced glomerulonephritis, with characteristic Ig granular deposits located in the glomeruli and in the vascular tree. Aleutian mink virus is found in serum, urine, and various organs. There is usually severe hypergammaglobulinemia, which is sometimes mono-clonal, associated with elevated free antibody titers against the virus. The antibodies are not neutralizing and do not confer protection. One also finds, in the serum and urine, immune complexes composed of DNA, anti-DNA anti-bodies, and antivirus antibodies. Free anti-DNA antibodies in the serum indicate that these complexes are in antibody excess. The presence of these complexes is compatible with the existence of GN and arteritis.

## INDUCED DISEASES

It is relatively easy to induce an autoimmune disease in various species by injecting organ extracts in the presence of adjuvant or certain viruses.

### Diseases Induced by Injection of Organ Extracts

#### EXPERIMENTAL THYROIDITIS

Injection of homologous thyroid extracts, emulsified in complete Freund's adjuvant, provokes the appearance of thyroiditis in guinea pigs and rats. This disease, which resembles Hashimoto's thyroiditis and the spontaneous thyroiditis of the obese chicken (described earlier), causes destruction of the normal follicular architecture and the appearance of mononuclear cell infiltrates. It is also associated with autoimmune signs of the human disease. Thus, there are autoantibodies and delayed hypersensitivity directed against thyroglobulin. At variance with obese chicken thyroiditis, induced thyroiditis is preventable by neonatal thymectomy. 6-mercaptopurine also prevents the disease by suppress-ing delayed hypersensitivity without altering antithyroglobulin antibody pro-duction. The pathogenic role of the autoantibodies is, nevertheless, suggested by the prevention of transfer of the disease by incubation of B cells with highly radiolabeled thymidine and the possibility of transferring the disease with serum, provided it is administered in sufficiently high doses. T cells also intervene, probably essentially as helper T cells for antibody production. The intervention of cytotoxic T cells has, however, recently been suggested by studies showing H-2 restriction in the effector phase of the disease (Cohen). The disease is controlled genetically both at the level of the antithyroglobulin-immune response (at a locus situated in the I region) and, more unexpectedly, at that of the thyroglobulin used for the autoimmunization. The thyroglobulin of certain strains more readily induce the appearance of the autoimmune disease than that of others.

EXPERIMENTAL ALLERGIC ENCEPHALOMYELITIS (EAE)

EAE is an autoimmune disorder that results in demyelinization of the central nervous system. It is obtained by the injection of central nervous homogenates together with adjuvant. The clinical and pathologic manifestations, which in many ways resemble those of multiple sclerosis, are secondary to the response that develops against the basic encephalitogenic protein of myelin (BEP). BEP is a protein whose primary structure has been entirely elucidated, with a molecular weight of 18,200 daltons and an isoelectric point greater than 10. It possesses several antigenic determinants that have been localized, sequenced, and synthesized in an active form. In particular, it has been possible to synthesize the peptide fragments that induce delayed hypersensitivity to BEP (and an EAE) without antibody production and, reciprocally, a peptide fragment that induces antibody formation without producing delayed hypersensitivity or EAE. Some of the antigenic determinants of basic protein are not encephalitogenic but may prevent the development of EAE following BEP injection.

Convergent arguments indicate that, contrary to other spontaneous or induced autoimmune disease, EAE is essentially mediated by T cells. The development of lesions is correlated with the existence of delayed hypersensitivity, both in vivo and in vitro, against BEP, whereas no such correlation has been found for anti-BEP antibodies. Injection of BEP with Freund's incomplete adjuvant, which diminishes the severity or even prevents EAE, is associated with a parallel depression of delayed hypersensitivity without inhibition of anti-BEP antibody production. Moreover, the transfer of lymphoid cells to healthy animals results in transfer of the disease (except after treatment of the cells with anti-T cell serum), whereas transfer with serum is not possible (although such transfer has been reported by a few workers). Both B and T cells bind labeled BEP, whereas only B cells bind labeled thyroglobulin. In cell transfer experiments in which the cells undergo a prior treatment with radiolabeled BEP, the "suicide" of B cells has no effect on EAE development, although this prevents the formation of anti-BEP antibodies. However, these data do not exclude the possibility that in addition to effector T cells, antibodies directed against antigens other than BEP may play a role, particularly locally secreted antibodies produced by B cells localized within the central nervous system itself.

The development of EAE is genetically controlled, being linked at least partially and polygenically to the major histocompatibility complex.

AUTOIMMUNE GLOMERULONEPHRITIS (GN)

When kidney extracts or purified preparations of glomerular basement membrane, either homologous or xenogeneic, are injected into sheep or rats in the presence of Freund's adjuvant, GN is produced. The GN is characterized histologically by cellular proliferation and subendothelial deposits. Immunofluorescence (anti-IgG sera) reveals linear deposits along the glomerular basement membrane. GN with linear Ig deposits may also be produced by injecting rats with serum from rabbits immunized with rat kidney extracts (Masugi's nephritis; see p. 830).

see p. 830

### EXPERIMENTAL ALLERGIC MYASTHENIA GRAVIS (EAMG)

Rabbits immunized with acetylcholine receptor (AchR) from eel electric organ in complete Freund's adjuvant develop a myasthenic syndrome (weakness, reversible with anticholinesterase treatment). EAMG has been produced in several other species including rats, mice and monkeys. In the latter species, the signs are very reminiscent of human MG with ptosis, disorders of ocular movement and dysphagia.

The disease is associated with the presence of antibodies directed to AchR. Developement of EAMG in mice is dependent on the major histocompatibility complex, but interestingly anti-AchR titers are similar in susceptible and resistant strains. EAMG clinical evolution is bimodal. The first wave may be fatal but most animals recover after a few days. The second wave is progressive and often ends in death. Monoclonal anti-AchR antibodies, have recently been produced using the hybridoma technique. Some (but not all) of these monoclonals induce a myasthenic syndrome when injected into mice in μg amounts.

## *Virus-Induced Diseases*

### MOUSE LYMPHOCHORIOMENINGITIS (LCM)

In the mouse, LCM virus induces an acute lethal disease characterized by facial edema and convulsions. At autopsy, there are diffuse necrotic lesions with cellular infiltrates, especially involving the central nervous system. However, some mice survive (paradoxically, those with the highest initial viremia), either because they eliminate the virus or because they become partially tolerant (induction of tolerance is favored by high virus dosage). Tolerance is particularly easy to produce in newborn or neonatally thymectomized mice; it is associated with intense viremia and several chronic immunologic manifestations, including GN and hepatitis. Tolerance is, nonetheless, incomplete, and one usually finds marked hypergammaglobulinemia with significant titers of antivirus antibodies, unless these antibodies are masked inside of immune complexes. The immune complexes are responsible for the GN.

The pathogenesis of acute lethal disease and chronic immune complex disease is related to the immune response of the host, as suggested by their prevention after administration of various immunosuppressive treatments, such as irradiation, amethopterin, cyclophosphamide, cortisone, or antilymphocyte serum (ALS). In this respect, it is of interest that in certain cases, particularly when ALS is used, antivirus antibody production is not altered. In the fatal form of the disease, observed after intracerebral injection in immunocompetent mice, the virus infects the cells without being directly cytopathic. In fact, it is the lymphoid cells sensitized against the virus that destroy the infected cells and the manifestations of LCM are due to this autoimmune reaction. The T cells of infected mice transmit the disease and result in the death of mice that carry the virus, even though not diseased. In addition, an increased number of cytotoxic T cells are found in the cerebrospinal fluid. The virus induces the formation of cellular neoantigens, as evidenced by the rejection of skin grafts from virus-bearing mice by noninfected syngeneic mice. The reaction against the host's own infected cells involves autologous transplantation antigens (see p. 482) since cytotoxic T cells only exert their cytotoxic effects on cells bearing H-2K or H-2D antigens in common with them. Cell-transfer experiments have shown that protection also undergoes H-2 restriction.

It is paradoxical that T cells, although responsible for the lesions are also responsible for protection against the disease, at least in the early phases of the viral infection. Subsequently, interferon-activated macrophages, neutralizing antibodies, and complement all intervene. The cytotoxic T cells appear to act by destroying the infected cells at the eclipse stage before the virus can multiply. Some time before the minimum number of cells necessary for the organism's function succumb to the infection, the destruction of infected cells is protective and beneficial to the host. Nonetheless, if too many cells are infected, the cellular destruction produces clinical consequences. Similar mechanisms are probably involved in human viral hepatitis, in the GVH response, and even in the rejection of virus-infected skin grafts.

Finally, it is apparent that any viral infection may be equally well explained by the presence of a weak cellular response against a cytopathic virus as by a strong immune response against a noncytopathic virus.

### OTHER PERSISTENT VIRAL DISEASES

Findings similar to those reported in the preceding paragraph (LCM) have been noted in Aleutian mink disease, in mouse infection by lactodehydrogenase virus, Moloney leukemia virus, and polyoma virus, and in infectious horse anemia.

# IV. ETIOLOGY AND PATHOGENESIS OF AUTOIMMUNITY

We have just discussed several types of very different experimental immune diseases, either spontaneous or induced. In man, a variety of possible autoimmune disorders exists. There is probably no point in proposing a unitary mechanism for all these diseases. We will rather discuss several hypotheses, some of which may be applicable in their original form, or after modification, to most human and animal autoimmune diseases. Before presenting these concepts, we will briefly discuss some general factors that favor development of autoimmunity, which may serve to vindicate our hypotheses.

## FACTORS THAT FAVOR AUTOIMMUNITY

Several factors favor the onset of autoimmunity in man and animals.

### Age

In animals, spontaneous autoimmune diseases, like the lupus syndrome in NZB mice or thyroiditis in obese chickens, do not begin until after the initial one-third of the species' life-span, and the severity increases with age. In aging mice of all strains (but with variable intensity, depending on strain), autoantibodies, in particular, antinuclear antibodies, appear along with IgG deposits in renal glomeruli, as detected by immunofluorescence. In man, autoimmune diseases often occur in relatively young subjects, but the incidence of pathologic serum autoantibodies in apparently healthy subjects sharply increases with age (Fig. 25.5).

### Sex

Females are more susceptible to autoimmune diseases than are males, as indicated by higher incidence and greater severity of NZB mouse disease and of obese chicken disease in females. Lupus is also more common in women than in men. These differences are probably not linked to genetic factors borne on, for example, sex chromosomes, but rather to differences in hormonal makeup. Androgen treatment of female NZB mice attenuates the disease, whereas castration of male NZB mice aggravates or accelerates it.

### Genetic Factors

The near relatives of patients with autoimmune diseases (parents, children, siblings) often show the same disease, sometimes in a patent form but more commonly as autoantibodies in apparently healthy subjects. This observation has been made for thyroiditis, pernicious anemia, biliary cirrhosis, and SLE; it suggests the intervention of a genetic factor in the pathogenesis of the disease. The autoimmune diseases of NZB mice and obese chickens are also genetically controlled. It has been possible to produce an experimental disease by genetic

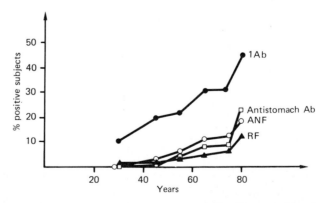

**Fig. 25.5** Increase in the level of various autoantibodies as a function of age in a rural Australian population (RF, rheumatoid factor; ANF, antinuclear factor; Antistomach: antiparietal cell antibodies; 1 Ab, at least one autoantibody). (From B. Hooper, S. Whittingham, J. D. Mathews, I. R. MacKay, and C. Curnow, Clin. Exp. Immunol. 1972, *12*, 79.)

selection based on the spontaneous appearance of antinuclear antibodies in Swan mice ( Monier ). The polygenic control of autoimmune diseases is, however, ill defined. Preliminary studies indicate two gene categories, one that controls the autoimmune condition and the other antibody specificity.

### Immunologic Background: Frequency of Cellular Immune Deficiency

We have already mentioned the existence of deficient cellular immunity and, more generally, deficient T-cell function in NZB mice. A comparable deficiency seems to be present in human lupus, although its reality is much less well established. A possible role of T-cell failure is supported by evidence that neonatal thymectomy aggravates NZB mouse disease and obese chicken thyroiditis (by contrast to the suppression of the latter disease after neonatal bursectomy). The effect of thymectomy in man is less well known, but several cases of autoimmunization and even lupus have been reported in subjects thymectomized for myasthenia gravis (however, interpretation of these reports is complicated by the fact that myasthenia gravis is itself associated with several immunologic abnormalities).

### Viral and Bacterial Infections

A role for infection in causing autoimmune diseases has been often suggested (type-C virus in lupus, slow virus in multiple sclerosis, streptococci in acute GN and rheumatic fever). We will later examine various mechanisms by which these microorganisms may act. In fact, there is considerable difficulty in establishing a cause and effect relationship between a given infection and an autoimmune disease. The infections suggested are often rather common, and the published correlations often lack use of control groups. Thus, these studies are subject to criticism. Direct demonstration of the presence of bacteria or viruses and demonstration of evidence of their passage (serodiagnosis) represent only indirect evidence; moreover, the recent demonstration of viral particles in various experimental and human autoimmune diseases is not very specific, because these particles have been found in numerous nonautoimmune diseases. Infections may, nonetheless, play an important role as a source of antigens for initiation of immune complex production, for example, of nuclear antigens in lupus and NZB mice.

### Relationship Between Autoimmunity and Immunoproliferative Syndromes

Numerous experimental and clinical arguments suggest that interrelations exist between autoimmunity, monoclonal Ig production, and malignant immunoproliferative syndromes. An undeniably increased frequency of autoantibodies is found in the monoclonal Igs of both man and mouse. The development of lymphoid neoplasia is common in some autoimmune diseases, particularly in Sjögren's syndrome and immunosuppressed subjects (whether due to a congenital immunodeficiency or following pharmacological immunosuppression). Conversely, it is not uncommon to see autoantibodies appear in patients suffering from lymphoma or chronic lymphatic leukemia. NZB and (NZB × NZW) $F_1$ mice develop, successively with age, autoantibodies, an immune complex GN, monoclonal macroglobulinemia, and malignant lymphoma. Finally, it is noteworthy that NZB mice together with BALB/c mice are the only mouse strains in which it is possible to induce monoclonal Ig-producing plasmocytomas by mineral oil injection. It is possible that an abnormality of the regulation undertaken by T cells on immune responses represents the common origin of these diverse abnormalities.

### Association of Autoimmune Diseases

Autoimmune diseases tend to be associated with each other more often than expected on the basis of chance. For example, pernicious anemia is 50 times more frequent in subjects with Hashimoto's thyroiditis than in normals (10% incidence versus 0.2%). A reciprocal correlation is seen in pernicious anemia. The association is still more frequent if the presence of autoantibodies is the criterion. Thirty percent of patients with Hashimoto's thyroiditis have antigastric parietal cell antibodies, and, conversely, 50% of patients with pernicious anemia show antithyroglobulin antibodies, even though the two antibodies do not cross react. It is interesting to note that most of these disease disorders are associated with the same HLA antigens (HLA-A1, B8, DR3, see p. 695). Similarly, one often notes associations and cases intermediate between SLE, hemolytic anemia, thrombocytopenic purpura, rheumatoid arthritis, and dermatomyositis. Interestingly, organ-specific autoimmune diseases (thyroiditis, pernicious anemia, Addison's disease) are rarely associated with nonorgan-specific diseases (like lupus). These data suggest a predisposition common to the diseases of each group. This suggestion is mostly conjecture, although, because both organ-specific spontaneous thyroiditis in the obese chicken, and NZB mouse disease are aggravated by neonatal thymectomy. Furthermore Sjögren's syndrome (see p. 819) associates a pseudolupus syndrome and organ-specific thyroid and salivary gland antibodies.

## THEORIES OF AUTOIMMUNITY

The theories of autoimmunity have wide theoretical implications for recognition of "self" and tolerance and also clinical applications, which probably explains why they have always intrigued immunologists. New theories appear now at a regularly increasing pace, which is associated with the rapid growth of knowledge about mechanisms of cellular immunity. We will deal successively with three main theories that, as we shall see, are not mutually exclusive.

### Forbidden Clones

In proposing the clonal theory for antibody selection, which implies that for each antigenic determinant there is a corresponding family, or "clone," of lymphoid cells that bear the corresponding receptors, M. F. Burnet gave a basis for the absence of autoimmunity in normal subjects and, therefore, a theory of autoimmunity. In this theory, initially there are lymphocytic clones for autoantigens, but the immature lymphocytes are destroyed or inactivated during fetal life on direct contact with the autoantigens. The only autoreactive cells that escape this elimination are those directed against sequestered autoantigens, namely, antigens that are not accessible to circulating lymphocytes (either because of a cellular barrier or because they appear late in development). These sequestered autoantigens could give rise, after fetal life, to true immune responses once introduced into the circulation, for example, after traumatic damage to the organ itself. This hypothesis has been confirmed for spermato-zoan antigens, which are sequestered in seminal tubes and appear late in fetal development. Metalnikoff demonstrated (in 1900) that guinea pigs immunized with their own sperm (without adjuvant) produced spermatozoa-immobilizing antibodies. Similarly, lens antigens are sequestered by absence of lymphatic drainage from the anterior chamber of the eye. After trauma these antigens are released into the circulation, with the appearance of a true autoimmune disease: sympathetic ophthalmia.

Except for these particular cases, the forbidden clone theory has very little evidence to support it, particularly for nuclear, erythrocytic or thyroglobulin antigens, responsible for the major human autoimmune diseases. These au-toantigens do not induce autoimmunization when injected into normal animals. In fact, there is no true sequestration of these antigens. This is obvious for red blood cells or nuclear antigens released by lysed cells but also true for other antigens usually considered as sequestered, including thyroglobulin (which is found in the serum of children or adults at concentrations on the order of 0.01–0.05 mg/ml). Moreover, thyroid trauma or partial destruction by $^{131}$I does not produce autoimmunization.

The hypothesis of elimination of autoreactive clones (the forbidden clones) is also contradicted by the demonstration of lymphocytic reactivity to autoan-tigens in adults. Lymphocytes bind on their surface labeled thyroglobulin or autologous red blood cells; 1–3% of lymphocytes in normal human peripheral blood bind labeled thyroglobulin, as detected by autoradiography. Interestingly, autologous serum albumin does not bind to the same lymphocytes under identical conditions. Another suggestion of potential lymphocytic autoreactivity comes from the work of Cohen and Feldman, who have shown that lymphocytes could be autosensitized in vitro on monolayers of thymic epithelial cells or fibroblasts. After a 5-day incubation, lymphoid cells become sensitized and are able to kill syngeneic fibroblasts in vitro (but not allogeneic fibroblasts) or to induce a graft-versus-host reaction after injection in syngeneic recipients. Autorosettes formed by normal lymphoid cells with autologous red blood cells, and autosensitization are blocked by the presence of syngeneic normal serum, a phenomenon that could be due to circulating autoantigens or autoantibodies, or to other factors.

Further evidence against the forbidden clone theory is suggested by the formation of autoantibodies in normal animals after injection of modified autoantigens or of substances that cross-react with autoantigens. This nearly immediate production of autoantibodies suggests the presence at all times of autoreactive B cells, which are nonfunctional in normals. In addition, loss of tolerance to a sequestered autoantigen does not explain very well the common association of several autoantibodies for different specificities in a given subject, the familial genetic factor, and increased autoimmune manifestations with age.

Furthermore, the existence of autoreactive T cells is suggested by (1) Cohen and Wekerle experiments, which have recently been confirmed for testicular and cerebral antigens, (2) the demonstration of autologous erythrocyte-binding T cells with H-2 specificity (Charreire) and T cells that bind myelin basic protein, and (3) the autologous-mixed lymphocyte reaction in which T cells transform in the presence of autologous B cells, by recognition of autologous Ia determinants.

The H-2 restriction of the recognition of non H-2 antigens by T lymphocytes has been described in detail in chapters 4 and 24. It is well recognized that viral or chemical antigens are identified in association with H-2 antigens. This self-recognition only occurs under strictly physiologic conditions and may not directly intervene in the pathogenesis of autoimmune disease. However, it is difficult to avoid drawing a comparison with the data described above on the role of viral-induced or chemically induced modifications of autoantigen molecules in the initiation of autoimmune reactions. Recent Cohen's data mentioned above, showing H-2 restriction in experimental allergic thyroiditis support such a comparison.

### Cross-Reactions With Autoantigens

It was mentioned earlier (chap. 20) that immunologic tolerance induced by low doses of antigens essentially involves T cells, whereas tolerance at high doses of antigens involves both B and T cells. Weigle proposed that the absence

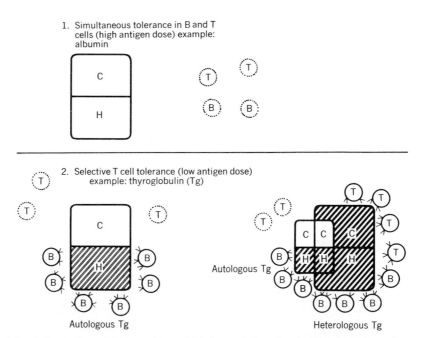

**Fig. 25.6** Schematic representation of high- and low-dose tolerance toward autoantigens. Elimination of autotolerance toward thyroglobulin by heterologous thyroglobulin (C, carrier; H, hapten). Nontolerant cells (complete circle) react against hapten or carrier determinants (cross-hatched). Tolerant cells (broken cricles) do not react against these determinants (white).

of autoimmunity in normal subjects could be due to a T-cell tolerance for the autoantigens present at low serum concentrations, for example, thyroglobulin, and to a B- and T-cell-type tolerance for antigens (like albumin) present in high concentrations. The onset of autoimmunity would be due to the loss of the T-cell-type tolerance or, more precisely, to a "bypassing" of tolerant T cells by T cells specific for another "carrier." This bypass can be obtained by a modification of autoantigen molecules that would induce the appearance of new carrier determinants toward which T cells are not tolerant or by use of substances that share determinants with autoantigens but that possess a sufficient number of differences to serve as carriers.

This autotolerance breakdown reminds one of termination of tolerance to bovine serum albumin (BSA) in the mouse by injection of human serum albumin (HSA), which shares antigenic determinants with BSA or by administration of arsanilated BSA (see p. 584). This mechanism does not apply to autoantigens present at high concentration like albumin. Injection of methylated or arsani-lated albumin does not induce the appearance of antialbumin antibodies, and albumin binding to lymphocytes has not been observed. B lymphocytes that bind thyroglobulin are not tolerant to this antigen, whereas B cells are tolerant to albumin, which probably involves tolerance at the level of both the T cell and the B cell. This hypothesis is consistent with the finding mentioned above that autoimmune diseases seem to be due to the pathogenic action of antibodies produced by B cells and not to the direct action of T cells, with the exception of experimental allergic encephalomyelitis. In addition, some workers have suggested the possibility that myelin basic protein is sequestered during development for a long period and does not therefore induce T-cell tolerance, but this remains to be confirmed. We shall now examine in more detail the two mechanisms whereby tolerant T cells are bypassed.

MODIFICATIONS OF THE AUTOANTIGEN MOLECULE

It is possible to modify the thyroglobulin molecule by various procedures and then induce an autoimmunization by injecting it alone without adjuvant. These modifications of the molecule may be achieved by proteolytic digestion, chemical treatment (addition of sulfanil, arsanil, or picryl groups), or physical treatment (heat, ultrasound), all of which alter the molecular conformation.

Changes in the autoantigen molecule probably explain the autoimmunization observed during some drug treatments. Thus, α-methyldopa (Aldomet) combines with Rhesus (Rh) antigens of red blood cell membranes, and this reaction leads to production of anti-Rh antibodies (Note, however, that according to a recent report Aldomet could also act by altering superior T-cell function). A similar mechanism may be the cause of lupus-like syndromes induced by procainamide or hydralazine. It might also explain the antierythro-cytic autoimmunization observed during *Mycoplasma pneumoniae* infection, by mycoplasma-induced modification of erythrocytic antigenicity.

ANTIGENS THAT GIVE RISE TO CROSS-REACTIONS

Certain hemolytic streptococci (in particular, the A 12 group) have antigenic determinants shared with the myocardium and with glomerular basement membranes. Other determinants, which are not possessed by myocardium, might serve as carriers for the shared determinants, thus leading to antiheart autoimmunization in rheumatic fever (see p. 929).

An identical mechanism was suggested for *Escherichia coli* 014 and some colon antigens and for the autoimmunization obtained after injection of heterologous organ extracts (species-specific determinants serving as carriers). The encephalitis that may follow antirabies vaccination (monkey cerebral tissue) may also be explained in this way. Playfair showed that it was possible to induce the appearance of antierythrocytic autoantibodies by injecting normal mice with rat erythrocytes (which possess both autoantigens, shared with the mouse and different determinants that can be used as carriers). The thyroiditis induced in the mouse or the rabbit by injecting heterologous thyroglobulin without adjuvant (bovine, porcine, or human) probably is caused by the same mechanism.

OTHER MECHANISMS

Viruses might be the source of autoantigens after induction of viral neoantigens on the cell surface. These neoantigens could then be carriers, leading to autoimmunization.

Adjuvants might act by several mechanisms: by binding to autoantigens and modifying them, by simply altering their configuration at the water-oil interface for Freund's adjuvant, or by nonspecific stimulation of T or B cells.

The allogeneic effect observed after injecting allogeneic cells may play a role that simulates the activity of the carrier-hapten system by bypassing tolerant T cells. This allogeneic effect probably explains the antierythrocytic autoimmunization observed in bone marrow grafts in man.

### Loss of Suppressor T-cell Function

The existence of a specific tolerance of T cells and its bypassing by various mechanisms represent an attractive theory of autoimmunity. However, some findings cannot be easily explained by it. For example, why the associations between various autoantibodies and why do these associations segregate into two groups, one for organ-specific and the other for nonorgan-specific diseases? Genetic and familial factors are also not well explained. Finally, least understandable of all would be the aggravating influence of thymectomy in NZB mice and in obese chickens: autoimmunity achieved through the activity of carrier-specific T cells should be decreased by thymectomy, but the opposite is observed. The abnormal onset of autoimmune manifestations in neonatally or adult thymectomized mice and in nude mice is also poorly explained.

An additional factor, loss of suppressor T-cell function, possibly linked to the premature thymus failure mentioned above, answers many of these objections (see p. 714). The failure of suppressor T cells (whether or not they are autoantigen-specific) will lead to a generalized hyperfunctioning of B cells, with preferential antibody production against (1) thymus-independent autoantigen (which do not need "helper" T cells). However, suppressor T cells are often deficient without alteration in helper T-cell function, and their deficiency may then lead to augmentation in helper function and thus to augmented response against thymus-dependent antigens, (2) antigens released in large quantities, for example, after trauma or bacterial or viral infection, and (3) antigens against which the subject is a good responder. One should recall that immune responses vary from one subject to another and that in the mouse, and probably also in man, these variations are controlled by immune response (Ir) genes.

This theory would explain not only the deleterious effects of thymectomy but also the frequent association of several categories of autoantibodies in one patient, the prevalence of a given antibody and of the corresponding clinical manifestations, and the role of genetic factors (Ir gene or others). One should note, however, that many of the arguments supporting the role of the loss of superior T-cell function are also compatible with other types of T-cell imbalance (e.g. excess of helper T cells or B cell intrinsic hyperactivity (see p. 715)

### Conclusions

The three theories discussed above each have experimental data that attest to their validity, but all are in some ways at odds with other clinical or experimental results. One could propose the forbidden clone theory for such autoimmune diseases as sympathetic ophthalmia and autoimmune sterility, a selective abnormality in T-cell tolerance for organ-specific autoimmune diseases, like Hashimoto's thyroiditis (in spite of the thymectomy data in obese chicken) and Aldomet®-induced autoimmune hemolytic anemia, and last, a loss of suppressor T cells in nonorgan-specific autoimmune diseases like SLE. In fact, these hypotheses are oversimplified, and it is likely that they all interrelate in some unknown way. In any case one may notice that in all three theories, a major role is given to a thymus or T-cell abnormality, which is reminiscent of Burnet's initial theory in which the thymus plays a crucial role in the elimination of the so-called forbidden clones.

## V. EXPERIMENTAL PATHOLOGY OF IMMUNE COMPLEXES

Deposition of antigen-antibody, or immune, complexes (IC) in organs and tissues provokes characteristic lesions that are thought to cause an ever-increasing list of pathologic conditions. IC may form locally in situ, as in Arthus's reaction, or appear as preformed circulating complexes. We will discuss here only the effects of circulating complexes and not the lesions of Arthus's reaction or the effects of antibodies directed against organs or vascular structures.

### EXPERIMENTAL MODELS OF IMMUNE COMPLEX DISEASES*

The most classic model of circulating IC disease is serum sickness, namely, "acute IC disease" (AICD). A chronic model of serum sickness disease has also been described. Recently, a new model of chronic IC disease has been reported that implicates living antigens, such as viruses.

* Section authored by J. Benveniste.

### Acute IC (Serum Sickness) Disease

Injection of high-dose heterologous proteins (for example, BSA, 250 mg/kg) into rabbits is followed most of the time by a series of very reproducible phenomena. BSA is eliminated in three phases, as described earlier (p. 330): equilibration for 2 or 3 days, followed by a catabolic phase of 3–4 days, and then immune elimination after 5–6 days. During the third phase, IC appear and are detectable in the serum. Simultaneously, arterial, articular, glomerular, cardiac, and cutaneous lesions develop that are characteristic of the disease. Glomerular lesions are modest (see p. 833), consisting of endothelial proliferation and slight thickening of basement membranes. One seldom finds neutrophils in the glomeruli. Proteinuria appears between Days 7 and 9 at levels as high as 1–2 g/24 hr. Arteritis is mainly localized to the coronary arteries and branches of the aorta or pulmonary artery. Initially, it consists simply of endothelial cell proliferation, but it progresses rapidly to fibrinoid necrosis with neutrophilic invasion. Immunofluorescence reveals antigen, C3, and Ig in the glomerular and arteriolar basement membranes with a characteristic granular aspect. However, these deposits are only detectable early in the disease. They disappear within 24–48 hr from the glomeruli and from the arterial lesions. The disease progresses to complete cure in 2–3 weeks.

### Chronic IC Disease

When a heterologous protein is injected daily in rabbits, some of them develop a membranous GN in 4–5 weeks, without simultaneous arterial lesions. GN appears only if a moderate amount of antibody is produced and when

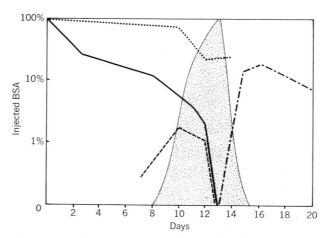

**Fig. 25.7** Acute serum sickness disease induced in the rabbit by injection of [131]I-labeled bovine serum albumin (BSA,—). Precipitation of labeled BSA by anti-Ig sera assesses the appearance of soluble immune complexes (– – –). Formation of complexes is associated with a decrease in the serum level of complement (·········) and with the appearance of clinical signs of serum sickness (proteinuria, renal, articular, and vascular changes; dark zone). Later, after the 14th day, one sees free antibodies in the serum (· – · – ·). (From F. J. Dixon. *In* R. A. Good and D. W. Fisher, Eds., Immunobiology, ed. 5. Stamford, Conn., 1973, Sinauer, p. 164.)

enough antigen is injected to produce soluble complexes in antigen excess. One may, however, provoke GN in hyperimmunized rabbits by increasing daily doses of antigen. If antigen dose is insufficient, few soluble complexes form, which neither circulate nor deposit. The course of disease may, however, be modified by injecting massive antigen doses. Recent studies have shown that when large antigen doses are given to rabbits as multiple daily injections, resulting in significant antibody production, diffuse lesions are produced throughout the entire arteriolar-capillary system that are comparable to human SLE. It seems probable that under these conditions, large quantities of IC of heterogeneous size have formed. In sum, these observations indicate that development of glomerular deposits and arteriolar lesions are dependent on the nature and quantity of the immune complexes.

Glomerular lesions of chronic IC disease have been studied in detail (p. 834). These lesions vary widely, depending on the immunologic situation, ranging from a slight thickening of glomerular basement membranes to epithelial proliferation with crescents. In the most severe forms, immunofluorescence and electron microscopy show deposits along the epithelial side of the basement membrane; these deposits contain C3, antigen, and Ig. These severe forms are observed in settings in which antigen injections are given on a very chronic basis. They may lead to death in renal failure after several weeks.

### Other Experimental IC Diseases

Experimental IC diseases in the mouse have already been described in the preceding pages: lymphochoriomeningitis, chronic infection by lactodehydrogenase virus, and NZB, B/W, and Swan mouse spontaneous diseases. Many species, such as mice, sheep, and rats, have Ig (and probably IC) deposits in their glomeruli during the last third of life. Aleutian mink disease is a spontaneous and transferable IC disease (see p. 716).

## MECHANISM OF COMPLEX DEPOSITION AND CREATION OF TISSUE LESIONS*

### Complex Deposition

The passage of large aggregates, like IC, across capillary walls had been widely studied, when it was realized that IC lesions in rabbits, mice, and guinea pigs could not be achieved by administering preformed IC. Similarly, antigen injection into immunized animals or antibody injection into animals with free antigen in circulation does not create IC deposition. These observations suggest that an active factor is necessary for IC deposition. Further experiments have shown that deposition does occur when IC are injected simultaneously with histamine, serotonin, or a mast cell degranulating agent (anaphylatoxin, octylamine). Conversely, antihistamine or antiserotonin administration prevents the usual IC deposition in serum sickness. Decreased circulating platelets, which

* Section authored by J. Benveniste.

represent the major histamine reservoir in the rabbit, is also associated with reduced IC deposition.

In vitro study of the immunologic mechanisms of vasoactive histamine release by platelets under the influence of IC showed that either complement up to C3 (immunoadherence) or up to C9 (lysis) and neutrophils were involved in IC deposition. Another mechanism, complement independent, has recently been described. This mechanism involves polymorphs sensitized by antigen injection. Its study was prompted by the observation that IC deposition is independent of C3, C6, and neutrophils in the rabbit and by the observed positive correlation between this mechanism and the appearance of AICD. The complement-independent mechanism requires the presence of basophils sensitized by IgE antibodies directed against the injected heterologous protein.

In vitro, at 37°C, in the presence of antigen, basophils degranulate and release histamine and platelet-activating factor (PAF-acether). The platelets then release vasoactive amines. PAF-acether, isolated from human and rabbit leukocytes, macrophages and platelets, is a phospholipid (1-0-alkyl-2-acetyl-glyceryl-3-phosphorylcholine). A good correlation has been observed between the presence of circulating basophils and the amount of PAF-acether extracted from human leukocyte preparations. Basophil number and PAF-acether amount are much decreased in SLE during its active phases (Benveniste). These results favor a role of the IgE-basophil system in human IC diseases.

The size of complexes play a critical role in deposition. Only soluble complexes formed in antigen excess in protein antigen-antibody systems with IC larger than 19S are capable of deposition and causation of lesions. AICD is seen only in rabbits that have complexes larger than 19S. Very large complexes, formed in antibody excess, are rapidly eliminated from the circulation, probably by the reticulohistiocytic system. Small complexes circulate for a long time without deposition. The role of complex size has also been documented in

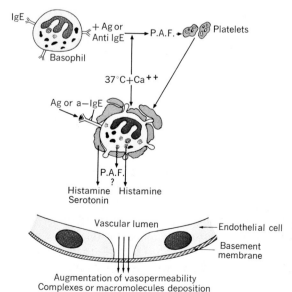

Fig. 25.8 Mechanisms of immune complex deposition under influence of the IgE-basophil-platelet-activating factor (PAF-acether) system.

chronic IC disease. Another important factor in IC deposition is the mode of blood flow in vessels: turbulence favors complex deposition, which may explain why IC-induced lesions preferentially develop at points of arterial branching and bifurcation. Experimentally, IC deposition may be enhanced by mechanical constriction around the aorta (rabbit).

These data suggest the following model of IC deposition in AICD: the circulating antigen stimulates IgG and IgE antibody production. Reaction with IgG in antigen excess provokes formation of soluble IC. Antigen reaction with IgE on basophil membranes induces degranulation with release of histamine and PAF from basophils. PAF causes platelet aggregation and induces release of histamine and serotonin. These reactions require contact between antigen and IgE and preferentially occur in turbulent blood flow. Increased capillary vasopermeability results in the deposition of large complexes by filtration along vascular walls. It is possible that other mediators, which may originate in basophils, are also involved indirectly in uptake of large complexes by endothelial cells of vessel walls. Finally, IC deposition depends on two requirements: (1) the quality of circulating complexes, for example, size and structure, which relates to the immune response (IC diseases probably occur selectively in animals, and perhaps in humans, who produce small amounts of antibodies and thus show relative antigen excess) and (2) the capacity to provoke an anaphylaxis-type IgE response that favors IC deposition.

### Lesions

Once deposited along the basement membranes, IC are capable of activating complement to release low-molecular-weight mediators (C3a, C5a) that are chemotactic for neutrophil polymorphs. The IC deposits, during phagocytosis, cause release of lysosomal proteolytic enzymes and produce characteristic IC lesions. There are, unfortunately, numerous exceptions to this scheme. For example, AICD GN has been observed in animals previously decomplemented and depleted of neutrophils. Certain forms of GN in experimental chronic serum sickness disease do not invoke a neutrophilic reaction.

### Resolution of Lesions

Neutrophils seem to play a major role in eliminating IC lesions through phagocytosis. Neutrophil-depleted animals eliminate deposited IC much more slowly than do normal animals. However, IC disappearance does not always cause clinical cure if the lesions are already well established.

## TECHNIQUES FOR DETECTING IMMUNE COMPLEXES

The role of IC in the pathogenesis of many immunologic diseases is now well established, and therefore IC detection would provide considerable diagnostic help. Several methods have been recently proposed that permit indirect demonstration of IC in settings where they are present in large amounts, for example, in SLE and rheumatoid arthritis (RA).

## Immunoglobulin Deposits (Immunofluorescence)

The demonstration of Ig deposits in tissues (usually by immunofluorescence) is suggestive of IC deposition, especially when the deposits appear to be granular and are associated with complement (C1q or C3). These Ig deposits are even more pertinent in the rare instances when an antigen may be demonstrated along with the corresponding antibody, by elution and antigen-antibody separation techniques. It must be recalled, however, that Ig in tissues may also be associated with autoantibodies directed against tissue structures or may sometimes, particularly when present in small quantities, represent non-specific Ig deposition.

## Direct IC Demonstration

In theory, detection of circulating IC requires isolation of the complex, followed by elution, and then recovery of both Ig that possesses antibody activity and the corresponding antigen. This is usually impossible since it can be performed only in situations in which the antigen is known. In some cryoglobulinemias, the antigen has been separated from antibody by lowering pH or elevating molarity (by urea or potassium iodiate solutes). It was then shown that DNA and anti-DNA antibodies, renal tubular antigens and corresponding antibodies or lymphocytotoxic antibodies could be demonstrated in some IC. It is important to note that the precipitate could not be shown to contain antigen or antibody prior to elution. In rare situations where antigen is particulate (e.g., HBs), demonstration of particles by electron microscopy after precipitation with anti-Ig serum indicates the presence of complexed HBs. Relative to the latter method, it should be recalled that the capacity of serum to transfer virus is suppressed after Ig precipitation in chronic viral IC diseases of the mouse. Note also that recent data indicate that a significant proportion of circulating IC are made of anti-idiotypic antibodies reacting with the idiotypes borne by autoantibodies or antibodies directed to infectious agents.

## Mixed Cryoglobulins

The serum of some patients precipitates in thermal cold (between 0 and 22°C). The cryoprecipitates (which redissolve at 37°C) may contain fibrin, monoclonal proteins like those seen in multiple myeloma, or nonmonoclonal Ig, often of several classes, as determined by immunoelectrophoresis. Mixed cryoglobulinemia refers to the presence of multiple Ig classes. By immunoelectrophoresis or radial immunodiffusion, IgM and IgG are seen in variable proportions, and less often IgA and complement (C1q, C3) are observed

It is of interest that many patients with cryoglobulinemia show circulating rheumatoid factors (RF). Sometimes RF is found only in the cryoprecipitate itself (and not free in sera). In other cases, the cryoprecipitate contains anti-DNA or antilymphocytic antibodies. Cryoprecipitability is usually determined by an interaction between two IgM and IgG components (neither of these components alone will cryoprecipitate). However, only individual IgM fractions

**Table 25.3   Immune Complex Diseases in Man**

| | | |
|---|---|---|
| Infection | Bacterial | Subacute bacterial endocarditis |
| | | Infectious meningitis |
| | Mycobacterial | Lepromatous leprosy |
| | Protozoal | Malaria |
| | Viral | Dengue fever, hepatitis B |
| Exogenous | Nutritional | Gluten sensitivity |
| | Environmental | Extrinsic alveolitis |
| | Drugs | Serum sickness (penicillin, sulfonamides) |
| | | Induced lupus (procainamide, hydralazine) |
| Autoantigens | IgG | Rheumatoid arthritis |
| | Nucleic acids | Lupus |
| | Tumor antigens | Lymphomas |
| | | Carcinomas |
| Others (unknown antigens) | Renal diseases | |
| | Gastrointestinal diseases | |
| | Crohn's disease | |
| | Ulcerative colitis | |

After A. M. Denman.

are potentially cryoprecipitable: although the IgG component in complex may be replaced by IgG from a normal subject, the IgM component must be the patient's own product.

Mixed cryoglobulinemia may be accidentally discovered in subjects without clinical manifestations (essential cryoglobulinemia). However, most often, mixed cryoglobulinemia is discovered in patients who present with purpura, Raynaud's syndrome, arthralgia, or renal tubular acidosis. It is commonly seen in SLE, rheumatoid arthritis, and Sjögren's syndrome and less often in membranoproliferative GN and thyroiditis. Mixed cryoglobulinemia may be present in specific infectious diseases, including infectious mononucleosis, syphilis, and bacterial infections, both subacute and chronic. Immunoproliferative disorders, such as myeloma and Waldenström's macroglobulinemia, in which monoclonal proteins can show anti-IgG activity, may also be associated with mixed cryoglobulinemia.

The presence of cryoglobulinemia during immunization of normal animals (at the phase of immunocomplexemia) and in human diseases in which IC are implicated suggests that mixed cryoglobulins may represent circulating antigen-antibody complexes. The frequent finding of complement components (C1q, C4, C3) within the precipitate (often associated with serum hypocomplementemia, as with anticomplementary activity of serum) along with demonstrated antibody activity and less common antigen, in the cryoprecipitate tend to corroborate the hypothesis that a high percentage of nonmonoclonal cryoglobulinemia represents circulating IC.

### Methods for Detecting Circulating Immune Complexes

The methods employed for the detection of circulating IC fall into two main groups. Those of the first group can be applied in the majority of cases and detect IC irrespective of the antigen they contain. Those of the second group attempt to demonstrate, in a specific manner, complexes involving a given antigen by evaluation of the relative proportions of free to Ig-bound antigen.

NONANTIGEN-SPECIFIC METHODS

These methods are based on differences in the properties between Ig molecules complexed with antigen and free Ig. These differences bear on the physical modifications involved in the formation of the complex and in the biologic activities of the complexes, particularly fixation of complement and binding of Fc fragment and complement receptors on present on certain cells.

*Methods Based on the Physical Properties of Complexes.*   The formation of IC leads to the formation of new molecular structures characterized with regard to free Ig by an increase in size, alterations of surface properties, alterations in solubility, and modification of the electrical charge.

Analytical ultracentrifugation enables the detection of large-sized complexes. Thus, the protein peaks with a sedimentation constant of 22S or 19S–17S are observed in certain patients suffering from rheumatoid arthritis. These are respectively IgM-IgG or IgG-IgG complexes. This method has the disadvantage of low sensitivity. When used alone without immunochemical characterization of the peaks, it does not allow the confirmation of the presence of IgG in the peaks. In a similar fashion, saccharose gradient fractionation, gel chromatography, or selective ultracentrifugation combined with immunochemical characterization may also be used, which permits the demonstration of Ig's of higher molecular weight than native Ig. These analytical techniques have theoretical interest but are too cumbersome for routine large-scale application.

Under certain conditions, the abnormal precipitation of serum proteins in a serum sample may be indicative of the presence of IC. Mixed cryoglobulins (IgG-IgM) represent, as has been seen, the most commonly encountered IC. Precipitation by polyethylene glycol (PEG) (molecular weight 6,000) may also be used, but proteins other than IgG may precipitate; it is preferable to characterize proteins precipitated by PEG (IgG, IgM, C1q, C4).

*Methods Based on Complement Fixation.*   The interaction of IC with complement is the basis of many techniques used to detect IC. Two large groups of techniques may be distinguished. First, those founded on competitive inhibition by complexes of complement hemolytic activity; second, those that involve the direct demonstration of C1q fixation on IC. The weakness common to all of these techniques lies in the possible fixation to C1q of substances other than IC, notably certain cell components or microbial products.

1.   Tests of C1q deviation. The measurement of anticomplement activity consists of the incubation of the serum sample with a source of complement and then followed by the measurement of the complement activity as evaluated by hemolytic capacity.

The C1q deviation test consists of measurement of the anticomplement activity restricted to C1q. The method depends on the competitive inhibition of the fixation of radiolabeled C1q on sensitized erythrocytes by IC. In the first stage, the test serum is incubated with the labeled C1q, then, the sensitized erythrocytes are added. The red cells are isolated by centrifugation and their radioactivity counted. This test is sensitive, and, unlike the preceding technique, it is not confused by products that exclusively activate the alternative pathway.

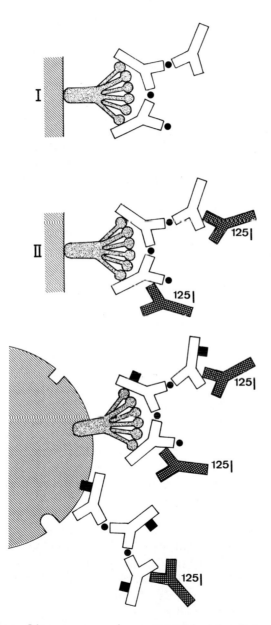

**Fig. 25.9** Detection of immune complexes. *Top*: Principle of the technique using the fixation of immune complexes on C1q in the solid phase. *Bottom*: principle of the technique using the fixation of immune complexes on "Raji" cells.

It is possible to replace the sensitized erythrocytes by IgG-coated latex particles or Sephadex.

The inhibition of IgG-coated latex particle agglutination by IC invokes the same principle. However, this latter method is influenced by the presence of rheumatoid factor.

2. Direct measurement of the interactions of IC with C1q. The C1q-in-agarose precipitation test, one of the first of this type to be described, is only positive with sera containing large quantities of IC. It is based on the diminution of IC solubility in the presence of high concentrations of C1q.

The C1q fixation test is more sensitive and more quantitative. It consists of incubating the serum under study with radiolabeled C1q and thus separating the free C1q from the IC-bound C1q by differential precipitation by PEG. The percentage of labeled C1q precipitated is directly dependent on the quantity of IC present. The test may also be performed in the solid phase. The serum to be tested is incubated in the polystyrene tube whose walls are coated with C1q. The quantity of IC fixed on the walls of the tube is evaluated after the addition of radiolabeled or enzyme-linked anti-immunoglobulin antibody.

In all these tests, the C1q present in the serum is inactivated by heating to 56°C or addition of EDTA.

*Methods Based on Interaction with Rheumatoid Factor (RF).*   Several techniques for the detection of IC use the property of rheumatoid factor of binding to IC. These techniques are analogous to the preceding ones, the RF playing the role of C1q. The principal tests are those of direct precipitation by RF in agarose gel and the inhibition by IC of the interaction between RF (subsequently bound to cellulose) and aggregated Ig. However, these tests are relatively insensitive even when improved by the use of monoclonal RF. In addition, they may not be employed when the serum to be tested contains RF and the results obtained depend on the serum level of free Ig, which may react with the RF.

*Methods Using the Binding of IC to Cellular Receptors.*   IC have the property of binding onto receptors for the Fc fragment of IgG or for complement (when they have fixed complement). Several methods capitalize on this property. They possess the inconvenience of employing living cells, which renders their standardization difficult.

Interaction with Fc receptors. The platelet aggregation test depends on the fixation of IC on platelets. Inhibition of the ADCC phenomenon (see p. 413) is linked with the combination of IC to the Fc fragment of IgG coating the target cells. The inhibition of IgG incorporation by macrophages is performed with labeled IgG and guinea pig peritoneal exudate cells.

Interaction with complement receptors. Several cells, particularly B lymphocytes and, cells from the continuous lymphoblastoid Raji cell line, possess receptors for C3 or its degradation products C3b and C3d (see p. 75). The test which employs Raji cells consists of incubating the test serum with the Raji cells. The cell suspension is then washed and the radiolabeled Ig fraction of a rabbit antihuman Ig is added to it. The IC, bound to the Raji cells by the C3 they bound in vivo and, to a lesser degree by their Fc fragments, fix the labeled antiserum. Aberrant results may be obtained in the presence of antilymphocytic antibodies.

Inhibition of EAC rosettes produced with red cells coated with antibody and complement is also used, but false results may be obtained because of the possible interference of free C3 and its degradation products.

*Conclusions.* The multiplicity of available methods makes the choice difficult. In theory, it is desirable to employ methods that are sensitive, specific, reproducible, and sufficiently easy to perform that they can be used routinely. The first three may be realized with simple methods, such as the search for mixed cryoglobulins (insensitive) or the PEG test (if possible combined with immunochemical characterization of the precipitates). It then seems preferable to employ several tests, for example, the solid-phase C1q fixation test and the Raji cell test. It must however be realized that all the methods described are subject to certain risks of error, particularly false-negatives—if the venopuncture is not performed at 37°C to avoid the loss of cryoprecipitable IC in the clot— or false-positives—if the Ig have been aggregated by freeze-thawing or heating above 56°C.

Some authors prefer to express their results in terms of mg of Ig aggregated, which, in fact, is somewhat illusory since the aggregates have heterogeneous sizes and in any case do not represent true IC.

SEARCH FOR ANTIGEN-SPECIFIC IC

When the antigen responsible for IC formation is known, it is possible to identify IC more directly. For particulate antigens (for example, HBs antigen), the serum may be examined by electron microscopy after centrifugation or precipitation by PEG. The presence of HBs antigen may also be detected by radioimmunoassay after dissociation of the IC by heating or through destruction of Ig by protease or by studying the percentage of antigens that can be precipitated by anti-Ig sera. In the case of DNA, the quantity of anti-DNA antibody liberated after DNAase treatment may be evaluated. One can also attempt to dissociate cryoglobulins at acid pH, to separate antigen and antibody and then test the activity of the anti-DNA antibody. These techniques can only rarely be applied, and their interpretation is often difficult.

# *BIBLIOGRAPHY*

ALLISON A. C. The roles of T and B lymphocytes in self-tolerance and autoimmunity. Contemp. Topics Immunobiol., 1974, *3*, 227.

ALLISON A. C. Auto-immune diseases: concepts of pathogenesis and control. *In* N. Talal, Ed., Auto-immunity: genetic, immunologic, virologic and clinical aspects. New York, 1977, Academic Press, p. 91.

ALLISON A. C. and DENMAN A. M. Self tolerance and autoimmunity. Brit. Med. Bull., 1976, *32*, 124.

AMOS B., SCHWARTZ R. S., and JANICKI B. W. Immune mechanisms and disease. Acad. Press, New York, 1979, 376 pp.

BACH J. F., BACH M. A., CARNAUD C., DARDENNE M., and MONIER J. C. Thymic hormones and auto-immunity. *In* N. Talal, Ed., Auto-immunity: genetic, immunologic, virologic and clinical aspects. New York, 1977, Academic Press, p. 91.

BURNET F. M. Autoimmunity and autoimmune disease. London, 1972, Medical and Technical Publ.

COCHRANE C. G. Mechanisms involved in the deposition of immune complexes in tissues. J. Exp. Med., 1971, *134*, 75s.

COCHRANE C. G. and KOFFLER D. Immune complex disease in experimental animals and man. Adv. Immunol., 1973, *16*, 186.

COCHRANE C. G. Immune complex mediated tissue injury. *In*: Mechanisms of Immunoatphology (S. Cohen, P. A. Ward, and R. T. McCluskey [eds.]). John Wiley & Sons. New York, 1979, 25.

DIXON F. J., THEOFILOPOULOS A. N., IZUI S., and MCCONAHEY P. J. Murine SLE aetiology and pathogenesis. *In*: Immunology 80 (M. Fougereau and J. Dausset eds.) Acad. Press, New York, 1980, 959.

GOLDSTEIN I. M. and WEISSMANN G. Cellular and humoral mechanisms in immune complex injury. *In* L. Brent and J. Holborow, Eds., Progress in immunology. II. Vol. 5. Amsterdam, 1974, North Holland, p. 81.

GREY H. M. and KOHLER P. M. Cryoimmunoglobulins. Semin Hemat., 1973, *10*, 87.

HAAKENSTAD A. O. and MANNICK M. The biology of immune complexes. *In* N. Talal, Ed., Auto-immunity: genetic, immunologic, virologic and clinical aspects. New York, 1977, Academic Press, p. 227.

HASHIM G. A. Myelin basic protein structure, function and antigenic determinants. Immunol. Rev. 1978, *39*, 60.

HOTCHIN J. Virus, cell surface and self: lymphocytic choriomeningitis of mice. Amer. J. Clin. Path., 1971, *56*, 333.

KRAKAUER R. S. and CATHCART M. K. Immunoregulation and autoimmunity. Elsevier, New York, 1980, 257 pp.

MÖLLER G. (Ed.) Auto-immunity and self non self determinants. Transpl. Rev., 1976, *31*.

PATERSON P. Auto-immune neurological disease: experimental animal systems and implications for multiple sclerosis. *In* N. Talal, Ed., Auto-immunity: genetic, immunologic, virologic and clinical aspects. New York, 1977, Academic Press, p. 644.

PROFFITT M. R., HIRSCH M. S., and BLACK P. H. Viruses, auto-immunity and murine lymphoma. *In* N. Talal, Ed., Auto-immunity: genetic, immunologic, virologic and clinical aspects. New York, 1977, Academic Press.

ROSE N. R., BACON L. D., SUNDICK R. S., KONG Y. M., ESQUIVEL P., and BIGAZZI P. E. Genetic regulation in auto-immune thyroiditis. *In* N. Talal, Ed., Auto-immunity: genetic, immunologic, virologic and clinical aspects. New York, 1977, Academic Press, p. 63.

ROSE N. R., BIGAZZI P. E., and WARNER N. L. Genetic control of autoimmune disease. Elsevier, New York, 1979, 466 p.

ROSE N. R. General aspects of autoimmune disease. *In*: Mechanisms of Immunopathology (S. Cohen, P. A. Ward, and R. T. McCluskey [eds.]). John Wiley & Sons. New York, 1979, 143.

TALAL N. Autoimmunity and lymphoid malignancy in NZB mice. *In* R. S. Schwartz, Ed., Progress in clinical immunology. New York, 1974, Grune & Stratton, p. 101.

TALAL N. Auto-immunity and lymphoïd malignancy: manifestation of immunoregulatory disequilibrium. *In* N. Talal, Ed., Auto-immunity: genetic, immunologic, virologic, and clinical aspects. New York, 1977, Academic Press, p. 183.

TALAL N. Tolerance and autoimmunity. *In*: Clinical Immunology. (C. W. Parker [ed.]). Saunders, Philadelphia, 1980, 86.

TALAL N., ROUBINIAN J. R., SHEAR H., HOM J. T., and MIYASAKA N. Progress in the mechanisms of autoimmune disease. *In*: Immunology 80 (M. Fougereau and J. Dausset [eds.]). Acad. Press, New York, 1980, 889.

THEOFILOPOULOS A. N., WILSON C. B., and DIXON F. J. The Raji cell radio-immune assay for detecting immune complexes in human sera. J. Clin Invest., 1976, *57*, 169.

WARNER N. L. Genetic aspects of auto-immune disease in animals. *In* N. Talal, Ed., Autoimmunity: genetic, immunologic, virologic and clinical aspects. New York, 1977, Academic Press, p. 33.

WEIGLE W. O. Cellular events in experimental auto-immune thyroiditis, allergic encephalomyelitis and tolerance to self. *In* N. Talal, Ed., Auto-immunity: genetic, immunologic virologic and clinical aspects. New York, 1977, Academic Press, p. 141.

WILLIAMS R. C. Immune complexes in clinical and experimental medicine. Harvard University Press, Cambridge, 1980, 565 pp.

ZUBLER R. H. and LAMBERT P. Immune complexes in clinical investigation. *In* R. A. Thompson, Ed., Recent advances in clinical immunology. Edinburgh, 1977, Churchill-Livingstone, p. 15.

## ORIGINAL ARTICLES

BENVENISTE J., HENSON P. M., and COCHRANE C. G. Leukocyte-dependent histamine release from rabbit platelets. The role of IgE, basophils and platelet-activating factor. J. Exp. Med., 1963, *118*, 503.

COHEN I. R. Autoimmunity and self-recognizing T-Lymphocytes. *In* L. Brent and J. Holborow, Eds., Progress in immunology. II. Vol. 5. Amsterdam, 1974, North Holland, p. 5.

DIXON F., CROKER B., DEL VILLANO B., JENSEN F., and LERNER R. Oncornavirus infection and «auto» immune complex disease of mice. *In* L. Brent and J. Holborow, Eds., Progress in immunology. II. Vol. 5, Amsterdam, 1974, North Holland, p. 49.

THEOFILOPULOS A. N., SHAWLER D. L., EISENBERG R. A., and DIXON F. J. Splenic immunoglobulin secreting cells and their regulation in autoimmune mice. J. Exp. Med., 1980, *151*, 446.

TRON F., CHARRON D., BACH J. F., and TALAL N. Establishment and characterization of a permanent murine hybridoma secreting monoclonal anti-DNA antibody. J. Immunol., 1980, *125*, 285.

Chapter 26

# HYPERSENSITIVITY STATES

Jean-François Bach

I.   INTRODUCTION
II.  ATOPIC DISEASES (TYPE-I HYPERSENSITIVITY)
III. ALLOIMMUNIZATION (TYPE-II HYPERSENSITIVITY)
IV.  EXTRINSIC ALLERGIC ALVEOLITIS (TYPE-III HYPERSENSITIVITY)
V.   CONTACT DERMATITIS (TYPE-IV HYPERSENSITIVITY)
VI.  ALLERGIC DRUG REACTIONS

## I.  INTRODUCTION

Antibody production and development of delayed hypersensitivity (DH) in response to allo- or heteroantigens may have unfavorable effects for the individual entirely independent of autoimmunization. These harmful reactions, which may induce diseases if they recur, define hypersensitivity. We will deal here with acute hypersensitivity states; chronic diseases like glomerulo-nephritis (GN) or systemic lupus erythematosus (SLE) are discussed elsewhere. It is in reference to hypersensitivity states that Gell and Coombs proposed a four-part classification of immune reactions (described on p. 5). This classi-fication, sometimes criticized as schematic for overall physiologic immune responses, finds here its best application.

Type-I hypersensitivities are linked to IgE and to the release of various mediators by mastocytes and basophils. This type includes, in addition to the generalized anaphylactic reaction, which may terminate as anaphylactic shock, all allergic (or atopic) states that are local anaphylactic reactions, including hay fever, asthma, and urticaria.

Type-II hypersensitivities relate to the direct binding of antibodies to cellular antigens (membrane antigens or antigens secondarily imbedded in the membrane). The most classic example is erythrocytic alloimmunization observed after incompatible blood transfusion or in newborn hemolytic disease. Some drug reactions are due to antibody reactions to the drug, which is bound to platelets or red blood cells. We should also mention here the possible effects of "lymphocyte-dependent antibodies." These antibodies lead to the destruction of IgG-coated target cells by K-cell action (see p. 413). However, to date no definite intervention of these antibodies in human immunopathology has been demonstrated.

Type-III hypersensitivities reflect the pathologic effects of immune complexes. We will not repeat our earlier discussion of circulating immune complex diseases like serum sickness disease and its equivalents, which is observed in certain drug-induced reactions (see p. 766), SLE, or GN (see chaps. 28 and 29). Rather, we will here limit ourselves to acute hypersensitivity reactions of type III, which relate to the action of immune complexes formed locally in the tissues (where antibodies bind to tissue antigens) and represent the human equivalent of Arthus phenomenon (see p. 361). The best known clinical example of this hypersensitivity is the interstitial pneumonitis observed in farmer's lung and pigeon breeder's disease after inhalation of antigens (certain actinomycetes or avian antigens). Some authors incorrectly relate to type-III hypersensitivity the endotoxinic shock (Shwartzman's phenomenon) which is not immunologic, in precise terms, except by the possible involvement of complement (see p. 363).

Type-IV hypersensitivities are associated with DH or, more generally speaking, with cell-mediated immunity defined by direct T-cell intervention. Allergic contact eczema is the purest clinical example of this type of hypersensitivity.

## II.  ATOPIC DISEASES (TYPE-I HYPERSENSITIVITY)

### INTRODUCTION: CONCEPT OF ATOPY

Under this category, various clinical manifestations that relate to "immediate hypersensitivity" have been described (chap. 11). The term "allergy" refers to these diseases (allergic rhinitis, asthma, atopic eczema); mecial allergology is a well-established discipline. The word allergy is sometimes used ambiguously and has even been considered synonymous with immunity.

The exact definition of atopy is debated. It is probably best to include hypersensitivity manifestations (whose various aspects we will examine later) related to abnormalities in IgE production. Nonetheless, recall that IgE is a normal circulating immunoglobulin and that specific IgE are produced in most normal subjects after adequate antigenic stimulation, especially in certain parasitic diseases. More precisely, Pepys defines atopy as an abnormal form of immunologic reactivity in which IgE reagins result from ordinary exposure to common environmental allergens (particularly when the allergen is inhaled or ingested). Abnormal reactivity is detected by cutaneous or inhalation tests. The major environmental allergens are found in house dusts, pollen, and hair of domestic animals. When tests that determine specific IgE responses are available in the future, atopy definition will probably improve.

### Atopic State

The atopic state is a relatively specific entity despite considerable hetero-geneity in clinical cases. Atopy ranges from single sensitization to a given allergen to polysensitization. Several factors explain this heterogeneity. The allergen obviously plays an important role (geographic). When a mesquite tree strain (*Prosopis*) was brought into Kuwait, it provoked the appearance of many atopy cases secondary to pollen from this tree. The geographic distribution of pollen allergies precisely corresponds with pollen tree distribution. Atopic subjects in Europe are not allergic to "ragweed" pollen, which is the most incriminated allergen in the United States. Several years are required to develop an allergy to this pollen, but sensitization may then last 10–20 years (even after the last exposure to the allergen). An especially intense exposure to an allergen may significantly increase the incidence of allergies, as in the case of those to bakers' and wheat flour.

### Multiple Sensitizations

The association of multiple sensitizations with clinically discrete manifes-tations (e.g., hay fever, asthma, or eczema) in one given subject is more frequent than would be expected on the basis of coincidence. Polysensitizations, especially common in children and young adults, suggests an abnormal immunologic reactivity. Deliberate nasal administration of protein (like ribonuclease) or polysaccharide antigens results in much greater sensitization (as measured by skin tests) in atopic than in nonatopic subjects, even when the latter show preexistent nonatopic asthma. Atopic and nonatopic subjects show the same response with respect to precipitating antibodies. The difference in IgE response is not observed after parenteral injection. It is not linked to an altered (inflammatory) mucosal reaction in atopic subjects that might enhance absorp-tion and availability of allergens, because antigenic stimulation remains inef-fective in nonatopic patients with rhinitis. It is possible that a deficiency of IgA mucous secretion may be implicated, because atopic subjects seem to produce less secretory IgA than do nonatopic subjects.

### Genetic Factor

A role of a genetic factor is controversial. A significant correlation is found between atopy and the presence of hay fever or infantile eczema in other family members. Monozygous twins are often, but not always, coallergic to the same allergens. A lesser correlation is found for asthma, probably because of the existence of many causes for asthma other than immediate hypersensitivity. The claimed existence of a genetic factor was recently supported by demon-stration that allergy to ragweed fraction is tightly linked to the HLA- B7 antigen and by demonstration of genetic control of reaginic antibody production in the mouse. However, the genes involved in human atopy are ill defined, and their number is in itself a matter of controversy.

### Other Factors

Additional factors may augment IgE production and reinforce atopy. Examples are certain parasitic and bacterial infections. Rat infestation by *Nippostrongylus brasiliensis* (a parasite) increases the production of reagins to allergens to which the rats were previously sensitized (e.g., ovalbumin or house dust; see p. 493). Adult thymectomy increases IgE production in the rat, probably because of loss of suppressor T cells, whereas, paradoxically, neonatal thymectomy depresses IgE production (loss of helper T cells).

### IgE

The role of IgE in atopy is well established. Circulating IgE (measured by radioimmunoassay) binds to tissues and there induces basophil and mastocyte degranulation by the mechanism described in chapter 11. IgE-producing cells are particularly prominent in lymphoid tissue within the tracheal, bronchial, and intestinal mucosae particularly in the tonsils and adenoidal tissues. High-affinity IgE antibodies are present in nasal washings, liquid tears, and in sputum of atopic subjects.

## CLINICAL MANIFESTATIONS OF ATOPY

The clinical manifestations of allergy vary with age.

In the newborn, the most common allergies develop in response to food antigens, including milk, eggs, and liver oils. In the children, atopy is very common in the form of eczema, which disappears between 4 and 5 years of age; children with prior atopic eczema often develop respiratory allergies in adult life. However, in the adult, allergy is generally fixed (chronic), with a tendency for progression with time, either in severity or in number of allergens involved. The most common clinical manifestations are hay fever (usually seasonal), bronchial asthma, atopic dermatitis, and urticaria, especially the acute form. Other clinical manifestations of atopy are less well documented and will not be discussed here. These manifestations include hyperplastic sinusitis, nasal polyps, vernal conjunctivitis, convulsions, and certain gastrointestinal disorders. Note that allergic reactions occurring in the gastrointestinal tract as a consequence of allergen ingestion is relatively frequent, particularly in children, toward cow's milk. Clinical features mainly include nausea, vomiting and diarrhea.

### Anaphylactic Shock

Although properly speaking this reaction is not an atopic manifestation (it is not commonly observed in atopic subjects), the mechanisms of action are the same as those in atopy.

A description of anaphylactic shock in man will be given in chapter 28. The main symptoms are discomfort, skin erythema or urticaria, pruritus, respiratory insufficiency, and hypotension, which may terminate in cardiac arrest. When anaphylaxis follows subcutaneous or intramuscular injection, erythema and edema may also be observed at the injection site. The main causes of anaphylactic shock in man are heterologous serum injections, drug intake, insect bites, rupture of hydatic cysts, and hyposensitization treatments.

### Allergic Rhinitis

This disease is provoked by exposure of the nasal mucosa to inhaled allergens. The clinical manifestations are hyperemia and edema of the nasal mucosa. Mucous hypersecretion and swelling of the mucosa may lead to obstruction of airways. Mucosal irritation causes frequent sneezing. One observes in the eye analogous reactions of redness, watering, and mild edema. Less commonly, there is a dry cough or actual asthma. Most often, the involved allergens are pollens and house dusts. There is some correlation between the frequency of attack of rhinitis and atmospheric pollen counts. Treatment includes antigen removal, antihistamines (especially effective at the beginning of the season), and symptomatic drugs, such as sympathomimetics, atropinic agents, and even steroids. It is also possible to hyposensitize by use of the suspected allergen.

### Bronchial Asthma

This clinical syndrome is characterized by paroxysmal bronchial obstruction, respiratory insufficiency, and mucous hypersecretion. The disease is initially acute and features long intervals without signs or symptoms. Chronicity develops associated with more frequent attacks and reduced periods of remission. Atopy is a common cause of asthma but is only involved in 60% or less of cases. Bacterial infections may be especially important in nonatopic asthma. Mixed forms are often observed, with both atopic and infectious asthma. It is important to recognize that many forms of asthma cannot be readily classified. Interstitial pneumonitis related to Arthus's phenomenon must be differentiated from asthma but is often not easily dissociable. Clinically, the asthmatic attack is characterized by expiratory dyspnea, accompanied by, a few hours later, the development of increased nonpurulent mucous expectoration. Auscultation supports the diagnosis by revealing ronchi and sibilant sounds. Blood and sputum contain excess eosinophils but eosinophilia may also be observed in infectious asthma. Morphologically, there is bronchial infiltration by mucus and eosinophils. However, there is no histologic distinction between atopic asthma, which has its onset in atopic subjects in relation to defined allergens and nonatopic asthma, which may follow infection.

The role of allergic phenomena in the pathogenesis of asthma in atopic subjects is likely but has not been absolutely demonstrated. Asthma is often preceded by atopic dermatitis or hay fever. One may also find allergens that cause cutaneous reactions after subcutaneous injection in asthmatic patients or asthma when they are introduced by inhalation of known allergens (in the form of aerosols). There is a highly significant association with seasonal rhinitis. Serum IgE is often elevated, whereas other immunoglobulins are normal. It has been possible to transfer the asthmatic reaction by blood removed from a subject sensitive to horse proteins. It has also been possible to demonstrate release of mediators of bronchoconstriction in the lungs of allergic subjects in response to a specific allergen.

However, there is still much to learn about the mechanisms by which contact with allergen provokes an asthmatic attack. Histamine, which is a bronchoconstrictor, is probably involved, but other mediators of immediate hypersensitivity may also be active. In fact, antihistamines are not effective for treating asthma, and serum histamine levels are not elevated during attacks. Slow-reacting substance of anaphylaxis (SRS-A) is also a bronchoconstrictor, even in the presence of antihistamines; however, SRS-A inhalation does not produce asthmatic attacks. It may, in fact, act by potentiating histamine's action. Serotonin, too, is bronchoconstrictive, but the serotonin level in human lungs is almost negligible.

The role of kinins as bronchoconstrictors is also hypothetical. Acetylcholine, to which the bronchial mucosa in asthmatics is strongly reactive (hence its former use for diagnosis), is not specific for asthmatics and is not a priori produced in immunologic reactions. This nonspecific reactivity of bronchial mucosa may perhaps be due to a block of β-adrenergic receptors. It certainly makes difficult the interpretation of a role for any given mediator in the pathogenesis of asthma. It is of interest that injection of human serum that contains reagins enhances bronchial sensitivity to acetylcholine (Mecholyl) injection entirely independent of the allergen administered. There are, in addition, many nonimmunologic factors that may provoke acute asthma, including inhalation of various irritants (e.g., dusts, certain gases) or cold air, both of which change pulmonary function in normal subjects. The role of hormones is very obscure. The existence of asthma aggravated by aspirin ingestion is definite, but sensitivity to aspirin does not seem to be immunologic.

Treatment of asthma should focus on the different pathophysiologic levels of allergen, mediator production and release and, most importantly, bronchoconstriction. The patient is advised to avoid contact with known allergens (e.g., food, drug, or domestic animals).

Hyposensitization may be useful in the case of airborne allergens (see p. 750). Histamine production may be inhibited by antihistamine drugs, but the results of this treatment are usually disappointing, except in childhood. Attempts to decrease reagin production by immunosuppressive treatments have also been disappointing. Conversely, suppression of basophilic and mastocytic mediator release by administration of sodium cromoglycate is definitely effective. Steroids or ACTH are still more effective, but, because of side effects, their use should be limited to aerosols in most subjects. Their mode of action in asthma is not understood.

A direct effect by lessening bronchoconstriction follows the use of sympathomimetic drugs (epinephrine, isoproterenol, ephedrine) administered orally or by aerosols. Their application must be limited by their propensity to cause alterations in myocardial function and blood pressure, especially because the patients themselves tend to increase their drug dosage. Xanthine derivatives like theophylline or aminophylline are less efficient bronchodilators but are also less dangerous. Sedatives may be prescribed in cases of anxiety, which frequently occurs in these patients, but respiratory function must first be evaluated (including blood gases). Antibiotics are used to treat acute infections, but penicillin must be avoided due to its high allergenicity; polymyxin should not be used because it causes histamine release. Expectorants and neuroleptics are occasionally employed.

### Atopic Urticaria

Urticaria is defined as a focal erythematous swelling of the skin with smooth surface and irregular borders. There is no preferential localization. Pruritus is often present. The lesion disappears 12–48 hr after onset without leaving scars. Acute and chronic urticarias should be differentiated on the basis of a 6-week break point. Morphologic features are venular and capillary dilatation, with an increase in dermal papillae. With time, lymphocytic and eosinophilic infiltrates appear.

A role of immediate hypersensitivity in the pathogenesis of urticaria is well established; urticaria is the human equivalent of the localized anaphylaxis reaction described on p. 349. It is a common finding in anaphylactic shock, for example, in acute serum sickness disease. Several anaphylaxis mediators enhance vascular permeability of the skin, such as histamine and serotonin. Histamine injection causes formation of a pruritic wheal. Injection of allergen causes a decrease in the local histamine content. The antigen may cause basophil degranulation in vitro. Lastly, antihistamines may induce the disappearance of urticaria.

It is important to differentiate IgE- from IgG-associated urticaria. The latter is seen in certain drug reactions (see p. 764) and in immune complex diseases like serum sickness disease. Atopic urticaria must be specially separated from nonimmunologic urticaria caused by pressure or cold, whether or not associated with cryoglobulinemia, urticaria secondary to solar exposure, urticaria secondary to histamine release (by such drugs as morphine, codeine, polymyxin B, or tubocurarine B) and idiopathic urticaria. The treatment of atopic urticaria is similar to that of other allergic phenomena described earlier. Treatment includes elimination of causative antigens (most often, food allergens or drugs and, rarely, pollens or bacterial antigens; see p. 350). In chronic or resistant cases, antihistamines, sympathomimetics, or even steroids may be helpful.

### Allergic Eczema

Atopic dermatitis has several other names, including diathesis prurigo, Besnier's prurigo, diathelic eczema, eczema pruriginosum allergicum, endogenous eczema, and allergic eczema. It progresses on to a lichenified dermatitis. Infantile eczema and atopic dermatitis often coexist but may represent two separate and unrelated diseases; individuals may develop only one of these two diseases.

Infantile allergic eczema must be differentiated from contact eczema (discussed on p. 759) and from allergic and seborrheic eczema. The eruption usually begins at about 3 months of life, often on the cheeks and scalp. The macules are initially pink, then dry and exfoliate (crusts). The lesions are very pruritic. They become pigmented (brown), dry, and lichenify at about 2–3 years. The eczema is progressive but also remits. It may heal completely at 5–10 years of age. In the adult, atopic dermatitis presents completely lichenified lesions with a slowly progressive course (chronic). Various complications ensue, including ocular cataracts and circulatory insufficiency in the extremities. Abnormal pharmacologic reactions may be noted, including a exaggerated local (vasoconstrictive) response to epinephrine and acetylcholine injections. Conversely, the skin of these subjects does not show the erythema normally seen after local injection of nicotinic esters, histamine, or bradykinin. The histology is not pathognomonic; in particular, chronic lesions cannot be differentiated from chronic contact eczema. In the acute form, the lesions include intraepidermal vesicles, dilated vessels, edema, and mononucleated cellular infiltrates; in the chronic form, hyperkeratosis and hyperplasia of Malpighi's layer and cellular infiltration are prominent.

Arguments in favor of the intervention of immediate hypersensitivity in infantile allergic eczema and atopic dermatitis are not very convincing. The association of eczema with asthma or allergic rhinitis is suggestive, as are the high hereditary incidence of the disease and exacerbation after contact with the presumed allergen. In fact, contact with suspected allergens causes only an exacerbation in preexisting lesions and no new lesions. In 20–30% of patients there is no personal or familial history of atopy. Cases of atopic dermatitis have been reported in agammaglobulinemic subjects. Skin lesions that occur after passive allergen injection or passive transfer of IgE antibodies and allergen do not resemble atopic dermatitis, particularly the lichenified form. Finally, immediate hypersensitivity does not adequately explain atopic eczema but other hypotheses are not more convincing, including psychosomatic theories or those which postulate a decreased threshold of cutaneous irritability as causing pruritus and secondary skin lesions. Purely symptomatic therapy is directed at relief of pruritus (local steroids, tranquilizers). Hyposensitization has been mostly ineffective.

### Gastrointestinal Allergy

Gastrointestinal and systemic reactions may appear in minutes or hours following the ingestion of certain foods. The most common causative foods are almonds, peanuts, shellfish, and certain berries, but, in fact, many other foods may be incriminated. Identification of the responsible agent may be determined by skin-testing. The symptoms may be gastrointestinal (diarrhea and vomiting), systemic (taking the form of anaphylactic shock), or less severe manifestations, such as urticaria or eczema. In children, the foods commonly responsible are cow's milk (the antigen concerned is $\beta$-lactoglobulin) and, to a lesser degree, flour, eggs, and fish oils. Diarrhea, usually chronic in nature, is often one of the earliest clinical manifestations. Depending on the case, food antigens react with IgE in the intestinal mucosa or with IgE localized outside the digestive tract.

## SEARCH FOR THE ALLERGEN

Separation of the environmental antigen from atopic subjects is the best therapy. When elimination is not feasible, specific allergen hyposensitization often results in long-term improvement with minimal side effects. These two approaches do, however, imply that the allergen responsible must be known.

### Patient's History

The patient's history often narrows the field of possible allergens, both in relation to seasonal rhinitis, asthma, and urticaria and, more rarely, to gastrointestinal disorders. A good inquiry must list all possible allergens and eventually exclude some.

### Tests

Certain data are only suggestive of atopy. They include eosinophilia and elevated serum IgE (radioimmunoassay, see Fig. 26.1), contrasting with normal concentrations of other immunoglobulins. However, these findings, especially eosinophilia, are nonspecific. Elevated IgE is, indeed, the rule, and very high levels are seen in atopy (in excess of 5,000 U/ml) but such levels are also observed in many nonatopic subjects, unfortunately.

A direct search for allergens requires skin tests, provocation tests, and, in selected cases, specific IgE detection in the serum or on circulating basophils. Tests that examine cell-mediated immunity are only in the experimental stage at present.

#### SKIN TESTS

Several allergens in various concentrations are applied topically (patch testing). The choice of the allergens employed may be guided by the patient's history, especially for rare allergens. Atopic reactions are characterized by their rapid onset, within a very few minutes.

Alternative techniques include the scratch test, intradermal allergen application, or the prick test. Various methods have been developed for preparation and standardization of allergenic extracts. We have discussed (p. 351) the promising results obtained in the isolation of the main determinants of a few common allergens. The reactions are evaluated semiquantitatively (from 1+ to 4+). Skin tests given clinically useful results, except for food allergens, for which disappointing results are usually obtained. Baker's asthma induced by barley flour inhalation is associated with positive skin reaction to barley, even when ingestion (not inhalation) of barley causes no symptoms. In theory, skin tests present the risk of anaphylactic shock. However, this risk is minimized by use of small amounts of allergens and by not studying obviously responsible allergens. It is noteworthy that corticosteroids do not suppress the skin reactions, except when administered locally.

#### PROVOCATION TESTS

In addition to being difficult to perform, provocation tests are time-consuming due to the need for multiple controls and represent a risk or discomfort to the patient. They are indicated, however, in cases where there remains a possibility that only one or several of multiple allergens giving positive skin tests are responsible for the clinical manifestations and in cases in which a positive reaction does not make sense clinically. They include inhalation tests (ventilatory function is measured, if possible, before the onset of acute asthma), mucosal application (the allergen is applied to the eye or nose), or allergen addition to food when there has been prior specific withdrawal of the incriminated "food allergens" from the diet.

DEMONSTRATION OF SPECIFIC IgE

The demonstration of specific IgE remains one of the best diagnostic criterion. Several methods have been proposed. (1) In the method that employs passive serum transfer from patients (Prausnitz-Küstner technique), described on p. 349, the patient's serum is injected subcutaneously into a nonallergic subject at multiple sites. Forty-eight hours later, the suspected allergens are deposited into the same sites, in a manner similar to the classic skin test just previously described. This technique raises tough ethical questions, and there is a risk of hepatitis transmission. Thus, it is now seldom used. It would be desirable to perform the technique in other primates than men, but monkeys, the only animals capable of fixing human IgE, are difficult to utilize. They may be sensitized at the level of the eye, lung, or skin. Shelley's test consists of fixing patient IgE to rabbit basophils and then provoking basophilic degranulation by the allergen. Unfortunately, the results of this technique have been disappointing, which could have been predicted because of the homocytotropy of human IgE, which binds only to human and monkey cells.

(2) The second method involves measurement of specific serum IgE by use of radioimmunoassays with certain well-defined allergens, such as penicillin. The allergen is first coupled to insoluble dextran particles, and patient serum is added. The patient's serum binds to dextran particles. After centrifugation of particles, labeled anti-IgE serum is added, followed by a repeat centrifugation, and the quantity of labeled Ig fixed is quantified. This is the radioallergosorbent test (RAST) (Fig. 26.1).

(3) Measurement of specific IgE on basophils or mastocytes or degranulation in the presence of allergen is, in theory, preferable to measurement of serum IgE, because the allergic phenomenon is linked to degranulation. Histamine release by circulating leukocytes in the presence of the allergen may be measured; basophils can be counted before and after exposure to allergen (basophils may be stained with toluidine blue). These methods may also be used to search for blocking antibodies produced during hyposensitization (see p. 750).

OTHER APPROACHES

Another approach is to look for specific lymphocytic sensitization to various allergens. Blast transformation in the allergen presence has been widely studied but has given contradictory and sometimes disappointing results. It is interesting to note, however, that blast transformation may remain positive a long time after the last exposure when specific IgE antibodies are not found any more. Solid data are not yet available on the (preliminary) use of leukocyte migration inhibition and the rosette tests.

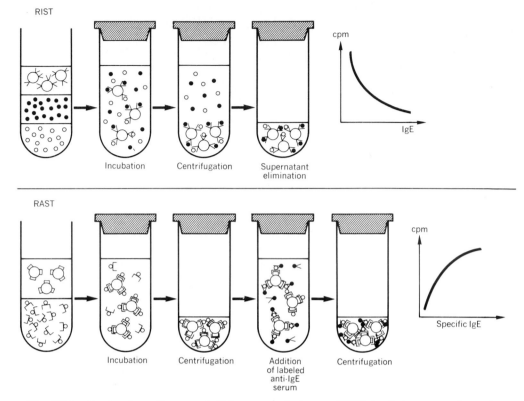

**Fig. 26.1** Evaluation of serum IgE by two techniques: RIST (radioimmunoadsorption test), which measures the total level of serum IgE ( $\overset{\curlyvee}{\varphi}$ , anti-IgE antibody; ●, labeled IgE; ○, cold IgE, to be dosed); RAST (radioallergosorbent test), which measures allergen-specific IgE ( $\overset{}{\varphi}$ , allergen bound to agarose beads, $\curlyvee$ , allergen-specific antibody, to be dosed; ●<, labeled anti-IgE serum).

## IMMUNOTHERAPY OF ATOPY

Treatment of allergic reactions first makes use of antigenic removal when possible. More commonly, hyposensitization is employed. Despite the long time that this method has been used, its therapeutic mechanism is still ill defined, and, more important, its efficacy, as attested to by randomized trials, has not been determined. However, recent well-controlled studies have indicated that this therapy is effective for allergies to ragweed pollen and house dust allergens.

The treatment consists of injecting increasing doses of allergen. At the beginning, specific IgE levels increase, followed by a decrease and, most noteworthy, no increase during the offensive season. The treatment must be prolonged at relatively high doses; however, there is no real agreement concerning the dose and nature of allergen to be administered, especially in regard to the frequency of injection. The method may be modified for treatment of asthma (allergen inhalation) or rhinitis (nasal instillations).

Hyposensitization sometimes causes production of "blocking" antibodies that depress the skin reactions that result from passive transfer of autologous serum. It is suspected that blocking antibodies may be responsible for favorable clinical effects of hyposensitization; this hypothesis, however, remains to be confirmed, especially since there is no correlation between the quantity of blocking antibodies detected by passive autotransfer and the degree of clinical improvement. There seems to be, however, a correlation between increased IgG antibodies, decreased IgE level, and clinical improvement. Blocking antibodies probably act by a negative feedback mechanism similar to that described on p. 340.

Hyposensitization is also associated with long-lasting decreased histamine release by the patient's leukocytes, which may reflect a decrease in histamine reserves due to degranulation induced by injection of allergen. This explanation is not entirely satisfactory, because the basophil's half-life does not exceed 8–12 days.

# III. ALLOIMMUNIZATION (TYPE-II HYPERSENSITIVITY)*

Alloimmunization results from introduction into the organism of an erythrocytic, leukocytic, or serum alloantigen, as defined in chapters 21–23. Alloimmunization occurs in three circumstances: pregnancies, during which fetomaternal alloimmunization occurs secondary to introduction of fetal cells into the maternal circulation, leading to the hemolytic disease of the newborn; blood transfusions; and skin or organ grafts.

Alloimmunization involves polymorphic systems that have immunogenic markers. It is important to understand that the protein allotypic markers, which define allotypy, are very poorly immunogenic. For this reason, antiprotein immunization is of little clinical consequence.

Also, some genetic systems are not immunogenic. For example, antiadenylate kinase or antihaptoglobin alloantibodies have never been reported. These genetic markers are not defined by an immunogenetic technique but by biochemical criteria. They do represent genetic variation within a species, as do blood groups, but they are not implicated in hemolytic disease of the newborn or iatrogenic disease (transfusion, transplantation).

In addition, the probability of alloimmunization depends not only on immunogenicity but also on gene frequency in the various polymorphic systems. One example is HLA system, which represents a balanced polymorphism, in which each genetic variant has a high probability of occurring in a given locus. Because most genetic variants are immunogenic, the probability of developing anti-HLA antibodies is, a priori, very high.

Fetomaternal alloimmunization and transfusional alloimmunization are not identical. In the present practice of transfusion there is minimal phenotypic selection (except, of course, for ABO and Rh groups). Many immune alloantibodies therefore develop, but it is very unusual to observe the appearance of

* Section authored by C. Salmon.

an alloantibody against a private antigen, which requires numerous transfusions. Conversely, fetomaternal alloimmunization against a private antigen occurs more frequently because of repeated exposure to the same paternal haplotypes. Thus, there is a higher probability of the appearance of an antibody to an antigen of low frequency.

## FETOMATERNAL ALLOIMMUNIZATION

### Hemolytic Disease of the Newborn

In end-stage pregnancy or during actual parturition, Rhesus-positive (Rh$^+$) fetal cells are released into the circulation of the Rh$^-$ mother, where they are recognized as foreign, and a primary antibody response is provoked. This response is initially slow. The first antibodies are only detected several weeks after birth of an unaffected child. A second pregnancy may repeat this immune stimulus. As soon as the first fetal cells reach the maternal circulation, a strong and rapid secondary response develops, with production of large amounts of anti-Rh antibodies. These antibodies are IgG and express on the Fc fragment (heavy chain) a device that permits passage through the placenta. Anti-Rh antibodies enter the fetal circulation and there act to destroy fetal red blood cells, whose degradation products contain bilirubin, which the immature liver of the newborn cannot rapidly remove. The newborn may then die of hemolysis or, if he survives, may present profound neurologic sequelae due to lesions of basal ganglia, which are sensitive to the toxic action of bilirubin.

This is the spontaneous course of newborn hemolytic disease (with its unrelenting progression). Exchange transfusion of the newborn, with appropriate blood, has represented an important therapeutic advance. Now available, however, is an invaluable prophylactic treatment, which consists of injecting Rh$^-$ mothers, newly delivered of an Rh$^+$ child, with anti-Rh antibodies. These antibodies eliminate fetal red blood cells, which were introduced into the mother's circulation at the moment of parturition. The mechanism of this specific immunosuppression has previously been discussed (p. 342).

### Newborn Hemolytic Disease May Be Due to Antibodies Other Than Anti-Rh

Fetomaternal immunization to Rh antigen is the most frequent cause of newborn hemolytic disease, but this disease is not limited to anti-Rh standard alloimmunization. Other antigens implicated include E and c, K of Kell's system, Fy$^a$ of Duffy's system, Jk$^a$ of Kidd's system, S and s antigens of the MNSs systems, and many other antigens from different blood group systems.

The only antibodies giving the hemolytic disease are IgG, because IgM alloantibodies, like anti-Le$^a$ or P$_1$, do not cross the placenta and thus are not clinically dangerous. Transplacental passage of maternal IgG autoantibodies has been observed in a few cases. The appearance in the fetus of anti-i antibodies, which recognize an antigen that is well developed in the fetus, may induce discrete hemolysis. The ABO system itself may be involved if the mother has a high titer of immune anti-A antibody produced by prior heterologous stimulation, especially vaccination. Finally, there are exceptional cases of fetomaternal alloimmunization linked to private antigens.

Allotypic standoffs between mother and child are not limited to erythrocytic antigens. Not infrequently, antileukocytic and antiplatelet alloantibodies or antibodies directed against IgA allotypes may occur during pregnancy. In a few cases, antiplatelet alloimmunization was responsible for neonatal thrombocytopenia.

# TRANSFUSIONAL ALLOIMMUNIZATION

## Alloimmunization to Cellular Membrane Antigens

This alloimmunization concerns blood-group and HLA antigens.

The frequency of alloantibody development correlates with transfusional frequency. About 8% of polytransfused (more than 20 transfusions) recipients are immunized to blood group antigens, and about 25% of them show alloantibodies to HLA antigens (as detected by lymphocytotoxicity). The high correlation between incidence of antibody appearance and number of transfusions indicates that these antibodies are definitely immune antibodies.

The appearance of the antibodies is coordinated. A subject with an anti-HLA antibody is more likely to produce an antierythrocytic antibody than is a subject without an anti-HLA antibody. The presence of an antileukocytic or antiplatelet antibody is evidence of the capacity of the subject to be immunized and urges for a very thorough search for antierythrocytic alloantibodies. The fact that in the same patient all sorts of antibodies against cellular antigens develop suggests that some subjects are easily immunized while others are difficult to immunize. Susceptibility to immunization is linked to sex, with immunization of the female twice exceeding that of the male (independent of pregnancies and of the number of transfusions). The appearance of antileukocytic and antiplatelet antibodies is particularly frequent in patients with alcoholic cirrhosis, a disease known to be associated with immune dysfunction.

Repeated transfusions permit to evaluate the relative antigenicity of the various blood group antigens in man; K antigens and, to a lesser extent, E and c antigens are particularly strong immunogens.

**Table 26.1  Frequency of Antierythrocytic, Antileukocytic, or Antiplatelet Alloimmunization in 639 Transfused Subjects**

| | |
|---|---|
| Cirrhosis | 49* |
| Hodgkin's disease | 21 |
| Hemophilia | 21 |
| Epitheliomas | 18 |
| Myeloid aplasia | 17 |
| Lymphocytic leukemias | 12 |
| Acute leukemia | 7 |

* All values are percentages and have been corrected in reference to the number of transfusions given.
After Salmon and Schwartz.

### Antiprotein Immunization

At variance with membrane alloantigens, allotypic markers of human proteins are very poorly immunogenic. Also, the conditions in which they give rise to antibodies differ from those for erythrocytes and leukocytes: antibody appearance is independent of the number of transfusions; antibodies do not appear more frequently in women; and anti-Gm antibody appearance in polytransfused subjects does not relate to the appearance of other antibodies (antired blood cell, antiplatelet, or antileukocytic).

One must differentiate these antiprotein alloantibodies that appear in polytransfused subjects from anti-IgA antibodies, which develop after transfusion in subjects with IgA deficiency (these antibodies may also have important clinical consequences).

### Applications for Transfusion

Recognition of transfusion-induced alloimmunization has important clinical consequences. It is known that, except for anti-IgA class-specific antibodies, transfusion accidents do not relate to antiprotein antibodies (including rare antiallotypic or other antibodies). Antileukocytic and antiplatelet antibodies are the cause of chills and fever during transfusion, and HLA immunized subjects must therefore sometimes be transfused with leukocyte-depleted blood. Obviously, antierythrocytic alloimmunization plays far the most important role in transfusion reactions. High-risk subjects are women, cirrhotic patients, subjects with antileukocytic antibody, those with prior antierythrocytic immunization, and those who lack a public antigen and are rapidly immunized. All of these subjects must be phenotyped in the Rh, Kell, Duffy, and Kidd systems.

Overall, it is wise to systematically phenotype subjects who are expected to receive multiple transfusions, such as patients with thalassemia, hemophilia, malignant hemopathies, and other diseases characterized by recurrent blood loss.

### Conclusions

Alloimmunization that occurs after transfusion raises the question of the genetic control of the immune responses to alloantigens. It is likely that the alloimmune response to repeated transfusions obeys the same laws as those described in mice or guinea pigs (see chap. 24). Clinical studies, such as those in volunteers who receive Rh+ red blood cell injections for harvesting anti-D serum, should help to test this hypothesis. Preliminary results show that anti-D antibody production is not linked to one HLA antigen.

### General Rules for Blood Transfusions

Information on erythrocytic blood groups is utilized in blood transfusion to avoid incompatibility between donor and recipient. Incompatibility is present if the transfusion juxtaposes an antigen and its specific corresponding antibody. This situation leads to binding of the antibody to the erythrocyte-borne antigen; erythrocytes thus sensitized by the antibody are destroyed by hemolysis. The possibility of contact between antigen and antibody has two mechanisms:

transfusion of an antigen into a recipient who possesses the corresponding natural antibody (hemolytic accidents by ABO or, more rarely, anti-Lewis incompatibility) or of an immune antibody (e.g., anti-Rh alloimmunization); less commonly, transfusion of an antibody that is capable of hemolyzing the recipient's red blood cells (dangerous donor).

### ABO INCOMPATIBILITIES

The natural antibody present in the recipient's serum is responsible for hemolytic accidents. Therefore, one must avoid transfusion of the antigen that corresponds to the recipient's antibody or antibodies; an O donor may theoretically donate blood to an A, B, or AB recipient, an A donor may give to an A or AB recipient, a B donor may donate to a B or AB recipient, and an AB donor can only give his blood to an AB recipient.

Conversely, there is a conflict between antigen and antibody which causes hemolysis if an A subject who possesses an anti-B agglutinin receives B or AB blood, if a B subject who possesses an anti-A agglutinin receives A or AB blood, and if an O subject who possesses anti-A and anti-B agglutinins receives A, B, or AB blood. Because the natural antibody is always present in individuals without the corresponding antigen, the risk of hemolytic accidents is immediate and constant in case of incompatibility.

However, experience shows that the donor's natural anti-A and B antibodies are usually not dangerous, probably because of dilution of the donor's antibody in the recipient's plasma or because of absorption onto tissue antigens.

### DANGEROUS UNIVERSAL DONORS

Hemolytic accidents may be observed after transfusion of whole blood from O to A recipients. These accidents are due to the presence in the donor of an anti-A antibody of the immune type added to the natural antibody. This immune anti-A antibody results from prior silent immunization by an environmental A substance, from pregnancy-induced immunization, or from any other stimulation (see p. 622).

### ALLOIMMUNIZATION

Any subject who does not possess a given antigen may develop an antibody to that antigen if it is repeatedly introduced into the circulation. Most often, the antigen involved is standard Rh, the importance of which in blood transfusion is such that it is imperative that Rh$^-$ subjects never receive Rh$^+$ blood.

However, antigens other than standard Rh may stimulate immune antibody formation (in order of frequency: K, E, c, Jk$^a$, Fy$^a$), either by repeated blood transfusions or in pregnancies. It is obvious that the risk of such stimulation increases with the number of transfusions or pregnancies. Nonetheless, an alloimmunization accident may be seen after only one transfusion in women sensitized by a previous pregnancy.

Polytransfused subjects must be subject to particularly intense serologic followup.

The situation is sometimes very complex. Some subjects have very exceptional blood groups, which means that they lack an antigen that "everyone" else possesses. For example, a Vel-negative subject recognizes virtually all donors as foreign and becomes immunized. Other subjects, especially cirrhotic ones, produce numerous antibodies that correspond to high-frequency antigens. For both subjects, very rare blood reserves are required, which may now readily be prepared by deep-frozen blood storage.

### NATURAL ALLOANTIBODIES OUTSIDE THE ABO SYSTEM

Natural alloantibodies may be seen in nontransfused subjects independent of the ABO system. These alloantibodies include anti-Le$^a$, anti-P$_1$, and, more rarely, anti-M and anti-Lu$^a$ antibodies. The presence of these antibodies, especially anti-Le$^a$ or anti-Le$^b$, may shorten Le(a+) or Le(b+) erythrocytic survival (inefficient transfusions), and if the antibody is active at 37°C and hemolyzes in vitro, it may cause true transfusional hemolytic accidents (dangerous transfusions). These subjects are in a sense "dangerous recipients." The same is true for certain subjects with exceptional phenotypes like Tj(a−), P$_k$, who have naturally dangerous antibodies.

### CONCLUSIONS

To avoid immediate transfusional hemolytic accidents, not only ABO and standard Rh compatibility must be considered but also the possibility of irregular antibodies, which may be natural, like anti-Lewis or anti-Tj$^a$, or result from immunization, like anti-K, anti-E, or anti-c. Dangerous O donors must be recognized and their blood should be reserved only for O-group recipients.

In practice, transfusional hemolytic accidents may be avoided by the following three rules: (1) Comparision of the ABO blood group of the patient and of that of the blood bottle at bedside prevents most ABO accidents. This comparison is a legal requirement in France and does not supplant the need for a compatibility slide test. (2) Screening for irregular agglutinins at the time of the first transfusion must be performed to avoid accidents due to a natural irregular alloantibody of the anti-Le$^a$ type or to unknown antibodies in women with multiple pregnancies. (3) Precise and adequate immunologic examination of polytransfused patients should be performed to detect immune alloantibodies.

## IV.  EXTRINSIC ALLERGIC ALVEOLITIS (TYPE-III HYPERSENSITIVITY)

Certain inhaled particles, which penetrate deeply into the lungs, stimulate production of precipitating antibodies, which cause localized hypersensitivity reactions, analogous to Arthus' reaction. These particles affect the alveoli and bronchioles, without, however, causing obstruction of the airways (unlike asthma).

The list of antigens, generally organic dusts and often proteins, capable of causing this type of reaction increases each year. In theory, any organic dust if inhaled in sufficient quantity should induce formation of precipitating antibodies and lead to extrinsic allergic alveolitis (Table 26.2).

**Table 26.2   Main Etiologies of Extrinsic Allergic Alveolitis**

| Name of disease | Antigen source | Precipitins against |
|---|---|---|
| THERMOPHILIC ACTINOMYCETE SPORES | | |
| Farmer's lung | Moldy hay and other moldy vegetable produce | *Micropolyspora faeni* and *Thermoactinomyces vulgaris* |
| Air-conditioning lung | Growth in humidified hot-air ventilation systems | *M. faeni* and *T. vulgaris* |
| Fog fever in cattle | Moldy hay | *M. faeni* |
| Bagassosis | Moldy sugar cane bagasse | *T. sacchari* |
| Mushroom worker's lung | Mushroom compost | *M. faeni? T. vulgaris?* |
| FUNGAL SPORES | | |
| Maple bark pneumonitis | Moldy maple bark | *Cryptostroma corticale* |
| Malt worker's lung | Moldy barley or malt dust | *Aspergillus clavatus* *A. fumigatus* |
| Cheese washer's lung | Moldy cheese | *Penicillium casei* |
| Suberosis | Moldy cork bark | *Penicillium frequentans* |
| Sequoiosis | Moldy redwood sawdust | *Graphium* *Aureobasidium pullulans* |
| Bird fancier's lung | Pigeon/budgerigar/parrot/hen droppings dust | Serum proteins and droppings antigen |
| Pituitary snuff taker's lung | Porcine and bovine posterior pituitary powder | Serum protein and pituitary antigens |
| Fish meal worker's lung | Fish meal | Fish meal extracts |
| Insect antigens | | |
| Wheat weevil | Infested wheat flour | *Sitophilus granarius* |
| POSSIBLE SIMILAR DISEASES (NOT PROVEN) | | |
| Thached-roof disease | Moldy thatch dusts | Thatch of huts |
| Smallpox handler's lung | | |
| Paprika splitter's lung | | |
| Furrier's lung | | |
| Coffee worker's lung | | |

After J. Pepys.

The best known pathologic situations are farmer's lung disease and pigeon breeder's disease.

## FARMER'S LUNG DISEASE

Spores of the thermophile actinomycete *Micropolyspora faeni* (Thermopolyspora) are the main agent that causes the disease. The actinomycetes are present in hay, especially when local temperatures exceed 40°C. The role of *M. faeni* is shown by gel immunoprecipitation; intense precipitation lines result from apposition of patient sera and *M. faeni* extracts. Spores about 1 μm in diameter penetrate the lungs (a farmer working with decaying hay may inhale up to 750,000 spores per minute). Other actinomycetes may also be causative in decaying hay and vegetable dust, and possibly also spores of certain fungi or bacteria, or even certain insect antigens.

Pulmonary and systemic symptoms begin 6–10 hr after inhalation of contaminated dust. A dry cough appears followed by severe dyspnea with associated crackling rales. Pulmonary evaluation reveals an alveolar -capillary block. Acute-phase x-rays show nodular infiltrates that persist for a few days to a few weeks. In chronic forms, fibrosis may appear. Anatomic examination reveals infiltrates of plasma cells, histiocytes, and, possibly, epithelial cell granulomas, hence the name used to describe the disease, "hypersensitivity granulomatous intestitial pneumonitis." *M. faeni* may be isolated from lung tissues and sputum. However, *M. faeni* is also seen in the expectoration of any exposed person who may not show the disease. Local symptoms are associated with fever, malaise, chills, diffuse pain, and emaciation. It is important to note that almost half of subjects who develop precipitins show no clinical disorder. Diagnosis may be difficult when clinical symptoms are mild.

The etiologic diagnosis may be corroborated by provocation tests, which involve inhaling aqueous solutions of actinomycete extracts. These tests produce exactly the systemic and pulmonary manifestations of the acute episode described above, with the same 6–8-hr time lag. Serologic tests confirm the diagnosis. Precipitin lines only disappear 2–3 years after exposure when the subject has long been exposed to the antigen. About 15% of farmers exposed to moldy hay show precipitin lines, and 50% of them present clinical symptoms. Precipitins are always absent in nonexposed control subjects. Interestingly, cattle who eat moldy hay may develop pulmonary diseases and associated *M. faeni* precipitins. *M. faeni* may be found in other vegetables that come into contact with excess temperature, such as mushroom compost (which can cause pneumonitis in subjects with contact). One may also mention allergic alveolitis due to fungi (*Cryptostroma corticale* is responsible for lung disease of maple tree barkers) and to *Aspergillus fumigatus*. In the latter case, one must differentiate hypersensitivity alveolitis from other immunopathologic disorders induced by *A. fumigatus* (atopic asthma, extrinsic asthma, pulmonary infiltrates, and circulating eosinophilia with low-titer anti-Aspergillus precipitins and reagins).


## PIGEON BREEDER'S DISEASE

Avian antigens may be the cause of an immunologic pneumonitis very similar to farmer's lung disease. Various species of birds may cause this disease: pigeon, parrot, parakeet, and, less commonly, chicken.

It is interesting that professional chicken breeders often show serum precipitins (in about 50% of cases) but very rarely develop pneumonitis. A single bird may suffice to cause disease, explaining certain cases observed in children. Precipitins to the serum or fecal extracts of the incriminated bird are seen, with cross-reactions between numerous species; the more intense precipitin lines develop to the species responsible. Also, hemagglutinins and complement-fixing antibodies can be shown. Antigens that precipitate in avian serum are localized in the γ-globulin fraction. Patient's antibodies are IgA, IgG, and IgM. Low titers of precipitins are found in 20–40% of bird breeders who have no clinical disorder, but they never occur in nonexposed subjects. Patient's serum transferred into rats may induce a passive Arthus reaction. Skin tests may give either a positive reaction of rapid onset (type I, anaphylactic reaction) or semidelayed reactions (type III, Arthus reaction). The type-I anaphylactic reaction is usually weak, whereas the semidelayed reaction is intense. The latter reaction has the same kinetics as does dyspnea, as assessed by tests performed by inhalation of avian antigenic extracts.

In this type of hypersensitivity, it is important to differentiate between type-I allergy to antigens present in feathers, which is an immediate and intense cutaneous reaction and may give an immediate asthmatic attack after inhalation, and type-III hypersensitivity associated with precipitins, which yields essentially semidelayed-type skin reactions. In the latter case, acute dyspnea may be induced by inhalation, but with an incubation period of 5–6 hr.

## CONCLUSIONS

The data available indicate that extrinsic allergic alveolitis (pigeon breeder's and farmer's lung diseases) relate to a hypersensitivity state similar to Arthus reaction. Certainly, the time lag (6–8 hr) is very suggestive. The presence of Ig and C3 deposits in the lungs, which has been demonstrated in farmer's lung disease, the characteristic symptomatology present after antigen inhalation, and especially the course of skin reactions are also highly suggestive. The postulated mechanism does not exclude, however, the existence of an associated delayed hypersensitivity, which is suggested indirectly by granuloma formation in chronic forms. In addition, lymphocytes from patients with pigeon breeder's disease undergo blast transformation in the presence of avian serum; this argument only indirectly favors associated DH, even though T lymphocytes respond better than do B lymphocytes in this test, B-cells may show a significant response. The rapid onset of skin reactions is probably not linked to IgE reagins, because inhalation tests do not cause early-onset asthma of the atopic type. The etiology of these skin reactions is not really understood.

## V.  CONTACT DERMATITIS (TYPE-IV HYPERSENSITIVITY)

Dermatitis (or, eczema, both words here being synonymous) may develop after skin contact with certain substances. This contact may be a simple irritation, when the substance causes physiochemical skin reactions (toxic dermatitis). However, the disease may also represent an immunologic conflict, and one speaks then of allergic contact dermatitis. These alternative mechanisms may, in certain patients, be associated. Numerous substances may induce allergic contact dermatitis. These substances are often organic and are encountered in the workplace, for example, chromates, formol, synthetic resins, antioxidants, terebentin, and nickel; other substances relate to the household situation, for example, cosmetics, some synthetic materials, rubber, certain stain removers, locally applied drugs, and, in the United States, the pentadecylcatechols in poison ivy. Sensitizing agents are generally of low molecular weight, but proteins may also be implicated.

Many of these substances, like chloro- and nitrobenzene, bind to proteins, usually to lysine amino groups. Other products bind to sulfhydryl cysteine groups. Still others, like picric acid, penicillin, and sulfonamides, bind directly to proteins. Sometimes a degradation product of the substance administered binds to proteins. Binding of drug to protein may, in certain cases, modify the protein's structure, for example, by destroying crucial disulfide bonds. The reaction specificity bears on both protein and hapten. The same hapten bound to another protein does not provoke the reaction. Recognition of this fact is important, because the interposition of groups between the hapten and the protein may diminish reactivity.

The problem is complicated by the existence of numerous cross-reactions and polysensitizations. Thus, sensitivity to $p$-phenylenediamine may be associated with sensitization to aniline, aminophenol, diaminophenol, methylaniline, and aminobenzene; however, all substances that possess a $p$-amino group may not cause reactions. The degree of cross-reaction is highly variable among patients. It has been proposed that cross-reactions may represent conversion of various allergens into a common haptenic substance, after chemical modification in the skin. A final question is the mysterious phenomenon of contact sensitivity induced by light exposure in subjects sensitized to sulfonamides or phenothiazine derivatives. Ultraviolet light may modify antigenic structure, thus making it more immunogenic. Nonimmunologic effects may also be involved (phototoxicity).

The acute reaction is characterized by erythema, edema, and the presence of vesicles. in chronic forms, the lesions thicken, increase in size, and lichenify. Both acute and chronic reactions show intense pruritus. The distribution of lesions corresponds to exposure zones; however, once sensitized, some subjects may develop lesions outside of the exposure zone or show accentuated lesions after a new contact. Lesions are minimal on strongly keratinized surfaces, such as the palms and soles; conversely, lesions are particularly marked on eyelids and in genital areas.

Induction of contact sensitivity takes 4–5 days. A shorter time lag indicates prior sensitization. Conversely, several months to even several years are sometimes required before reactions to weak immunogens develop. Once established, hypersensitivity is very long-lasting, sometimes enduring for several years.

Immunologic mechanisms of contact allergic eczema are established on a solid experimental basis. Landsteiner first demonstrated that contact sensitivity induced in the guinea pig by dinitrochlorobenzene (DNCB) requires DNCB conjugation to skin proteins, apparently through covalent bonds. Transfer experiments have shown that contact hypersensitivity is transferable by lymphoid cells (well demonstrated in the guinea pig but still unproven for man) but not by serum. Such eczema may be induced in the presence of Freund's complete adjuvant by antigens that do not need coupling to skin proteins like picryl chloride conjugated to erythrocytic stromas. These lesions occur normally in agammaglobulinemic subjects but are considerably diminished in T cell-type immune deficiencies. The local histologic findings (edema, mononucleated cell infiltrates with alterations in tonofilaments and desmosomes of epithelial cells) and regional lesions (hypertrophy of paracortical zones of lymph nodes) simulate cell-mediated immunologic reactions. Contact hypersensitivity to hapten-epidermal protein conjugates appears to proceed via mechanisms identical to those of classic DH reactions to hapten and dermal protein complexes (as described on p. 368). The only difference is the difficulty of demonstrating the immunogen formed in the skin after coupling to skin proteins; perhaps for this reason, it is difficult to show in vitro lymphocytic hyperactivity by classic tests of leukocyte migration inhibition or blast transformation.

This difficulty, partly answered by studies that involve metabolic transformations in the skin of radiolabeled haptens, explains why the only method that permits identification of the responsible substance in skin tests, are either epi- or intradermal tests. The epidermal reaction is most often utilized and involves application of test substance directly to the skin without penetration. A reaction is sought 48 hr later. A positive reaction represents erythema associated with edema and often vesicles and papules. Interpretation of these tests is difficult and there are numerous false positive and false negative readings.

The individual's susceptibility to contact hypersensitivity is governed by genetic control mechanisms. This hypothesis is suggested in man by the fact that only a very small percentage of subjects exposed to a substance known to induce contact hypersensitivity develop clinical eczema. In the guinea pig, the response to DNCB or to beryllium fluoride is a function of a dominant mendelian gene.

Lastly, one should note that the exacerbation that occurs after new contact has an experimental equivalent: a generalized rash may develop in the sensitized guinea pig after intradermal injection of 150 μg of Neosalvarsan, followed by intravenous injection of 6 mg of the same product. This rash looks like that seen in serum sickness disease; thus, there is posed the question of intervention of immune complexes in the pathogenesis of the lesions. Similar results may be obtained by intravenous potassium bichromate injection or by use of the same compound applied to the skin previously treated by glass paper. Here, one observes an exacerbation in the preexisting lesions that were induced by the previous topical application. This exacerbation is immunologically specific: increase of preexisting lesions is only observed when the antigen is the same as in the primary sensitization. Exacerbation reactions usually take 4 hr to appear (versus 24 hr for local application) and are associated with polymorph infiltrates (as contrasted with mononucleated cell infiltrates observed after local application).

It is possible to eliminate contact hypersensitivity to a given substance. A specific tolerance is induced when the hapten is injected in high dose or intravenously prior to attempted sensitization. Guinea pigs previously sensitized to potassium bichromate may be desensitized by intravenous injection of bichromate given concurrently with an epicutaneous application of the same product. Repetitive contact with the antigen may sometimes also induce tolerance. To desensitize, one must inject the hapten in a form that binds to host proteins or as the hapten-protein conjugate. These experimental data indicate a promising future for hyposensitization treatment, aided perhaps by supplemental immunosuppressive agents that seem to favor induction of tolerance in animals. At the present time, however, treatment of contact dermatitis is limited to elimination of contact with potentially responsible antigens and corticosteroids if the subject is very sick. Steroids are ineffective in preventing onset of sensitization but are (moderately) effective in reducing the inflammatory reaction in man.

# VI.  ALLERGIC DRUG REACTIONS

Allergic reactions are very common and may sometimes represent severe side effects of drug treatment. They must be distinguished from such side effects as overdosage, normal pharmacologic effects on target cells other than those for which the drug is prescribed (for example, leukopenia associated with alkylating agents), the placebo effect, and reactions linked to an enzymatic malfunction in the patient receiving the drug (e.g., primaquine-induced hemolytic anemia). Also, idiosyncrasy must not be confused with an allergic reaction. Idiosyncrasy, in fact, includes all unusual responses that occur in only a limited number of subjects, in contrast to overdosage and pharmacologic effects, which are regularly observed. Idiosyncrasy includes particularly enzymatic deficiencies. On the other hand, drug allergy must not be taken too literally. All immunologic side effects of drugs are not allergy in the purely restrictive sense (type-I, IgE-mediated reaction). We will show that cytotoxic (type II), immune complex (type III), DH reactions (type IV) may also be encountered. Before describing these respective mechanisms, let us briefly discuss the immunogenicity of the main classes of allergizing drugs, which generally have such a low molecular weight that they are nonimmunogenic when not complexed to a carrier.

## DRUG IMMUNOGENICITY

Most drugs with a molecular weight of 500–1000 daltons only become immunogenic after binding irreversibly (covalent bonds) to autologous proteins. It is frequent that only degradation products that react with these proteins induce immune reactions. In fact, drugs essentially behave like haptens. Nonconjugated drugs are, under certain conditions, able to inhibit the immune response against the drug-protein conjugate, by a mechanism similar to that described for haptenic inhibition (see p. 564). This phenomenon explains the virtual absence of sensitization to certain drugs, which bind to protein, and the fact that skin tests are frequently negative.

Some products do not themselves bind to proteins, for example, sulfonamides, salicylic acid, barbiturates, and quinidine. But their degradation products have this property. Thus, several penicillin G degradation products (not necessarily derived from enzymatic degradation) give rise to hapten-protein conjugates. These products include benzylpenicillenic acid, benzylpenicilloic acid (BPO), and benzylpenamaldic acid. In man, the BPO group is the major haptenic determinant (95% of penicillin G transforms into penicilloic acid). Benzylpenamaldic acid is, quantitatively, a minor determinant. Metabolic drug transformation ensures drug elimination from the circulation but may also be necessary for conjugation to a carrier. These conjugates are often produced by normal metabolic pathways and their formation cannot be prevented. Genetic control of certain drug reactions may relate to the individual capability of subjects to transform drugs into metabolites. Conversely, extrinsic factors that modify drug metabolism, especially by enzymatic induction, may modify formation of metabolites. The haptenic determinants of other allergenic drugs than penicillin that are allergizing have not yet been identified. Progress in this field is awaited. Covalent binding of drugs to proteins is not an absolute rule, because some drugs (e.g., Sedormid) do not form strong bonds with proteins. Although one cannot exclude that drug metabolites react with proteins, it is likely that these products act according to another unknown mechanism. It is interesting to note, in this respect, that haptenic inhibition cannot be obtained in vitro by use of any of these drugs.

## NORMAL IMMUNE RESPONSE TO DRUGS

An immune response to a drug is not necessarily associated with allergy. Most subjects treated for a sufficient period of time by a drug that produces hapten-carrier immunogenic conjugates show an immune response. The antibodies produced are variable, both quantitatively and qualitatively, concerning Ig class (IgG, IgE, IgM) and specificity for the different determinants. IgE antibodies, detected by Prausnitz-Küstner's test, have been reported to be much more common in atopic subjects (80%) than in those with no antecedent of allergy (25–30%), but the higher incidence of drug reactions in atopic subjects is controversial. IgE antipenicillin antibodies are found even in subjects not previously treated by the antibiotic. These subjects may have been stimulated by penicillin traces present in their food.

Antibodies to chloramphenicol or streptomycin are present in subjects who are not hypersensitive to these drugs. One may also observe DH reactions and positive blast transformation tests in subjects treated with penicillin who show no clinical reactions, in particular, no skin reaction. The only exceptions to this finding of immune reactions usually developing during treatments but not leading to allergic reactions are products that cause purpura or hemolytic anemia after noncovalent binding to platelets or red blood cells. Antibodies against these drugs are rarely found unless purpura or anemia is present.

## ANAPHYLACTIC DRUG REACTIONS (TYPE I)

These reactions occur within minutes or seconds after administration of the agent. They are characterized by a generalized urticaria often associated with asthma. In severe cases, a lethal anaphylactic shock may be observed. More rarely, there is delayed and transient urticaria (24–48 hr).

Products that are most often involved are the penicillins. Antipenicillinic antibodies produced by allergic patients belong to various immunoglobulin classes (IgG, IgM, IgE). IgG and IgM antibodies may be detected by passive hemagglutination. IgE antibodies specific for the major penicilloyl determinant may be detected by skin tests or by radioimmunoassay (RAST; see p. 749). Seventeen to 91% of patients, depending on the investigator, show reactive skin tests in response to penicilloyl polylysine. However, many patients develop positive skin tests during penicillin treatment without any side effects. The reciprocal is very unusual but does occur. By studying minor determinants, the specificity of skin tests is improved, but this procedure may expose the subject to anaphylaxis during the test. Penicillin anaphylactic reactions might thus relate to sensitization to the minor determinant, perhaps because IgG antibodies directed against the major determinant are blocking antibodies. Measurement of specific serum IgE (by RAST) by use of phenoxymethylpenicilloyl polylysine, benzylpenicilloyl polylysine, or penicilloyl polylysine reveals the presence of antibodies of very high specificity in the vast majority of allergy cases while nearly all exposed patients who do not present with allergic reactions are negative.

## CYTOTOXICITY-TYPE REACTIONS (TYPE II): THROMBOCYTOPENIC PURPURA AND HEMOLYTIC ANEMIA

Some drugs bind to blood cells, forming hapten-carrier antigenic conjugates. Antibodies to these complexes may cause thrombocytopenia, anemia, or leukopenia, depending on the cell involved.

### *Thrombocytopenic Purpura*

The serum of some patients with thrombocytopenic purpura occurring during drug treatment, especially with Sedormid or cephalothin, agglutinates the patient's platelets but only if the drug remains present. In the presence of complement, platelet lysis may even occur. The serum factor responsible is a γ-globulin, probably an antibody. This antibody is not directed against platelet antigens (it does not agglutinate platelets alone) but reacts with determinants formed after drug binding to platelets. The bond formed is very weak—when platelets are incubated with the patient's serum in the presence of drug and are then washed, both antibody and drug are eluted from platelets unless the platelets are washed in a drug-saturated solution. Dialysis of sensitized platelets against saline without drug elutes both antibody and drug. These data confirm the importance of the bond interposed by the drug between the antibody and platelets. The drug may bind to platelets other than those of the patient which suggests that most patients given the sensitizing drugs have drug-coated platelets. The platelet-drug complex is probably a weak immunogen, because very few patients become sensitized. The marked lability of the drug-platelet complex probably explains this weak immunogenicity.

In other cases, especially thrombocytopenic purpura due to antazoline, immune precipitates are formed after drug addition to the serum of the thrombocytopenic patient. These precipitates involve conjugates of the drug with certain serum proteins. The significance and effects of drug binding to proteins are unknown. It is noteworthy that excess circulating free drug does not inhibit the interaction of the antibody with the drug complex or with the platelets.

This weak drug binding to platelets suggested to Shulman a hypothesis according to which antibody is directed not against the drug-platelet complex but against a stable conjugate of the drug with a soluble noncellular macro-molecule. This immune complex, of antibody and conjugate, would then passively and secondarily bind to platelets, causing agglutination and lysis. In the same hypothesis, the antibody could also bind to the drug itself, and the immune complex would then bind to platelets and provoke agglutination. This hypothesis would explain why high concentration of circulating unbound drug does not inhibit agglutination. The recognized phenomenon of agglutination of platelets (or leukocytes) by immune complexes favors this hypothesis; this mechanism may explain the transient thrombocytopenia or granulocytopenia that occurs about 1 hr after the onset of anaphylactic shock. One may, however, question the validity of this model in reference to long-term thrombocytopenia induced by some drugs.

### Hemolytic Anemia

Hemolytic anemia may be induced by numerous drugs that act by multiple mechanisms. Some drugs bind to red blood cells. Patient's serum agglutinates the patient's red blood cells (and red blood cells from other subjects) in the presence of the drug. Complement addition sometimes causes hemolysis. The antiglobulin Coombs' test (performed after incubation of erythrocytes with patient's serum and drug, followed by washing) is positive. Drug binding to red blood cells is often weak, simulating Sedormid binding to platelets. Examples include stibophen, *p*-aminosalicylic acid, and chlorpropamide. Positive Coombs' tests could be, then, explained by complement fixation. These cases should be compared to cases of hemolytic anemia caused by insulin where (analogous to Shulman's hypothesis for thrombocytopenia) binding of drug-antibody immune complexes onto red blood cells plays an important role. For other products (penicillin, cephalothin, amidopyrine), the finding of an antidrug antibodies does not prove the cause of the anemia because such antibodies are present in drug-treated subjects who do not show anemia or allergic reactions. Final proof requires a reversal of anemia after cessation of drug treatment and its recurrence when the drug is readministered. In vitro absorption experiments suggest that the hemolytic anemia provoked by penicillin may especially relate to the minor benzylpenamaldic determinant. Only a minority of antipenicillin antibodies are responsible for hemolytic anemia. IgG antibodies are more often involved than IgM.

Some drugs may induce hemolytic anemia by means of true autoantibodies, as in the case of α-methyldopa (Aldomet). About 20% of patients chronically treated by α-methyldopa (for more than 1 year) show positive Coombs' tests. Unexpectedly, the autoantibody has Rh specificity. The antibody reacts with the patient's own red blood cells (collected when Coombs' test has become negative) and with red blood cells from normal subjects of the same Rh phenotype as the patient. One conceives of α-methyldopa modifying Rh antigens, which then become immunogenic by the mechanism of autotolerance breakdown first described by Weigle (see p. 725). Other products also seem capable of inducing a hemolytic anemia by means of anti-Rh autoantibodies. They include L-Dopa (used for Parkinson's disease) and mefenamic acid. In addition, α-methyldopa and L-Dopa also stimulate production of antinuclear antibodies.

Lastly, some drugs provoke hemolytic anemia by nonimmunologic mechanisms, as in the case of primaquine and other products, which cause hemolysis in subjects who present with certain enzymatic deficiencies. This is true also of cephalosporins, which bind to β- and γ-globulins and form complexes which bind, in turn, to the red blood cells and induce their elimination. A direct positive Coombs' test may then be observed by use of anti-β- and anti-glo-γ-bulin, which can be a cause of errors of interpretation. Cephalothin may also bind to β- and γ-globulins of the erythrocytic membrane. Anemia associated with chronic interstitial nephritis due to phenacetin treatment is of unknown origin but is probably nonimmunologic. The direct Coombs' test is generally negative, with a few exceptions, in which autoantibodies and antiphenacetin antibodies are present.

### Allergic Drug-Induced Leukopenia

Data similar to those described above for hemolytic anemia and thrombocytopenic purpura have been reported in certain drug-induced leukopenias. Leukoagglutinins to normal leukocytes may often be demonstrated in the absence of the drug but drug addition often enhances agglutination; in unusual cases, agglutination is only observed in the presence of the drug. Such leukoagglutinins are only found during the acute phase of agranulocytosis. It may be that only during the acute phase are drug concentrations sufficient to sensitize leukocytes. In any case leukoagglutinins are only transient and often disappear as soon as treatment stops. In addition to its transient nature, the presence of leukoagglutinins in drug-induced leukopenia is very rare. Thus, it is important to establish other methods for detecting antileukocytic antibody in the presence of the drug (cytotoxicity, antiglobulin or complement fixation, immunofluoresence). As discussed for thrombocytopenic purpura, one does not know whether the drug binds to leukocytes directly or by means of the intermediary of immune complexes. As was also discussed in regard to purpura, there is no leukoagglutination inhibition by circulating unbound drug. The main agents responsible for drug-induced allergic leukopenia are sulfonamides, amidopyrine, noramidopyrine, chlorpromazine, promazine, hydroxychloroquine, and propranolol.

## DRUG-INDUCED REACTIONS THAT IMPLICATE IMMUNE COMPLEX FORMATION (TYPE III)

Reactions induced by some drugs in many ways resemble serum sickness disease, in that they feature arthralgia, fever, and urticaria within a few days after the onset of treatment. This type of reaction is particularly frequent with penicillin. Both serum IgG and IgM antibodies are involved.

Drug-induced Arthus reactions are probably very unusual, except for extrinsic allergic alveolitis caused by hypophyseal powders; (see p. 757). It is also possible that some penicillin reactions proceed via this mechanism.

Lastly, one should recall the possible intervention (mentioned earlier) of immune complexes formed by drugs which passively fix to blood cells and lead to their elimination.

# DRUG-INDUCED REACTIONS THAT IMPLICATE DELAYED HYPERSENSITIVITY (DH) (TYPE IV)

Intradermal injection of penicillin may cause a skin reaction that cannot be distinguished from classic DH reactions. Levine showed that there is strict specificity for the carrier: patients treated by benzylpenicillin develop skin reactions only to benzylpenicillin conjugated to human γ-globulins but not to benzylpenicilloyl conjugated to polylysine or human serum albumin. Some authors wonder whether DH to penicillin may be responsible for clinical reactions. There is little doubt that some drugs used topically or frequently handled by nurses or drug workers may cause allergic contact eczema, a true DH reaction (an example is streptomycin).

# OTHER POSSIBLY IMMUNOLOGICALLY INDUCED DRUG REACTIONS

Allergic drug reactions are not only restricted to the four main groups of response that have just been described. Other situations exist in which drug hypersensitivity may precipitate clinically detectable pathologic manifestations. These reactions are less well recognized than the ones previously described, and, for certain even more poorly documented instances, their very existence has been doubted.

Some acute interstitial nephritides appear to be linked with a drug hypersensitivity. The most commonly incriminated products are the sulfonamides and methicillin. In the case of the latter, recent studies have suggested that it may bind to the antigen of the tubular basement membrane, thus modifying it and making it immunogenic, the nephritis being due to an antitubular autoimmunization. Antitubular basement membrane antibodies are often found in the serum and glomeruli (linear deposits along the tubular basement membrane).

Certain drugs seem to be causally related to acute interstitial alveolitis associated with the presence of eosinophils. Furantoin, para-aminosalicylic acid (PAS), penicillin, sulfonamides, hydralazine, aspirin, and hydrochlorothiazide are the most often incriminated drugs. the intervention of antidrug antibodies and sensitized T cells has been suggested but remain to be demonstrated.

The development of an acute immunoproliferative syndrome, immunoblastic angioma has been reported following the taking of certain drugs, particularly the hydantoins.

Finally, it should be remembered that some connective tissue disorders may be aggravated or even initiated by certain drugs. Lupus in particular may be induced by numerous products, and some cases of periarteritis nodosa can be secondary to the ingestion of certain hydantoin derivatives. Also, some cases of hypersensitivity angiitis have been described after taking certain drugs, such as sulfonamides, hydralazine, chloramphenicol, penicillin, tetracycline, barbiturates, hydantoins, guanethidine, thiazides, certain metals, phenylbutazone, quinine and its derivatives, aspirin, phenacetin, and ε-aminocaproic acid.

# *BIBLIOGRAPHY*

ACKROYD J. F. Immunological mechanisms in drug hypersensitivity. *In* L. P. G. H. Gell, R. R. A. Combs, and P. J. Lachmann, Eds., Clinical aspects of immunology, ed. 3. Oxford, 1975, Blackwell, p. 877.

ASSEM E. S. K. and VICKERS M. R. Serum IgE and other in vitro tests in drug allergy. Clin. Allergy, 1972, *2*, 325.

DASH C. H. and JONES H. E. H. Mechanisms in drug allergy. Edinburgh, 1972, Churchill.

DE WECK A. L. Penicillin allergy as a model for the study of immediate hypersensitivity in man and animals. *In* T. E. MANDEL, C. CHEERS, C. S. HOSKING, I. F. C. MC KENZIE, and G. I. V. NOSSAL, Eds., Progress in immunology III. Proc. 3rd Intern. Cong. Immunol. Sylney. Amsterdam, 1977, North Holland.

GLEICH G. J. and MULLER S. A. Atopic dermatitis: a review with emphasis on pathogenesis. *In* Clinical Immunology (C. W. Parker [ed.]). Saunders, Philadelphia, 1980, 1316.

GLEICH G. J., SACHS M. A., and O'CONNELL E. J. Hypersensitivity reactions induced by foods. *In* Clinical Immunology (C. W. Parker [ed.]). Saunders, Philadelphia, 1980, 1261.

GUPTA S. GOOD R. A. Cellular, molecular and clinical aspects of allergic disorders. *In*: Comprehensive Immunology. Plenum Press, New York, London, 1979, 628 p.

HONG R., AMMANN A. J., CALN W. A., and GOOD R. A. The biological significance of IgE in chronic respiratory infections. *In* D. H. Dayton, Ed., The secretory immunologic system. U.S. Publ. Health Service, Gov. Printing Office, 1969, DC 20-402 p. 433.

JOHANSSON S. G. O., FOUCARD T., and DANNAEUS A. IgE in human disease. *In* L. Brent and J. Holborow, Eds., Progress in immunology. II. Vol. 4. Amsterdam, 1974, North Holland, p. 61.

MIESCHER P. A. and MÜLLER-EBERHARD M. J. Textbook of immunopathology, ed. 2, section II. New York, 1976, Grune of Stratton, p. 369.

MOLLISON P. L. Blood transfusion in clinical medicine. ed. 5. Oxford, 1972, Blackwell, p. 516.

PARKER C. W. Systemic anaphylaxis. *In*: Clinical Immunology (C. W. Parker [ed.]). Saunders, Philadelphia, 1980, 1208.

PARKER C. W. Drug Allergy. *In*: Clinical Immunology (C. W. Parker [ed.]). Saunders, Philadelphia, 1980, 1219.

PARKER C. W. Asthma and Rhinitis. *In*: Clinical Immunology (C. W. Parker [ed.]). Saunders, Philadelphia, 1980: 1372.

PEPYS J. Atopy. *In* L. P. G. H. Gell, R. R. A. Coombs, and P. J. Lachmann, Ed., Clinical aspects of immunology, ed. 3. Oxford, 1975, Blackwell, p. 877.

PERKINS H. A. Immunologic hazards of blood transfusion. *In* E. Nykänen, Ed., Transfusion and immunology. Helsinki, 1975.

PINEDA A. A. and TASWELL H. F. Transfusion reactions association with anti-IgA antibodies. Report of four cases and review of the literature. Transfusion (Phila.), 1975, *15*, 10.

PLATTS-MILLS T. A. E. Desensitization Treatment for hay fever. Immunology Today, 1981, 2, 35.

REED C. E. Allergic mechanisms in extrinsic allergic alveolitis. *In* L. Brent and J. Holborow, Eds., Progress in immunology. II. Vol. 4. Amsterdam, 1974, North Holland, p. 271.

McVIE J. G. Drug-induced thrombocytopenia. *In* R. H. Girdwood, Ed., Blood disorder due to drugs and other agents. Amsterdam, 1972, Excerpta Medica.

VYAS G. N. and FUNDENBERG H. H. Isoimmune anti-IgA causing anaphylactoid transfusion reactions. New Engl. J. Med., 1969, *280*, 1075.

## ORIGINAL ARTICLES

BERG T., BENNICH and, JOHANSSON S. G. O. In vitro diagnostic of atopic allergy I. A comparison between provocation tests and the radio-allergic adsorbent test. Int. Arch. Allergy, 1971, *40*, 770.

FAUX J. A., WIDE L., HARGREAVE F. E., LONGBOTTOM J. L. and PEPYS J. Immunological aspects of respiratory allergy in budgerigar (*Melopsittacus undulatus*) fanciers. Clin. Allergy., 1971, *1*, 149.

LICHTENSTEIN L. M., NORMAN P. S., and WINKENWERDER W. L. Immunologic and clinical studies of a single year of immunotherapy for ragweed hay fever. J. Allergy, 1969 *43*, 180.

ROCKLIN R. E., SHEFFER A. L., GREINEDER D. K., and MELMON K. L. Generation of antigen-specific suppressor cells during allergy desensitization. New Engl. J. Med., 1980, 302, 1213.

# Chapter 27

# AUTOIMMUNE HEMOLYTIC ANEMIA

## Charles Salmon

I.   INTRODUCTION
II.  SEROLOGIC TECHNIQUES
III. NATURE AND SPECIFICITY OF AUTOANTIBODIES
IV.  IMMUNOLOGIC CLASSIFICATION
V.   MECHANISMS OF HEMOLYSIS
VI.  CLINICAL ASPECTS
VII. MODERN PATHOGENETIC HYPOTHESES

## I.  INTRODUCTION

Autoimmune hemolytic anemias (AHA) are defined by the presence of either an immunoglobulin or complement on the erythrocyte surface. AHA is differentiated from two other immunologic hemolytic anemias, alloimmune fetomaternal hemolytic anemia (see p. 752), in which IgG antierythrocytic antibodies cross the placenta to induce newborn hemolytic disease, and immunoallergic hemolytic anemia (see p. 765), in which an antigen, usually a drug, is responsible for formation of an immune complex (IC) on the red blood cell surface. In the latter case, the erythrocytic surface also has antidrug Ig (penicillin) or complement (rifampicin). α-Methyldopa-induced hemolytic anemia represents a unique case. This drug induces formation of an IgG autoantibody, which is then found on the red blood cell surface. Thus, a true autoimmune hemolytic anemia can be drug induced.

AHA present several unique features. In many cases, autoantibody specificity is known, the antigen being a blood group antigen of high frequency. In addition, a pathogenic role of the autoantibody can often be demonstrated, especially for IgG. In this respect, AHA represents a privileged model of autoimmune pathology. The mechanisms of hemolysis in AHA are relatively well understood. Hemolysis generally occurs in tissues and relates to opsonic adherence or immunoadherence, whether or not sensitization is caused by IgG alone or combined with complement.

Clinical aspects of AHA largely depend on the immunologic type of the anemia. The presence of IgG only or IgG plus complement represent the classic two main categories. They differ in terms of hemolysis mechanism, incidence of associated diseases, and sensitivity to steroid therapy. Recent immunologic observations have made possible a better appraisal of the etiologic mechanisms of autoimmunity. Several antibodies may be found on the erythrocytic surface, each of which sensitizes its individual target antigen. Furthermore, it is not uncommon to see over a long period of time, or during exacerbations, the appearance of antibodies of different specificities or nature (IgG or IgM). Overall, antierythrocytic autoantibodies probably represent only one element of a more generalized immunologic disorder that includes various other antibodies, autoantibodies, alloantibodies, and heteroantibodies. Note lastly that physicochemical studies of the antibody reaction with the patient's target antigen indicate that these antigens are normal and cannot be differentiated from those of normal subjects.

## II. SEROLOGIC TECHNIQUES

The simple techniques of classic immunohematology identify both the nature and the specificity of autoantibodies and are the basis for the immunologic (AHA) classification.

## COOMBS' TEST

The direct Coombs' test defines the presence of AHA by demonstrating erythrocytic sensitization by either immunoglobulin or complement. Originally, polyvalent antiglobulin sera were used to detect globulins present on red blood cells without identification of their specific nature. Methodologic progress was first made by Dacie, who developed the neutralization test. If antiglobulin is neutralized by addition of purified IgG, the red blood cell must be coated with IgG antibody; conversely, if the antiglobulin is not absorbed but still reacts with the patient's red blood cells, a non-IgG-type Coombs' test is defined. It is now known that, in most of the latter cases, complement (C3—especially C3d—and C4) is present on the erythrocytic surface. The differentiation of IgG from non-IgG represented significant progress in our understanding of AHA, and subsequent developments have verified the meaningfulness of differentiating IgG-positive from non-IgG-positive Coombs' tests.

The availability of purified anti-IgG, -IgM, -IgA, -C3, and -C4 antisera has permitted definition of the nature of autoantibodies that sensitize red blood cells. It generally suffices, in clinical practice, to recognize whether the red blood cell is sensitized by an IgG antibody or by complement, by use of specific anti-IgG or anticomplement antibodies. Sensitization by IgA is exceptional. IgM sensitization is difficult to prove by the Coombs' test. Even the purest anti-IgM-precipitating reagents only rarely agglutinate in the Coombs' test.

## ELUTION

The Coombs' test recognizes the nature of sensitization. Elution defines autoantibody specificity. Elution by means of heat or ether separates the antibody(ies), which are then exposed to a panel of red blood cells, including exceptional human red blood cells deprived of public antigens and, sometimes, animal red blood cells. To recognize IgM specificity, human, monkey, rabbit, rat, and sheep erythrocytes must be used. To identify IgG specificity, the panel includes silent Rh phenotype cells, and Pk and Tj(a−) type erythrocytes.

Other techniques may also be used to confirm the nature of the eluate. An example is treatment of the eluate by monospecific precipitating antisera, which eliminate antierythrocytic antibody activity, thus confirming the results of the Coombs' test. Similarly, positive IgM Coombs' tests may be verified by anti-$\mu$ antibodies, which specifically inhibit IgM in the eluate. Other techniques, including the use of proteolytic enzymes (bromelin, trypsin, or papain), are used to detect the presence of patient red blood cell sensitization, but these methods, of course, do not provide any additional information about the nature of the antibodies in question.

## SERA STUDIES

Direct study of the patient's serum is required to complete the evaluation initiated by red blood cell testing. The antibodies found on red blood cells may also be present in the circulation, but antibodies with a specificity different from those bound to red blood cells may also be found. A case in point is IgG autoantibodies. One particularly searches for cold agglutinins, the presence of which is suggestive of certain associated diseases and for hemolyzing activity.

# III. NATURE AND SPECIFICITY OF AUTOANTIBODIES

## IgG AUTOANTIBODIES

IgG autoantibodies are either IgG1 or IgG3. They are most often specific for high-frequency antigens of the Rh system, in particular Hr (Rh 18, Ee, or nl) antigens. Table 27.1 shows an identification procedure for anti-Hr specificity. All erythrocytes that have normal Rh phenotypes for the E or e zone, that is, E antigen, e antigen, or both E and e, are agglutinated. Erythrocytes from the rare subjects with the silent Rh complex, in connection with the production of Cc, compound antigens, or Ee, and Rh-null erythrocytes, are not agglutinated.

**Table 27.1    Identification of anti-Hr Specificity (or nl) of IgG Autoantibody**

|  | Autoantibody eluted from red blood cells of a subject with AHA | Alloantibody responsible for newborn hemolytic disease; $[D^{IV}(C)^-/D^{IV}(C)^-]$ mother |
|---|---|---|
| Normal Rh phenotypes |  |  |
|   ddccee | + | + |
|   DCCee | + | + |
|   DccEc | I | + |
|   DccEE | + | + |
| Exceptional Rh phenotypes |  |  |
|   D−/D− | − | − |
|   $D^c$−/$D^c$− | − | − |
|   $D^{IV}$ (C)−/$D^{IV}$ (C)− | − | − |
|   Rh null | − | − |

The Ee-zone products are absent in $D--$, $Dc-$, and $D^{IV}(C)-$ complexes. These three red blood cell types (of which only a few cases are known) are not agglutinated by the IgG-type antibody eluted from the erythrocytic surface. The anti-Hr antibody thus reacts with an antigen produced by the Ee zone of the Rh complex.

Anti-Hr specificity is most frequently encountered but is not the only autoantibody specificity in AHA. In one study of 55 successive cases, isolated anti-Hr antibody was implicated in 25. In the others, anti-Hr was associated with anti-E, anti-ce, anti-Ce, or anti-D antibodies. Specificity of anti-Hr autoantibodies seems no different from that of anti-Hr alloantibodies observed in subjects with silent Rh $D--/D--$, $Dc-/Dc-$, or $D^{IV}C-/D^{IV}C-$ phenotypes, which may be responsible for newborn hemolytic disease (see Table 27.1).

Similarly, anti-e or anti-LW autoantibodies have a specificity similar to that of the alloantibodies present in some $R_2R_2$ or LW subjects. Therefore, both of the antibody types, allo and auto, recognize the same cells. Another autoantibody of complex specificity is the anti-$Hr_0$ or $Rh_{17}$ antibody. Schematically, this antibody seems to recognize an antigen produced within the Dd or Cc zone. Table 27.2 indicates the main specificities of IgG autoantibodies.

The entire profile of IgG antibody specficities is not yet resolved. Recently, antibodies obtained in eluates from several patients with IgG AHA were found to be completely absorbed by Rh-null erythrocytes, which indicates that their antibody specificity did not relate to Rh-system antigens.

**Table 27.2    IgG Autoantibody Specificity**

|  | Auto | $R_2R_2$ | $D--$ | Rh-null |
|---|---|---|---|---|
| Anti-e | + | − | − | − |
| Anti-nl (Ee) | + | + | − | − |
| Anti-pdl | + | + | + | − |
| Anti-dl (non-Rh) | + | I | + | + |

It is also important to recognize that in many cases, the eluates contain an antibody mixture (e.g., anti-Hr and anti-e antibodies). It is usually possible to separate out the specific antibodies. Identification techniques for these mixtures follow the same principles as do studies of serum antibodies from polytransfused subjects. For example, a mixture of anti-Hr + e absorbed onto $R_2R_2$ erythrocytes (which have the Hr antigen but are deprived of the e antigen) still contains the anti-e antibody. It is also possible to eluate the anti-Hr antibody from the surface or erythrocytes used for absorption.

## ANTI-P IgG AUTOANTIBODIES

This autoantibody deserves specific mention because it has an original specificity. It recognizes $P_1$ and $P_2$, but not pp, $Pk_1$, or $Pk_2$ red blood cells (exceptional red blood cells). The biochemical structure of P activities suggests that the target antigen has a glucidic nature. Once again, this specificity is analogous to the anti-P antibody of Pk subjects as well to the anti-P antibody component of Tj(a−) subjects, which are both alloantibodies. However, a critical difference is that the autoantibody is IgG, whereas the alloantibodies are IgM. Anti-P autoantibody binds complement; it elutes at 20°C but as the complement remains on the erythrocytic surface at 37°C, hemolysis may occur. The term "biphasic hemolysis" has been used to underscore this characteristic. An IgG antibody of similar specificity is seen very early in the course of certain acute steroid-sensitive hemolytic anemias. It is also present in children after various nasopharyngeal viral infections with positive Coombs' test (complement type).

## IgM AUTOANTIBODIES

In the great majority of cases, IgM autoantibodies are cold agglutinins, that is, antibodies with a greater affinity for antigen at low temperatures than at 37°C. Not uncommonly the antibody does not bind to its antigen at 37°C. Such an antibody is therefore very exothermic; when it combines with specific antigen, much heat is released (see p. 603). In many cases, these agglutinins are present in high concentration in serum. They define then a separate category of AHA, cold agglutinin disease. In other cases, when the autoantibodies are present in low concentration, they may be responsible for the presence of complement on erythrocytic surfaces although, in these cases, IgM on the erythrocytic surface is difficult to detect by means of the Coombs' test alone. If, however, the erythrocytes are washed in saline at 4°C, an anti-I or -i IgM antibody may sometimes be eluted at 56°C. Cold agglutinins may be classified on the basis of their specificity (Table 27.3).

### Ii Specificity

The I antigen, recognized by classic anti-I cold agglutinins, is a high-frequency antigen, only absent in about one of 5000 subjects and transiently in newborns. I antigen develops during the first few months of life, at the same time that i antigen (a possible substrate) disappears. i Antigen, to which cold

**Table 27.3   Specificity of Cold Agglutinins**

| Specificity | Human I+ | I− | Monkey | Rabbit | Rat | Comments |
|---|---|---|---|---|---|---|
| Anti-I | + | − | − | + | − | Titer often aug- |
| Anti-i | − | + | + | − | ou ± | mented by pro- |
| Anti-Ii | + | + | + | + | ou ± | teases |
| Anti-Pr1 |  |  |  |  |  | Titer diminished by |
| (Sp1/HD₁) | + | + | − | − | − | proteases and neur- |
| Anti-Pr2 |  |  |  |  |  | aminidase |
| (HD₂) | + | + | − | − | + |  |
| Anti-Prᵃ | + | + | − | − | − | Titer only diminished by protease and not by neuraminidase |

agglutinins are more rarely directed, is present in large amounts on newborn erythrocytes and in small amounts in adults. Certain IgM autoantibodies agglutinate all human or animal red blood cells that contain either I or i antigen. It is convenient, for the moment, to suppose they have both anti-I and anti-i specificities. These specificities are outlined in Table 27.3. They represent glucidic determinants, the intimate structure of which is currently under investigation.

### Pr1, Pr2, and Prᵃ Specificities

In about 3% of cases, cold agglutinins are directed toward antigens that disappear when the erythrocyte is treated by protease, neuraminidase, or both. These isotypic specificities have been found in all human red cells tested. Examples are anti-Pr1 (or Sp1 or HD), anti-Pr2, and anti-Prᵃ antibodies. The anti-Pr1 antibody is defined as recognizing an antigen present in man but not in monkey, rabbit, or rat. Anti-Pr2 antibody has the same properties but, in addition, recognizes an antigen present in the rat. Anti-Prᵃ antibody recognizes an antigen that disappears after protease treatment but is unaffected by neuraminidase treatment. Thus, unlike Pr1 and Pr2 antigens, Prᵃ is probably not associated with sialic acid molecules.

### ABO Cold Agglutinins

Anti-A, and anti-B cold IgM autoantibodies were recently described. These antibodies are highly exothermic IgM ($-\Delta H = 35$ kcal/mol) and are therefore very different from IgM alloantibodies, which have the same anti-B specificities but cause a heat-producing reaction, in $A_1$ subjects, of only 16 kcal/mol. Here, too, the target antigen seems to be perfectly normal.

### Mixed Specificities

In certain cases, the specificity of IgM cold autoantibodies corresponds to complex antigens that participate in several independent genetic structures. These antibodies include anti-HI, anti-AI, and anti-BI autoantibodies. In a recent case (Doinel), the antibody was isolated, purified, and hydrolyzed. All subunits, including Fab, separated by enzymatic hydrolyses had the same specificity, recognizing a reactive structure due to the vicinity of A and B common part, and the I antigen. This finding also illustrates how analysis of IgM autoantibodies of complex specificity may further define chemical relationships of antigens on the erythrocytic surface.

### IgM Antibodies Active at 37°C

IgM autoantibodies as a group show considerable diversity of activity, depending on termperature, pH, and erythrocyte tested. Most interesting of all are the IgM autoantibodies active at 37°C, which may be responsible for the presence of complement on the erythrocytic surface in the absence of high titers of cold agglutinins in serum. However, in some cases, these autoantibodies represent anti-I and anti-i antibodies, which are less exothermic than are cold agglutinins. As an example, during the course of an AHA associated with ovarian tumors, a positive Coombs' test, and low cold agglutinin titer (<1/8), the tumor extract contained a 19S IgM κ autoantibody of anti-I specificity. This autoantibody had a maximum titer at 4°C (1/256) but did agglutinate at 37°C normal erythrocytes treated with proteolytic enzymes.

## OTHER ANTIERYTHROCYTIC AUTOANTIBODIES

It is extremely uncommon to observe autoantibodies of other classes or specificities than those just mentioned. IgA autoantibodies are extremely rare, but IgA anti-Rh autoantibodies have been described. They may be detected by a direct Coombs' test by use of an anti-IgA or polyvalent antiglobulin. Specificities of these antibodies are anti-e and anti-Hr, similar to those of IgG antibodies. Several cold IgA agglutinins have also been reported, with essentially anti-Pr1 specificity.

Anti-U or -N autoantibodies of the MNS system and an anti-Xg$^a$ autoantibody have also been described. Bird has described "pseudoautoimmune" hemolytic anemia, in which a hidden T or Tn antigen was uncovered by bacterial action; the specific antibody present in all adult human sera sensitized the red blood cell thus modified. The presence of T or Tn polyagglutinability is not, however, constantly associated with an hemolytic anemia.

## SIGNIFICANCE OF THE DIRECT COMPLEMENT COOMBS' TEST

Complement is present on the red blood cell surface in almost 80% of hemolytic anemias. The nature of complement factors present on red blood cells in vivo may be recognized by monospecific antisera. C3 and C4 factors are, for example, bound to complexes of P antigen and anti-P IgG or of I antigen and anti-I IgM. These complexes bind complement in vivo where C3 is mostly inactivated by C3b inactivator and converted to C3c ($\beta_1$A) and $\alpha_2$-D. In IgG-type hemolytic anemia, it has not been possible to fix complement in vitro on the eluted

**Table 27.4  Immunologic Classification of 786 Cases of Autoimmune Hemolytic Anemia***

| Thermal classification | | Classification according to nature and specificity of sensitizing agent | | | | | | | Number | Frequency (%) |
|---|---|---|---|---|---|---|---|---|---|---|
| | Class | IgG | IgA | IgM | C | Elution (%) | Serum | | Number | Frequency (%) |
| **Warm antibody** | | | | | | | | | | |
| γ | IgG | + | Some-times+ | − | − | Anti-Rh (85) | Free anti-Rh | | 192 | 25 |
| Inter-mediate | "Mixed" | + | Some-times+ | Some-times+ | + | Anti-Rh (60) | Free anti-Rh, CA (7%), warm BH | | 166 | 22 |
| Non γ | Comple-ment | − | − | − | + | Sometimes IgM active at 37°C | CA, 1/32. Some-times IgM ac-tive at 37°C | | 235 | 30.5 |
| **Cold antibody** | | | | | | | | | | |
| CA | Cold agglutinins | − | − | − | + | − | CA ≥ 1/32 | | 165 | 21 |
| BH | anti-P IgG | − +4°C | − | − | + | − | anti-P BH | | 8 | 1 |

Rare antibodies: IgA, anti-Rh, IgG anti-i

*CA, cold agglutinin; BH, biphasic hemolysin; H: hemolysin.

autoantibody bound on specific erythrocytes. For this reason, the meaning of a positive IgG-complement Coombs' test in autoimmune hemolytic anemia of the mixed type is unclear at present.

In hemolytic anemia of the complement type, it is even more difficult to understand how sensitization of red blood cells precisely occurs. Jandl has shown that positive Coombs' tests of the complement type represent binding of very small amounts of IgG antibodies. With a very sensitive technique, Jandl has been able to detect IgG excess on red blood cells in 29 of 30 subjects with positive Coombs' test of complement type. The direct complement Coombs' test requires 60–200 IgG molecules per red blood cell, in contrast to the 20–30 molecules present in subjects with negative Coombs' test. It is possible that this small amount of IgG explains why a positive reaction with an anti-IgG antiglobulin does not usually occur. It may also explain the exclusive presence of complement on the erythrocytic surface. In a few cases, it has been possible, by washing erythrocytes at 4°C and then eluting at 56°C, to show an anti-I or an anti-i antibody in the eluate. Whether this occurs in vivo remains unknown.

Even more rarely, the presence of warm hemolysin has been observed. It is possible that some of the "complement" Coombs' tests actually represent transient binding of an antigen-antibody complex, which is then rapidly eluted from the red blood cells. Clear proof of this hypothesis is still lacking; the antigen involved is unknown.

The immunologic and clinical significance of isolated complement Coombs' tests is not clear in all cases. In our series (see Table 27.4), positive complement Coombs' tests without obvious clinical hemolysis were not uncommon. If more extensive clinical study is performed, other clinicopathologic abnormalities may be seen, including various lymphoreticulopathies or lymphoid infiltration of the bone marrow detected by biopsy or lymphangiography. If the Coombs' test is performed by use of opalin slide and not centrifugation (as in some English series), the direct Coombs' test is not positive in most healthy subjects.

## IV.  IMMUNOLOGIC CLASSIFICATION

The identification of the nature of globulins present on the erythrocytic surface and of the antigenic specificities of autoantibodies in eluates or serum has permitted the proposal of an immunologic classification of autoimmune hemolytic anemia (see Table 27.4):

*IgG-type AHA.*   The Coombs' test is positive with anti-IgG and negative with anticomplement antibodies. In most cases, antibody specificity is anti-Rh.

*Mixed-type AHA.*   The Coombs' text is positive with both anti-IgG and anticomplement antibodies. Here again, the IgG antibody most often has anti-Rh specificity.

*Complement-type AHA.*   The anti-IgG Coombs' test is always negative, whereas the anticomplement Coombs' test is always positive. If anti-IgM antiglobulins are used, the Coombs' test may be positive.

*Cold agglutinin AHA.*   These anemias are characterized by serum cold agglutinin titers in excess of 1/32. The antibodies most often responsible are anti-I. Coombs' test, performed after red blood cells are washed at 37°C, is negative for anti-IgG and positive for anticomplement.

*Anti-P IgG AHA.* This AHA is very rare and corresponds to the bithermic hemolysin of Donath-Landsteiner. There is anti-P specificity; the positive direct Coombs' test is of the complement type.

Other types of AHA (e.g., anti-Rh IgA and anti-i IgG) are even less commonly seen.

This simple and precise classification has superseded the prior terminology of cold and warm antibodies. It is especially important to differentiate AHA and IgG (pure and mixed IgG) from AHA with complement sensitization (i.e., complement and cold agglutinin types).

# V.  MECHANISMS OF HEMOLYSIS

One of the rewards of studying AHA autoantibodies is to demonstrate the direct involvement of the autoantibody in the disease pathogenesis. Such a demonstration, not usually evident for antibodies involved in other autoimmune pathology, makes AHA a particularly attractive pathophysiologic model.

Once autoantibody specificity has been identified, red blood cell survival studies permit one to show, by use of selected $^{51}$Cr-labeled erythrocytes, that red blood cells that bear the specific antigenic target have a shortened life-span, while, at the same time, red blood cells without the antigen maintain a normal survival. Antibody binding onto the erythrocytic surface and formation of a specific complex on the membrane precede hemolysis.

Data from two studies are presented in Tables 27.5 and 27.6. In the first patient, anti-e and, particularly, anti-Hr antibodies are implicated in the hemolysis. In the second patient (Table 27.6), only anti-e antibody is responsible for hemolysis. Such studies have real practical applications, for example, in the blood selection for transfusion. Unless the patient is Rh negative, $R_2R_2$ red blood cells can be prescribed if necessary.

In IgG AHA in which antibodies have an Rh specificity, it has been possible to show the toxicity of the specific (anti-Rh, -e, -D, -c, and -Ce) antibodies; the pattern, of course, varies according to patient. Because clinical hemolysis may occur intermittently, comparative study of target and nontarget erythrocytes may be very difficult. Serial isotopic measurements cannot be performed without an interval between injections of labeled red blood cells. It can, however, be shown that the autoantibody is responsible for hemolysis.

The participation of anti-I cold agglutinins in hemolysis is not as clear. The

**Table 27.5   Half-Life of $^{51}$Cr-Labeled Red Blood Cells in a dce/dce Patient With Anti-e + nl Autoantibodies**

D--/D-- red blood cells: (e – nl – ) = 23 days
DcE/DcE red blood cells: (e−nl+) = 24 days
dce/dce red blood cells: (e+nl+) = 12.5 days
The anti-e appears to be responsible for half-life diminution

**Table 27.6    Half-Life of $^{51}$Cr-Labeled Red Blood Cells in a CDe/cde Patient With Anti-e + nl Autoantibodies**

DcE/DcE red blood cells: (e−nl+) = 14 days
DCe/dce red blood cells: (e+nl+) = 4 days
The anti-nl is less hemolytic in vivo than is anti-e

degree of reactivity in the antiglobulin test and the intensity of hemolysis do not necessarily correlate, and a red blood cell sensitization may sometimes be seen and confirmed by antibody elution, without hemolysis. Most chronic autoimmune AHA show exacerbations separated by remissions, in the course of which autoantibodies are still present on erythrocytic surfaces. This fact may possibly relate to quantitative variations, but the sensitization threshold (for hemolysis) cannot be readily defined.

Several observations indicate that erythrocytic destruction in AHA involves additional factors. It is not enough for a red blood cell to be sensitized, it must also be prematurely destroyed. Engelfriet has shown that the pathologic role of autoantibodies of various IgG subclasses is not equal. IgG3 is almost always hemolytic, but hemolysis is variable for IgG1, and nil for IgG2 or IgG4. We shall later see that these differences relate to the ability of phagocytic cells to recognize the Fc fragment of the various IgG.

Despite these limitations, it is, nonetheless, established that the autoantibody is the main factor responsible for hemolytic anemia. In animal experiments the degree of hemolysis is proportional to the total amount of human anti-I cold agglutinins injected. IgG-type AHA are usually more severe when free auto-antibodies are present in serum. Lastly, there is a correlation between the thermal amplitude of hemolyzing antibodies and the intensity of hemolysis seen.

## INTRAVASCULAR HEMOLYSIS

Hemolysis of circulating red blood cells is very uncommon, and only observed during acute exacerbations of the disease. It is due to a complete activation of all complement components, C1–C9, leading to rupture of erythrocytic membranes, hemoglobulin release, and hemoglobinuria when the hemoglobin concentration in the blood reaches the threshold of glomerular filtration (and therefore urinary excretion). Such a mechanism is observed only in cases in which the autoantibody binds complement in vitro and is strongly hemolyzing (Donath-Landsteiner's biphasic hemolysin, warm hemolysin with positive direct complement Coombs' test, and, least often, cold hemolysin).

## INTRATISSUE, OR EXTRAVASCULAR HEMOLYSIS

The destruction of sensitized red blood cells is in the vast majority of cases due to phagocytosis by fixed cells. The organ sites of destruction depend on the nature of erythrocytic sensitization (IgG versus complement factors). Phagocytosis has therefore at least two aspects. In the first case (IgG on the surface), there is opsonic adherence; in the second case (complement factors), immune adherence is critical (see p. 268). These two mechanisms result in either total phagocytosis of sensitized red blood cells or morphologic changes that probably shorten erythrocyte life-span.

## SITE OF SEQUESTRATION

Radioactive ($^{51}$Cr) labeling of red blood cells permits one to localize sequestration within various organs. External counting enables to study the fate of labeled antibody-sensitized erythrocytes. Table 27.7 shows data obtained in 55 AHA cases from two Parisian laboratories. For IgG autoantibodies, sequestration is predominantly splenic. In complement-mediated AHA, there is diffuse sequestration, but the liver predominates.

Clinical and experimental observations confirm the central role of the spleen when erythrocytes are sensitized by IgG. Furthermore, survival of erythrocytes previously sensitized by anti-Rh IgG is restored to normal after splenectomy. Consistent with this finding is evidence that in splenectomized mothers, fetal Rh+ erythrocytes show normal red blood cell survival after injection of anti-D immunoglobulin. These facts may explain the relative effectiveness of splenectomy in IgG AHA, even when antibody titer and degree of sensitization are unaltered by surgery.

## OPSONIC ADHERENCE

Opsonic adherence requires warm IgG anti-Rh autoantibodies, which generally do not fix complement, even in high autoantibody concentrations. The absence of complement fixation may be due to the peculiar location of antigenic determinants on the red blood cell surface, which may not allow two molecules of the same specificity to form the "doublet" required for complement binding. Lo Buglio has demonstrated in vitro formation of rosettes between circulating monocytes, or splenic macrophages, and IgG-coated erythrocytes. Opsonic adherence represents interaction between the macrophage membrane and the Fc fragment of IgG1 and IgG3 subclasses. Electron microscopy reveals a close

**Table 27.7 Sequestration Site of $^{51}$Cr-Labeled Erythrocytes in 55 Autoimmune Hemolytic Anemias With a Half-Life of Less Than 18 Days**

| Sequestration | Anti-Rh IgG | Mixed | Complement without cold agglutinin | Cold agglutinins |
|---|---|---|---|---|
| Splenic | 11 | 9 | 1 | |
| Predominantly splenic | 1 | 9 | | 1 |
| Hepatosplenic | 2 | 4 | 1 | 1 |
| Predominantly hepatic | | 4 | 2 | 3 |
| Diffuse (spleen, liver, sacrum) | 9 | 2 | 2 | 1 |

After Y. Nagean and A. Combrisson.

adherence between the macrophage and red blood cell, with membranocyto-plasmic strips (from the macrophage) partly or totally surrounding the erythrocyte.

Erythrocytic destruction seems first to involve adherence of sensitized erythrocytes to macrophages, followed by complete or, more often, partial phagocytosis. There also occurs a decrement in membrane lipids, acetylcholin-esterase, and intracellular potassium. The loss of part of the membrane changes the volume to surface ratio of red blood cells and produces spherocytes. The newly formed spherocytes have a shortened life-span; they are sequestered in the spleen because of their stiffness. There is an excellent correlation between the degree of spherocytosis and the $^{51}$Cr-labeled red blood cell half-life.

## IMMUNOADHERENCE

The intensity of hemolysis during the course of cold agglutinin AHA depends in part on their thermal amplitude and the exterior temperature. It is important to recognize that even though erythrocytic autoagglutination in peripheral vessels explains such symptoms as acrocyanosis and Raynaud's syndrome, hemolysis is not always seen. Tissue sequestration of red blood cells seems to be the critical hemolytic mechanism in chronic cold agglutinin disease.

Immune adherence involves interaction between macrophages (especially hepatic) and the C3 factor of complement. Brown, Lachmann, and Dacie have shown that adherence to Kupffer cells of rabbit erythrocytes sensitized by human cold agglutinins occurred in C6-deficient rabbits, but did not occur in C3-deficient rabbits. A small number of C3-coated erythrocytes is retained in the liver, and some of them are phagocytosed. Most of them reappear in the circulation, but their transient adherence to macrophages may explain the microcytosis observed in certain complement-type AHA.

Resistance to hemolysis of cold agglutinin AHA red blood cells probably explains why these erythrocytes show better survival. In vivo C3 inactivation to $\alpha_2$-D is probably protective, in that immune adherence is diminished. An erythrocyte previously sensitized by $\alpha_2$-D will continue to bind anti-I cold agglutinins but cannot be coated by C3.

## PRESENT CONCEPTS ON HEMOLYSIS MECHANISMS

The present concepts of the respective role of intravascular hemolysis and various types of phagocytosis (immunoadherence, opsonic adherence) are summarized in Table 27.8.

For an IgG-sensitized erythrocyte (especially IgG3, or IgG1) and particularly when the antibody does not fix complement, the erythrocyte is recognized by splenic phagocytes by opsonic adherence, and is then partially or completely phagocytosed. If the IgG binds complement with activation of all components through C9, the sensitized erythrocyte (EAC) is hemolyzed within the vessel. This phenomenon occurs when the autoantibody is a biphasic anti-P hemolysin. If complement activation stops at C3, the red blood cell is phagocytosed after immunoadherence, especially in the liver.

**Table 27.8   Mechanisms of Hemolysis in Autoimmune Hemolytic Anemia**

All IgM autoantibodies fix complement. Here again, when complement is activated to C9, the erythrocyte is lysed within the circulation; otherwise, and more often, the same immunoadherence phenomenon is observed. Erythrocytes coated with the initial complement components acquire relative protection against phagocytosis; a transient recirculation of $\alpha_2$-D coated erythrocytes occurs.

## VI.  CLINICAL ASPECTS

We have seen how AHA may be classified according to the nature of the autoantibodies present. We shall now describe the clinical circumstances in which hemolytic anemia occurs.

### INCIDENCE

Acquired autoimmune hemolytic syndromes may occur at any age but predominate in children before 4 years and in the adult after 50 years (Fig. 27.1). This double-frequency peak, which is not always obvious in some series, may represent immaturity or fragility of the immune system occurring at the two extremes of the normal life-span, early childhood and old age.

Inclusion of subjects with various lymphoid neoplasias, in whom hemolysis is often subclinical, is justified by the presence of obvious signs of erythrocytic autosensitization.

### CLINICAL INTEREST OF IMMUNOLOGIC CLASSIFICATION

Immunologic classification based on the nature of antierythrocytic autoantibodies and the Coombs' test is widely used. IgG, mixed, complement, and cold agglutinin classes occur with a similar frequency. Only a few exceptional cases are not classifiable, particularly those associated with hemolysins. (In our

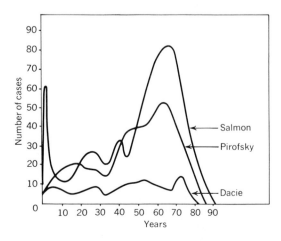

**Fig. 27.1** Incidence of hemolytic anemia according to age.

**Table 27.9   Etiologic Data in 510 Cases of Autoimmune Hemolytic Anemia (AHA)**

| | | Warm antibody AHA | | | Cold antibody AHA |
|---|---|---|---|---|---|
| | | IgG | Mixed | C | |
| Infections | | 4 | 8 | 4 | 52 |
| Diseases of the lymphoid system | Chronic lymphocytic leukemias | 31 | 22 | 22 | 5 |
| | Sarcomas | 3 | 6 | 14 | 16 |
| | Others | 11 | 14 | 13 | 11 |
| Miscellaneous | Systemic lupus erythematosus | 5 | 10 | 7 | 1 |
| | Connective tissue diseases | | | 8 | |
| | Cirrhosis | | | | 17 |
| | α-Methyldopa treatment | 3 | | | |
| | Others | 13 | 12 | 23 | 5 |
| Cold agglutinin disease | Chronic | | | | 33 |
| Idiopathic AHA | | 59 (46%) | 54 (43%) | 13 (10%) | 15 (12%) |

experience, totaling more than 1000 cases, the Coombs' test was negative in only one subject.) Immunologic classification is of considerable clinical importance. The proportion of subjects in whom clinical hemolysis is observed varies according to AHA types (approximating 100% in IgG and mixed types, 80% in complement type, and only 60% in cold agglutinin type) and also the clinical circumstances in which AHA is discovered. Table 27.9 summarizes data from 510 AHA cases in which precise clinical information was obtained, which include lymphangiography or bone marrow biopsy.

This table shows that antierythrocytic autoantibodies may appear in many conditions including infectious diseases, lymphoid system disorders, especially lymphoreticular diseases, connective tissue diseases, and sometimes drug reactions (α-methyldopa). Bacterial or viral infections (e.g., mumps, measles, and, especially, mycoplasma pneumoniae) are often associated with cold agglutinin AHA. They are usually self-limited, even though they respond poorly to corticosteroids. Acute AHA in children probably represents a particular case of curable AHA, which will be discussed later. Lymphoreticulopathies are associated with all of the above types of AHA, with IgG and mixed types occurring in chronic leukemia and complement and cold agglutinin types in sarcomas. Systemic lupus erythematosus (SLE) is usually of the mixed or IgG-type AHA. One should also note that 141 of 510 cases in Table 27.9 were considered idiopathic.

In nearly half of the cases of the mixed type, there is no apparent underlying disease, despite extensive clinical and laboratory examination.

Conversely, in complement and cold agglutinin types (independently of "cold agglutinin disease," which appears to be similar to Waldenström's macroglobulinemia), clinical and laboratory tests reveal an underlying disease in about 90% of cases. The onset of AHA may permit discovery of a previously unrecognized reticulopathy. Finally, two main forms of AHA can be contrasted. The first is represented by an IgG-type autoantibody (IgG and mixed type); hemolysis is long-lasting and progressive, sequestration of radiolabeled red blood cells is often predominantly splenic, corticosteroids are often effective, and in half of the cases the hemolytic syndrome is idiopathic. The second type is associated with complement on the surface of red blood cells with or without cold agglutinins; overt hemolysis is less common, labeled red blood cell sequestration is diffuse, steroids are less often effective, and an associated viral or lymphorecticular disease is often present.

## CLINICAL FORMS

In addition to the distinction between IgG and complement types, differentiation among acute, transient, and prolonged (chronic) AHA is useful for the clinician.

### Acute Forms

These forms more often occur in the young and less commonly in the adult. They have a rapid onset, which is often acute involving intravascular hemolysis. One often notes the coincidence of hemolytic crisis with clinical, viral, or bacterial infection (nasopharyngitis, mycoplasma pneumonia, infectious mononucleosis, varicella, measles) or vaccinations. Often, however, no obvious infection is found. In addition, the relationship between the infecting agent and hemolysis remains to be demonstrated.

### Prolonged or Chronic Forms

These forms are observed at all ages but especially in adults. Onset may be acute, but more often the anemia is progressive and insidious. Half of the time (secondary type), these forms are associated with other diseases, including complex clinical or biologic disorders, such as malignant hemopathies, systemic diseases, autoimmune disorders like SLE or pernicious anemia, liver cirrhosis, ulcerative colitis, or immune deficiencies. The intimate relationships between the latter disorders and autoantibody production is complex and often obscure.

In other cases, anemia seems clinically isolated ("idiopathic"), sometimes associated with thrombocytopenia which defines the classic Evans' syndrome. In this category is included the very peculiar AHA caused by prolonged administration of $\alpha$-methyldopa, which occurs in 0.8% of patients who receive the drug.

### Curable Acute Hemolytic Anemia of Childhood

The prognosis of AHA in childhood largely depends on the immunologic type. It has been observed that in complement-type AHA, anemia resolves completely and has a peculiar clinical course. Hemolysis appears suddenly 5–10 days after the onset of nasopharyngeal infection, with acute onset of fever and hemoglobinuria. If early examination is performed, a hemolyzing autoantibody with anti-P specificity similar to the biphasic hemolysin of Donath-Landsteiner is detected. High-dose steroid therapy works rapidly to achieve complete resolution within a few days or weeks. On the other hand, if the disease is of the IgG type, anemia will very likely be chronic, and in mixed-type cases of chronicity anemia is even more frequent (Table 27.10).

### AHA and Tumors in the Adult

The relationships between AHA and certain malignancies remain relatively obscure. There are definite cases in which ablation of benign or malignant tumors considerably improves AHA; a dramatic example is dermoid cysts of the ovary. Similarly, clinical improvement has been reported after removal of an ovarian teratoma. In this case, an anti-I antibody of the IgM type was identified in the tumor extract. It has also proven possible to ameliorate AHA occasionally by colectomy for treatment of ulcerative colitis. These cases are, however, exceptional, and, in fact, AHA is most often associated with diffuse involvement of lymphoreticular tissues (reticular or lymphoid malignant sarcomas, bone marrow infiltration by lymphocytes, chronic lymphocytic leukemia, more rarely myeloproliferative disorders).

## TRANSFUSIONAL THERAPY

The first rule is to transfuse only if clinically symptomatic anemia is present, for example, with symptoms of cerebral or myocardial ischemia. In most cases, the very wide specificity of the autoantibodies make it nearly impossible to find a compatible donor. Transfused erythrocytes will be rapidly destroyed. Therefore, transfusions must be reserved for hematologic emergencies and does not represent primary treatment.

It is, however, possible when the autoantibodies are IgG, with anti-e, anti-Ce, and anti-ce specificities, to use $R_2R_2$ blood (2% frequency in Caucasian populations). But in this case the transfusion must be evaluated in terms of the patient's phenotype. For an Rh− subject, it is better not to transfuse $R_2R_2$ blood because of the very high risk of anti-D alloimmunization. If the patient is Rh+, there is less risk, although anti-c or anti-E antibodies may develop. In any case, if there is a choice to be made between an autoantibody and an alloantibody directed against an antigen of rather high frequency (for example,

**Table 27.10  Course of 80 Cases of Autoimmune Hemolytic Anemia (AHA) in Children**

|  | Number of cases | Rapid progress toward cure | Chronic progressions |
|---|---|---|---|
| IgG AHA | 20 | 7 | 13 |
| Mixed AHA | 30 | 4 | 26 |
| Complement AHA | 30 | 23 | 7 |
| Total | 80 | 34 | 46 |

between an autoanti-e and an alloanti-c in an $R_1R_1$ subject), the best rule seems to first consider the alloantibody compatibility. Unlike alloantibodies, antiery-throcytic autoantibodies are practically never the cause of anuric transfusion accidents. Let us also mention that the use of frozen blood facilitates transfu-sional treatment.

# VII.   MODERN PATHOGENETIC HYPOTHESES

Autoimmune hemolytic anemia constitutes a privileged research tool for the immunopathologist. It permits a precise clinical evaluation of the general theories discussed in chapter 25. Autoantibodies show a well-defined specificity. Except for isotypic specificities (Spl, Pr, etc.), these specificities are blood group antigens that correspond to antigens (generally allotypes) of high frequency and of monomorphic specificity, such as Hr, LW, or I. These antibodies can be analyzed by classic immunogenetic techniques and may even be used in blood grouping (e.g., anti-e, anti-LW, anti-Hr, or anti-I antibodies).

Other antibodies, such as anti-I(A + B), allow investigation of topochemical relationships between normal antigenic determinants on the red blood cell surface. In addition, the recent demonstration of binding and elution from Rh-null red blood cells of certain IgG autoantibodies that correspond to high-frequency antigens suggests that new specificities, different from the Rh system, may be discovered by the use of these privileged IgG reagents.

Despite many similarities to alloantibodies, autoantibodies often have physicochemical properties different from those of their alloantibody analogs. Thus, biphasic anti-P hemolysin is a complement-fixing IgG, whereas the anti-P antibody of Pk subjects and the anti-P component of Tj(a−) subjects are IgM. Similarly, very few anti-B autoantibodies, despite their precise B-reactive specificities, even up to the weak $B_3$ phenotype, are actually exothermic antibodies ($-\Delta H = 35$ kcal/mol) and thus, in the strict sense, are cold antibodies. Conversely, IgM alloantibodies of A subjects have enthalpy variation of the order of 15 or 20 kcal/mol.

## AUTOANTIGENS OR TARGET ANTIGENS

The knowledge of autoantigens structure is limited, compared to that of antigens in normal subjects. However, at the present time, no differences have been recognized between autoantigenic and alloantigenic specificities and it is even possible, in certain cases, to use autoantibodies to characterize normal antigens. Wurmser used a thermodynamic method to study B-specific reactive antigenic structures present in subjects with anti-B autoantibodies. In at least two cases, the B antigen was completely normal ($-\Delta H = 16$ kcal/mol against an anti-B antibody of an A subject). This finding indicates that the binding forces of the antigen with anti-B alloantibody (hydrogen bond, Van der Waals forces, ionic attraction) are those of normal B antigens. Since the autoantigen does not appear to be modified, it is probably not in itself responsible for AHA induction but only represents the autoantibody target.

**Table 27.11  Specificity Variations of Autoantibodies**

| Dates | | | | Specificities | | |
|-------|---|---|---|---|---|---|
| 9/7/64 | | | | nl | + | "pdl" |
| 3/8/64 | e | + | | nl | | |
| 22/9/64 | | | | nl | | |
| 25/4/66 | | | | nl | | |
| 7/5/66 | | | | nl | + | c |
| 20/7/66 | e | + | | nl | + | c |
| 27/10/66 | e | | | | | |

Autoantibody formation therefore probably results from an abnormality of the immune system, without a primary role for autoantigen changes or from stimulation by an environmental antigen that cross-reacts with the erythrocytic membrane antigens of the patient. This antigen is unknown in the precise case of the anti-B antibody mentioned previously.

## MULTIPLE SPECIFICITIES AND VARIATIONS OF SPECIFICITY OR NATURE

Autoantibodies on the erythrocytic surface are sometimes multiple, each fixed to its own antigen. One example is a mixture of anti-c and anti-Hr + ce antibodies. Adsorption or elution-refixation tests on appropriately selected red blood cells permits easy separation of the various autoantibodies in the eluate.

Similarly, one sometimes sees different specificities in the serum and on the erythrocytic surface (anti-I serum and anti-e antibodies in the eluate) or antibodies of different nature. It is not uncommon to observe changes with time in antibody specificity (Table 27.11) or in antibody nature (Table 27.12). Thus, targets may be multiple at one given moment and may also change with time or between relapses. One example is an anti-e antibody appearing after an earlier anti-Hr antibody.

The wide variety in autoantibody specificities, the simultaneous presence of several distinct molecules of different specificities on the erythrocytic surface, their serial appearance during exacerbations, and the coexistence or serial

**Table 27.12  Variations in Nature of Autoantibodies**

| Dates | IgG | Specificity | C | Eluate specificity | Cold agglutinins |
|-------|-----|-------------|---|--------------------|------------------|
| 28/10/67 | — | — | + + | Anti-I | 1/8 |
| 16/11/67 | — | — | + | Anti-I | 1/4 |
| 3/1/68 | — | — | + | — | 0 |
| 28/1/69 | + + + | Anti-nl | + | — | 0 |
| 3/2/69 | + + | Anti-nl | (+) | — | 0 |
| 10/10/69 | + | Anti-nl | + | — | 0 |
| 15/1/70 | — | — | — | — | 0 |

appearance of different IgG autoantibodies suggest that several clones of immunocompetent cells are simultaneously implicated in one given patient.

## SATELLITE ANTIBODIES

One may ask whether autoantibody production is associated with alloantibody production in abnormally high concentration or with production of other autoantibodies. Fig. 27.2 shows that a large variety of satellite antibodies is seen in AHA. In one-third of the cases, antinuclear antibodies, blood group allo-hemagglutinins in abnormally high concentration, or alloantibodies to private blood group antigens are present. Additionally, it is possible, by immunofluorescence, to demonstrate antismooth muscle antibodies, antithyroglobulin antibodies, and antigastric antibodies in IgG-type AHA. The variety and intensity of these immunologic abnormalities indicate that antierythrocytic autoantibodies are only one manifestation of a more fundamental disorder of the immune system.

Two of these findings merit further comment. The large excess of ABO allohemagglutinins occasionally observed is not explained by specific antigenic stimulation because of the nonimmune character of these antibodies. Even more importantly, in one-third of patients, alloantibodies are directed against private blood group antigens. Such antibodies are only seen in about 2% of normal subjects. It would seem most unlikely that both normal subjects and patients with hemolytic anemia are submitted to extrinsic stimulation by these rare antigens the more so since the environmental presence of these antigens has not been demonstrated. In particular, the role of transfusion is excluded. In addition, there are usually two or three antibodies of this type in a given patient. The normal frequency of these antigens being about 1/1000, the probability of these three antigens occurring in a single transfusion is very low, of the order of $10^{-9}$. It seems more likely that these antibodies represent activation of normally silent clones in response to nonspecific stimulation. The nature of the hypothetical nonspecific stimulation is unknown. One should note that there is no cross-reaction between antibodies to these private antigens and autoantibodies directed against Hr or I antigens.

Thus, AHA is not only characterized by antierythrocytic autoantibodies

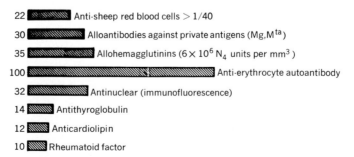

**Fig. 27.2** Autoantibodies in hemolytic anemias (percentage of patients studied); for defintiion of $N_4$, see p. 622.

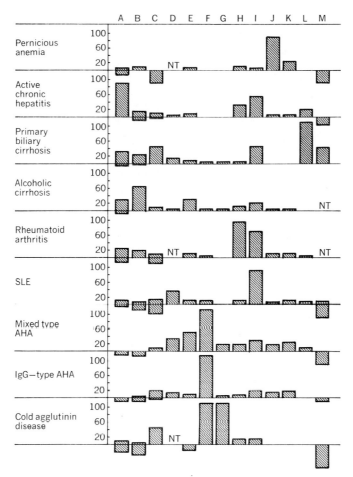

**Fig. 27.3** Incidence (%) of immunologic abnormalities in various autoimmune nonrelated syndromes. Increases in antibody levels are represented by the bars above the horizontal lines; decreased levels are shown below the horizontal lines. A, serum IgG; B, serum IgA; C, serum IgM; D, antibody against private antigen; E, ABO allohemagglutinins; F, Coombs' test; G, cold agglutinins; H, rheumatoid factor; I, antinuclear factors (immunofluorescence); J, antistomach; K, antithyroid, L, antimitochondria antibodies; M, total complement; NT: not tested.

but, similar to many other autoimmune diseases, also by other antibodies. Each autoimmune disease has its own immunologic profile. For example, the distinctive antibody is anti-intrinsic factor antibody in pernicious anemia, anti-DNA antibody in SLE, antimitochondrial antibody in biliary cirrhosis, antithyroid antibody in Hashimoto's thyroiditis, and rheumatoid factor in rheumatoid arthritis. In addition to these predominant autoantibodies, a whole series of satellite antibodies are usually present. Systematic analysis of these abnormalities shows interesting convergences: antibodies directed against private antigens are seen not only in idiopathic acquired hemolytic anemia of the mixed or IgG type but also in SLE and, unexpectedly, in primary biliary cirrhosis (Fig. 27.3).

Similarly, an abnormal production of anti-ABO alloantibodies is present in mixed AHA and alcoholic cirrhosis (Fig. 27.3).

## HYPOTHESES

Recent biologic data have modified hypotheses of the pathophysiology of autoimmune hemolytic anemia.

The oldest theory specified changes occurring in erythrocytic antigens. This possibility seems unlikely since no differences between erythrocytic antigens in the patients and their homologs in normal subjects have been detected. The special case of AHA with polyagglutinability has been linked to the presence of antibodies directed against hidden T or Tn antigens. Bird has proposed that these hemolytic anemias be called "pseudoautoimmune." Note that, conversely, the appearance of nonconverted acceptors in subjects with myeloproliferative disorders (an example is H substrate in $A_1$ subjects) is not associated with antibody formation.

A second classic theory, similar to the preceding one. states that the causal agent binds to the erythrocytic antigen or modifies its degradation. This hypothesis probably explains the anti-I cold agglutinin production (Feizi) that occurs in the rabbit after injection of human erythrocytes that were previously incubated with *Mycoplasma pneumoniae* (no response is observed after injecting erythrocytes or *M. pneumoniae* alone). This hypothesis might also explain AHA due to α-methyldopa (binding of drug to red blood cells).

A third theory involves cross-reactions. The causal agent is supposed to have an antigenic structure similar to that of the target antigen recognized by the autoantibody. This theory could explain Feizi's studies mentioned above, because of the possible antigenic similarity between *M. pneumoniae* and the I antigen of human red blood cells.

Another theory is based on the not infrequent occurrence of unrelated alloantibodies or heteroantibodies along with antierythrocytic autoantibodies. Stimulation by an alloantigen could cause a general stimulation of the antibody-forming system. This theory would explain the appearance of autoantibodies in subjects with prior immune alloantibodies secondary to incompatible blood transfusions. The allostimulation-induced transient appearance of autoantibodies, could relate to a phenomenon of cellular cooperation analogous to the allogeneic effect described on p. 538.

None of the above theories explains the numerous cases in which several autoantibody systems coexist, directed, for example, against Rh antigens (lipoprotein), ABH antigens (glycoprotein), or nonerythrocytic autoantibodies, such as anti-DNA or anti-immunoglobulin antibodies. The existence of these satellite antibodies is suggestive of a constitutional or acquired malfunction of the antibody-forming system (see p. 722). It is noteworthy that more than one-third of AHA patients have lymphoproliferative diseases. Proof that the malignant cells effectively produce autoantibodies has, however, only rarely been obtained. Such examples include clonal macroglobulins with cold agglutinin activity and IgA myeloma with anti-Pr$^a$ activity.

# BIBLIOGRAPHY

ATKINSON J. P. and ROSSE W. F. Immunohematology. *In*: Clinical Immunology (C. W. Parker [ed.]). Saunders, Philadelphia, 1980, 930.

DACIE J. V. The haemolytic anemias, congenital and acquired. Part 2: The autoimmune anemias, ed. 2. London, 1962, Churchill.

DACIE J. V. and WORLLEDGE S. M. Autoimmune hemolytic anemias. Progr. Hemat., 1969, 6, 82.

ENGELFRIET C. P., BORNE A. E. G., BECKERS D., and LOGHEM J. J. Autoimmune haemolytic anemia. Serological and immunochemical characteristics of the autoantibodies. Mechanisms of cell destruction. Serol. Haemat., 1974, 7, 328.

HABIBI B., HOMBERG J. C., SCHAISON G., and SALMON C. Autoimmune hemolytic anemia in children; review of 80 cases. Amer. J. Med., 1974, 56, 61.

HARBOE M. Cold autoagglutinins. Vox Sang. (Basel), 1971, 20, 289.

MOLLISON P. L. Measurement of survival and destruction of red cells in haemolytic syndromes. Brit. Med. Bull., 1959, 15, 59.

MOLLISON P. L. Blood transfusion in clinical medicine, ed. 4. Philadelphia, 1967, Davis, p. 496.

PIROFSKY B. Autoimmunization and the autoimmune hemolytic anemias. Baltimore, 1969, Williams & Wilkins.

VOS G. H., PETZ L., and FUDENBERG H. H. Specificity of accquired haemolytic autoantibodies and their serological characteristics. Brit. Haemat., 1970, 19, 57.

WOLF W., ZUELZER M. D., RENATO MASTRANGELO M. D., CYRIL S., STULBERG P., POULIK M., ROBERT H., PAGE M. S., RUBY I., and THOMPSON M. S. Autoimmune hemolytic anemia. Natural history and viral immunologic interactions in childhood. Amer. J. Med., 1970, 49, 80.

WORLLEDGE S. Immune drug induced haemolytic anemia. *In* R. H. Girdwood, Ed., Blood disorders due to drugs and other agents. Amsterdam, 1973, Excerpta Medica.

## ORIGINAL ARTICLES

BROWN D. L., LACHMANN P. J., and DACIE J. V. The in vivo behaviour of complement coated red cells. Studies in C6-deficient, $C_3$-depleted and normal rabbits. Clin. Exp. Immunol., 1970, 7, 401.

DOINEL C., ROPARS C., and SALMON C. Anti-I (A + B): an autoantibody detecting an antigenic determinant of I and a common part to A and B. Vox Sang. (Basel), 1974, 27, 515.

KIRTLAND H. M., MOHLER D. N., and HORWITZ D. A. Methyldopa inhibition of suppressor lymphocyte function: A proposed cause of autoimmune hemolytic anemia. New Engl. J. Med., 1980, 302, 825.

LOBUGLIO A. H., COTRAN R. S., and JANDI S. H. Red cell coated with immunoglobulin G. Binding and sphering by mononuclear cells in man. Science, 1967, 158, 1582.

ROECKLE D. Serological studies on the Pr1/Pr2 antigens using dog erythrocytes. Vox Sang. (Basel), 1973. 3, 206.

Chapter 28

# PATHOLOGY OF IMMUNE COMPLEXES AND SYSTEMIC LUPUS ERYTHEMATOSUS

**Jean-François Bach**

I.   GENERAL CONSIDERATIONS
II.  HUMAN SERUM SICKNESS: A MODEL FOR ACUTE
     IMMUNE COMPLEX DISEASE
III. SYSTEMIC LUPUS ERYTHEMATOSUS: A MODEL FOR
     CHRONIC IMMUNE COMPLEX DISEASE
IV.  PRESUMED PRESENCE OF IMMUNE COMPLEXES IN
     OTHER DISEASES

## I.  GENERAL CONSIDERATIONS

### EXPERIMENTAL MODELS

We have already discussed (chap. 25) several experimental immune complex (IC) diseases, including experimental serum sickness, lymphochoriomeningitis, and lactodehydrogenase virus disease. We have also described spontaneous IC diseases in NZB mice and Aleutian minks. In all of these cases, IC provoke multifocal lesions and, in particular, glomerulonephritis (GN), associated with Ig deposits visible by immunofluorescence. These experimental situations have their human equivalent; for example, serum sickness observed after injecting antitetanus serum very much resembles the experimental disease. Systemic lupus erythematosus (SLE) resembles, in many respects, the chronic viral diseases mentioned above, especially the autoimmune disease of NZB and B/W mice. Periarteritis nodosa features vascular lesions similar to those of Aleutian mink disease.

## CRITERIA FOR A PATHOGENETIC ROLE OF IMMUNE COMPLEXES

IC deposits have been implicated in and may be causative of numerous human pathologic lesions. Similarities, both clinical and immunologic, to experimental diseases in which IC intervention has been proven are apparent. However, proof of the involvement of IC requires direct demonstration of IC in the lesion plus evidence of its pathogenicity.

To demonstrate the presence of IC in organs or in the circulation it is necessary to show that antibody and antigen are both present and are associated. The existence of Ig deposits in the kidneys suggests the presence of antibody but is not definitive, because the precise antibody activity is not known and combination with the corresponding antigen is not proven. Antibody activity of Ig deposits in the kidney (in particular, antibodies against Australia antigen or DNA) has only been obtained rarely in individuals with GN by elution of Ig at the time of nephrectomy, biopsy, or autopsy. The presence of antigen has been even more difficult to demonstrate; unsubstantiated results have been obtained by immunofluorescence, suggesting the presence of streptococcal antigens in acute GN and DNA in lupus. Study of circulating IC poses the same problems as mentioned for tissue Ig deposits. Here, too, the most convincing results have been obtained in SLE with DNA-anti-DNA antibody complexes.

Demonstration of pathogenicity of IC is even more challenging. The similarity of the symptoms observed to those seen in experimental IC diseases or to those of acute serum sickness is very important evidence. Thus, the coexistence of IC with arthralgia, Raynaud's syndrome, or with lesions of GN similar to those seen in serum sickness disease suggests that IC are involved in the pathogenesis of the disease. However, because of the frequent absence of such clinical similarities to IC disease and of the relative lack of specificity of IC disease symptoms, evidence for the pathogeneticity of IC is usually only indirect.

## II. HUMAN SERUM SICKNESS: A MODEL FOR ACUTE IMMUNE COMPLEX DISEASE

Serum sickness is defined as a series of reactions that occur after administration of heterologous serum. Although clinical interest in this disease has diminished, due to the fact that less serotherapy (in particular, antidiphtheria serotherapy) is now prescribed, from a theoretical point of view, the model of acute serum sickness is still very interesting. Serotherapy is still used for treating tetanus, rabies, snake-bites, gas gangrene, and botulism, and heterologous antilymphocytic sera, which may cause serum sickness, are used as immunosuppressive agents.

### DESCRIPTION

The reactions that occur after injection of heterologous sera may be differentiated into two categories: serum sickness, properly speaking, which is due to

IC, and anaphylaxis, which is due to IgE antibodies. The former will nearly always occur if the amount of serum administered exceeds 200 ml, and its frequency is still high for 10 ml of serum, approximately 10%. Its incidence is decreased if purified γ-globulin is used instead of whole serum. Seven to 12 days after injection of serum, fever, urticaria, lymphadenopathy, and myalgia are noted. Simultaneously there may occur arthralgia, or even arthritis, and characteristic neurologic, vascular, and glomerular lesions develop after a short time. These lesions become symptomatic usually after fever and articular symptoms. Neurologic lesions mainly affect the motor nerves, particularly the brachial plexus. They may produce a Guillain-Barré syndrome. Vasculitis may be observed in the heart, pancreas, testicles, liver, muscles, and skin. Renal lesions resemble acute GN, with proteinuria and hematuria. Renal biopsy reveals diffuse extramembranous deposits that include IgG and C3 (immunofluorescence). The serum levels of hemolytic complement and C3 are reduced.

A second serum injection provokes the same symptoms, which occur significantly more rapidly. Injection of serum into a subject previously sensitized by earlier immunization (sometimes decades previously) with a related antigen may lead additionally to a severe anaphylactic reaction that is characterized by shock, hypotension, urticaria, dyspnea, nausea, vomiting, and asphixia and that may be fatal. Anaphylaxis is associated with the presence of IgE antibodies (reagins), with antibody activity directed against heterologous serum proteins. IgE may be demonstrated by intradermal injection of serum, which produces a local erythematous reaction; sometimes the same phenomenon occurs spontaneously at the site of the initial injection.

## IMMUNOPATHOLOGY

Serum sickness is associated with production of antibodies directed against heterologous proteins, which may be detected by various techniques. Precipitation may be used but is often insufficiently sensitive. Reaginic antibodies may be detected by passive cutaneous anaphylaxis. The most sensitive technique is passive hemagglutination, using tanned red blood cells coated with horse serum. Hemagglutination titers often exceed 1/10,000, even reaching $1/10^6$ at the apogee of antibody production. An excellent (but not absolute) correlation has been demonstrated between the titer of hemagglutinating antibodies and the onset of clinical signs; antibody titers do not, however, predict clinical severity. Injection of horse serum may sometimes give rise to anti-Forssman antibody production, detectable by a sheep red blood cell agglutination test.

Precipitating and hemagglutinating antibodies are mostly IgG and have two effects: they diminish the biologic activity of the injected heterologous proteins by accelerating their elimination, and they combine with the circulating antigen to form immune complexes. IC are responsible for certain clinical manifestations, especially arthralgia, GN, and neurologic or vascular lesions. The presence, in the glomeruli of subjects with serum sickness secondary to horse serum injection, of human IgG and horse Ig deposits (immunofluorescence) documents IC deposition in the kidney. The decrease in serum complement level also suggests pathophysiologic mechanisms analogous if not identical to those of experimental serum sickness disease and poststreptococcal acute GN.

## III.   SYSTEMIC LUPUS ERYTHEMATOSUS: A MODEL FOR CHRONIC IMMUNE COMPLEX DISEASE

### PROBLEMS OF DEFINITION

SLE is a disease characterized by multifocal clinical manifestations, especially involving the skin, joints, and kidneys, associated with numerous biologic signs of autoimmunity, including very specific anti-DNA antibodies. Changes in the skin gave the disease its name, after their initial description by two Frenchmen, Cazeneuve and Chausit. None of these factors considered alone suffices to make a definitive diagnosis of SLE.

It is possible to define SLE on the arbitrary basis of the presence of antinative DNA antibodies. This definition has had particular merit since the introduction of specific, reproducible, and sensitive techniques, such as the Farr assay. However, it is perhaps unwise to define a syndrome on the basis of biological characteristics that have not been shown to directly cause the disease: anti-DNA antibodies may not be exclusive to the disease; moreover, some subject with anti-DNA antibodies show no clinical manifestations.

Another approach to diagnosis consists of defining lupus on the basis of clinical signs (GN with Ig deposits, arthritis, skin lesions) or biologic features (antinuclear factors or antileukocytic antibodies, hypocomplementemia, false VDRL reaction, the presence of circulating IC, or cryoglobulinemia) and then identifying the disease when some or all of these items are present. This approach is that proposed by Dubois and the American Rheumatism Association (Table 28.1). It was a realistic approach several years ago; it is less acceptable now that specific anti-DNA antibodies can be measured by sensitive techniques. This approach, however, is useful in benign forms with few symptoms and has the merit of not being committed to any pathogenetic theory.

An intermediate approach to delineation of the disease state consists of defining lupus in two dimensions, the presence of one or more of the clinical manifestations mentioned above and the presence, at some point in time, of

**Table 28.1   Criteria of SLE Diagnosis (American Rheumatism Association)**

| | |
|---|---|
| Facial erythema (butterfly wings) | LE cells |
| Discoid lupus erythematosus | False-positive syphilis reaction |
| Raynaud's syndrome | Proteinuria (3.5 g/24 hr) |
| Alopecia | Urinary cylinders |
| Photosensitivity | Pericarditis, pleuritis, or both |
| Oral or nasopharyngeal ulceration | Psychosis, convulsions, or both |
| Arthritis without deformation | Hemolytic anemia, leukopenia, thrombocytopenia, eventually associated |

antinative DNA antibodies. This approach implies that in some patients suspected of having the disease, diagnosis will be made only after several years, for example, after discontinuing therapy if a search for antinative DNA antibodies had not been undertaken before treatment. It is justified because of the not uncommon delayed appearance of clinical sings that were initially absent.

## CLINICAL DESCRIPTION

Clinical manifestations of SLE are characterized by involvement of multiple organs at distant foci and by multiple exacerbations interrupted by remissions. The various clinical manifestations show widely variable incidence and significance in terms of morbidity and mortality. The three most common localizations are renal (also potentially the most life-threatening), articular, and cutaneous. Other sites of lupus localization are indicated in Fig. 28.1.

### Kidneys

Glomerular lesions are extremely variable from one case to another, both in nature and intensity, regardless of the presumed identity of the pathophysiologic mechanism involved. The frequency of renal changes in SLE is difficult to estimate, because the patients initially consult specialists as the first symptoms of the disease appear, and the presumed expertise of the consultant may therefore influence the assessment of the overall frequency of involvement of a given organ. A high incidence of 46% renal involvement was reported by Dubois in 1964 in a series of 520 patients. Much higher incidences are reported in subjects subjected to systematic renal biopsies with immunofluorescence techniques: 75–80%. The clinical picture is not pathognomonic but resembles that of many chronic GN. Proteinuria is of variable intensity and is sometimes massive (nephrotic syndrome). Hematuria, generally microscopic, is very com-

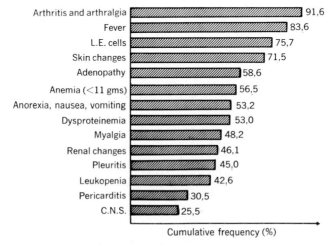

**Fig. 28.1** Symptoms of systemic lupus erythematosus (SLE). (From E. L. Dubois. Lupus erythematosus, ed. 2. Berkeley, 1974, University of Southern California Press.)

Patholo

Nucle:
becom
ment :
LE cel
pheno
after !
surrou
phase
cells w
(2
used f
of kid
substr
applyi
ultrav
clear :
Its wi(
not h:
classif
nucle(
exam|
and a
severa
cence
antibo
bodies
cell's r
be du(
antige
(!
or syr
fying
from
overn
and a
itates
sera g
of a s(
(Fig. !
heatir
Farr 1
sulfat(
filter,
(4
antinu
tinatic
compl
latter

mon. Renal insufficiency is frequent and tends to spontaneously worsen. Arterial hypertension is also common, and its incidence is exaggerated by corticosteroid treatment.

There is a great histologic polymorphism, even though one patient often shows the same types of lesions throughout the course of the disease. The kidney may be normal by light microscopy or show only minimal glomerular changes, best seen on electron microscopy. In many of these cases, immunofluorescence reveals weak fixation of anti-IgG serum along the glomerular basement membrane or in the mesangium. In other cases, the appearance is that of typical membranous GN, with Ig and complement deposits on the epithelial surface of the basement membrane. A third profile is membranoproliferative glomerulitis, in which, occasionally, the rigid appearance of glomerular basement membranes confers the term "wire loop." Immunofluorescence here reveals granular IgG, IgA, IgM, and C3 deposits. Another type is focal GN, which presents many of the above features but not uniformly. When the kidney is normal or has undergone only minimal changes, the outcome is generally favorable. As in the idiopathic form, extramembranous glomerulitis has a relatively good prognosis in general, because renal failure is unusual, but the glomerulonephritis is generally steroid resistant. Focal GN has also a good prognosis. The outcome of diffuse proliferative GN is most often unfavorable, characterized by an early onset of renal failure.

### Joints

Joints are the most common site of localization of SLE (in nearly 92% of Dubois' cases). Arthritis occurs particularly in acute phases and tends to fall into the clinical background when systemic illness and cutaneous and renal lesions develop. Arthritis is usually transient and migratory but is sometimes associated with serious effusion. Pain may be very intense or mild (simple arthralgia). Myalgia is often associated. Acute joint lesions usually regress rapidly during corticosteroid treatment and do not leave sequelae. Subacute forms resemble other states of persistent inflammatory arthritis. Chronic forms may appear as monoarthritis of the knee, ankle, or elbow or may present symmetrically; in these cases, deformations and radiographic abnormalities are very similar to the features of rheumatoid arthritis and pose a problem of differential diagnosis. These problems can usually be resolved by demonstrating SLE-specific immunologic abnormalities. Examination of the synovial fluid may facilitate diagnosis, especially when the exudate contains LE cells and shows reduced level of intrasynovial complement.

### Skin

In acute forms, erythema begins in the face, most often as small red or purple spots with induration that may rapidly extend to impart a diffuse erythema throughout the face. The eruption stops at the hairline, excludes the eyes, and disappears around the chin and ears. It may rapidly extend, in a series of exacerbations, to the limbs, involving the dorsal part of the hands and feet, forearms, legs, and shoulders and the trunk, breast, and back. Alopecia is frequent, and there may be lesions that appear as red patches or rapidly

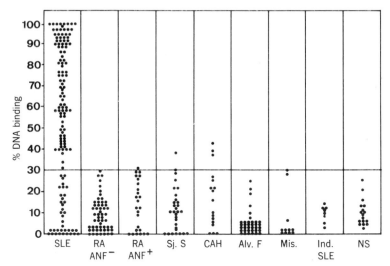

**Fig. 28.2** Antinative DNA antibodies detected by the Farr test. (From G. R. V. Hughes and P. J. Lachmann. In P. G. H. Gell, R. A. Coombs, and P. J. Lachmann, Eds., Clinical aspects of immunology. Oxford, 1975, Blackwell, p. 117.) Key: SLE: Systemic lupus erythematosus; RA: rheumatoid arthritis; ANF: antinuclear factor; Sj. S: Sjögren's syndrome; CAH: chronic active hepatitis; Alv. F: alveolar fibrosis; Mis.: miscellaneous diseases; Ind. SLE: drug-induced SLE; NS: normal subjects.

migration of nucleic acids that do not readily spontaneously migrate in a gel (counterimmunoelectrophoresis or electrosyneresis; see p. 317). These methods can be applied to the detection of anti-DNA antibodies but are, in general, less lupus specific and less sensitive than is the Farr test.

*Different Antibody Categories.* Antinuclear antibodies are the autoantibodies most characteristic of SLE. Their presence in large amounts was unexpected, because DNA is weakly immunogenic in the animal where it requires coupling to a carrier to produce large antibody amounts.

(1) *Anti-DNA antibodies.* Antibodies against endogenous DNA generally react with denatured DNA. There are, however, determinants specific of native DNA or of denatured DNA. The anti-DNA activity of Fab and $F(ab')_2$ fragments confirms that binding between lupus serum and DNA does, indeed, relate to the presence of anti-DNA antibodies; this confirmation is important because normal Ig, IC, and some complement factors (like C1q) interact nonspecifically with DNA. The size of DNA antigenic determinants that react with anti-DNA antibodies is approximately that of oligonucleotides with five purine or pyrimidine bases.

(2) *Anti-RNA antibodies.* Antibodies directed against double-stranded RNA may be demonstrated in more than two-thirds of SLE patients' sera. These antibodies also react with RNA virus. The antibody shows higher affinity for viral RNA than for mammalian RNA. Anti-RNA antibodies also react with synthetic polyribonucleotides, such as polyinosinic polycytidylic acid (rl-rC).

(3) *Antinucleoprotein antibodies.* Antinucleoprotein antibodies react with many still ill-defined antigens, in particular, with an antigen isolated from calf thymus called "sNP" (soluble nucleoprotein).

(4) *Other antibodies.* There are also antibodies directed against histones (basic proteins of nucleoproteins) and nuclear glycoproteins, which include, in particular, the sM antigen mentioned above.

(5) *Antinuclear antibody classes and subclasses.* Classes and subclasses of antinuclear antibodies are easily studied (immunofluorescence) by use of class-specific anti-Ig sera. All Ig classes are represented (IgM, IgE, IgA, IgG). The same is true for subclasses; there are often particularly high levels of IgG3 and especially IgG1, the two subclasses that bind complement. The presence of IgG antinative DNA antibodies, measured after fractionation of serum IgG and IgM on a sucrose gradient, are more often associated than IgM antibodies with severity and a bad prognosis.

*Seroclinical Correlations.* Seroclinical correlations again pose the dilemma of the definition of SLE. It is difficult to evaluate the frequency of anti-DNA antibodies in SLE, when the definition of the disease often includes, for many authors, the presence of the said antibodies. It is particularly difficult to distinguish SLE with clinically predominant articular localization from rheumatoid arthritis with anti-DNA antibodies; true rheumatoid arthritis may transform several years later into SLE with polyvisceral lesions (especially renal lesions). In addition to this problem, "mixed connective tissue diseases," apparently of benign evolution, have been described in which antibodies may be present that precipitate thymic extract (giving a speckled aspect on immunofluorescence). With these reservations noted, Table 28.2 lists the frequencies of each antibody category in the various disease states.

Examination of the data (Table 28.2) reveals the relative absence of specificity of antinuclear antibodies, as determined by immunofluorescence. Complement fixation reactions are more often positive for nucleoproteins than for DNA. The Farr test is of particular interest; it is very often positive in SLE and, furthermore, is relatively specific for the disease. Reactivity in the Farr test shows a direct correlation with disease outcome; increase in binding level usually precedes clinical activation. Compared to immunofluorescence, the Farr test is nearly as sensitive but is much more specific. It may be positive in some cases prior to positive immunofluorescence. It may however be frankly positive in a few patients with apparently benign outcome.

Not shown in Table 28.2 but noteworthy is evidence that anti-RNA antibodies, as detected by precipitation, complement fixation, or, especially, the Farr test, are found in about 50% of SLE patients, 7% of normal subjects, and in numerous other diseases, including rheumatoid arthritis (10–15%), psoriasis (10%), myasthenia gravis (15–20%), and scleroderma (10%). Although these antibodies have less diagnostic relevance than do native anti-DNA antibodies, the anti-RNA antibodies are interesting in that they react with RNA virus. A further point worth emphasizing is the high incidence of anti-RNA antibodies in discoid lupus (about 40% positive) compared to the usual absence of anti-DNA antibodies.

### ANTILYMPHOCYTIC ANTIBODIES

Antilymphocytic antibodies (AL) are often present in SLE. They are detected by lymphocytotoxicity in the presence of complement at 15°C (antibodies are much more active at this temperature than at 37°C, in contrast to anti-HLA lymphocytotoxic antibodies observed after transfusion, pregnancy,

DEMONSTRATION OF IMMUNE COMPLEXES

Immune complexes in serum can be detected by several techniques. Positive results are particularly seen during active phases. The presence of mixed cryoglobulins is already suggestive. More direct evidence for IC may be obtained by various methods based on evidence (1) that complexes precipitate under circumstances in which free Ig does not (in particular, in the presence of polyethylene glycol and rheumatoid factor), (2) that they bind C1q (which is the basis of techniques of C1q precipitation in gel, C1q binding, and measurement of anticomplementary activity of the serum) (3), that they expose Fc fragments of IgG and thus bind to Raji cells or inhibit EAC rosettes formed by B cells with complement-coated erythrocytes, or (4) that they possess peculiar properties, such as the ability to aggregate platelets or be phagocytosed by macrophages. Complexes may be isolated by chromatography or ultracentrifugation on sucrose gradients, which demonstrates immunologic IgG at molecular weights higher than for native IgG. All of these methods, strictly speaking, do not prove the existence of IC, which requires demonstration of the presence of the antigen (e.g., DNA) linked to Ig. This demonstration has been seemingly accomplished in rare cases after elution of antibodies and antigens at low pH or high molarity, particularly in studying cryoglobulin precipitates.

The presence of IC deposits in tissues, particularly in skin and kidney, is suggested by the presence of Ig and complement by immunofluorescence techniques. Kidney eluates taken at autopsy from SLE patients may contain DNA in high titers or antinucleoprotein antibodies. Here, too, DNA antibodies may only be demonstrable after dissociation of complexes by low pH, high ionic strength, or by DNase treatment.

CRYOGLOBULINS

Mixed cryoglobulins are commonly seen in SLE. Cryoglobulins may cause a specific symptomatology, which is initiated by exposure to cold. Mixed cryoglobulins contain both IgG and IgM; they also often contain complement factors (C1q and C3). The presence of mixed cryoglobulins is generally associated with high levels of circulating IC (see p. 732). In some cases, antibody activity can be shown within cryoglobulins, sometimes only after low-pH elution. These antibodies include rheumatoid factor, lymphocytotoxic, antinuclear, and anti-DNA antibodies.

COMPLEMENT ABNORMALITIES

The level of serum complement in terms of hemolytic activity is decreased in nearly 50% of lupus subjects and even more often in active disease. At the same time, various individual components of complement, C2, C3, C4, and, less frequently, C1q, are decreased (Fig. 28.3). Complement consumption by IC is most often responsible for hypocomplementemia, even when the alternative pathway is involved, as suggested by C3PA and properdin deposition in kidneys and skin and low levels of serum C3PA in many cases of lupus. One may also recall that certain lupus sera have anticomplementary activity and that C3 and C4 may be present in cryoglobulins and glomerular deposits.

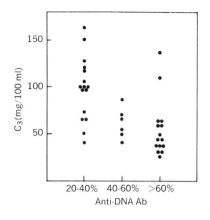

**Fig. 28.3** Correlation between serum level of C3 (mg %) and titer of the antinative DNA antibody activity, as evaluated by the Farr test. (From J. F. Bach and F. Tron, 1975.)

SLE may sometimes be associated with selective deficiencies in certain complement components. These deficiency states are often hereditary and not a consequence of the disease. They are perhaps the cause or at least contribute to its etiology. For example, hereditary deficiencies in C1q, C1r, C1s, C2, C3, and C4 have been described in patients with SLE or in subjects who present a closely similar clinical picture. These patients may also show decreases in other complement factors during the course of their disease. The most commonly observed abnormality is a deficiency of C2, which is often associated with the HLA antigens A10, B18, and DW2. Again, despite the fact that these patients have a single complement-factor deficiency, they may also develop decreased levels of other factors during the course of their disease.

### Abnormalities of Cell-Mediated Immunity

Although cell-mediated immunity has been the subject of extensive experimental studies, contradictory findings have been reported. Delayed hypersensitivity to nuclear antigens has been demonstrated by skin tests, leukocyte migration inhibition, and lymphocytic transformation tests. It is, however, difficult to exclude the possibility that these positive findings (skin and migration tests) are due to DNA reacting with anti-DNA antibodies and, therefore, to formation of IC. Independent of immunosuppressive treatment, some authors have observed a diminution in skin reactions to tuberculin, depressed development of primary delayed hypersensitivity reactions against dinitrochlorobenzene or keyhole limpet hemocyanin, a decrease in the in vitro response to phytohemagglutinin or in the mixed-lymphocyte reaction, a diminished number of T cells, as evaluated by the spontaneous sheep red blood cell rosette test, and a decreased serum level of thymic hormone. Many of these observations are controversial, and therefore it cannot be definitely stated that in SLE a T-cell deficiency exists that is analogous to that present in NZB mice; however, the present data are very suggestive of such deficiency, particularly during the active phases of the disease.

At autopsy, SLE patients often show thymic abnormalities, with many germinal centers containing plasma cells. These thymic abnormalities are, however, not specific for SLE and may be secondary to it, a hypothesis that should be kept in mind with respect to all of the findings mentioned above.

# ETIOLOGIC STUDIES

Numerous factors seem to favor the onset of SLE. It is likely that the development of SLE requires the simultaneous involvement of more than one factor. In some cases, however, one factor, if present at a particularly high level, may itself cause the disease.

## Search for Viruses

Because it is possible that a virus causes NZB mouse autoimmune disease, a thorough search for a viral etiology of SLE has been underway, but the results are still inconclusive. Two findings are of interest and serve to stimulate continued investigation: antiviral antibodies present in the serum and viral inclusions seen in tissues.

### VIRAL SEROLOGY

Some antinuclear antibodies, particularly anti-RNA, react better with viral than with mammalian RNA. Significant increases in antiviral antibody titers, particularly those of antimeasles antibodies, are often seen in lupus. These increases, however, are modest in degree and often represent augmented levels of antibodies to several different viruses in a given patient.

### VIRAL INCLUSIONS

Tubular structures, 20–25 nm in diameter, grouped together, simulating the appearance of myxovirus, are often observed in lymphocyte, kidney, and epithelial cell cytoplasm of lupus patients. However, these inclusions are not SLE specific, because they are also found in discoid lupus, Sjögren's syndrome, some neoplasias, scleroderma, dermatomyositis, and subacute sclerosing pan-encephalitis. These inclusions are also seen in many continuous lymphoblastoid cell lines. The structures initially aroused interest because they resemble nucleocapsids of myxo- and paramyxoviruses. Nonetheless, the viral nature of these inclusions has not been proven. It has not been possible to show that they contain viral RNA, and antimyxovirus sera do not bind to them. In addition, virus from inclusion-containing tissues has not been isolated. These inclusions are of limited interest at the present time because of uncertainty about their origin and because they are not specific, even though they are very frequently seen in SLE.

## Immunologic Factors

We have discussed the multiple immunologic abnormalities encountered in SLE. Autoantibodies are very numerous but are usually not organ specific (antinuclear, antierythrocytic, antileukocytic, and anticardiolipin antibodies); organ-specific antibodies, like antithyroglobulin and antigastric, are much less frequent, not occurring more frequently than in normal subjects. A cell-mediated immune deficiency is not as well established in SLE as in NZB mouse disease. It does, however, probably exist in SLE, as indicated by a decrease in the T-cell population and in the lymphocytic response to phytohemagglutinin. Finally, a deficiency of T cell-mediated immunity occurs along with hyper-production of autoantibodies. These autoantibodies are probably responsible for the major manifestations of the disease through the intermediary of IC deposits. But the T-cell deficiency has not yet been shown to be responsible for the B-cell abnormality, in the manner suggested experimentally in NZB mice, which lack suppressor T-cell function.

Some cases of SLE are also associated with hereditary deficiencies of complement components (C1q, C2, C4). And, hereditary deficiencies of complement are very often associated with a lupus-like syndrome. The relationship between complement deficiencies and SLE is difficult to understand. The complement deficiency could be secondary to SLE, for example, by IC consumption. If so, it is not clear why only selected complement components would be depleted. In addition, one could not explain the intermittent transmission of the familial complement deficiencies without any of the signs and symptoms characteristic of SLE. Perhaps complement deficiency is integral to the etiology of the lupus syndrome, because of enhanced susceptibility to infection or impaired elimination of normally formed IC.

### Genetic Factors

Many findings suggest an essential role of genetic factors in the etiology of SLE.

#### FAMILIAL LUPUS

It is not rare to observe multiple cases of lupus in one family. Because of female preponderance, the sister-sister and sister-mother associations are most frequently encountered. When a monozygotic twin has the disease, the other twin is almost always involved, with very rare exceptions. In many cases, members of the patient's family do not show overt clinical SLE but only suggestive manifestations of autoimmunity, such as hypergammaglobulinemia (5–20% versus 3–4% in normal subjects) or false-positive serologic results for syphilis. There is an increased frequency of rheumatoid arthritis in these families.

#### SLE AND HLA GROUPING

The study of HLA groups in SLE has shown variable results. Several authors have reported an increased frequency of HLA-B8, DR3 (and DR2) groups. These findings have not always been confirmed. One should also note that many mouse strains (e.g., DBA/2 mice) that possess the same H-2 as that of NZB mice ($H-2^d$) do not exhibit autoimmunity.

#### RACIAL FACTOR

SLE seems to occur more frequently among black people than among whites in the United States, apparently independently of social and economic factors.

ENVIRONMENTAL FACTORS

The contribution of environmental factors, in a large sense, has been suggested by the discovery of a lupus microepidemic in a Nevada community in which a common blood ancestry was excluded and by high incidence of antinuclear antibodies found in personnel who regularly study sera of SLE patients in immunologic laboratories.

## Endocrine Factors

FEMALE PREVALENCE

SLE predominates in women (90%). The explanation for this high prevalence in females is probably represented by the action of female hormones, as suggested by improvement in the disease of female NZB mice by androgens and aggravation in male NZB mice after castration. In addition, it should be noted that oral contraceptives have also been accused of favoring the development of lupus-like syndromes or aggravating the progression of already-established disease and that recent studies indicate an endocrine predisposition to SLE estrogen anomalies in some patients.

SLE AND PREGNANCY

Pregnancy may aggravate SLE, particularly in its renal manifestations during the first half of gestation. Subsequently, the increased levels of plasma corticosteroids effectively explain the usual absence of relapses. In fact, it is during the days following parturition that relapses most commonly occur, probably as a result of a sudden reduction in the plasma cortisol. Thus, the general rule is to administer relatively high doses of corticosteroids in the weeks following delivery.

## Drug-Induced Lupus

Certain drugs may induce de novo biologic or even clinical lupus. Induced or "iatrogenic" lupus raises interesting theoretical and clinical questions.

INDUCING DRUGS

Numerous drugs have been incriminated. Those most often implicated include hydralazine, isoniazid, antiepileptic drugs, particularly hydantoins, and a procaine derivative (procainamide); other drugs are more rarely incriminated, including α-methyldopa, sulfonamides, oral contraceptives (which might act by accentuating the endocrine factor), penicillamine, and tetracycline (Table 28.4).

CLINICAL AND IMMUNOLOGIC ASPECTS

The clinical picture generally resembles that of moderately severe SLE, usually appearing after prolonged treatment with the drug. Joint pains initiate the syndrome and are almost always present. Fever is also common, especially in the early stages of the disease. The skin and lungs are commonly involved.

## Table 28.4   Lupus-Inducing Drugs

| | |
|---|---|
| Anticonvulsants | Mephenytoin, diphenylhydantoin, trimethadione, primidone, ethosuximide, carbamazepine, phenylethylacetylurea |
| Antituberculous | *Isoniazid\**, *p*-aminosalicylic acid, streptomycin |
| Antihypertensives | *Hydralazine,* α-methyldopa, L-dopa, guanoxan |
| Phenothiazines | *Chlorpromazine,* perphenazine, promethazine, perazine, thioridazine, levopromazine |
| Anti-infectious agents | Penicillin, tetracycline, sulfamethoxypyridazine, sulfadimethoxine, griseofulvin |
| Miscellaneous | D-Penicillamine, quinidine, oxyphenazine, phenylbutazone, methylthiouracil, propylthiouracil, *procainamide*, amoproxan, tolazamide, methysergide, antiomaline, oral contraceptives |

\* Products in italics are those with the best documented lupus-inducing action.
After E. J. Dubois, Lupus erythematosus, 2nd ed. University of Southern California Press, 1974.

However, renal lesions (especially clinical) are unusual. One generally finds LE cells and antinuclear antibodies by immunofluorescence; antinative DNA antibodies are less commonly seen. The clinical abnormalities occur sporadically; however, systematic studies of patients regularly taking SLE-inducing drugs (such as procainamide or hydralazine) reveal up to a 30% incidence of developing antinuclear antibodies. The prognosis is usually favorable: the syndrome regresses when treatment is stopped, either spontaneously or after steroid treatment.

Antiepileptic drug-induced lupus seems most similar to idiopathic SLE. It is possible that some subjects treated by the drug in question may actually have had prior isolated neurologic symptoms of SLE. Similarly, renal symptoms may be difficult to evaluate in hydralazine-induced lupus, because the hypertension for which the drug is prescribed might possibly be a part of a lupus syndrome, with hydralazine merely aggravating the biologic syndrome.

### NATURE OF INDUCED LUPUS

There is obviously great interest in determining the mechanism responsible for induction of lupus. Clinical and biologic resemblances to idiopathic lupus are striking. Perhaps drug-induced lupus unmasks a true lupus diathesis in genetically or immunologically predisposed patients. This hypothesis would explain why lupus-inducing drugs aggravate the disease in NZB mice. On the other hand, this hypothesis would only apply to lupus-like syndromes that show clinical symptoms, because antinuclear factors are found in a very high percentage (approximately 30%) of asymptomatic drug-treated patients.

Experimentation has not produced a definite answer. It is difficult to provoke experimental SLE in animals with drugs known to induce lupus in man, even though positive results have been reported with hydralazine in dog, guinea pig, and rat. Both isoniazid and hydralazine administered chronically in the mouse lead to the appearance of antinuclear antibodies. The mechanism of induction is obscure; possible mechanisms are release or denaturation of nuclear antigens, in particular DNA; drug autoantigenicity after coupling to serum proteins; viral activation; or modifications of the lymphoid system by, for example, depression of suppressor T cells. It is interesting to note that some inducing drugs (like hydralazine and procainamide) can bind to DNA and then modify its physical and chemical properties.

### Conclusions

It is at present difficult to integrate the multiple factors that may initiate or aggravate lupus in man. Factors other than those discussed will undoubtedly be recognized in the future, for example, the effect of certain bacterial infections that release endotoxin or the existence of an impaired capacity to repair DNA after nuclear damage, which might cause increased release of DNA. At present, it is impossible to state whether one or more of the factors mentioned above are necessary for the disease to express itself in the severe form.

## THERAPEUTIC ASPECTS

Effective treatment of lupus is now available, for both its clinical and biologic manifestations; selection of the best therapeutic method would be mere speculation, however.

### Main Treatments

#### STEROIDS

Glucocorticoids represent a very effective treatment. In high doses (0.8–1.0 mg/kg), definite clinical improvement and attenuation of biologic abnormalities occur, with a decrease in serum levels of anti-DNA autoantibodies, the disappearance of circulating IC, and an increase in serum complement levels. Clinical disease in the absence of renal lesions is generally improved by doses of 0.3–0.5 mg/kg of prednisone, whereas renal disease usually requires a higher dosage (0.7–1 mg/kg) over a period of several weeks. A longer duration of treatment may be the cause of severe side effects, particularly infections in these patients who are already spontaneously immunosuppressed by the disease process.

#### IMMUNOSUPPRESSIVE AGENTS

The use of immunosuppressants would seem logical in a disease characterized by exaggerated production of antibodies. Azathioprine (Imuran) and cyclophosphamide (Cytoxan) are most often used. On a theoretical basis, cyclophosphamide is a more logical choice than azathioprine, because it affects both B cells and T cells, whereas azathioprine essentially acts mainly on T cells (see chap. 33) and it has been shown that SLE is often associated with T-cell deficiency, which probably plays a role in the pathogenesis of the disease. Thus, a drug that depresses T-cell function is not a priori to be recommended. In addition, cyclophosphamide has proven superior to azathioprine in NZB mice. In human lupus, favorable effects have been reported with both products; however, recent comparative trials seem to give the edge to cyclophosphamide.

Less toxic drugs (than corticosteroids and immunosuppressive agents) may be used in between exacerbations, particularly antimalarial and anti-inflammatory agents like indomethacin. However, there have been few objective documentations of their effect on the prognosis of disease.

PLASMAPHERESIS

Some groups have recently proposed that plasmapheresis is indicated in acute, rapidly progressive forms of the disease. It is not, as yet, possible to be sure of the real benefits of this new treatment.

### Results

The long-term course of SLE is extremely variable. Some patients not treated by corticosteroids or immunosuppressants survive many years without exacerbation, either clinical or biologic, and might be considered "cured." Other cases progress inexorably, despite treatment, with only transient remissions. Renal failure or central neurologic lesions may then cause death. In other cases, the disease will progress in the form of intermittent, repeated relapses, over many years. These exacerbations are responsive to corticosteroid treatment in low doses if symptoms are articular or cutaneous; high- or moderate-dose treatment with corticosteroids plus an immunosuppressive agent is usually necessary when renal or neurologic alterations occur.

### Interpretation

The mode of action of corticosteroids in SLE is not well established. They probably do not simply act as anti-inflammatory agents, because diminution in levels of antinuclear antibodies usually occurs concurrently with clinical improvement. Corticosteroids and immunosuppressive agents possibly act by diminishing IC production, as suggested by the disappearance of serum cryoglobulins. However, the various etiologic factors in SLE are not a priori modifiable by immunosuppressive treatment. It is possible that in the future, treatment will include immunostimulation or, more precisely, T-cell stimulation to restore suppressor T-cell function and eliminate potential viruses.

# IV.  PRESUMED PRESENCE OF IMMUNE COMPLEXES IN OTHER DISEASES

We have reviewed two diseases, serum sickness and SLE, in which IC involvement is well demonstrated. We shall see later (chap. 29) that IC are probably implicated in the majority of GN. There are other diseases in which a role of IC is highly suspect, but the evidence in these cases is less well documented. Arguments that favor the involvement of IC derive from demonstration of Ig deposits in tissues, from serum abnormalities that suggest the presence of IC, or from the similarity of the symptomatology with that of the classic IC diseases, represented by SLE and serum sickness. All of this evidence is, however, indirect, and there is no direct proof for IC responsibility in the diseases' pathogenesis. Note that diseases caused by locally formed IC (Arthus' phenomenon) such as extrinsic allergic alveolitis (see p. 756) will not be discussed in this chapter.

## RHEUMATOID ARTHRITIS

### Introduction: Problems of Definition

Rheumatoid arthritis (RA) is an inflammatory polyarticular disease usually easily distinguishable clinically from other inflammatory arthritides (acute rheumatic fever, gout, ankylosing spondylitis, psoriatic arthritis). The protean nature of its clinical and biologic manifestations makes definition difficult, the more so since there are cases in which the biologic and clinical symptomatologies overlap with those of other immunologic diseases, such as SLE or scleroderma. A given patient who presents with typical RA signs plus anti-DNA antibodies may be considered to have SLE complicating RA, SLE that primarily involves the joints, or RA with antinuclear antibodies but not SLE. The absence of specific clinical and biologic features in RA makes absolute definition impossible. For this reason, rheumatologists have proposed a fairly arbitrary definition of RA. Furthermore, it is not clear whether one disease, RA, has multiple clinical forms or whether several diseases exist with different mechanisms. This dilemma is particularly troublesome in subjects who present with juvenile-onset arthritis.

### Clinical Features

Clinical manifestations are essentially, and often exclusively, articular. More women (75%) than men are affected at all ages; there are, however, two peaks of incidence, one between 30 and 40 years and the other between 50 and 60.

This disease is characteristically an inflammatory arthritis that features stiffness, pain (maximum in the morning, decreasing during the day), swelling, and erythema. Localization is often symmetric and predominates in the metacarpophalangeal, interphalangeal, and wrist joints. Knees are also often affected. Synovial fluid can be easily studied in the latter site; the liquid is sterile and may contain numerous cells, including polymorphs, which show phagocytosed immunoglobulins (RA cells). After several years, radiologic abnormalities may be seen, due to osteoporosis of contiguous bone, destruction of cartilage, and, finally, bone resorption and displacement with ankylosis. At this point, the disease may be extremely incapacitating and require major therapy. Histologically, the synovium exhibits inflammation, characterized by polymorph and plasma cell infiltrates and by thickening of the cartilage. Acute phases are generally associated with very large elevations in sedimentation rate.

The clinical picture of RA may also include extra-articular manifestations. Subcutaneous nodules at pressure points, particularly the anterior side of the forearms, are not uncommon (15–20% of cases), generally associated with high seropositivity. The nodules have a distinctive histologic appearance, characterized by central necrosis surrounded by granulomatous and inflammatory reactions. In severe forms of RA, it is not unusual to observe other sites of localization in various organs (lungs, pleura, pericardium, myocardium, eyes, and central nervous system). These sites of involvement, which are often subclinical, may be found in more than 50% of cases at autopsy.

The outcome of the disease is extremely variable, ranging from nearly complete quiescence to rapid progression and total incapacitation within a few years. Early seropositivity (rheumatoid factor) has statistically a worse prognosis than do seronegative cases. In certain cases, amyloidosis may occur (10–20% of cases autopsied) or severe vasculitis may develop.

Polyarthritis in childhood merits particular comment. The disease may resemble adult RA but is often less painful. Articular deformations are less marked, but cervical spine lesions are more frequent. In other cases (Still's disease), juvenile arthritis may be distinguished from adult RA by the presence of multiple extra-articular manifestations, particularly intermittent fever, cutaneous rash, adenopathy, splenomegaly, or iridocyclitis. The prognosis for children is variable but generally is better than in adults.

### Immunologic Abnormalities

The numerous immunologic abnormalities observed in RA suggest an immune basis for the disease.

#### RHEUMATOID FACTORS

Rheumatoid factors (RF) are anti-Ig antibodies. RF detected by the Rose-Waaler reaction and the latex test are usually IgM anti-IgG antibodies that react with the Fc fragment of altered IgG (after combination with antigen or after aggregation). The Rose-Waaler test consists of agglutination by RF of sheep (or human) red blood cells previously coated with hyperimmune hemagglutinins (IgG) produced in the rabbit. The latex test involves agglutination of latex particles coated with Cohn's fraction II (immunoglobulin) of normal human serum. By use of specific anti-D antisera, such as "Ripley" serum (named after the patient source), RF may be evaluated by the agglutination of Rh + D erythrocytes coated with anti-D antibody. However, one must distinguish between agglutination obtained with Ripley-type antiserum (which agglutinates all RF-containing sera) and agglutination reactions observed against Ig alloantigens (Gm antigens; see p. 632).

All RF are not anti-IgG IgM. Some RF are of the IgG class, as shown by binding of RA sera on anti-IgG antibody immunoadsorbents or by immunofluorescence of IgG preparations (for example, IgG-coated red blood cells). IgM RF detected by the Rose-Waaler test and the latex test are found in about 70% of adult RA cases. Seronegativity is frequent in juvenile RA. RF of the IgG class are often seen in classic seronegative RA. The presence of RF is not specific for RA; significant levels of RF are seen in 5% of normal subjects (the frequency increases with age) and in other diseases, particularly connective tissue diseases, acute or chronic infections, and liver diseases (Table 28.5). The presence of anti-IgG activity in low titers in many normal sera necessitates the delineation of a pathologic threshold for the Rose-Waaler test ($\geq \frac{1}{32}$) and the latex test ($\geq \frac{1}{160}$),

**Table 28.5   Rheumatoid Factor in Nonrheumatic Diseases**

| | F II Latex (% positive) | Rose-Waaler (RW) (% positive) | Concordance |
|---|---|---|---|
| Pulmonary fibrosis | 61 | 61 | |
| Virus A$_2$ influenza | | | |
|    With antivirus antibodies | 14.8 | 14.8 | |
|    Without antivirus antibodies | 2.3 | | |
| Aged subjects | 10.9 | 12.5 | |
| Leishmaniasis | + | + | |
| | | | |
| Subacute bacterial endocarditis | 48 | 27 | |
| Leprosy | 33 | 14.7 | F II + ⎫ |
| Secondary syphillis | 26 | 14 | RW − ⎭ |
| | | | |
| Tuberculosis | 13 | 5 | |
| | | | |
| Alcoholic cirrhosis | 60 | <5 | |
| Viral hepatitis | 40 | <5 | F II + ⎫ |
| Tertiary syphilis | 11 | 0.7 | RW − ⎭ |
| Sarcoidosis | 9.9 | <5 | |
| | | | |
| Trypanosomiasis | 0 | + | F II − ⎫ |
| | | | RW + ⎭ |
| | | | |
| Normal subjects | 1.1 | 1.1 | |
| Aged subjects | 28 | 2 | |

After A. P. Peltier, in J. Pillot and A. P. Peltier, eds., Techniques en Immunologie, Paris, 1973, Flammarion Médecine Sciences, p. 122.

which explains why some patients with relatively low RF titers pass from positivity to negativity.

### Ig AND COMPLEMENT ABNORMALITIES

Hypergammaglobulinemia is frequently seen in RA and usually represents increased serum IgG. Serum complement is usually normal, whether assessed by total hemolytic complement (CH50), C1q, C3 or C4. There is, however, an interesting and important reduction in synovial fluid levels of CH50 and C3.

### CRYOGLOBULINS AND IMMUNE COMPLEXES

Cryoglobulins are often found in the serum and synovial fluid of RA patients. These cryoglobulins are usually mixed (IgG-IgM) and also contain IgM RF. Ig and C3 deposits are visible by immunofluorescence in the synovial tissues, suggesting IC deposits. Final suggestive evidence of IC in RA is the occasional finding of circulating (serum) or synovial IC, by means of the C1q-binding technique.

Sera from RA patients often show Ig peaks between 7S and 19S (ultracentrifugation), which relate to RF-IgG complexes, dissociable by low pH; at other times, complexes are larger than 19S.

ANTINUCLEAR SEROLOGY

LE cells and antinuclear antibodies detected by immunofluorescence are frequently detected in otherwise clinically typical RA. These antibodies are antinucleoprotein in nature but more rarely may be antinative DNA antibodies in low concentration.

CELL-MEDIATED IMMUNITY

Study of cell-mediated immunity in RA has produced conflicting results, both for in vivo delayed hypersensitivity and in vitro tests (E rosettes, mixed-lymphocyte reaction, phytohemagglutinin response). At variance with SLE, RA patients most often have normal T-cell function. There may be, however, delayed hypersensitivity toward IgG, as assessed by leukocyte migration inhibition in the presence of IgG and perhaps by the rheumatoid rosette test that use the same red blood cells employed in the Rose-Waaler test (however this test may also recognize B, or even K cells, with Fc receptors). Finally, it should be mentioned that recently, in juvenile RA, autoantibodies directed against certain T-cell subpopulations (suppressor T cells?) have been described. The effects of these remain to be clarified.

## Etiology

EXPERIMENTAL ARTHRITIS

There is no good experimental model of human RA. Most similar to human RA is the experimental arthritis provoked by infectious agents or immunologic phenomena. Injection of pleuropneumonia-like organisms (PPLO) or infection by *Erysipelothrix rhusiopathiae* or *Streptobacillus moniliformis* induce an inflammatory reaction in the rat that superficially resembles RA. *Bedsonia* injection may also produce polyarthritis in sheep. Immunologic models also include a polyarthritis provoked by Freund's complete adjuvant or by injection of autologous or heterologous fibrin or *Streptolysins* S.

BACTERIAL AND VIRAL INVESTIGATIONS

The presence of RF and IC in RA suggests the existence of a chronic antigenic stimulation. Many studies have been performed in a search for infectious agents in the synovium, in parallel with tests for serum antibodies or cell-mediated immunity. Positive findings have been reported for *Bedsonia* and, especially, for *Mycoplasma (M. fermentans)*. However, claims of demonstration of cell-mediated immunity to *M. fermentans*, as shown by leukocytic migration inhibition, appear to be actually due to contamination of *Mycoplasma* preparations by IgG.

CONCLUSION

Theories of pathogenesis abound. An infectious etiology was long considered most likely, and at one time RA was termed an "infectious" arthritis rather than "rheumatoid." Studies of the relationship between RA and streptococci, initiated in the 1930s, led current immunologic research in RA. Ten to 20 years later, because of the favorable effects of steroids, an endocrine origin was suggested. Today, the multiple immunologic abnormalities observed suggest an immunologic mechanism, with possibly an infectious agent as an antigenic source.

The existence of a chronic immunologic response is suggested by the presence of RF, which is found in other situations characterized by chronic stimulation (see Table 28.5). The frequent coexistence of hypergammaglobulinemia, cryoblobulins, and IC provides similar suggestive evidence. The presence of IC in the synovial fluid associated with decreased local complement levels (contrasting with normal serum concentrations) suggests a possible immune reaction developing inside the synovium, which may also contain numerous plasma cells. However, the antigen that elicits antibody and IC production has not been found. The existence of necrotic rheumatoid nodules and vasculitis is compatible with an IC mechanism. Cryoprecipitable complexes might also explain the common occurrence of Raynaud's syndrome in RA. Note that in this setting, RF would then be the consequence of IC production rather than a direct etiologic factor. In fact, immunization by heterologous Ig and RF transfusions do not produce arthritis; many subjects with high RF titers do not show articular manifestations.

Other hypotheses invoke abnormalities of thymus-derived cells: failure of T cell-mediated immunity, which would favor IC production (as in SLE) or, conversely, hyperfunctioning T cells, whose local mediators secreted in the synovial fluid would cause arthritis. In partial support of the latter hypothesis, it is interesting to note that numerous T cells are found in the synovial fluid and that injection of T-cell culture supernatants may induce an inflammatory arthritis that closely resembles RA. In this proposed scheme, IC production might be favored by T-cell hyperfunction through a helper effect. The IC would be responsible for certain symptoms (nodules, vasculitis, Raynaud's syndrome) but not for the arthritis itself. Evidence for a role of T-cell hyperfunction is a demonstrated clinical efficacy of thoracic duct cannulation, which essentially eliminates T cells, and of azathioprine administration, which selectively alters T-cell function (see chap. 33). This hypothesis would have the merit of explaining the RA cases observed in agammaglobulinemic patients.

### Treatment

Steroids are very effective but may produce severe side effects when given at high doses. It is difficult to determine whether they act as anti-inflammatory agents or as true immunosuppressants. Therapeutic success reported with antimetabolites (such as azathioprine) or alkylating agents (cyclophosphamide or chlorambucil) does not resolve this question, because these products are also anti-inflammatory (see p. 954).

Penicillamine, antimalarial agents, and gold salts are also used. Their mode of action and their long-term benefits are uncertain. Their utilization has been advocated because of the risks involved with long-term steroid treatment. Symptomatic treatment consists of anti-inflammatory agents (salicylates, indomethacin, phenylbutazone), surgical or isotopic synovectomy, functional reeducation, and orthopedic surgery.

# SJÖGREN's SYNDROME

Sjögren's syndrome consists of keratoconjunctivitis sicca, xerostomia with or withiout parotid gland hypertrophy, and polyarthritis. The sicca syndrome (kerato conjunctivitis and xerostomia) may be isolated but in other cases is associated with arthritis very similar to RA or with symptoms suggestive of periarteritis nodosa, SLE, or scleroderma. Keratoconjunctivitis is observed in 10–30% of subjects with RA.

## Clinical Picture

Sjögren's syndrome is a relatively benign disease that particularly affects 40–60-year-old women. Keratoconjunctivitis is sympomatic of a "burning" or sandy sensation in the eyes and the inability to produce tears, which may be documented by applying filter paper to the corner of the eye (Schirmer's test). Slit lamp examination demonstrates corneal debris, including filaments. Xerostomia is symptomatic of oral dryness, with inability to produce saliva and increased thirst. Dental caries are common, as is bilateral parotid hypertrophy. Technetium scintigraphy allows quantification of the functional changes in salivary glands. In addition, increased levels of $\beta_2$-microglobulin may also be found in the salivary juice. On histologic examination, salivary and lacrimal glands show a lymphocytic and plasma cell infiltration, with acinar atrophy and cellular proliferation along the canaliculi. Articular signs mimic RA. Renal lesions are very rare, except when Sjögren's syndrome is associated with SLE, periarteritis nodosa, or scleroderma. However, renal tubular abnormalities may be unmasked by oral acid administration tests.

Waldenström's macroglobulinemia, chronic lymphocytic leukemia, certain lymphomas, and sarcoidosis may be associated with Sjögren's syndrome. Conversely, one may see the onset of lymphoid system diseases, especially reticulum cell sarcoma, Hodgkin's disease, or lymphomas, during the chronic course of an otherwise typical Sjögren's syndrome.

## Immunologic Abnormalities

Hypergammaglobulinemia is common; Rose-Waaler test and the latex test are almost always positive. Antinuclear antibodies are seen, by immunofluorescence, in more than half of the cases; these antibodies are sometimes antinucleolar but usually give a homogeneous or speckled reaction. One may find antinative DNA antibodies by the Farr test. Mixed cryoglobulinemia is frequent and may be responsible for purpura. Antibodies that react with the cytoplasm of epithelial cells that border the salivary ducts may be detected by immunofluorescence, especially when polyarthritis is present. However, these antibodies are seen in 25% of RA patients without the sicca syndrome. Lastly, at variance with RA or SLE, antithyroglobulin antibodies are frequently seen (35–50%), sometimes along with Hashimoto's thyroiditis.

Recent studies suggest that two forms of Sjögren's syndrome can be distinguished by clinical, immunogenetic and serologic criteria. Primary form is not associated with RA, is associated with HLA B3DR3 and with the presence of a precipitating antinuclear antibody called SS-B. The secondary form occurs in RA and is associated with HLA-DR4 and the autoantibody "RAP" reacting with a nuclear antigen "RANA" which is related to infections with the Epstein-Barr virus.

### Etiology

The etiology of Sjögren's syndrome may represent the intersection of SLE, RA, and other connective tissue and even organspecific autoimmune diseases. This syndrome is probably immunologic in origin, but the exact mechanism is unknown. Experimental models are of no great help. However, guinea pigs injected with submaxillary gland extracts, in the presence of Freund's complete adjuvant, develop submaxillary lesions and, to a lesser degree, parotiditis, featuring lymphocytic infiltration. Also, abnormalities of salivary glands (chronic inflammation and degenerative lesions with atrophy) are observed in autoimmune NZB and (NZB × NZW) $F_1$ mice and in the South African rodent *Praomys* (*Mastomys*) natalensis, which, in addition, may have thymoma and polymyositis. The possible etiologies for Sjögren's syndrome are numerous: (1) IC pathology is suggested because of the frequent findings of RF, antinuclear antibodies, cryoglobulins, association with other connective tissue diseases, and analogy to salivary lesions observed in NZB mice; (2) autoantibodies; (3) direct cellular lytic mechanisms involving T cells, as has been discussed in the section dealing with RA. Finally, it should be noted that Sjögren's syndrome is significantly associated with antigens HLA-A1, B8, and DR3.

## POLYARTERITIS NODOSA AND NECROTIZING ANGIITIS

### Classification

Polyarteritis nodosa was initially described as a disease with necrotic and nodular lesions in small and medium arteries, and with multiple clinical symptoms, particularly neurologic and renal. The term "polyarteritis nodosa" was based on the observation that all three arterial layers were affected. Nodules are rarely seen, and therefore one could simply call this disease "polyarteritis." In fact, there are many arterial diseases that have the common feature of necrotizing angiitis, differing in their distribution, biologic signs, and clinical course. An etiology or association with immunologic mechanisms is very hypothetical, even though the angiitis resembles that observed in aleutian mink disease and serum sickness (see pp. 716 and 728).

## Polyarteritis Nodosa

Polyarteritis nodosa occurs at any age but is especially common between the ages of 40 and 50. The lesions are panarterial and sometimes focal. They are characterized by fibrinoid necrosis associated with intima rupture and leukocytic infiltration (initially neutrophils and eosinophils, later plasma cells). Immunofluorescence shows fibrin, IgG, and complement but often also albumin, thus suggesting nonspecificity of the deposits. It has never been possible to demonstrate binding of γ-globulin from polyarteritis patients onto arteries of healthy subjects, which suggests that Ig deposits do not correspond to antiarterial antibodies. The outcome of the disease may represent healing, but it may also result in unfortunate sequelae, such as fibrosis, nodule formation, aneurysmal dilatation, and even thrombosis or arterial dissection. Any artery may be affected, particularly those of the kidney, heart, lung, pancreas, liver, spleen, digestive tract, testicles, muscles (hence the usefulness of muscle biopsy), peripheral nerves, and brain.

### CLINICAL PICTURE

The clinical course may be insidious or, on the other hand, rapid, even explosive. The multifocal nature of the disease by itself suggests the diagnosis. Frequent manifestations include renal (ischemic lesions rather than GN with Ig deposits), cardiac (myopathy or coronary insufficiency), peripheral nerve (polyneuritis), lung (asthma), muscle (myopathy), and skin (cutaneous nodules). Arterial hypertension is often very severe and may be "idiopathic" or secondary to renal involvement.

Abdominal pain is common, usually due to mesenteric arteritis. Gastrointestinal bleeding may occur. Symptoms may suggest a "surgical" abdomen. Other localizations are more rare (hepatitis, pancreatitis, pneumonia, pulmonary infarction, lung abscess). Of note is the rarity of arthritis, in which IC intervention is frequent. Diagnosis is difficult when specific symptoms and biologic signs are absent. Eosinophilia is common, especially in cases that simulate asthma. Serologic abnormalities are rare; hypergammaglobulinemia is modest or absent. The diagnosis is essentially histologic, requiring renal or muscle biopsy but it is not unusual, because of the focal nature of lesions, to see authentic polyarteritis nodosa (subsequently verified by evolution or autopsy) associated with negative biopsy. The long-term outcome is often unfavorable, although some forms of the disease have a favorable prognosis. In most cases, steroids have an immediate, favorable effect on clinical symptoms, but this effect is not long-lasting. The response to immunosuppressive agents is not well established; in a recent series (Mayo Clinic) of 110 patients, 48% survived 5 years from the time of diagnosis.

### ETIOLOGY

An immunologic origin for polyarteritis nodosa is suggested by the existence of angiitis in experimental IC diseases, such as serum sickness, Aleutian mink disease, and the disease seen in an albino strain derived from NZB mice and aged Sprague-Dawley rats. The presence of Ig and complement in arterial lesions is also suggestive (with the reservations discussed earlier). The existence of allergic vasculitis, closely simulating polyarteritis, seen secondary to some drug allergies (in particular to thiouracil, bismuth, sulfonamides, penicillamine, and hydantoins) is somewhat supportive. In addition, it has recently been reported that patients with polyarteritis have a very high incidence of circulating Australia antigen ($HB_s$). This observation raises the possibility that $HB_s$-containing IC may sometimes be involved in the pathogenesis of the disease. Demonstration of $HB_s$ antigen in the lesions would corroborate this hypothesis. All of these findings provide only indirect evidence. Overall, there are only few immunologic abnormalities in patients with polyarteritis, in contrast with the multiple abnormalities seen in SLE. Note, however, the presence in some cases of circulating IC and hypocomplementemia, which are suggestive of IC involvement.

### Other Angiitides

#### CHURG AND STRAUSS SYNDROME

This syndrome is similar to polyarteritis nodosa in all regards. It is characterized by lung involvement and intense eosinophilia.

#### WEGENER'S GRANULOMATOSIS

Wegener's granulomatosis is characterized by necrotic granulomas in the upper and lower respiratory tract and lesions of necrotic focal vasculitis that affect arteries and veins of the lungs, kidneys, and occasionally other organs. Clinically, there is sinusitis, rhinitis with septal perforation, pneumonia, or peripheral neurologic lesions. Renal involvement leads to renal failure. Anemia and eosinophilia are more frequent than in polyarteritis. The outcome is usually unfavorable; mortality often occurs in 4 months. As in polyarteritis, the affected arteries may contain IgG. Corticosteroids are not very effective, highly encouraging results have been reported with cyclophosphamide.

#### ACUTE VASCULITIS

One must also metnion, at this stage, the acute "hypersensitivity vasculitis" sometimes observed 3–6 weeks after an infection or drug intake. As other necrotizing angiitides, vasculitis is defined by the lesion of leukocytoclastic vasculitis (fibrinoid necrosis of the vessel wall, infiltrates of pyknotic polymorphs, and cellular debris). Clinical signs essentially include indurated purpura and erythema. Hypocomplementemia and circulating IC, Ig, and C3 deposits in vessel walls (seen by immunofluorescence) may be present. The clinical outcome is usually favorable. Schönlein-Henoch purpura is a clinically different syndrome, associating arthralgia, abdominal pain, and eventually glomerular lesions with the purpura. The skin lesion is also that of a leukocytoclastic vasculitis.

#### GIANT-CELL ARTERITIS

Giant-cell arteritis (temporal arteritis or Horton's disease) usually affects aged subjects, particularly women (75%). The arterial lesions affect all three arterial walls, beginning in the intima and leading to arterial fibrosis and obstruction. The inflammatory reaction is intense, especially in the media, where giant cells appear. The disease usually remains localized in the carotid vessels (temporal, retinal, and cerebral arteries). Headache is frequent and very severe, and pain in the back of the neck, jaws, and tongue is not uncommon. The temporal artery may be inflamed, prominent, tender, and contain nodules. Ocular symptoms are common (photophobia, pain) and are often associated with retinal arteritis. Systemic symptoms are not unusual (fever, asthenia, cachexia, muscle and bone pains). The clinical course may often be chronic, and there is a significant risk of blindness. The disease may also regress, especially after steroid treatment. The etiology of the disease is unknown.

TAKAYASU'S ARTERITIS

Takayasu's arteritis is characterized by segmental lesions (arteritis) of the aorta and its branches, along with granulomas and diffuse inflammation (lymphocytic and plasma cell infiltrates). Necrosis is often prominent in the media and leads to thrombosis, which is the cause of several clinical manifestations, including absent pulses with unobtainable blood pressure in the upper limbs, limping, alopecia, syncope, seizures, and mental confusion. The disease is rapidly fatal because of cardiac failure, coronary insufficiency, or cerebrovascular accidents. Immunologic abnormalities occur frequently and include increased Ig levels (IgG, IgA, IgM). Antiaortic antibodies have been found in some series (Japanese patients). The presence of antinuclear antibodies and, in some cases, RF also suggests immunologic mechanisms.

# POLYMYOSITIS AND DERMATOMYOSITIS

## Clinical Picture

Polymyositis and dermatomyositis are myopathies that, like all diseases classified by these names, feature muscle weakness. The definition of polymyositis is unsatisfactory: some authors use the word polymyositis to describe all myopathies in aged subjects, while others, like Denny Brown, reserve its use for cases associated with inflammatory lesions as opposed to necrotizing myopathies (with or without myoglobinuria), such as progressive chronic vacuolar myopathy or progressive degenerative granular myopathy. Others prefer the use of a purely clinical definition: Pearson distinguishes five types that are not necessarily related to each other.

*Type I: Idiopathic polymyositis.* Type I is the most common form, affecting primarily 30–50-year old women. Polymyositis is often insidious in onset, and typical skin lesions, Raynaud's syndrome, and arthritis may be found in association.

*Type II: Idiopathic dermatomyositis.* A cutaneous erythematous rash appears on the face, particularly on paraorbital, neck, and shoulder areas. The rash is occasionally widespread. The cutaneous lesions are associated with extreme muscular weakness and myalgia. Relatively benign arthritis is often also observed. Women are more usually affected, between 20 and 70 years of age. The evolution is either acute or subacute.

*Type III: Dermatomyositis (or polymyositis) associated with malignant tumor.* This form is seen in men 40 years or older and clinically resembles type I or II in association with a malignant tumor.

*Type IV: Childhood polymyositis-dermatomyositis.* This type occurs most often as a chronic disease and more rarely is acute. The predominant clinical findings, in addition to polymyositis (type I), include contractures, skin ulcerations, and calcifications in affected muscles. Histologically, vasculitis is present, featuring ischemic necrosis of vessels.

*Type V: Intermittent acute myositis.* This type is acute and rapidly progressive. Myoglobinuria is often present, and differentiation from sporadic myoglobinuria may be difficult. Type V shows repeated exacerbations, which are more frequent than in myoglobulinuria; myolysis is not provoked by vigorous exercise but, instead, probably by viral infections.

*Type VI: Sjögren's syndrome with polymyositis.* Muscles show progressive infiltration by plasma cells and lymphocytes. The typical symptoms of Sjögren's syndrome plus muscle weakness suggest the diagnosis.

In summing up, the protean nature of polymyositis manifestations is evident. The common denominator is muscular weakness, sometimes associated with dysphagia (recognized by esophageal hypotonia by radiography) or a reduction in vital capacity.

Myalgia is common but not constant. Laboratory help establish the diagnosis. An increase in serum levels of certain muscle-produced enzymes, including serum oxaloacetic transaminase (SGOT) and aldolase, is often observed during acute phases. Electromyography reveals abnormal electric potentials, which are not absolutely specific. If performed in these muscles, muscle biopsy (which may be guided by electromyography) in clinically asymptomatic forms reveals degenerative lesions (focal or diffuse), vacuolization of muscle fibers, associated necrosis, fibrosis, and regeneration. There may be lymphocytic and plasma cell infiltrates. One also finds increase in serum Ig level in about 50% of cases, a positive Rose-Waaler reaction or latex test in more than one-third of cases, and occasionally antinuclear factors.

Guided by repeated serum measurements of enzymes, the treatment essentially consists of use of corticosteroids, avoiding those products particularly toxic to muscles like dexamethasone and triamcinolone. The best responses are obtained in types I and II.

### Etiology

An immunologic origin of polymyositis is suspected by indirect evidence, such as the presence of lymphocytes and plasma cells in the muscles, hypergammaglobulinemia, RF and antinuclear antibodies. The presence of Ig in muscle lesions has not been well established. The search for infectious agents has not been conclusive, except for, perhaps, the finding in a few cases of tubular structures in the muscles that resemble certain myxoviruses. Drug allergy has been incriminated in some cases (sulfonamides and penicillin). The association of polymyositis with malignant tumors does not have a satisfactory explanation. The myopathy might be secondary to a toxic product or might result from hypersensitivity to antigens common to muscles and tumor. The latter hypothesis is supported by a few examples of autosensitization: in patients with dermatomyositis and breast cancer, an immediate cutaneous reaction may develop after intradermal inoculation of tumor extracts, and the same reaction may be transmitted by the patient's serum. The presence of antimyosin autoantibodies was reported by Caspary in about half of a series of 25 patients; however, numerous control sera were also positive. There are usually no antistriated muscle antibodies detected.

The best arguments in favor of the immunologic origin of polymyositis are suggested by experimental data: injection of rabbit muscle extracts in the presence of Freund's complete adjuvant produces a myopathy in guinea pigs very similar to polymyositis. The guinea pigs develop a delayed hypersensitivity response to muscle tissue, and the disease can be transferred by cell injections. Lymph node cells of these animals may be lymphocytotoxic toward muscle tissue in vitro. Myositis is also observed after injecting xenogeneic thymus extracts into guinea pigs (see p. 928), and the disease occurs spontaneously in a small South African rodent simultaneously with thymoma and elevated antimuscle antibody titers. It is, nonetheless, difficult to be certain that an immunologic mechanism is the cause of polymyositis, and whether IC or antimuscle autoantibodies are involved.

## SCLERODERMA

Scleroderma (systemic sclerosis) is a generalized disease of the connective tissue characterized by inflammatory, fibrous, and degenerative alterations of the skin (hence scleroderma) that also affect the synovium, kidneys, heart, lungs, and digestive tract. It is often rapidly fatal, with death due to recurrent complications, myocardial infarctions, or renal failure.

### Clinical Picture

The disease begins between 30 and 50 years of age, particularly in women. Cutaneous lesions are nearly always present, on the hands, face, neck, thorax, abdomen, and back, but lower limbs are usually not involved. Fingers may be shiny, swollen, and stiff; the skin is thickened, dark, and fixed to subcutaneous tissue. The lesions are complicated by contractures, ulcerations, and infections. Skin biopsy reveals increased collagen deposition, atrophied epidermis, and arteriolar hyalinization (immunofluorescence is usually negative), Raynaud's syndrome is present in more than 90% of cases. Articular localization is similar to that of rheumatoid arthritis, both clinically and histologically. Synovial biopsy reveals lymphocytic and plasma cell infiltrates. Muscle lesions are similar to those in polymyositis but less marked, and there is no elevation in serum muscle enzymes. Esophageal lesions are very common. Symptoms of the latter vary from simple dysphagia to major involvement that causes severe cachexia. Pulmonary fibrosis is the cause of dyspnea. Chronic respiratory insufficiency may develop with diminished transcapillary diffusion (which relates to thickening of alveolar basement membranes). Heart lesions may cause pulmonary arterial hypertension, with chronic cor pulmonale, left ventricular insufficiency, arhythmias, and pericarditis. Intestinal involvement is frequent, causing impaired motility and often symptomatic malabsorption. Renal localization is common, with a severe associated arterial hypertension, proteinuria, and rapidly progressive renal failure. Histologically, the kidney shows fibrinoid necrosis, along with intimal (intralobular) arterial hyperplasia. Ig and C3 deposits may be present in these arterioles. There may also be liver and neurologic lesions (polyneuritis or lesions of the central nervous system). The disease may progress rapidly with a poor prognosis; long survivals have also been observed. The response to steroids is disappointing. Numerous other treatments (alkylating agents, sodium versenate, potassium *p*-aminobenzoate, penicillamine, aminocaproic acid) have not produced convincing remissions.

### Etiology

Scleroderma displays a characteristic fibrosis associated with hyperproduction of collagen tissue, but collagen is not qualitatively abnormal, at least in regard to its amino acid composition and physicochemical properties. Increased hydroxyprolinuria occurs in severe cases, as does increased local synthesis of mucopolysaccharides, but the etiologic significance of these manifestations is unknown. An immunologic basis for scleroderma has been suggested because of the frequent association of the disease with other presumptive immunologic disorders, including RA, Sjögren's syndrome, polymyositis, and SLE. In addition, cutaneous lymphocytic and plasma cell infiltrates are seen along with IgG and complement deposits (kidney). Hypergammaglobulinemia is observed in nearly half of the cases, and RF is also often noted; other findings are false-positive syphilis reactions and antinuclear antibodies (40–90%). The latter antibodies usually show a speckled aspect by immunofluorescence, occasionally homogeneous or diffuse patterns, and more rarely, but very suggestive, nucleolar pattern. Serum hemolytic complement is normal; however, there may be anticomplementary activity of the serum, mixed cryoglobulins, and circulating IC.

## BIBLIOGRAPHY

ANDRES G. A., SPIELE H., and McCLUSKEY R. T. Virus-like structures in systemic lupus erythematosus. *In* Progress in clinical immunology. Vol. 1. New York, 1972, Grune & Stratton, p. 23.

BACH J. F., BACH M. A., and TRON F. New conceptions of autoimmunity and of systemic lupus erythematosus. Adv. Nephrol. Vol. 6. Chicago, 1976, Yearbook, p. 5.

BACH J. F. Systemic lupus erythematosus (SLE). In: Nephrology (J. Hamburger J. Crosnier, and J. P. Grunfeld [eds.]). John Wiley & Sons, New York, 1979, 597.

BOHAN A. and PETER J. B. Polymyositis and dermatopolymyositis. New. Engl. J. Med., 1975, *292*, 344.

CLOT J. and SANY J. Immunological aspects of rheumatoid arthritis. Rheumatology. Basel, 1975, Karger, 369 p.

DUBOIS E. L. Lupus erythematosus, ed. 2. University S. California Press, 1974, 798 p.

ESTES D. and CHRISTIAN C. L. The natural history of systemic lupus erythematosus by prospective analysis. Medicine, 1971, *50*, 85.

FAUCI A. S., HAYNES B. F., and KATZ P. The spectrum of vasculitis. Clinical pathologic, immunologic and therapeutic considerations. Ann. Int. Med., 1978, 89, 660.

GLASS P. and SCHURR P. Auto-immunity and systemic lupus erythematosus. *In* N. Talal, Ed., Auto-immunity: genetic, immunologic, virologic and clinical aspects. New York, 1977, Academic Press, p. 531.

HALL C. L., COLVIN R. B., and MCCLUSKEY R. T. Human immune complex diseases. In: Mechanisms of immunoapthology (S. Cohen, P. A. Ward, and R. T. McCluskey [eds.]). John Wiley & Sons, New York, 1979, 203.

HUGHES G. R. V. and LACHMANN P. J. Systemic lupus erythematosus. *In* P. G. H. Gell, R. R. A. Coombs, and P. J. Lachmann, Eds., Clinical aspects of immunology. Oxford, 1975, Blackwell, p. 1117.

LAWLEY T. J. and FRANK M. M. Imune complexes and immune complex diseases. In: Clinical Immunology (C. W. Parker [ed.]). Saunders, Philadelphia, 1980, 143.

MESSNER R. P. Polymyositis. In: Clinical Immunology (D. W. Parker [ed.]). Saunders, Philadelphia, 1980, 677.

MIESCHER P. A. and MÜLLER-EBERHARD M. J. Textbook of immunopathology, ed. 2., section II. New York, 1976, Grune & Stratton, p. 369.

NYDEGGER U. E., KAZATCHKINE M. D., and LAMBERT P. H. Involvement of immune complexes in deseases. In: Immunology 80 (M. Fougereau and J. Dausset [eds.]). Acad. Press, New York, 1980, 1025.

PERPER R. J. (Ed.) Mechanisms of tissue injury with reference to rheumatoid arthritis. Ann. N.Y. Acad. Sci., 1975, *256*.

PHILLIPS P. E. The virus hypothesis in systemic lupus erythematosus. Ann. Intern. Med. 1975, *83*, 709.

RODNAN G. P. Progressive systemic sclerosis (scleroderma). In: Clinical Immunology (C. W. Parker [eds.]). Saunders, Philadelphia, 1980: 784.

SILVESTRI L. G. The immunological basis of connective tissue disorders. Proc. 5th Lepetit Colloquium. Amsterdam, 1975, North Holland.

THEOFILOPOULOS A. N. and DIXON F. T. The biology and detection of immune complexes. Adv. Immunol. 1979, 28, 89.

WEISMAN M. and ZVAIFLER N. Cryoglobulins in rheumatoid arthritis. *In* J. Clot and J. Sany, Eds., Immunological aspects of rheumatoid arthritis. Basel, 1975, Karger, p. 60.

WHALEY K. and BUCHANAN W. W. Sjogren's syndrome and associated diseases. In: Clinical Immunology (C. W. Parker [ed.]). Saunders, Philadelphia, 1980, 632.

WILLIAMS R. C. Immune complexes in clinical and experimental medicine. Harvard University Press, Cambridge, 1980, 565 p.

ZVAIFLER N. J. and GREENBERG P. D. Immunopathology of rheumatoid arthritis. In: Mechanisms of immunoapthology (S. Cohen, P. A. Ward, and R. T. McCluskey [eds.]). John Wiley & Sons, New York, 1979, 247.

ZVAIFLER N. J. The immunopathology of joint inflammation in rheumatoid arthritis. Adv. Immunol., 1973, *16*, 265.

ZVAIFLER N. J. Rheumatoid arthritis. *In* N. Talal, Ed., Auto-immunity: genetic, immunologic, virologic and clinical aspects. New York, 1977, Academic Press, p 569.

## ORIGINAL ARTICLES

AGNELLO V., KOFFLER D., EISENBERG J. W., WINCHESTER R. J., and KUNKEL H. G. Clq precipitins in the sera of patients with SLE and other hypocomplementaemic states: characterization of high and low molecular weight types. J. Exp. Med., 1971, *134*, 2280.

ANDREWS B. S., EISENBERG R. A., THEOFILOPOULOS A. V., ISUI S., WILSON C. B., MCCONAHEY P. J., MURPHY E. D., ROTH J. B., and DIXON F. J. Spontaneous murine lupus-like syndromes. Clinical and immunopathological manifestations in several strains. J. Exp. Med., 1978, *148*, 1198.

FRANK M. M., HAMBURGER M. I., LAWLEY T. J., KIMBERLY R. P., and PLOTZ P. H. Defective reticuloendothelial system Fc receptor function in systemic lupus erythematosus. New Engl. J. Med., 1979, 300, 518.

GOCKE D. J., MORGAN C., BOMBARDIERI S., LOCKSHIN M., and CHRISTIAN C. L. Association between polyarteritis and Australia antigen. Lancet, 1970, *ii*, 1149.

HILL G., HINGLAIS N., TRON F., and BACH J. F. Systemic lupus erythematosus: morphologic correlations with immunologic and clinical data at the time of biopsy. Am. J. Med., 1978, *64*, 61.

KOFFLER D., AGNELLO V., THOBURN R., and KUNKEL H. G. Systemic lupus erythematosus prototype of immune complex nephritis in man. J. Exp. Med., 1971, *174*, 169s.

PINCUS T., SCHUR P., ROSE J. A., DECKER J. L. and TALAL N. Measurement of serum DNA-binding activity in SLE. New Engl. J. Med., 1969, *281*, 701.

SAKANE T., STEINBERG A. D., and GREEN I. Studies of immune functions of patients with SLE: Complement dependent TgM anti T cells antibodies preferentially inactivate suppressor cells. J. Clin. Invest., 1979, 63, 945.

TORRIGIANI G., ROITT I. M., LLOYDS K. M., and CORBETT M. Elevated IgG antiglobulins in patients with seronegative rheumatoid arthritis. Lancet, 1970, *I*, 14.

## Chapter 29

# IMMUNOPATHOLOGY OF GLOMERULONEPHRITIS

**Jean-François Bach**

I.   INTRODUCTION
II.  EXPERIMENTAL MODELS
III. ANATOMOCLINICAL CLASSIFICATION OF HUMAN
     GLOMERULONEPHRITIS
IV.  MECHANISMS INVOLVED IN HUMAN
     GLOMERULONEPHRITIS
V.   THERAPEUTIC ASPECTS

## I. INTRODUCTION

Glomerular nephropathies are an exceptionally interesting topic for the immunologist. Glomerulonephritis (GN) provoked by antikidney antibodies, such as that of Goodpasture's syndrome, is one of the purest models of autoimmune diseases caused by antiorgan autoantibodies. Above all, most human GN are seemingly associated with the presence of immune complexes (IC; discussed in chap. 28), and therefore provide an ideal model for the study of IC-induced lesions. For these reasons, we will devote a large place to a detailed discussion of the immunologic aspects of human GN. There are important immunologic and even clinical analogies between experimental and human GN. This favorable situation, too rare in other fields of immunopathology, accounts for the important place given in this chapter to experimental GN models.

## II. EXPERIMENTAL MODELS

Glomerular lesions may be induced in numerous experimental models. All of them are not immunologic, for example, a nephrotic syndrome may be induced

The author thanks J. Berger for his critical appraisal of this chapter.

by certain toxic substances, such as mercury. However, we will discuss here only immunologically induced experimental GN, which are the best studied and closest to human GN. These experimental GN may be classified, as mentioned above, into two main groups according to the different mechanisms involved: GN due to antiglomerular basement membrane (anti-GBM) antibody and immune complex GN.

## EXPERIMENTAL GLOMERULONEPHRITIS INDUCED BY ANTI-GBM ANTIBODY

### *Glomerulonephritis Induced by Passive Injection of Nephrotoxic Antibodies*

In 1900, Lindemann was the first to describe a nephritis produced in the rabbit by injection of antikidney serum (serum of a guinea pig immunized by rabbit kidney extracts), but it was Masugi who, between 1929 and 1935, provided the best clinical and anatomopathologic description of this type of experimental nephritis.

DESCRIPTION

The severity of GN is strictly dependent on the amount of serum injected. At high and medium doses, GN occurs within 5–8 days, with evidence of proteinuria, nephrotic syndrome, and renal failure, linked to the direct action of antikidney antibodies on glomeruli. At low doses, there is no GN or a mild form due to the immune reaction of the organism to the heterologous proteins contained in the injected serum which, independently of its anti-GBM nature, leads to the formation of IC. In fact, the disease develops in two phases, a heterologous phase linked to the action of anti-GBM antibodies and an autologous one linked to IC formation. The autologous reaction actually corresponds to IC deposits, as demonstrated by the presence of autologous Ig in the glomeruli (by immunofluorescence).

The autologous phase starts on the seventh day and significantly modifies the lesions and symptoms of the heterologous phase observed at high and intermediate doses. This autologous reaction is responsible for GN chronicity, because, when the autologous phase is absent, clinical signs and anatomic lesions rapidly attenuate and then disappear. It is interesting to note, for comprehension of Goodpasture's syndrome observed in clinical practice, that the chief extrarenal manifestations of nephrotoxic antibody nephritis are pulmonary.

Glomerular lesions are fairly stereotyped during the heterologous phase. On light microscopy, the basement membrane is thickened by endomembranous deposits, associated with moderate proliferation. In addition, glomeruli are infiltrated by numerous polymorphs. On electron microscopy, one finds irregular endomembranous deposits and polymorphs, whose contact with endothelial cells and GBM may be distinguished. Immunofluorescence permits the precise anatomic localization of nephrotoxic antibodies in glomeruli: the anti-GBM antibody localizes exclusively on GBM. It is essential to note that deposits are endomembranous and linear, that is, continuous.

MECHANISMS

The immunologic mechanisms of nephrotoxic antibody-induced GN have been well delineated. Antikidney antibodies deposit in the glomeruli within 15 min after injection of nephrotoxic serum. Obstruction of the renal artery for 25 min protects the corresponding kidney from GN. Low-affinity circulating anti-GBM antibodies remain, however, in the circulation after this 25-min period. Interestingly, when one transplants a kidney from a rat with Masugi's GN to a normal animal, the transplanted kidney, rapidly loses its deposits, which indicates that the antibodies not localized in the kidney play a role in the persistence of glomerular deposits. Complement binds to anti-GBM antibodies deposited in the kidney (except if the nephrotoxic serum has been obtained in the duck, because avian antibodies do not bind mammalian complement). The level of serum complement decreases rapidly after injection of nephrotoxic serum, and complement is found in the glomerular deposits by use of immunofluorescence with anti-C3 and anti-C4 sera. Complement plays a crucial role in GN onset, because pepsin or papain fragments of anti-GBM sera, which keep their specific antibody sites but lose the ability to fix complement, do not induce any true GN, although their fixation on GBM has been proven. At best, one may observe at high doses transient proteinuria for 2 or 3 days, perhaps explained by an incomplete action of proteolytic enzymes. The role of complement is confirmed by the absence of GN in animals in which complement activity has been diminished prior to antikidney serum injection (for example, by injection of anticomplement antibodies, heat-aggregated γ-globulin, antigen-antibody soluble complexes, or zymosan particles). Decomplementation is, however, incomplete, which probably explains why its effect may be overcome by increasing nephrotoxic serum doses. In addition, regardless of the dose of serum injected, decomplementation does not suppress the autologous phase.

It has been noted that polymorphs accumulate in the glomeruli in the hours following injection of antikidney serum, more so with higher doses. This accumulation of polymorphs is probably linked to release of C3a and C5a and fixation of C5, C6, and C7 complement factors, known to possess chemotactic activity for polymorphs. The precise mode of action of polymorphs has not been determined, but it is possible that, as in the Arthus reaction, they release hydrolytic enzymes, a hypothesis supported by the absence of granules in polymorphs that infiltrate the glomeruli. If complement plays a fundamental role in the genesis of Masugi's GN by locally attracting polymorphs, one should note, however, that antikidney sera produced in the duck provoke a GN without binding mammalian complement. This indicates that in certain conditions GN may occur without complement intervention or polymorph infiltration. Recent data suggest that complement mainly acts in cases where the antibodies are not available in optimal quantities. Proteinuria observed in the presence of massive concentrations of anti-GBM antibodies is not increased by the action of complement.

The immunologic mechanisms of the autologus phase are those of IC-induced GN described below. The autologous phase may be suppressed by induction of tolerance toward proteins of the species that provides the antikidney serum.

anti-BSA antibody production). The maximal intensity of glomerular lesions is observed on the 12th or 13th day, when BSA becomes practically undetectable in the serum. For secondary immunization, GN begins earlier, on about the fifth day. In both cases, GN onset coincides with a drop in complement levels During this period, one may detect high amounts of circulating IC by using radiolabeled BSA as the antigen and precipitating it with immunoglobulins by ammonium sulfate at concentrations that do not precipitate free uncomplexed BSA.

The size of IC may be evaluated by ultracentrifugation on sucrose gradients. IC generally have a molecular weight between 300,000 and 500,000 daltons, which suggests an $Ag_2Ab$ structure (two antigen molecules per antibody molecule) or $Ag_2Ab_2$ or $Ag_3Ab_2$. More rarely, one may also observe larger IC that contain IgM. IC are also found in glomeruli by immunofluorescence, as assessed by the presence of Ig, BSA, and complement in the form of granular deposits. These weak and transient deposits are found on the 10th day, when IC are found in the circulation and before the development of glomerular lesions.

On light microscopy, these glomerular lesions appear as a diffuse cellular proliferation (involving all glomeruli) of endothelial and mensangial cells, associated with hypertrophy of endothelial and epithelial cells. Numerous polymorphs are less consistently seen. GN is generally reversible within 2–3 weeks; the reversal of disease process is first revealed by disappearance of the inflammatory infiltrate; the mesangial hypercellularity often disappearing last. The reversible nature of GN is probably linked to the rapid disappearance of IC in the serum. One may note that the disappearance of glomerular lesions coincides, on light microscopy, with that of deposits seen by immunofluorescence.

### BSA CHRONIC SERUM SICKNESS

The repeated (daily, for example) injection of low doses of protein antigens may induce a chronic GN, whereas repeated high-dose administration causes the appearance of vascular lesions. According to experimental protocols, but also unexpectedly according to individual animals, three types of situations may be observed. Some animals do not form antibodies and do not develop GN. Others form large amounts of antibodies and develop reversible GN, similar to that of acute serum sickness at the immune phase of antigen elimination. These animals often die from anaphylactic shock when antigen is reinjected. The third situation is represented by animals that form low amounts of antibodies. These animals are the only ones to develop chronic GN, probably because they are the only ones to possess antibody concentrations appropriate for the formation, with the repeatedly injected antigen, of IC in sufficient amounts and of sufficient duration to produce the lesions. GN lesions consist of hypertrophy and proliferation of mesangial cells, possibly associated with inflammation of the juxtamesangial segment of the glomerulus.

The use of radiolabeled BSA permits, as in acute serum sickness, the evaluation of the size of complexes (here all are formed by IgG). In animals that form low amounts of antibodies (and develop chronic GN), one finds IC of 500,000–700,000 daltons between 5 and 24 hr after antigen administration.

These complexes correspond to structures that vary in size from $Ag_3Ab_2$ to $Ag_4Ab_3$. In animals that produce moderate amounts of antibodies, antigenic elimination is more rapid, and IC are of larger size (from 500,000 to several million daltons, with an average size of about $10^6$ daltons). When animals produce very large amounts of antibodies, the injected antigen is eliminated within a few minutes, and IC are few and of large size ($>10^6$ daltons).

The nature of the glomerular lesions varies with the rate of antibody production. In animals that produce little antibody, with small-sized complexes, one may note thickening of GBM (membranous GN aspect), often with intense proteinuria but no renal failure, or diffuse cellular proliferation, occasionally accompanied by local necrosis and frequently associated with renal failure. Membranous GN are especially observed when injecting low antigen doses, whereas proliferative GN are observed when injecting high doses. These differences may probably be explained by the amount of size of IC produced. Immunofluorescence confirms the presence of granular deposits of antigen Ig, and complement in the glomeruli. Coalescence of deposits may produce the chracteristic picture of "humps." Electron microscopy shows the IC deposits in more detail, revealing their localization on the external part of the basement membrane, associated with proliferation of endothelial cells and fusion of the foot of epithelial cell podocytic processes. Membranous GN is reversible if antigen injections are discontinued. Antigen disappears first (probably masked by antibody and complement); Ig deposits then disappear, before those of complement, which may persist for several months. The half-life of IC deposits is about 5 days (versus 10 days in acute serum sickness). Administration of high doses of antigen shortens this half-life, which, in theory, could have a therapeutic application. When intermediate amounts of antibodies are produced, lesions are generally moderate (proliferation and hypertrophy of mesangial cells) and are not accompained by clinical signs (no proteinuria). Immunofluorescence, then, shows essentially mesangial deposits in which the antigen is not demonstrable but could again be masked within IC by excess antibody.

### INTERPRETATION

The differences in GN incidence according to immunization protocol suggest that IC size and quantity influence the onset and pattern of GN. To summarize, small size and relatively soluble complexes observed in cases of weak antibody production give membranous GN in the presence of low antigen concentrations and proliferative GN in the presence of higher antigen concentrations. Complexes of larger size, which are more transient, are found in animals that produce intermediate amounts of antibodies and provoke mild mesangial lesions. Very transient complexes of large size observed in situations where large amounts of antibodies are produced do not cause GN.

In other words, small-sized soluble complexes (Germuth's class I, $< 10^6$ daltons) give rise to diffuse membranous GN, sometimes associated with cellular proliferation when IC are abundant; intermediate-sized complexes (class II, $\sim 10^6$ daltons) produce focal mesangial lesions. Large-sized complexes (class III) are rarely localized in glomeruli. We should mention here that small-sized complexes are responsible for acute serum sickness disease. Note also that to that of collagen, and epithelial cells (or podocytes), which surround the GBM externally.

### Principal Pathologic Aspects

On light microscopy, several characteristic glomerular lesions may be distinguished. Nearly all cases of GN belong to one of these categories, with a few exceptions, which combine several lesions. The principal basic lesions are the following.

#### DEPOSITS

Deposits may be extramembranous along the GBM externally, beneath the epithelial cells. When deposits coalesce along a GBM segment, they may appear as a hump. They may also be endomembranous, mesangial, or occur within the GBM itself.

#### PROLIFERATION

Glomerular cell proliferation is most often diffuse and involves all glomeruli. It may be purely endocapillary, affecting both mesangial and endothelial cells, endo- and extracapillary, or endocapillary associated with endomembranous fibrinoid desposits (membranoproliferative or mesangiocapillary proliferative GN). In certain cases, one may observe dense deposits inside the GBM and tubular basement membranes, which are better seen by electron microscopy. Occasionally, one discerns membranoproliferative GN type II from type I in which no dense deposits are seen.

#### FOCAL AND SEGMENTAL LESIONS

These lesions involve only a portion of some glomeruli (proliferation, deposits, or necrosis).

#### SEGMENTAL AND FOCAL HYALINIZATION

In these lesions, capillaries are thickened irregularly by a hyalinlike substance.

## IMMUNOFLUORESCENCE (Figs. 29.1 and 29.2)

The use of immunofluorescence for the study of renal biopsies has been the source of important progress in the classification of human GN. The technique generally consists of direct immunofluorescence with fluorescein-labeled sera directed against various Ig classes, complement components, or other proteins, such as fibrin.

## OTHER INVESTIGATIONS

New immunologic techniques, both humoral and cellular, have recently opened a very promising field of investigation. Study of the complement system has

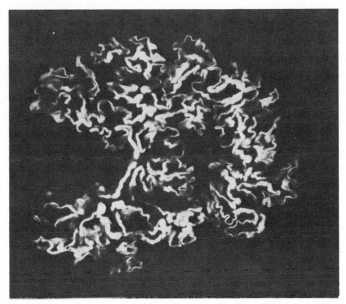

**Fig. 29.1** Linear glomerular IgG deposits seen by immunofluorescence. (From J Berger.)

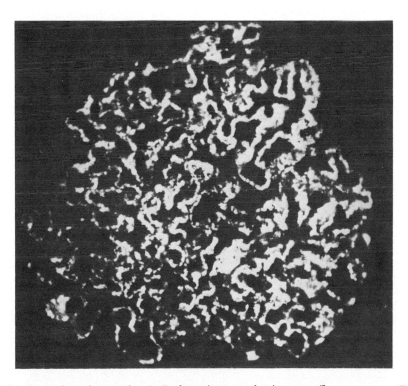

**Fig. 29.2** Granular glomerular IgG deposits seen by immunofluorescence. (From J. Berger.)

**Table 29.1  Classification of Human Glomerular Diseases**

| Usual designation | Pathologic aspects | Immuno-fluorescence | Complement | Evolution | Comments |
|---|---|---|---|---|---|
| Acute GN | Endocapillary proliferation. Extramembranous "hump" deposits | IgG, C3 (granular) | Low C3 | Reversibility | Frequency of streptococcal etiology |
| Membranous GN | Extramembranous deposits | IgG along external side of GBM (granular). C3 in weak amounts | Normal | Chronic course GN but favorable course in 1–3 years in many cases | |
| Membranoproliferative (or mesangiocapillary) GN | Endomembranous deposits (sometimes dense deposits). Endothelial and mesangial proliferation. Sometimes lobular aspects | IgG, C1q, and C3 or C3 alone in mesangium and in deposits | C3 more or less decreased. Normal C4 | Chronic GN. Progressive and irreversible aggravation | Presence of nephritic factor in cases with hypocomplementemia |
| Rapidly progressive GN | Endo- and extracapillary proliferation or isolated extracapillary proliferation | Fibrin without Ig or IgG, C1q, C3, and fibrin | Variable | Rapid aggravation | Reversibility in some cases associating endo- and extracapillary proliferation |
| GN with linear deposits | Proliferative segmental endo and/or extracapillary GN | Linear deposits of IgG and C3 along internal side of GBM | Normal | Variable course but often toward irreversible aggravation | Anti-GBM antibodies in serum. Frequency of pulmonary manifestations (Goodpasture's syndrome) |

| Disease | Histology | Immunofluorescence deposits | Complement | Clinical course / prognosis | Serology / origin |
|---|---|---|---|---|---|
| GN with IgA-IgG deposits (Berger's disease) | Normal kidney or segmental and focal GN | IgA, IgG, and C3 deposits in the mesangium of all glomeruli | Normal | Most often benign but sometimes possible evolution toward renal failure | Augmentation of serum IgA |
| Henoch-Schönlein purpura | Segmental and focal GN | IgA, IgG, and fibrin deposits | Normal | Chronic GN. Frequent degradation | |
| SLE GN | Normal kidney. Extra-membranous GN. Focal GN. Membrano-proliferative GN | Endo and/or extra-membranous deposits of IgG, IgA, C1q, and C3 | Low C1q, C3, and C4 | Variable. Unfavorable for membranoproliferative GN | Anti-native DNA antibodies in the serum |
| Nephrotic syndrome with minimal glomerular changes | Normal kidney | Negative | Normal | Corticosteroid-sensitive nephrotic syndrome | Uncertain immunologic origin |
| Nephrotic syndrome with focal sclerosing GN | Segmental and focal hyalinosis | Negative (or minimal IgG, IgM, and C3 in areas of sclerosis) | Normal | Often corticosteroid-resistant nephrotic syndrome. Frequent progression toward renal failure | Uncertain immunologic origin |
| Amyloidosis | Deposits of amyloid substance | | Normal | Progressive degradation | |

been particularly rewarding in numerous forms of GN, especially in acute GN, membranoproliferative GN, and SLE (see chap. 8).

## ANATOMOIMMUNOCLINICAL CORRELATIONS

Before discussing immunologic mechanisms of human GN, it is useful to summarize the main correlations observed among the four approaches just mentioned. The existence and consistency of correlations are by themselves a very striking argument in favor of the diversity of human GN and of the autonomy of the clinical forms that have been distinguished (Table 29.1).

# IV.  MECHANISMS INVOLVED IN HUMAN GLOMERULONEPHRITIS

We have previously seen that experimental immunologic GN can be classified into two categories; anti-GBM antibody-induced GN and IC-induced GN. Clearly, one may ask whether any of human GN can be included in one of these two categories. The investigations just mentioned provide a promising approach (but not yet definitive). Arguments can be collected that relate, quite plausibly, certain forms of GN to one or the other mechanism mentioned above, without however, specifying in these special cases the etiology of the disease.

## ANTI-GBM GLOMERULONEPHRITIS

The experimental nephrotoxicity of heterologous anti-GBM antibodies and the induction of GN by autoimmunization to kidney extracts suggest that anti-GBM autoantibodies, the existence of which has been demonstrated in some patients with GN, could be the origin of certain forms of human GN. We will review the immunologic tests that demonstrate the existence of sensitization to GBM in certain cases of human GN and will then dicuss the role of such anti-GBM immunity in the pathogenesis of certain GN.

### Methods for Studying Anti-GBM Immunity

Numerous methods have been utilized to study anti-GBM immunity in man. The antigens used have varied widely according to type, from one worker to another. Because of the differences in antigens, comparisons of results are difficult, especially with respect to degree of solubility and method of GBM fractionation. Studies on purified GBM are a priori more reliable than those on total kidney extracts. The techniques employed for detection of anti-GBM immunity may be grouped into three categories: serum antibodies, immunofluorescence, and cell-mediated immunity.

### DIRECT DETECTION OF SERUM ANTI-GBM ANTIBODIES

Several techniques have been used to detect anti-GBM antibodies in serum. Some of these techniques are sensitive but do not permit analysis of antigenic determinants, such as passive hemagglutination or agglutination of GBM-coated latex particles or collodion. Conversely, other methods, such as immunoprecipitation, are less sensitive but allow analytic study. Passive hemagglutination has been employed for study of experimental and human GN. In animals, hemagglutination titers do not correlate with the nephrotoxic activity of heterologous sera. However, it has been demonstrated in man that while the titer is effectively of no diagnostic value (significant titers are observed in membranoproliferative GN or in cases of cortical necrosis), the avidity of antibodies for GBM, as measured by inhibition of hemagglutination, enables the detection of sera whose anti-GBM antibody activity could be responsible for GN; by this method, only cases with linear Ig deposits are positive. The recent application in several laboratories of the Farr test to purified $^{125}$I-labeled GBM represents significant progress.

### IMMUNOFLUORESCENCE

Immunofluorescence may be performed directly on kidneys or after transfer of the patient's serum previously labeled with fluorescein on a normal kidney section. Deposits observed in experimental GN provoked by nephrotoxic serum injection, or in Goodpasture's syndrome, are characterized by the presence of IgG and C3 and especially by a linear distribution along the GBM.

Defining linearity is not always easy. Some extramembranous IC deposits may, indeed, be incorrectly considered linear when they are small, numerous, and almost contiguous. In uncertain cases, transfer of the patient's serum onto a normal kidney section often helps, although the patterns observed are sometimes difficult to interpret because deposits are of weak intensity. Only high-affinity anti-GBM antibodies will bind during transfer, whereas complexes or anti-GBM antibodies of low affinity will not bind. When working with nephrectomy or autopsy material, it is often possible to elute the antibodies found in deposits in an acid medium (pH 3.2) after kidney homogenization. One should note, finally, that immunofluorescence only demonstrates, in principle, antibodies directed against antigenic determinants accessible to circulating antibodies, whereas the serologic reactions mentioned above, which employ kidney extracts, may give positive reactions with "hidden" antigens, which are protected in vivo from the action of antibodies.

### STUDY OF CELL-MEDIATED IMMUNITY

Leukocyte migration inhibition has recently been applied to human GN. The two-phase technique consists of studying inhibition of guinea pig macrophage migration in the presence of a supernatant of the patient's lymphocyte culture incubated with the antigen (GBM or streptococcal antigens); the one-phase technique involves direct incubation of peripheral leukocytes with antigen in a capillary tube. The immunologic significance of the leukocyte migration inhibition test is still controversial in man (see p. 394), especially for the one-phase technique, but some data suggest, however, that the sensitization detected is probably effectively related to delayed hypersensitivity.

### Goodpasture's Syndrome

In 1919, Goodpasture described the association of GN and hemorrhagic lung disease. Numerous cases have been reported since, usually in young men, with no obvious hereditary factor, except in a few isolated cases.

The lung disease is generally the first clinical event, but it may also occur after renal disease. The clinical picture is characterized by hemoptysis, which is often repetitive. X-ray examination reveals bilateral infiltrates with a mottled or finely reticular appearance, localized most often in the central pulmonary fields. These x-ray aspects generally rapidly regress after cessation of hemoptysis. Renal disease is manifest in the form of renal failure, often rapidly progressing to irreversible damage. Proteinuria and hematuria are associated with renal failure but there is no arterial hypertension in the majority of cases. Renal biopsy reveals necrotic GN, sometimes diffuse but often segmental or focal. The earliest manifestation is focal fibrinoid necrosis. Endo- and extra-capillary proliferation (with crescents) occurs concomitantly when lesions become diffuse. Lastly, and importantly for differential diagnosis, there is usually no vascular lesion.

The tests described above for the study of anti-GBM immunity are all positive. Immunodiffusion may show the presence of anti-GBM antibodies; passive hemagglutination inhibition by soluble GBM shows that these antibodies are of high affinity. The leukocyte migration inhibition test is regularly positive, by either the one-phase or the two-phase technique. Immunofluorescence detects in all cases linear IgG deposits along the inside of the GBM and, more inconsistently, $\beta_1$C-globulin. Complement deposits are usually linear, like those of IgG, but sometimes also granular. It is possible to transfer the linear IgG deposits onto a normal kidney section. This transfer assesses the presence in the serum of anti-GBM circulating antibodies of high affinity. The fixation occurs in vitro, both on glomerular and on tubular basement membranes, whereas the original section shows linear deposits only on GBM and much more rarely on tubular basement membranes (antibodies bind in vivo to GBM before reaching tubular basement membranes). In addition, it is possible to eluate antibodies present in deposits. The antibodies eluted have the same properties as do those found in serum but represent a higher percentage of IgG (1.5 versus 0.05%). In some cases, antibodies are only found in the eluate, their concentration being too weak to be detected in the serum.

The spontaneous outcome of Goodpasture's syndrome is very often unfavorable. Renal failure progresses within a few weeks, while hemoptysis persists. Numerous cases of stabilization or even cure have, however, been reported. Renal transplantation and chronic hemodialysis may be applied successfully, with, however, a risk of recurrence when transplantation is employed. Chemotherapy has on the whole proven disappointing.

We thus may summarize the main elements of Goodpasture's syndrome:

association of hemoptoic pneumopathy, without a detectable cause, and rapidly progressive renal failure; segmental and focal necrotic GN; presence of high-affinity anti-GBM antibodies in the serum; and linear IgG deposits visible by immunofluorescence and transferable to normal kidney sections. By this definition, Goodpasture's syndrome appears to be a very rare if not exceptional entity (1–5% of GN according to statics).

The pathogenesis of Goodpasture's syndrome must be envisaged in relation to the immunologic data mentioned above. The presence of anti-GBM antibodies in serum and glomeruli (studied after elution) and the Ig and linear complement deposits on the GBM suggest convincingly that anti-GBM antibodies are responsible for the GN, by analogy with Masugi's experimental GN. Antigenic determinants shared by lungs and GBM (demonstrated by antilung antibody fixation in the kidney and by induction of pulmonary lesions after antikidney autoimmunization and of glomerular lesions after antilung autoimmunization) explain the double pulmonary and renal disease. This hypothesis is corroborated by the possibility of obtaining linear deposits on GBM after injection of a single dose of serum from patients with Goodpasture's syndrome in the monkey. Conversely, nonrecurrence of the disease after transplantation, observed on several occasions, opposes this hypothesis. The starting point of the disease (pulmonary or renal) is not determined. The usual initial occurrence of pulmonary lesions might indicate that pulmonary antigens induce autoimmunity, but we have seen that renal lesions might also be observed first. Perhaps the responsible autoantigens are neither renal nor pulmonary but are microbial, with determinants shared with basal membranes. Note that, contrary to the

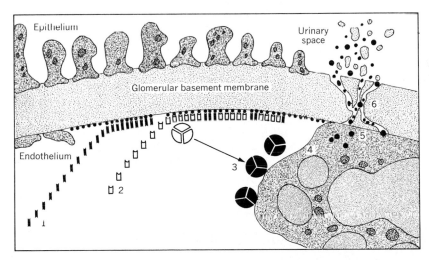

**Fig. 29.3** Schematic representation of lesions induced by antiglomerular basement membrane (anti-GBM) antibodies. (1) Anti-GBM antibody binds to GBM; (2) complement (C3) attaches to GBM receptors for C3 and activates C5, C6, and C7; (3) C567 generates a chemotactic factor that attracts polymorphs; (4) polymorphs attach to GBM; (5) polymorphs release proteolytic enzymes; (6) enzymes injure GBM, which becomes permeable to proteins. (From F. J. Dixon. *In* R. A. Good and D. W. Fisher, Eds., Immunobiology, ed. 5. Stamford, Conn., 1973, Sinauer, p. 168.)

suggestions of certain authors, bilateral nephrectomy does not seem to produce a reduction in the level of anti-GBM antibodies.

### Other Glomerulonephritides With Anti-GBM Immunity

Circulating antikidney antibodies, as detected by passive hemagglutination, agglutination of latex particles or collodion, immunodiffusion, and especially by the Farr test and immunofluorescence (linear Ig deposits along the GBM), have been demonstrated in certain cases of GN not clinically linked to Goodpasture's syndrome; there are cases with or without linear Ig deposits on the GBM.

#### CASES WITH LINEAR DEPOSITS

In these cases, antibodies detected in serum or after kidney elution show little differences from those found in Goodpasture's syndrome. It is usually a rapidly progressive GN. The pattern of deposits by immunofluorescence is identical, and practically the only difference from Goodpasture's syndrome is the absence of lung disease. Whatever the cause of such a clinical difference, one may a priori equate these cases of GN with linear deposits with Goodpasture's syndrome on a clinical and immunopathologic basis.

#### CASES WITHOUT LINEAR DEPOSITS

GN cases without linear deposits, despite the presence of anti-GBM antibodies in the serum, are more complex. Passive hemagglutination with purified GBM is positive in some cases of severe proliferative GN without linear deposits. The leukocyte migration inhibition test is often positive in the presence of GBM but also in the presence of streptococcal membranes. The role of anti-GBM immunity in these GN without linear deposits is uncertain. The granular pattern of Ig deposits and the merely moderate affinity or specificity of circulating anti-GBM antibodies are not in favor of a direct action of these antibodies on glomeruli. It is, however, possible that anti-GBM antibodies intervene through complex deposits in glomeruli. These complexes would be composed of anti-GBM antibodies and GBM itself, or of an antigen that shares determinants with GBM, such as the streptococcal antigen. One may also mention the possible role of autoimmunization secondary to GBM release associated with GN lesions. This hypothesis cannot be excluded, but it would then be necessary to explain why only proliferative GN give positive results, while they do not necessarily correspond to the most severe glomerular lesions.

### Secondary Anti-GBM Autoimmunization

Low-affinity anti-GBM antibodies are found in patients with severe renal vascular lesions (cortical necrosis, periarteritis nodosa, thrombotic microangiopathy). These anti-GBM antibodies are probably linked to autoimmunization secondary to glomerular necrosis. A similar autoimmunization has been described against liver antigens in the course of hepatic necrosis in viral hepatitis and against heart antigens after myocardial necrosis following myocardial infarction.

# IMMUNE COMPLEX GLOMERULONEPHRITIS

It is often suggested, or implied, that all human GN may be explained by one or the other immunopathologic mechanisms described above in relation to experimental GN, namely, the nephrotoxic action of anti-GBM antibodies or of IC. The very low incidence of anti-GBM GN in man would imply, in that scheme, that the vast majority of human GN is linked to IC deposition. We shall see in the following pages that this IC intermediary is quite likely for numerous GN, but that it does not explain all cases that are not linked to anti-GBM antibodies. Some forms of GN could very well be due to other mechanisms or even to nonimmunologic causes. This is the case in particular of nephrotic syndromes with minimal glomerular changes or with focal and segmental hyalinization, for which there is no argument that indicates an immunologic origin. Arguments that implicate IC in the pathogenesis of certain human GN may be grouped under five headings: Ig and complement deposits in kidneys, serum protein abnormalities identical to those induced by IC, demonstration of antigen within glomerular deposits, recurrence of certain GN after transplantation, and analogies of human GN with experimental models.

### Ig and Complement Deposits

Ig and complement deposits are found (by immunofluorescence) in a large percentage of GN (Table 29.1). These deposits may be granular on the internal or external surface of GBM or diffuse in the mesangium. We have already seen GN with linear deposits due to anti-GBM antibodies, the significance of which is very different. The nature of deposits is quite variable (see Table 29.1) but in most cases involves IgG, IgM, IgA, and complement (C1q, C3, C4). Demonstration of IgE in lipoid nephrosis has not been confirmed.

### Detection of Circulating IC

Detection of low amounts of IC present in serum of GN subjects is difficult. Ultracentrifugation on sucrose gradients and gel chromatography, which isolate "complexed" Ig at an elution volume that corresponds to a molecular weight higher than that of native Ig, are generally insufficiently sensitive and of little clinical value. Other methods (described on p. 734) give positive results in certain clinical forms (SLE, acute GN, GN due to chronic septicemia, such as subacute bacterial endocarditis), in particular, the detection of cryoglobulins or tests of labeled C1q fixation. Mixed cryoglobulins have been observed in membranoproliferative GN in a few cases, but generally tests searching for IC are negative in membranoproliferative GN and in extramembranous or focal GN. In addition, even in positive cases, proof has not been obtained for the presence of antigen within IC, and the significance of IC detected by these techniques remains uncertain, as is the role of these IC in the pathogenesis of the disease.

### Antigen Demonstration

We have just seen the importance of demonstration of the antigen inside IC to assess the "complexed" nature of Ig within high-molecular-weight aggregates. The discovery of antigens responsible for chronic GN should permit the development of new approaches in etiologic research and might, in addition, improve the still very speculative therapeutic approach to chronic GN.

One must first recognize that the percentage of GN where a specific antigen may be incriminated is yet very limited (less than 5% for all GN cases). This percentage is even lower if strict criteria are used to assess the role of the antigen. However, because of the theoretical importance of these cases, we will briefly review them. Antigens that have been best documented are serum proteins and bacterial, parasitic, or viral antigens.

Serum sickness disease, observed in man after injection of vaccines or especially heterologous sera, is frequently associated with GN. Such quasiexperimental GN has all of the characteristics of experimental serum sickness GN, that is, an acute GN, with endocapillary proliferation and, more rarely, membranoproliferative GN if serum injections are repeated.

Among GN due to IC involving microbial antigens, one must first mention poststreptococcal acute GN. Epidemiologic data that incriminate streptococci are relatively solid statistically but less convincing in individual cases. The notion of recent streptococcal infection (such as tonsilitis) and increase in antistreptolysin titer is, in fact, questionable. Demonstration of streptococcal antigens in kidneys by use of labeled antistreptococcal sera has been reported, but this isolated observation is a matter of controversy. Perhaps such studies are performed too late, when the antigens is already coated with Ig and complement. Bacteria have also been incriminated during certain septicemic states, for

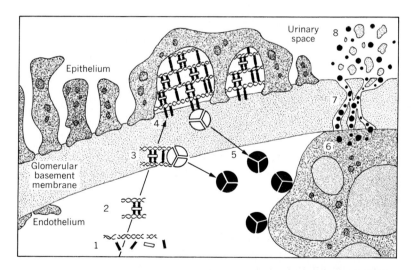

**Fig. 29.4** Schematic representation of glomerular lesions induced by soluble immune complexes of DNA and anti-DNA antibodies in extramembranous lupus glomerulonephritis. (1) Free DNA, anti-DNA antibody, and complement; (2) immune complex forms; (3) the complex crosses the GBM; (4) it is trapped on the epithelial side of the GBM; (5) complement releases a chemotactic factor; (6) polymorphs attach to GBM; (7) polymorphs release enzymes; (8) the injured GBM becomes permeable to proteins. (From F. J. Dixon. *in* R. A. Good and D. W. Fisher, Eds., Immunobiology ed. 5. Stamford, Conn., 1973, Sinauer, p. 170.)

example, in the course of staphylococcemia observed in hydrocephalic children bearing atrial-ventricular shunts. In one of these cases, staphylococcal antigens have been identified in glomerular deposits. A role for IC has also been suggested in subacute bacterial endocarditis and syphilis.

Parasitic nephropathies have been extensively studied. Malarial antigens have been demonstrated in the glomerular deposits of malaria patients with the nephrotic syndrome. These antigens were associated with anti-*Plasmodium* antibodies, as shown after kidney elution. It is possible that GN observed in certain cases of intestinal or urinary schistosomiasis are linked to the same mechanisms.

Viral antigens have also been the subject of numerous studies. The presence of Australia antigen in glomeruli has been noted in certain GN patients carrying the Australia antigen, but the specificity of such observations remains to be demonstrated. The most convincing data have been reported in SLE. Nuclear antigens, in particular, native and denatured DNA, and the corresponding antibodies may be eluted from the kidney. Even in these cases, however, the pathogenetic nature of IC in GN genesis has not been adequately proven. Other antigens have been discovered within Ig deposits in some GN cases. One may observe thyroglobulin in certain thyroiditis with GN, and renal tubular antigens in some cases of sickle-cell disease; reminiscent of Heymann's experimental GN (see p. 836).

### Glomerulonephritis Recurrence After Renal Transplantation: Problem of Rejection Glomerulonephritis

IC-induced GN often lead to renal failure, justifying renal transplantation. It is not rare that GN may then recur in the transplant. This recurrence is more frequent when the kidney is taken from a homozygous twin rather than from a genetically different donor, probably because in the latter case the immuno-suppressive treatment given to prevent rejection has a preventive therapeutic effect on GN recurrence.

The most remarkable fact about such a recurrence is the similarity of anatomoclinical findings between initial and recurrent diseases. A membrano-proliferative GN with dense deposits will recur in the form of dense deposits, and the same is true for lobular membranoproliferative GN or GN with IgG-IgA deposits. This similarity is a strong argument to assert that these diseases are, indeed, recurrent GN, because otherwise one could also propose in allograft recipients the possibility of "rejection GN." Such rejection GN is seen in chronic allogeneic disease after repeated injections of allogeneic cells. It is probably due to IC formed by transplantation antigens and antibodies. Rejection GN may be observed in certain patients whose initial nephropathy was not a GN but a chronic interstitial nephritis or congenital nephropathy. They are associated with mesangial proliferation and endomembranous deposits.

### Conclusions: Analogies With Experimental Models

All of the arguments discussed in the preceding pages indicate that numerous human GN are probably linked to IC deposits. Analogies are numerous with acute serum sickness for acute GN or with chronic serum sickness for membranous GN (light microscopy and immunofluorescence). However, numerous differences persist, and, except in the very rare cases mentioned above, the antigen is not found. In addition, the analogy with experimental models is much less striking in focal GN or in GN associated with dense deposits. In the latter case, notably in Berger's disease (mesangial deposits of IgG and IgA), the pathogenic role of large size IC formed in the presence of antibody excess is suggested by the mesangial localization of the deposits and by the short delay usually seen between infection and episodes of hematuria.

In fact, the precise mechanisms of formation of deposits and the action of IC remain to be determined. It is probable that in the majority of cases the deposits are derived from circulating IC. The roles of the IC uptake by the mesangium of mediators secreted by basophils (see p. 731), of complement and glomerular C3 receptors, or even of the intervention of complexes formed locally on an antigen 'planted' in the mesangium or fixed by GBM are difficult to delineate in any particular case.

## HYPOCOMPLEMENTEMIC GLOMERULONEPHRITIS

Hypocomplementemia is common in acute GN, either poststreptococcal or not, and in SLE. A very severe hypocomplementemia is also observed in certain membranoproliferative GN (about 30–40% of cases of membranoproliferative GN and still more frequently in GN with dense deposits). However, at variance with what is observed in SLE (in which the level of all complement factors is diminished, probably due to consumption by IC), only C3 and further factors (C5–C9) are decreased. C1, C2, and C4 levels remain normal. These data suggest that the alternative complement pathway may be activated, the more so since, by immunofluorescence, all patients have C3, and only a fraction of them have Ig, C1q and C1r. It is interesting here to recall that activation of the alternative pathway of complement may be obtained by nonimmunoglobulinic factors. The presence of a "nephritic factor" (C3NeF) has been described in the serum of some of these patients; C3NeF is not produced by the kidney, because it persists after nephrectomy. It is capable of activating C3 in vitro (in vitro, C3NeF inactivates the complementary activity of normal human serum). The CeNeF factor, which is an immunoglobulin (probably an immunoglobulin with autoantibody activity directed against C3b-Factor B complex), inactivates C3 in the presence of $Mg^{++}$ by stabilizing the C3 convertase of the alternating pathway (C3b, Bb). There is no proof, however, that these complement abnormalities are responsible for the GN. In fact, recurrence of GN with dense deposits is seen in transplanted patients irrelevant to the presence of C3NeF and decrease in C3 level. Although the reduction of C3 levels is predominantly due to hypercatabolism, it is usually associated with impaired synthesis. Membranoproliferative GN without major hypocomplementemia and without C3NeF factor are no different clinically from hypocomplementemic membranoproliferative GN.

Hypocomplementemia is almost always observed in dense deposit GN and it is only this particular type of GN (membranoproliferative, type III) that is

associated with the presence of C3NeF and, in rare cases, with partial lipodystrophy. Close pathogenetic links have been suggested between partial lipodystrophy and membranoproliferative GN. In fact, although the simultaneous
presence of C3NeF and lowered C3 levels are observed relatively frequently in
partial lipodystrophy, urinary signs (that is overt GN) are only seen in about
half the cases. In addition, it is known that the appearance of C3NeF is almost
certainly secondary to the GN and it is therefore improbable that it plays a
significant role in the pathogenesis of partial lipodystrophy. In addition to
membranoproliferative GN, it is not rare in acute or in certain chronic GN to
observe C3 deposits without C1q and C4 deposits, and even sometimes without
Ig. One may also imagine here intervention of the alternative pathway activation,
perhaps through IC, which may also activate it (see p. 261). This activation
could be maintained by C3b, which is a degradation product of C3 that activates,
in turn, the alternative pathway by a feedback mechanism.

## CONCLUSIONS

Although there is a vast literature on the immunopathology of human GN, and
despite a frequent belief, one must admit that the mechanisms, and therefore
the cause, of most human GN remain to be found. The usual nonrecurrence
of Goodpasture's syndromes after transplantation, the uncertain nature of the
antigen, and the diversity of anatomoclinical syndromes for IC-induced GN
argue against direct extrapolation to man of experimental models. On the other
hand, however, analogies with such experimental models are striking, and it is
likely that progress in immunologic techniques will make the elimination of
uncertainties a reality. It is probable that numerous forms of GN will, then, be
related to IC with certainty and that knowledge of the responsible antigen will
permit the development of new therapeutic approaches. It is also possible that
certain forms of GN, now thought to be related to IC, will appear to be linked
to other mechanisms, possibly not immunologic ones.

# V.  THERAPEUTIC ASPECTS

The likelihood of immunologic mechanisms in the pathogenesis of GN is the
basis for the use of immunosuppressive treatments in these diseases. It is,
however, raher paradoxical to note that, except for SLE, GN associated with
relatively clear immunologic mechanisms are usually unresponsive to immunosuppressive treatment, whereas nephrotic syndromes with minimal changes,
in which the role of immunologic factors is not well documented, are responsive
to corticosteroids and alkylating agents. This relative inefficacy of immunosuppressants in chronic GN might be explained by the relative resistance of
antibody production to immunosuppressants (only cell-mediated immunity is
clearly altered by these products; see chap. 33). In addition, one may imagine
that in certain cases, immunosuppression may aggravate GN, either by T-cell
depression and an increase in the autoimmune potential, as in SLE, or, as has

**Table 29.2   Provisional List of Antigens That Are Strongly Suspected of Inducing GN via Immune Complexes in Man***

|  | *Antigens* | *Clinical situation* |
|---|---|---|
| Iatrogenic agents | Drugs | Drug-induced GN, gold-salt nephritis |
|  | Antitoxins ⎫<br>Xenogeneic sera ⎭ | Serum sickness |
| Bacteria | *Streptococcus nephritogenes* | Post streptococcal GN |
|  | *Staphylococcus albus* | GN of ventriculoatreal shunts |
|  | *Corynebacterium bovis* ⎫<br>Enterococci ⎭ | Endocarditis |
|  | *Streptococcus pneumoniae* | Pneumonia |
|  | *Treponema pallidum* | Syphilis |
|  | *Salmonella typhi* | Typhoid fever |
| Viruses | Hepatitis B | Hepatitis |
|  | Oncornavirus | Leukemias |
|  | Measles |  |
|  | Epstein-Barr | Burkitt's lymphoma |
| Parasites | *Plasmodium malariae* ⎫<br>*Plasmodium falciparum* ⎭ | Malaria |
|  | *Schistosoma mansoni* | Bilharziasis |
|  | *Filaria loa* | Filariasis |
| Other agents | Nondeterminate | Endocarditis, leprosy, kala-azar, mumps, chicken pox, infectious mononucleosis, Guillain-Barré syndrome |
| Autoantigens or antigens of exogenous origin | Nuclear antigens | SLE |
|  | Immunoglobulins | Essential cryoglobulinemia |
|  | Tumor antigens (carcinoembryonic antigen) | Neoplasms |
|  | Thyroglobulin | Thyroiditis, certain extramembranous GNs |
|  | Renal tubular antigen | Sickle cell disease, renal carcinoma |

* After C. B. Wilson.

been shown in rabbit chronic serum sickness with cortisone, by diminution of antibody production and formation of IC more nephrotoxic than those produced with high antibody titers. In conclusion, except for SLE, nephrotic syndromes with minimal changes, and certain rapidly progressive GN (for which cyclophosphamide and corticosteroids are more indicated than is azathioprine; see p. 962), there is no clear indication for the use of immunosuppressive agents or steroids in the treatment of acute or chronic GN. It is too early to evaluate the recent trials of plasmapheresis performed in some forms of GN with anti-GBM antibody or large amounts of circulating IC.

# BIBLIOGRAPHY

DIXON F. J. The pathogenesis of glomerulonephritis. Amer. J. Med., 1968, *44*, 493.

FRANKLIN E. C. Cryoproteins. In: Clinical Immunology (C. W. Parker [ed]). Saunders, Philadelphia, 1980:534.

GERMUTH F. G. Immunopathology of the renal glomerular immune complex deposits and anti-basement membrane diseases. Boston, 1973, Little, Brown.

HAMBURGER J., BERGER J., HINGLAIS N., DESCAMPS B. New insights into the pathogenesis of glomerulonephritis afforded by the study of renal allografts. Clin. Nephrology, 1973, *1*, 1.

HAMBURGER J., HINGLAIS N., and DE MONTERA H. Renal biopsy in 1000 cases of chronic glomerular disease. *In* E. Lovell-Becker, H. O. Heinemann, and R. L. Shermann, Eds., Nephrology-Cornell Seminars. Baltimore, 1971, Williams & Wilkins, p. 63.

KINCAID-SMITH P., MATHEW T. M., and LOVELL BECKER E. (Ed.). Glomerulonephritis morphology, natural history and treatment. 2 vol. New York, 1973, Wiley.

METCOFF J. (Ed.). Acute glomerulonephritis. Boston, 1967, Little, Brown.

RAIJ L. and MICHAEL A. F. Immunologic aspects of kidney disease. In: Clinical Immunology (C. W. Parker [ed]). Saunders, Philadelphia, 1980:1051.

WEST C. D., RULEY E. J., FORRISTAL J., and DAVIS N. C. Mechanism of hypocomplementemia in glomerulonephritis. Kidney Intern., 1973, *3*, 116.

WILSON C. B. Immune complex glomerulonephritis. *In* Proc. 5th Int. Cong. Nephrology. Basel, 1971, Karger, p. 68.

WILSON C. B. Immunopathology of glomerulonephritis. *In* P. A. Miescher and H. J. Müller-Eberhard, Eds., Textbook of immunopathology, ed. 2. New York, 1976, Grune & Stratton, p. 529.

WILSON C. B. Immunopathology of antibasement membrane antibodies. In: Mechanisms of Immunopathology (S. Cohen, P. A. Ward, and R. T. MacCluskey [eds]). John Wiley & Sons, New York, 1979:181.

## ORIGINAL ARTICLES

BERGER J. IgA glomerular deposits in renal disease. Transpl. Proc., 1969, *1*, 939.

BHAN A. K., COLLINS A. B., SCHNEEBERGER E. E., and McCLUSKEY R. T. A cell-mediated reaction against glomerular-bound immune complexes. J. Exp. Med., 1979, 150, 1410.

LEIBOWITCH J., HALBVACHS L., WATTEL S., GAILLARD M. H., and DROZ D. Recurrence of dense deposits in transplanted kidneys. II: Serum complement and nephritic factor profiles. Kidney Intern., 1978, in press.

Mc CLUSKEY P. T. The value of immunofluorescence in the study of human renal disease. J. Exp. Med., 1971, *184*, 242s.

SUTHERLAND J. C. and MARDINEY M. R. Immune complex disease in the kidneys of lymphoma-leukemia patients. The presence of an oncornavirus-related antigen. J. Nat. Cancer Inst., 1973, *50*, 533.

WILSON C. B. and DIXON F. J. Antigen quantitation in experimental immune complex glomerulonephritis. I. Acute serum sickness. J. Immunol., 1970, *105*, 279.

Chapter 30

# IMMUNOPROLIFERATIVE DISORDERS

**Jean-Louis Preud'homme**

I. INTRODUCTION

II. CONCEPT OF MONOCLONAL IMMUNOGLOBULIN AND OF MONOCLONAL LYMPHOCYTIC PROLIFERATION

III. B-LYMPHOCYTE PROLIFERATIONS AND RELATED DISORDERS

IV. T-LYMPHOCYTE PROLIFERATIONS

V. PROLIFERATIONS OF UNCERTAIN CLASSIFICATION

## I. INTRODUCTION

Immunoproliferative disorders (IPD) represent a nosology that is complex, has imprecise boundaries, and includes extremely different diseases. Generally included under the term IPD are proliferative diseases that affect cells derived from lymphoid cells or cells that resemble, by morphologic or functional criteria, those involved in immune responses (except monocytes). Such a definition will depend obviously on the criteria used for identification of these cells. In recent years, immunochemical analysis of sera has enabled recognition of monoclonal Ig secretion. This finding has been extremely useful for the characterization of such diseases as multiple myeloma. Recently, new methods that permit study of lymphocytic surface markers allowed an approach at the cellular level toward identification of proliferative diseases. The insights gained have provided a better understanding of the pathophysiology of certain lymphoid proliferative disorders by recognition of their B- or T-cell nature and their degree of differentiation. These studies have resulted in a reclassification as immunoproliferative syndromes of disorders that had not been included in this nosology previously, Note, however, that lymphocytic markers in man are far from satisfactory. Therefore, exact classification of some of these syndromes is still imprecise, and their inclusion in the present chapter may be transient. Before discussing IPD (particularly B lymphocyte-derived IPD, which are best characterized and most common), two concepts must be clarified before we can attempt to evaluate pathogenetic mechanisms; "monoclonal immunoglobulin" and "monoclonal lymphocytic proliferation."

## II. CONCEPT OF MONOCLONAL IMMUNOGLOBULIN AND OF MONOCLONAL LYMPHOCYTIC PROLIFERATION

### CONCEPT OF MONOCLONAL IMMUNOGLOBULIN

Unlike the extreme heterogeneity of normal Ig, monoclonal Ig is homogeneous. Homogeneity of monoclonal Ig results from the fact that all molecules possess the same heavy and light chains. They may therefore be typed for their heavy chain class and subclass and their light chain type, by immunologic methods. These molecules all bear the same allotypic markers, which correspond to determinants coded for by a single chromosome. Moreover, all molecules of a monoclonal Ig have the same amino acid sequence. The identity of the variable region of the heavy and light chains confers on each monoclonal Ig an individual antigenic specificity.

This structural homogeneity is expressed as an identical electric charge on the monoclonal Ig molecules and explains the appearance of a narrow peak (spike) on electrophoresis. This spike of monoclonal Ig contrasts with the diffuse (heterogeneous) nature of normal Ig. In addition to its purely diagnostic impact, the electrophoretic spike permits quantitation of circulating monoclonal Ig. This quantification has considerable practical importance, because measurement of monoclonal Ig by radial immunodiffusion gives unreliable results. However, the electrophoretic spike may not always be visible, either because the amount of monoclonal Ig is minimal, or because Ig is complexed to other serum proteins. In addition to electrophoresis, immunoelectrophoretic analysis is necessary because it permits typing of the monoclonal Ig and proves homogeneity by use of antisera specific for the various heavy and light chains. It is sometimes necessary to first isolate the monoclonal Ig to perform typing. This is often the case for IgM, which, due to its high molecular weight, migrates less well in agarose than does IgG and is therefore not accessible on immunoelectrophoresis to antilight-chain antibodies, which are precipitated in the more external (mobile) IgG precipitation line. One should note also that some IgM may precipitate in the application reservoir and must therefore first be depolymerized (cysteine, mercaptoethanol) before gel immunodiffusion study.

### NORMAL NATURE OF MONOCLONAL IMMUNOGLOBULIN

Monoclonal Ig was long considered abnormal (hence the former name paraprotein, which is now obsolete) because some chemical studies indicated differences between monoclonal and normal Ig (these studies, in fact, compared homogeneous and heterogeneous Ig populations), and also because there is a specific antigenicity for each monoclonal Ig. Actually, an antiserum obtained by monoclonal Ig immunization, followed by adequate absorption by normal Ig does not precipitate normal Ig or any other monoclonal Ig, but only the monoclonal Ig used in immunization. This individual antigenic specificity, similar to idiotypy, is linked to determinants borne by the variable parts of the monoclonal Ig. In fact, this antigenicity is not peculiar to monoclonal Ig: the precipitation reaction of an immune serum with an individual specificity of the homologous monoclonal Ig may be inhibited by the addition of large quantities of normal Ig (or Fab fragment taken from a normal IgG pool). These data show that some determinants on the variable regions of each monoclonal Ig are also present on small numbers of Ig molecules from normal subjects.

Further evidence for the normality of monoclonal Ig has been provided by studies of antibodies of narrow specificity. If one looks at heterogeneous antibodies from animals immunized with certain antigens, one may isolate, by various methods (affinity chromatography, isoelectric focusing), homogeneous antibody populations that have one given specificity and affinity for one antigen. These homogeneous populations may be completely analogous, according to the various criteria just mentioned, to monoclonal Ig. In addition, monoclonal antibodies that show electrophoretic spikes have been obtained in several species after immunization with certain antigens, such as pneumococcal or streptococcal polysaccharides. This production of monoclonal antibodies, which disappears when immunization stops, is genetically controlled.

In man, too, monoclonal Ig are present (sometimes transiently) in the absence of malignant disease, both in pathologic circumstances and in apparently healthy subjects (vide infra). Another argument that favors the normal nature of monoclonal Ig is the fact that various biologic functions of normal Ig, including antibody activity, are present in monoclonal Ig. For all of these reasons, monoclonal Ig should not be considered an abnormal protein and a malignancy marker, but rather a protein synthesized by a single plasma cell clone; this concept does not prejudge and benign or malignant nature of the clone. This hypothesis of Ig synthesis by a single clone easily explains the homogeneity of monoclonal Ig.

However, recent study have shown that monoclonal Ig may be structurally abnormal. Indeed, the study of murine plasmacytoma cells has shown that mutations affecting Ig production spontaneously occur at a very high rate. The frequency of such mutations is considerably increased by mutagenic drugs, including those commonly used for the chemotherapy of human patients with myeloma. These mutations may result in a loss of the ability to synthesize one or both Ig chains, or in the production of Ig chains with various structural abnormalities (deletions, heavy-chain class switch, etc.). The production of similar altered immunoglobulin chains has not only been documented in patients affected with immunoproliferative disorders but also in patients with apparently benign monoclonal plasma cell populations, either spontaneously or as a result of chemotherapy. It must be pointed out that the secretion of structurally abnormal Ig molecules may have severe consequences. In certain cases, structurally abnormal Ig may precipitate in various organs resulting in a severe systemic disease.

# ANTIBODY ACTIVITY OF MONOCLONAL IMMUNOGLOBULINS

When considering the vast number of possible antigens, it is not surprising that only a small number of antibody activities have been identified in monoclonal Ig, despite detailed search. In addition, because of its structural homogeneity, all molecules of a monoclonal Ig react with the same determinant of the antigenic molecule. Thus, some reactions, like precipitation and agglutination, are only observed if the determinant is repetitive on the antigenic structure or if the monoclonal Ig is polyvalent (IgM or polymeric IgA). On the other hand, the antibody activity of monoclonal Ig is often observed at very high dilutions, which explains why fortuitous discovery within a monoclonal Ig-containing serum of antibody activity at very high titers (e.g., $10^6$) may lead to the discovery of antibody activity in monoclonal Ig. It must be stressed, however, that some monoclonal Ig react with some antigens independently of specific antibody activity to the antigen. It is necessary, to prove the immunologic nature of the interaction, to show that the activity is borne on the Fab fragment of the monoclonal Ig and to demonstrate that there is a definite specificity and a stoichiometric relationship.

Antibody activities that have been identified for human monoclonal Ig are listed in Table 30.1. Some of these antibody activities occur with a very high frequency. An example is antidinitrophenyl activity, which often has a weak affinity constant and may only represent a cross-reaction with the true antigen, which has not been identified. This is also true for anti-IgG activities, the incidence of which is remarkably high (close to 10% of monoclonal IgM).

Many of the monoclonal Ig antibody activities that have been recognized are autoantibody activities (Table 30.1). This fact has led to the hypothesis that autoantibody-producing cells are particularly sensitive to neoplastic transformation. Conversely, a specificity to heterologous antigens has sometimes been linked to exogenous stimulation: antistreptolysin antibody activity of monoclonal Ig developed in a myeloma patient who presented with several attacks of rheumatic fever; in another case, antihorse $\alpha_2M$ activity has been found in a subject who received several injections of horse serum. In these cases, the antigenic stimulation occurred several decades before clinical appearance of the myeloma. This fact suggests a biphasic evolution: immune response to the antigenic stimulation with proliferation of stimulated clones, followed (second phase) by malignant transformation of one of these clones (perhaps induced by an oncogenic virus).

# CONCEPT OF MONOCLONAL LYMPHOCYTIC PROLIFERATION

In most cases of malignant proliferation of cells of B-lymphocyte origin, the cells bear surface Ig. Surface Ig are synthesized by all proliferating cells and contain only one heavy chain and one light chain. There is also a restriction on the heavy chain subclass which means that all heavy chains are of the same subclass. The allelic exclusion phenomenon has also been found. A still stronger

**Table 30.1   Antibody Activities of Human Monoclonal Immunoglobulins**

| Activity anti- | Ig class | Consequences |
|---|---|---|
| Erythrocyte antigens | IgM, IgA | Cold agglutinin diseases |
| Ii | IgM | |
| Sp 1 | IgM | |
| A$_1$ | IgM | |
| Stored erythrocytes | | |
| Bacterial, viral, and fungal antigens | IgG | |
| Streptolysin | IgG | |
| Staphylolysin | IgM | |
| Klebsiella | IgG | |
| Brucella | IgG | |
| Rubella | IgG | |
| Candida | IgG | |
| Plasma proteins | | |
| IgG | IgM, IgG, IgA | Mixed cryoglobulinemia (and hyperimmunoglobulinemic purpura) |
| IgG complexed to antigen | IgM | |
| Lipoprotein | IgA, IgM | |
| Fibrin monomer | IgG | |
| Transferrin | IgG | Hemochromatosis |
| Horse $\alpha_2$M | IgG | |
| Serum albumin | IgM | |
| Dinitrophenyl | IgM, IgG, IgA | |
| Lecithin | IgM | False syphilis reaction |
| Heparin | IgM | |
| Phosphorylcholine | IgM | |
| Tissue antigens | | |
| Gastric parietal cells | IgA | |

After M. Seligmann and J. C. Brouet, Sem. Hematol. 1973, *10*, 163.

argument in favor of the monoclonal nature of surface Ig in lymphocytic proliferation comes from the observation that when antibody activity of surface Ig is detectable, the same antibody activity is present in the surface Ig of all proliferating lymphocytes. The same argument applies to idiotypic determinants that are shared by all surface Ig molecules of one given proliferating clone. Antibody activities described so far for surface monoclonal Ig are limited in number: antierythrocytic activity, anti-Forssman antigen activity, and anti-IgG activity (the latter is not uncommon). The monoclonal nature of proliferating B lymphocytes has also been demonstrated by criteria other than homogeneous surface Ig, for example, by the synthesis of only one isomeric enzyme form.

There seems to be one apparent exception to the class restriction rule in the study of surface Ig in monoclonal proliferation. This exception occurs when μ and δ chains are present simultaneously on the surface of a single cell. These findings simulate the case of normal B lymphocytes, since the majority of normal B cells synthesize both surface IgM and IgD as in most patients with chronic lymphocytic leukemia. It must be remembered that surface IgM and IgD of monoclonal lymphocytes share (as do normal B lymphocytes) the same light chain, the same idiotypic specificity, and, eventually, the same antibody activity, which probably reflects the identity of variable regions of both Ig.

One may then apply to surface monoclonal Ig, considered to be a cellular marker of lymphocytic clone proliferation, a line of reasoning analogous to that used when examining serum monoclonal Ig. Circulating monoclonal Ig has provided abundant amounts of homogeneous molecular populations, the study of which has been crucially important in our understanding of structure and function of Ig. One may hope that homogeneous cellular populations of monoclonal lymphocytes will also contribute to our knowledge of immunocompetent cell physiology.

# III.  B-LYMPHOCYTE PROLIFERATIONS AND RELATED DISORDERS

Cellular studies permit a tentative classification of proliferating B lymphocytes according to the exact nature of the proliferating cell and with respect to the presence or absence of cell maturation. monoclonal B-lymphocyte proliferations may be associated with maturation arrest (most cases of chronic lymphocytic leukemia) or may show persistent differentiation toward plasma cells (macroglobulinemia). The proliferation may affect a clone of the most mature cells in the B-cell line (myeloma).

## MULTIPLE MYELOMA

Multiple myeloma is a malignant plasma cell proliferation that affects mainly the bone marrow, usually beginning in old age. The etiology is unknown. Whereas genetic factors have not been implicated in human disease, such factors have been shown in animal myeloma. Only certain species are affected. In the mouse, the disease occurs spontaneously in some strains (C3H), while in others (BALB/c), it is easily induced by intraperitoneal introduction of mineral oil or plastic disks. Plasmacytoma induction is practically impossible in axenic BALB/c mice, which suggests the need for a certain degree of proliferation and clonal expansion after antigenic stimulation. This may mean that genetically sensitive hosts must first produce a sufficiently large cell population before an appropriate oncogenic stimulus can transform them into myeloma cells. The nature and localization (bone marrow) of the proliferation easily explain the clinical and biologic manifestations of the disease.

### Secretion of Monoclonal Ig

A direct consequence of monoclonal plasma cell proliferation in myeloma is monoclonal Ig secretion. The immunochemical study of serum and urine permits differentiation of several patterns.

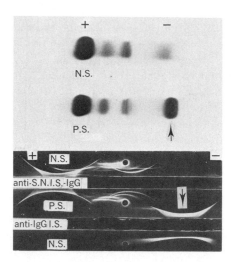

**Fig. 30.1**  IgG myeloma. Electrophoresis (*top*) reveals a narrow spike of γ mobility. By immunoelectrophoresis (*bottom*), the precipitation arc of monoclonal Ig (arrow) is symmetric, with a characteristic "shiplike" appearance. Analysis by use of monospecific antisera reveals that it is a monoclonal IgG. Note the very clear diminution in the precipitation line of normal nonmonodonal, IgG in the pathologic serum. Precipitation lines of IgA and IgM from the pathologic serum are not visible, thereby confirming the important decrease in serum levels of these immunoglobulins. NS, normal serum; PS, pathologic serum; anti-SN-IS-IgG, antihuman normal serum absorbed by IgG; anti-IgG IS, anti-IgG antiserum (reacts with γ, λ, and κ chains).

#### MYELOMA WITH ENTIRE MONOCLONAL Ig

This type is characterized by a monoclonal Ig spike without detectable free light chains (Fig. 30.1). It usually represents equilibrated synthesis of heavy and light chains by proliferative plasma cells. Normal serum Ig levels are usually decreased (see below).

#### MYELOMA WITH ENTIRE MONOCLONAL Ig AND BENCE-JONES PROTEINURIA

This pattern is more common. In the serum, an electrophoretic spike of monoclonal Ig is sometimes associated with circulating monoclonal light chains (Fig. 30.2). The urine contains free light chains of one type (Bence-Jones protein), which are identical to the light chains of the circulating monoclonal Ig. Bence-Jones light chains are usually present as monomers and/or dimers. They often exhibit classic thermolability: acidified urine is heated to 50–60°C,

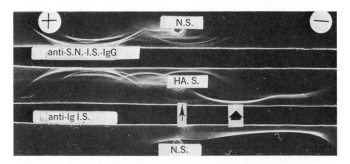

**Fig. 30.2**  IgG myeloma with serum Bence-Jones protein. NS, normal serum; HAS, patient's serum; anti-SN-IS-IgG, antihuman serum absorbed by IgG; anti-Ig-IS, anti-IgG serum (reacts with γ, λ, and κ chains). The anti-IgG serum produces two abnormal precipitation lines, the nature of which has been specified by study of monospecific sera. The most cathodal abnormal line (large arrow) is a κ IgG; the most anodal one (narrow arrow), in partial identity with the previous one, is a Bence-Jones protein of the κ type.

and a precipitate appears; this precipitate solubilizes at 100°C and again reappears on cooling. Urinary Bence-Jones proteins often show an electrophoretic mobility that differs (distance from application well) from that of serum monoclonal Ig. Under certain conditions (especially severe renal failure), the quantity of Bence-Jones protein in the circulation is so large that it produces a discrete electrophoretic spike.

These cases represent an unbalanced synthesis of heavy and light chains by myeloma plasma cells. Light chains synthesized by plasma cells in excess are excreted as free light chains.

### MYELOMA WITH ISOLATED BENCE-JONES PROTEIN

In about 20% of cases, no entire monoclonal Ig is detected, and the serum shows only hypogammaglobulinemia. Here, the only detectable monoclonal Ig is Bence-Jones protein. These forms are an expression of an even more profound imbalance in regulation of Ig chain synthesis. Malignant plasma cells secrete only light chains. However, the finding by immunocytochemical methods of an apparently unreleased intracellular heavy-chain in the plasma cells of patients with Bence-Jones myeloma is not uncommon. Recent study of Ig biosynthesis in one such case showed the production of abnormally short gamma chains (lacking one domain). The synthetic rate of these abnormal heavy chains was normal, their assembly with light chains was partially blocked, their secretion was delayed, and they were degraded after secretion. Such findings well explain the absence of detectable entire monoclonal IgG in the patient's serum. In a very few cases, Bence-Jones protein in polymerized form is present only in the serum.

### NONSECRETORY MYELOMA

In about 1% of cases, the most careful immunochemical analysis shows no monoclonal Ig in the serum or urine. However, monoclonal Ig synthesis may easily be demonstrated at cellular level by immunofluorescence study of bone marrow plasma cells in most cases (Fig. 30.3).

The mechanism responsible for this apparent nonsecretion is probably complex. It may include true nonsecretion, with either intracellular accumulation of Ig chains or intracytoplasmic degradation of structurally abnormal chains and secretion of abnormal (deleted) Ig molecules that are then rapidly degraded and are therefore not detectable by immunochemical methods. The latter situation probably corresponds to the majority of patients. In very rare cases, it seems that the plasmocytes have lost all their capacity for immunoglobulin synthesis.

### IMMUNOCHEMICAL DISTRIBUTION OF MYELOMATOUS PROTEINS

The relative frequency of the various classes and subclasses of heavy and light chains in the monoclonal myeloma Ig correlates, in general, with the concentration of the various Ig types in normal serum. Thus, IgG myeloma with κ light chains occurs most frequently (with respect to γ-chain subclasses, the order of decreasing frequency is γ1, γ2, γ3, γ4). IgA myeloma is less

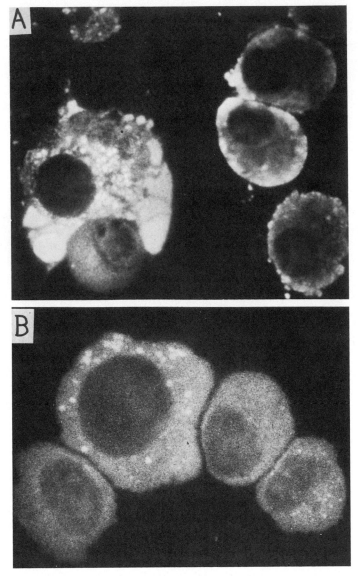

**Fig. 30.3** Nonexcreting myeloma; medullary plasma cells seen by cytoplasmic immunofluorescence. In some cases (A), plasma cells contain round structures, strongly positive by immunofluorescence, which correspond to very swollen ergastoplasmic cisternae. The aspects of these cells is not specific. In other cases (B), The plasma cell appearance is not very unusual.

frequent and is most often of the $\alpha 1$ subclass. IgD myeloma is rare and IgE myeloma exceptional. The distribution of electric charges of myeloma proteins is also the same as that of normal serum Ig molecules. The diagram of the incidence of myeloma proteins plotted as a function of their electrophoretic mobility looks very similar to that of normal serum Ig.

The exception is IgM myeloma, which has a much lower incidence (about

1% of the total cases) than would be expected from its normal serum levels. One should note that IgM and IgD myelomas undergo especially severe course (often accompanied by considerable Bence-Jones proteinuria). The majority of IgD myeloma proteins have light chains of the λ type. There is, lastly, a high incidence of leukemic forms in the rare cases of IgE myelomas. However, overall, there is no absolute correlation between immunochemical type of myeloma proteins and clinical course of the disease.

CONSEQUENCES OF THE PRESENCE OF A SERUM MONOCLONAL Ig

The presence of circulating monoclonal Ig at high concentrations may cause significant but nonspecific symptoms (sharply elevated sedimentation rate, red blood cell rouleau formation, hyperproteinemia), which may antedate other disease symptoms. Hypocholesterolemia, of uncertain origin, is common when the monoclonal Ig spike is very large. Hypoalbuminemia is sometimes observed and has complex etiologies.

Hyperviscosity syndrome is seen much less often than in macroglobulinemia (see p. 873). Its presence relates to several factors, including the absolute monoclonal Ig concentration, the Ig molecular form, and its state of aggregation. Monoclonal IgG3 may cause hyperviscosity syndromes, even at relatively modest serum levels, because of the high tendency of IgG3 molecules to form aggregates.

Monoclonal Ig may also be a cryoglobulin. Because monoclonal cryoglobulins are often present in high concentration and because they often precipitate at a relatively high temperature (sometimes close to 37°C), these cryoglobulins may have dramatic clinical consequences. Conversely, the pyroglobulin nature of monoclonal Ig (irreversible precipitation at 56°C) is rare and has no clinical manifestations.

Although their actual mechanism of action is not unequivocal (capillary lesions, possible thrombocytopenia), hemorrhagic complications often relate directly to monoclonal Ig. This relationship might represent platelet function abnormalities secondary to monoclonal Ig adsorption on the platelet surface, an inhibitory action by monoclonal Ig on fibrin monomer polymerization, or an antifactor VIII circulating anticoagulant. An interaction between high serum levels of monoclonal Ig and polymorphs may be responsible for their diminished phagocytic capacity, rate of migration, and adhesive properties.

One should note that all these abnormalities, which relate to serum monoclonal Ig, are not peculiar to myeloma. Recognition of these symptoms is important, because removal of significant quantities of monoclonal Ig by plasmapheresis is often remarkably effective in reversing clinical signs and symptoms that may be life threatening. Other consequences of monoclonal Ig secretion, such as amyloidosis, will be discussed below.

### Bone and Tumor Involvement

Because plasma cell proliferation mainly occurs in bone marrow, it is not surprising that bone lesions are present in the majority of cases. In addition to monoclonal Ig, myeloma cells secrete various substances, including interferon (whose role in human disease has not been shown) and a polypeptide that activates osteoclasts and thereby mobilizes bone calcium. X-ray studies reveal bone lesions of two main types, which are often associated. The characteristic osteolytic (punched-out) lesions are mostly seen in flat bones (skull, ribs, pelvis) and the long bone diaphysis. Diffuse or localized osteoporosis often predominates and is seen especially in vertebral bodies. Clinically, the bone symptoms often represent the major complaints. Pain may be intense and chronic. Pathologic fractures (particularly vertebral collapse) are more common than are palpable bone tumors. Hypercalcemia is inconstant but often present; it can be so severe that it produces characteristic signs or symptoms.

The high incidence of vertebral lesions explains why the most common neurologic complication is spinal cord compression (which, alternatively, can be caused by paraspinous plasmacytic tumors). Plasma cells may also be proliferative in other organs (hepatomegaly, splenomegaly, and, occasionally, other viscera), especially in the final stages of the diseases.

### Hematologic Aspects and Lymphocyte Marker Study

Bone marrow examination demonstrates plasmacytic proliferation. The plasmacytic infiltration on bone marrow smears is of variable morphology; in some cases, the cells are almost normal, but more often they are dystrophic and show cytoplasmic and nuclear aberrations. The high percentage of plasma cells in bone marrow aspirates constitutes a major diagnostic clue, because bone marrow plasmacytosis of greater than 20% is rarely observed, except in myeloma. When plasmacytosis is less profound, morphologic abnormalities, especially nuclear, may suggest the diagnosis. In some cases where cytologic study of bone marrow smears is not conclusive, pathologic examination of specimens obtained by needle biopsy may enable demonstration of plasma cell proliferation. The common triad of the three disease signs, bone marrow plasmacytosis, monoclonal Ig, and bone lesions, establishes a diagnosis that must be certain because of the invariably fatal course of the disease.

As a consequence of bone marrow invasion by proliferating plasma cells, marrow insufficiency of variable degree results, usually manifest as a more or less severe anemia. Neutropenia and thrombocytopenia are less common, at least prior to chemotherapy. The disease is only rarely leukemic and, if so, shows circulating plasmacytosis and polyvisceral lesions, either in the end stages of the disease or as its initial manifestation (plasma cell leukemia).

Study of lymphocytic markers commonly shows the existence of a monoclonal B-lymphocyte population that carries surface Ig with the same heavy and light chains as those of the myeloma proteins. These lymphocytes are thought to belong to the proliferating clone. Studies performed with anti-idiotypic antisera have shown in several patients the presence of a relatively large percentage of blood lymphocytes that express the idiotypic specificity of the monoclonal Ig. In most cases, these idiotypic lymphocytes are B-lymphocytes. Recent study of the bone marrow cells using highly specific antiidiotypic antibodies has shown that pre-B-cells already express the same idiotype as the myeloma protein. These results show that although the proliferation appears to be purely plasmacytic upon morphologic grounds, the proliferative process, in fact, affects early precursors. This concept is applicable to many instances of malignant diseases. Conversely, it has been demonstrated in a few cases that a large percentage of blood lymphocytes expressing membrane receptors with the same idiotype and the same antibody specificity as the myeloma protein were T cells. The interpretation of these findings is not yet clear but it raises the question of the origin of the proliferation in a stem cell that has not been committed toward the B line. It is noteworthy that the availability of a homogeneous population of T lymphocytes with membrane receptors of known specificity has allowed one of the first characterizations of T-cell antigen receptors; molecules made of two chains of about 70,000 daltons.

### Secondary Immunodeficiency

A profound deficiency of humoral immunity is usually observed in myeloma. Normal Ig are decreased in concentration in 90% of cases; low levels of circulating antibodies occur, and the primary response to various antigenic stimulations is strongly depressed. In contrast with these findings, cellular immunity is normal or little affected prior to cytotoxic treatment.

The humoral deficiency is due mainly to a diminished synthesis of normal immunoglobulins. In addition, hypercatabolism of normal IgG probably plays a role in IgG myelomas. Normal B lymphocytes are decreased in number, and normal plasma cells are very rare. Recent data strongly suggest that myeloma cells secrete a humoral factor that depresses synthesis of normal Ig, probably by inhibiting normal B-lymphocyte proliferation in response to antigenic stimulation. This factor does not appear to be directly suppressor. It activates adherent cells (probably macrophages) which, as a result, suppress normal B cells.

The importance of this immunodeficiency, subsequently aggravated by chemotherapy and neutropenia along with functional abnormalities of polymorphs explains the frequency and the gravity of infectious complications (mainly respiratory), which are the chief cause of death from myeloma in man.

### Other Manifestations

Secretion of excess free light chains is implicated in two other manifestations of myeloma, amyloidosis and renal failure and in a recently recognized syndrome (light chain deposition disease).

#### AMYLOIDOSIS

This manifestation is present in 10–25% of cases in autopsy series, but it appears to occur less frequently in recent series. Its topography is mainly vascular, lingual, cardiac, muscular, digestive, and pulmonary. These localizations are identical to those of primary amyloidosis, which some authors consider to be a latent plasmacytic dyscrasia. The role of free light chains in the pathogenesis of amyloid deposits in immunoproliferative diseases and in primary amyloidosis now seems well established. Study of the primary structure of amyloid substances from such patients has shown that the amino acid sequences are identical to those of the variable portion of Ig light chains. In addition, enzymatic treatment of certain Bence-Jones proteins, especially λ type, has made possible the in vitro production of an amyloid material. Amyloidosis in immunoproliferative diseases seems to be due to deposition of light-chain fragments, including the variable part and probably also limited segments of the constant region.

RENAL DISEASE

Progressive renal failure is observed in more than 50% of cases. Acute renal failure with anuria is also seen but is rare. The close correlation between renal insufficiency and Bence-Jones proteinuria, the anatomic characteristics of myeloma nephritis (tubular prominence with obstruction by voluminous, stratified cylinders composed of Bence-Jones protein associated with other plasma proteins, and significant atrophy of the tubular epithelium), and some experimental data suggest that Bence-Jones proteins directly cause the renal lesions. The precise mechanism is still uncertain. The primary lesions might be epithelial atrophy due to nephrotoxicity of Bence-Jones proteins (which are filtered by the glomeruli but, in addition, are secreted by tubules) or obstructive cylinder formation favored by local pH conditions and hyperconcentrations of Bence-Jones protein in tubules.

Other factors also contribute to the onset of myeloma renal failure: amyloidosis, calcium excess, cryoglobulinemia, interstitial nephritis linked to urinary infections, plasmacytic infiltrates, and hemodynamic factors (hyperviscosity, reduced renal blood flow, and anemia). These many factors probably explain the high frequency and the severity of renal disease in myeloma.

LIGHT CHAIN AND MONOCLONAL Ig DEPOSITION DISEASE

Although this syndrome has only very recently been recognized, its frequency is possibly higher than that of amyloidosis. It is characterized by predominantly renal or polysystemic (liver, heart, nervous system, vessels, lungs, etc.) deposition of an amorphous nonamyloid material that contains monoclonal Ig detectable by immunofluorescence. The monoclonal Ig determinants found in the tissue deposits (and in monoclonal plasma cell populations in the bone marrow) most often consist of light chains (of the kappa type in the majority but not all cases). However, in several cases, the deposits contained both a heavy and a light chain. Although the major clinical manifestation is a progressive renal failure with frequent nephrotic syndrome, the hepatic or cardiac manifestations may be predominant. The underlying immunoproliferative disease is often myeloma. It may also be a pleomorphic proliferation similar to macroglobulinemia. In several patients, there is a monoclonal plasma cell population with no evidence of malignant disease after several years of followup examinations.

Biosynthesis experiments, in several cases, have shown the secretion of structurally abnormal Ig chains (abnormally short or elongated light chains which polymerized into high molecular-weight covalent polymers known as deleted heavy chains). Several arguments strongly suggest that the structural abnormalities are directly responsible for tissue deposition. These altered Ig molecules are usually not detectable (or in very small amounts) in serum and urine. It is noteworthy that, in two cases, the disease has probably resulted from the emergence of a mutant clone-producing abnormal Ig induced by chemo-therapy in patients first affected with common myeloma. Conversely, a few patients presented with common Bence-Jones myeloma with no obvious abnor-mality of their Ig chains and the mechanism of precipitation in such cases still unclear.

# CHRONIC LYMPHOCYTIC LEUKEMIA

Whereas myeloma represents proliferation of the most mature cells of the B-cell lineage that secrete serum monoclonal Ig, chronic lymphocytic leukemia (CLL) provides (in most cases) the best example of monoclonal proliferation of B lymphocytes. At the cellular level, one finds a surface monoclonal Ig not usually seen in the serum by immunoelectrophoretic analysis, although a recent work performed with antiidiotypic antibodies, has shown that a significant proportion of serum IgM represents the secretion product of the proliferating clone. By still unknown mechanisms, the lymphocytic proliferation significantly alters the patient's immune state, resulting in immunodeficiency and, frequently, autoimmune manifestations.

The disease affects elderly, predominantly male, subjects. It occurs rarely before the age of 50. Its distribution is worldwide, but it is very rare in Japan and China. This fact, and the occasional existence of familial forms, suggests that genetic factors play a role in the incidence of the disease.

## *Lymphocytic Proliferation*

### ANATOMIC CHARACTERISTICS

CLL was first defined by the pathologic features of lymphocytic prolifer-ation. An absolute blood lymphocytosis, usually modest (20,000–50,000 cells/mm$^3$) but sometimes very marked, is most often observed. This lymphocytosis by itself nearly suffices for the diagnosis if it is clear-cut (5,000–10,000 cells/mm$^3$) and found repeatedly on serial examination over a period of several months in subjects older than 50. CLL lymphocytes do not divide much; thus, hyperlymphocytosis represents, in part, accumulation of leukocytes secondary to an alteration in cell traffic, including a decrement in recirculation from the blood to the lymph nodes and other tissues.

The bone marrow is very cellular, and lymphocytosis usually exceeds 30%. Histologic examination of the bone marrow (biopsy) reveals a diffuse or nodular lymphocytic infiltration in a hypercellular marrow. This examination is neces-sary if the bone marrow aspirate shows a less suggestive pattern of lymphocytosis (<30%).

Lymph node involvement is common. Lymphadenopathies are generally symmetric, both superficial and deep (especially abdominal, as shown by lymphangiography). Lymph node biopsy is of interest in disease forms that have no other localizations and shows the architecture to be obliterated by a uniform lymphocytic proliferation. Splenomegaly is less common; however, the lymphocytic proliferation may infiltrate any tissue.

The morphologic features of CLL lymphocytes (by light or electron microscopy) do not usually differentiate them from normal small lymphocytes, but sometimes the proliferation includes atypical lymphocytes.

IMMUNOLOGIC CHARACTERISTICS

Chronic lymphocytic leukemia has been the subject of numerous studies of lymphocytic markers. In most cases, the proliferating cells are B lymphocytes. Leukemic lymphocytes synthesize surface Ig, express C3 and IgG Fc receptors, possess specific B-lymphocyte antigens, bind aggregated IgG, and lack T-lymphocyte markers. Normal T lymphocytes are present in a reduced percentage in the blood and dilution of T lymphocytes by B lymphocytes probably explains the weak or delayed response to phytohemagglutinin. Actually, the absolute number of circulating normal T cells is often normal or increased. Normal T-lymphocyte numbers have been considered as having a good prognostic significance. A T-cell origin of the proliferation is envisaged in rare cases in which no surface Ig is detected. In fact, in most cases, other B-cell markers are present, and there are no T-cell markers. However, a definite T-cell origin of proliferation has been demonstrated in a few cases (see below).

The B-lymphocyte proliferation of CLL is monoclonal: all lymphocytes from a given patient synthesize homogeneous surface Ig, which show heavy-chain class and subclass restrictions and allelic exclusion and share light chains of a single type and the same idiotype and antibody activity. On freshly drawn lymphocytes, one sometimes detects the simultaneous presence of μ, δ κ, and λ chains. The surface Ig synthesized is, however, always monoclonal, and this false polyclonal pattern represents anti-IgG activity of monoclonal surface IgM (with serum IgG binding), fixation of circulating immune complexes onto the lymphocytic surface, or the combined presence of surface Ig and of antibodies directed against surface lymphocytic determinants. (Biclonal proliferations are discussed below.)

As with normal lymphocytes, IgM is the predominant surface Ig of leukemic lymphocytes. Light chains are most often of the κ type (Table 30.2). In most cases, an IgD that has the same light chain is associated with the surface IgM. As discussed above, the simultaneous presence of surface IgM and IgD does not argue against the monoclonal nature of the B-cell proliferation. Although their incidence may be overestimated in studies that do not include in vitro study of surface Ig synthesis, cases in which surface Ig is really of the IgG class are not uncommon. In contrast, chronic lymphocytic leukemia characterized by surface IgA is very exceptional (Table 30.2).

In the majority of cases, the monoclonal surface Ig is not detectable in the serum by conventional immunochemical methods, and one does not find plasma cells containing the monoclonal Ig. The quantity of surface Ig (generally less than on normal lymphocytes) is very similar for all lymphocytes in a given patient, which results in a very homogeneous pattern on immunofluorescence. One may, thus, consider that CLL lymphocytes show a block in differentiation since they are incapable of normal maturation to plasma cells. Conversely, most cases of CLL with serum monoclonal Ig correspond to some degree of persistent maturation. In about 10% of cases, a serum Ig spike is present. A monoclonal

**Table 30.2  Distribution of Surface Immunoglobulins in 124 Cases of Chronic Lymphocytic Leukemia**

| Serum monoclonal immunoglobulin* | Number of cases | Biclonal surface immunoglobulins | | | | | | | |
|---|---|---|---|---|---|---|---|---|---|
| | | μ | | γ | | α | | μγκλ | Non-detectable |
| | | κ | λ | κ | λ | κ | λ | | |
| None | 97 | 42 | 15 | 10 | 7 | 1 | 1 | 15† | 6 |
| IgM | 11 | 6 | 2 | 6 | 4 | | | 3† | |
| IgG | 14 | 1‡ | 1‡ | | | | 2 | | |
| IgA | 2 | | | | | | 2 | | |
| Total | 124 | 67 | 27 | 1 | | 1 | 5 | 18 | 6 |

* This study includes a high number of serum monoclonal immunoglobulins because of a deliberately biased patient recruitment.

† Synthesis of a monoclonal IgM in all cases studied.

‡ Surface immunoglobulins really synthesized by cells whereas IgG were found on cells studied immediately after collection. IgG (probably antilymphocytic antibodies) were bound in vivo on cells and thus masked the presence of IgM.

IgM is more often present but in amounts not sufficient to produce an electrophoretic spike.

The concept of persistence of some differentiation toward plasma cells does not apply to every case of CLL with serum monoclonal Ig. In some cases, the proliferative process affects a clone of Ig-secreting lymphocytes that themselves actively secrete the monoclonal Ig in the serum. In other cases, the serum monoclonal Ig is unrelated to the proliferation and may result from the conjunction of repeated antigenic stimulations with the immunodeficiency state that is most common in CLL patients. Finally, the serum monoclonal Ig may be the product of a second proliferating clone. As discussed below, biclonal proliferative processes are not exceptional. In such cases of biclonal CLL with a serum Ig spike, the major cell population is usually composed of the usual CLL B lymphocytes, which are blocked in their maturation and do not secrete their Ig products, whereas the second clone, which is the origin of the serum Ig, accounts for a minority of the cells in the blood and bone marrow.

### Secondary Immunodeficiency

Humoral deficiency is frequently present in CLL. It is usually better demonstrated by studying antibody production than by looking for the presence of hypogammaglobulinemia. The latter is an inconstant finding, particularly at the onset of the disease; it may even be replaced by a diffuse hyperimmunoglobulinemia. In many cases, hypoimmunoglobulinemia occurs during the course of the disease and then progressively worsens. The Ig deficiency may be global or selective for one or two Ig classes. The antibody response is depressed, with low levels of isohemagglutinins and diminished response to vaccination. One should note that preexisting antibody production is usually well maintained, whereas the patients have become incapable of immunization by new antigens.

The latter dichotomy is still more clear-cut for cellular immunity, which is normal for antigens previously experienced, whereas primary immunization to new antigens (like dinitrochlorobenzene) is suppressed.

This immunodeficiency explains the high frequency of infections, not only bacterial but also viral and fungal. It probably plays a role in the high incidence of epithelial carcinomas (6–10% of cases) compared to the frequency in normal subjects of the same age.

### Autoimmune Manifestations

Immune abnormalities are also manifest by the high incidence of autoimmune abnormalities, the manifestations of which may be clinical or merely biologic (autoantibody presence). Autoimmune hemolytic anemia is one of the major complications of chronic lymphocytic leukemia, observed in about 20% of cases. Other clinical manifestations of autoimmunity may be seen, although more rarely, including immunologic thrombocytopenic purpura, Sjögren's syndrome, and less commonly rheumatoid arthritis and systemic lupus erythematosus. The relatively high frequency of these manifestations justifies the systematic search for latent lymphoid proliferation in aged subjects who present with those, or other, autoimmune abnormalities.

### Modification of the Cellular Nature of the Disease

The course of chronic lymphocytic leukemia is often prolonged and relatively peaceful for several years. Any exacerbation should initiate a search for a more malignant hemopathy, in addition to the complications already mentioned. Relatively frequently, lymphoid proliferation is replaced, or associated, with proliferation that resembles that of histiocytic sarcoma or Hodgkin's disease. This proliferation is, in fact, an immunoblastic sarcoma due to transformation of the lymphoid proliferation: in the cases studied for lymphocytic markers, cells of reticulosarcomatous aspect were, indeed, B cells with the same surface Ig chains as lymphocytes and thus probably derived from the latter cells.

At variance with chronic myeloid leukemia, which usually progresses to acute leukemia, acute blastic transformation is extremely rare in CLL. In the very rare cases of acute transformation that have been studied immunologically, lymphocytes of the chronic phase and blast cells of the acute phase were shown to belong to the same clone. They contained the same surface Ig, and, in one case, it was even shown that surface Ig of both lymphocytes and blast cells had the same antibody activity.

## MACROGLOBULINEMIA AND RELATED DISEASES

### Waldenström's Macroglobulinemia

Waldenström's macroglobulinemia is characterized by the association of a pleomorphic lymphoid proliferation with a serum monoclonal IgM spike. This disease is the best example of monoclonal B-lymphocyte proliferation with persistent maturation, a concept already considered for most cases of CLL with serum monoclonal Ig. Both diseases are, in fact, very similar. The differences between CLL with an IgM spike and hyperlymphocytic macroglobulinemia are only semantic; chronic lymphocytic leukemia is diagnosed when a relatively monomorphous lymphocytic proliferation, intense hyperlymphocytosis, and an IgM spike of less than 10 g/liter are observed; macroglobulinemia is diagnosed if monoclonal IgM concentrations are high and hyperlymphocytosis is moderate or absent. It is therefore not surprising that both diseases show common characteristics. The presence of high concentrations of IgM in macroglobulinemia, however, does bestow significant additional clinical consequences.

As in chronic lymphocytic leukemia, macroglobulinemia more often affects males than females, at ages 50–70. Studies of families of patients with macroglobulinemia have shown a genetic predisposition. In these families there is either a high incidence of serum monoclonal IgM or abnormalities of serum IgM levels (without monoclonal Ig) and of rheumatoid factors.

#### LYMPHOID PROLIFERATION IN WALDENSTRÖM'S MACROGLOBULINEMIA

The sites of localization of lymphoid proliferation (bone marrow, lymph node, spleen) are very similar to those of CLL. The proliferation is pleomorphic and consists of polymorphic lymphocytes, with all intermediate forms between small lymphocytes and plasma cells, and of moderate percentages of plasma cells. Immunologic studies indicate that these cells are of B-cell lineage and belong to the same clone (since all of them from small lymphocytes up to plasma cells, synthesize a monoclonal surface IgM with the same light chain and eventually possess the same antibody activity as those of the serum monoclonal IgM). Most of these cells also synthesize a surface IgD identical to the IgM in light-chain type, idiotypy, and antibody activity (and, therefore, probably in variable region). However, IgD is absent from the plasma cell surface, which suggested that surface IgD disappears during the course of terminal maturation of B lymphocytes that contain surface IgM; an hypothesis supported by the study of normal differentiation in mice and men. Only plasma cells and a variable but generally low percentage of lymphocytes contain intracytoplasmic IgM in amounts sufficient to be detectable by the usual immunocytochemical methods. It is probable that only these cells secrete IgM. One should note that there is no clear-cut correlation between serum monoclonal IgM level and the extent of the proliferation.

In the blood, hyperlymphocytosis is inconstant and usually moderate. However, even when lymphocyte counts are normal, study of lymphocytic markers shows that the majority of circulating lymphocytes belong to the same B-lymphocyte clone as that of marrow cells, thus explaining the abnormalities seen in mitogen responses analogous to those in CLL. One may therefore consider Waldenström's macroglobulinemia to be a monoclonal proliferation of B lymphocytes with persistence of cellular maturation up to the IgM-producing plasma cells. The analogy to a leukemic process, even in the absence of hyperlymphocytosis is obvious.

As in CLL, the lymphoid proliferation may undergo a modification into immunoblastic sarcoma with the same surface markers as those of the lymphocytic clone. Features of the secondary immunodeficiency, which is at the origin of infectious complications, the high incidence of cancer and autoimmune disorders, and the possible development of bone marrow insufficiency, are very similar to those described for CLL.

PROTEIN ABNORMALITIES

A very high sedimentation rate and hyperproteinemia are generally observed. Electrophoresis shows an abnormal spike in the β2 or γ position. Immunoelectrophoretic analysis of the patient's serum usually permits easy identification of the monoclonal IgM (Fig. 30.4). However, if the IgM is euglobulinic, it may precipitate within the application well and therefore require depolymerization before immunochemical study. The euglobulinic nature of IgM is the basis of the inconstantly positive and nonspecific Sia test (formation of a white flocculent precipitate when a drop of serum is added to distilled water). One should also note that to type its light chains, it may be necessary to isolate the monoclonal IgM by gel filtration or ultracentrifugation on a density gradient. Analytic ultracentrifugation may yield quantitative data on the proportions of high molecular weight constituents. Rarely, serum monoclonal IgM is a monomeric 8S form. Conversely, it is not unusual to find small amounts of subunits associated with the 19S IgM. The urinary output of large quantities of

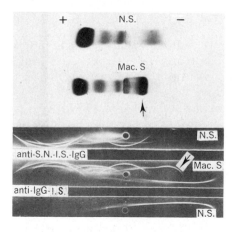

**Fig. 30.4** Macroglobulinemia. Note the existence of a $\beta_2$ peak by electrophoresis. Immunoelectrophoresis (*bottom*) reveals an abnormal line (arrow), the IgM nature of which is revealed by use of a monospecific anti-$\mu$ serum. Study of this IgM, isolated by ultracentrifugation in a density gradient, confirmed its monoclonal nature. NS, normal serum; Mac. S, pathologic serum; anti-SN-IS-IgG, antihuman serum antiserum absorbed by IgG; anti-IgG IS, anti-IgG serum (reacts with $\gamma$, $\lambda$, and $\kappa$ chains).

Bence-Jones protein is very rare, whereas minimal amounts of free urinary monotypic light chains are found relatively frequently.

The consequences of serum monoclonal IgM may be severe and may require repeated plasmapheresis. The hyperviscosity syndrome includes sensory symptoms (ocular, sometimes even amaurosis, hypoacousia), neurologic signs (psychomotor slowing, somnolence, possibly coma), and, occasionally, myocardial failure. Retinal examination shows characteristic lesions. This syndrome is related to IgM intrinsic viscosity and to its serum levels. Hemodilution is usually seen when IgM levels are high and can be documented by radioisotopic measurement of blood volumes. Hemodilution causes a false anemia; however, true anemia (production defect, autoimmune hemolysis) is very common. Hemorrhagic phenomena are also common, observed especially on mucosal surfaces, and relate directly to the serum macroglobulinemia.

When the IgM is a cryoglobulin, clinical manifestations may be severe. Cryoblobulins are of two types. The monoclonal type consists exclusively of IgM. Mixed cryoglobulinemia associates a monoclonal IgM with polyclonal IgG; it actually represents cryoprecipitation of immune complexes in which IgM is an anti-IgG antibody.

### Nonmacroglobulinic Pleomorphic Lymphoid Proliferation

The monoclonal B-lymphocyte proliferation syndrome with persistence of maturation is not limited to macroglobulinemia but may involve surface IgG or IgA lymphocytes. In fact, in certain cases, the proliferation is identical to that of a macroglobulinemia, but the serum monoclonal Ig is an IgG or an IgA. At the cellular level, the findings are similar to those in macroglobulinemia, except for the class of the heavy chain of the monotypic Ig on the lymphocytic surface and in the plasma cell cytoplasm.

In some cases with a similar pleomorphic proliferation, there is no monoclonal Ig in serum or urine or eventually only a urinary Bence-Jones protein, but a monoclonal IgM is present at the cellular level. The results of immunocytochemical studies are identical to those described in macroglobulinemia. Here the questions raised are similar to those mentioned above regarding nonsecretory myeloma.

### Cold Agglutinin Disease

This disease is distinguished by the special antibody activity of the monoclonal serum Ig, which is an antierythrocytic autoantibody (generally of anti-I specificity), active at 4°C. The monoclonal Ig is most often an IgM κ. The bone marrow lymphoid proliferation is usually limited, perhaps because hemolytic anemia permits recognition of the disease at a very early stage. However, a definite number of circulating lymphocytes contain surface Ig (monoclonal IgM and IgD) with antierythrocytic antibody activity.

## BICLONAL PROLIFERATIONS

Combined immunologic study of serum and cells in immunoproliferative diseases has revealed the existence of biclonal proliferation. In most cases, monoclonal Ig light chains are of the same type, suggesting a common origin for both clones. This hypothesis has been confirmed in certain cases where a minor population synthesized both monoclonal Ig and in other cases where the identity of light chains and of variable portions of heavy chains of both Ig was proven.

All combinations with respect to type of proliferation and possible maturation of one or the other clone are possible (Table 30.3). One should note that in double serum monoclonal Ig, when one of the Ig is an IgM, the proliferation is usually pleomorphic, as in macroglobulinemia (Table 30.3, example A3). For some yet unknown reason, when CLL is associated with myeloma (example B in Table 30.3), the myeloma protein often belongs to the IgA class.

Biclonal processes consisting of one B-cell clone and one T-cell clone are not exceptional. In addition, the frequency of the association between a T-cell proliferation (T-CLL or Sézary's syndrome) is too high to be merely coincidental. Studies with antiidiotypic antibodies failed to show a common clonal origin of the two clones. The significance of this peculiar association is not yet known.

**Table 30.3   Examples of Immunoproliferative Syndromes With Double Proliferation**

| Proliferation characteristics | Surface immunoglobulins | Intracytoplasmic immunoglobulins (plasma cells) | Serum monoclonal immunoglobulins |
|---|---|---|---|
| A. Biclonal lymphocytic | | | |
| 1. Cessation of maturation of both clones | IgM κ + IgG κ | 0 | 0 |
| 2. Persistent maturation of one clone | IgM κ + IgG κ | IgG κ | IgG κ |
| 3. Maturation of both clones | IgM κ + IgG κ | IgM κ + IgG κ | IgM κ + IgG κ |
| B. Lymphocytic and plasmacytic | IgM λ + (IgA λ)* | IgA λ | IgA λ |
| C. Biclonal plasmacytic | (IgG κ) + (IgA κ) | IgG κ + IgA κ | IgG κ + IgA κ |

* Parentheses indicate inconsistent detection of immunoglobulins on the plasma cell surface.

# HEAVY-CHAIN DISEASES

Heavy-chain diseases are known for the three main Ig heavy-chain classes, $\alpha$, $\gamma$, and $\mu$. They are characterized by the presence in the serum of a pathologic Ig deficient in light chains and comprising only part of the heavy chains. The absent portion is always located in the Fd region and has a length that varies among patients. Chain deletion has been demonstrated, or at least strongly suggested, in a few cases in which pathologic proteins have been subjected to intense structural study.

Abnormal proteins in heavy-chain diseases are likely to be monoclonal; they belong to one single heavy chain subclass, always $\alpha1$ in $\alpha$-chain disease, and show structural homogeneity. However, they are rarely homogeneous by electrophoresis and usually give rise to broad bands. These abnormalities may be located in the $\alpha$- or $\beta$-globulin area and are often difficult or even impossible to detect by simple electrophoresis, especially if present in small quantity. The same is true for standard immunoelectrophoresis performed with polyvalent antisera. These proteins are often very rich in carbohydrates. They are observed in large amounts in the urine of certain patients with $\gamma$-heavy-chain disease. In $\alpha$- and $\mu$-heavy-chain diseases, they occur in the serum as polymers of variable size.

Biosynthetic studies have shown that the cells synthesize abnormal heavy chains in a form very similar to that of serum Ig. The messenger-RNA coding for the heavy chain is itself abnormally short. However, in the absence of studies at the DNA level, the precise mechanism responsible for this abnormality is still unclear. Recent studies suggest that an abnormal processing (splicing) of pre mRNA, perhaps secondary to a limited defect of the heavy-chain gene located in an area involved in the splicing process (J region?), may play a role in the deletion of a large segment of the polypeptide chain. In addition, a limited post synthetic proteolysis of the amino-terminal part of the heavy chain is probable in some cases and may also account for the amino-terminal heterogeneity of certain heavy-chain disease proteins. There is generally no light-chain synthesis detectable by sensitive biosynthesis experiments. However, monotypic light chains are synthesized by the same cells as those which produce the abnormal heavy chain in about one half of $\mu$-chain disease patients. These light chains do not assemble with heavy chains and are secreted independently as Bence-Jones proteins. Monoclonal light-chain synthesis was also found recently in a few cases of $\gamma$- and $\alpha$-heavy-chain diseases. This observation and the result of the study of murine models of heavy-chain diseases suggest that the light-chain gene might be present and transcribed, but that its translation might be altered in most cases.

The clinicopathology of heavy-chain diseases is different from that of myeloma and is fairly characteristic for each type of disease. In common forms of $\gamma$-heavy-chain disease, men older than 35 are usually affected, with a pleomorphic lymphoplasmacytic proliferation that involves lymph nodes, liver, spleen, and bone marrow. Sometimes tonsillar erythema and uvular edema may suggest the diagnosis; these signs are inconstant, though. Alpha-chain disease involves the secretory IgA system. The gastrointestinal form is the most common type, with lymphoplasmacytic proliferation throughout the small intestine and mesenteric lymph nodes. Intestinal villous atrophy and a severe intestinal malabsorption syndrome usually develop. An immunoblastic transformation has been observed in several patients. In others, simple antibiotic treatment has had a remarkable effect, and the existence of apparently complete remissions without further therapy raises the question of whether the initial stages of the disease correspond to a malignant process. The gastrointestinal form affects young subjects in particular geographic areas, namely, North Africa, the Middle East, Far East, southern Europe, and South America. This geographic predilection possibly indicates an antigenic stimulation by intestinal microorganisms. Respiratory forms are rare but can be observed in Caucasian populations. Mu-chain diseases generally present a symptomatology of CLL. The bone marrow may contain vacuolated plasma cells of a peculiar aspect.

The individual clinicopathologic pattern is not necessarily this clear-cut. For instance, in a patient whose age, geographic origin, and anatomoclinical symptoms suggested gastrointestinal α-chain disease, it was actually diagnosed as γ-heavy-chain disease.

## CRYOGLOBULINEMIAS

Cryoglobulins are serum globulins that precipitate at temperatures below 37°C. The precipitation temperature is highly variable, however; sometimes it is very close to the internal temperature of the organism, thus necessitating collection and separation of serum at 37°C. The amount of cryoglobulins is also highly variable; to demonstrate certain small cryoglobulins, prolonged storage at 4°C may be required.

### Immunochemical Characteristics

Immunochemical studies of purified cryoglobulins enable one to distinguish three types.

Group-I cryoglobulin is exclusively a monoclonal Ig, usually IgM or IgG, but occasionally IgA or Bence-Jones protein. The mechanism of cryoprecipitation is poorly understood but probably relates to the molecular structure of the monoclonal Ig.

Group-II cryoglobulins are mixed and have two Ig constituents, one of which is monoclonal. These cryoglobulins are generally IgM-IgG complexes in which the monoclonal IgM has anti-IgG antibody activity, and the IgG is polyclonal. The isolated IgM does not cryoprecipitate; cryoprecipitation reoccurs when normal IgG is added. Less commonly, the anti-IgG antibody is a monoclonal IgA or IgG.

Group-III cryoglobulin is mixed, polyclonal, and usually contains heterogeneous IgM and IgG (sometimes IgM, IgG, and IgA). These cryoglobulins may represent immune complexes of immunoglobulins (polyclonal IgG) and anti-immunoglobulins (IgM). One may sometimes also demonstrate antigens other than Ig within these cryoglobulins, such as polysaccharides or nucleic acids. The cryoprecipitate may then be constituted of antibodies of various classes that react with the antigen. There may also be an interaction between polyclonal rheumatoid factors and IgG antibodies, which are themselves complexed to the antigen (see p. 732).

### Clinical Signs

In view of this immunochemical heterogeneity, it is not surprising that patterns of clinical symptoms of cryoglobulins are complex. One must differentiate signs due to cold exposure from those common to immune complex diseases, in which the contribution of cold is most inconstant. The most common symptoms are cutaneous (vascular purpura, necrosis of exposed parts) and vasomotor (Raynaud's syndrome, erythrocyanosis). Less frequently, arthralgia is seen. Most worrisome are the renal and neurologic lesions (usually chronic renal failure and sometimes acute glomerulonephritis).

Accidents due to cold exposure (severe Raynaud's syndrome, necrotic purpura, gangrene) are usually observed in the monoclonal cryoglobulins with high serum levels. Mixed cryoglobulin accidents are represented especially by chronic vascular purpura; other vasomotor signs are inconspicuous. A cryoglobulin may be discovered because of a systematic examination or because of biologic abnormalities like variations in sedimentation rate according to temperature, erythrocytic autoagglutinability, unexpected variations in serum proteins or low $\gamma$-globulin levels.

### Associated Diseases

The immunochemical characterization of cryoglobulins has a definite interest in terms of etiology, because associated diseases are clustered according to the type of cryoglobulin. It is not surprising, thus, that monoclonal cryoglobulins and those with a monoclonal constituent are observed mostly in immunoproliferative diseases (myeloma, macroglobulinemia, CLL, sarcomas). Conversely, polyclonal cryoglobulins are associated with autoimmune diseases (Sjögren's syndrome, rheumatoid arthritis, systemic lupus erythematosus), with diseases commonly associated with autoimmune abnormalities (thus, during the course of CLL, one may observe various cryoglobulin varieties), and with certain bacterial, viral, and parasitic infections.

Finally, in some cases, the cryoglobulin is idiopathic. This label is only applied after extensive examination and several years' follow-up because symptoms secondary to the presence of cryoblobulin may lead to its early discovery at a time when the disease responsible for the cryoglobulin is still completely latent.

## NON-HODGKIN'S LYMPHOMAS

As a result of lymphocytic marker studies, the great majority of lymphomas may be classified as monoclonal proliferations of B-lymphocyte origin. This is the case for nodular lymphomas, irrespective of their pathological type.

### Well-Differentiated Lymphocytic Lymphomas

It is not surprising that this process is B cell in origin, because it is very similar to CLL. This disease is considered by most authors to be a form of lymphocytic leukemia localized in lymph nodes.

### Burkitt's Lymphoma

Burkitt's lymphoma is composed of cells of B-lymphocyte origin, both in the African form of the disease (in which a close relationship to Epstein-Barr virus is known) and in cases observed in America and Europe (in which Epstein-Barr virus is often absent from the cellular genome). In about 2% of patients with acute lymphoblastic leukemia, the blast cells appear to be identical to Burkitt's cells and may be immunologically classified as B cell in orgin.

### Poorly Differentiated Lymphocytic Lymphomas

In most cases, blast cells express various B-cell markers, especially surface monoclonal Ig, which here, as in Burkitt's lymphoma, is present in high density. In some cases, no lymphocytic markers are found, and cells in a few rare cases have a T-cell origin.

## SERUM MONOCLONAL IMMUNOGLOBULINS IN THE ABSENCE OF IMMUNOPROLIFERATIVE DISEASES

This definition should exclude this case from our immediate consideration. However, its clinical importance justifies brief mention. It turns out that serum monoclonal Ig spikes are seen not infrequently in the absence of the above-described diseases. They may be found in patients affected with various diseases (primary immunodeficiency, Gaucher's disease, papulous mucinosis, certain cases of connective tissue diseases, cirrhosis, bacterial or viral infections) and even in apparently normal individuals, especially the elderly (3% of subjects older than 70).

There are at least three findings that are useful in distinguishing "benign monoclonal gammopathies" from "malignant gammopathies": a small quantity of circulating monoclonal Ig (less than 1 g%), the absence or only minimal amounts of Bence-Jones protein (Bence-Jones proteinuria in excess of 1 g/liter is seldom observed in the absence of immunoproliferative diseases), and normal levels of normal Ig. None of these features is absolute, however. Even when all three are present, they do not guarantee diagnosis of benign gammopathy. One is therefore often hesitant to accept this diagnosis, despite thorough hematologic exploration. The tests must be serially repeated, and the evolution of the disease must be carefully studied. If the monoclonal Ig concentrations clearly increase during the subsequent months or within one year, there is probably an underlying proliferative disorder. Stability of monoclonal Ig concentrations is a good prognostic finding. Regression or spontaneous disappearance of a spike strongly suggests that malignant proliferation is not present.

## IV.   T-LYMPHOCYTE PROLIFERATIONS

These proliferations are much rarer than B-lymphocyte proliferations. A monoclonal nature is likely but cannot be proven due to a lack of clonal markers for T lymphocytes.

## SÉZARY'S SYNDROME

This syndrome is clinically characterized by a significant erythrodermia that features edema, pigmentation, and cutaneous infiltration. The blood and skin contain very peculiar cells that have been well characterized morphologically and cytogenetically. These cells may infiltrate lymph nodes, bone marrow, and various tissues but are especially attracted to the epithelium. Sézary cells are sometimes stimulated by phytohemagglutinin, form spontaneous rosettes with sheep red blood cells, and react with specific immune anti-T sera. They do not express any B-lymphocyte markers. Sézary cells correspond to relatively mature T cells since they are capable of expressing the functions of differentiated T cells, such as "helper" function.

Mycosis fungoides is similar to and may be a simple clinical variant of Sézary's syndrome. The immunologic characteristics of the two diseases are, indeed, very similar.

## CHRONIC LYMPHOCYTIC LEUKEMIA AND LYMPHOMAS

Recall that the proliferating lymphocytes in CLL are very rarely of T-cell origin. The incidence of these minority cases is very small in Caucasians (only 2 in a series of 130 random patients). However, T cell-derived CLL is perhaps not as rare as was first believed, since 23 cases were recently observed in the same hematology department. The clinical features are often peculiar and consist of splenomegaly, moderate blood and bone marrow involvement, skin lesions, and unusual cytologic and cytochemical characteristics of the lymphocytes. Interestingly, the majority of the unusual cases of chronic lymphocytic leukemia seen in Japan represent T-cell proliferation. T-cell origin has also been documented in rare cases of diffuse poorly differentiated lymphocytic lymphoma, especially in children (lymphoblastic lymphoma in recent classifications) in whom the disease appears to be closely related to acute lymphocytic leukemia (ALL). As discussed below, ALL is clearly of T-cell origin, in about 25% of cases.

A few cases have been reported in which CLL lymphocytes express both T- and B-cell lymphocytic markers. Such findings require careful study because of possible errors in evaluating the lymphocytic markers (Table 30.4). In addition, one must take into account the fact that there is no absolute specificity of some B-lymphocyte markers (IgG Fc receptors, C3 receptors).

## MONONUCLEAR SYNDROMES

Although these syndromes are not, properly speaking, proliferative, for the sake of completeness, it is noteworthy that most large mononucleated cells in infectious mononucleosis and related syndromes are T lymphocytes, most of which express a suppressor phenotype.

**Table 30.4   Examples of Leukemic Lymphocytes Which Appear to Express Both B- and T-Cell Markers**

| Disease | Sheep red blood cell rosettes | Surface immunoglobulins | Binding of aggregated IgG | T-lymphocyte specific antiserum |
|---------|-------------------------------|-------------------------|---------------------------|---------------------------------|
| A*      | +                             | +                       | +                         | —                               |
| B†      | +                             | +                       | —                         | +                               |
| C‡      | +                             | +                       | +                         | +                               |

\* In patient A, a B-lymphocyte proliferation synthesized a monoclonal surface IgM with anti-Forssman antigen antibody activity. This antigen is borne by sheep red blood cells and lymphocytes formed immune rosettes with sheep red blood cells.

† In patient B, proliferation was of T-lymphocyte origin, and immunoglobulins found on the cell surface were not synthesized by lymphocytes.

‡ In patient C, a very unusual case, the cells have expressed both B- and T-cell characteristics.

# V.   PROLIFERATIONS OF HETEROGENEOUS OR UNCERTAIN CLASSIFICATION

Either because of insufficient study or of discrepancies in results of lymphocytic marker studies, the exact classification of some proliferative disorders is uncertain. Thus, indications for inclusion of some malignant diseases as immunoproliferative syndromes are still not well established. In addition, lymphocyte marker studies revealed the heterogeneity of certain diseases which appeared to be homogeneous upon morphological criteria.

## ACUTE LYMPHOBLASTIC LEUKEMIA (ALL)

### B-Derived ALL

A B-lymphocyte origin is rare among unselected cases of ALL (about 1% of cases) and it correlates with a very poor prognosis. More frequently (2% of ALL cases), the blast cells present the cytological, cytochemical, and electron microscopic characteristics of Burkitt lymphoma cells (ALL of the L3 type in the recent FAB classification). Cytogenetic studies have demonstrated the same characteristic translocations as in classical Burkitt lymphoma. The homogeneity of this syndrome is also outlined by immunological studies. In virtually every case, the blast cells are B-cells bearing high density surface IgM with little or no surface IgD (sIg belonging to the IgG or the IgA classes feature very rare cases). IgG Fc receptor is lacking in about one half of cases. Small amounts of serum monoclonal Ig of the same type as the monoclonal surface Ig were recently found in several cases. In one case, where the cells lacked B-cell markers, it was, in fact, a pre-B leukemia (see below). The identification of this subgroup of ALL, which is easy upon morphologic and immunologic grounds, is of clinical importance because of the very poor prognosis with a medium survival of 4 months.

### T-Derived ALL

The cells from approximately 20% of patients with ALL belong to the T-cell lineage. These T-blasts are E-rosette positive (although this is not a constant feature), they react with xeroantisera to T cells or with monoclonal anti-T cell antibodies and they often show particular cytochemical features (acid phosphatase positivity). T-derived ALL is more often observed in boys aged 6–10. It may present a distinct clinical picture with mediastinal mass, higher white cell counts and tumoral presentations, shorter remissions, and poorer prognosis than in common ALL.

### Non-T Non-B ALL and Pre-B ALL

In the majority of cases, the lymphoblasts do not express any of the usual lymphocytic markers leading to the designation of non-T, non-B ALL. Positive findings in this group is that of antigenic determinants, recognized by xeno-antisera or monoclonal antibodies (common ALL antigen), of the enzyme terminal deoxynucleotidyl transferase (TdT), which is normally found in immature cells (and also in T-ALL). The exact nature of the blast cells has been a matter of controversy but it is now clear that most cases are related to the B-cell line. Indeed, in a significant proportion of the cases (16.7% in a series of 311 ALL cases), the blast cells resemble pre-B cells. Pre-B cells are the first cells in the B-line to be identifiable by cytochemical methods. Both normal and leukemic pre-B-cells contain intracytoplasmic μ-chains, most often without light chains, in the absence of surface Ig. Intermediate pre-B/B phenotype (with scant amounts of surface μ-chains) has been observed in a few cases. Rarely, intracytoplasmic Ig in pre-B leukemia may belong to the IgG class which suggests that isotype switching may be operative at a very early stage of the B-cell development. Pre-B leukemia does not differ significantly from the other cases of non-T, non-B ALL in terms of clinical parameters and survival. In fact, common non-B, non-T ALL lymphoblasts (without intracytoplasmic Ig) probably correspond to a more immature stage in the B-line as shown by the finding of specific B-cell antigen identified by monoclonal antibodies and by the study of Ig gene rearrangement.

Recent work has provided new insight into the immunological nature of the blast cells in ALL. It is now clear that ALL may be divided in several groups according to the immunological nature of the cells, and that this immunological classification has a prognostic significance.

## POORLY DIFFERENTIATED HISTIOCYTIC LYMPHOMA LARGE CELL LYMPHOMA

This tumor probably represents a heterogeneous group, because in the few cases studied, surface markers have been very variable. There is no lymphocytic marker in the majority of cases, and, only rarely, has a monocytic, B-lymphocyte, or T-lymphocyte origin been demonstrated. In most cases with B-cell features, the lymphoma was supervening on a well-characterized B-lymphocyte proliferation (CLL, Waldenström's macroglobulinemia, heavy-chain disease, or no-dular lymphoma). It is worth mentioning that in the mixed small and large cell lymphoma (mixed lympho-hystiocytic lymphoma) all proliferating cells display the same phenotype, and, therefore, probably correspond to the same clone. This phenotype is variable and the results of immunological study are quite similar to those obtained in large cell lymphomas.

## HODGKIN'S DISEASE

Contradictory findings have been reported in Hodgkin's disease. Three hy-potheses have been suggested, giving a monocytic or a B- or T- lymphocyte origin to Reed-Sternberg's cells. Recent data strongly argue against a lympho-cytic origin. Hodgkin's disease is often associated with a severe deficiency of cellular immunity.

## HAIRY CELL LEUKEMIA (LEUKEMIC RETICULOENDOTHELIOSIS)

This disease is characterized by huge splenomegaly, commonly a pancytopenia, a characteristic monocytopenia and the presence in the blood, spleen, and bone marrow of particular cells with a hairy appearance. The nature of these cells is a matter of controversy, because they appear to show both monocytic (phagocytic properties, high-affinity Fc receptors), B-lymphocyte (synthesis of monotypic surface Ig) characteristics, and even T-cell markers in some cases. In fact, the properties of hairy cells vary from patient to patient and also possibly from time to time and from organ to organ in the same patient. In vitro stimulation of hairy cells by various mitogens leads to striking phenotypic changes (switch from a B- to a T-phenotype, for instance) and this probably explains the controversies in the literature.

## *BIBLIOGRAPHY*

AZAR H. A. and POTTER M. Multiple myeloma and related disorders. New York, 1973, Hagerstown, Harper & Row.

BERGSAGEL D. E. Plasma cell myeloma. An interpretation review. Cancer, 1972, *30*, 1588.

BRODER S. and WALDMANN T. A. Immunologic defects in patients with plasma cell neoplasms. *In*: Clinical Immunology Update. Elsevier, New York, 1979, p. 1.

BROUET J. C., CLAUVEL J. P., DANON F., KLEIN M., and SELIGMANN M. Biological and clinical significance of cryoglobulins. Amer. J. Med., 1974, *57*, 775.

DURIE B. G. and SALMON S. E. Cellular kinetics, staging and immunoglobulin synthesis in multiple myeloma. Annu. Rev. Med., 1975, *26*, 283.

FRANGIONE B. and FRANKLIN E. C. Heavy chain diseases: clinical features and molecular significance of the disordered immunoglobulin structure. Semin. Hemat., 1973, *10*, 63.

FRANKLIN E. C. Mu chain disease. Arch. Intern. Med., 1975, *135*, 71.

MACKENZIE M. R. and FUDENBERG H. H. Macroglobulinemia: an analysis of 40 patients. Blood, 1972, *39*, 874.

MOLLER G. (Ed.) T and B lymphocytes in humans. Transpl. Rev., 1973, *16*.

MOLLER G. Activation and regulation of immunoglobulin synthesis in malignant B-cells. Immunol. Rev., 1979, vol. 48.

PREUD'HOMME J. L., BROUET J. C. and SELIGMANN M. Lymphocyte membrane markers in human lymphoproliferative diseases. *In* M. S. Seligmann, J. L. Preud'homme, and F. M. Kourilsky, Eds., Membrane receptors of lymphocytes. Amsterdam, 1975, North Holland, p. 417.

PREUD'HOMME J. L. and SELIGMANN M. Surface immunoglobulins on human lymphoïd cells. Progr. Clin. Immunol., 1974, *2*, 121.

SELIGMANN M. B and T cell markers in lymphoïd proliferations. New. Engl. J. Med., 1974, *290*, 1483.

SELIGMANN M. The main immunochemical, clinical and pathological features of alpha chain disease. Arch Intern. Med., 1975, *135*, 78.

SELIGMANN M. and BROUET J. C. Antibody activity of human myeloma globulins. Semin. Hemat., 1973, *10*, 163.

TWOMEY J. J. and GOOD R. A. The immunopathology of lymphoreticular neoplasms. Comprehensive Immunology, Vol. 4, Plenum Press, New York, 1978, 763 p.

WARNER N. L. Membrane immunoglobulins and antigen receptors and B and T lymphocytes Adv. Immunol., 1974, *19*, 67.

WARNER N. L., POTTER M., and METCALF D. (Eds.). Multiple myeloma and related immuno globulin-producing neoplasms. UICC Technical Rep. Ser., 1974, *13*, 1.

WILLIAMS R. C. and MESSNER R. P. Alterations in T and B cells in human disease states. Annu. Rev. Med., 1975, *26*, 181.

ZAWADZKI Z. A. and EDWARDS G. A. Non-myelomatous monoclonal immunoglobulinemia. Prog. Clin. Immunol., 1972, *1*, 105.

# Chapter 31

# IMMUNE DEFICIENCY STATES

## Claude Griscelli

I.   PRIMARY LYMPHOCYTE IMMUNODEFICIENCIES
II.  PHAGOCYTIC CELL DEFICIENCIES
III. SECONDARY IMMUNODEFICIENCIES

# I. *PRIMARY LYMPHOCYTIC IMMUNODEFICIENCEIS*

## INTRODUCTION

Since the first observation of agammaglobulinemia by Bruton in 1952, more than a thousand cases that represent more than 20 distinct types of immunodeficiencies (ID) have been reported. The vast majority are hereditary diseases. Their classification is in a state of constant change according to our improving knowledge of applied and basic immunology. Important new information has been gained by demonstration of thymus- and bone marrow-dependent pathways of immunity, recognition of markers that differentiate these two populations, and increased understanding of the maturation of T- and B-lymphocytes and of the regulatory function of T cells on B-cell activity (see chap. 4). The discovery of an enzymatic abnormality [adenosine deaminase (ADA) deficiency] associated with an immune deficiency has led to new approaches to elucidate the intrinsic abnormalities.

The present ID classification is based on the specific immunologic abnormalities, genetic transmission, and clinical symptoms (see Table 31.1 and Fig. 31.1).

## ABNORMALITIES OF THE LYMPHOID STEM CELL

Some deficiencies are characterized by abnormalities that affect both B- and T-cell lines. Because of the complex symptoms seen, they are usually designated

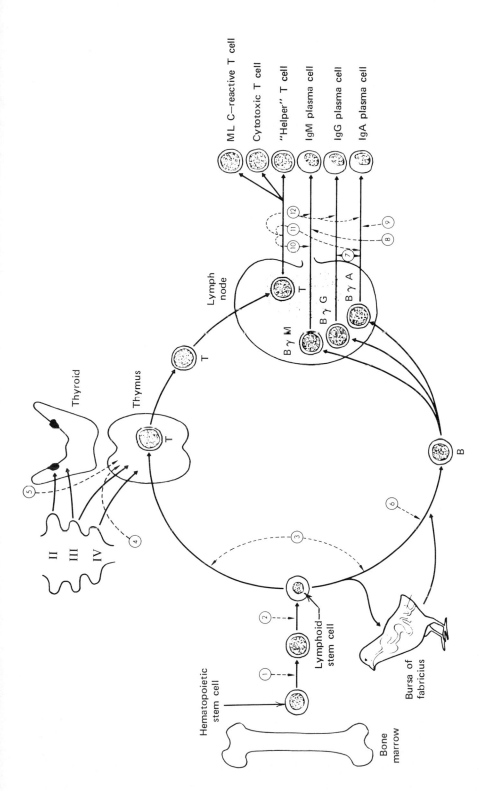

**Fig. 31.1** Mechanisms of the main lymphocytic immunodeficiencies. 1, Reticular dysgenesis; 2, alymphocytosis with agammaglobulinemia; 3, SCID; 4, Di George's syndrome; 5, Nezelof's syndrome (?); 6, agammaglobulinemia with absence of B cells; 7, sex-linked IgG deficiency with increased levels of IgM; 8, dissociated IgM deficiency; 9, IgA dissociated deficiency; 10, Wiskott-Aldrich's syndrome; 11, ataxia telangiectasia; 12, combined partial variable immunodeficiencies.

885

**Table 31.1   Primary Lymphocytic Immunodeficiencies (See Fig. 31.1)**

Abnormalities of the lymphocytic stem cell
  Reticular dysgenesis or global hematopoietic hypoplasia
  Severe combined immunodeficiencies (SCID)
    Alymphocytosis and agammaglobulinemia
    Selective abnormality of T-cell precursors with secondary agammaglobulinemia
    SCID associated with other genetic abnormalities
    SCID with deficient adenosine deaminase
Abnormalities in T lymphocytes (cellular deficiency)
  Absence of thymus and parathyroids (Di George's syndrome)
  Thymic hypoplasia and hypoparathyroidism (partial Di George's syndrome)
  Lymphocytopenia with lymphocytotoxins
  Deficiency in inosine phosphorylase
Abnormalities in B lymphocytes (humoral deficiencies)
  Agammaglobulinemia with B-cell absence
  Sex-linked deficiency of IgA and IgG with hyper IgM
  Dissociated deficiencies in IgM or IgA
Partial T- and B-lymphocyte abnormalities
  ID with thrombocytopenia and eczema (Wiskott-Aldrich's syndrome)
  ID with cerebellar ataxia and telangiectasia
  Hypogammaglobulinemia or variable partial combined deficiency
    Intrinsic B-cell abnormality
    Excess in supressor T cells
Unclassifiable immunodeficiencies
  ID with achondroplastic dwarfism
  ID with effector cell deficiency and melanization abnormalities
  Hypogammaglobulinemia with transcobalamin II deficiency

as "severe combined immunodeficiencies" (SCID). The abnormality occurs at an early stage in differentiation of stem cells to pre-T and pre-B cells. Three types of disorders are recognized (Table 31.1).

### Reticular Dysgenesis

Reticular dysgenesis is characterized not only by major lymphocytic abnormalities but also by hematologic disorders that affect other blood cell types.

### Alymphocytosis with Agammaglobulinemia

Alymphocytosis with agammaglobulinemia is the most severe isolated lymphocytic abnormality, with total absence of cell-mediated and humoral immunities. This is a genetically acquired disease transmitted by an autosomal recessive gene (Glanzman and Rimiker) or by a sex-linked recessive gene. The abnormality occurs at the level of the lymphoid stem cell, which is incapable of differentiating into T and B cells. The blood film reveals a profound lympho-penia ($<500$ lymphocytes/mm$^3$). The thymus is embryonic in type, containing very few lymphocytes and no formation of Hassall's corpuscles is seen. The lymph nodes are very hyperplastic and lymphocyte-depleted, more so in the superficial cortex (B zone) than in the deeper (T zone) cortex. The medulla is absent and the only cells recognizable are histiocytes. The splenic white pulp is extremely reduced.

### SCID With B Cells Present

SCID with B cells present corresponds to a very different situation defined by a profound deficiency of the T-cell population with retention of B cells. Two main syndromes are observed. These are: (1) selective T-lymphoid precursor deficiency and (2) primary thymic epithelium deficiency

#### SELECTIVE T-LYMPHOCYTE PRECURSOR DEFICIENCY (GRISCELLI)

Selective T-lymphocyte precursor deficiency is a genetic disorder transmitted by an autosomal recessive or sex-linked recessive gene and characterized by the complete absence of T lymphocytes and the exclusive presence of B lymphocytes. The number of circulating lymphocytes is either normal or reduced (1000 to 2500/mm$^3$). Membrane-marker studies reveal the absence of E rosette-forming cells and of cells recognized by anti-T antisera, whereas there is a greatly increased percentage (90 to 100%) of cells bearing the B-cell markers (surface Ig, C3, and Fc receptors). The B lymphocytes of these patients appear to be present in very much increased numbers in absolute terms. Although the majority (60 to 70%) possess both membrane IgM and IgD, a considerable percentage (20 to 30%) only possess membrane IgD. Those membrane IgG that are present are mainly cytophilic (maternal IgG). A few B lymphocytes possess IgA. Despite the presence of B lymphocytes, these patients are usually agammaglobulinemic. In some, the serum levels of IgM are normal or elevated. Antigenic stimulation, even with polysaccharide antigens, fails to induce any antibody production, even when serum IgM is present. There is no proliferative response to mitogenic stimulation, attesting to the absolute deficiency of T lymphocytes, although an MLC response is observed. This is attributable to B lymphocytes, which are capable of proliferation in an allogeneic situation with the help of irradiated stimulator T lymphocytes. Restoration of B-lymphocyte proliferative capacity in response to pokeweed mitogen (PWM) is also observed when the patient's lymphocytes are cocultured with normal T lymphocytes. During these cocultures, the patient's B lymphocytes become capable of maturing into plasmocytes. Nevertheless, after 7 days of culture with PWM, the plasmocytes generated from the B lymphocytes from such patients, with the help of normal T lymphocytes, contain IgM or both IgM and IgD but no IgG or IgA. Such presence of two Ig classes, IgM and IgD, in the same cell is never observed in the normal situation. This may be interpreted as an abnormal state of differentiation, probably linked to the ontogenic development achieved in the complete absence of T lymphocytes. Two to 3 months after an HLA-A-B and D-identical bone marrow graft, the thymus of these patients becomes radiologically visible. T cells appear in the blood and antibodies are produced after stimulation in all the systems so far tested. The immunologic reconstitution is entirely attributable to the T-cell precursors from the donor, which are capable of migrating into the recipient's thymus and undergo maturation with the help of hormonal factors from the patient's thymic epithelium. The serum levels of thymic factor in these patients (M. Dardenne and J. F. Bach) are normal in the first months of life and before marrow transplantation. Studies of cellular chimerism after marrow transplantation from a donor of the opposite sex to the recipient demonstrate that the restitution of humoral function is due to the patient's own B cells. These studies, based on the detection of the Y chromosome by quinacrine fluorescence and examination of the karyotype, reveal, in fact, that only the donor's T cells are detectable in the recipient, whereas the B cells of the patient, which were present before the graft, persist. Study of immunoglobulin allotypes shows that the Ig and subsequently produced antibodies carry the recipient's Gm allotype. These findings suggest that the humoral deficiency is linked to a fault in B/T cooperation resulting from a selective abnormality of T-cell precursors.

### PRIMARY DEFICIENCY OF THE THYMIC EPITHELIUM (PYKE AND GELFAND)

Primary deficiency of the thymic epithelium, suggested by the initial observations of Nezelof, has been developed by Pyke and Gelfand on the basis of a collection of arguments resulting from a study, performed in vitro, in two patients in the same family. The marrow lymphoid precursors of these patients were capable of differentiating into T (E rosettes) and B (antiovalbumin or anti-SRBC plaque-forming cells) lymphocytes when they were cultured on monolayers of normal thymic epithelial cells. Conversely, the patient's own thymic epithelial cells, cultured in vitro, were incapable of inducing the differentiation of normal bone marrow lymphoid precursors. Although these observations suggest the possibility of a primary functional deficiency of the thymic epithelium as the basis of the immune deficiency, confirmation, based on a parallel study of the levels of serum thymic factor (facteur thymique sérique [FTS]) and on immunologic reconstitution by an injection of this factor or by a fetal thymus graft, is awaited.

### SCID With Adenosine Deaminase Deficiency (Giblett)

SCID with adenosine deaminase deficiency is an autosomal recessive-transmitted genetic disorder characterized by an enzyme deficiency of purine metabolism. Adenosine deaminase deficiency affects the erythrocytes and platelets whose functions remain unimpaired as well as the T and B lymphocytes whose functions are severely affected. The levels of intralymphocytic enzyme are less than 0.5% of normal. The functional abnormality seems to be linked with the accumulation of upstream substrates: adenosine, AMP, ADP, ATP, and their respective reduced derivatives. The accumulation of ATP produces a fault in lymphocytic multiplication and differentiation.

The first infections develop at the age of 3 to 6 months. Their severity and type are similar to those seen in other SCIDs. The hemogram shows a lymphocyte count that varies from patient to patient. In general, there is a profound lymphopenia (100–500 mm$^3$). Examination of the membrane markers shows, in some patients, the presence of a reduced number of T and B lymphocytes. There is no proliferative response to mitogenic stimulation, but, in certain cases, the response in MLC and the production of cytotoxic cells is retained. This dissociation is taken as an argument in favor of an abnormality of lymphocyte differentiation caused by the enzymatic deficit whose effect is only expressed beyond the acquisition of MLC responsiveness and cytotoxic cell production. Ig levels vary from patient to patient. The usual persistance of very low Ig levels, especially IgM, and the subnormal production of antibodies in certain patients indicate a residual enzyme activity in B lymphocytes.

Adenosine deaminase (ADA) deficiency is suspected by the presence of morphologic skeletal abnormalities, such as short ribs with concave ends, poorly developed iliac crests, bony metaphyseal spicules on long bones, and the particular appearance of the epiphyseal plate of the inferior part of the descending limb of the ischium. Investigatory studies of enzyme concentration, performed on erythrocytes and then confirmed in lymphocytes, reveal almost absent levels of ADA in the patient and close to 50% of the normal level in the parents, both being heterozygotic. The levels of adenosine and desoxyadenosine in serum and urine are elevated in the patient.

### Diagnosis of SCID

All the different varieties of SCID have in common the same suceptibility to infections and a fatal outcome before the age of 1 year. The most commonly encountered infections are bacterial, viral, or mycotic. Their localization is most often gastrointestinal, giving rise to acute recurrent diarrhea, which then becomes chronic (candidiasis), or pulmonary, taking the appearance of an interstitial mycotic pneumopathy, a viral infection, or an infection with *Pneumocystis carnii*. Attention is usually drawn to the repetitiveness of the infections, their resistance and dissemination under treatment, or by the development of a generalized "BCG-itis" or generalized vaccinia as a result of the profound cell-mediated immunodeficiency. In other cases, the diagnosis is made when the signs of a graft-versus-host (GVH) reaction supervene after an allogeneic blood transfusion. These signs are a morbilliform skin eruption, profuse diarrhea, and pancytopenia with a variable eosinophilia. This picture can also be produced by a disseminated viral infection and only the demonstration of a double lymphocyte population allows the confirmation of a GVH reaction. The presence of a profound lymphopenia, the absence of a thymic opacity on X-rays, and the absence of serum IgM in an infected patient also constitute strongly presumptive evidence for a SCID. The diagnosis is confirmed by the absence of cutaneous reactions after intradermal injection of phytohemagglutinin (PHA), (1 to 3 $\mu$g/0.1 ml), the absence of a small percentage of E rosette-forming cells, and the complete absence of the proliferative response in vitro in the presence of mitogens. The absence of a marked lymphopenia and the presence of serum IgM does not, however, exclude the diagnosis of SCID with B cells present.

The occurrence of one or several deaths before the age of 1 year among the siblings or among the ancestors and maternal family suggests a sex-linked form. Consanguinity is in favor of an autosomal recessive transmission. In a family that has already had a child suffering from SCID, this usually leads to conducting the next childbirth under axenic conditions with protection of the child in a sterile airproof enclosure. In this latter eventuality, the diagnosis may be made after birth by examination of the umbilical cord blood. The study of membrane markers and lymphocyte capacity to respond to mitogens and the estimation of the level of serum thymic factor (FTS) allows confirmation of the presence or absence of the deficiency. In the rare families with ADA deficiency it is theoretically possible to measure the concentration of ADA in cells from the amniotic fluid, with the aim of possibly terminating the pregnancy in cases where the fetus is certainly homozygotic.

### Treatment of SCID

In the case of a generalized disorder of lymphoid stem cells, a selective abnormality of T-lymphoid precursors or ADA deficiency, the most effective treatment is an HLA-A-B-D bone marrow transplant. The chances of finding an HLA-A-B-D genoidentical donor among the siblings is, in fact, reduced because of previous deaths. In the absence of a compatible donor among the siblings, current practice is to look for an HLA-A-B-D-identical donor, whether related or not to the prospective recipient. The chances of finding a suitable donor among the family are greater when consanguinity exists. The chances of finding a nonrelated donor are greater when the histocompatibility groups are of the more frequently occurring types. Considering the risks of a GVH reaction, even when a minimum difference in histocompatibility exists, the choice of donor must be made very carefully, especially when the donor is chosen from outside the family. The study of HLA-A-B-D antigens is completed by a mixed lymphocyte culture (MLC), using irradiated recipient lymphocytes as the stimulator, and by determination of the DR groups, using anti-DR serum-mediated cytotoxicity. In rare cases, it may be useful to examine the production of cytotoxic cells during an MLC between the future donor and the recipient to further evaluate the histocompatibility.

The actual transplantation consists of an intravenous injection of $10^8$ to $10^9$ marrow cells per kg. No particular preparation of the transfused cells is necessary apart from filtration to remove the fatty islets. The patient whose cellular immunity is profoundly affected requires only anti-infectious treatment as preparation. When the graft "takes," it leads to a complete immunologic reconstitution, although this may be delayed for 1 to 6 months, during which serious infections may supervene. The anti-infectious protection may be ensured by confinement of the child in an airproof sterile enclosure or exposure to a laminar air flow. Decontamination of an airproof enclosure by the use of appropriate nonabsorbable antibiotics is justifiable when one or several highly pathogenic bacterial strains are present in the enclosure. Gastrointestinal lesions, observed in a GVH reaction, even when apparently perfect histocompatibility exists, may actually favor the development of an enterobacterial septicemia. The success rate of bone marrow transplantation for SCID is currently greater than 70%, when ideal conditions for the choice of donor and bacterial protection exist. Ten years experience since the earliest bone marrow grafts (Good et al) give good reason to hope that under ideal conditions such grafts will become increasingly successful.

In the absence of a histocompatible marrow donor, it has, in the past, been necessary (in certain cases), to transfuse semi-identical marrow or blood stem cells, purified on an albumin gradient (Dicke and Van Bekkum), provided by one of the two parents. This practice has now been abandoned because of the grave risks of a fatal GVH reaction. The transplantation of lymphoid tissue (liver and/or thymus) from a 9- to 12-week fetus in the form of an intraperitoneal injection of dissociated cells for thymus and transfusions of suspended liver cells may produce immunologic reconstitution with the establishment of chimerism. The outcome of these grafts, however, is risky. The reconstitution obtained is, in fact, only partial, usually being limited to cellular immunity (even when fetal liver is used). The risks of acute or chronic GVH disease are not negligible and a progressive exhaustion of the grafted cell population is frequently observed.

In those cases in which a primary failure of the thymic epithelium is diagnosed, one may attempt to perform a fetal thymus transplant, a transplant of cultured thymic epithelial cells (Hong et al), or inject bovine thymic extracts, such as thymosin (described on p. 951) (Wara and A. Goldstein). These attempts are faced with the difficulties involved in determining with any certainty the existence of the failure of the thymic epithelium in a given SCID. The results so far obtained are still very limited and poorly documented.

## ISOLATED T-LYMPHOCYTE ABNORMALITIES

### Di George's Syndrome

Congenital absence of the thymus and parathyroids defines Di George's syndrome. This syndrome is an embryopathy in which abnormal development of the third and fourth branchial arches occurs. The existence of possible hereditary transmission is suggested by family studies. Immunologically, it is characterized by complete absence of T-cell function, as observed in mice after neonatal thymectomy (see p. 61). T cells, recognized by their various markers, are not present in the peripheral blood, in paracortical thymus-dependent zones of lymph nodes, and in the periarteriolar zone of the splenic white plup (which is very hypoplastic). Conversely, B cells are present in these organs and in the blood.

B-cell maturation is normal, and plasma cells are observed. Antibody synthesis after antigenic stimulation is normal. This normal reaction was not anticipated, because neonatally thymectomized and nude mice (nu/nu), which lack a thymus, show maturation abnormalities of B cell-derived IgG and IgA plasma cells, which are correctable by thymus grafting. Despite the absence of T cells, lymphocytopenia is not severe (between 1500 and 3000/mm$^3$); circulating lymphocytes are null or B lymphocytes. The bone marrow contains T-cell precursors capable of expressing T-cell markers after incubation with thymic extracts (specific heteroantigens detected by a cytotoxicity test using an anti-T cell serum or E rosette formation). The diagnosis is usually made on the basis of neonatal tetany secondary to parathyroid absence. The association of other malformations, including abnormalities of the thoracic arch vessels, Fallot's tetralogy, retrognathism, or hypertelorism is also very suggestive. Absence of the thymic shadow is also confirmatory but may be difficult to perceive in cases with an associated cardiomyopathy (which may give a false thymic shadow).

Lymphocytopenia is variable. Immunologic studies show absence of delayed hypersensitivity (DH) reactions, and negative phytohemagglutinin (PHA) intradermoreaction. T-cell deficiency is confirmed by in vitro tests that show no rosette formation and an absence of lymphocytic response to PHA or con A and in the mixed-lymphocyte reaction. The levels of serum immunoglobulin are normal or elevated. Antibody synthesis varies from patient to patient and shows a dissociated pattern, being null for some antigens but moderate or normal for others. The percentage of B lymphocytes is increased (30 to 60%), and B cells express all the appropriate membrane markers and are capable of proliferation and maturation into plasmocytes in the presence of PWM and of allogeneic T cells. These patients suffer severe viral, fungal, bacterial, or parasitic infections leading to death, despite the presence of antibodies. Nephrocalcinosis is observed in 50% of autopsied cases.

In addition to these complete forms, partial Di George's syndromes exist (Table 31.2) that are characterized by the presence of an ectopic thymus in the cervical region that is sometimes palpable. In these cases, a partial deficiency in T-cell function is observed. The parathyroids may also lie in an ectopic position and exhibit impaired function. The abnormalities vary from case to case, and diagnosis is much more difficult to make than in the complete form. In the majority of cases, it is the association of a transitory or persistent neonatal hypoparathyroidism together with a cardiac malformation that leads to the search for a cellular immune deficiency. Immunologic investigation then reveals weak or normal cutaneous responses to PHA, a percentage of E rosette-forming cells of 15 to 50%, and a high percentage of "null" cells (30 to 40%). These "null" cells do not express any of the classical T- or B-cell markers and correspond to pre-T cells, as is revealed by an anti-T cell serum and their capacity, in vitro, to acquire E rosette-forming capacity in the presence of thymic extracts. Proliferative responses to mitogenic stimulation or in MLC are normal and the production of cytotoxic cells is obtained in mixed-lymphocyte culture. Often a hypergammaglobulinemia is seen, mainly due to IgA and IgE, but also to IgG, antibody synthesis being normal or even excessive in all the systems studied. B-cell hyperactivity may be a reflection of a fault in suppressor function exerted physiologically by T cells in the neonatal period. The leukocytes of infants suffering from a partial Di George's syndrome differentiate with abnormal rapidity into IgM, IgA, and IgG plasmocytes when cultured for 7

**Table 31.2  Comparison of Complete and Partial Di George's Syndromes**

|  | T cells evaluated by sheep red blood cell rosettes (%) | Cardiac malformations | Parathyroid abnormalities | Spontaneous correction of T-cell abnormalities |
|---|---|---|---|---|
| Complete Di George's syndrome | <2 | Variable | Constant | Possible within a few years |
| Partial Di George's syndrome | 15–30 | Variable | Variable (deep or moderate) | Frequent |

days in the presence of PWM. The T cells of these patients do not appear to exert their usual suppressor effect when cocultured with allogeneic B cells and PWM. Finally, it can be seen that the immunologic abnormalities are relatively modest, especially when current investigations are employed. The diagnosis of thymic hypoplasia is difficult and only detectable by using a number of criteria among which the detection of a low level of serum thymic factor (FTS) is particularly valuable.

The natural history of partial Di George's syndrome is difficult to predict in any individual case. The immediate prognosis is predominantly determined by the severity of the possible cardiac malformation. There is some degree of susceptibility to infection, particularly during the first few months of life in a hospital environment, infection with resistant organisms being especially severe. The partial deficiency in cellular immunity persists for several years. The concept that a spontaneous progressive correction of the deficiency occurs in certain patients has not been documented in any publication.

Treatment of Di George's syndrome requires one or several fetal thymus transplants. Correction of some of the immunologic abnormalities is extremely rapid, taking only a few hours, as is shown by lymphoblastic proliferation in the presence of PHA. The rapid response to treatment is compatible with the action of a hormonelike substance secreted by the thymic epithelium. This hypothesis suggests that Di George's syndromes might be corrected by substitution therapy with purified thymic extracts. We have observed, in one case of Di George's complete syndrome treated with bovine thymus fraction V (A. Goldstein), full normalization of the number of E rosette-forming cells and restoration of the capacity to proliferate in response to mitogenic stimulation and in MLC (Griscelli et al). The treatment of the cardiac malformation is determined by the type of anomaly that is present. It is usual to advise no treatment in those cases suffering from a complex cardiac malformation. Hypoparathyroidism is corrected by the use of vitamin D and calcium. In the neonatal period, injections of parathormone are often necessary.

### Other Syndromes

Lymphocytopenia with lymphocytotoxin is a rare syndrome characterized by hypergammaglobulinemia and lymphocytopenia (T lymphocytes). It relates to the presence of a complement-dependent lymphocytotoxin. A D-chromosomal abnormality is observed. A fatal outcome may be due to infection or to development of reticulosarcoma.

Inosine phosphorylase (IP) deficiency, of which there are three recorded cases, occurs, like ADA deficiency, at the level of purine metabolism, affecting the transformation of inosine into hypoxanthine. It causes an apparently isolated deficiency of cellular immunity. The first signs of infection appear late after the first year of life. In one case, the administration of BCG at the age of 3 months provoked a positve cutaneous tuberculin response without the dissemination of the BCG. The same child died of generalized vaccinia at the age of 17 months. The observation of a progressive "malignant" chickenpox in another patient appears to indicate a particular susceptibility to viral infections. The association of an anemia of central origin has been observed in one of the recorded cases.

Immunologic investigation reveals a moderate lymphopenia that mainly involves the T-cell population. The percentage of E rosette-forming cells is low, being of the order of 15 to 20%. The capacity to proliferate in response to mitogenic stimulation and MLC (allogeneic) is low but not completely absent. The B-cell populations appear to be unaffected, and they are present in normal numbers in the peripheral blood. The levels of serum immunoglobulins are normal as is the capacity for antibody synthesis. Anatomical study of one case (Nezelof and Griscelli) has shown a hypoplastic thymus containing few thymocytes but Hassall's corpuscles were present. The thymus-dependent zones of the splenic white pulp and the deeper cortex of lymph nodes are hypoplastic, but the B-zones and plasmocytes containing the three main classes of Ig appear to be normally developed.

IP deficiency, whose metabolic consequences are comparable with those described in ADA deficiency, is transmitted in an autosomal recessive manner. It affects both lymphocytes and erythrocytes. The heterozygotic subjects, whose enzyme levels are about 50% of the normal level, are readily detectable. It is possible that in the future it will be possible to detect the abnormality prenatally.

## B-LYMPHOCYTE ABNORMALITIES

### Sex-Linked Agammaglobulinemia (Bruton's Disease)

In principle, sex-linked agammaglobulinemia is defined by the absence of B lymphocytes from blood and peripheral lymphoid organs, associated with a total agammaglobulinemia in a boy. The existence of familial cases involving a brother or a maternal uncle, provides an important argument in favor of the diagnosis. The absence of B lymphocytes from the blood is demonstrated by the study of all the B-lymphocyte markers, including surface Ig, IgG, Fc, and C3 receptors and B lymphocyte-specific xenoantigens. In the peripheral lymphoid organs, the B zones of the splenic white pulp and superficial cortex are atrophic. There are no germinal centers and plasmocytes are absent, as much from these organs as from the gastrointestinal tract. However, immunofluorescent studies of the medullary lymphoid cells reveal the presence of a small number of lymphocytes containing traces of intracytoplasmic IgM (Cooper). These cells are normally detected in the bone marrow. They are thought to be pre-B-cell precursors. The cellular abnormality in sex-linked agammaglobulinemia therefore occurs at the early stages of B-lymphocyte maturation. It is possible that this abnormality is due to a microenvironmental deficiency that is necessary for this maturation, comparable with that which exists at the level of the bursa of Fabricius in birds. These B-cell abnormalities are associated with major alterations in antibody synthesis.

The T-cell population is normal in number, representing almost all of the peripheral blood cells. The E-rosette percentage is greater than 85 to 90%. T-lymphocyte functions are normally expressed, both in vivo and in vitro. However, the presence of T lymphocytes and non-T cells (macrophages or null cells) has been described in peripheral blood, which have a suppressor effect on the maturation of B lymphocytes into plasmocytes when cocultured in the presence of PWM (Siegal). This observation is reminiscent of the suppressor-cell population that seems to be present in excess in certain chickens rendered agammaglobulinemic by bursectomy.

The first infections occur around the age of 3 months when most of the maternal IgG has disappeared. These infections are mainly bacterial and usually confined to the ear, nose, and throat region, bronchial tree, and digestive tract. They may be the origin of the development of septicemia or meningitis. Recurrent bronchial infections are responsible for bronchiectasis that are initially localized but later more diffuse, causing respiratory insufficiency in adolescence. Certain viruses, such as enterovirus may give rise to serious infections. Vaccinial poliomyelitis has been described and echovirus neuromeningitis has also been observed. Intestinal infections with *Giardia* is often seen and, when untreated, may result in intestinal malabsorption. The treatment of these infections is initially performed by means of preventive intramuscular injections of gammaglobulins (0.5 ml/kg of a 16% preparation) given twice monthly. Intravenous administration is generally reserved for acute infectious episodes treated in hospital. Curative treatment requires bactericidal antibiotics appropriate to the causative organisms. In some cases with frequent infections and recurrent bronchitic episodes, preventive therapy with alternating use of three antibiotics, prescribed individually for 15 to 20 days per month, may be advised. Regular respiratory physiotherapy reduces the ill effects of bronchial hypersecretion. Intestinal infections due to *Giardia* are treated with repeated doses of metronidazole or quinacrine.

The absence of B lymphocytes may be seen in conditions other than sex-linked agammaglobulinemia. Some of these conditions involve girls and imply other forms of genetic transmission. Isolated humoral deficiencies are also observed, characerized by the total absence of B lymphocytes, contrasting with the presence of low concentrations of serum IgM and normal or elevated levels of IgD and IgE. Although the mechanisms of these deficiencies are certainly different from those of Bruton's disease, the clinical manifestations and prognosis are very similar. It seems as though the allergic manifestations occasionally described in Bruton's disease are more readily observed in those forms in which IgD and IgE are present.

### IgA and IgG Deficiency With Increased Circulating IgM

IgA and IgG deficiency with increased circulating IgM is transmitted by an autosomal recessive gene and is much rarer than complete agammaglobulinemia. Its prognosis is also less severe. IgM-type antibody synthesis is normal. The pathophysiology of this syndrome remains unknown. It may be linked with a maturation abnormality of B-cell populations of the $\mu$ into $\alpha$ and $\gamma$ types.

### Dissociated Deficiencies

Serum IgM deficiency is usually complete without any abnormality of the other Ig class levels. In certain cases, however, it involves a single isolated diminution of IgM levels. B lymphocytes are present in the blood, and cells bearing membrane IgM and IgD are found in normal numbers. The production of antibodies directed against polysaccharidic antigens, such as pneumococcal SIII antigen, is profoundly disturbed. The T lymphocytes are normal in number and quality. The infections observed are usually localized to the ear, nose, and throat, respiratory tract, and meninges and are due to pneumococci, *Hemophilus*, or meningococci. In view of the impossibility of preventing the infections by IgM-class immunoglobulin injections, whose half-life is known to be very short (4 to 5 days), antibiotic therapy with oral penicillin is occasionally prescribed and is given in a continuous manner when the deficiency gives rise to frequent and/or serious infections.

IgA deficiency is common, affecting about 1 individual in 800. Very often asymptomatic and discovered fortuitously, IgA deficiency may, however, be responsible for repeated respiratory, and intestinal infections. These infections are usually only of modest frequency and severity. Allergic manifestations are occasionally seen, in which case elevated levels of serum IgE are frequently present. There is also an abnormal incidence of autoimmune disorders or immunologically based abnormalities (1 to 3% of patients suffering from SLE or rheumatoid arthritis possess an IgA deficiency). IgA deficiency is also frequently associated with gluten intolerance. An explanation for these associations is not yet clearly defined, but they probably do not have a single common origin. The absence of IgA in the gut may explain the abnormal absorption of certain antigens, such a gliadin, responsible for celiac disease. The partial deficiency of T function, sometimes detected in IgA-deficient patients may be the cause of autoimmune processes by reduction of suppressor T cell activity.

IgA-bearing B lymphocytes are normal or increased in number in the peripheral blood. Their presence contrasts with the absence of IgA plasmocytes in all the lymphoid organs, including the tonsils and intestinal mucosa. IgA deficiency is often complete, involving both monomeric IgA, normally synthesized in the bone marrow and tonsils, and dimeric IgA synthesized in the mucosa and tonsils (Brandzaeg). In certain patients, membrane IgA-bearing lymphocytes are capable of maturing into IgA-containing plasmocytes after coculture with normal T lymphocytes in the presence of PWM. This observation suggests that the maturation abnormality of the IgA system may be, at least in those patients, linked to a failure of B-cell and T-cell cooperation. This interpretation appears to be corroborated by the demonstration of excessive suppressor-cell function by the T cells of IgA-deficient patients on the in vitro maturation of normal B lymphocytes into IgA plasmocytes in the same coculture system in the presence of PWM. (Waldmann). Actually, the various IgA deficiencies do not constitute a homogeneous group. The abnormality of T-cell and B-cell cooperation is not found in all the cases, and although certain IgA deficiencies are familial, others appear to be sporadic and acquired, notably after congenital German measles. Finally, the partial deficit in T-cell function is inconstant.

An isolated monomeric IgA deficiency has been reported in some cases (Griscelli and Brandzaeg). Serum IgA, in these circumstances, is present in traces, and medullary IgA plasmocytes are absent. Dimeric IgA are synthesized normally by the IgA plasmocytes of the intestinal mucosa and are secreted normally in the saliva. This observation confirms that the IgA system is composed of two subsystems, one monomeric, the other dimeric, of which only one may be deficient. So far, however, there has been no recorded case of isolated dimeric IgA deficiency.

IgA deficiency with elevated IgE levels may be seen in young children who have repeated infections of the upper respiratory tract. This type of deficiency, apparently associated with microbial allergy, is still incompletely investigated and remains poorly understood.

Deficiency of the secretory component of IgA, described by Strober et al, may have, at the mucosal level, consequences comparable to the abnormalities seen in cases of general IgA deficiency, resulting from a fault in the secretion of dimeric IgA. The two cases described had chronic intestinal candidiasis.

## PARTIAL B- and T-LYMPHOCYTE ABNORMALITIES

This is a group of immunodeficiencies represents a vast panorama of diseases with undetermined nosologic limits and poorly understood pathogenesis.

### Combined Immunodeficiency with Thrombocytopenia and Eczema (Wiskott-Aldrich's Syndrome)

Wiskott-Aldrich's syndrome is transmitted via a sex-linked recessive mode and exhibits symptoms that are difficult to relate to each other. Neonatal thrombocytopenia is peripheral in type and is associated with a thrombopathy with deficient platelet aggregation, abnormal $\alpha$ corpuscles, and, possibly, enzymatic abnormalities in the citric acid cycle. Death occurs in about one-third of cases before the age of 3–4 years. Eczema is chronic but of variable intensity, both among patients and during the life-span of any one patient. The eczema is associated with increased IgE levels. The immune deficiency consists of a deficit in IgM (in 50% of cases), increased serum IgA levels, and, sometimes, decreased IgG levels.

B cells that bear $\mu$ chains are present, even when IgM is deficient. There is also decreased antibody production against some polysaccharide antigens and a decreased number of receptors on monocytes membranes for the Fc fragment of IgG. There is lastly a progressive cellular deficiency, which culminates within a few years in lymphocytopenia, predominately of the T-cell type. Functional T-cell abnormalities involve DH reactions and in vitro lymphoblastic proliferation in response to mitogens and antigens or in mixed-lymphocyte reaction. This partial combined immunodeficiency is responsible for bacterial, fungal, viral, and parasitic infections that may be fatal before 10–15 years of age. The frequency of leukemia and cancer is abnormally high in these subjects.

Substitution treatment is thwarted by thrombocytopenia, which hinders intramuscular γ-globulin injection, which is a rather ineffective treatment for this syndrome, anyway. Steroid therapy does not appear to be particularly effective. Only one bone marrow transplantation has been attempted, but the long-term response to this treatment is not known. Lawrence's transfer factor (see p. 376), which restores DH reactions and in vitro mitogen responses, has been used by numerous investigators, with variable but generally favorable results. The mechanism of action of transfer factor is considered to be both specific for the antigen to which the donor has been immunized and nonspecific, in that DH may be conferred toward antigens apparently not already experienced by the donor.

### Combined Immunodeficiency with Ataxia and Telangiectasia

This autosomal recessive hereditary disease presents three types of abnormalities that are apparently unrelated: cerebellar ataxia, the initial symptoms of which occur at about 2 years of age, is associated with an absence or severely decreased numbers of Purkinje cells; telangiectasias easily visible on the conjunctiva but also present on the skin; and combined partial progressive immunodeficiency, with deficits in IgA (50% of cases) and IgG (3%) in the presence of normal IgM levels. In those cases of deficient serum IgA, the intestinal mucosa contains no IgA but does possess significant amounts of IgM. The cellular deficiency is represented by lymphocytopenia and progressive lymphoid hypoplasia, which worsen with time. The thymus is hypoplastic. The immunodeficiency facilitates bacterial infections, particularly those of the ear and lung, and leads to bronchiectasis. Gastrointestinal infection does not occur. Autoimmune manifestations are very frequent. The syndrome features a high incidence of lymphosarcoma, Hodgkin's disease, and reticulosarcoma. Ten percent of patients afflicted with the disorder die of cancer. In these patients, the recent observation of faults in DNA repair and an abnormal chromosomal sensitivity to x-rays may explain the frequent chromosomal breaks detected by examination of the karyotype. This also suggests that the development of neoplasia involving a leukocyte population may be due to a cellular mutation that more easily occurs because of the abnormalities of DNA repair.

### Hypogammaglobulinemia with Variable Expression

Second only to isolated IgA deficiency, hypogammaglobulinemia with variable expression is the most common ID. It is a heterogeneous entity in the process of diversification and probably consists of several syndromes. These syndromes have several features in common in addition to the association of hypogammaglobulinemia with the persistance of peripheral blood lymphocytes. Thus, this is a very different situation from that in Bruton's disease since the deficiency of Ig production is a consequence of the failure of B lymphocytes to mature into plasmocytes and not of the absence of B lymphocytes.

The syndrome manifests itself, usually by infections or autoimmune phenomena, either early around 2 to 4 years of age, or later in adulthood. Familial cases may be found, but the mode of transmission is not precisely known. Most cases are sporadic. Some types seem to be secondary to a viral infection, such as congenital German measles, HB virus infection, or Epstein-Barr virus. A sex-linked recessive familial susceptibility has been described for EB virus, which is responsible for severe infectious mononucleosis, sarcomas or hypogammaglobulinemia in boys belonging to the same family (Purtillo).

The hypogammaglobulinemia varies from one patient to another and at different times in the same patient. The capacity for antibody synthesis is also variable, and generally dissociated, normal for some antigens, weak or absent for others. The number of circulating B lymphocytes is normal and increases normally during infection (Preud'homme). B cells are also present in the peripheral lymphoid organs. Spleen and lymph-node germinal centers are either absent or present in an exaggerated state of development, but plasmocytes are rare. In some patients splenic and lymph-node hyperplasia are seen that may also involve the intestinal lymphoid tissue. This is probably a reactive hyperplasia in response to antigenic stimulation resulting from chronic or repeated infections. It may disappear with appropriate treatment when it occurs with a bacterial infection that responds to antibiotic therapy. There is an abnormally high incidence of neoplasia, in particular, lymphosarcomas, which develop from B lymphocytes.

The B lymphocytes of these patients are generally incapable of in vitro maturation in response to PWM. The underlying mechanisms for this do not appear to be simple. An intrinsic B-cell abnormality, excessive suppressor T cell, or insufficient helper T-cell activity have all been cited. In the two latter cases, the patient's B lymphocytes are capable of in vitro maturation into plasmocytes when cocultured with normal T lymphocytes and PWM. Conversely, such patients' T lymphocytes, when cocultured with normal leukocytes, may exert a suppressor effect on the plasmacytic maturation of B lymphocytes (Waldmann). The possible inhibition of the suppressor effect by hydrocortisone in vitro has resulted in therapeutic trials of steroid therapy in this condition; but, as yet, the results are difficult to evaluate. The efficacy of other T-cell functions varies from patient to patient. In general, there is a partial deficiency that can only be appreciated by means of more extensive investigation of T-cell function. The individual variations are such that no dissection can be made of T-cell function in a given subject.

The infective complications (bacterial, viral, fungal, or parasitic) are of variable gravity and frequency in different patients. Repeated bronchial infections result in bronchial dilatation and bronchiectasis. Numerous immunologic manifestations, such as rheumatoid arthritis, granulomatous ileitis or colitis, gluten intolerance, polyradiculoneuritis, and, finally, thymoma are often associated with the hypogammaglobulinemia. They may be due to complement-fixing aggregated Ig in the injected preparations or to isoimmunization against Ig (mainly IgA). Immunostimulatory treatment with transfer factor or levamisole may produce some biologic improvement, but the clinical benefits are difficult to establish in a condition with such a varying natural history, and the risks of initiating autoimmune complications must be considered.


# UNCLASSIFIABLE IMMUNODEFICIENCIES

Some immunodeficiencies cannot readily be categorized within the syndromes presented in the preceding pages. We will discuss only four of these unclassifiable immunodeficiencies.


### Immunodeficiency Associated with Achondroplastic Dwarfism

Achondroplastic dwarfism immunodeficiency is an autosomal recessive hereditary syndrome that exhibits variable characteristics, namely, partial combined deficiency, isolated cellular deficiency, or isolated humoral deficiency. A variant of this syndrome features cartilage and integumental abnormalities (cartilage-hair hypoplasia). In the latter, the immunodeficiency is either combined or purely cellular.

### Immunodeficiency with Hypopigmentation

Immune deficiency with hypopigmentation, recently described in four families (Griscelli et al), combines an immune deficiency with a partial oculo-cutaneous albinism. It is a disorder that is transmitted by an autosomal recessive gene and is easily recognized by the accompanying silver coloration of the hair and eyebrows, susceptibility to infection, and a complex hematologic syndrome with pancytopenia and recurrent hypofibrinogenemia, which occurs either spontaneously or is provoked by an infection. This syndrome is reminiscent of Chediak-Higashi disease (CH, see p. 905), whose natural history is subjected to "accelerated phases." Immune deficiency with hypopigmentation is distinct from CH disease, however, since: (1) It is not accompanied by giant leukocyte granulations, such as occur in CH disease. (2) It has the peculiarity of hypopigmentation, linked to an abnormality of melanosome transfer from melanocytes to keratinocytes. This transfer is normally accomplished by the phagocytosis of melanocyte dendrites by keratinocytes and does not occur in this disorder because of the failure of melanocytes to develop dendrites. Because of this, mature melanosomes (stages III and IV) accumulate in the melanocytes, which appear black when stained with Fontana's reagent. (3) The immune deficiency is different. The sensitivity to infectious complications only appears to be partially attributable to a granulocytic abnormality, which, in this case, is characterized by a polar distribution of membrane receptors for Concanavalin A and a moderate deficiency of bactericidal activity. T and B populations are present but possess a complete functional deficiency that is associated with diminished antibody-producing capacity with, in one case, hypogammaglobu-linemia and a defect in cellular immunity. Delayed cutaneous hypersensitivity reactions are absent despite normal in vitro proliferative responses to antigens that induce delayed hypersensitivity. Responses to mitogens in culture and the MLC response are normal, but skin graft rejection studied in one case was extremely retarded. The leukocytes of these patients do not stimulate (in a normal fashion) normal leukocytes in MLC and the production of cytotoxic cells has been found to be profoundly altered in the two patients studied. Finally, the T-cell helper function appears normal, more with regard to normal lymphocytes than those of the patient himself. All these abnormalities suggest the presence of a membrane deficiency involving granulocytes, monocytes, melanocytes, and lymphocytes. Correction of the Con A receptor-distribution abnormality by in vitro incubation with cyclic GMP or one of its activators, carbamyl choline, suggests the existence of a deficiency that affects the intra-cellular metabolism of cyclic GMP.

### Chronic Mucocutanous Candidiasis. A Selective Cellular Deficit

The chronic candidiases are a heterogeneous group in which mucocuta-neous candidiasis occurs, characterized by a selective immune deficiency, apparently isolated, marked by a deficiency of delayed hypersensitivity, prolif-eration, lymphokine production (MIF) in response to *Candida* antigens, and by the presence of large quantities of anti-*Candida* antibodies in the serum. The deficiency appears to vary with time and is particularly evident during relapses of candidiasis, disappearing or at least diminishing during remissions. Recently, the characterization of a specific inhibitor of lymphoblastic proliferation in response to *Candida* antigens has led to the suggestion that the cellular ID may be secondary to the infection and not primary. This inhibitor, which is present in the patient's serum during relapses, is, in fact, composed of the polysaccharide antigens of *Candida* (Fischer et al). This observation is suggestive of a macrophage abnormality in which the macrophages are incapable of effectively catabolizing *Candida* antigens.

Treatments rest principally on the eradication of *Candida* by the use of antifungal agents. Prolonged treatment is often necessary (i.e., several months). The study of in vitro sensitivity of *Candida* to antifungal agents is rendered necessary by the frequency of organism resistance. Immunostimulants alone appear to have no effect, and it is by no means certain that they are beneficial even in combination with antifungal drugs.

### Hypogammaglobulinemia Associated with Transcobalamin II Deficiency

This recently described deficiency (one case) establishes a relationship between vitamin $B_{12}$ metabolism and Ig synthesis. Vitamin $B_{12}$ injection corrected the hypogammaglobulinemia of the patient in question.

## THE IMMUNE DEFICIENCY OF AGING (J. F. BACH)

For several years, there has been a growing interest in the study of changes that occur in the immune system during aging. The immune deficiency observed is not a major one and consequently does not predispose to abnormally frequent or serious infections, although a greater sensitivity to infections in aged persons has been clearly established. Nevertheless, there exist some arguments that suggest that the immune deficiency may play a role in the development of certain disorders in the aged, particularly certain malignancies and autoimmune disorders.

The lymphoid organs involute with age. This evolution is quite clear for the thymus whose weight progressively diminishes after puberty (see p. 20). The diminution in size of the spleen (mainly the white pulp) and lymph nodes is much less obvious. The relative number of B and T cells, as estimated by membrane markers, has been variously estimated. Although such changes occur (for certain authors), the variations remain only moderate and consist of an increased number of membrane Ig-bearing cells and a reduced number of θ-positive cells in the mouse and E rosette-forming cells in man. Perhaps more obvious differences will become apparent when it becomes possible to study lymphocyte subpopulations. The recent demonstration in the mouse of a frank decrease of Lyt 123$^+$ T lymphocytes is interesting in this regard. Clearer results are obtained when one examines lymphocyte functions. Reduced response to PHA, Con A, and in MLC are frequently observed, although the differences observed are relatively modest and the techniques themselves have a very great variability whether employed in young or old subjects. Diminished generation of cytotoxic cells (very early in the mouse) and delayed hypersensitivity reactions are also noted. Finally, concomitant with the diminution of thymic weight with age, there also occurs a fall in the levels of circulating thymic hormone.

Antibody production is less obviously affected, although a diminution in the primary responses to thymus-dependent antigens is observed. The very frequent appearance of autoantibodies, which are often nonpathogenic, is almost certainly linked with the T-cell immune deficiency.

The exact mechanism whereby immune function declines with age is poorly understood. The involvement of serum factors, as suggested by some workers, has not been clearly established. A stem-cell deficiency, notably in their capacity to multiply, may occur. In contrast, impaired phagocytic function cannot be incriminated since their number and function appear to be normal. Although the B-cell number is not altered, their intrinsic function, considered independently of T-cell regulatory activity, tends to diminish with age. In particular, the number of antibody-forming cell precursors against a given antigen is reduced. In fact, it appears that it is at the level of the thymus and T cells that one must look for the causes of age-induced immunologic abnormalities. Adult thymectomy accelerates their development. Conversely, thymus grafts from aged mice are less effective (although still significantly so) in restoring T-cell function in irradiated, thymectomized mice than are thymus grafts from young or newborn mice. Conflicting data has been reported on suppressor T-cell function, which is either augmented or diminished according to different authors. The progressive cessation of thymic hormone and T-cell production may produce a preferential disappearance of the most recently thymic-produced cells, the Lyt $123^+$ cells. The important and complicated role of these cells in regulation of the immune response may explain the sometimes paradoxical variations that have been observed.

## II.   PHAGOCYTIC CELL DEFICIENCIES

### THE NEUTROPENIAS AND AGRANULOCYTOSES

The congenital neutropenias are a group of genetically derived or constitutional disorders that have varying mechanisms and prognoses. About 200 cases have now been recorded.

Their symptomatology is generally that of recurrent bacterial infections of the ear, nose, throat, lung, and skin. The cutaneous lesions are inflamed, painful, slightly purulent, and are complicated by regional lymphadenitis or subcutaneous flares with massive edema, often localized in the cervical or perineal regions. Painful sterile ulcers occur in the oral cavity, throat, or tongue and are frequent and/or repetitive in a cyclical fashion. Physical examination often reveals splenomegaly, even in the absence of infection. Hypogammaglobulinemia and thrombocytopenia are commonly present. Examination of blood and bone marrow films allow the distinction of five main conditions.

#### Congenital Granulocytic Aplasia

Congenital granulocytic aplasia is a deficiency of differentiation characterized by an almost complete absence of medullary granulocytes.

### Deficiency in Granulocyte Proliferation (Kostman)

In deficiency in granulocyte proliferation, the characteristic marrow film reveals the presence of young granulocytes as far as the promyelocyte stage, a few myelocytes, and complete absence of more mature cells. It is a disorder that is transmitted by means of a dominant gene.

These two forms have in common an early onset, in the first few months of life; a serious prognosis; and resistance to all forms of therapy, with corticosteroids and androgens being inactive. The blood film reveals eosinophilia, monocytosis, plasmacytosis, and thrombocytosis (poor prognostic sign) in both types of disease. An HLA-identical bone marrow transplant may correct the agranulocytosis.

### Deficiency of Granulocyte Maturation

In deficiency of granulocyte maturation, the marrow film shows a normal pattern of young granulocytes as far as, and including, metamyelocytes, and almost complete absence of polynuclears. This situation, which is the most common form of constitutional neutropenias, is probably due to a central fault of the granulocyte line because of a maturation deficiency, or it may be a result of an autoimmune peripheral destruction with the reduction of the reserve compartment of the bone marrow, this being reflected in the periphery. The blood film reveals a neutropenia that is less severe than in the first two types but accompanied by a lymphocytosis. The first infections occur early in life (sixth month), but the apparent onset of hematologic abnormalities is difficult to detect. In fact, the early blood films may be normal, and it is only much later, when infection supervenes, that a transitory diminution in the blood granulocyte number is noted. It is only logical that one initially thinks of a drug-induced or infectious neutropenia; but, over the course of several years, the constitutional nature of the disorder becomes evident. The familial incidence has been mentioned but is, in fact, rare. The prognosis is clearly less grave than in the first two forms. Infections are less serious and also less frequent. Spontaneous resolution may take place after several years or after treatment with corticosteroids.

### Deficiency of Polynuclear Migration from the Marrow

Deficiency of polynuclear migration from the marrow is a rare situation characterized by a profound peripheral blood neutropenia and the presence of large number of granulocytes in the marrow. The bone marrow polynuclears may be vacuolated and multisegmental. These abnormalities are due to the aging of the polynuclear cells in the bone marrow and their inability to enter the circulation. The neutropenia is chronic and is responsible for frequent, although moderate, bacterial infections. During each infective episode, in fact, a moderate granulocytic response cooperates with antibiotic therapy to limit the spread of infection. A granulomatous ileitis or colitis may be seen in this form of disorder, although their mechanisms are not, at present, clear. It is probable that this neutropenia is related to the so-called lazy-leukocyte syndrome described by Miller et al. This disorder is characterized by a chronic neutropenia with a bone marrow that is rich in granulocytes of all stages. The peripheral blood granulocytes retain their phagocytic and bactericidal functions but appear to be incapable of responding to chemotactic factor. However, these are hypotheses that remain to be confirmed.

### Cyclic Neutropenia

Cyclic neutropenia is also a rare disorder, characterized by a cylic deficiency of granulocyte production. Myelograms show granulocytic depopulation, followed by an increase in the number of young granulocytes and a transient normalization of the granulocyte cell line. This cycle, which is of 21 to 28 days duration, is echoed in the hemogram, which reveals a transient agranulocytosis that lasts about a week, followed by an almost complete correction of the granulocyte level. During each episode of neutropenia, the patient develops an infection of which the most characteristic feature is stomatitis. The etiology is completely unknown and the disorder may evolve over several years. A chronic neutropenia may follow the cyclic phase by several months or years.

## QUALITATIVE GRANULOCYTE ABNORMALITIES

Since the description of chronic septic granulomatosis by Berendes in 1957, several other distinct granulocytic abnormalities have been described. Some result from a distinct enzymatic defect, whereas others are linked with a functional abnormality whose mechanism is not yet clear.

### Chronic Septic Granulomatosis

Chronic septic granulomatosis is a rare disorder transmitted in a sex-linked recessive mode or, more rarely, by an autosomal recessive gene, of which about 150 cases have been described. The clinical picture is dominated by repeated bacterial infections of the skin, lymph nodes (suppurative adenitis), lungs (pneumonias or pulmonary abcesses), bones and liver (recurrent hepatic abcesses). The causal organisms are most commonly *Staphylococcus aureus* or *S. albus, Serratia marescens*, enterobacilli, or salmonellae. *Candida* and *Aspergillus* infections are also seen. A few cases of disseminated BCG infection and infestation with *Pneumocystis carinii* have also been described.

Clinical examination discloses an almost constant hepatosplenomegaly and polylymphodenopathy, residuals of lymphoid stimulation by numerous infections, as in hypogammaglobulinemia. Some misleading sites of the disease should be appreciated. Granulomatous lesions of the bladder may simulate bladder tumors. Pyloric granulomas may give the picture of pyloric stenosis.

The hemogram always shows a neutrophil polynucleocytosis, which is occasionally very high (20 to 80,000/mm$^3$) and frequently associated with an eosinophilia. The diagnosis may be indicated by the study of the reduction of nitroblue tetrazolium (NBT) in the course of latex phagocytosis in the presence of this dye. In septic granulomatosis, the reduction of NBT is markedly decreased. This is, however, a relatively coarse colorimetric test. Metabolic study of the polynuclears in vitro (showing a reduced oxygen utilization and breakdown of hydrogen peroxide and superoxide ions during phagocytosis) and the study of polynuclear bactericidal activity in vitro are much more precise and reproducible investigations. The study of bactericidal activity of *staphylococci* or *S. marcescens* shows an important diminution of bacterial lysis and permits the recognition of heterozygotes in whom these functions are on the order of 50% of those of controls. The bactericidal activity exerted by macrophages is also abnormal in these patients and partially altered in those suffering from the sex-linked form. The bactericidal deficiency appears to be linked with a granulocytic deficit of NADPH oxidase. The other functions of granulocytes, chemotaxis and phagocytosis, are normal. Histologic examination of lymph nodes demonstrates the presence of lipid pigments in macrophages, demonstrating an abnormality of the catabolism of ingested bacterial antigens.

Antibiotic and antifungal therapy represent the mainstays of treatment during an overt infection. Continuous prophylactic antibiotic therapy is dangerous because of the risk of developing infections with resistant organisms. The use of cell-penetrating antibiotics (tetracycline and isoniazide, for example), which have the advantage of destroying nonkilled phagocytized bacteria, do not seem to be very effective. Corticosteroids, prescribed as anti-inflammatory agents with the aim of reducing phagocytic capacity and therefore permitting more effective antibacterial activity against extracellular organisms by antibiotics, are probably dangerous in the long term. The natural history of the disease, which is normally fatal within a few years (less than 20% of patients reach the age of 20 years), has resulted in attempts at bone marrow transplantation in a few cases. The follow-up is not yet long enough to enable an appreciation of the results of this form of reconstitution.

### Other Enzymatic Deficiencies of Granulocytes That May Give Rise to Infections

Other rare granulocytic enzyme deficiencies produce diminished bactericidal capacities. These are myeloperoxidase deficiency, described by Lehrer and Cline in patients having *Candida* infections; G6PD-deficiency, described by Cooper and Brehner; and secondary granulocytic deficiency, which produces a deficiency in lactoferrin and alkaline phosphatase, described by Strauss in a patient who was subject to repeated staphylococcal infection.

### Chediak-Higashi Disease

Chediak-Higashi disease is an autosomal recessive-transmitted disease, of which 100 recorded cases exist. It is characterized by an abnormality of the membranes of certain intracellular organelles that fuse to give rise to the giant intracellular inclusions that are typical of this disorder. This syndrome consists of a partial oculocutaneous albinism and a susceptibility to bacterial infections that are linked with granulocytic functional abnormalities. The albinism is due to pigment dilution. The intramelanocytic melanosomes of large size are poorly transferred to the surrounding keratinocytes. Albinism is particularly well seen in the hair, which takes on a silvery appearance. The disorder produces a cutaneous and ocular photosensitivity. Infections are mainly bacterial and situated in the ear, nose, and throat regions and in the skin and lungs.

Hematologic study reveals characteristic giant cytoplasmic granulations in leukocytes that are more plainly visible in granulocytes. Functional study of granulocytes shows complex abnormalities: deficiency of chemotaxis (Clark and Kimball), impaired early bactericidal activity (Root), partial deficits in certain enzymes (β-glucuronidase, myeloperoxidase), marked elastase deficiency (Vassalli and Griscelli), faulty membrane-receptor distribution for Con A receptors that spontaneously adopt a polar distribution, this being corrected by cyclic GMP activators (Oliver). A profound defect of natural killer (NK) activity has been observed in this disease.

The natural history of the disease is characterized by bacterial infection and episodes of the so-called accelerated phase, typified by pyrexia, which cannot always be explained on the basis of infection; increased splenomegaly; and pancytopenia, which is dominated by agranulocytosis and severe thrombocytopenia. Neurologic signs with alteration of the level of consciousness may be seen. Major electrolytic and water disturbances may be seen and hypofibrinogenemia is occasionally observed in the terminal phase. The accelerated phases are very often fatal. Considered for a long time to be lymphosarcomatoses, they probably represent a response to infection with complex metabolic consequences. Apart from symptomatic treatment (antibiotic therapy for an overt infection, corticosteroids during an accelerated phase) no satisfactory treatment exists. There has been some hopeful progress with the recent demonstration of the correction of some of the granulocytic abnormalities by the use of vitamin C (Boxer). However, these observations remain to be confirmed.

One patient (a boy) received an HLA-identical bone marrow graft after a total body irradiation which resulted in a complete reconstitution (Griscelli, et al). Two months after bone marrow transplantation, leukocytes which were all of donor origin (sister) did not contain giant granules and normally expressed NK activity.

### Eczema, Elevation of IgE Levels and Susceptibility to Infections

This syndrome described by Buckley, which probably corresponds with Job's syndrome, is characterized by eczema that becomes infected with cold cutaneous staphylococcal abcesses, recurrent bacterial (staphylococcal) or fungal lung abcesses with pleural complications, and slightly inflamed suppurative adenitis. The infections are generally only slightly febrile and have a torpid evolution. Hematologic investigation reveals a marked eosinophilia and occasional polymorphonuclear cytosis without any other quantitative abnormality. There is a significant elevation of IgE levels ($\geq$ 5000 IU/ml). The first observation described the existence of diminished granulocyte bactericidal activity, but this abnormality has not been confirmed. In contrast, there is an impaired granulocyte response to chemotactic factors. This abnormality may be linked to serum factors that inhibit granulocytic chemotaxis. The evolution of the disease is punctuated with frequent infective incidents. Prolonged symptomatic treatment (antibiotics and antifungal agents) together with intramuscular gammaglobulin injections, prescribed despite the hypergammaglobulinemia, and levamisole may diminish the frequency of infections to some degree.

Other chemotactic problems, either in isolation or associated with other polymorphonuclear functional abnormalities, have been described. They are all characterized by the occurrence of repeated bacterial infections. Some are associated with Leiner-Moussus-type skin lesions with reduced C5 levels (Miller) or ichthyosis. The granulocytic chemotactic disturbance found in all these disorders is probably linked with diverse intrinsic or extrinsic abnormalities, detailed knowledge of which will permit a coherent discrimination of all these syndromes.

# III.  SECONDARY IMMUNODEFICIENCIES (J. F. BACH)

Immune deficiencies may be observed during a large number of disorders. These deficiencies are often dissociated, involving, more commonly, cell-mediated immunity than the humoral one; and collectively they are less dramatic in their effects than the primary deficiencies, which have just been described. They may, however, play an important role in the progression of the diseases with which they are associated, either by modifying their symptomatology and natural history, or, occasionally, by predisposing to severe infections. These secondary immune deficiencies are quite diverse. We shall consider them under four headings.

## DEFICIENCIES ASSOCIATED WITH MALIGNANT BLOOD DYSCRASIAS AND CANCERS

Deficiencies of cell-mediated immunity are seen in a number of disorders of the lymphoid system.

### Leukemias

A large number of patients suffering from chronic lymphatic leukemia develop hypogammaglobulinemia and chronic infections. Despite this hypogammaglobulinemia, many of these patients have the capacity to produce de novo antibodies against an antigenic stimulus. Cellular immunity, however, is often abnormal. Other myeloid or lymphatic leukemias may be associated with deficiencies of cellular or humoral immunity, but the derangements are often overshadowed by the primary clinical picture.

### Myeloma and Other Dysglobulinemias

Most patients suffering from myeloma have a deficiency of antibody production after stimulation with an antigen, such as KLH. Although the patients have elevated serum immunoglobulin levels, many of them have lowered "normal" immunoglobulin levels that are not of the monoclonal proliferative origin. This immune deficiency may explain the abnormal incidence of septicemia and pneumonia seen in these patients. Cellular immunity is only slightly altered, if at all. Similar abnormalities are seen in Waldenström's macroglobulinemia.

### Hodgkin's Disease

For many years, it has been known that patients suffering from Hodgkin's disease express negative delayed sensitivity skin reactions to antigens that, in the majority of healthy individuals, elicit positive responses. These patients suffer from an abnormal incidence of diverse bacterial, viral, or fungal infections, many of which are possibly due to "opportunisitic" organisms. Humoral immunity is normal. In contrast, cell-mediated immunity is impaired, and this occurs very early in the disease. Deficient PHA responses are seen, and there is prolongation of skin-graft survival in these patients. Recent studies have shown, in the blood of such patients, the presence of prostaglandin-producing adherent cells, which suppress the response to PHA of normal lymphocytes. The role of these cells in the mechanisms of the immune deficiency remains to be proved.

### Cancers

Impaired cellular immunity has been incriminated as a factor in the development of certain cancers. In fact, although deficiencies of cutaneous hypersensitivity reactions and reduced numbers of E rosette-forming cells and, even, in some cases, impaired responses to mitogenic stimulation have been demonstrated, this depression of immune responses seems to be secondary to the cancerous affliction rather than a causative factor. In favor of this interpretation is the observation that these abnormalities may disappear after surgical ablation of the tumor. This factor is important from the point of view of discussing the timing of immunotherapy, for example by BCG, in the treatment of certain cancers. Finally, it should be recalled that thymomas (benign or malignant) may be associated with an immune deficiency, such as hypogammaglobulinemia (primary variable hypogammaglobulinemia described above) or a cellular immune deficiency.

## DEFICIENCIES ASSOCIATED WITH AUTOIMMUNE DISEASES

For some years, the role of cellular immunity disorders in the connective tissue disorders has been the subject of contradictory reports. In general, it has generally been considered that the cutaneous-delayed hypersensitivity responses and certain T-cell parameters are diminished in patients suffering from SLE and to a lesser degree, Sjögren's syndrome and rheumatoid arthritis. However, these changes are not usually severe and their relationship with lymphocytotoxic antibodies has not been excluded. In addition, lowered levels of thymic hormone are seen in cases of SLE, which may explain certain of the anomalies that have just been described. It should also be recalled that there exist more general links (discussed on p. 721) that seem to combine certain autoimmune diseases, immunoproliferative syndromes and immune deficiencies. These links are illustrated in animals by the NZB mouse model, in which the mice successively develop an immune deficiency (at the T-cell level), an autoimmune disease, and a monoclonal macroglobulinemia, and in man, by Sjögren's syndrome, in which very often autoimmune manifestations and lymphoid neoplasia are associated. Also, it should be remembered that there is an increased incidence of autoimmune phenomena in primary immune deficiency cases.

## DEFICIENCIES ASSOCIATED WITH INFECTIOUS DISEASES

The primary immune deficiencies are manifested essentially by the occurrence of severe and frequent infections. Conversely, certain infections occur against an apparently normal immunologic background and may induce an immune deficiency state, particularly of cellular immunity. It may result from bacterial infection. Thus, acute miliary tuberculosis may cause a transitory anergy toward tuberculin, the mechanism whereby this is accomplished being obscure (serum factor or suppressor T cells?). Lepromatous leprosy is also often associated with a T-cell deficit, although it is difficult to know whether this is a primary or secondary deficit. Whooping cough (pertussis) is associated with hyperlymphocytosis and may cause the cutaneous tests of delayed hypersensitivity to become transiently negative. This may also occur in some parasitoses where, quite frequently, an immune deficiency and reduced antibody production occurs in malaria and trypanosomiasis. In fact, the most common agents that cause a secondary immune deficiency are the viruses.

The immunosuppressive phenomena induced by viral infections are now well documented in both man and the laboratory animal. During the 4 to 6 weeks that follow a spontaneous or induced experimental viral infection, certain immunologic parameters may be modified. These modifications vary in type and intensity and appear to depend as much on the causal virus as the particular susceptibility of the host. In animals, numerous studies have shown that experimental infection with viruses (whether oncogenic or not) produce profound deficiencies of humoral immunity. Specific antibody production in response to antigens, such as sheep red cells, bovine albumin, or viral or bacterial extracts is markedly diminished when the antigen is administered several days after virus infection. However, in certain experimental models, such as infections with murine hepatitis virus, the effect of the viral infection depends on the timing of virus administration. If the virus is given before the antigen, immunosuppression is seen. If the virus is injected together with, or shortly after, antigen administration, the production of antibodies is, in contrast, increased. Cellular immunity may also be depressed by viral infections as exemplified by lymphopenia and diminution of the in vitro proliferative response induced by mitogens or antigens. Finally, nonspecific immunity is not spared since impaired neutrophil polynuclear responses to chemotactic factors have been described during viral infections in man. The mechanisms underlying these transitory immunosuppressed states are still poorly understood and probably vary from one model to the other. In some instances, the infection may induce aberrations of one or several of the three cell types responsible for immune responses, that is, at the T-lymphocyte level (measles virus), B-lymphocyte level (infectious mononucleosis), or macrophage level (poliomyelitis).

In other cases, it is possible that circulating soluble substances, such as adrenal hormones or interferon, may have an immunosuppressive effect. Whatever their nature, the study of these phenomena have a dual interest. From the fundamental point of view, they permit a new approach to the study of different lymphocyte subpopulations and their interactions, such as the effects of diverse soluble mediators of immunity. From the practical point of view, they enable a better understanding of the serious superinfections encountered during viral infections, especially measles infection in tropical regions, and a better grasp of the complexities of persistent immunologic abnormalities in certain fetal infections. Finally, it raises the still unresolved problem of the role of repeated or persistant viral infections in the genesis of certain "acquired" prolonged states of immunosuppression.

## DEFICIENCIES ASSOCIATED WITH METABOLIC DISORDERS

States of protein malnutrition, such as kwashiorkor, may result in complex immunodeficiencies with, in particular, a common diminution of thymic size and of T-cell number and function. Antibody responses are less commonly diminished depending on the antigen involved. The number of circulating B cells is normal or subnormal. The levels of the various complement factors may be reduced as well as phagocytic function. All these abnormalities rapidly become corrected when the protein status becomes normalized. Finally, a paradoxical situation occurs when modest caloric restriction takes place, in which case immunity against certain infections is augmented and the life-span of autoimmune mice is prolonged.

Diabetes mellitus also often causes frequent infections that are usually systemic. The underlying cellular basis and the precise role of the abnormal glucose metabolism remains unknown.

Major renal failure, even when partially corrected by intermittent hemodialysis, causes an immune deficiency involving both cellular and humoral immunity. Some infectxons are abnormally frequent, such as tuberculosis, and the percentage of HBs antigen carriers is very much higher in this patient population, although they have few signs of hepatitis. This is also the case with other disorders associated with deficiencies of cellular immunity. The few cases undergoing renal transplantation before 1960 without immunosuppression demonstrated a relative incapacity of these patients to reject the grafts that functioned for several weeks, despite the absence of therapeutic immunosuppression. Numerous in vitro studies of B and T lymphocytes have not yet allowed a precise determination of the exact cellular basis of this deficiency. The markers and functions of T cells (particularly delayed hypersensitivity reaction) are more often abnormal than is antibody production (humoral response to certain vaccines, however, is diminished).

The various nephrotic syndromes and certain enteropathies may result in a deficiency of humoral and/or cellular (generally modest) immunity by the protein depletion (notably Ig) they cause.

## OTHER SECONDARY IMMUNE DEFICIENCIES

Diverse other disorders may cause general immune deficiencies that may also be limited to a single particular antigen. Mention should particularly be made of sarcoidosis (see p. 938), subacute sclerosing panencephalitis (see p. 935), sickle cell disease, burns, alcoholic cirrhosis, and iron-deficiency anemia.

Finally, a further possible cause of transient immune deficiency is pregnancy. Cell-mediated immunity, evaluated by cutaneous-delayed hypersensitivity reaction and the mitogen-induced lymphocyte transformation test, is depressed during pregnancy. This deficiency is partly linked with the existence in the serum of inhibitors, such as chorionic gonadotropins that inhibit the in vitro lymphocyte transformation induced by PHA. A factor liberated by fetal lymphocytes has also been described that may also have an inhibitory effect on lymphocyte transformation.

# *BIBLIOGRAPHY*

ADLER N. H., JONES K. H., and NAZIUCHI H. Aging and immune function. *In* R. A. Thompson, Ed., Recent advances in clinical immunology. Edinburgh, 1977, Churchill-Livingstone, p. 77.

BEKKUM D. W. VAN. Use and abuse of hemopoietic cell grafts in immune deficiency states. Transpl. Rev., 1972, *9*, 3.

BELLANTI J. A. and SCHLEGEL R. J. The diagnosis of immune deficiency diseases. Pediat. Clin. Amer., 1971, *18*, 49.

BERGSMA D. Immunodeficiency in man and animals. Sunderland, 1975, Sinauer.

BJÖRKSTEIN B. and QUIE P. G. Abnormalities of circulating phagocyte function. *In* R. A. Thompson, Ed., Recent advances in clinical immunology. Edinburgh, 1977, Churchill-Livingstone, p. 181.

BLAESE R. M. T and B cell immunodeficiency diseases. *In*: Clinical Immunology (C. W. Parker [ed]). Saunders, Philadelphia, 1980, 314.

BUCKLEY R. H. Replacement therapy in immunodeficiency. *In* R. A. Thompson, Ed., Recent advances in clinical immunology, Edinburgh. 1977, Churchill-Livingstone, p. 219.

COOPER M. D., KEIGHTLEY R. G., WU L. Y. F., and LAWTON III A. R. Developmental defects of T and B cell lines in humans. Transpl. Rev., 1973, *16*, 57.

COOPER M. D., LAWTON A. R., MIESCHER P. A., and MULLER-EBERHARD P. Immune deficiency. Springer Berlin, 1979, 184 p.

DENT P. B. Immunodepression by oncogenic viruses. Prog. Med. Virol., 1972, *14*, I.

DOUGLAS S. D. Immunological aspects of protein malnutrition. *In* R. A. Thompson, Ed., Recent advances in clinical immunology. Edinburgh, 1977, Churchill-Livingstone, p. 15.

FUDENBERG H., GOOD R. A., GOODMAN H. C., HITZIG N., KUNKEL H. G., ROITT I. M., ROSEN F. S., ROWE D. S., SELIGMANN M., and SOOTHILL J. F. Primary immunodeficiencies: report of a world health organization committee. Pediatrics, 1971, *47*, 927.

GATTI R. A. On the classification of patients with primary immunodeficiency disorders. Clin. Immunol. Immunopath., 1974, *3*, 243.

GOOD R. A. Immunologic reconstitution: the achievement and its meaning. *In* R. A. Good and D. W. Fischer, Eds., Immunobiology. Stanford, Conn., 1971, Sinauer, p. 231.

GOOD R. A. The lymphoid system, immunodeficiency and malignancy. *In* Advances in the biosciences. Vol. 12. New York, 1974, Pergamon Press, p. 123.

GOOD R. A. and BACH F. H. Bone marrow and thymus transplants: cellular engineering to correct primary immunodeficiency. Clin. Immunol., 1971, *2*, 65.

Good R. A. and Bergsma D. (Eds.) Immunologic deficiency diseases in man. New York, 1974, National Foundation Press.

Good R. A., Kappor N., Pahwa R. N., West A., and O'reilly R. J. Current approaches to the primary immunodeficiencies. *In*: Immunology 80 (M. Fougereau and J. Dausset [eds]). Acad. Press, New York, 1980, 906.

Hitzig W. M. and Grob P. J. Therapeutic uses of transfer factor. *In* R. S. Schwartz, Ed., Progress in clinical immunology. Vol. 2. New York, 1974, Grune & Stratton, p. 69.

Hong R. Immunodeficiency: enigmas and speculations. *In* R. S. Schwartz, Ed., Progress in clinical immunology. Vol. 2. New York, 1974, Grune & Stratton, p. 1.

Kay M. M. B. and Makinodan T. Immunobiology of aging; evaluation of current status. Clin. Immunol. Immunopath., 1976, *6*, 394.

Notkins A. L., Mergenhagen S. E., and Howard R. J. Effect of virus infections on the function of the immune system. Annual Rev. Microbiol., 1970, *24*, 525.

Pollara B., Pickering R. J., Meuvissen M. J., and Porter I. H. Inborn errors of specific immunity. Acad. Press, New York, 1979, 469 p.

Rosen F. Immunological deficiency diseases. *In* F. H. Bach and R. A. Good, Eds., Clinical immunobiology. Vol. 1. New York, 1972, Academic Press, p. 271.

Rosen F. S. Immunodeficiency diseases. *In*: Mechanisms of Immunopathology (S. Cohen, P. A. Ward, and R. T. MacCluskey [eds]). John Wiley & Sons, New York, 1979, 307.

Santos G. W. Application of marrow grafts in human diseases: its problems and potentials. Contemp. Topics Immunobiol., 1972, *I*, 143.

Stiehm E. R. and Fulginiti V. (Eds.). Immunologic disorders in infants and children. London, New York, 1973, Saunders.

Stossel T. P. Disorders of phagocytic effector cells. *In*: Mechanisms of Immunopathology (S. Cohen, P. A. Ward, and R. T. MacCluskey [eds]). John Wiley & Sons, New York, 1979, 271.

Thomas E. D., Storb R., Clift R. A., Fefer A., Johnson F. L., Neiman P. E., Lerner K. G., Glucksbert H., and Buckner C. D. Bone marrow transplantation. New. Engl. J. Med., 1975, *292*, 832, 895.

Turner-Warwick M. Immunology of the lung. Arnold, London, 1978, 326 p.

Yunis E. J., Handwerger B. S., Hallgren H. M., Good R. A., and Fernandez G. Aging and immunity. *In*: Mechanisms of Immunopathology (S. Cohen, P. A. Ward, and R. T. MacCluskey [eds]). John Wiley & Sons, New York, 1979, p. 91.

## ORIGINAL ARTICLES

August C. S., Rosen F. S., Filler R. M., Janeway C. A., Markowski B. and Kay H. Implantation of a foetal thymus, restoring immunological competence in a patient with thymus aplasia (Di George's syndrome). Lancet, 1968, *2*, 1210.

Cooper M. D., Lawton D. R., and Bockman D. E. Agammaglobulinemia with B-lymphocytes. Lancet, 1971, *2*, 791.

Fischer A., Ballet J. J., and Griscelli C. Specific inhibition of in vitro *Candida*-induced lymphocyte proliferation by polysaccharidic antigens present in the serum of patients with chronic muco-cutaneous candidiasis. J. Clin. Invest., 1978, *62*, 1005.

Gatti R. A., Dilen A. D., Meuwissen H. J., Kong R. A., and Good R. A. Immunological reconstitution of sex-linked lymphopenic immunological deficiency. Lancet, 1968, *2*, 1366.

Geha R. S., Schneeberger E., Merler E., and Rosen F. Heterogeneity of «acquired» or common variable agammaglobulinemia. New Engl. J. Med., 1976, *295*, 1273.

Giblett E. R., Anderson J. E., Cohen F., Pollara B., and Meuwissen H. J. Adenosine desaminase deficiency in two patients with severely impaired cellular immunity. Lancet, 1972, *2*, 1067.

Griscelli C., Durandy A., Virelizier J. L., Ballet J. J., and Daguillard F. Selective defect of precursor T cells associated with apparently normal B lymphocytes in severe combined immunodeficiency disease. J. Pediat., 1978, *93*, 404.

GRISCELLI C., DURANDY A., GUY-GRAND B., DAGUILLARD F., HERZOG C., and PRUNIERAS M. A syndrome associating partial albinism and immunodeficiency. Amer. J. Med., 1978, *65*, 691.

PREUD'HOMME J. L., GRISCELLI C., and SELIGMANN M. Immunoglobulins on the surface of lymphocytes in fifty patients with primary immunodeficiency diseases. Clin. Immunol. Immunopathol., 1973, *1*, 241.

PURTILO D. T. Epstein-Barr virus induced ontogenesis in immune deficient individuals. Lancet, 1980, *9*, 300.

SELIGMANN M., GRISCELLI C., PREUD'IIOMME J. L., SASPORTES M., HERZOG C., and BROUET J. C. A variant of severe combined immunodeficiency with normal in vitro response to allogenic cells and an increase in circulating B-lymphocytes persisting several months after successful bone marrow graft. Clin. Exp. Immunol., 1974, *17*, 245.

VIRELIZIER J. L. Mechanisms of immunodepression induced by viruses: possible role of infected macrophages. Biomedicine, 1975, *22*, 255.

# Chapter 32

# EXTENSION OF THE SCOPE OF IMMUNOPATHOLOGY

## Jean-François Bach

I.   INTRODUCTION
II.  ORGAN-SPECIFIC AUTOIMMUNE DISEASES
III. POSTINFECTIOUS IMMUNOPATHOLOGY
IV.  UNCLASSIFIABLE DISEASES

## I.  INTRODUCTION

We have already described three classic autoimmune diseases: systemic lupus erythematosus (SLE), hemolytic anemia, and Goodpasture's syndrome. We have also discussed diseases associated with the presence of immune complexes: SLE, rheumatoid arthritis, and glomerulonephritides. The major hypersensitivity states have been reviewed. An immunopathologic nature is probably not limited to only these diseases. Table 32.1 lists the diseases for which immune phenomena are either proven or suspected. Note the variety of mechanisms involved (some of which are very hypothetical). In this chapter, we will briefly outline the main arguments that suggest immunologic origins for the pathophysiology of these disorders. We shall not, however, provide a full clinical description of these diseases, which is more a concern of internal medicine than of immunopathology, even if this distinction is, of course, only arbitrary, as it is obvious that clinical immunology, because of the myriad of disciplines involved, is an integral part of internal medicine.

## II.  ORGAN-SPECIFIC AUTOIMMUNE DISEASES

We have already discussed in considerable depth two organ-specific autoimmune diseases, autoimmune hemolytic anemia (chap. 27), and Goodpasture's syndrome (p. 844), because these two diseases, like SLE (chap. 28), are the only ones for which a solid autoimmune pathogenesis has been well established. Numerous other diseases are probably autoimmune in orgin, as suggested by the presence of autoimmune manifestations and by analogy to experimental models. This is particularly true for several endocrine diseases.

## HASHIMOTO'S THYROIDITIS

Hashimoto's throiditis usually affects females rather than males (5 to 10 females are affected for every male afflicted). It is histologically characterized by lymphocytic infiltration and glandular destruction, and resultant myxedema. The thyroid gland's attempts to regenerate (new acini formation), together with lymphoid hyperplasia, explains the usual presence of a goiter. In severe forms, fibrosis and epithelial atrophy develop. Separate from these histologic features is thyroiditis in which there is no regeneration. Atrophic thyroiditis, also sometimes associated with goiter, shows moderate plasma cell infiltration. The latter disease is very rare, compared to Hashimoto's thyroiditis, and is associated with slightly different immunologic abnormalities. Clinically, goiter coexists with myxedema.

Autoantibodies in thyroiditis are directed against four principal autoantigens. (1) Thyroglobulin (which constitutes 75% of the gland proteins) has a molecular weight of 650,000 daltons and contains most of the body iodine. Antithyroglobulin antibodies are detected by precipitation (especially in the atrophic variant) radioimmunoassay, agglutination of thyroglobulin-sensitized latex particles, or by passive hemagglutination with tanned red blood cells. The latter is the most sensitive technique. In fact, it is overly sensitive, because antibodies in high titer are detected by this technique in most thyroid diseases (especially in primary adult myxedema: 90% positivity). (2) Microsomal antigens, associated with lipoproteins, are detected by immunofluorescence on thyroid slices, complement fixation, and, more rarely, by passive hemagglutination, cytotoxicity on trypsinized thyroid cells, or radioimmunoassay. Some antimicrosomal antibodies are specifically antithyroid, while others react with microsomal extracts from other organs. (3) The "second" colloid antigen, detected by immunofluorescence, has been isolated by chromatography and does not contain iodine. (4) Surface antigens of thyroid cells against which antibodies are also detected by immunofluorescence or mixed hemabsorption.

Practically all patients with Hashimoto's thyroiditis have circulating anti-thyroid antibodies. In the atrophic variant, antibodies are found in high concentration: antithyroglobulin precipitins are observed in more than 90% of such patients and passive hemagglutination titers exceed 1/10,000, ranging up to several millions. Antimicrosomal antibodies with complement fixation titers of 1/128 to 1/2000 are also present, as are antibodies against the second colloidal antigen. In the hypercellular form of the disease, precipitating antibodies are usually absent (positivity in about 5% of patients). Passive hemagglutination to thyroglobulin is negative or slightly positive, but complement fixation to microsomal antigens is strongly positive, and there may be antibodies against the second colloidal antigen. The presence of these antibodies is helpful in

**Table 32.1  Classification of Diseases Considered Immunologic or Including Immunologic Phenomena**

| | Proven | Suspected | Hypothetical |
|---|---|---|---|
| Autoimmune diseases | Hemolytic anemia<br>Hashimoto's thyroiditis<br>Graves' disease<br>Sympathetic ophthalmia<br>Goodpasture's syndrome<br>Systemic lupus erythematosus | Addison's disease<br>Some infertilities<br>Pemphigus<br>Pernicious anemia<br>Myasthenia gravis | Some pulmonary fibroses<br>Insulin-dependent diabetes<br>Ulcerative colitis<br>Crohn's disease<br>Hypoparathyroidism |
| Secondary autoimmune reactions | Autoimmune neutropenia<br>Certain thrombocytopenic purpuras | Dressler's syndrome | |
| Immune complex diseases | Serum sickness disease, acute glomerulonephritis, systemic lupus erythematous, chronic glomerulonephritis, rheumatoid arthritis | Essential cryoglobulinemia, Sjögren's syndrome, necrotic angiitis, scleroderma, dermatomyositis and polymyositis | Primary biliary cirrhosis |
| Diseases by hypersensitivity state | I. Anaphylactic shock (serum sickness, insect bites, drug reactions, ruptures of hydatid cysts), atopy (hay fever, urticaria, certain asthmas), drug allergy<br>II. Newborn hemolytic disease, transfusional incompatibilities, some drug reactions (Sedormid, α-methyldopa)<br>III. Farmer's lung disease, bird-breeder's disease<br>IV. Some drug allergies (contact dermatitis) | Milk intolerance, eczemas, some erythrodermas | |

| | | | |
|---|---|---|---|
| Postinfectious immunopathology | Subacute bacterial endocarditis | Acute hepatitis, chronic hepatitis, hepatosplenic schistosomiasis | Rheumatic fever, multiple sclerosis, Guillain-Barré's syndrome |
| Immunoproliferative disorders | Myeloma, Waldenström's macroglobulinemia, Sezary's syndrome | Hodgkir's disease, some acute leukemias | |
| Rejection pathology | Skin and organ allograft rejection, rejection of certain tumors, fetomaternal relationships | | |
| Immunodeficiencies | Congenital immunodeficiencies, Secondary immunodeficiencies: immunosuppressive treatment, hemopathies, infections (measles, whooping cough) | | |

diagnosing Hashimoto's thyroiditis, even if they are not specific for the disease, since diffuse (colloid) goiters are associated with high antibody titers in about 2% of cases and with moderate titers in 40% cases, while precipitation is always negative. Thyroid cancer may cause significant antibody production (in about 10% of cases); histologic verification of questionable cases is therefore necessary. Antibodies are also found in subacute thyroiditis in low titer, and are especially elevated in Graves' disease (where high titers are seen in about 20% of patients). Passive hemagglutination against thyroglobulin is weakly positive in about 50% of cases.

Some in vitro studies have shown the existence of cell-mediated immunity to thyroid antigens in Hashimoto's thyroiditis. Lymphoblastic transformation and leukocyte migration inhibition with thyroglobulin and microsomal antigens are often positive. A direct lymphocytic cytotoxicity to monolayers of thyroid cells has been demonstrated. It is still too early to say whether these results relate to the action of T cells or K cells (the cytotoxicity of which would be exerted in the presence of antibodies secreted by B cells), the more so because ADC-inducing antibodies (see p. 413) are present in Hashimoto's thyroiditis.

In summary, the presence of autoantibodies in almost all cases of Hashimoto's thyroiditis, the extensive cell infiltration, the common association with other autoimmune diseases (e.g., pernicious anemia: 30% of thyroiditis patients have antibodies to gastric mucosa, 1–3% possess anti-intrinsic factor antibodies, while, conversely, 50% of pernicious anemia patients have antithyroid antibodies), and its analogy to experimental thyroiditis (see p. 716) or spontaneous thyroiditis (see p. 715) indicate that Hashimoto's disease is probably of autoimmune etiology. The causative mechanisms are unknown (i.e., antibodies, cytotoxic T cells, K cells?). It is important to recall that spontaneous thyroiditis in the obese chicken is suppressed by neonatal bursectomy and is exacerbated by neonatal thymectomy; conversely, neonatal thymectomy prevents the onset of experimental allergic thyroiditis induced with thyroglobulin in Freund's adjuvant. Note also that experimental allergic thyroiditis can be transferred with cells and not with serum. It may be that deposition of immune complexes, whose presence in the blood has been suggested also plays a role, at least in maintaining the disease. It is important to recognize that antithyroid antibodies are present in 5–10% of normal subjects, particularly those over 50 (>20% in subjects over 70). Some focal thyroiditis may be found in aged subjects at autopsy in the absence of clinical thyroid dysfunction.

## GRAVES' DISEASE (DIFFUSE TOXIC GOITER)

Much evidence suggests that thyrotoxicosis is an autoimmune disease. Some of the evidence is indirect: Graves' disease often occurs in families in which Hashimoto's thyroiditis or goiter also occurs. An association with pernicious anemia, myasthenia gravis, thrombocytopenic purpura, SLE, Sjögren's syndrome, and autoimmune hemolytic anemia occurs as frequently as in Hashimoto's thyroiditis. In 30% of cases, antigastric antibodies are also present. The finding of an IgG factor that stimulates thyroid release (similar to thyroid-stimulating hormone), the "long-acting thyroid stimulator" (LATS), represents an even more direct argument. LATS is detected by McKenzie's assay, which consists of measuring the serum level of $^{131}$I in mice before and after injection of serum from thyrotoxic patients or their immunoglobulins. LATS is found in 20–40% of subjects; the highest concentrations are found in patients refractory to $^{131}$I treatment or in those afflicted with pretibial myxedema. A role for LATS in the pathogenesis of the disease is suggested by the presence of thyrotoxicosis in hypophysectomized patients and also by the transference of thyrotoxicosis to newborns of mothers with Graves' disease for a time that approximates IgG half-life. LATS apparently is an autoantibody that binds to thyroid membrane antigens close to thyroid-stimulating hormone (TSH) receptor sites, where it activates the adenyl cyclase system. The absence of LATS in some patients with thyrotoxicosis and the presence of LATS in some euthyroid subjects are not well understood but may simply relate to the use of a xenogeneic species (mice) for its detection. An in vitro assay for LATS has recently been developed. This assay involves measurement of colloidal drops in cultured human thyroid slices after addition of TSH or LATS. This test detects a "human-specific thyroid stimulator" (HTS) and is positive in most patients. It is partially species specific. Performed on mouse thyroid, this test is only positive with sera that are positive in the in vivo mouse test. The relative species specificity of LATS explains its absence in a significant proportion of patients. TSH, and, indeed, thyroid stimulating antibodies in general, act by stimulating TSH receptors. In practice, three in vitro techniques have replaced McKenzie's test. They measure (1) the

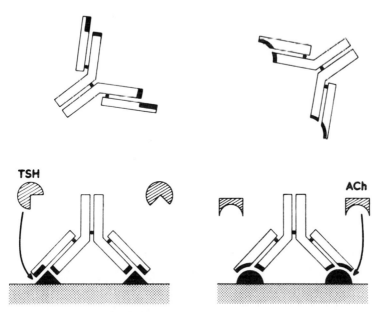

**Fig. 32.1** Antireceptor autoantibodies. The autoantibody competes with the hormone or mediator, causing (depending on the situation) either stimulation (left, in the case of hyperthyroidism) or blockade (right in the case of myasthenia gravis). (After I. R. Mackay. *In* Progress in immunology, III, Proc. 3rd Int. Cong. Immunol. Sydney. Amsterdam, 1977, North Holland, p. 490.)

increase in thyroid colloid, (2) the activation of adenylcyclase, or (3) the displacement of radiolabeled TSH from thyroid cell membranes. 80% of patients suffering from thyrotoxicosis are positive with this latter technique. Thyroid-stimulating antibodies have effects on other tissues. They may notably be responsible for pretibial myxedema and exophtalmos by stimulating metabolism of the retro-orbital tissues. In addition they stimulate lipolysis. These antibodies seem to be distinct from HTS since this latter antibody has extra-thyroid effects. Conversely, HTS is not the only antibody that reacts with TSH receptors. Finally, there appears to be a group of antibodies, which may or may not be biologically active, directed against different antigenic determinants of these receptors. It should also be remembered that Graves' disease is significantly associated with the presence of HLA antigens B8 and DR3 (see p. 695).

## ADDISON'S DISEASE

Addison's disease is primary adrenal insufficiency. Tuberculosis was formerly usually causative, but idiopathic Addison's disease (probably autoimmune) is now more often etiologic (in 80% of cases). The actual incidence of tuberculous etiology is difficult to assess because it is usually difficult to diagnose, We will not herein describe acute adrenal insufficiency and the clinical presentation of shock nor will we discuss chronic adrenal insufficiency with its concomitants of asthenia, hypotension, and other characteristic biochemical abnormalities. We shall, however, recall the distinction between primary and secondary adrenal insufficiencies based on the response to ACTH or Synacthen stimulation, both of which give positive responses only in cases of secondary adrenal insufficiency. Histologically, Addison's disease is characterized by fibrosis with significant lymphocytic infiltration.

An autoimmune basis for Addison's disease was suspected following the demonstration of antiadrenal autoantibodies by complement fixation or immunofluorescence techniques. Immunofluorescence is positive for these antibodies in about 65% of idiopathic Addison's disease patients, but it is nearly always negative for a tuberculous etiology and in normal subjects, as well as in most other organ-specific autoimmune diseases. Knowledge of the biochemical nature and of the distribution of adrenal antigens is lacking. Antigens are essentially cytoplasmic and localized in the mitochondrial fraction. The leukocyte migration inhibition test may also be positive, but interpretation is difficult in man. In addition, idiopathic Addison's disease is often associated with other autoimmune diseases, including Hashimoto's thyroiditis; diffuse toxic goiter; pernicious anemia, sometimes limited to only achlorhydria (in 20–30% of cases); diabetes mellitus (8% to 20% of cases); hypoparathyroidism; and ovarian insufficiency. The three latter diseases are also often associated with antibodies directed against the organs involved, in particular, antibodies to gonadal steroid-producing cells. The incidence of various autoantibodies, especially those to thyroglobulin, stomach wall, and intrinsic factor, is abnormally high. All of these data, as well as allergic experimental adrenalitis and the appearence of antiadrenal antibody after injection of adrenal extracts in the presence of Freund's adjuvant, suggest that idiopathic Addison's disease is probably autoimmune in origin. Finally, it is worthwhile remembering that, like several other autoimmune diseases, Addison's disease is associated with HLA antigens HLA-B8 and DR3 (see p. 695).

## DIABETES MELLITUS

An autoimmune origin has been suggested for some juvenile-onset insulin-dependent forms of diabetes mellitus. Arguments in favor of this hypothesis are mostly indirect, namely, the association of other autoimmune diseases, such as thyroiditis, Addison's disease, myasthenia, or pernicious anemia, the frequent presence of various autoantibodies, especially antithyroid and antigastric, and lymphocytic infiltrates in the islets of Langerhans. Experimental insulinitis obtained after immunization with pancreatic extracts in the presence of Freund's adjuvant gives a picture that is quite distant from that of human diabetes. Anti-islet antibodies are found by immunofluorescence in about two-thirds of cases of insulin-dependent diabetes. It is possible to demonstrate lymphocyte transformation and inhibition of leukocyte migration in the presence of pancreatic extracts. The existence of anti-insulin antibodies, although demonstrated by some workers, is less certain. In some cases of extreme insulin resistance, diverse organ-specific antibodies may be demonstrated and occasionally antibodies directed against insulin-receptors are seen. In addition, there is a very significant association between insulin-dependent juvenile-onset diabetes and HLA antigens A1, B8, DR3, and B15; this association is even more clear if one includes those patients with anti-islet autoantibodies.

Finally, insulin-dependent juvenile-onset diabetes is associated with significant stigmata of autoimmunity that may play an etiologic role. It is, however, difficult to visualize the role of this mechanism in comparison with other mechanisms that have been incriminated (viruses, obesity, etc.), occurring on a predispositional genetic background.

## HYPOPARATHYROIDISM

Hypoparathyroidism may be associated with antiparathyroid antibodies, demonstrable by immunofluorescence. The disease is also unusually associated with Addison's disease. Finally, lymphocytic infiltrates are commonly observed in the atrophic gland. Several arguments thus suggest the possibility of an autoimmune etiology.

## MALE STERILITY

Spermatozoa bear auto-and alloantigens, which may be responsible for auto-or alloimmunization, leading to sterility. The existence of autoantigens was shown by induction of allergic orchitis following injection of autologous testicular extracts in the presence of Freund's adjuvant. Antibodies that reacted to spermatozoa, as detected by immobilization, agglutination, cytotoxicity, or immunofluorescence, were noted. Several autoantigen categories were demonstrated. In addition, other specific antigens may be seen in the seminal fluid. One so-called spermatozoa-coating antigen (SCA) binds to the surface of spermatozoa. The fixation of antigens present in seminal fluid onto spermatozoa is not limited to SCA. This is the case of other purely seminal antigens and for antigens of the AB group in secretor subjects (see p. 616; note that anti-A and anti-B antibodies do not agglutinate spermatozoa).

Some sterile men (about 3%) have antispermatozoa autoantibodies in their serum and seminal fluid that can be detected by agglutination (micro- or macroscopic) or immobilization (complement dependent). The presence of higher titers of antibodies in the seminal fluid than in the serum has suggested that antibody production is localized in the former. It is of interest that spermagglutinins can be found in obstructive azoospermia, in inflammatory lesions of the epididymal epithelium characterized by spermatozoan extravasation, and also after vasectomy. These findings suggest that internal retention of spermatozoa may cause autoantibody formation. The absence of fetal autotolerance is due to the late development of spermatozoa-specific antigens in ontogenesis. The pathogenetic nature of antispermatozoa autoantibodies has not been demonstrated. Indeed, spermagglutinins can be present in normal fertile men who have normal numbers and forms of spermatozoa. The possibility that antibodies are cytotoxic has, however, not been ruled out.

## FEMALE STERILITY

Female antispermatozoa alloantibodies might cause sterility. Foreign proteins are absorbed across vaginal walls and the cervical mucosa. Experiments in the guinea pig indicate that the vagina is not a good site for inducing antispermatozoa primary responses; however, when immunity develops after parenteral injection, the antigens placed into the vagina may cause a secondary response. Thus, it is possible that inflammatory or mechanical alterations in the vagina may relate to significant antispermatozoa immunization. Indeed, agglutinating and immobilizing spermatozoa antibodies may be detected in the serum of some sterile women but usually not in fertile women (further data are, however, needed). In sterile women, antispermatozoa antibodies may also be demonstrated by passive hemagglutination or immunofluorescence techniques. The significance of these antibodies is uncertain. Immunization with spermatozoa of female guinea pigs or mice reduces their fertility. However, antispermatozoa antibodies are found in the serum of certain fertile women (although in low titers). Correlations between the various tests mentioned above and the search for serum antibodies are weak. The latter test, which is the only one performed routinely, for practical reasons, may not be adequate, because the critical factor may be localized genital antibody secretion, particularly of secretory IgA.

Histocompatibility antigens in the form of single haplotypes are present on spermatozoa. However, anti-HLA antibodies are not the cause of female sterility. Indeed, one of the best sources of anti-HLA antisera is serum from multiparous women.

Little is known about possible relationships between ovarian insufficiency and autoimmune etiology. There is a frequent association of amenorrhea and

Addison's disease with antibodies directed against ovarian (steroid) secretory cells (see p. 920). It is possible that in the future, better techniques for detection of antiovary (possibly antisteroid) antibodies may increase our understanding and recognition of autoimmune ovarian insufficiency.

## PERNICIOUS ANEMIA

Pernicious anemia is a megaloblastic anemia characterized by decreased vitamin $B_{12}$ absorption secondary to atrophy of the gastric mucosa. This atrophy and achlorhydria probably have an autoimmune origin.

Antigastric antibodies are of two types. Antibodies may be directed against gastric parietal cells, as detected by complement fixation or immunofluorescence; the antigen is located on the microvilli membrane. A second antibody is directed against intrinsic factor, a glycoprotein secreted by parietal cells whose function is to bind vitamin $B_{12}$ and thus permit its intestinal absorption. The binding of anti-intrinsic factor antibody to its target prevents fixation of vitamin $B_{12}$ onto its binding site. This antibody is detected by blocking vitamin $B_{12}$ binding and is alternatively called "blocking antibody," "antibinding site antibody," or "type-1 antibody." Indeed, there is a second antibody that reacts with the vitamin $B_{12}$-intrinsic factor complex without actual binding to the vitamin $B_{12}$ binding site.

In the laboratory, the antibinding site antibody is detected by virute of its inhibition of radiolabeled vitamin $B_{12}$ fixation on liquid gastric extracts. The second antibody is detected by studying physicochemical changes in the vitamin $B_{12}$-intrinsic factor complex induced by antibody binding (variations in electrophoretic mobility, for example). Antigastric wall antibodies occur in about 2% of normal subjects younger than 20 years old, in 6–8% of middle-aged subjects (up to 60 years), and in 15% of those older than 60. However, they are found in 80%–90% of pernicious anemia patients, 30–40% of related family members, 30% of subjects with myxedema or Graves' disease, 25% of idiopathic Addison's disease patients, and in 20% of patients with insulin-dependent diabetes. They are also very common in atrophic gastritis (20% incidence) or total gastric atrophy (50% incidence). On the other hand, anti-intrinsic factor antibodies are usually only seen in pernicious anemia.

Patients with pernicious anemia present with severe atrophic gastritis or complete gastric atrophy. Antigastric parietal cell antibodies are found in about 60% of cases studied by complement fixation but are detected in 90% of the same subjects when immunofluorescence techniques are applied. Anti-intrinsic factor antibodies are found in the serum or gastric fluid in 60–70% of cases, but there is no apparent relationship between the antibody titers present in these two fluids. Interestingly, administration of radioactive vitamin $B_{12}$ mixed with anti-intrinsic factor antibody (serum) inhibits vitamin $B_{12}$ absorption, in both healthy and diseased subjects. When the antibody is not present in the serum or gastric fluid, immunofluorescence may reveal the presence of immunoglobulins in mononucleated cells, which are found throughout the gastric mucosa. In addition, it is possible that cellular hypersensitivity to intrinsic factor, suggested by a positive lymphoblastic transformation test or leukocytic migration inhibition test in the presence of gastric extracts, also plays a role, which would explain the onset of pernicious anemia in agammaglobulinemic subjects.

All of these data suggest a probable autoimmune origin of pernicious anemia and atrophic gastritis; other evidence that favors this conclusion is the frequent association of thyroiditis, thyrotoxicosis, Addison's disease, hypoparathyroidism, and antithyroid, antiadrenal, or antidermal antibodies. Gastric parietal cells secrete both hydrochloric acid and intrinsic factor (pepsin is secreted by other cells). Achlorhydria precedes a loss or decrease in intrinsic factor secretion. Antigastric wall antibodies might be responsible for gastric atrophy and achlorhydria. Anti-intrinsic factor antibodies in pernicious anemia might act by inactivating intrinsic factor or by altering its secretion. However, note that gastric atrophy, and even atrophic gastritis, may be observed in the absence of autoantibodies. Conversely, antigastric parietal cell autoantibodies may be observed in the absence of gastritis, even if gastritis is abnormally common in subjects with autoimmune endocrinopathy who possess antigastric parietal cell autoantibodies.

## AUTOIMMUNE CYTOPENIAS

In the preceding chapters, we have already discussed the idiopathic autoimmune hemolytic anemias as well as the drug-induced immunologically mediated hemolytic anemias, thrombocytopenic purpuras and neutropenias. Autoimmune phenomena may also explain certain drug-induced neutropenias and thrombocytopenias, which may occur either in isolation or in the context of a preexisting autoimmune disease, such as SLE or Felty's syndrome (rheumatoid arthritis with splenomegally and neutropenia).

**Table 32.2  Frequencies of Antibodies Directed Against Thyroid and Gastric Parietal Cells**

|  | Antigastric parietal cell antibody (%) | Antithyroid antibody (%) |
|---|---|---|
| Normal subjects | <10 | 0–15 |
| Pernicious anemia | 84 | 55 |
| Atrophic gastritis | 20 | — |
| Gastric atrophy | 50 | — |
| Primary myxedema | 32 | 87 |
| Hashimoto's thyroiditis | ? | ? |
| Thyrotoxicosis | 28 | 53 |
| Iron-deficiency anemia | 24 | — |
| Addison's disease | 23 | 31 |
| Rheumatoid arthritis | 5–11 | <10 |
| Diabetes mellitus (insulin dependent) | 18 | 14 |
| Subjects related to a patient with |  |  |
|   Pernicious anemia | 36 | 50 |
|   Severe atrophic gastritis | 20 | — |
|   Thyroid disease | 20 | 46 |

After I. Chanarin.

Autoimmune neutropenias may or may not predispose to infections. Leukoagglutinins are often, though not always, found, but their titers do not correlate with the degree of neutropenia. Antibodies may also be found by antiglobulin consumption. As a rule, the bone marrow is normal although, in rare cases, autoantibodies have been found to be capable of suppressing the growth of medullary cells in vitro and in vivo. A role for immune complexes and antibodies that mediate ADCC has also been suggested. Treatment requires steroids and immunosuppressive agents.

Idiopathic thrombocytopenic purpuras are linked with the destruction of circulating platelets by antiplatelet antibodies. When the thrombocytopenia is severe, hemorrhages are seen. The thrombocytopenia often follows a viral infection, especially in children, and a possible role for virus fixation onto platelets has been raised. In other cases, the thrombocytopenic purpura is only one facet of an autoimmune disease. The immunologic diagnosis of the disease is confirmed by the demonstration of antiplatelet antibodies by agglutination or complement fixation. The presence of Ig on the patients' platelets may also be sought by the use of an anti-Ig serum. In fact, these techniques are insensitive and often negative. The presence of autoantibodies may be detected in specialised laboratories by more refined tests based on the liberation of $^{14}$C-serotonin or platelet factor III, or, even more sensitive, the action of antiplatelet/platelet-immune complexes on granulocytes or lymphocytes. Study of the in vivo half-life of radiolabeled platelets shows considerable curtailment of the half-life. Splenectomy is indicated in persistant thrombocytopenia. Steroids are also effective but usually only transiently. Vincristine is used in certain resistant cases.

## PEMPHIGUS VULGARIS AND BULLOUS PEMPHIGOID

Pemphigus is a cutaneous disease characterized by the widespread occurrence of bullae that destroy intercellular bridges between epidermal cells (acantholysis). An autoimmune origin of the disease is suggested by the presence of cutaneous immunoglobulin and complement deposits (detected by immunofluorescence), and, in most patients, serum antibodies directed against epidermal intercellular antigens. These antibodies are not specific for human skin (they react with esophageal epithelium and tongue in several species). Their titer correlates with the severity of the disease. They are also present in myasthenia gravis and in severe burn patients (the latter suggests that they may be secondary to skin lesions). Human skin fragments cultivated in vitro are not altered histologically by these antibodies; however, the antibodies may have an essential action on intercellular connections. Acantholysis may be induced by injecting rabbits with serum from pemphigus patients (but only if they also receive chemical treatment simultaneously). A high incidence of rheumatoid factors and antinuclear antibodies is also characteristic and suggests that the disease has an immunologic etiology.

Other bullous diseases (bullous pemphigoid and dermatitis herpetiformis) are also associated with various immunologic abnormalities, particularly with antiskin antibodies and cutaneous immunoglobulin deposits. In pemphigoid, the antibody is directed against the basement membrane of the dermoepidermal junction. IgA deposits are especially common in dermatitis herpetiformis, as is the presence of HLA-B8 and DR3 antigens.

## ALLERGIC EYE DISEASE (IDIOPATHIC UVEITIS)

Ocular trauma may release autoantigens that may cause autoimmunization. Eye wounds may result in phacoanaphylaxis, uveitis, and sympathetic ophthalmia.

Phacoanaphylaxis follows ocular injury, including cataract surgery. It is usually unilateral. Lens antigens have two roles: they stimulate the autoimmune response and are also targets once sensitization has been established. The disease may also occur bilaterally if antigens are exposed in the contralateral eye. Lens antigens are sequestered in fetal life; this sequestration probably explains why they are considered foreign substances when released by trauma. Experimental guinea pig immunization with lens antigens induces a uveitis similar to the human disease, both clinically and pathologically.

Sympathetic ophthalmia is a granulomatous uveitis that occurs as a consequence of ocular perforation and affects the uveal tract. Lesions become bilateral after variable periods (3 weeks to several years). Circulating antiuvea antibodies are associated with delayed hypersensitivity to uveal tissue (skin tests). It is possible to induce uveitis or choroiditis in the guinea pig by injecting uveal tissue in Freund's adjuvant. However, these histologic lesions differ from human uveitis. An autoimmune origin of this lesion is not as well established as it is for phacoanaphylaxis.

## POSTMYOCARDIAL INFARCTION AND POSTCARDIOTOMY SYNDROME

Myocardial necrosis caused by myocardial infarction or trauma (after open heart surgery or pericardectomy) may lead to a syndrome that features fever, chest pain, and pleural or pericardial effusion (Dressler's syndrome). Arthralgia, leukocytosis, and increased erythrocytic sedimentation rate are also common. The syndrome begins a few days after myocardial infarction or trauma. Since antimyocardial antibodies have been detected (by immunofluorescence, complement fixation, or passive hemagglutination), this syndrome may have an autoimmune etiology. These antibodies also react with striated skeletal muscle but not with smooth muscle. They may be a cause, or a consequence, of Dressler's syndrome. They are not very specific, because they are also found in idiopathic pericarditis and endomyocardial fibrosis. At best, a pathogenic role is suggested by the fact that their appearance correlates with development of the clinical syndrome. A role for cell-mediated immunity may also be envisaged.

## MYASTHENIA GRAVIS

The symptoms of myasthenia gravis are muscular weakness and easy fatigua-bility; the former is due to a partial neuromuscular block, demonstrable by

**Table 32.3   Autoantibodies in Myasthenia Gravis**

| Antibodies | Early-onset myasthenia (%) | Families of these patients (%) | Late-onset myasthenia (%) | Controls (%) |
|---|---|---|---|---|
| Antistriated muscle | 5.6 | 13.4 | 40 | 3.8 |
| Antinuclear | 14.8 | 8.7 | 39.2 | 3.5 |
| Antimitochondria | 5.6 | 4.0 | 3.8 | 0.6 |
| Antismooth muscle | 9.2 | 12.1 | 10.1 | 1.9 |
| Antithyroid | 44.4 | 34.9 | 36.7 | 14.2 |
| Antigastric parietal cell | 11.3 | 9.5 | 21.5 | 4.6 |

After W. J. Irvine and J. R. Kalder.

electromyography, which can be provoked by giving antichoinesterase agents. The neuromuscular block may be presynaptic (affecting acetylcholine production) or postsynaptic (affecting motor plate receptors). Myasthenia gravis is excessively associated with many autoimmune diseases, including thyrotoxicosis, thyroiditis, pernicious anemia, Addison's disease, SLE, and Sjögren's syndrome. In addition, there are many autoantibodies present (antinuclear in 10% to 40% of cases, antithyroid in 40%, rheumatoid factor in 5% to 10%; Table 32.3) and the disease is significantly associated with HLA-A1 and B8 antigens that are markers of several immunologic diseases (see p. 695).

The presence of thymic abnormalities also suggests an immunologic etiology. One may find a thymoma (epithelial, lymphoid, or, more often, lymphoepithelial), or there may be simple hyperplasia characterized by numerous germinal centers (which are nonspecific for the disease). In some cases, the thymus is normal. Thymectomy is therapeutically effective (in 60% to 80% of cases); this fact, along with the presence of thymic abnormalities, has prompted a search for the existence of a circulating thymic factor that might depress neuromuscular transmission. G. Goldstein has now isolated a polypeptide factor (with a molecular weight close to 6000 daltons, called "thymopoietin") from calf thymus. This factor was later shown to induce the appearance of alloantigens on the surface of T-lymphocyte precursors (see p. 96). The significance of this observation remains uncertain, however.

In fact, another theory, implicating another type of humoral factor seems to be operative. This factor is an antibody-directed to the acetylcholine receptor on the motor end plate which is found in the serum of almost all myasthenic patients. This antibody is detected by an immunoprecipitation reaction mixing a human receptor preparation, the serum of the patient being investigated and labeled α-bungarotoxin, which has a high affinity for the receptors. The antibody titer is grossly related to the severity of the disease. Placental transmission of the antibodies explains the occurrence of neonatal myasthenia in the newborn of myasthenic mothers and the beneficial effects of plasmapheresis. Antiacetylcholine receptor antibodies are essentially species specific and may or may not disappear after thymectomy.

Myasthenic patients also show a high incidence of striated antimuscle antibodies, generally IgG, detectable by immunofluorescence, complement fixation, or passive hemagglutination. These antibodies react with cardiac muscle and, in fact, have two specificities: S, associated with complement-fixing antibodies directed against striated muscles, and SH, associated with noncomplement fixing antibodies, which react with striated muscle and heart. The latter antibody is detected by passive hemagglutination. S antibodies also bind to the cytoplasm of thymus epithelial cells, onto muscle structures present in some of these cells. The incidence of antimuscle antibodies is higher in cases with thymoma, and these antibodies may, in fact, be found in cases of thymoma without myasthenia. Subjects with very severe stages of the disease have antibodies more often than do those with less advanced forms. Antistriated muscle antibodies are, however, probably not the cause of neuromuscular blockade, because they do not fix onto the motor plate, are not present in myasthenic newborns, and are often absent in myasthenia without thymoma.

An experimental disease reminiscent of myasthenia occurs after injection of heterologous thymus or muscle or of isolated acetylcholine receptors in the presence of Freund's adjuvant. Cross-reactions between antithymus and antistriated muscle antibodies probably explain why either thymus or muscle immunization produces thymitis (defined as aggregates of small lymphocytes around Hassall's corpuscles) and a partial neuromuscular block. This neuromuscular block bears no relation to the presence of antistriated muscle antibodies but correlates with thymitis. Thymectomy performed in the guinea pig before immunization with muscle extracts prevents neuromuscular blockade. Thymectomy performed after the onset of the blockade diminishes its intensity. It should be mentioned that mastomys (South African rodents), which have a high incidence of thymoma, develop myositis, atrophy of striated muscles, and myocarditis and also have antistriated muscle antibodies.

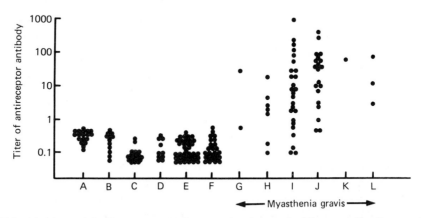

**Fig. 32.2**  Antiacetylcholine receptors in myasthenia gravis. These antibodies are found in the vast majority of myasthenias (G: in remission; H: exclusively ocular myasthenia; I: moderate form; J: moderately severe form; K: severe acute form; L: chronic severe form). In contrast, these autoantibodies are not found in the various control groups (A: normal subjects; B: Lambert-Eaton syndrome; C: amyotrophic lateral sclerosis; D: polymyositis; E: various neurologic abnormalities; F: nonneurologic diseases). (After J. M. Lindstrom, M. E. Scybold, V. A. Lennon, S. Whittington, and D. D. Duane, Neurology, 1976, 26, 1054.)

In conclusion, numerous arguments favor an autoimmune origin for myasthenia gravis, probably through antibodies, but its mechanisms remain unclear. The autoimmune reaction may cause secretion of humoral factors that suppress neuromuscular transmission. Antiacetylcholine receptor antibody is an appealing explanation. A pathophysiologic role for antistriated muscle antibodies and antithymus antibodies is less clear. The favorable therapeutic effects of thymectomy and plasmophoresis and the prevention of experimental "paramyasthenic" syndromes by thymectomy show that humoral factors secreted by the thymus, perhaps influenced by antithymus antibodies, have a role. Unexplained is the cross-reactivity between thymic and antistriated muscle antibodies.

# III.  POSTINFECTIOUS IMMUNOPATHOLOGY

In this section, we will describe clinical features or diseases that follow bacterial or viral infections in which the infection, however, is probably not the direct cause of the disease. Systemic lupus erythematosus (virus?), acute, and certain poststreptococcal glomerulonephritides have already been discussed (see pp. 797 and 840).

## RHEUMATIC FEVER

Rheumatic fever is a polyarthritis that is usually self-limited, abating within a few days and leaving a risk of cardiac complications (valvular, myocardial, or pericardial). In rare cases, the disease may reappear and aggravate cardiac lesions. Histologically, one may recognize the presence of quasiconstant characteristic Aschoff's nodules, which are cell aggregates that surround eosinophilic material. The causative role of β-hemolytic streptococci is well established. Rheumatic fever usually occurs 1–3 weeks after a febrile sore throat. The *Streptococcus* may be cultured, and various types of β-hemolytic streptococci are etiologic. There is usually a high titer of antistreptolysin O (>500 Todd units) concurrent with antibodies directed toward other streptococcal products (e.g., hyaluronidase or streptokinase). It is important to note that a simultaneous search for several antibodies almost always yields positive results for at least one antibody.

The basis of the relationship between streptococcal infection and rheumatic fever remains speculative. Generally, no streptococci are found in heart lesions. Direct participation of streptococci or their exotoxins is, moreover, improbable because of the time lag between infection and clinical onset of the disease, and because antibiotic administration has no beneficial effect on the course of the disease if given several days after symptomatic sore throat. Production of antistreptococcal antibodies is only slightly higher than that observed in other streptococcal infections. Apparently, there is no overall immunologic hyperreactivity that causes antibody production to antigens other than streptococcal ones. It seems possible that antistreptococcal antigens may function as immune complexes (antigen excess), simulating serum sickness disease (which may also cause heart lesions). This hypothesis obviously does not explain why the heart is selectively affected, nor does this mechanism explain why there is β-hemolytic streptococcal specificity. It is possible that the streptococci induce formation of antibodies directed against autoantigens released by infected tissues or against autoantigenic determinants present in the streptococci (myocardial cross-reactions). A cross-reaction has been demonstrated between streptococcal membranes and heart tissues: such antibodies do occur in the serum of rheumatic fever patients. These antibodies (shown by immunofluorescence) may selectively bind sarcolemma or cause diffuse binding, as in postinfarction and postcardiotomy syndromes (see p. 926). They may be found in 40–60% of subjects with heart lesions. Moreover, Ig and C3 deposits (detected by immunofluorescence) are found on auricular biopsy of mitral valve surgery patients.

Interestingly, antiheart antibodies in rheumatic fever may be absorbed by streptococci (unlike autoantibodies in Dressler's syndrome). Serum absorption by streptococci completely suppresses cardiac binding. Conversely, absorption by heart tissue diminishes antistreptococcal activity. It is still difficult to determine the clinical role of the antibodies that react with both streptococci and heart tissue; they are also found in benign (nonrheumatic fever) streptococcal infection. The titer of these antibodies may be higher in the early phases of rheumatic fever; late-phase antibodies seem to be more easily absorbed by heart tissue than by streptococci and could be secondary to late autoimmunization. In addition, there may be antigenic determinants shared by streptococci and cerebral neurons, which could explain the chorea observed in rheumatic fever. In conclusion, the data available suggest that heart antibodies produced during the initial response to streptococcal antigens may be responsible for the disease. We have already discussed mechanisms by which foreign antigens may induce cross-reacting autoantibodies (see p. 724). It is, nonetheless, surprising that no clear distinction between rheumatic fever patients and common streptococcal infection patients exists in terms of antibody titers; it is nearly impossible to reproduce acute rheumatic fever by experimental immunization with streptococci. Heart and streptococcal antigens, in addition, are extremely complex and poorly understood. We may not yet be able to recognize antibodies that are actually involved in the disease (cross-reacting antibodies); cell mediated immunity may be involved but, alternatively, anti-heart autoimmunity may not be pathogenic. The intervention of cell-mediated immunity has also been seriously considered.

## HEPATITIS

Knowledge about acute and chronic hepatitis was boosted by the discovery of Australia antigen (HBs) by Blumberg in 1965. Discussion continues as to whether particles visible on electron microscopy are the actual virus of hepatitis B or one of its metabolic products. It is believed that the 40-nm particles (core) may be the actual virus, while the smaller particles may represent its degradation products. It is now known that the 42 nm diameter Dane particles, or more precisely their central zone or core, may represent the virus, whereas the small particles represent some of their products. The cores also possess antigens

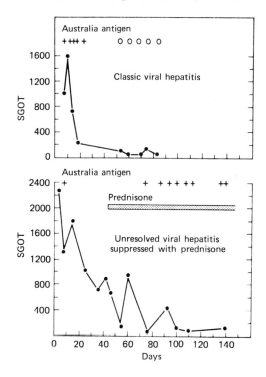

**Fig. 32.3** Evolution of Australia antigen (HBs) antigenemia (0/+) during ordinary viral hepatitis (*top*) and complicated hepatitis treated with prednisone (*bottom*). (From R. Wright, R. W. McCollum, and G. Klatskin, Lancet, 1969, *2*, 117.)

(HBc) that are distinct from the surface antigens (HBs). A further antigen, HBe, has recently been described and is separate from HBs and HBc; it appears transiently before the onset of the clinical symptoms of acute hepatitis. Its persistance is a poor prognostic sign. It should also be noted that several subtypes of HBs antigens exist that are useful in epidemiologic studies.

### Acute Hepatitis

We differentiate between epidemic hepatitis (due to virus A) and inoculation hepatitis (due to virus B); the latter may be transmitted by other routes (e.g., gastrointestinal). Icterus follows a long incubation time (15–50 days for virus A, 50–100 days for virus B). The prodrome is reminiscent of acute serum sickness, because urticaria and arthralgia are usually present. Icterus is then seen most often associated with the symptoms of hepatocellular failure (retained sulfobromophthalein) and cytolysis (increased transaminase level). In virus B hepatitis, HBs antigen appears in the serum before the elevation of transaminases and disappears a few days later, except in a few patients, in whom it persists for months to years without necessarily causing overt clinical or biologic hepatic disease. It is, then, usual but not constant for anti-HBc antibodies to occur.

The mechanisms responsible for the development of liver lesions remain obscure. The host's response to the virus is an important factor: immunosuppressed hosts (chronic hemodialysis or renal transplantation) show an increased HBs antigen incidence and do not always eliminate it (40% to 50% of hemodialyzed patients in France have the HBs antigen). These subjects only rarely show the characteristic clinical signs of hepatitis (e.g., icterus) and rarely develop chronic hepatitis despite persistence of the HBs antigen. In normal subjects, a transient depression of T-cell function occurs during the acute phase of the disease (the significance of this depression is controversial). However, during acute hepatitis, cell-mediated immunity to HBs antigen (lymphoblastic transformation test or leukocyte migration inhibition) is seen. At the beginning of the acute phase of hepatitis, hypocomplementemia and elevated serum IgG levels are observed. Various autoantibodies are found in most cases of acute hepatitis (in nearly 80% of cases), in particular, antismooth muscle antibodies and rheumatoid factor.

### Chronic Active Hepatitis

Chronic active hepatitis (CAH) is one form of chronic hepatitis characterized by progressive course, accompanied by numerous immunologic abnormalities (the so-called lupoid hepatitis, autoimmune hepatitis, or plasmacytic hepatitis). Clinically, CAH causes slight if any icterus and splenomegaly. Transaminases are elevated during exacerbations. Hepatocellular insufficiency is significant but is highly variable from case to case. It may evolve to cirrhosis. Prior to cirrhosis, the histologic features are hepatocellular necrosis and lymphocytic and plasmacytic infiltration.

Immunologic abnormalities include hypergammaglobulinemia, antinuclear antibodies (in 20% to 50% of cases), which may induce an in vitro LE cell phenomenon, rheumatoid factor, smooth muscle antibodies (apparently directed against structures similar to actomyosin), and antibodies to biliary canaliculi. Antibodies directed against various bacteria and viruses may also be observed. IgG levels are elevated in about 70% of cases, and hypocomplementemia is common (the latter may be due to consumption by immune complexes or decreased synthesis).

Significant inhibition of leukocyte migration in the presence of hepatic antigenic extracts has been reported. The presence of serum HBs antigen is highly variable (5% to 25% of cases). Thus, one refers to seropositive and seronegative CAH. Antismooth muscle IgG antibodies are only present in the

**Table 32.4   Comparison of Chronic Active Hepatitis (CAH) With and Without HBs**

|                              | CAH with HBs                 | CAH without HBs              |
|------------------------------|------------------------------|-----------------------------|
| Age                          | Predominant in aged subjects | Predominant in young subjects |
| Sex                          | Usually affects men          | Usually affects women       |
| Extrahepatic manifestations  | Rare                         | Frequent                    |
| Various autoantibodies       | Rare                         | Frequent                    |
| Hypergammaglobulinemia       | Moderate                     | Important                   |
| Geographic distribution      | Localized to certain regions | Apparently universal        |
| Response to corticosteroids  | Not well established         | Favorable                   |
| Prognosis                    | Unknown                      | Usually mediocre            |

seronegative form of the disease. Generally speaking, autoantibodies (especially antinuclear) and hypergammaglobulinemia occur only in seronegative CAH. The latter disease is more common in young women, whereas seropositive hepatitis more often affects males over 40. Seronegative forms show significant association with HLA-A1 and -B8 antigens.

In conclusion, acute hepatitis and CAH (which may or may not be interrelated) are associated with important immunologic abnormalities. The available data are compatible with a concept of immunologic aggression of virus-infected hepatocytes producing neoantigens that cause antibody formation and lymphocytic sensitization (whether to HBs or other antigens, in particular a membrane lipoprotein antigen). Immune complexes, notably HBs antigen and its corresponding antibody, may explain most of the extrahepatic manifestations, particularly the prodromal phase of acute hepatitis, but doubtless play a minor role in the pathogenesis of the hepatitis itself. Their intervention in the pathogenesis of certain cases of polyarteritis nodosa has been discussed. This hypothesis, which remains to be documented, states that the hepatitis virus is not in itself pathogenic or that pathogenicity may not be the primary factor in the disease.

These data concern the B virus. Analogous mechanisms may almost certainly be envisaged for epidemic acute hepatitis due to A virus, but, in the absence of markers (like HBs antigen), the immunopathology of this form of hepatitis is much less well documented. A new hepatitis virus has recently been isolated, the non-A non-B virus. Its involvement in the onset of acute hepatitis and chronic active hepatitis is now demonstrated, but its prevalence among hepatitis patients still remains to be determined.


## LEPROSY

Leprosy is caused by Hansen's bacillus (*Mycobacterium leprae*). Tuberculoid leprosy resembles cutaneous tuberculosis and is only slowly progressive. This form of the disease must be differentiated from lepromatous leprosy, which affects bones, nerves, and mucosal membranes. In the latter, enormous numbers of bacilli are present, and there is an unfavorable prognosis. There are, however, intermediary states, and the disease may vary from one form to another. The existence of cell-mediated immunity to the bacillus can be demonstrated in tuberculoid leprosy by positive skin reactions to lepromin (an emulsion of the bacteria). This reaction is usually negative in lepromatous leprosy.

Lepromatous leprosy is characterized by many immunologic abnormalities. There is a generalized loss of delayed hypersensitivity cutaneous reactivity to mycobacterial and nonmycobacterial antigens. At the same time, in vitro blast cell responses to PHA are decreased, and there is a reduced number of T cells (as assessed by the sheep red blood cell rosette test). A circulating factor may depress DNA synthesis in lepromatous patients. Such decreased cell-mediated immunity is associated with elevated serum Ig titers, the presence of cryoglobulins and of immune complexes (detected by the techniques described on p. 734), and with the presence of numerous autoantibodies. Anticardiolipin antibodies may cause false positive syphilis reactions. These abnormalities may either be secondary to the disease or indicators of a peculiar immunologic background that favors development of the disease. This immunologic picture resembles systemic lupus erythematosus (SLE), since B-cell hyperfunction is associated with T-cell depression (see p. 713).

## GUILLAIN-BARRÉ SYNDROME

Some infections may be complicated by an acute polyneuritis that may involve all the peripheral nerves but particularly affects those nerves supplying the muscles of respiration and the cranial nerves with corresponding threat to the prognosis. This is notably the case with some respiratory infections and a number of acute viral infections, such as measles, infectious mononucleosis, and hepatitis. Recovery begins after the third week of the syndrome and complete cure often, but not always, occurs in several months. Guillain-Barré's syndrome is a demyelinating disorder of the peripheral nerves characterized by a mononuclear cell infiltrate similar to that seen in experimental allergic neuritis obtained by the injection into an animal of a preparation of peripheral nerve myelin in the presence of Freund's adjuvant. By comparison with the data obtained with this experimental model, it has been suggested that cell-mediated immunity, transmissible by means of lymphoid cells, plays the essential role rather than antimyelin antibodies. In addition, lymphocyte transformation and lymphokine production can be observed in response to peripheral nerve extracts by lymphocytes from patients suffering from the Guillain-Barré syndrome. On the other hand, the specificity of the demyelinating activity observed in the serum of these patients is not demonstrable any more than is that of the IgM and C3 deposits seen along these nerves by the use of immunofluorescent techniques. The frequent presence of circulating IC and, possibly, an acute glomerulonephritis, confirms the existence of humoral abnormalities but does not provide any direct evidence in favor of their pathogenic role in peripheral neuritis. The treatment of the Guillain-Barré syndrome requires the use of corticosteroids and possibly immunosuppressants, but their therapeutic efficacy is still uncertain.

# IV.   UNCLASSIFIABLE DISEASES

Under this heading, we have placed several diseases that are not readily classifiable. However, these disorders possess immunologic abnormalities that may partially explain their pathogenesis.

## MULTIPLE SCLEROSIS AND OTHER DEGENERATIVE DISEASES OF THE CENTRAL NERVOUS SYSTEM

The pathogenesis of multiple sclerosis remains speculative. Demonstration of several immunologic abnormalities has suggested an immunologic origin, perhaps associated with viral infection. Cerebrospinal fluid IgG level may be elevated without a rise in serum IgG, suggesting local IgG synthesis. Lymphocytes may also be increased in number in the cerebrospinal fluid but are of unknown nature and origin. A possible analogy with experimental allergic encephalomyelitis (see p. 717) has prompted study of humoral immunity and delayed hypersensitivity to cerebral tissue, but the results have been generally negative. The only positive results show cytotoxic antibodies to glial cells and cultivated myelinized nerve fibers; however, these antibodies are not specific for multiple sclerosis. Preliminary studies that demonstrate a cytotoxic action of lymphocytes toward cerebral tissue have yet to be repeated. Studies that show a specific depression of leukocyte migration inhibition to measles virus have not been confirmed. The search for a virus has been disappointing. The sera of patients with multiple sclerosis may contain, however, high titers of antimeasles antibodies, which are also present in the cerebrospinal fluid. Analogies with experimental neurologic diseases in the sheep caused by slow viruses (scrapie and visna) are not too impressive. Although an immunologic basis for multiple sclerosis is suspected because of these immunologic abnormalities, and because of the partial analogy to allergic encephalomyelitis, the mechanisms involved and the role of a virus remain to be determined. A now well-established association is known to exist between the presence of the disease and the histocompatibility groups, HLA-B7 and DR2, and the observation of a deficiency of certain subpopulations of T cells, in particular suppressor T cells (as assessed by functional analysis or by using monoclonal anti-T cell antibodies). This may be the basis of new theoretical and experimental approaches.

Several other degenerative diseases of the central nervous system seem to be linked with a chronic viral infection. Subacute sclerosing panencephalitis is due to measles virus. Progressive multifocal leukoencephalopathy is due to a papaovirus. The subacute spongiform encephalopathies, such as kuru and Jakob-Creutzfeldt disease in man and scrapie in sheep, seem to be due to transmissible agents that can be isolated from the brain and are probably slow viruses. Although the role of the host's immune response in the genesis of these diseases is not very clear, it is tempting to suggest that a cellular immune deficiency may contribute to the pathogenesis of these diseases. This would particularly explain the persistence of measles virus in the presence of high antibody titers in subacute sclerosing panencephalitis. Furthermore, in vitro tests of delayed hypersensitivity against measles virus are generally negative.

## CROHN'S DISEASE (REGIONAL ENTERITIS)

Crohn's disease is a chronic inflammatory condition of the intestine, especially severe in the terminal ileum, that has no known etiology. The main symptoms are diarrhea, emaciation, and abdominal pains that may sometimes simulate acute appendicitis. Several extraintestinal manifestations may complicate the disease. These concomitants include polyarthritis, ankylosing spondylitis, erythema nodosum, oral ulcers, and liver dysfunction. Histologic examination reveals inflammatory features, diffuse hyperemia, ulcers, mononuclear cell infiltration, and granuloma.

Several immunologic abnormalities have been described in Crohn's disease, for example, a positive Kweim test (intradermal reaction toward extracts of sarcoid lymph nodes) and depressed phytohemagglutin (PHA) or delayed hypersensitivity reactions. These data require more study, however. Circulating lymphocytes from Crohn's disease have been claimed to be cytotoxic for colonic epithelial cells, and the serum of these patients may inhibit K-cell cytotoxicity (see p. 413), perhaps through immune complexes. These data are much too preliminary to suggest a significant contribution of immunologic phenomena to the pathogenesis of the disease. However, Crohn's disease is sometimes associated with other diseases also suspected to have an immunologic origin. There are also great similarities to ulcerative colitis, for which an immunologic basis is more firmly established.

## ULCERATIVE COLITIS

Ulcerative colitis is a chronic inflammatory colonic disease characterized by diffuse inflammation of all or part of the mucosa. The major symptoms are diarrhea and colonic hemorrhage. The disease progresses despite many remissions. As in Crohn's disease, extraintestinal complications, such as uveitis, arthritis, ankylosing spondylitis, erythema nodosum, and liver dysfunction, are not uncommon. The histologic features include deep ulcerations and lymphocytic infiltrates.

Numerous etiologies for Crohn's disease have been proposed, namely, infectious, nutritional, psychosomatic, and immunologic. The latter has been proposed based on demonstration of various immunologic abnormalities. Serum anticolon antibodies have been demonstrated in affected patients by passive hemagglutination. Similar results are also obtained with immunofluorescence techniques. However, positive results are found in only about 20% of subjects, with either of these techniques, and there is no correlation with the severity of the disease. Colonic antigens are lipopolysaccharides similar to gram-negative bacteria; anticolon autoantibodies cross-react with anti-*Escherichia coli* lipopolysaccharide antibodies. Interpretation is complicated by the existence of colonic alloantigens because anticolon alloantibodies may incorrectly be considered to be autoantibodies.

Lymphocytes from patients with this disease have been reported to cause a colon-specific cytotoxic reaction that disappears after colectomy. This reaction may be inhibited by homologous (but not by autologous) serum and by *E. coli* lipopolysaccharides. However, the specificity of these observations has not yet been clearly demonstrated. Other data, now well established, include a depressed response to PHA and the presence of immune complexes, detected by inhibition of K-cell cytotoxicity.

## CELIAC DISEASE

Celiac disease is a disorder of the small intestine characterized by steatorrhea due to malabsorption and infiltration of the jejunal lamina propria by lymphocytes and plasmocytes. The digestive symptoms are due to gluten ingestion. Exclusion of gluten from the diet produces clinical remission from the disease.

It was initially thought that patients suffering from celiac disease were congenitally deficient in a peptidase necessary for the hydrolysis of a toxic degradation product of gluten. Biochemical studies of the jejunum have not confirmed this hypothesis. These days one rather leans towards an immunologic pathogenesis based on the existence of several converging pieces of evidence. First, the lymphoplasmocytic infiltration mentioned above. Second, if gluten is regiven to someone who was sensitive and abstained from it, anaphylactic shock may occur. In addition antigluten antibodies may be found in the serum and intestinal secretions. The serum levels of IgA-, IgD-, and IgM-bearing cells in the jejunum is increased and antireticulin antibodies and IC are seen in the serum. Finally, as with many other autoimmune diseases, this disorder is associated with antigens HLA-A1, B8, DR3. It is also associated with an increased incidence of dermatitis herpetiformis, which is itself associated with the same HLA antigens A1, B8, and DR3.

## BILIARY CIRRHOSIS

Biliary cirrhosis is characterized by intrahepatic cholestasis, pruritus, icterus, steatorrhea, and hepatosplenomegaly. The prognosis is unfavorable once hepatic failure ensues. The histologic hallmark is mononuclear cell infiltration, concurrent with granulomatous and postnecrotic cirrhosis. Numerous immunologic abnormalities have suggested an autoimmune origin. Antismooth muscle and antinuclear antibodies are frequently found, simulating chronic active hepatitis (see p. 932). A more characteristic antibody is antimitochondrial, detectable by immunofluorescence; this antibody is not organ or species specific. It is present in 90% of biliary cirrhosis cases and in less than 10% of patients with active chronic hepatitis and other varieties of cirrhosis. The mitochondrial antigens have not yet been defined. Delayed hypersensitivity is often depressed, as assessed by globally negative skin tests and a depressed T-cell function in the in vitro lymphocyte response to PHA. Australia antigen is generally absent. All of these facts suggest that primary biliary cirrhosis may be autoimmune in origin; however, definitive evidence is lacking. Its relationship to active chronic hepatitis remains to be determined.

## BEHÇET'S SYNDROME

Behçet's syndrome is a chronic inflammatory disorder that manifests itself by mucosal ulcers (notably of the mouth and genital organs), vasculitis, arthritis, gastrointestinal symptoms and ocular effects that may, in the long term, result in blindness. Its pathogenesis is unknown. A role for a virus has been suggested as well as the implication of autoimmunization against mucosal antigens on the basis of the demonstration of antimucosal cell antibodies detected by immunofluorescence and the presence of lymphocytes and plasmocytes around the vessels. There is also lymphocytic hyperreactivity in response to mucosal antigens. The syndrome is associated with the HLA-B5 antigen.

## SARCOIDOSIS

Sarcoidosis is a systemic granulomatous disorder involving mainly the respiratory system (dyspnea), the skin (erythema nodosum), the eyes (iritis), and the lymphoid system (splenomegaly, lymphadenopathy). The disease is often asymptomatic and diagnosed fortuitously on thoracic x-rays, which show mediastinal lymphadenopathy and pulmonary infiltration. The Kveim test consists of an intradermal injection of a splenic extract from a patient with sarcoidosis. A positive test occurs when the inoculation site becomes nodular and histology shows that this nodule contains granulomas analogous to those seen in cutaneous lesions. The test is positive in 80% of patients and only in 2% of the normal population. The significance of this test is, however, limited by the lack of precision in defining what exactly constitutes a granuloma microscopically and the complexity of preparing the antigen. Its significance is further obscured by the fact that attempts to analyze the lymphocytic response of such patients to splenic extract have given conflicting results. More interesting, from the immunologic point of view, are the abnormalities of cellular immunity seen in these patients. Depression of delayed-hypersensitivity responses almost amounting to anergy, diminution of T-cell number (E rosette test), diminished lymphocyte responses to mitogenic stimulation (even though this is quite variable from one patient to another) have all been described. At the same time, one may see increases in the Ig levels and the presence of certain autoantibodies (notably antinuclear, antithyroid, and antigastric) and circulating immune complexes. It is tempting, in view of all this data, to incriminate immunologic phenomena to explain the granuloma, but no simple etiologic schema that includes all the multiple immunologic abnormalities can readily be proposed.

## AMYLOIDOSIS

This is a systemic disease caused by the deposition in various organs of a proteinaceous substance, termed amyloid, which is easily recognized on light microscopy. The main clinical manifestations of this disorder are renal (the most serious), cutaneous, cardiac, hepatic, neurologic, muscular, and gastrointestinal.

Primary amyloidosis, which has no known cause and occasionally has an hereditary link, is distinguished from secondary amyloidosis, which is secondary to myeloma or other dysglobulinemia, rheumatoid arthritis, familial mediterranean fever, of chronic infections, particularly tuberculosis. It should be noted that all these disorders are associated with significant immunologic abnormalities, from which arises the concept that amyloidosis has a relationship with the immune system.

In actual fact, the solubilization of the fibrils of amyloid substance and analysis of their amino acid sequences show that, in numerous cases, amyloid substance is composed of Ig light chains, particularly of their variable parts (Glenner). In other cases, however, analysis of amyloid substances fails to reveal any Ig fragments but shows the presence of a substance with a molecular weight of about 8,000 that is unrelated to Ig and is known as substance A (Franklin).

The serum level of substance A is elevated in many cases of amyloidosis and also in rheumatoid arthritis or inflammatory disorders as well as in the elderly.

Several mechanisms may serve to explain the deposition of Ig in the form of amyloid substance in the tissues, for example, the abnormal catabolism of immune complexes by macrophages, a de novo synthesis of Ig with reduced solubility, production of Ig with abnormal light chains (deletion), or an abnormal and isolated synthesis of light chains.

## OTHER DISEASES

Certain poorly characterized immunologic abnormalities may be observed in disorders as diverse as polychondritis, Weber-Christian disease, or idiopathic pulmonary fibrosis. It may be an elevation in serum Ig levels, the presence of circulating immune complexes, the presence of lymphoplasmocytic infiltrates in the lesions, the (unconfirmed) presence of autoantibodies (by immunofluorescence), or a significant association between the disorder and either an abnormal incidence of autoimmune diseases or HLA antigens. These data must be interpreted with care and await more extensive information before concluding that an actual relationship exists between the immunologic phenomenon and its role in the pathogenesis of the disease.

## BIBLIOGRAPHY

ALLISON A. C. Self tolerance and auto-immunity in the thyroïd. New Engl. J. Med., 1976, 295, 821.

ARNASON B. Idiopathic polyneuritis as an autoimmune disease. In: Immune mechanisms and disease (D. B. Amos, R. S. Schwartz, and B. W. Janicki [eds.]). Acad. Press, London, 1980, 179.

CHAJEK T. and FAINARU M. Behçet's disease. In: Clinical Immunology (C. W. Parker [ed.]). Saunders, Philadelphia, 1980, 632.

DONIACH D. Autoimmunity in liver diseases. In R. S. Schwartz, Ed., Progress in clinical immunology. Vol. I. New York, 1972, Grune & Stratton, p. 45.

DONIACH D. and MARSHALL N. J. Autoantibodies to the thyrotropin (TSH) receptors on thyroid epithelium and other tissues. In N. Talal, Ed., Autoimmunity: genetic, immunologic, virologic and clinical aspects. New York, 1977, Academic Press, p. 621.

DONIACH D. and ROITT I. M. Thyroid and autoallergic disease. In P. G. H. Gell, R. R. A. Coombs, and P. J. Lachmann, Eds., Clinical aspects of immunology. ed. 3. Oxford, 1975. Blackwell, p. 1355

DONIACH D. and ROITT I. M. Autoimmune thyroid disease. In P. Miescher and H. Müller-Eberhard, Eds., Textbook of immunopathology, ed. 2, New York, 1973, Grune & Stratton.

EDDLESTON A. L. W. F. Immunology and the liver. In: Clinical Immunology (C. W. Parker [ed.]). Saunders, Philadelphia, 1980, 1009.

FAMBROUGH D. M. Control of acetylcholine receptors in skeletal muscle. Phys. Rev., 1979, 59, 165.

FRANKLIN E. C. and GOREVIC P. D. The amyloid diseases. In: Immunology 80 (M. Fougereau and J. Dausset [eds.]). Acad. Press, New York, 1980: 1219.

GLENNER G. G., TERRY W. D., and TSERSKY C. Amyloïdosis. Its nature and pathogenesis. Seminars in Hematology, 1973, 10, 65.

GLENNER G. G. Amyloid deposits and amyloidosis (Part I and Part II). New Engl. J. Med., 1980, 302, 1283, 1333.

HARBOE M. and GLOSS O. Immunological aspects of leprosy. In: Immunology 80 (M. Fougereau and J. Dausset [eds.]). Acad. Press, New York, 1980: 1231.

IRVINE W. J. Autoimmunity in endocrine diseases. In T. E. Mandel, C. Cheers, C. S. Hosking, I. F. C. Mc Kenzie, and G. J. V. Nossal, Eds., Progress in immunology III. Proc. 3rd Intern. Cong. Immunol. Sydney. Amsterdam, 1977, North Holland.

IRVINE W. J. and KALDER J. R. Muscle in allergic disease. Myasthenia gravis and polymyositis. In P. G. H. Gell, R. R. A. Coombs et P. J. Lachmann, Eds., Clinical aspects of immunology. Oxford, 1975, Blackwell, p. 1467.

IRVINE W. J. and BARNES E. W. Addison's disease and associated conditions. In P. G. H. Gell, R. R. A. Coombs, and P. J. Lachmann, Eds., Clinical aspects of immunology, ed. 3. Oxford, 1975, Blackwell, p. 1301.

JEFFREY W. and PARISH W. E. Allergic infertility: laboratory techniques to detect antispermatozoal antibodies. Clin. Allergy, 1972, 2, 261.

JOHNSON M. H., HEKMAN A., and RUMKE P. The male and female genital tracts in allergic disease. In P. G. H. Gell, R. R. A. Coombs, and P. J. Lachmann, Eds., Clinical aspects of immunology, ed. 3. Oxford, 1975. Blackwell, p. 1509.

LEVO Y. and FRANKLIN E. C. Systemic immunologic complications of hepatitis B virus infection. In: Clinical Immunology Update. Elsevier, New York, 1979, 161.

LINDSTROM J. Autoimmune response to acetylcholine receptors in myasthenia gravis and in animal models. Adv. Immunol., 1979, 27, 1.

McGUIGAN J. E. and LEIBACH J. R. Immunology and diseases of the gastro intestinal tract. In: Clinical Immunology (C. W. Parker [ed.]). Saunders, Philadelphia, 1980, 867.

Mc KAY I. R. and CARNEGIE P. R. Cell-surface receptors and auto-immune response. In N. Talal, Ed., Autoimmunity; genetic, immunologic, virologic and clinical aspects. New-York, 1977, Academic Press, p. 569.

MIESCHER P. A. and MÜLLER-EBERHARD H. J. (Eds.) Textbook of immunopathology, section II, ed. 2. New-York, 1976, Grune & Stratton, p. 369.

NEUWELT E. A. and CLARK N. Y. Clinical aspects of neuroimmunology. Williams and Wilkins, Baltimore, 1978, 277 p.

PATERSON P. Y. Auto-immune neurological diseases: experimental animal systems and implication of multiple sclerosis. In N. Talal, Ed., Autoimmunity: genetic, immunologic, virologic and clinical aspects. New-York, 1977, Academic Press, p. 643.

ROSE N. R., BACON L. D., SUNDICK R. S., KONG Y. M., ESQUIVEL P., and BIGAZZI P. E. Genetic regulation in auto-immune thyroiditis. In N. Talal, Ed., Auto-immunity: genetic, immunologic, virologic and clinical aspects. New-York, 1977, Academic Press, p. 141.

ROSE F. C. Clinical neuroimmunology. Blackwell, Oxford, 1979, 526 p.

ROSENTHAL C. J. and FRANKLIN E. C. Amyloidosis and amyloid proteins. In R. A. THOMPSON Ed., Recent advances in clinical immunology. Edinburgh, 1977, Churchill-Livingstone, p. 41.

RUMKE P. H. Auto- and isoimmune reactions to antigens of the gonads and genital tract. In: Immunology 80 (M. Fougereau and J. Dausset [eds.]). Acad. Press, New York, 1980: 1065.

SHORTER R. G. Immunological aspects of gastrointestinal disease: an up-to-date account of inflammatory diseases such as ulcerative colitis and Crohn's disease. In L. Brent and J. Holborow, Eds., Progress in immunology. II. Vol. 4. Amsterdam, 1974, North Holland, p. 209.

TRUELOVE S. C. and DEWEL D. P. The intestine in allergic diseases. In P. G. H. Gell, R. R. A. Coombs, and P. J. Lachmann, Eds., Clinical aspects of immunology, ed. 3. Oxford, 1975, Blackwell, p. 1441.

WEIGLE W. O. Cellular events in experimental auto-immune thyroïditis, allergic encephalomyelitis and tolerance to self. In N. Talal, Ed., Autoimmunity: genetic, immunologic, virologic and clinical aspects. New York, 1977, Academic Press, p. 141.

WHITNACK E. and BISNO A. L. Rheumatic fever and other immunologically mediated cardiac diseases. In: Clinical Immunology (C. W. Parker [ed.]). Saunders, Philadelphia, 1980, 894.

ZUCKERMAN A. J. Human viral hepatitis. Hepatitis-associated antigens and viruses. ed. 2. Amsterdam, 1975, North Holland, 422 p.

## ORIGINAL ARTICLES

AHARONOV A., ABAMSKY O., TARRAB-HADZAI R., and FUCHS S. Humoral antibodies to acetylcholine receptors in patients with myasthenia gravis. Lancet 1975, *1*, 346.

BACH M. A., PHAN DINH TUY F., TOURNIER E., CHATENOUD L., BACH J. F., MARTIN C., and DEGOS D. Deficit of suppressor T cells in active multiple sclerosis. Lancet, 1980, 2, 1221.

BLUMBERG B. S., SUTNICK A. I., and LONDON W. T. Australia antigen as a hepatitis virus: variation in host response. Amer. J. Med., 1970, *48*, 1.

GOLDSTEIN G., STRAUSS A. J. L., and PICKERAL L. S. Antigens in thymus and muscle effective in induction of experimental autoimmune thymitis and the release of thymin. Clin Exp. Immunol., 1969, *4*, 3.

HAAS G. G., CINES D. G., and SCHREIBER A. D. Immunologic infertility: Identification of patients with antisperm antibody. New Engl. J. Med. 1980, 303, 727.

JENSEN D. M., MC FARLANE I. G., PORTMANN B. S., EDDLESTON A. L. W. F., and WILLIAMS R. Detection of antibodies directed against a liver-specific membrane lipoprotein in patients with acute and chronic active hepatitis. New Engl. J. Med., 1978, *299*, 1.

KAPLAN M. H. and MEYESERIAN M. An immunologic cross-reaction between group A streptococcal cells and human heart tissue. Lancet, 1962, *1*, 706.

LERNMARK A., FREEDMAN J. F., HOFFMANN C., RUBENSTEIN A. H., STEINER D. F., JACKSON R. I.., WINTER R. J., and TRAISMAN H. S. Islet-cell surface antibodies in juvenile diabetes mellitus. New Engl. J. Med., 1978, *299*, 375.

LINDSTROM J. M., EINARSON B., LENNON V. A., and SYBOLD M. E. Pathological mechanisms in experimental auto-immune myasthenia gravis. I. Immunogenicity of syngeneic muscle acetyl-choline receptors and quantitative extraction of receptor and antibody-receptor complexes from muscles of rats with experimental auto-immune myasthenia gravis. J. Exp. Med., 1976, *144*, 685.

McKAY I. R. and MORRIS P. J. Association of auto-immune active chronic hepatitis with HL-A, 1,8. Lancet, 1972, 2, 793.

PAPATESTAS A. E., ALPERT I. I, OSSERMAN K. E., OSSERMAN R. S., and KARK A. E. Studies in myasthenia gravis: effects of thymectomy. Amer. J. Med., 1971, *50*, 465.

ZABRISKIE J., HSU K. G., and SEEGAR B. C. Heart-reactive antibody associated with rheumatic fever: characterization and diagnostic significance. Clin. Exp. Immunol., 1970, 7, 147.

ZEROMSKI J., PERLMANN P., LAGERCRANTZ R., HAMMARSTRÖM S., and GUSTAFSON B. E. Immunological studies in ulcerative colitis. VII. Anticolon antibodies of different immunoglobulin classes. Clin. Exp. Immunol., 1971, 7, 469.

# Chapter 33

# IMMUNOMANIPULATION

## Jean-François Bach

I.   INTRODUCTION: CLASSIFICATION
II.  ADJUVANTS AND IMMUNOSTIMULANTS
III. IMMUNOSUPPRESSANTS
IV.  CONCLUSION: A NEW CONCEPT OF IMMUNOLOGIC
     THERAPY

# I.  INTRODUCTION: CLASSIFICATION

It is possible to modify positively or negatively the spontaneous course of immune reactions. Immunostimulation is possible at several levels. In some cases of immune deficiencies, the stimulation may involve reconstitution of the impaired element by grafting bone marrow or thymus cells or by injecting of thymic extracts (see chap. 31) One may also use biologic products that are the normal mediators of immune reactions, such as antibodies (γ-globulins) for humoral immunity or, more hypothetically, transfer factor for cell-mediated immunity. In addition, it is also possible to augment the intensity of an immune response without producing lasting modification in the immune system. Such stimulation may be antigen specific, that is, only produced to a given antigen, as in the case of adjuvants, which stimulate responses to the antigen placed at their contact. When stimulation is nonantigen specific, the treatment, then, affects all responses induced during the phase of activity of the material used. These agents are classified as "immunostimulants."

Immunosuppression may be nonspecific, applying simultaneously to all immune responses induced during the action of the agent used. This type of immunosuppression may be the result of destruction of lymphoid cells, irradiation, or injection of certain chemical products (antimetabolites, alkylating agents) or biologic agents (antilymphocyte serum, asparaginase). Immunosuppression may also be antigen specific, in which case it is essentially a form of tolerance. This form of immunosuppression is reminiscent of the specific

**Table 33.1    Immunomanipulation**

Immunostimulation
   Reconstitution of a deficient immune system
      Cell grafts (bone marrow, thymus)
      γ-globulins
      Transfer factor
   Antigen-specific stimulation
      Adjuvants in the presence of the antigen
   Nonspecific stimulation
      Immunostimulants
Immunosuppression
   Nonspecific immunosuppression
      Inactivation or elimination of lymphoid cells by thymectomy, irradiation (eventually
      extracorporeal), thoracic duct cannulation, antimetabolites, antilymphocyte sera
   Specific immunosuppression
      Tolerance and facilitation
      Passive antibody injection
      Desensitization

suppression of antibody production obtained by passive injection of antibody simultaneous with the antigen, or shortly thereafter. Hyposensitization therapy, employed by allergologists by injecting increasing doses of antigen, represents a peculiar aspect of specific immunosuppression, the mechanism of which is still obscure (see p. 750).

We will not discuss, in this chapter, bone marrow or thymus grafts and transfer factor, which have been described in man under the topic of immunodeficiencies (see chap. 31) and which have also been mentioned with respect to animal models (see chap. 4). Likewise, previous chapters have already discussed serotherapy (see p. 494), tolerance (see chap. 20), passively injected antibodies (see pp. 340 and 752), and hyposensitization treatment (see p. 750). This chapter will be limited to a discussion of adjuvants, immunostimulants, and immunosuppressants. This classification into immunostimulants and immunosuppressants is both classic and convenient. However, it must be appreciated that it is a schematic classification. We shall see that certain sitmulants may have suppressor effects and vice versa.

# II   ADJUVANTS AND IMMUNOSTIMULANTS

## INTRODUCTION: DEFINITIONS

In 1925, Ramon described the first adjuvant. It was then known that some horses immunized repeatedly by diphtheria toxoid produced progressively increasing titers of antitoxin antibodies, whereas antibody titers in other horses were stabilized after a few injections. Ramon observed that particularly good responders showed an intense inflammatory reaction at the last injection site; from this observation, he formulated the hypothesis that such abscesses could be responsible for the particularly intense immune response. He proved this hypothesis by showing that addition of pus to toxoid augmented the production of antitoxin antibodies. Soon after, it was shown that the same effects could be obtained with tapioca or bread crumbs.

We have seen that numerous proteins are weak immunogens when injected alone. Thus, injection of diphtheria toxoid leads to the production of very low levels of antibody in the rabbit, when it is injected alone intravenously. When incorporated in a water-oil emulsion that contains mycobacteria and injected intradermally, toxoid provokes the production of significant levels of antibody. Substances that augment the specific immune response to an antigen when mixed or combined with the antigen, or at least injected simultaneously with it are defined as "adjuvants." Adjuvants act essentially by increasing antigen immunogenic potency. Thus, they act most often by increasing globally the various types of immune responses. However, this global augmentation may sometimes selectively favor a particular category of response by modifying regulatory mechanisms, particularly antigenic persistence and antibody feedback (see p. 340). Immunostimulants have a more general action on immunity: they may simultaneously modify several immune responses by causing a nonspecific and transient increase in immune reactivity. This stimulation may be global or limited to a single type of response.

Adjuvants are used experimentally to augment antibody production or to favor the development of delayed hypersensitivity. In man, they are generally employed in vaccinations. Immunostimulants have regained interest because of their potential use for the treatment of certain cancers, especially leukemias.

In fact, numerous products have both adjuvant and stimulant properties, such as Freund's complete adjuvant or endotoxins. For this reason, we will discuss together adjuvants and immunostimulants. These very diverse products will be grouped into five categories (Table 33.2): oil adjuvants, mineral salts, double-stranded nucleic acids, natural substances (fungi, parasites, and, especially, bacteria), thymic extracts, and, lastly, other substances (vitamin A, tapioca).

## OIL SUBSTANCES: FREUND'S ADJUVANTS

### Description

It was Freund who, in 1947, was the first to demonstrate the capacity of oil in water emulsion, or especially water in oil emulsion, to enhance immunologic responses. Numerous oil adjuvants with various compositions have been studied; one of the most active substances, Bayol F, is composed of paraffin (42.5%), monocyclic naphthalene (31.4%), and polycyclic naphthalene (26.1%). Adjuvant 65, which consists of a water-in-oil emulsion that contains aluminum monostearate, has been used in man for antiinfluenza vaccination. The discovery that addition of mycobacteria considerably increased the adjuvant activity of oil substances represented important progress; this discovery led to the development of Freund's complete adjuvant, the most widely used adjuvant in animal studies.

Freund's incomplete adjuvant (IFA) is a simple water emulsion that contains

**Table 33.2   Adjuvants and Immunostimulants**

| Oil adjuvants | Natural substances |
|---|---|
| Freund's complete adjuvant | Bacterial endotoxins, bacterial phospho- |
| Freund's incomplete adjuvant | lipid extracts, whole bacteria |
| Mineral salts | Fungal |
| Aluminum phosphate or hydroxide | Parasitic |
| Beryllium sulfate | Other substances |
| Calcium alginate | Vitamin A |
| Double-stranded nucleic acids | Tapioca |
| Poly(IC) | Saponin |
| Poly(AU) | Levamisole |

antigen in mineral oil. The emulsifying agent may be lanolin or Arlacel A, which is a mannide monoleate. It appears as a creamy emulsion, with very tiny water drops containing the antigen surrounded by mineral oil. Complete Freund's adjuvant (CFA) is essentially IFA with killed mycobacteria added to it.

### Active Principle of Complete Freund's Adjuvant

Extensive studies were undertaken to characterize the active principle of mycobacteria. First, it has been shown that the active principle, known as the wax D, was contained in fractions extracted from *Mycobacterium tuberculosis* by chloroform. Wax D is composed of glycolipids and peptidoglycolipids; the latter are responsible for the adjuvant activity. These peptidoglycolipids are composed of mycolic acids esterified to a polysaccharide (arabinose, galactose, or mannose), itself linked to a peptide fragment composed of D-and L-alanine, D-glutamic acid, and $\alpha,\epsilon$-diaminopimelic acid. The active principle of CFA also includes glucosamine, galactosamine, and muraminic acid. The intact molecule is highly tensioactive: it hydrolyzes into lipophilic mycolic acid and hydrosoluble glyco-peptides, separately inactive. Lederer has recently isolated, from delipidated mycobacterial walls treated by lysozyme, a hydrosoluble product, called "water-soluble adjuvant" (WSA). This component, which proved to be an arabino galactan linked to a peptidoglycan does not provoke arthritis and does not stimulate phagocytosis, as does the wax D, although it maintains the activity of the adjuvant. Most recently it was demonstrated that (synthetic) N-acetyl-muramyl-L-alanyl-D-isoglutamine (muramyl dipeptide, MDP) had the minimal structure required for adjuvant activity.

### Effects of Freund's Adjuvants on Immunity

CFA and IFA augment antibody production and render subimmunogenic doses of antigen immunogenic. The mixture of adjuvant and antigen must be injected subcutaneously or, better, intradermally, because the adjuvant loses its action when administered intravenously. The adjuvant and the antigen may be injected separately at an interval of a few days if both injections are made at the same site. CFA is particularly effective at low antigen doses. Freund's adjuvants are effective with haptens and various antigens (polypeptides, proteins, bacteria, viruses), thus disproving the belief that antigenic determinants shared between mycobacteria and the antigen are responsible for the action of these adjuvants. However, CFA is only active on immune responses to thymus-dependent antigens.'

CFA may modify the class of antibodies normally produced in its absence by favoring IgG production over that of IgM, or of IgG2 rather than IgG1 in the guinea pig. CFA and IFA are necessary for the production of cytophilic antibodies, which are essentially IgG2. Freund's adjuvants also stimulate secondary responses and may inhibit induction of tolerance or even lead, in certain cases, to tolerance breakdown (see p. 584). CFA favors, often dramatically, the development of delayed hypersensitivity (DH) reactions. CFA is indispensable for the development of DH toward simple antigens, such as synthetic polypeptides. It can also accelerate rejection of skin grafts, tumors, and lymphoid cells. IFA, conversely, has no effect on the development of DH reactions and more generally on cell-mediated immunity. Note lastly, that the presence of CFA is required for the production of experimental immune diseases, such as experimental encephalomyelitis or allergic thyroiditis (see p. 716). The repeated injection of CFA may also induce arthritis.

The action of CFA, and particularly of Bacillus Calmette-Guérin (BCG), on tumors has recently been studied extensively in man and in animals. The incidence of leukemia is lower in children previously vaccinated with BCG. Syngeneic grafts of methylcholanthrene-induced sarcoma or of tumors induced by type-12 adenovirus are rejected by BCG action. Such effects on tumors have also been obtained with a purified fraction of BCG, the "methanol-extractable residue" (MER), used in oil. A final, and unexpected, property of CFA is the induction of plasmacytomas. Munoz showed, in 1957, that inoculation of paraffin oil that contained *Mycobacterium phlei* and a protein antigen could, in certain cases, lead to the production of ascites that contain large amounts of antibody. In 1960, Potter and Robertson showed that intradermal injection of a mixture of IFA and staphylococci (or, more simply, Bayol F) three times at 2-month-intervals induced the appearance of plasmacytomas that synthesized a monoclonal immunoglobulin with possible antibody activity directed against staphylococci. These monoclonal immunoglobulins have proven very useful in the study of immunoglobulin primary structure.

### Mechanisms of Action

Actually, the adjuvant effect of IFA is twofold: it delays antigenic destruction and increases antigenic dispersion. The delay in local destruction (by macrophages) and in elimination has been well studied. Thus, *Shigella* antigens are still detectable at their inoculation site 22 weeks after CFA injection. The local half-life of labeled antigen is considerably increased (1–14 days). The augmentation of antigenic dispersion observed is also involved since excision of the inflammatory granuloma after 14 days does not diminish antibody production, and excision at 30 min does not completely prevent antibody synthesis. In conclusion, IFA action is apparently linked to the progressive and intermittent release, in lymphatic channels and lymph nodes, of the antigen from multiple microfoci formed by the drops of water in oil emulsion.

The action of CFA, which is linked to the presence of the mycobacteria added to the effects of IFA, is obscure and apparently complex. CFA induces lymphocytic proliferation, as assessed by lymphoid organ hyperplasia. Cannulation of regional lymphatics shows that the granuloma is the site of intense lymphocytic traffic, possibly with sequestration. The preferential effects of CFA on cell-mediated immunity and on antibody production against thymus-dependent antigens suggest that CFA more specifically stimulates T-lymphocyte proliferation. In this regard, it is significant that the adjuvant effects of CFA (and even of IFA) on antibody production are not observed in T cell-depleted mice after thymectomy, irradiation, and restoration by bone marrow cells. Recent studies have suggested that CFA may also stimulate suppressor T cells and, thus, in certain protocols, favor the development of some tumors. Other recent studies with MDP have shown that it acts both on macrophages and T cells.

The possible role of antigenic stimulation by mycobacteria must be considered in light of Maillard and Bloom's experiments, which demonstrated that spleen cells from mice stimulated in vivo by *M. tuberculosis* and incubated in vitro with BCG had an increased in vitro response to sheep red blood cells (SRBC), probably linked to a secondary in vitro response to BCG. It might be that, in this experimental system, T cells sensitized to tubercle bacillus produce mediators analogous to those observed in the allogeneic effect (see p. 538). In fact, supernatants from spleen cells sensitized in vivo and incubated in vitro with BCG, added to cultures of normal spleen cells, increase the immune response to RBC.

Finally, it has been reported that CFA stimulates macrophages which phagocytose it (enhancing, in particular, the clearance of colloidal carbon), and cells implicated in antibody-dependent cellular cytotoxicity (ADCC). It would also increase interferon synthesis by macrophages.

## MINERAL SALTS AND TENSIOACTIVE SUBSTANCES

### *Mineral Salts*

Numerous mineral salts possess adjuvant properties, for example aluminum hydroxide and phosphate, which have been used in animals and in man (particularly for antidiphtheria vaccination), calcium phosphate, silica, iron oxide, and beryllium sulfate.

Solutions of alum-precipitated antigens provoke the development of local granulomas at the site of injection, essentially composed of macrophages. The antigen is slowly released from this deposit, giving rise, after the sensitization period, to a true secondary reaction. The effect of alum is much less obvious, if not absent, for classic secondary reactions induced by a booster injection. Alum preferentially stimulates the production of IgG1 rather than IgG2 antibodies, in contrast to the action of CFA.

Beryllium sulfate has an exclusive adjuvant effect on antibody production but no effect on DH. Its action on T cells is, however, suggested by the absence of an adjuvant effect on antibody production in "B" mice. Its action on macrophages is probably more important. Beryllium sulfate and circulating phosphates form complexes that are phagocytosed by macrophages. In addition, incubation of peritoneal cells, which have previously phagocytosed *Maia squinado* hemocyanin (MSH), with beryllium significantly enhances the production of antibodies induced by the transfer of these macrophages to a nonantigen-stimulated host.

Silica, kaolin, and carbon are also good adjuvants for the production of antibodies. Paradoxically, stimulation of antibody production is more clear-cut if these adjuvants are injected a long time prior to antigen injection (up to 120 days for ovalbumin in the rabbit). Aluminum silicate also favors development of DH.

### Tensioactive Substances

Numerous emulsifying substances augment antibody synthesis; these substances include colloidometallic hydroxides, alginate, lanolin, quaternary ammonium salts, certain phospholipids, certain proteins, and sulfur derivatives of guanidine. The mechanism of action of these products is not well known but appears to be localized in the cell membranes.

## MICROBIAL EXTRACTS

We have already described the adjuvant role of mycobacteria in CFA. Other bacteria contain active adjuvant, or immunostimulant principles; examples are corynebacteria, *Bordetella pertussis*, and brucellae. These bacteria may be used in unaltered form or as extracts, such as endotoxins, which are both powerful adjuvants and major immunostimulants. Their use, however, is now entirely restricted to experimental purposes because of the highly toxic nature of the majority of these products, especially the endotoxins.

### Bacterial Endotoxins

Endotoxins can be contrasted with exotoxins, which diffuse outside of bacteria. Their action on immunity is complex, because they act as antigens, adjuvants, immunostimulants, neurotropic toxins, and pyrogens.

#### CLASSIFICATION: BIOCHEMICAL ASPECTS

It had been known for many years that addition of typhoid vaccine to another vaccine enhanced very significantly the efficiency of the resultant vaccination. The active adjuvant principle of *Salmonella* and, more generally, of gram-negative bacteria (*Salmonella typhi*, *B. pertussis*, *Brucella melitensis* is contained in the lipopolysaccharide (LPS) fraction of bacterial extracts. It is not necessary to administer endotoxin at the antigen injection site to obtain the stimulating effect. A maximal effect can, however, only be obtained when endotoxin is administered at the same time or less than 6 hr after antigen injection. The association of stimulating and toxic activities is made plausible by the fact that rabbits made tolerant to endotoxin by repeated injections of this toxin are no more sensitive to the toxic or to the stimulating effects of the toxin. Antigenic determinants that confer serospecificity to endotoxins are borne by lateral-chain oligosaccharides. Incubation of endotoxins with antisera directed against them does not detoxify LPS. At variance with neurotropic exotoxins, which are thermolabile proteins, lipopolysaccharide endotoxins of gram-negative bacteria are heat resistant. Their molecular weight is about $10^6-10^7$ daltons. The active principle responsible both for their adjuvant and for their toxic effects has been isolated and is called "lipid A."

Normal serum is capable of deteriorating and detoxifying endotoxins in vitro by means of factors called "endotoxin-detoxifying components" (EDC). These factors include a thermostable calcium-dependent factor, which degrades LPS into smaller sized molecules, which are then degraded and eliminated. They also include a thermolabile calcium-independent factor.

### TOLERANCE TO ENDOTOXINS

Resistance of the host to a small dose of endotoxin is increased by previous injection of a small quantity of another endotoxin that lacks antigenic determinants in common with the first one. This phenomenon of "tolerance" to endotoxins is not linked to active immunization but, rather, appears to be due to stimulation of the reticulohistiocytic system.

Indeed, tolerance is accompanied by augmentation of phagocytosis, whereas blocking of the reticulohistiocytic system by thorostrast sensitizes the animal to endotoxins. This mechanism, however, does not explain why BCG and zymosan, which very strongly stimulate phagocytosis, sensitize the host to the action of endotoxins, whereas cortisone, which exerts a protective effect, has no macrophage-stimulating action but has rather a suppressive effect. Whatever its mechanism of action, tolerance to endotoxins does not seem to be a immunologic phenomenon. It is not prevented by neonatal thymectomy.

### EFFECTS OF ENDOTOXINS ON IMMUNITY

Endotoxins clearly have adjuvant effects; when added to the antigenic preparation, they increase antibody production. They may break tolerance states. Endotoxins are, however, without effect on delayed hypersensitivity (DH) reactions, although this point is still debated. In addition, they have a general immunostimulating activity. Thus, endotoxin injection increases the nonspecific resistance to bacterial infections (gram positive or gram negative) and to various viruses. For this effect to be achieved, however, there must be an interval of a few hours between endotoxin injection and infectious agent administration. When administered at the same time as antigens, endotoxins may, conversely, depress the resistance. There probably is a relationship between this immunostimulating action and the recent demonstration of an antitumor effect, although this effect is much less marked than that obtained with corynebacteria and mycobacteria.

### MODE OF ACTION

Endotoxins act both on B lymphocytes and on macrophages. The action on B lymphocytes has been well demonstrated; it explains their clear effect on antibody production, which contrasts with the absence (at least relative) of an effect on DH. Their action on antibody production is obtained in the absence of T cells in "B" mice. A direct action on B cells is also demonstrated by the capacity of LPS to stimulate B-cell proliferation, at least in the mouse, although this effect is not found in man (see p. 76). An action on macrophages is suggested by the capacity of LPS (and lipid A) to activate macrophages in vitro to make them cytotoxic for lymphoma cells. Transfer to irradiated hosts of macrophages that have incorporated both *E. coli* LPS and bovine serum albumin (BSA) confers a better anti-BSA immunity than does transfer of macrophages that have only phagocytosed the BSA. In addition, endotoxins augment the production of interferon by macrophages.

### Corynebacteria

Several corynebacteria, particularly *Corynebacterium parvum* and *C. rubrum*, are potent adjuvants. *C. diphtheriae* is, however, inactive. Corynebacteria are especially potent adjuvants of antibody production. Their action on DH is much less clear. They also have an immunostimulant action: they augment the resistance to bacterial infections and the development of certain tumors.

Live *C. parvum* injected intravenously provokes generalized lymphoid hyperplasia and stimulates the reticulohistiocytic system, as assessed by enhancement of colloidal carbon clearance. The latter activity may be responsible for the adjuvant activity, although there is no absolute correlation between the intensity of stimulation of the reticulohistiocytic system and the adjuvant effect of the various corynebacteria strains. T cells are not necessary for the adjuvant action because this effect may develop in the absence of T cells. Corynebacteria may, in addition, stimulate antibody production against thymus-independent antigens. When injected intravenously at high doses, corynebacteria even inhibit some T-cell functions (response to PHA or the mixed-lymphocyte reaction) but here, again, perhaps via an action on macrophages.

### Bordetella pertussis

*Bordetella pertussis* is a potent adjuvant, a property that has been long attributed to its content of endotoxin. Apparently, however, there is also a thermolabile adjuvant protein that augments sensitivity to histamine, hence its name "histamine-sensitizing factor" (HSF). *B. pertussis* is an adjuvant of antibody production equally effective against thymus-dependent and thymus-independent antigens. The mode of action of *B. pertussis* is not clear. It induces lymphocytosis. Its action on macrophages (which phagocytose it) appears to be important also, as assessed by the increased capacity of peritoneal macrophages that have phagocytosed an antigen like MSH in the presence of *B. pertussis* to stimulate anti-MSH antibody production after transfer to unimmunized animals.

### Other Substances

Injection of phospholipid extracts of *Salmonella typhimurium* into mice renders them resistant to various infections and enhances the blood clearance of bacteria. The phospholipid bacterial extract isolated by Fauve from *Salmonella* is also mitogenic and induces the release by lymphocytes of mediators that inhibit macrophage spreading. Ubiquinone, isolated from lipid extracts of *E. coli* is also an immunostimulant.

Some parasites may nonspecifically enhance immune defenses, particularly those against intracellular agents, such as *Listeria, Salmonella,* and *Brucella.* Infection by *Benoista jellisoni* delays the evolution of Friend's leukemia and of the spontaneous leukemia of AKR mice; *Toxoplasma gondii* inoculation increases resistance to Friend's leukemia, L 1210 leukemia, and sarcoma 180. Similar results have been reported with *Nippostrongylus brasiliensis* and *Schistosoma mansoni.*

Lentinan is a polysaccharide extracted from a comestible mushroom, *Lentinus elodes,* endowed with antitumor activity. Its action, which has been demonstrated toward sarcoma 180 in the mouse, is apparently mediated by T cells because it is not observed in neonatally thymectomized mice. Lentinan has no adjuvant effect on antibody production, on DH reactions, and graft rejection and does not increase colloidal carbon clearance. Lentinan might act by increasing sensitivity to histamine and serotonin.

## POLYRIBONUCLEOTIDES AND INTERFERON INDUCERS

Double-stranded nucleic acids, such as the synthetic polyribonucleotide inducers of interferon, for example, polyinosinic-polycytidilic acid [poly(IC)] or poly-adenylic-polyuridylic acid [poly(AU)], are potent immunostimulants. They enhance antibody production in the adult and newborn. They may favor rejection of certain tumors (sarcoma, lymphoma, leukemia). Their action seems to be exerted essentially on immature T cells. Poly(AU) action is very diminished in neonatally thymectomized mice treated by antilymphocyte serum (ALS). Poly(AU) also enhances the T-cell proliferative response to tuberculin and in the mixed-lymphocyte culture. An action on macrophages could also occur, as suggested by the augmentation by poly(AU) of the capacity of macrophages that have phagocytosed an antigen to stimulate antibody production to this antigen after transfer to a nonimmunized animal. These actions seem to be independent of interferon induction observed with certain polynucleotides. Poly(AU), is, in addition, a better immunostimulant than poly(IC), which is the only one of the two that induces interferon synthesis. But other interferon inducers are also immunostimulants, in particular tilorone, pyran and poly-acrylic acids.

## THYMIC EXTRACTS

The thymus exerts many of its functions by means of the intermediary of thymic hormones. It was therefore tempting to use these hormones in the immunologic reconstitution of certain immune deficiencies or even as phar-macologic stimulation of T lymphocytes. Synthetic thymic factors are now available and have been shown capable of normalizing certain T-cell functions in thymus-deprived or autoimmune mice and even to stimulate suppressor T cells in normal mice. These synthetic factors have not yet been employed in a controlled manner in man. In contrast, more gross thymic extracts, particularly Goldstein's fraction V, have been administered to patients suffering from immune deficiency or certain malignant tumors, with promising results, both at the clinical level and on immunologic parameters. There is, as yet, insufficient follow-up on these preliminary results, however, to appreciate their significance fully.

## LEVAMISOLE

Levamisole is a synthetic derivative of tetramisole. Initially employed as an antihelminthic agent, it was found to possess interesting immunostimulating properties in animals and perhaps even in man. In particular, it increases the number of T cells as assessed by the E rosette test and may transform negative delayed cutaneous hypersensitivity reactions into positive responses. Experimentally, and perhaps also in man, it can stimulate antitumor immunity. Finally, it has been reported by several groups that levamisole has a favorable therapeutic effect on rheumatoid arthritis. Its mechanism of action is uncertain. It seems, however, that it essentially acts at the level of the T lymphocyte and, to a lesser degree, on macrophages.

## CONCLUSIONS REGARDING MECHANISMS OF ACTION OF ADJUVANTS

From this review of the mode of action of the main adjuvants, the reader is probably struck by the wide diversity of sites of action. The augmentation of antigenic potency is reminiscent of the increase in immunogenicity linked to aggregation of certain soluble proteins (see p. 577). The use of adjuvants is, in fact, required to obtain antibodies against deaggregated proteins. Antigens may be retained at the inoculation site, as has been demonstrated for CFA. Adjuvants may also lead to lymphoid hyperplasia in regional lymph nodes, where lymphoid cells are exposed to high antigen concentrations. They may directly stimulate immunocyte proliferation and differentiation (as is the case for LPS for B lymphocytes). These mitogenic actions are probably responsible for some immunostimulating effects. At the cellular level, numerous mechanisms have been mentioned, for example, adenyl cyclase stimulation [for poly(AU)], formation of bridges between macrophages and lymphocytes, and release of various soluble factors.

## III.  IMMUNOSUPPRESSANTS

Immunosuppressants are used in immunologic diseases to suppress immunologic reactions that may be responsible for certain clinical signs. The choice of the agent and the dose employed is generally rather arbitrary due to ignorance of the mode of action of each product and of the pathophysiology of the disease being treated. Recent data on the mechanism of action of the main immuno-suppressants at the cellular level and on the immunologic reactions responsible for certain diseases, in addition to new pharmacologic approaches toward an understanding of the metabolic pathways of immunosuppressants, should in the future enable a more rigorous immunosuppressive treatment of some immunologic diseases.

## PROBLEMS OF DEFINITION

Immunosuppressants may be defined as agents that depress or suppress immune responses. This definition is simple but is, in fact, very imprecise because of the great polymorphism and complexity of immune responses.

Knowledge of the mechanism of action of immunosuppressants should help in their definition, but, as we shall see, this knowledge is still very preliminary, both at the chemical and cellular levels. However, we know already that all immunosuppressants do not have a similar action on T cells responsible for DH and graft rejection or on B cells implicated in antibody production. Thus, ALS and azathioprine (AZ) seem to have a preferential action on T cells, whereas alkylating agents act on both B and T cells. In addition, all immuno-suppressants do not have the same cytologic action. Some agents, such as cyclophosphamide, are essentially cytolytic; others, such as methotrexate, may be antimitotic, while still others may provoke lymphocytic elimination by opsonization in the liver, as in the case of ALS. Lastly, some might act by a reversible action on the lymphocytic membrane, for example, AZ. It is not surprising, regarding this diversity of action, that the various categories of immune responses demonstrate different sensitivities to each of these agents. In addition, it is not surprising that very few immunosuppressive agents show an optimal immunosuppressive activity in all immune responses. It should also be remembered that according to the administration protocol and type of immune response being studied, some products, such as cyclophosphamide or ALS, may depress or augment the intensity of the immune response. Definition of immunosuppressants may be improved by considering the existence of these various categories of immune responses, and a new definition of immunosup-pressants could be "products capable of suppressing or depressing the devel-opment of at least one type of immune reaction." This definition is more restrictive than the previous one, in which the totality of immune responses was considered, but it does not, however, solve all problems.

Two aspects of immunosuppression remain difficult to approach: (1) the anti-inflammatory action of numerous immunosuppressants, that is, their action on symptomatic manifestations of immunologic sensitization, which is often difficult to distinguish from the action on specific sensitization of lymphocytes to the antigen, and (2) the narrow margin between toxic and biologically active doses, which makes the definition of an immunosuppressant especially difficult when the product in question has a weak therapeutic index. These two aspects are sufficiently important pharmacologically to merit further discussion.

## ANTI-INFLAMMATORY EFFECT

Clinical manifestations of immune responses are often the consequence of inflammation secondary to action of antibodies or of various mediators secreted by T lymphocytes or macrophages (see p. 453). One may thus suppose that, in effect, anti-inflammatory substances may depress the expression of immune responses without, however, modifying the specific sensitization of lymphocytes, which retain their complete pathogenic potential, as demonstrable by cellular transfer experiments in untreated animals. This hypothesis applies, in particular, to indomethacin, which is a prostaglandin synthesis inhibitor that may, under certain circumstances, delay skin graft rejection in the guinea pig. Conversely, true immunosuppressive products often exert an anti-inflammatory action (as tested on inflammations not induced by immunologic phenomena) that may be very intense in certain cases and that does not always seem to correlate with immunosuppressive activity. This possibility explains the difficulty of relating the global effect of a product on immune responses to a true immunosuppressive action rather than to an anti-inflammatory effect. It is, however, an essential question clinically and experimentally. Indeed, if a product known to be immunosuppressive in animals acts essentially as an anti-inflammatory agent in man, it is, then, better to use anti-inflammatory agents exclusively, for example, acetylsalicylic acid or indomethacin, because of freedom from all of the side effects linked to immunosuppression, such as bone marrow aplasia and infections. In experimental studies, it may be unwise to use a product as an immunosuppressant when the interpretation of its effects may be biased by anti-inflammatory effects. This problem is difficult to approach in man but may be studied in animals by comparing the activities of the products considered, administered during the first days after antigenic stimulation, for example, at the time of lymphocytic proliferation and sensitization, or, conversely, in the few days prior to reaction evaluation, for example, immediately prior to graft rejection or at the time of test antigen challenge for a DH reaction.

## THERAPEUTIC INDEX

The immunosuppressive action of numerous products is often obtained only at doses close to toxic levels. In man, a regular clinical and biologic follow-up is always undertaken to detect side effects and lower the dosage as soon as possible. In view of the narrow margin between effective and toxic doses, it is crucial to determine for each product the best treatment regimen, which will give the best immunosuppression with the least toxicity. The search for the best treatment protocol, which can be performed in animals, is very difficult to achieve in man. The problem is complicated by significant variations in metabolism of immunosuppressants among species, which represent a handicap for extrapolation of experimental data to man. This variation explains why we still do not know, for most products used clinically, whether a single dose or fractionated doses represent, for the same total dose, an equivalent risk of toxicity or equivalent immunosuppression. Because there are now several methods available for studying the serum level of metabolites of most products used clinically, this search should be easier in the future.

In vitro studies are interesting in this context because they provide information on the action of the drugs on lymphocytes, independent of their metabolism and of their general toxicity. Such studies, however, represent an imperfect approach, because in vitro activities do not necessarily correspond to in vivo activities: products very active in vivo may be inactive in vitro when they require, for their activation, certain metabolic transformations. In addition, some products may act on a stage of the immune response that is not represented in in vitro reactions, even when using very sophisticated tests, such as Mishell and Dutton's technique or the mixed-lymphocyte reaction, which are fairly complete immunologic reactions. Conversely, some agents may exert an immunosuppressive action in vitro at noncytotoxic concentrations but may not show any immunosuppressive action in vivo because the serum level of active metabolites is not adequate at nontoxic doses, either due to an insufficient activity or to an agent half-life that is too short. Therefore, these agents should rather be considered "potential immunosuppressants"; the term "immunosuppressants" would, then, be reserved for products that possess in vivo immunosuppressive activity at nontoxic doses.

In conclusion, and in view of these data, one may propose the five following criteria for an ideal immunosuppressant: there must be an important security margin between toxic and beneficial doses; the agent must have a selective effect on lymphoid cells and not be toxic for other cells; as far as possible, the agent must affect only cells specifically implicated in the immune response under treatment; the immunosuppressant should be administered for only a short time, until the foreign antigen is no longer recognized as foreign and, thus, after a certain time, it should be possible to reduce the dosage and possibly stop the treatment, which would circumvent further depression of defenses against infectious agents; the agent must be effective against preexisting immune responses. At the present time, none of the known agents meets all of these requirements.

## MODE OF ACTION OF THE MAIN IMMUNOSUPPRESSANTS

### Thiopurines (Azathioprine, 6-mercaptopurine)

Thiopurines, which are analogues of hypoxanthine, depress antibody production and DH reactions in numerous species, including man. They are used successfully for the prevention of organ graft rejection. Their toxicity is modest, essentially bone marrow aplasia and hepatitis.

The biochemical impact of thiopurines is not unequivocal; AZ inhibits RNA, DNA, and protein synthesis. When considering the mode of action of thiopurines on these processes at the molecular level, numerous possibilities may be envisaged: interference with coenzymes, incorporation into nucleic acids, enzyme inhibition, alteration of purine interconversions, inhibition of de novo purine synthesis, and fixation onto amino acids. These actions explain the observed inhibition of nucleic acid synthesis but are also compatible with numerous other subcellular actions, which might be the basis of immunosuppressive effects of these products. One might thus explain why AZ inhibits rosette formation by quiescent lymphocytes in less than 60 min, an action difficult to explain by DNA synthesis inhibition.

The fact that the best time for administration of a single AZ dose is 24 hr after antigen administration has been considered a particularly important argument in favor of the antiproliferative effect of thiopurines. In fact, this argument is not absolute, and AZ might just as well act on the first phases of the immune response. This possibility is compatible with the fact that the action of thiopurines is rapidly reversible in vivo, first because they are rapidly metabolized and, second, because their cellular action is not long lasting: if antigenic recognition occurs throughout the first 2–3 days after antigen administration, as suggested by the immunosuppressive effect of passively administered antibodies until the third day, one may suppose that thiopurines are not active if they are given before the antigen because their activity has disappeared when the antigen is still recognized and may induce a nearly normal immune response. The fact that AZ inhibits mixed-lymphocyte reactions only when added to the culture during the first 24 hr, while DNA synthesis is not yet detectable, favors such an interpretation.

In conclusion, the action of thiopurines on proliferation of immunocompetent cells by inhibition of DNA synthesis does not seem to represent their only mode of action. Other biochemical impacts and cellular actions, such as suppression of antigenic recognition, suggested by inhibition of SRBC recognition (tested by rosette formation), may be envisaged.

The target cells of thiopurines have been the object of numerous recent investigations. Macrophages are probably not the preferential target of AZ, because thiopurines do not modify the clearance of labeled antigens and do not alter phagocytosis in vitro. The only data that suggest the possibility of thiopurine action on macrophage function are those that show significant monocytopenia in the rat after treatment with low AZ doses. These observations, however, have yet to be confirmed. In addition, the anti-inflammatory effect of AZ, which is genuine, does not seem an essential concomitant for its immunosuppressive action.

Among lymphocytes, T cells seem to be a preferential target for AZ. Thus, T cell-dependent immune responses, such as DH, graft rejection, or in vitro mixed-lymphocyte reactions, are particularly sensitive to AZ action. The effect on antibody production is much less clear: at the usual doses (less than 3 mg/kg/day for AZ in man), there is no depression of antibody production. Doses of about 5–6 mg/kg/day are necessary to obtain suppression of antibody production in man. The preferential action of AZ on T cells is confirmed by its specific action on T-cell markers (rosette formation, θ-antigen). Thiopurines alleviate selectively the course of experimental immunologic diseases that are caused by T cells (suppressed by neonatal thymectomy), such as experimental allergic encephalomyelitis and thyroiditis. In the latter case, it is noteworthy that antithyroglobulin antibody production is not depressed by thiopurines, whereas there is suppression of DH. Lastly, AZ given alone preferentially favors the development of viral infections and, among bacterial infections, tuberculosis and salmonellosis, all of which are infections against which immune defenses involve essentially T cells (see p. 471). This preferential action on T lymphocytes, seen at moderate doses as used clinically, is rapidly reversible, the T cells being more inactivated rather than eliminated, which could explain why the profile of B- and T-cell markers is not modified during AZ treatment in patients.

### Alkylating Agents (Cyclophosphamide, Chlorambucil)

Cyclophosphamide is probably the most potent chemical immunosuppressant. It suppresses antibody production and induces tolerance to numerous antigens. Its action on cell-mediated immunity is genuine, although less dramatic than its action on antibody production. The toxicity of cyclophosphamide (bone marrow aplasia, hemorrhagic cystitis, alopecia, sterility) limits its use.

Alkylating agents function by substituting chemical groups at the level of nucleic acids and proteins. Their main biochemical impact is on DNA synthesis. Such alkylation does not necessarily lead to death or inactivation of cells when it occurs before the cell enters the cell cycle phase of DNA synthesis because alkylated DNA is still biologically active (although less active than native DNA) and also has a tendency to repair itself. The time at which an alkylating agent should be administered to obtain maximal immunosuppressive action is important: repair of DNA lesions is possible before the onset of cellular proliferation and after antigen administration; such proliferation compensates for the loss of the few immunocompetent cells initially destroyed. Given at the time of cellular differentiation and proliferation, cyclophosphamide may kill a significant number of DNA-synthesizing immunocompetent cells and thus may have a particularly clear immunosuppressive action. It may even lead to total clone destruction and tolerance. At the highest doses used (300 mg/kg), cyclophosphamide loses its specific effect and not only acts on rapidly proliferating cells but, more generally, on all cells with high rates of RNA and protein synthesis. This general action probably explains the greater sensitivity of lymphoid cells than other cells to alkylating agents.

High cyclophosphamide doses alter more B cells than T cells, probably because B cells have a more intense metabolic activity than do T cells. The preferential action of cyclophosphamide on B cells, when given at a high dose, is well established: injection of high doses of cyclophosphamide in the mouse induces a relative decrease in B-cell marker-bearing lymphocytes and short-lived cells known to contain a large proportion of B cells. Given in ovo or to newborn chickens, cyclophosphamide induces atrophy of the bursa of Fabricius, with subsequent complete agammaglobulinemia. Cyclophosphamide is one of the most potent inhibitors of antibody production in most species, whereas its effects on skin and organ graft rejection are much less spectacular. Cyclophosphamide also exerts a remarkable immunosuppressive action on the autoimmune disease of NZB mice, which show a T-cell deficiency associated with an exacerbation of B-cell function (see p. 714). T cells are, however, also affected by cyclophosphamide given at high doses, as indicated by the (selective) action on suppressor T cells and the need for both thymus and bone marrow cells to reconstitute the immunologic competence of mice injected with 300 mg/kg of cyclophosphamide. In some situations, T cells might be even more sensitive than B cells, particularly in tolerance. The action on suppressor cells must not be neglected in the interpretation of the effects of cyclophosphamide in various systems. It may thus increase the intensity of delayed hypersensitivity reactions or permit mice that are "nonresponders" against certain antigens to produce antibodies against such antigens (see p. 689). This effect on suppressor T cells may be obtained with lower doses of cyclophosphamide than those required to suppress antibody production. Thus, one may conclude that with short-term high-dose treatment, B cells are more sensitive to cyclophosphamide than are T cells, but with chronic treatment, T cells are just as sensitive as B cells, if not more so.

In contrast to the thiopurines, alkylating agents seem to exert their immunosuppressive action via destruction of proliferating cells. Cell lysis is, in fact, compatible with exponential dose-response curves, which contrast with the hyperbolic curves observed with thiopurines. This does not mean, however, that the immunosuppressive effect of cyclophosphamide should be assessed by total lymphocyte count, because, as has been seen, some lymphocytic populations are more sensitive than others to the lytic action of the product.

´Chlorambucil is sometimes used in place of cyclophosphamide because it causes fewer side effects, although both agents have a priori the same mechanism of action, DNA alkylation and an antiproliferative effect. Since the side-effects (alopecia, hemorrhagic cystitis, azoospermia), however, are linked to the mechanism of action of the product itself, one may wonder to what extent the lower toxicity of chlorambucil at doses used in man is not associated with a lower biologic activity. If that was the case, the immunosuppressive activity of chlorambucil would also be weaker, a conclusion not incompatible with experimental data and clinical observations (in fact, very few) published on that topic; that is, one cannot exclude the hypothesis that chlorambucil, at the usual doses of 0.1–0.2 mg/kg, is, in fact, equivalent to cyclophosphamide at doses of 0.5 or 1 mg/kg, much lower than what is commonly employed clinically (2–3 mg/kg). It would thus be important, in this respect, to obtain objective documentation to prove that chlorambucil is truly immunosuppressive in man.

### Corticosteroids

Corticosteroids are good immunosuppressants in the mouse when administered at high doses. Their action on antibody production is more obvious than that on cell-mediated immunity. Their immunosuppressive activity in man is much less well documented than that in the mouse and can even be considered questionable. In addition, their strong toxicity when given chronically (severe infections, diabetes, psychoses, osteoporosis, necrosis of femoral heads) limits their clinical use.

Steroids probably provoke several biochemical changes in lymphocytic membranes. Although this hypothesis is not definitively established, it is likely that all of these effects are secondary to steroid binding to specific cytoplasmic receptors. Steroid-receptor complexes interact with DNA and lead to changes in protein synthesis. The link between interaction with DNA and subsequent biochemical events is, however, still poorly understood. In particular, it is difficult to determine whether the diminution in glucose incorporation observed after steroid treatment is primary or, more likely, secondary to changes in protein synthesis. Cell lysis does not represent the final result of all actions of steroids on lymphocytes because steroids also inhibit cell metabolism and seem to alter lymphocyte traffic. In particular, steroids induce a redistribution of lymphocytes out of the circulation with a resulting accumulation in other body compartments such as the bone marrow.

The steroid target cell has not been precisely defined. Action on macrophages has long been considered predominant, but if steroids do alter macrophage functions, perhaps by lysosome stabilization, this action is, in fact, difficult to evaluate: steroids induce significant monocytopenia and inhibition of numerous macrophage and polymorph functions, but the link between these actions and the immunosuppressive effect remains difficult to establish.

A preferential action of steroids on B or T cells is also not well established. Hydrocortisone suppresses the graft versus host reaction when administered after induction of the reaction, but it has no effect on precursor cells. Interestingly, hydrocortisone depresses lymphocytotoxicity but does not destroy precursors of lymphocytic cells. The effect of steroids on T cells is, in fact, extremely complex. Among quiescent T lymphocytes (not engaged in a specific immune response), only thymus cortical lymphocytes (and possibly a subpopulation of PHA-reactive spleen cells) are sensitive to the action of steroids. Among lymphocytes engaged in an immune response, cytotoxic lymphocytes seem to represent a rather selective target; this hypothesis could explain some of the actions of steroids on grafts. For antibody-producing B cells, it seems that steroids do not affect precursors but, rather, act on precursor differentiation into antibody-producing cells.

In conclusion, it is difficult to determine the cellular basis of the immunosuppressive action of steroids. The problem is compounded in man, in whom lymphocytes are relatively resistant to the lytic action of steroids. There is actually little firm evidence of suppression of immune responses in man, and the role of an anti-inflammatory action must always be kept in mind.

### Antilymphocyte Sera

Antilymphocyte sera (ALS) are heterologous sera prepared by injecting rabbits or horses with purified lymphocytic preparations, preferentially thymocytes or lymphocytes from the thoracic duct. Their immunosuppressive effect is particularly dramatic on skin graft rejection: almost indefinite survival can be obtained in mice. ALS facilitate induction of tolerance to skin allografts when administered concomitantly with donor cells. ALS also have a depressive effect on antibody production, but this activity is more modest and only obtainable when treatment is initiated before antigen injection. An immunosuppressive effect of ALS has been demonstrated in man, but use of these sera is limited due to their side effects. ALS provoke sensitization against heterologous proteins contained in the antisera, which exposes the recipient to the risk of anaphylactic shock and diminishes the biologic activity of the injected antibodies. Contaminating antibodies (antired blood cell, antiplatelet, and antikidney), which cannot be eliminated completely, often cause problems. In addition, the immunosuppressive activity of ALS varies considerably among batches, and one must test each batch before using it in man, either in vivo, by skin graft survival in monkeys, or in vitro, by rosette formation with SRBC. It has been demonstrated that the rosette inhibition test is directly related to the in vivo immunosuppressive activity of ALS, at variance with leukoagglutination and lymphocytotoxicity. All of these difficulties probably explain the mediocre and disappointing clinical results, particularly in renal transplantation, as compared to the impressive results in the mouse. Nevertheless, it is to be expected that, in the light of recent data, a better choice of antigens used for ALS production, the use of more purified antibodies, and the immunologic surveillance of the immunosuppressive effect on each patient will permit better use of ALS in man.

ALS seem to act essentially by two mechanisms, T-cell depletion (the predominant effect) and inactivation of lymphocytic recognition receptors (Table 33.3).

T-CELL DEPLETION

ALS induce lymphocytopenia and lymphocytic depletion in lymphoid organs, exclusively in thymus-dependent areas. Thus, a global depletion of lymphocytes does not seem to be required for ALS to exert their immunosuppressive activity. The mechanism of depletion of long-lived recirculating lymphocytes is not completely understood. A direct cytotoxic action by lympholysis is not the major mechanism, because C5-deficient mice are sensitive to the immunosuppressive action of ALS. In fact, the main mechanism of T-lymphocyte elimination appears to be opsonization in the liver, with involvement of the

**Table 33.3   Main Arguments in Favor of a Selective Action, in Vivo, of Antilymphocyte Sera on T cells**

ALS-induced immunosuppression is partially corrected by injection of thymocytes (but not bone marrow cells)

ALS eliminate selectively carrier-specific T cells without altering hapten-specific B cells

Adult thymectomy very significantly enhances ALS-induced immunosuppression (at least for antilymph node sera)

Thymic extracts may diminish the immunosuppressive effect of ALS

ALS induce, in vivo, a decrease in the lymphocytic response to phytohemagglutinin and in the mixed-lymphocyte reaction and also a decrease in the number of θ antigen-bearing cells in the mouse

θ-Positive rosette-forming cells are more sensitive to ALS in vitro than are θ-negative cells

ALS are more active on cell-mediated immunity than on antibody production; ALS only depress humoral responses toward thymus-dependent antigens

ALS induce a selective depletion of thymus-dependent areas of the spleen and lymph nodes

Antibodies directed against T cell-specific antigens exert a particularly strong immunosuppressive action

ALS deplete long-lived lymphocytes, as does neonatal thymectomy

ALS augment the frequency of viral infections (which involve T cells) without diminishing significantly antiviral antibody production first four components of complement. The veracity of such opsonization has been directly demonstrated in various species.

### INACTIVATION OF SURFACE RECEPTORS

Antilymphocyte antibodies bind to the lymphocytic surface, as has been demonstrated directly by immunofluorescence. The lymphocytic surface coating may prevent recognition receptors from coming into contact with the antigen, which explains why ALS are only effective when administered before the antigen and why spleen cells from ALS-treated mice may regain their immunocompetence after treatment with trypsin. Complement might also participate in lymphocytic coating, as has been shown in the rosette inhibition test. It is possible to reconcile these two theories of the mode of action of ALS by suggesting that ALS might act, in the first few hours after their administration, by inactivating circulating lymphocytes, which would ultimately be eliminated by opsonization in the liver.

### Promising Recent Developments

Few new immunosuppressive agents have been developed in the course of the last 10 years. However, mention should be made of the encouraging results obtained recently with Cyclosporin A and total lymphoid irradiation.

Cyclosporin A is a cyclic peptide fungal extract. Initially used as an antifungal agent, Cyclosporin A was found to be a remarkable suppressor of T-cell mediated immune reactions. In particular, it suppresses lymphocyte proliferation in response to T-cell specific mitogens (PHA, Con A) and the production of antibodies against thymus-dependent antigens. It delays allograft rejection and may even induce the appearance of specific tolerance. Recent studies indicate that it acts selectively on helper T-cells with relative protection of suppressor T-cells. The toxicity of Cyclosporin A is slight in animals but may be more significant in man. Cyclosporin A appears to be immunosuppressive in man, but as yet there is insufficient follow-up to enable a satisfactory evaluation of its future potential clinical role.

Total lymphoid irradiation consists of selective irradiation of all the lymphoid organs but with protection and sparing of the bone marrow. This type of irradiation, which has already been used in a similar form in man for the treatment of Hodgkin's disease, produces a state of profound immunosuppression with an especially noted prolongation of allograft survival. When associated with an injection of allogeneic bone marrow cells, it is even possible to obtain tolerant states with long-term survival or chimerism and the possibility of almost indefinite survival of skin or organ grafts from the bone marrow donor. The mode of immunosuppressive action of total lymphoid irradiation is still largely unknown but may induce the preferential regeneration, after irradiation, of suppressor T cells, which should inhibit the immune response.

## CLINICAL APPLICATIONS

### Choice of Immunosuppressant

This choice depends on the disease; it is made difficult because of incomplete knowledge of the pathophysiology of most immunologic diseases.

However, some recent data, reviewed in the preceding chapters, enable formulation of an approach that may guide this choice.

Humoral immunity appears to be the primary causative factor, acting through the intermediary of autoantibodies or immune complexes in SLE, periarteritis nodosa, hemolytic anemia, and chronic glomerulonephritis. The use of immunosuppressants active on B cells (cyclophosphamide) seems to be justified for treatment of such diseases. Steroids have also been shown to be effective in these diseases, but their basic mechanism of immunosuppression is still so poorly understood that a precise mode of action cannot be proposed.

Cell-mediated immunity apparently plays a predominant role in rejection of transplanted organs and also perhaps in rheumatoid arthritis. Agents active on T cells, such as ALS, AZ, or cyclophosphamide (which also acts on B cells), are justified in such cases. Of interest is the dramatic improvement in the clinical status of patients with rheumatoid arthritis after thoracic duct cannulation, which selectively eliminates T cells. AZ and ALS are particularly effective in organ transplantation, probably because they depress T cells without affecting B cells, which produce facilitating antibodies, possibly favoring graft survival.

This choice of immunosuppressants based on the presumed mechanism of the disease is corroborated by the favorable action of cyclophosphamide in the autoimmune disease of NZB mice, an analog of human lupus, or in Aleutian mink disease, an analog of periarteritis nodosa, diseases in which AZ is inactive.

### Choice of Dosage and Treatment Follow-up

The dosage of immunosuppressants should represent a compromise that takes into account the immunosuppression desired and attempt to control its intensity to avoid the onset of severe infections and bone marrow toxicity, which is usual at high doses. Although one may try to define, in a series of patients, the dose that provides sufficient immunosuppression, it is generally difficult in a given case to measure the intensity of immunosuppression; in general, only the follow-up of the blood count will help to guide posology. One may, however, hope for progress in this field, both in evaluation of the active metabolite serum level and in the immunologic follow-up of patients subjected to chemical immunosuppression.

The serum levels of the active metabolites of certain immunosuppressants may be determined by chemical or radioimmunologic methods. Determination of serum levels is now possible for steroids and cyclophosphamide. Unfortunately, these methods are relatively tedious and may not be applied routinely. Biologic tests (rosette inhibition, mixed-lymphocyte culture inhibition) are easier to perform (Fig. 33.1) but also difficult to apply to each patient.

Immunologic follow-up of patients subjected to immunosuppressive treatment has not yet reached clinical practice, although such follow-up should be feasible. Thus, the number of B and T cells may be evaluated by counting the various rosette types (T cells, SRBC rosettes, or B cell-complement rosettes), by the mixed-lymphocyte reaction or the response to PHA (T cells), or by study of surface immunoglobulins (B cells). The specific response to an antigen is more difficult to measure with the techniques available (blast transformation in the presence of antigen, leukocyte migration inhibition). Significant progress

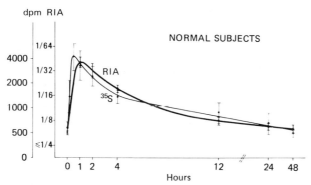

**Fig. 33.1** Serum level of azathioprine metabolites, measured by evaluation of the serum-specific $^{35}$S activity (bound to the azathioprine molecule) or by the inhibition of rosette formation (RIA). (From J. F. Bach and M. Dardenne, Proc. Roy. Soc. Med. 1972, 65, 260.)

has recently been achieved in the field of organ transplantation, particularly with respect to lymphocytotoxicity techniques (see p. 410) and the different humoral inhibitors (blocking antibodies) or cellular inhibitors (suppressor T cells, see p. 586). These tests of immunologic surveillance are useful in cases of strong immunosuppression as administered to patients undergoing bone marrow or organ grafting or during relapses of certain connective tissue or autoimmune diseases. Apart from these instances, immunosuppression remains moderate and its effects are not readily appreciable by means of the usually employed cell markers, which are probably somewhat crude. More detailed studies of lymphocyte function would be interesting and perhaps useful but much to cumbersome for routine use.

## IV. CONCLUSION: A NEW CONCEPT OF IMMUNOLOGIC THERAPY

Until recently, the treatment of immune diseases has been approached in very simple terms. Patients suffering from immune deficiency justified immunostimulation, those with a hyperimmune state were submitted to immunosuppressive treatment. However, the problem is complicated at several levels.

It is no longer easy to classify disorders into immune deficiency states or hyperimmune conditions. Certain autoimmune states seem to be secondary to, or associated with, an immune deficiency (mainly of T cells). The abnormal production of antibodies (and, subsequently, of immune complexes) or autoantibodies is subjected to subtle and variable regulatory mechanisms, which may be amplifier or suppressor. Graft rejection and cell-mediated immunity in general also involve the intervention of multiple effector cells (T, K, NK cells, macrophages, etc.) and regulatory cells.

In addition, the concepts of immunosuppressors and immunostimulants vary simultaneously with the growth in number and variety of drugs available.

Some immunostimulants may have a suppressor effect (such as BCG or thymic extracts); in contrast, certain immunosuppressants may selectively inhibit (during certain administration protocols) the suppressor T-cell population and augment some immune responses. This is the reason why, occasionally, all these products are grouped under a more operational term, immunomodulators.

In view of these data, it is clear that great caution must be excercised in the clinical use of these diverse methods. In the light of these considerations, it is difficult to know, a priori, which product is indicated above others in a given immune disease whose pathophysiology is often poorly understood. The most reasonable attitude is pragmatic: all the available immunomodulators must be tested in rigorous, randomized controlled clinical trials after having undergone equally rigorous investigation of their experimental effects.

## BIBLIOGRAPHY

BACH J. F. The mode of action of immunosuppressive agents. Amsterdam, New York, 1975, North Holland, 379 p.

BACH J. F. The use of regulatory biological products to manipulate immune responses. In: Immunology 80 (M. Fougereau and J. Dausset [eds.]). Acad. Press, New York, 1980, 1171.

BARNER A. D. The clinical use of antilymphocytes globulins. In R. A. Thompson, Ed., Recent advances in clinical immunology. Edinburger, 1977, Churchill-Livingstone, p. 203.

BAXTER J. D. and FORSHAM P. H. Tissue effect of glucocorticoids. Amer. J. Med., 1972, 53, 573.

BERENBAUM M. C. Comparison of the mechanisms of action of immunosuppressive agents. In L. Brent and J. Holborow, Eds., Progress in immunology. II. Vol. 5. Amsterdam, 1974, North Holland, p. 233.

BRAUN W. and UNGAR J. Non-specific factors influencing host resistance: a reexamination. Basel, 1973, Karger.

BRENDEL W., RING J., and SEIFERT J. Experimental and clinical aspects of ALG. In L. Brent and J. Holborow, Eds., Progress in immunology. II. Vol. 5. Amsterdam, 1974, North Holland, p. 245.

CHEDID L. L'immunostimulation. Cours de l'Institut Pasteur.

CLAMAN H. N. Corticosteroids and lymphoid cells. New Engl. J. Med., 1972, 21, 225.

COHEN J. J. The effects of hydrocortisone on the immune response. Allergy, 1971, 29, 358.

ELION G. B. Significance of azathioprine metabolites. Proc. Roy. Soc. Med., 1972, 65, 257.

FELDMAN D., FUNDER J., and EDELMAN I. S. Sub-cellular mechanisms in the action of adrenal steroids. Amer. J. Med., 1972, 53, 545.

FOURNIER C., DARDENNE M., BACH M. A., and BACH J. F. The selective action of azathioprine on T cells. Transpl. Proc., 1973, 5, 523.

Immunopotentiation. Ciba Found. Symp. 18. Amsterdam, 1974, Excerpta Medica.

KRAKAUER R. S. and CATHCART M. K. Immunoregulation and autoimmunity. Elsevier, New York, 1980, 257 pp.

LANCE E. M. The selective action of ALS on recirculating lymphocyte: a review of the evidence and alternatives. Clin. Exp. Immunol., 1970, 6, 789.

LEDERER E. Immunostimulation: Recent progress in the study of natural and synthetic immuno-modulators derived from the bacterial cell wall. In: Immunology 80 (M. Fougereau and J. Dausset [eds.]). Acad. Press, New York, 1980, 1194.

MORRISON D. and RYAN J. L. Bacterial endotoxins and host immune responses. Adv. Immunol., 1979, 27, 294.

SCHWARTZ R. S. Immunosuppression and neoplasia. In L. Brent and J. Holborow, Eds., Progress in immunology. II. Vol. 5. Amsterdam, 1974, North Holland, p. 229.

SLAVIN S., YATZIV S., ZAN BAR I., FUKS Z., KAPLAN H. S., and STROBER W. S., Non specific and specific immunosuppression by total lymphoid irradiation. In: Immunology 80 (M. Fougereau and J. Dausset [eds.]). Acad. Press, New York, 1980, 1160.

TAUB R. N. Biological effects of ALS. Progr. Allergy, 1971, *14*, 208.

WERNER G. H. Immunopotentiating substances with antiviral activity. Pharmacol. Ther., 1979, 6, 235.

WHITE R. G. Adjuvant stimulation of antibody synthesis. *In* P. A. Miescher, Immunopathology. 6th Int. Symp. Basel, 1970, Schwabe, p. 91.

# ORIGINAL ARTICLES

AISENBERG A. C. and MURRAY C. Cell transfer studies in cyclophosphamide induced tolerance. Cell. Immunol., 1973, 7, 143.

BACH J. F. In vitro assay for ALS. Fed. Proc., 1970, 29, 120.

BACH M. A. and BACH J. F. Activities of immunosuppressive agents in vitro. II. Different timing of azathioprine and methotrexate in inhibition and stimulation of mixed lymphocyte reaction. Clin. Exp. Immunol., 1972, *11*, 89.

BRENT L. Unresponsiveness to skin allografts induced by tissue extracts and ALS. Transpl. Proc., 1971, *3*, 684.

CHEDID L., AUDIBERT F., LEFRANCIER P., CHOAY J., and LEDERER E. Modulation of the immune response by a synthetic adjuvant and analogs. Proc. Nat. Acad. Sci. USA, 1976, *73*, 2473.

HALPERN B. N., BIOZZI G., STIFFEL D., and MOUTON D. Inhibition of tumor growth by administration of killed *Corynebacterium parvum.* Nature (London), 1966, *212*, 863.

KOTZIN B. L. and STROBER S. Reversal of NZB/NZW with total lymphoid irradiation. J. Exp. Med., 1979, 150, 371.

LARSSON E. L. Cyclosporin A and dexamethasone suppress T cell responses by selectively acting at distinct sites of the triggering process. J. Immunol., 1980, 124, 2828.

PENN I. and STARZL T. E. Immunosuppression and cancer. Transpl. Proc., 1972, 5, 943.

ROLLINGHOFF M., STARZINSKI-POWITZ A., PFIZENMAIER K., and WAGNER H. Cyclophosphamide sensitive T lymphocytes suppress the in vivo generation of antigen specific cytotoxic T lymphocytes. J. Exp. Med., 1977, 145, 455.

ROUTHIER G., EPSTEIN O., JANOSSY G., THOMAS H. C., SHERLOCK J., KUNG P. C., GOLDSTEIN G. Effects of cyclosporin A on suppressor and inducer T lymphocytes in primary biliary cirrhosis. Lancet, 1980, 2, 1223.

STAVY L., COHEN I. R., and FELDMANN M. The effect of hydrocortisone on lymphocyte mediated cytolysis. Cell. Immunol., 1973, 7, 302.

TURK J. L., PARKER D., and POULTER L. W. Functional aspects of the selective depletion of lymphoid tissue by cyclophosphamide. Immunology, 1972, *23*, 493.

**Appendix**

# INVESTIGATION OF IMMUNITY IN MAN

**Jean-François Bach**

I. HUMORAL FACTORS OF IMMUNITY

II. CELLULAR FACTORS OF IMMUNITY

III. SEARCH FOR AUTOIMMUNIZATION

IV. SEARCH FOR THE AGENT RESPONSIBLE FOR HYPERSENSITIVITY

V. STUDY OF IMMUNOGENETIC MARKERS

VI. OTHER TECHNIQUES

Progress in basic immunology in the past few years has led to remarkable developments in clinical immunology techniques. Most of these techniques have been described in the preceding chapters. In conclusion, we would like to present a synthesis of all techniques that may be used clinically. Some of them have been used routinely for a long time, while others still performed by only a few specialized laboratories but shall certainly become generalized in the near future.

We will not deal here with immunologic techniques used for diagnosis in numerous diseases of a priori nonimmunologic origin, as employed in microbiology (serodiagnosis) or endocrinology (radioimmunoassay of most hormones). We will limit ourselves to techniques that evaluate the levels of humoral and cellular immunity, distinguishing nonspecific factors, which control the general level of immune responses, from factors specific for a given antigen, which ensure the response toward that antigen (which is often an autoantigen).

## I. HUMORAL FACTORS OF IMMUNITY

Humoral immunity is mainly due to immunoglobulins and complement; numerous techniques, most notably Mancini's radial immunodiffusion, provide a method for the quantitation of the different immunologic constituents of serum and other biologic fluids. Techniques for detecting circulating immune complexes and cryoglobulins may also be included here.

## IMMUNOGLOBULIN EVALUATION

IgG, IgA, IgM, and IgD are quantified by radial immunodiffusion. IgE is generally evaluated by radioimmunoassay, less commonly by radioimmunodiffusion. It is possible but rarely useful, in clinical practice, to evaluate the levels of the various IgG subclasses. Immunoelectrophoresis permits the simultaneous semiquantitative evaluation of the three main immunoglobulins (IgG, IgA, and IgM). Immunoelectrophoresis is valuable, in parallel with zone electrophoresis, for the diagnosis of dysproteinemia and the characterization of monoclonal proteins, particularly urinary Bence-Jones proteins.

## COMPLEMENT STUDIES (see chap. 8)

Global complement activity is evaluated by total hemolytic complement (CH50). Several complement factors may be quantitated routinely by radioimmunodiffusion or by Laurell's rockett technique (for example, C1q, C3, and C4). Factor B may also be quantified in the same way. Assessment of nephritic factor may be performed after preincubation of the test serum with a standard serum, followed by quantification of C3 degradation products. Finally, a diagnosis of angioneurotic edema may be helped by the C1 esterase inhibitor assay (see p. 281). Evaluation of the hemolytic activity of all factors of the complement system and of their inhibitors is possible in specialized laboratories (see chap. 8).

## CRYOGLOBULINS (see pp. 732 and 876)

Cryoglobulins are detected by incubation of serum at 4°C after collection and coagulation at 37°C. These cryoglobulins may be quantitated and identified by their immunoglobulin class and the eventual presence of a monoclonal immunoglobulin. One distinguishes monoclonal and mixed cyoglobulins.

## DETECTION OF CIRCULATING IMMUNE COMPLEXES
(see p. 734)

Numerous techniques have recently been described for the detection of immune complexes or at least of protein abnormalities suggestive of their presence (direct demonstration of immune complexes requires the demonstration of the antigen and of its binding to antibody). The main techniques are C1q or C4 precipitation by polyethylene glycol, labeled C1q fixation, direct polyethylene glycol precipitation, inhibition of ingestion of aggregated immunoglobulin by macrophages, or binding of IC to Fc or C3 receptors on B lymphocytes or lymphoblastoid cell line (Raji cells), studied by radioimmunoassay or rosette formation. We should also include tissue immunofluorescence, performed in particular in the kidney, which enables demonstration of immunoglobulin deposits, most likely associated with immune complexes.

# II.   CELLULAR FACTORS OF IMMUNITY

Serial enumeration of lymphocytes, neutrophil polymorphs, basophils, and monocytes is generally of little value, although persistently decreased numbers of these elements may indicate general trends.

The T-lymphocyte enumeration is achieved by means of the sheep rosette test (see p. 69) or by cytotoxicity tests that use heterologous antilymphocyte sera rendered T-cell specific. Recently it has become possible to evaluate the number of total, suppressor/cytotoxic or helper/inducer T-cell subsets by using monoclonal anti-T cell antibodies (by indirect immunofluorescence). B lymphocytes may be counted by evaluation of membrane immunoglobulin or by the complement rosette test, although such tests are often difficult to interpret because contaminating monocytes (and sometimes polymorphs) may produce falsely elevated values. The erythrocyte-antibody (EA) rosette test or binding of aggregated immunoglobulin is even more difficult to interpret. T-cell function (which is not necessarily directly linked to T-cell number) may be evaluated by the response to T cell-specific mitogens (phytohemagglutin, concanavalin A) or by the mixed-lymphocyte reaction rendered one-way by inactivation of the stimulating lymphocytes by irradiation or mitomycin treatment. It is also possible to evaluate the capacity of blood lymphocytes to produce cytotoxic cells, as generated in a mixed-lymphocyte reaction, in the cell-mediated lympholysis (CML) reactions. Suppressor or helper T cells may be evaluated in coculture assays eventually after mitrogen polyclonal activation (see p. 550). Finally, one may quantitate the serum level of circulating thymic hormone by the rosette test, which evaluates the level of thymic epithelial function.

B- and T-cell functions may also be assessed in vivo. The induction of a primary cellular response to dinitrochlorobenzene or of a secondary response to tuberculin, *Candida*, or streptodornase-streptokinase may be demonstrated by skin tests or lymphocyte cultures in the presence of antigen, occasionally by the release of chemotactic factors by sensitized lymphocytes. Second-set humoral responses may be studied by booster vaccinations with diphtheria or tetanus toxoid or antipoliomyelitis vaccine. More rarely, one uses primary stimulation to antigens not previously encountered, such as hemocyanin.

The recently described K-cell population may be studied in various systems. As target cells, one may use heterologous red blood cells, tumor cells, or lymphocytes typed for the HLA antigens and coated with specific IgG antibodies.

Polymorph function may be studied by the nitro blue tetrazolium (NBT) reduction test, which is often difficult to interpret, or, better, by studying phagocytic or bactericidal activity (see chap. 5). These tests are essentially useful for the diagnosis of septic granulomatosis.

## III.   SEARCH FOR AUTOIMMUNIZATION

Antibodies may be demonstrated against numerous autoantigens.

Antithyroid autoantibodies are directed against several determinants, the majority localized in thyroglobulin or microsomes. They are detected by passive hemagglutination (for antithyroglobulin antibodies), complement fixation, or immunofluorescence. Antithyroid antibodies are nearly always found in Hashimoto's thyroiditis but also in numerous other thyroid diseases and even in other autoimmune diseases, such as pernicious anemia.

Antistomach autoantibodies may be directed against parietal cells (detected by immunofluorescence, complement fixation, or passive hemagglutination) or against the gastric intrinsic factor (detected by blocking of radiolabeled vitamin $B_{12}$ fixation). Antistomach antibodies are found essentially in pernicious anemia and atrophic gastritis and, to a lesser degree, in other autoimmune diseases, such as thyroiditis.

Antimitochondria antibodies are detected by immunofluorescence. They are found mainly in primitive biliary cirrhosis, more rarely in active chronic hepatitis and Sjögren's syndrome.

Antimuscle antibodies are also detected by immunofluorescence. One may distinguish antismooth muscle antibodies, frequently found in chronic active hepatitis, from antistriated muscle antibodies, present in nearly half of myasthenia gravis cases and in certain thymomas. These antistriated muscle antibodies give cross-reactions with antithymus antibodies, also found in myasthenia gravis. They must be distinguished from antiacetylcholine receptors, which are specific for myasthenia gravis.

We should also include, among other organ-specific antibodies detected by immunofluorescence, antiliver antibodies (found in primitive biliary cirrhosis, post necrotic cirrhosis, and in certain cases of drug-induced hepatitis), antiadrenal antibodies, found in Addison's disease, antimyocardium antibodies, found after myocardial infarction and certain commissurotomies and in rheumatic fever, and antiskin antibodies, characteristic of pemphigus vulgaris and bullous pemphigoid. Anti-intercellular substance antibodies, found in pemphigus, are distinguished from antidermoepidermal basement membrane antibodies, found in bullous pemphigoid.

Among nonorgan-specific autoantibodies, we should mention antinuclear, antierythrocyte, antileukocyte, antiplatelet, and antibasement membrane antibodies.

Antinuclear antibodies include a group of antibodies directed against the different antigenic constituents of cell nuclei. The test for LE cells, which detects antinucleoprotein antibodies, is simple but relatively insensitive and nonspecific of SLE (it is also positive in other diseases). Immunofluorescence, which permits the detection of most antinuclear antibodies, is almost always positive in lupus but also in numerous other immune diseases. Only the demonstration of antinative DNA antibodies is specific for lupus. These antibodies may be shown by passive hemagglutination, precipitation, or complement fixation; the best technique, however, in terms of sensitivity and specificity, is Farr's test, which utilizes radiolabeled DNA.

Antierythrocyte antibodies are detected by Coombs' tests by means of sera directed against the various immunoglobulin classes and C3, at 37 or 4°C. Several categories of hemolytic anemia are defined according to the immunologic type of antibodies involved.

Antileukocyte autoantibodies are detected by means of lymphoagglutination, lymphocytotoxicity, or complement fixation. The cytotoxicity test, performed at 15°C, permits detection of cold lymphocytotoxins (which are auto- or alloantibodies). Antileukocyte antibodies, particularly cold lymphocytotoxins, are found in lupus and numerous autoimmune diseases.

Antiplatelet autoantibodies are difficult to detect. The techniques used are thromboagglutination and complement fixation on platelets.

Antibasement membrane antibodies should be assayed when Goodpasture's syndrome is suspected. Immunofluorescence performed on the patient's kidney or on a normal kidney section after transfer of the patients' serum is the most commonly used method; the antibodies induce formation of linear deposits along the glomerular basement membrane. These antibodies, however, are not glomerulus specific because they react generally with tubular and pulmonary basement membranes. One may also detect antibasement membrane antibodies by passive hemagglutination and radioimmunoassay, but we do not yet know the true specificity of these tests (antibasement membrane antibodies of low affinity may be produced under numerous circumstances).

Anticardiolipin autoantibodies, which are responsible for a "false-positive" syphilis reaction, are observed in certain autoimmune diseases, especially in early lupus.

Rheumatoid factors are anti-immunoglobulin antibodies. They are usually detected by the Rose-Waaler reaction (which is an agglutination reaction that employs sheep or human red blood cells coated with rabbit IgG antibodies) or by the latex test (which utilizes latex particles coated with human IgG). One may also detect rheumatoid factors of the IgG type by fixation, followed by elution on heterologous immunoglobulin-coated columns.

The detection of autoimmunization at the cellular level is theoretically possible by various techniques, such as blast transformation, rosette or leukocyte migration inhibition (in one or two steps; see p. 394), or the lymphocytotoxicity assay. However, none of these techniques gives results interpretable as direct correlates of the involvement of cell-mediated immunity, because antibodies of different types may produce false-positive results. This important reservation, added to the difficulty and tediousness of these tests, explains why none of these techniques has been used routinely in studies of autoimmune diseases, despite the publication of promising results, especially with the leukocyte migration inhibition test, in numerous organ-specific autoimmune diseases.

## IV. SEARCH FOR THE AGENT RESPONSIBLE FOR HYPERSENSITIVITY

This topic has been developed in chapter 26. We will only recall here the main methods used to study each hypersensitivity type.

**Table 1  Investigation of Immunity in Man**

| Parameters of humoral immunity | Parameters of cellular immunity | Autoantibodies |
|---|---|---|
| IgG (Mancini) | Sheep red blood cell rosettes | Antithyroglobulin |
| IgM (Mancini) | Anti-T cell sera | Antithyroid microsome |
| IgA (Mancini) | Membrane Ig | Antistomach parietal cell |
| IgE (Radioimmunoassay) | Complement rosettes | Antiintrinsic factor |
| Immunoelectrophoresis | EA rosettes | Antimitochondria |
| Bence-Jones proteins | PHA response | Antismooth muscle |
| CH50 | Con A response | Antistriated muscle |
| C1q | Mixed-lymphocyte reaction | Antithymus |
| C4 | CML | Antiliver |
| C3 | Thymic hormone evaluation | Antisalivary gland |
| C1 esterase inhibitor | DNCB stimulation | Antiadrenal |
| Nephritic factor | Tuberculin skin tests | Antimyocardium |
| Properdin | Tuberculin in vitro responses | Antiepidermis |
| C3 proactivator | Chemotactic factors | LE cell |
| Cryoglobulins | | Antinuclear factor (IFI) |
| PEG precipitation | | Farr test (with native DNA and RNA) |
| Labeled C1q fixation | | Antierythrocyte autoantibodies |
| | | Leukoagglutinins |
| | | Lymphocytotoxins |

| Tests for hypersensitivity | Immunogenetics | Miscellaneous |
|---|---|---|
| Skin tests | Blood group antigens | Australia antigen: counterimmunoelectrophoresis, radioimmunoassay |
| RAST | SD (HLA) antigens | Carcinoembryonic antigen, α-feto protein |
| Sensitization of monkey lungs | LD antigens | Serum evaluation of immunosuppressants |
| Basophil degranulation | Ig allotypic antigens | In vitro evaluation of ALS activity |
| Antifungi precipitins | | |
| Antiavian precipitins | | |
| Antiavian hemagglutinins | | |
| Antidrug antibodies | | |
| Irregular agglutinins | | |
| Anti-HLA cytotoxic antibodies | | |
| Anti-HLA blocking antibodies | | |
| Anti-HLA LDA antibodies | | |
| Lymphocytotoxicity | | |
| Inhibition of leukocyte migration | | |

Cold lymphocytotoxins
Antiplatelet autoantibodies
Syphilis reaction
Rose-Waaler reaction
Latex test
Antibasement membrane antibodies (passive hemagglutination, radioimmunoassay)

In atopy, skin tests remain the best method (epi- or intradermal reactions). Provocation tests (per os or by inhalation) may also be used in certain cases. Lastly, and probably the most promising orientation for the future, one may demonstrate the existence of IgE allergen-specific antibodies by radioimmunoassays (RAST), when they are available, in vitro sensitization tests on monkey lungs, or tests of human basophil degranulation in the presence of allergen (but not by Shelley's test with rabbit basophils, because human reagins show little or no binding to heterologous basophils). Finally, it should also be remembered that global quantification of IgE (RIST) provides only indirect and nonspecific evidence in favor of an "atopic background."

In allergic interstitial pneumonia, antibodies directed against quite diverse antigens (mycotic agents, avian antigens) are generally detected by immunoprecipitation or hemagglutination.

In contact dermatitis, skin tests are mainly used.

Lastly, in drug allergies, the best test is function of the drug and its mechanism of action. Here, we include RAST and cutaneous tests for anaphylactic hypersensitivities, especially to penicillin, Coombs' test and leukoagglutination or thromboagglutination in the presence of the drug in cases of hemolytic anemia, leukopenia, or thrombocytopenia, and skin tests for products responsible for delayed hypersensitivity reactions.

Alloimmunizations and graft rejections give rise to the production of various alloantibodies. Antierythrocyte alloantibodies are detected by hemagglutination (using Coombs' tests) and anti-HLA antibodies are detected by microcytotoxicity techniques. In both cases, a battery of test cells is used, which enables definition of the specificity of the antibodies involved. In graft rejection, it may also be useful to demonstrate and quantitate blocking antibodies (for example, by inhibition of the mixed-lymphocyte reaction, inhibition of leukocyte migration, or lymphocytotoxicity) and antibodies that cause antibody-dependent cellular cytotoxicity (ADCC) by K cells. Attempts to more clearly quantitate cell-mediated immunity have generally proven disappointing, except for a few isolated cases, by means of lymphocytotoxicity and leukocyte migration inhibition.

## V.  STUDY OF IMMUNOGENETIC MARKERS

Immunologic techniques permit the definition of a great number of immunogenetic markers. Examples are the antigens of erythrocytic blood groups (ABO, Rh, MNS) the HLA A, B and DR antigens, and lastly, immunoglobulin allotypes (Gm, Inv.).

## VI.  OTHER TECHNIQUES

Clinical immunology laboratories may also perform other tests, in particular: assay for HBs, HBc and HBe antigens and corresponding antibodies by means of counterelectrophoresis or, better, by radioimmunologic dosage; assay for α-fetoprotein in hepatomas and carcinoembryonic antigens in cancers of the colon; serum levels of immunosuppressants, for example, by rosette inhibition; and in vitro evaluation of antilymphocyte sera activity (by cytotoxicity or, better, by rosette inhibition).

# GLOSSARY

Included below are definitions of the most commonly used terms in immunology. The reader is referred to the list of abbreviations and the index for symbols, acronyms, and abbreviations (H-2, Fab, Gm, MIF, etc.).

Reference: N. J. Herbert and P. C. Wilkinson, A dictionary of immunology. Blackwell, Oxford, 1971.

**Activation (macrophage)**    Augmentation of the level of macrophage function, especially under the action of mediators produced by sensitized T cells in the presence of antigen (MAF, macrophage-activating factor). One must distinguish this "functional activation" from the augmentation in number of peritoneal macrophages that occurs after injection of irritating substances, such as sodium thioglycollate, sometimes also called "activation."

**Adjuvant**    Preparation that when administered simultaneously with antigen increases the immune response to this antigen.

**Affinity**    Intrinsic association constant of an antibody toward an antigen, measured at equilibrium. It measures the binding strength and stability between antigen and antibody.

**Agglutinin**    Antibody whose fixation onto the corresponding antigen is expressed in vitro by an agglutination reaction. An antibody is said to be "agglutinating" (red blood cells) when it leads to hemagglutination in saline (0.15 M NaCl). In the opposite case, one speaks of "nonagglutinating" antibody.

**Agglutinin (cold)**    Antibody only or essentially agglutinating at low temperature.

**Allele**    A group of genes situated at one locus and having different effects on the same character.

**Allergen**    Any substance capable of provoking an allergic reaction.

**Allergy**    *Former meaning*: Abnormal reactivity of a subject to an antigen; *present meaning*: Synonymous with hypersensitivity, particularly immediate hypersensitivity.

**Allogeneic**    Describes genetically different individuals from the same species.

**Allogeneic effect**    Nonantigen specific immunopotentiation secondary to T-cell activation (probably mediated by soluble factor(s) / allogeneic effect factor(s)).

**Allotype**    Designates the existence of different antigenic determinants on immunoglobulins from normal individuals in the same species.

**Alternative pathway**    Activation pathway of complement that involves the direct stimulation of C3, without previous activation of C1, C4, and C2. Activation of the alternative pathway may be provoked by numerous substances, in particular, polysaccharides, endotoxins, and immune complexes.

**Amyloidosis**    Disease characterized by deposits, in numerous organs, of proteinlike material, the amyloid substance, defined by staining properties and fibrillar ultrastructure and tending to invade and destroy some organs, in particular, the kidneys.

**Anaphylaxis**    IgE-mediated hypersensitivity provoked by a previous injection of an antigen (preparing injection), followed by a later injection of the same antigen (provoking injection) and expressed in its acutest and clearest forms by anaphylactic shock.

**Anaphylatoxin**    Substance produced in the course of complement activation (C3a, C5a) that induces manifestations related to those provoked by mastocytic and basophilic degranulation and histamine release.

**Anatoxin (toxoid)**    Toxin that has lost, through heat or formol action, its toxic activity but that has retained its antigenic properties.

**Anergy**    State of an organism that has lost the ability to specifically react to an allergen to which it was previously sensitized.

**Antibody**    Plasma protein (immunoglobulin) that reacts specifically with an antigen.

**Antibody (anti-)**    Antibody produced in response to a protein antigen that is itself an antibody.

**Antibody (natural)**    Antibody found in serum without apparent preimmunization by the corresponding antigen (for example, antibodies against erythrocytic antigens of ABO blood groups).

**Antibody-dependent cellular cytotoxicity (ADCC)**    Cytotoxicity exerted by mononucleated cells (in particular K cells) toward target cells coated with small amounts of IgG antibody (lymphocyte-dependent antibodies, LDA).

**Anticomplementary**    That which inhibits complement action.

**Antigen**    Substance that provokes production of an antibody able to react specifically with it.

**Antigen (histocompatibility)**     Membrane antigen, common to all nucleated cells of the same organism, responsible for allograft rejection.

**Antigen (private)**     Antigen present on cells of only one or a few individuals, as opposed to public antigens, present on the cells of a large number of individuals.

**Antigenic determinant**     Structure present on the antigenic molecule surface and capable of combining with a specific antibody molecule. In his new terminology, Jerne speaks of epitope (antigen) as opposed to paratope (antibody; see p. 142).

**Antigenic modulation**     Loss of antigenic expression of membrane antigens secondary to antibody-induced redistribution of antigenic receptors.

**Antiglobulin test**     See Coombs' test.

**Arthus phenomenon**     Inflammatory reaction associated with edema, hemorrhage, and necrosis, occurring a few hours after intradermal administration of an antigen into an animal that possesses precipitating antibodies against this antigen.

**Atopy**     Constitutional or hereditary predisposition to develop immediate hypersensitivity reactions (asthma, hay fever, or other allergic reactions) to allergens that do not provoke any reaction in normal subjects.

**Autoantibody**     Antibody produced by an organism in response to an antigen from the same individual. By extension, in human disease, one refers to an autoantibody as an antibody active against antigens common to the human species without group or individual specificity.

**Autoantigen**     Substance capable of eliciting the appearance of an autoantibody within its host.

**Autoimmunity**     Immunization state toward the self-antigenic constituents of a given subject.

**Avidity**     Measurement of the binding strength of an antiserum toward macromolecular or particulate antigens. The avidity depends on the affinity of the various antibodies present in the antiserum, on the pattern of antigenic determinants, and on the physicochemical parameters of the medium.

**Axenic**     Description of an animal that does not bear any foreign host, equivalent to "germ free."

**B (cell or lymphocyte)**     Antibody-producing cell (and its precursors), which differentiates under the influence of the bursa of Fabricius in birds, and perhaps of its (unknown) equivalent in mammals.

**BCG (Bacillus Calmette-Guérin)**     *Mycobacterium bovis* strain of bovine origin, attenuated by serial cultures, that has lost its virulence but has retained its antigenic and immunogenic properties.

**Bence-Jones protein**     Monoclonal light chain, κ or λ, present in blood and urine of patients with multiple myeloma or Waldenström's macroglobulinemia.

**Blocking antibody**   Antibody capable of blocking the biologic activity of other antibodies or of lymphocytes in vivo or in vitro.

**Capping**   Process of redistribution of membrane determinants to one limited part of the cell surface under the influence of (generally divalent) antibody.

**Carrier**   Protein or polysaccharide to which haptens must be complexed for antibody production to result.

**Cell-mediated immunity**   T cell-mediated immunity transmissible by lymphoid cells (and macrophages) and not by serum. Cell-mediated immunity includes delayed hypersensitivity and graft rejection.

**Chimera**   Organism that possesses a foreign cell population.

**Clonal selection theory**   Theory of antibody formation according to which for any antigen there is a corresponding preformed clone (see "clone" below) of lymphoid cells that react specifically to that antigen. Autoantigen-reactive clones (forbidden clones) are eliminated in fetal life.

**Clone**   Set of cells derived from a single initial cell and therefore having the same genetic constitution.

**CML (cell-mediated lympholysis)**   Specific lymphocytotoxicity reaction generated in vitro during a mixed lymphocyte reaction.

**Co-isogenic**   Describes two individuals (or strains) that are genetically identical except for one locus.

**Competition (antigenic)**   Nonspecific immunosuppression toward an antigen, which occurs when this antigen is administered shortly after another antigen that does not share common determinants with it.

**Complement**   Complex enzymatic system of plasma proteins capable of binding to a large number of antigen-antibody systems and playing an essential role in immune effector mechanisms. Complement consists of nine components, respectively classified C1 through C9. The sequential intervention of these components does not follow this numeration. Activation of a given component is indicated by a horizontal line above the symbol that designates the component ($C\bar{3}$) or group of components ($C\bar{4}\bar{2}$).

**Complex (immune)**   Macromolecular complex of specifically linked antigen and antibody.

**Congenic**   Partially co-isogenic (differing not only at one locus, but also probably with respect to a chromosomal segment of undetermined length adjacent to this locus).

**Congenic resistant**   Describes congenic individuals (or strains) that differ at a histocompatibility locus and reject mutual tissue grafts.

**Contact hypersensitivity**   Delayed hypersensitivity caused by contact of skin with various antigens or haptens.

**Coombs' test**   Technique that enables detection of nonagglutinating antibodies through the action of a heterologous anti-Ig serum that causes agglutination.

**Cross (back)**    Mating of an $F_1$ individual with one of its parents.

**Cross-match**    Serologic technique used for the detection of antired blood cell or antileukocytic alloantibodies between two given individuals, before blood transfusion or allografting.

**Cross-reaction**    Reaction of antibody with an antigen other than the one which induced its formation but which possesses determinants identical or close to one of its own determinants.

**Cryoglobulin**    Immunoglobulin that precipitates in the cold, at variable temperatures below 37°C according to the type of cryoglobulin, and redissolving at 37°C. There are monoclonal cryoglobulins and mixed cryoglobulins (of the IgM-IgG type), where IgG is usually the antigen and IgM an anti-IgG antibody (IgM may or may not be monoclonal).

**Cytophilia**    Property of some antibodies to bind to the surface of certain cells, generally on appropriate receptors. Numerous antibodies are cytophilic for macrophages, which possess a receptor for the Fc fragment of IgG. IgE are cytophilic for mastocytes and basophils of the species to which they belong. They are "homocytotropic antibodies."

**Delayed hypersensitivity**    Hypersensitivity whose manifestations only appear 24 hr after contact with the antigen.

**Desensitization**    Technique used to alleviate or suppress hypersensitivity of an individual to a given allergen by repeated administration of this allergen at increasing doses.

**Deviation (immune)**    Immune paralysis selective of a category of immune responses that affects, for example, one class or subclass of antibody.

**Domain**    Homologous region of Ig molecules, stabilized by a disulfide bridge, that possesses thermodynamic and, possibly, functional autonomy. One distinguishes $V_L$ and $C_L$ domains on light chains and $V_H$, $C_H 1$, $C_H 2$, and $C_H 3$ domains on heavy chains.

**Endotoxin**    Bacterial wall toxin (lipopolysaccharide) released during lysis of some gram-negative bacteria.

**Enhancement (immunologic)**    Phenomenon by which a "facilitating" or "enhancing" antibody protects the corresponding antigen and the integrity of cytologic structures that bear it, thus preventing this antigen from inducing or being the target of an immune reaction.

**Epitope**    See antigenic determinants.

**Equivalence**    Situation in which the ratio of antigen and antibody concentrations ensures maximum precipitation, consuming all antibodies and antigens.

**Farr test**    Method for detecting antibodies or antigens, by use of antigens labeled with a radioactive isotope, in which antibody-bound antigen is isolated by precipitation with ammonium sulfate.

**Flagellin**    A major antigenic constituent (protein) of bacterial flagella.

**Forssman antigen**    Polysaccharide erythrocytic antigen common to some animal species (guinea pig, sheep) and microbes, the structure of which is similar to that of the human A antigen.

**Freund's adjuvant (CFA) (complete)**    Water-oil emulsion that contains killed mycobacteria in the oil phase.

**Freund's adjuvant (IFA) (incomplete)**    Water-oil emulsion without mycobacteria.

**Genotype**    Set of genetic material borne by an individual, including nonexpressed genes, as opposed to phenotype, which describes expressed genes.

**Germline theory**    Theory according to which the genetic information that corresponds to all antibodies is contained in the genetic heritage.

**Germinal center**    Aggregation of lymphocytes, lymphoblasts, and macrophages within primary follicles of lymphoid organs; develops after antigenic stimulation.

**Graft versus host reaction (GvH)**    Reaction observed after injection of allogeneic lymphocytes into an animal or a subject whose immune functions are depressed or genetically unable to reject the injected cells.

**Haplotype**    A set of genes present on a single chromosome.

**Hapten**    Substance, generally of low molecular weight, incapable of eliciting antibody formation by itself but able to react with an antibody and to become immunogenic and acquire true antigenic properties when coupled to a carrier.

**Helper (T cell)**    T cell that cooperates with B cells in antibody production and with other T cells in cell-mediated immunity. This cooperation is called the "helper effect."

**Hemagglutination**    Red blood cell agglutination under the action of specific agglutinins (antigen-antibody reactions) or bacterial or viral hemagglutinins or lectins, such as phytohemagglutinin, or occurring spontaneously under certain physicochemical conditions.

**Histocompatibility**    Degree of similarity of antigenic characters of graft-donor and recipient tissues.

**Homocytotropic (antibody)**    See cytophilia.

**Hybridoma**    Hybrid cell obtained by fusing a myelomatous cell and a B cell immunized against a defined antigen. Hybridomas are stable in culture and produce monoclonal antibody directed against a single determinant of the antigen.

**Idiotypy**    Antigenic determinants of an immunoglobulin borne by the variable part and linked to the antibody specificity toward the antigen.

**Immediate (hypersensitivity)**    Immunologic reaction due to IgE antibodies linked to the release of histamine or other vasoactive substances after antigenic administration.

**Immune adherence**    Agglutination between C3-coated cells and indicator cells bearing C3 receptors (e.g., human red blood cells).

**Immunity**    Initially reserved to describe the acquisition by the organism of new and specific defense properties after infection. By extension, this word describes all humoral and cellular factors that protect the organism against infectious agents or the effects of toxic antigens (except for tolerance phenomena).

**Immunofluorescence**    Method based on coupling of antibodies to a fluorochrome (usually fluorescein isothiocyanate), which makes their binding to the corresponding antigen detectable by immunofluorescence.

**Immunogenicity**    Capacity of a substance to elicit an immune response.

**Immunoglobulin**    General term that describes all serum globulins that are antibodies, presently divided into five classes: IgG, IgA, IgM, IgD, and IgE. Immunoglobulins are composed of two symmetric heavy and light chains.

**Immunology**    Discipline that studies normal and pathologic immune responses.

**Immunosuppressant**    Any substance that diminishes or suppresses an immune response.

**Immunostimulant**    Any substance capable of stimulating immune responses, even when administered at a distance from antigen.

**Incomplete antibody**    Used incorrectly to designate nonagglutinating antibodies.

**Instructive theory**    Theory of antibody formation according to which immunocompetent cells do not have any preformed specificity toward antigens but acquire it after contact with antigen.

**Interleukin 1**    (IL1) Lymphocyte activating factor (formerly LAF) produced by macrophages.

**Interleukin 2**    (IL2) Soluble mediator produced by T cells and acting on other T cells. Formerly known as T-cell growth factor (TCGF) and thymocyte stimulating factor (TSF) (see p. 386).

**Isoantibody**    Antibody elaborated by an organism in response to an antigen from other individuals of the same species. To be replaced by alloantibody.

**Jones-Mote (hypersensitivity)**    Delayed hypersensitivity reaction of weak intensity observed a few days after a first injection of protein antigen in aqueous solution.

**K cell**    Mononucleated cell population apparently neither B nor T that kills target cells coated with small amounts of antibodies.

**Lectin**    Plant substance that is not an antigen but that is, however, capable of provoking, in vitro, some phenomena that resemble immunologic reactions, such as lymphocytic blast transformation or erythrocytic agglutination.

**LE cell or Hargraves' cell**    Leukocyte (most often granulocyte or monocyte) that has phagocytosed the nucleus of another cell and that contains a large phagosome stained by May-Grünwald-Giemsa and gives a positive Feulgen reaction.

**Lymphocytotoxicity**     Cytotoxicity effect directly exerted by lymphocytes on a target cell, independent of complement.

**Lymphokine**     Soluble factor released during cell-mediated immunity by sensitized lymphocytes when the latter are incubated with antigen. Examples are macrophage-inhibitory factor (MIF), lymphotoxin, and chemotactic factor.

**Lysosome**     Cytoplasmic organelles with variable morphology, limited by a membrane and containing hydrolytic enzymes, which play an essential role in intracellular digestion and cell autolysis.

**Macroglobulin**     Serum globulins of high molecular weight ($>$400,000) with a sedimentation constant of 19S in ultracentrifugation and consisting of two proteins, $\alpha_2$-macroglobulin, or $\alpha_2$M, and $\beta_2$-macroglobulin, or $\beta_2$M or IgM.

**Macrophage migration-inhibitory factor (MIF)**     Protein factor that inhibits normal macrophage migration, secreted by lymphocytes from an animal sensitized to this antigen and released when these lymphocytes are incubated in vitro with the antigen. The MIF test consists of introducing into a capillary tube macrophages and lymphocytes in a culture medium. Migration outside the tube is inhibited if the medium contains an antigen to which the animal that has provided the lymphocytes is sensitized.

**Marker (lymphocyte)**     Property of a lymphocyte subpopulation that allows direct determination of the subpopulation to which a given lymphocyte belongs.

**Mastocyte**     Cells whose cytoplasm contains numerous basophilic granules, rich in mediators (heparin, serotonin, histamine) and whose release is provoked by various factors, in particular, homocytotropic antibodies. Mastocytes play an important role in immediate hypersensitivity.

**Memory (immunologic)**     Concept that expresses the capacity of an organism or of immunocompetent cells to respond in an accelerated and, particularly, intense way to new stimulation by an antigen previously introduced.

**Mishell and Dutton's technique**     Technique that enables one to obtain primary and secondary antibody responses in vitro by dissociated lymphoid cells.

**Mixed-lymphocyte reaction (MLR)**     Blast transformation in vitro (appearance of lymphoblasts and mitoses, increased thymidine incorporation) of lymphocytes in the presence of allogeneic lymphocytes. One distinguishes two-way MLR, in which both lymphocytic population react against each other, from one-way reactions, in which one of the two populations (the stimulating one) is inactivated by irradiation or mitomycin treatment.

**Multiple myeloma**     Malignant dysproteinemia characterized by bone pains (with x-ray picture of bone lysis), anemia, with IgG, IgA, more rarely IgD or IgE monoclonal immunoglobulin, and often thermosoluble Bence-Jones proteinuria. The disease is due to the proliferation of abnormal plasma cells within the bone marrow.

**Network theory**     Theory proposed by Jerne according to which there would normally exist at equilibrium a network of antibodies (with idiotypic determinants) and anti-idiotypic antibodies. The onset of an immune response would be linked to the rupture of this equilibrium by antigen introduction.

**Nude**     Mutant mouse strain, deprived of hair (hence its name) and showing congenital absence of the thymus.

**Null cells**     Lymphoid cells showing none of the B- and T-cell markers.

**Opsonin**     Antibody whose binding to the corresponding antigen facilitates its uptake by phagocytosis.

**Original antigenic sin**     Phenomenon according to which, after vaccination or primary infection by a virus, a second vaccination or reinfection by a virus related to the initial one, gives rise to a high antibody response against the first virus.

**Parabiosis**     Situation involving two or more individuals that have been connected in such a way that their circulation is linked at the level of peripheral vessels.

**Paracortical**     Deep cortex of lymph nodes that contains nearly all lymph node T cells.

**Paralysis (immune)**     Synonymous with "tolerance."

**Paratope**     Synonymous with "antibody" in Jerne's terminology. See epitope.

**Phagocytosis**     Engulfment and ingestion by a cell of inert or living solid particles from the environmental medium.

**Phenotype**     Set of characteristics of an individual that corresponds both to the expressed part of the genotype and to phenomena determined by the external medium.

**Pinocytosis**     Uptake and absorption by a cell of liquid droplets of the extracellular medium, without release of lysosomal enzymes.

**Plaque-forming cells**     Cells producing antibodies against erythrocytes, and forming a hemolytic plaque in gel medium in the presence of complement and erythrocytes.

**Polyclonal activator**     Substance activating some functions of lymphocyte subsets independently of their specificity for antigen. Phytohemagglutinin and concanavalin A are polyclonal T-cell activators. *E. coli.* lipopolysaccharide is a polyclonal B-cell activator (PBA).

**Pyroglobulin**     Monoclonal immunoglobulin which precipitates when heated at 56°C.

**Pyroninophilic**     Describes any cell whose cytoplasm becomes red after use of Unna-Pappenheim's stain with methyl pyronin green. This test suggests the presence of large amounts of RNA and thus active synthesis of proteins.

**Reagin**     Antibody (IgE in man) responsible for immediate hypersensitivity.

**Rheumatoid factor**     An antibody directed against IgG. Found in the majority of patients with rheumatoid arthritis and in some individuals with other diseases.

**Rose-Waaler test**    Reaction for detection of rheumatoid factor in serum based on agglutination of sheep (or human) erythrocytes previously incubated with a subagglutinating dose of serum from rabbits immunized against these red blood cells.

**Rosette**    Structure formed by adherence of erythrocytes around a lymphocyte (sometimes a macrophage).

**Russel body**    Acidophilic, very refringent inclusion that appears occasionally in the cytoplasm of degenerating plasma cells.

**Secretory piece**    Protein formed by epithelial cells that links two IgA molecules to form a dimer.

**Serum sickness**    Set of cutaneous, articular, and renal changes that appear 8–10 days after the first injection of heterologous serum.

**Shwartzman's reaction**    Synonymous with the Shwartzman-Sanarelli phenomenon. The reaction (apparently nonimmunologic) is necrotic, local, or systemic (involving kidneys, lungs, liver, and heart) and occurs after administration of endotoxin in a subject sensitized by a first injection of the same or another endotoxin.

**Site (antibody)**    Part of the antibody molecule with antigen recognition function.

**Site (antigenic)**    Formerly used to designate "antigenic determinant."

**Suppressor T cell**    Cell that exerts a negative control on the function of B cells, helper T cells, and effector T cells of cell-mediated immunity.

**Surveillance (immunologic)**    Concept proposed by Burnet according to which there exist immunocompetent cells (probably thymus dependent) that continuously eliminate abnormal cells produced by somatic mutations or maligant transformations.

**Syngeneic**    Describes all individuals who are genetically identical (for example, monozygous twins); in animals, this term describes individuals that, by successive consanguinous matings, form pure strains (inbred strains). Their genetic composition is practically identical, and graft rejection does not occur between them.

**T cell (T lymphocyte)**    Effector cell in cell-mediated immunity and regulatory cell (helper and suppressor) in antibody production, the differentiation of which is under the influence of the thymus.

**T-cell antigens**    T cell-specific antigens. One distinguishes alloantigens, such as the θ antigen in the mouse, from heteroantigens, defined by heterologous antisera absorbed by B antigen-bearing cells.

**Theta (θ) antigen**    Mouse alloantigen present in thymocytes, peripheral T lymphocytes, brain, and skin.

**Thymic hormone**    Polypeptides secreted by the thymus and intervening in differentiation of bone marrow precursors into T cells. Thymosin (A. L.

Goldstein), thymic humoral factor (N. Trainin), thymopoietin (G. Goldstein), and serum thymic factor, or FTS (J. F. Bach) presently designate the various preparations used, the interrelationships of which are unclear.

**Thymopoietin**    See thymic hormone.

**Thymosin**    See thymic hormone.

**Thymus dependent**    Depending on the thymus or on T cells. Thymus-dependent lymphocytes or thymus-derived lymphocytes are T cells (see "T cell" above). Thymus-dependent areas are regions in peripheral lymphoid organs where T cells selectively migrate. Thymus-dependent antigens are those against which antibody production (IgG and, to a lesser degree, IgM) requires T-cell intervention.

**Thymus independent**    Not depending on the thymus or on T cells. Thymus-independent areas are regions in peripheral lymphoid organs where B cells selectively migrate. Thymus-independent antigens are those toward which antibody production (essentially IgM) does not require the presence of T cells. Production of these antibodies is, however, not strictly thymus independent, because it may be under the regulatory influence of suppressor and amplifier T cells.

**Tolerance (immunologic)**    Central suppression of an immunologic reaction specific to a given antigen that occurs after previous contact with that antigen.

**Transfer factor**    Low-molecular-weight and dialyzable factor extracted from lymphocytes of subjects with cell-mediated hypersensitivity to a given antigen that, when injected into unsensitized subjects, confers on them the same hypersensitivity.

**Tuberculin**    Product of spontaneous autolysis of tubercle bacilli in their medium. Purified protein derivative (PPD) is a soluble protein fraction of tuberculin obtained after precipitation by trichloroacetic acid.

**Vaccine**    Antigenic preparation that prevents microbial infections by vaccination.

**Valence**    For an antibody, the number of accessible antibody sites per molecule. IgG antibodies are bivalent; IgM antibodies are usually penta- or decavalent. The valence of an antigen is the number of antigenic determinants present on the antigen molecule accessible to antibodies.

**Variable part**    N-terminal part of an immunoglobulin molecule, which contains the antibody site and possesses an amino acid sequence different for each specificity.

**Xenogeneic**    Describes individuals belonging to different species.

# ABBREVIATIONS USED IN THE TEXT

| | |
|---|---|
| ACTH | adreno corticotrophic hormone |
| ADA | adenosine deaminase |
| ADCC | antibody-dependent cell-mediated cytotoxicity |
| AFC | antibody-forming cells |
| AHA | autoimmune hemolytic anemia |
| ALG | antilymphocyte globulin |
| ALL | acute lymphoblastic leukemia |
| ALS | antilymphocyte sera |
| AMP | adenosine monophosphate |
| ANF | antinuclear factors |
| ASO | antistreptolysin O |
| | |
| BAF | B-cell activating factor |
| BCF | basophil chemotactic factor |
| BCG | Bacillus Calmette Guérin |
| BSA | bovine serum albumin |
| B/W | $(NZB \times NZW)F_1$ |
| | |
| C | constant |
| C3NeF | C3 nephritic factor |
| C3PA | C3 proactivator |
| CAH | chronic active hepatitis |
| CEA | carcino embryonic antigen |
| CFC | colony-forming cells |
| CFU | colony-forming unit |
| CH50 | complement hemolysing 50 |
| CLL | chronic lymphocytic leukemia |
| CML | cell-mediated lympholysis |
| Con A | concanavalin A |
| CSF | cerebrospinal fluid |
| CSF | colony-stimulating fluid |
| | |
| DEAE | diethylaminoethyl |
| DH | delayed hypersensitivity |
| DLA | dog leukocyte A antigen |
| DNA | deoxyribonuclease acid |
| DNCB | dinitrocholrobenzene |
| DNFB | dinitro-fluoro-benzene |
| DNP | dinitrophenyl |
| DR | D-related |
| | |
| E | erythrocyte |
| EA | erythrocyte antibody |
| EAC | erythrocyte antibody complement |
| EAE | experimental allergic encephalomyelitis |
| EBV | Epstein-Barr virus |
| ECF | eosinophil chemotactic factor |
| ECF-A | eosinophil chemotactic factor of anaphylaxis |
| EDTA | ethylediamine tetraacetate |
| ENA | extractable nuclear antigen |
| | |
| $F_1$ | first generation |
| Fab | antigen-binding fragment |

| | | | | |
|---|---|---|---|---|
| Fc | crystallizable fragment | | MA | membrane antigen |
| FTS | facteur thymic sérique | | MAF | macrophage activating factor |
| GBG | glycine-rich beta-globulin | | MBLA | mouse bone marrow leukocyte antigen |
| GBM | glomerular basement membrane | | MDP | muramyl dipeptide |
| GN | glomerulonephritis | | MER | methanol extractable residue (BCG) |
| GRF | genetically related factor | | MF | mitogenic factor |
| GVH | graft versus host reaction | | MHC | major histocompatibility complex |
| HBs | hepatitis B surface antigen | | MIF | migration inhibitory factor |
| HLA | human leukocyte A antigen | | MLC | mixed lymphocyte culture |
| HSA | human serum albumin | | MLR | mixed lymphocyte reaction |
| 5-HT | 5-hydroxytryptamin (serotonin) | | MSF | macrophage spreading factor |
| | | | MSV | murine luekemia and sarcoma virus |
| IBF | immunoglobulin binding factor | | 6-MP | 6-mercaptopurine |
| IC | immune complexes | | NBT | nitroblue tetrazolium test |
| ID | immunodeficiencies | | NF | nephritic factor |
| IF | initiating factor | | NIP | 4-hydroxy-3 iodo-5 nitrophenyl acetic acid |
| IFA | incomplete Freund's adjuvant | | NK | natural killer (cells) |
| IH | immediate hypersensitivity | | NZB | New Zealand black (mice) |
| IL | interleukin | | OAF | osteoclast activating factor |
| Ir | immune response (genes) | | | |
| KAF | conglutinogen activating factor | | PAF-ace-ther | platelet-activating factor |
| KLH | keyhole limpet hemocyanin | | PBA | polyclonal B cell activator |
| | | | PCA | passive cutaneous anaphylaxis |
| LAF | lymphocyte activating factor | | PEC | peritoneal exudate cells |
| | | | PEG | polyethylene glycol |
| LATS | long-acting thyroid stimulator | | PFC | plaque-forming cells |
| LCM | lymphochoriomeningitis | | PGE | prostaglandin E |
| LD | lymphocyte defined | | PHA | phytohemagglutinin |
| LDA | lymphocyte-dependent antibodies | | PIF | proliferative inhibitory factor |
| LDH | lactodehydrogenase virus | | PK | Prausnitz-Küstner |
| LE | lupus erythematosus | | PPD | purified protein derivative |
| LPS | lipopolysaccharide | | PVP | polyvinylpyrrolidone |
| | | | PWM | pokeweed mitogen |

| | | | |
|---|---|---|---|
| RA | rheumatoid arthritis | SNagg | serum normal agglutinators |
| Ragg | rheumatoid agglutinator | SRBC | sheep red blood cells |
| RAST | radio-allergosorbent test | SRF | skin reactive factor |
| RES | reticulo-endothelial | SRS-A | slow reactive substance of anaphylaxis |
| RF | rheumatoid factor | | |
| RFC | rosette-forming cells | Ss | serum serologic (protein) |
| Rh | rhesus | SSPE | subacute sclerosing panencephalitis |
| RIA | radioimmunoassay | | |
| RIST | radioimmunosorbent test | | |
| RNA | ribonuclcic acid | T cell | thymus derived cell |
| RNase | ribonuclease | TCGF | T-cell growth factor |
| RPCA | reverse passive anaphylaxis | Tdt | terminal deoxyribonucleotidyl transferase |
| RSV | Rous sarcoma virus | | |
| | | TF | transfer factor |
| SC | secretory component | THF | thymic humoral factor |
| SCID | severe combined immunodeficiency | TIP | translation inhibitory protein |
| SD | serologically defined | TL | thymus leukemia |
| SIRS | soluble immune response suppressor | TRF | T cell replacing factor |
| | | TSA | tumor specific antigen |
| SKSD | streptokinase streptodornase | TSTA | tumor associated transplantation antigen |
| SLE | systemic lupus erythematosus | | |
| | | V | variable (gene) |
| SIP | sex-limited protein | VCA | viral capsular antigen |
| SMAF | specific macrophage arming factor | WSA | water soluble adjuvant |

# INDEX

Page numbers in *italics* indicate major discussion of the entry.

A (substance), 938–939
A₁A₂ erythrocytes, 596, 614
ABO groups, 152, 593, 601, 603–609, *611–623*, 636–640
  hemolytic disease, 752
  incompatibilities, 753–756
Absorptions, 132
Acetylcholine receptors, 718, 926–929
Achondroplastic dwarfism, 899
ACTH, 303
Activation:
  lymphocytes, *51–58*, 544–545
  macrophages, 387, 403, 474
Actynomycetes, *757–758*
Acute anterior uveitis, 697
Acute glomerulonephritis, 796, 837, 840, 848
Acute hepatitis, 931–932
Acute lymphoblastic leukemia (ALL), 622, 880–881
Acute vasculitis, 822
ADA, *see* Adenosine deaminase
ADCC, *see* Antibody-dependent cell-mediated cytotoxicity
Addison's disease, 920–921
Adenosine deaminase (ADA), 886, *889*
Adenovirus, 477, 479
Adherence, lymphocyte, 47, 79
Adhesion, macrophages, 116–117
Adjuvants, 532, 726, *943–951*
  arthritis, 946
  defined, 978
Adrenal hyperplasia, 696–697
Adrenal reactive antibody, 920–921
Adrenergic receptors, 359, 745
Adsorbed antigens, 600
Adult thymectomy, *61,* 65, 98, 545, 546, 552, 586, 960
Affinity, 131, *286–292*, 312, 334, 339–341, 363, 563–564
  defined, 977
  labelling, 185–188
Agammaglobulinemia, 100, 551, *884–891, 894–897*
Agar, *see* Gel
Ag-B locus, 658, 660
Ageing, 20, 21, 720, 743, *901–902*, 918
Agglutination reactions, *319–321*, 324, *605–607*, 636–640

Agglutinator(s) rheumatoid serum (Ragg), 632
  serum normal (SN agg), 632
Agglutinogens, 320
Aggregated IgG, 76
Ag system, 635
Air-conditioning lung, 757
Alcoholic cirrhosis, 622, 753, 816
Aldomet, 725, 765, 770, 810–811
Aleutian mink disease, 484, 485, *716*
Alginate, 948
Alkylating agents, 392, *957–958*
ALL, *see* Acute lymphoblastic leukemia
Allelic exclusion, *219–220*, 240, 857
Allergens, *349–353*, 748–751, 977
Allergic:
  asthma, 744–746
  contact dermatitis, 759–762
  drug reactions, 762–767
  eczema, 746
  extrinsic alveolitis, 756–759
  orchitis, 921
  rhinitis, 744
  thyroiditis, 716–717, 918
Allergy, 740–751
  defined, 347, 366, 978
  to drugs, 762–767
Alloantigens, 598–599, 645–675
  defined, 133
Allogeneic, 400, 401
  defined, 401, 978
  disease, 423
  effect, *538–540*, 546, 584, 688
  effect factors (AEF), 388, 538, 539
  inhibition, 646
  restriction, 12, 87–88, 444, 482, 690, 691–692
Allografts:
  defined, 400
  immunosuppressants in, 421–422, 586–587
  rejection, 400–406, 421–422
  renal, 402, 406, 673–674
  tolerance, 586–588
Alloimmunization, 593, 602, 622–623, 751–756
Allophenic mice, 588, 688
Allopurinol, 352

Allotypes, 81, *217–224*, 548–550, 597,
        632–635
    defined, 597, 978
    human Ig, 220–224, 632–635
    membrane Ig, 82
    mouse Ig, 224
    rabbit Ig, 217–220
    restriction, 82
    suppression, 548–549
Alpha chain, *see* IgA
Alpha chain diseases, 875–876
Alpha feto protein, 434–435
Alpha-methyldopa, 725, 765, 770
Alpha 2 D, 782
Alpha-2 globulins, 635
Altered self, *87–88*, 691–694
Alternative pathway, of complement
        activation, *261–264*, 850–851
    defined, 978
Aluminum, 499, 947
Alveolar macrophages, 107
    basement membranes, 833
Alveolitis, allergic extrinsic, 756–759
Alymphocytosis, 886–887
Amidopyrin, 766
Ammonium sulfate precipitation, 299, 801
AMP, cyclic, 56, 97, 358, 359, 412
Amyloidosis, 815, 841, 865, *938–939*
    defined, 978
Anaphylactic shock, *347–348*, 743–744,
        763–764, 796
Anaphylatoxin, 257, 266, 354, 358, 361
    defined, 978
Anaphylatoxinic inhibitor, 266
Anaphylaxis:
    defined, 978
    history, 3, 346–347
Anatoxins, diphtheria, 469, 497, 622, 943
    defined, 978
Anemias:
    autoimmune hemolytic, 770–793
    drug induced, 765–766
    pernicious, 923–924
Anesthetics, 462
Angiitis, 716, 728, *820–823*
Angioneurotic edema, 266
Ankylosing spondylitis, 695–697
Antazoline (induced purpura), 764
Anti-ABH antibodies, 600–607, *620–623*,
        753–756
Anti-arterial antibodies, 820–823
Antibasement membrane antibodies,
        830–833, 838–839, 842–846, 925
Anti-B cell serum, 74
Antibiotics, 122, 123, 451
Antibody, *163–251*
    in allograft rejection, 405–406, 417
    in antibacterial defense, 468–471

    in antiviral defense, 478–480
    B cell origin, 535
    biosynthesis, 515–516
    classes, 191–199
        *see also* IgA; IgD; IgE; IgG; IgM
    defined, 978
    detection, 285–326, 505–520
    diversity, 232–249, 556–574
    in parasite elimination, 489
    site, 184–190
    in tumor rejection, 437–439
Antibody-dependent cell-mediated
        cytotoxicity (ADCC), 76–77, 413–415,
        440–442, 485, 918
    defined, 978
Antibody-producing cells, 505–528
Anticoagulants, 805, 863
Anticomplementary activity, 274, 322, 734
    defined, 978
Anti-DNA antibodies, 712, 716, 732,
        *800–803*, 836
Antiepileptic drugs, 811
Antierythrocytic antibodies, 751–756,
        *770–793*, 804–805, 858
Anti-GBM antibody induced
        glomerulonephritis, 830–833,
        838–839, 842–846
    antibody detection, 842–844
    autoimmunization, 832
Antigen, 129–161
    antibody reaction, 285–326
    binding cells, 83–88, *508–514*, 566,
        585–586, 688
    bridge theory, 541
    charge, 149, 292–293, 564
    competition, *343–344*, 551
        defined, 980
    defined, 129, 142, 978
    degradation, 115
    determinants, 132, 138–141, 151–153
    induced lymphocyte transformation, 72,
        378–379
    modification by antibody, 297–298
    molecular weight, 150
    sensitive cells, 511–512, 563
    specific receptors, 74, 81–85, 562
Antigen antibody complexes, interaction,
        285–326
    *see also* Immune complexes
Antigenic modulation, *83*, 437, 445
    defined, 979
Antigenic original sin, 131, *336–337*, 482,
        486
Antiglobulins:
    and immune complexes, 479, 732
    tests, *see* Coomb's test
Antihistamines, 347, 357–358, 729, 745
Anti-idiotype antibodies, 86, 215–216

Anti-immunoglobulin column, 79
Anti-inflammatory agents, 392
Anti-inflammatory effects of
    immunosuppressive agents, 954
Anti-intrinsic factor antibody, 923–924
Antilink antibodies, 139
Antilung immunization, 842–846
Antilymphocyte antibodies, 713, 803–804,
    893
Antilymphocyte sera (ALS), 51, 69, 74, 78,
    392, 421–422, 481, 546, 586, 795,
    *959–961*
Antimacrophage serum, 531
Antimalarial agents, 813
Antimetabolites, 392, 812, 818, *955–956,
    962–963*
Antimyosin antibodies, 825
Antinuclear antibodies, *800–803*, 817, 826,
    932
    *see also* Anti-DNA antibodies
Antiprotein immunization, 754
Antireceptor antibodies, 89, 718, 918–919,
    921, 926–929
Anti-Rh antibody, 628, 751–756, *772–774*
Anti-RNA antibody, 801–802, 808
Anti-smooth muscle antibody, 932, 937
Antistreptolysin, 929–930
Anti-T cell antisera, *64–69*
Antithyroglobulin antibody, 715, 716–717,
    724, *915–918*
Antithyroid antibody, 715, 716–717, *915–920*
Antitoxins, 468–469
Antitumor antibodies, 437, 439
    immunity, 430–448
    vaccination, 436–437
Antiviral antibodies, 478–480, 495, 808
Ap antigen, 598
Appendix, 31
Arteritis, 716, 728, *820–823*
Arthritis:
    acute hepatitis, 931
    adjuvant, 946
    rheumatic fever, 929
    rheumatoid, 814–819
    SLE, 799
Arthus reaction, 272, *361–362*, 370,
    754–759, 766
    defined, 320, 361, 979
Artificial antigens, 134
Ascaris, 486, 546
Aschoff body, 929
Aspergillus fumigatus, 758
Aspirin, 352, 357, 745, 819
Assembly, immunoglobulins, 524–525
Association constant, 286–291, 296
Asthma, 744–746
Ataxia telangiectasia, 898
Athymic mouse, *see* Nude mouse

Atopy, 740–751, 762–767
    defined, 740, 979
Atrophic gastritis, 923–924
Australia antigen, *see* HBs antigen
Autoantibodies, 708–710
    defined, 708, 979
Autoantigens, 133, 599, 708–710, 724–726
    defined, 979
Autografts, 400–401
Autoimmune cytopenias, 924–925
Autoimmune hemolytic anemia (AHA),
    *770–793*, 804, 870
    clinical aspects, 784–788
    immunologic classification, 778–779
    pathogenesis, 779–784, 788–790
    and tumors, 787
Autoimmune neutropenias, 925
Autoimmunity, 708–727
    defined, 708, 979
    *see also Chapters 27, 28, 29, 32*
Autologous rosettes, 509, 724
Autoradiography, 48, 87, 330, 514, 688
Autoreactivity, 723–724
Avian antigens, 758–759
Avidity, *296–297*, 469
    defined, 296, 979
Axenic, 332–333, 451, 507
    defined, 979
Azathioprine, 812, 818, *955–957*, 962–964

Bacillus Calmette Guérin, *see* BCG
Bacteria:
    defense against, 466–476
    endotoxins, 76, *270*, 361 362, 462, 578,
        584, 948–950
Bacterial adherence, 514
Bacterial antigens, 578
Bacterial colony inhibition, 514
Bacterial immobilization, 514
Bacteriolysis, 121–122, 471, 905
Bacteriophage neutralization, 324, 478, 514
Basement membrane:
    kidney, 830–832, 838–839, 842–846
    skin, 925
Basic proteins, 452
Basophil, 107, 198, 354–355, 730, 749
    chemotactic factor (BCF), 388
    cutaneous hypersensitivity, 368–369
    degranulation, 358–361, 730, 749
B cell, *60–67, 74–85, 99–102*
    activating factor (BAF), 386, 533
    activation, 76, 540–545
    alloantigens, 74, 662–664
    colonies, 40
    defined, 60–64, 979
    differentiating factor (BDF), 386
    differentiation, 99–102, 515–520
    hyperactivity, 714

immunodeficiencies, 885–891, 894–899
markers, 74–76
maturation, 99–102
mitogens, 76
ontogeny, 99–102
purification, 79–80
specific heteroantigens, 74
specificity for antigen, 83–84, 536–537
tolerance, 581
BCF, see Basophil, chemotactic factor
BCG (Bacillus Calmette Guérin), 367, 393,
     447, 462, 472, 497, 498, 889, *944–947*
defined, 979
infection, 889
Bedsonia, 817
Behçet's syndrome, 697, *937–938*
Bence-Jones proteins, 168, *860–861*, 873,
     979
Benign monoclonal gammapathies, 878
Berger's disease, 841
Beryllium sulfate, 947
Beta lipoproteins, 635
Beta lysin, 452–453
Beta 2 microglobulin, 228–229, 665
Bg antigens, 630
Biclonal proliferation, 874
Biliary canaliculi, reactive antibody, 932
Biliary cirrhosis, 937
Billroth's cords, 29
Biosynthesis of antibodies, 515–520
Biozzi's mice, *699–700*
Biphasic hemolysin, 774, 777
Bird fancier's lung, 758–759
Blast cells, see Lymphoblastic transformation
Blastogenic factor, 387, 390
Blocking antibodies:
     cytotoxic T cells, 406, 419, 441, 442–445,
         *586–588*
     defined, 980
     IgE, 750–751
B-locus, chicken, 658
Blood groups:
     ABO, see ABO groups
     rhesus, see Rhesus, grouping
B mice, defined, 61–63
Bombay phenotype, *601*, 614–615
Bone marrow, *23–24*, 60, 67, 93, 102
     grafts, 887, 890
     ontogenesis, 23
     structure, 23–24
Bordetella pertussis, 950
Botulism, vaccine, 497
Bradykinin, 151, 358, 459
Breakdown, tolerance, 584, 725
Bromelin, 640
Bronchial asthma, 744–746
Bruton's disease, 894–895
Budgerigar fancier's lung, 758–759

Bullous pemphigoid, 925–926
Burkitt's lymphoma, 433, 438–439, 477, *878*
Bursa of Fabricius, 20–23, 100
     equivalent in mammals, 23, 100
     involution, 22–23
     ontogenesis, 20–21, 100
     structure, 21–22
Bursectomy, 62, 100
B/W mice ((NZB × NZW) F1), 548, 712–715,
     836–837
BXSB mice, 715

C (constant):
     gene, 237–249, 567–568
     region, 174, 191–199, 217–224
C1, 253–257
     esterase inhibitor, 270, 280
C1q binding tests, 734–735, 806, 816
C2, deficiency, 280–283
C3, 257–284
     feedback cycle, *263–264*, 850
     NeF, 850–851
     pro-activator (C3PA), *261*, 269, 671
     receptors, 75, 544
C4, 236–259
C5, 256–260
C6, 256–260
     deficiency, 269
C7, 256–260
C8, 257–260
C9, 257–260
CAH, see Chronic active hepatitis
Calcium, 56, 358
Cancer, immunology of, 430–448
Candida, 900–901, 905
Capillary permeability, 356–357, 457
Capping, 43, 58, *82–85*, 649
     defined, 82, 980
Carbodiimides, 136, 147
Carbohydrate residues, Ig, 182, 197, 526
Carbon uptake, 111, 947
Carcinoembryonic antigen (CEA), 432,
     434–435
Cardiac infarction, 926
Cardiolipin, 155, 805
Carditis, rheumatic, 929–930
Carrier:
     coupling, 134–137
     defined, 130, 980
     effect, 114, *138–139*, 535–536, 687–688
Cartilage hair hypoplasia, 899
Cc antigens, 624–628
CEA, see Carcinoembryonic antigen
Celiac disease, 697
Cell-mediated immunity, 5, 61, *365–367*, 545
     defined, 980
     in RA, 817
     in SLE, 807

Cell-mediated lympholysis (CML), *410–413,*
  545, 667
  defined, 980
Cellular cooperation, 62, *530–552,* 582–584,
  687–691
  between B and T cells, *532–552,* 582–584,
    687–691
  between macrophages and lymphocytes,
    530–534, *689–690*
  between T cells, 545–546
Cephalosporins, 764, 766
Cerebral antigens, 65, 69, 717
Cerebrospinal fluid, complement, 278
CFC, *see* Colony forming cells
CFU, *see* Colony forming unit
CH 50, 273–274
Chediak-Higashi syndrome, 124, 463,
  *905–906*
Chemotactic factor, 387, 390, 395
Chemotaxis, 267
Chicken:
  bursa of Fabricius, 20–23
  obese, thyroiditis, 715–716
Chicken pox, 893
Chido, 671
Chimeras, 72, 608–609
Chlorambucil, 818, 957–958
Chloramphenicol, 352, 767
Chlorpromazine, 766
Cholera, vaccine, 324, 344, 497
Chorea, 930
Chorionic gonadotropins, 911
Chromium ($^{51}$Cr), 50, 410, 439–441, 482
  release, 647
Chronic active hepatitis (CAH), 697, 932–933
Chronic allogeneic disease, 423
Chronic granulomatous disease, 462,
  904–905
Chronic lymphocytic leukemia (CLL),
  867–871, 879
Chung and Strauss syndrome, 822
Circulating immune complexes, 727–737,
  806, 816, 847–850
Circulating thymic factor, 97
Circulation of lymphocytes, 49–51, 77–78
Cirrhosis, 622, 816, *937*
Clasmatosis, 526
Class, 191–199
  restriction on surface Ig, 82
  variation, 338–339, 508
Classical pathway of complement activation,
  252–261
Clonal selection:
  defined, 980
  theory, 560–561
Clones:
  defined, 980
  forbidden, 561, 722–724

of immunoglobulins, 168–169, 855–856
of lymphocytes, 149, 563–565, 855–856
Cloning inhibition factor, 388
Clonotype, 564–565
CML, *see* Cell-mediated lympholysis
Coagulation, 269–270, 363, 457
Cobra venom factor (CoF), 261, 266, 272
Coisogenic:
  defined, 980
  mice, 651
Cold agglutinin, 320, 603, 639, 774–777
  disease, 774–777, 785, 874
Collagen, 826, 833
Collagen producing factor, 388
Colloidal gold, 423
Colon:
  alloantigens, 133
  antibodies, 708
Colonic CEA, 434–435
Colony forming cells (CFC), 40
Colony forming units (CFU), 40
Colony stimulating factor (CSF), 40, 106,
  388
Colostrum, 468
Competition, antigenic, *343–344,* 551
  defined, 980
Complement, 252–284, 451
  activation, 252–264
  alternative pathway, *261–264,* 850–851
  biological role, 264–270
  classical pathway, 252–261
  components, 259
  Coombs' test, 776–778
  conversion products, 275
  deficiencies, 271, *277–278,* 451, 696, 807
  deposits, 275, 838, 840
  evaluation, 273–278, 968
  fixation, 253–254, 321–324
  fixation site, Ig, 253
  genetics, 271, 671
  in glomerulonephritis, 850–851
  hypersensitivity, 271–273, 361–362
  in Masugi's glomerulonephritis, 273, 831
  and phagocytosis, 118
  receptors, 74, 102
  in rheumatoid arthritis, 816
  in systemic lupus erythematosus, 806–807,
    809
Complex, immune, *see* Immune complexes
Compound antigen, 625
Concanavalin A (Con A), 52–58, 72, 540,
  548, 550, 837
Conformation of Ig, 181–182
Congenic mice, 65, 651, 683
  defined, 980
  resistant mice, 651
Congenital granulocytic aplasia, 902
Conglutinin, 269, 322–323

Conglutinogen activating factor (KAF), 262, 281
Connective tissue diseases, 794–828
Constant regions, 174, 191–199, 227–228
Contact allergic dermatitis, 368–369, 759–762, 767
Contact sensitivity, 368–369, 550, 759–762
defined, 980
Coombs' test, *320*, 642–643, 765, *771*, 776–778, 804
defined, 980
Cooperation, cellular, 62, *530–552*, 582–583, 687–691
between B and T cells, *532–552*, 582–584, 687–691
between macrophages and lymphocytes, 530–534, *689–690*
between T cells, 545–546
Copolymers, aminoacids, 146–147, 560, 679
Coprecipitation, 299
Corpuscles, Hassal's, 18–19
Cortical necrosis, renal, 363, 402
Corticosteroids, 93, 392, 462, *958–959*, 962–964
Corynebacteria, 463, *950*
Cot, 241–243
Cotton filtration, 47
Counter immunoelectrophoresis, 317, 802
Coxsackie virus, 478, 481
Crises, rejection, 402
Crohn's disease, 935–936
Cromoglycate, 361, 745
Crossed electrophoresis, 317
Cross-match, 648, 673
defined, 981
Cross reactions, 132, 141, *315–316*, 648, 724–726, 760, 792
defined, 981
Cryoglobulins, *732–733*, 806, 816, 863, 873, *876–877*, 968
defined, 981
CSF, *see* Colony stimulating factor
CTL, *see* Cytotoxic T lymphocytes
C-type viral particles, 808
Cunningham's technique, 506
Cutaneous reaction, *see* Skin, tests
Cyclic AMP, 56, 97, 358, 412
Cyclic antibody production, 342, 358–359, 412, 900, 906
Cyclic GMP, 52, 358–359, 412, 900, 906
Cyclic neutropenia, 904
Cyclophosphamide, 392, 478, 579, 582, *957–958*, 962–964
in glomerulonephritis, 852
in lupus, 812
in rheumatoid arthritis, 818
in Wegener's granulomatosis, 822

Cyclosporin A, 961
Cytolysis, 323, 410–416
Cytomegalovirus, 477, 480, 484–485
Cytopenias, autoimmune, 924–925
*see also* Autoimmune hemolytic anemia; Purpura
Cytophilic antibody, 118, 179–180, 512
defined, 981
Cytotoxic antibodies, 406, 417, 647
Cytotoxicity index, 323
Cytotoxic K cells, *see* Antibody-dependent cell-mediated cytotoxicity
Cytotoxic macrophages, 415, 443
Cytotoxic NK cells, 416, 443–444
Cytotoxic T lymphocytes (CTL), *410–412*, 439–441, 482, 666–668
Cytotropic antibodies, *see* Homocytotropic antibodies

Dangerous donor, 755
D antigen, 624–628
Danysz phenomenon, 311
Dash phenogroup, 625–626
Deaggregation, 577, 580
Dean and Webb's technique, 313
Deficiency, 232–240
of cell-mediated immunity, 885–894, 897–902
of complement, 271, *279–283*, 451, 696, 807
granulocyte, 902–907
of humoral immunity, 885–891, 894–899
in CLL, 870
in multiple myeloma, 865
Degalan, 79
Degranulation, 358–361, 730, 749
Delayed hypersensitivity (DH), 365–398
defined, 7, 365–367, 981
drug-induced, 767
immunogenicity, 155–158
and macrophages, 533
in RA, 817
in SLE, 807
suppression, 389–393
and suppressor T cells, 392–393, 551
transfer, 373–378
in vitro correlates, 378–389, 393–396
Delta chain, *see* IgD
Denaturation-renaturation, 144, 561
Dendritic cells, 332
Dense deposits, GBM, 838, 840, 850–851
Density gradient, 47, 78–79
Dermatitis:
atopic, 746
herpetiformis, 697, 926
Dermatomyositis, 823–825
Dermatophagoides pteronyssimus, 352

Desensitization, 391, 750–751, 761
  defined, 981
Desmosomes, 18
Detection of immune complexes, *731–737*,
    806, 816, 847–850
Determinants, antigen, 132, 138–141,
    150–151, 153
Deviation, immune, 391, 576
  defined, 981
Dextran, 48, 152, 158, 184
DH, *see* Delayed hypersensitivity
Diabetes mellitus, 462, 697, 910, *921*, 924
Dialysis, equilibrium, 287–291, 301
Diapedesis, 107, 111, 458
Diazotation, 135
Dick's reaction, 322
Diego antigen, 599, 629
Differentiation antigens, 65–69, 74, 90–91,
    435
Differentiation of lymphocytes, *see*
    Maturation
Diffusion, 305–318
Di George's syndrome, 891–893
Digoxin, 140
Dimeric IgA, 195–196, 344–345, 525
Dinitrochlorobenzene (DNCB), 369
Dinitrofluorobenzene (DNFB), 369
Diphtheria toxin, 311, 334, 495
  toxin (suppress) neutralization, 321, 469
  toxoid, 469, 497, 622, 943
Discoid lupus, 800, 803, 804
Dissociation of immune complexes, 167,
    *293–294*
Dizigotism, 608
DLA, 658
DNA, 233, 805, 837
  cell-mediated hypersensitivity, 807
  deletions, 237–238
  reactive antibodies, 712, 716, 732,
    *800–803*, 836
  repair, 812, 957
  *see also* Anti-DNA antibodies
DNCB, *see* Dinitrochlorobenzene
DNFB, *see* Dinitrofluorobenzene
Domains, 174–183, 193–198
  defined, 981
Donor:
  dangerous, 755
  graft, 400, 656, 672–674
  transfusion, 754–756
Double antibody production, 566, 874
DR antigens, 74, *663–664*, 695–698
D region, H-2, 648–653
Dressler's syndrome, 926
Drugs:
  immunogenicity, 352, *762–763*
  immunostimulating, 943–952

immunosuppressive, 577, 812, 818,
    851–852, *952–964*
  inducing lupus, 810–811
  reactions, 762–767
D segments, DNA, 233
DTH (delayed type hypersensitivity), *see*
    Delayed hypersensitivity
$D^u$, 624, 625, 640–642
Dual erythrocyte populations, 638
Duffy, 612, 630, 643
Dust, house, 351–352

Ea-1 antigen, 681
EAC, rosettes, 75–77
EAE, *see* Experimental allergic
    encephalomyelitis
Early antigen (EA), 438
EA rosettes, 76–77
EBNA, *see* Epstein-Barr nuclear antigen
EB virus, *see* Epstein-Barr virus
ECFA, *see* Eosinophil, chemotactic factor of
    anaphylaxis
*E. coli* lipopolysaccharide, 76, 158–159, 540,
    544–545, 578, 584, *948–950*
Ecotaxis, 35
Ectromelia, 124, 481
Eczema, 746, 759–762, 767, 897, 906
  allergic, 746
  contact, 759–762, 767
Edema, angioneurotic, 266
Educated T cells, 512, 537, 543
Ee, 624, 628
Eggs as allergens, 352
Electroimmunodiffusion, 318
Electrophoresis, 302
  Ig, 165–166, 198, 856, 860
  lymphocytes, 47, 79
Electrostatic forces, 292
Elution, 167, 293–296, 412, 732, 772, 806,
    843, 848–849
Encephalitis:
  experimental allergic, 695, 717–718
  vaccination-induced, 499
Encephalomyelitis, 717–718
Endocapillary proliferation, 838, 840–841
Endocrine factors in SLE, 720, 810
Endocytosis, lymphocytes, 45
Endogenous pyrogen activating factor
    (EPAF), 389
Endoplasmic reticulum, 43, 53, 54, 109,
    517–519
Endothelial cells, glomeruli, 837
Endotoxins, 75, 270, 362–363, 462, 578, 584,
    *948–950*
  defined, 981
Enhancement, 419, 422, 445, *586–588*
  defined, 981

Enzyme neutralization, 321
Eosinophil, 107, 124, 491, 744
  chemotactic factor (ECF), 387
    of anaphylaxis (ECF-A), 357–358
  promoting factor, 387
Eosinophilia, 821, 822
Epidermal reactive antibodies, 925–926
Epinephrine, 359
Epithelial cells:
  glomeruli, 837
  intestine, 31–34, 525
  thymic, 17–19, 93, 96–97, 691–692, 888
Epitope, 142
Epsilon chain, see IgE
Epstein-Barr nuclear antigen (EBNA), 438
Epstein-Barr virus (EBV), 73, 169, 433,
    438–439, 477, 898
Equilibrium dialysis, 287–289, 301
Equivalence, 305–310
  defined, 981
Ergastoplasm, 43, 53, 54, 517–519
E rosettes, 69–70, 72, 509
Erythroblast, 612–615
Erythroblastosis fetalis, 5, 752–753
Erythrocyte grouping, 636–643
Erythrophagocytosis, 119, 780–782
Estrogens and immunity, 461, 714
Evans blue, 349–350
Evans syndrome, 786
Evolution of immune responses, 225–232
Exon, 237
Exophtalmos, 920
Exotoxin, 468–469
Expansion-contraction hypothesis, 237
Experimental allergic encephalomyelitis
    (EAE), 695, 717–718
  thyroiditis, 716–717
Extracapillary proliferation, 838, 840–841
Extrathymic maturation, 97, 98
Extrinsic allergic pneumonitis, 756–759

Fab, 170–171, 178
Fab', 178
Fabricius, bursa of, see Bursa of Fabricius
Facilitation, 419, 422, 445, 586–588
FACS, see Fluorescence-activated cell system
Facteur thymique sérique (FTS), 97
Factor B, complement (C3PA or GBG),
    261–264, 671
Factor D, complement, 261–264
Farmer's lung disease, 756–758
Farr test, 299
  defined, 981
  DNA, 801–804
Fatty acids, 450
Fc, 170–171, 178, 193, 195, 225
  receptors, 70–71, 76, 99, 269, 736
Fd, 171, 178

Feedback, antibody, 340–343, 563
Felty syndrome, 924
Female sterility, 922–923
Ferritin, 136, 330, 515
Fetal liver, 90, 93, 94, 100, 891
Fetomaternal immunization, 752–753
α-Feto protein, 432, 434–435
Fetus as allograft, 424–427
$F_1$ human serum albumin fragment, 144–145
$F_1$ hybrid, 648
Fibrillar protein, 142
Fibrinogen, 216
Fibrinolysis, 269
Ficoll gradient, 47
Filariasis, 486, 492
First set rejection, 400
Fixation, complement, 253–257, 322–323
Flagellin, 84, 99, 158–160, 331, 540, 576,
    578–580, 584
  defined, 981
Flocculation, 312, 313
Flour allergy, 748
Fluorescein, 136, 304
Fluorescence:
  augmentation, 301
  polarization, 301
  quenching, 300
Fluorescence-activated cell system (FACS), 80
Fluorochromes, 136, 304
Focal GN, 799, 838, 840–841
Follicles, 25–28, 30, 332
Food allergy, 747
Forbidden clones, 561, 722–724
Forces linking antigens and antibodies,
    292–296
Formaldehyde, 142, 469, 497
Forssman antigen, 133, 598, 623, 796, 880
  defined, 982
Fragments, Ig, 178
Free radicals, 121
Freund's adjuvants, 944–947
  defined, 982
Friend's virus, 685, 695
FTS, see Facteur thymique sérique
Fusion, 523
Fv, 178, 188, 211

Galactosidase, 514
β-Galactosidase, 160
Gall body, 43
Gamma chain, see IgG
Gamma chain diseases, 875–876
Gammaglobulins, 165, 166
  as antigen, 576, 577
G antigen, 625
Gastric reactive antibody, 923–924
  parietal cells, 923–924
Gastrointestinal allergy, 747

GBG, *see* Glycine rich beta globulin
GBM (glomerular basement membrane):
  antigenic structure, 832–833
  reactive antibodies, 830–833, 838–839,
    842–846
Gc globulins, 635
Gel:
  filtration, 302
  precipitation, 313–319
Gelatin, 146
Gell and Coombs' classification, 5–8, 740–741
Genetically related factor (GRF), 533
Genetic control:
  of antibody formation, 232–249, 567–573,
    677–703
  of IgE production, 742
  of non-specific immunity, 461–462
  of tumor rejection, 444
Genetic factors in SLE, 809
Genetic selection, 629, 699–701
Genotype, defined, 982
Germinal centers, 25–33, 332
  defined, 981
Germ-line theories, 244, 568–569
  defined, 982
Giant cell arteritis, 822–823
G IX antigen, 65, 695
Glomerular basement membrane, *see* GBM
Glomeruli, 837
Glomerulonephritis (GN), 829–853
  anti-GBM induced, 830–833, 838–839,
    842–846
  complement in, 840–841, 850–851
  experimental, 829–837
  human, 840–841, 842–852
  immune complex induced, 728–729,
    833–837, 847–850
  recurrence, transplantation, 849
Glutaraldehyde, 167, 364
Glycine rich beta globulin (GBG), 259, 291
Gm system, 200, 220–224, 632–635, 719
GN, *see* Glomerulonephritis
Goiter, 915–920
Gold salts, 819
Golgi apparatus, 41–45, 52, 82, 516–517,
  526
Goodpasture's syndrome, 697, 838–839,
  842–846
Graft, 399–429
  defined, 982
  *vs.* host reaction (GvH), 422–424, 545–546,
    572, 890
  rejection, 399–422, 672–675
Granulocyte deficiencies, 902–907
Graves' disease, *918–920*, 924
Gross' virus, 381, 670, 685
Guillain-Barré syndrome, 934
  in serum sickness, 796

Gut associated lymphoid system, 31–34, 99,
  100
GvH, *see* Graft, *vs.* host reaction

H-1, locus:
  mouse, 651, 653
  rat (Ag-B), 658
H-2:
  antigens, 228, *649–651*, 652–653, 658–659,
    691–694
  complex, 646–654, 683–686
  defined, 650
  region, 646–671, 683–686
  restriction, 12, *87–88*, 444, 482, 690,
    691–694
Hageman's factor, 270
Haploidy, functional, 634
Haplotype, 595, 651
  defined, 982
Haptens, 129, *134–141*, 535–538, 579, 762
  antibody reaction with, 138–141
  defined, 129, 982
  haptenic groups, 138–141
  inhibition, 176, 563, 761
Hashimoto's thyroiditis, 820, *915–918*, 924
Hassal's corpuscles, 18–19
Hay fever, 744
Hayry cell leukemia, 882
Hazerick's phenomenon, 801
HBs antigen, 485, 695, 732, 822, 849,
  *930–933*
Heart, reactive antibodies, 926, 929–930
Heavy chain diseases, 875–876
Helper factors, 541–544
Helper T cells, 69, 71, 160, 420, 534–545,
  687–689
  defined, 982
Hemagglutination:
  defined, 982
  inhibition, 632
  *see also* Agglutination reactions
Hematoxylic body, 801
Hemochromatosis, 696
Hemocyanin, 547, 969
Hemolysin, 622, 637, 777
Hemolysis, 323, 779, 784
Hemolytic activity of complement, 273
  anemia, 751–756, 765–766, *770–793*
  index, 323
  plaques, 506–508
Henoch-Schönlein purpura, 822, 841
Hepatitis, 930–933
Hereditary complement deficiencies,
  279–283, 697, 807, 809
Herpes virus, 433, 477–478, 480–482, 484
Heteroantigens, 133, 598
Heterogeneity of antibodies, 167–168, 190,
  289–291

Heterokaryotic monozygotism, 609
Heteroligating antibodies, 141
Heterophile antibodies, 133
Heymann's glomerulonephritis, 836
Hh-1 factor, 670
Hh system, 612–622
Hidden antigens, 600
Hirst's reaction, 322
Histamine, 267, 347–349, 354–359, 459, 460,
    743–750
Histiocytes, 107
Histocompatibility:
    antigens, 228, 572, 594–610, 648–653,
        692–694
    chemistry, 645–676
    defined, 982
HLA, 594, 655–658, 661–662
    and allergy, 742
    alloimmunization, 753, 922
    antigens, 228, 630, 655–658, 661–662
    and complement, 271, 671
    and diseases, 695–698
    region, 671
    and renal grafts survival, 673–674
    and SLE, 697, 809
H2O2, 121
Hodgkin's disease, 819, 882, 908, 961
Hom-I genes, 670
Homing phenomenon, 34–35, 77, 78
Homocytotropic antibodies, 353–354
    see also IgE
Homogeneous antibodies, 167–168, 213,
        289–291, 855–859
Homogeneous pattern, ANF, 801
Homologies, Ig, 174–177, 200–207
Hormone, thymic, 95–96, 547, 712–713, 888,
        893, 927, 951–952
    and autoimmunity, 712, 807
    defined, 986–987
Horton's disease, 822–823
House dust, 351–352
H-substance, 614–615
Human glomerulonephritis, 837–852
Humps, 838, 840
Hyaluronidase, 459
Hybrid:
    antibodies, 184, 241–243, 509, 515
    cells (hybridomas), 12, 68, 69, 169–170,
        523, 548
    resistance, 646, 650
    RNA-DNA, 232
Hybridization, RNA-DNA, 241–243
Hybridomas, 12, 66, 69, 169–170, 523, 548
Hydantoins, 767, 810–811, 822
Hydralazine, 810–811
Hydrocortisone, see Corticosteroids
Hydrogen bonds, 292
5-Hydroxytryptamine (5 HT), see Serotonin

Hyperacute rejection, 402–404
Hypercomplementemia, 276
Hypersensitivity, 740–769
    cutaneous basophil, 368
    delayed type, 7–8, 365–398, 759–762, 767
        defined, 981
    immediate, 5–6, 347–364, 741–751
        defined, 982
    type I, see Immediate hypersensitivity
    type II, 6, 751–756
    type III, 6–7, 756–759
    type IV, see Delayed hypersensitivity
Hypervariable zones, Ig, 174, 208–209, 213
Hyperviscosity syndrome, 863, 873
Hypocomplementemia, 276–277
    in glomerulonephritis, 850–851
Hypogammaglobulinemia, see
        Agammaglobulinemia
Hypoparathyroidism, 921
Hypopigmentation, 900, 905
Hyposensitization, see Desensitization


Ia antigen, 74, 87, 532, 540, 544, 588, 650,
        662–663, 665–666, 690–691
    like antigens (DR antigens), 663–664,
        695–698
IA locus, 662–663, 684–685, 690–691
I antigen, 612, 615, 623, 774–775, 858,
        874
IB locus, 684–685
IC, see Immune complexes
IC locus, 684–685
ID, see Immunodeficiencies
Identify, reaction of, 315–316
Idiotypes, 86, 209–216, 236–237, 856, 859,
        864, 868
    defined, 982
    and network theory, 572, 573
    restriction, 82, 86
    suppression, 215, 490, 549–550
    on T cells, 82, 216
IE locus, 684–685
IFA, see Incomplete Freund's adjuvant
IgA, 195–196
    anti-IgA, antibodies, 754
    cell cycle, 33–34
    deficiency, 551, 895–898
    deposits, 841
    dimeric, 195, 344–345, 525
    local immunity, 344–345
    metabolism, 224–225
    nephropathy, 697, 841
    plasma cells, 31–34
    secretory, 344–345, 468, 525
    secretory component (SC), 34, 195, 525
    serum levels, 196, 230
    subclasses, 178, 635

IgD, 196, 887
  membrane IgD, *82*, 101, 868, 872
  metabolism, 224–225
  myeloma, 862
  serum levels, 196, 230
  surface IgD, *82*, 101, 770, 868, 872
IgE, *196, 353–354*, 741–751, 763–764
  and atopic diseases, 741–751
  metabolism, 224–225
  myeloma, 862
  in nephrotic syndrome, 847
  radioimmunoassay, 750
  serum levels, 196, 230
  specific, 749–750
IgG, *170–183*, 197, 289–290, 338, 508
  deficiency, 894–897
  metabolism, 224–225
  serum levels, 196, 230
  subclasses, 362
  surface IgG, 82, 101
Ig-1 locus, 214–215
IgM, *193–194*, 289–290, 338, 415, 416, 450
  deficiency, 897
  metabolism, 224–225
  polymeric, 195, 476
  serum levels, 196, 230
  surface IgM, 82, 101
IgM/IgG switch, 338, 508, 522, 687
IgND, *see* IgE
IgT, 543
IH, *see* Immediate hypersensitivity
I-J locus, 547, 650, 687
Immediate hypersensitivity (IH), 5–6,
    *346–363*, 741–751
  defined, 982
Immune adherence, 268, 323, 782
  defined, 982
Immune anti-A antibodies, 602, 622, 623,
    755
Immune complexes (IC):
  complement fixation, 253–257, 264
  defined, 980
  deposition, 275, 485, 729–731
  detection, 731–737, 806, 816, 847–850
  experimental pathology, 727–731
  and hypersensitivity, 271, 361–362
  induced GN, 727–729, *833–837*, 847–850
  pathogenicity, 795
  and rheumatoid arthritis, 816–817
  size, 834–835
  and SLE, 806
Immune deviation, 391, 576
Immune paralysis, 575
Immune response genes, *see* Ir genes
Immunity, 1, 396, 465–466
  active, 495–500
  defined, 465–466, 982
  passive, 494–495

Immunization, 329–339, *495–500*
Immunoadherence, 268, 323–324, 782
  defined, 982
Immunoadsorbents, 79, 80, 135, 138, 412
Immunochemistry, 129, 326
Immunoconglutinin, 269, 323
Immunocytes, 38–58, 505
Immunocytologic techniques, 515–520
Immunodeficiencies (ID), 477, *884–913*
  B cell, 894–899
  mixed, 887–891, 897–901
  secondary, 865, 870
  severe combined, 887–891
  stem cell, 885–891
  T cell, 891–894
Immunodeviation, 391, 576
Immunodiffusion, 305–318
Immunodominant sugar, 153
Immunoelectrophoresis, 317
Immunoenzymatic technique, 305
Immunofluorescence, 74, 80–85, 304–305,
    515–516, 801
  defined, 983
  glomeruli, 838  841
Immunogen, 130–162, 577
  defined, 130
Immunogenetics, defined, 594
Immunogenicity, 130–134, 155–158, 577
  defined, 983
Immunoglobulins (Ig), 163–249
  allotypes, *217–224*, 548, 632–636
  aminoacid sequences, 172–177
  antibody site, 184–190
  binding factor (IBF), 388
  chains, 170–171
  classes, 191–199
  conformation, 181–183
  defined, 983
  deletion, 526–527
  deposits, 729–732, 795, 799, 834, 838–841,
    847, 925
  domains, 174–183, 194–198
  fragments, 170–171, 178
  genes, 232–240
  genetic basis of diversity, 232–249,
    556–573
  idiotypes, 82, 86, *209–216*, 487, 573
  isolation, 165–169
  membrane Ig, *see* Immunoglobulins,
    surface Ig
  metabolism, 224–225
  ontogeny, 229–231
  phylogeny, 225–229
  surface Ig, 74, 80–84, 101, 239–240
  synthesis, 521–528
Immunologic surveillance, 443
  defined, 986
Immunologic tolerance, 575–588

Immunology, 1–11
    defined, 983
Immunomanipulation, 942–965
Immunopathology:
    experimental, 707–738
    human, 740
Immunopotentiation, 943–952
Immunoprecipitation, 305–319
Immunoproliferative disorders, 854–893
Immunostimulants, 943–952
    defined, 983
Immunosuppression:
    by antibodies, *340–341,* 752
    and cancer, 436
    by drugs, 953–964
Immunosuppressive agents, 392, 436, 577,
        586, *953–964*
    defined, 983
Immunotherapy:
    of atopy, 750–751
    of cancer, 446–447
Incomplete antibody, defined, 983
Incomplete Freund's adjuvant, 944–947
Indomethacin, 813, 819, 954
Infectious mononucleosis, 438, *879,* 909
Inflammation, 453–461
Influenza, 336, 497, 816
Inosine phosphorylase, 893
Insect bites, 368
Instructive theories, 559–560
    defined, 983
Insulin, hemolytic anemia caused by, 765
Insulinitis, experimental allergic, 921
Insulin receptor, reactive antibody, 921
Intercapillary tissue, 837
Interferon, 388, 389, *452–453,* 482, 951
Interleukin 1, LAF, 533
Interleukin 2, TCGF, 97, *386, 388,* 410, 537,
        539
Internal image, 573
Intestinal IgA, 33–34, 344–345
Intracellular bacteria, 471–472
Intrinsic association constant, 286–291
Intrinsic factor, reactive antibody, 918,
        *923–924*
Inv, 220–222, 632
Iodination, protein, 137
I region, 650, 658–664, *683–686,* 689–690
Ir genes, 660, 670, 678–698
Ir-IA, 684
Ir-IB, 684
Iridocyclitis, 815
Irregular agglutinins, 642
Irregular natural antibodies, 601
ISf, 635
Islet cell reactive antibody, 921
Isoantibody, defined, 983

Isoantigen, 133
Isocyanate, 136
Isogeneic, defined, 400–401
Isograft, defined, 400–401
Isoimmune, *see* Alloimmunization
Isolation, lymphocytes, 47–48
Isoproterenol, 359
Isothiocyanate, 136, 304
Isotypes, 170, 191–199

Jakob-Creutzfeldt's syndrome, 477, 935
J chain, 194, 196, 525
Jerne network theory, 572–573
Jerne plaque technique, 506–508
Jerne selective theory, 560, 572
Jk antigens, Kidd, 630
Jones-Mote reaction, 368, 392
    defined, 983
J piece, *see* J chain
J sequence, 233–235
Junction sequences, 233–235
Juvenile rheumatoid arthritis, 815

KAF, *see* Conglutinogen activating factor
Kallidin, 459
Kallikrein, 270, 459
Kaolin, 948
Kappa chains, *see* Light chains
K cells, 76–77, *413–415,* 440–442, 485, 918
    defined, 983
Kell, 612, 629, 643
Kennedy's technique, 40
Keratoconjunctivitis, 819–820
Kern factor, 191, 228
Keyhole limpet hemocyanin (KLH), 547
Kidd system, 630
Kidney:
    grafts, 402–404, 672–673
    reactive antibodies, 830–833, 838–839,
        842–846
Kinins, 270, 358, 360, 459, 745
    defined, 983
Klotz's representation, 288
K region, H-2, 648–653
Kupffer cells, 107
Kuru, 477, 935
Kveim test, 938
Kwashiorkor, 910

Lactodehydrogenase (LDH) virus, 484, 719
β-Lactoglobulin, 747
Lactoperoxidase, 80, 85
Lambda chains, *see* Light chains
Lamina propria, 33
Laser, 80
Latex test, 815–816
LATS, *see* Long-acting thyroid stimulator

Lattice theory, 307
Laurell's techniques, 317
LCM, *see* Lymphochoriomeningitis
LDA antibodies, *see* Antibody-dependent cell-mediated cytotoxicity
LD antigens, 647, 648–662
LDH, *see* Lactodehydrogenase virus
L Dopa, 765
LE cells, 800–801, 817
    defined, 983
$Le^a$ (or $Le^b$) substance, 612, 616–620, 623
Lectins, 51–58, 72
    defined, 983
Leishmaniasis, 486, 487, 490, 816
Lens antigens, 723, 926
Lentinan, 951
Lepromatous leprosy, 933–934
Lepromin, 933
Leprosy, 816, 909, 933–934
Leukemias, 432, 440, 638, 639, 907
    acute, 880–881
    chronic lymphocytic (CLL), 867–871, 879
    mouse, 695
Leukoagglutination, 647, 766
Leukocyte:
    antigens, *see* Histocompatibility, antigens
    inhibitor factor (LIF), 387
    migration inhibition test, 382–385, 394–396
Leukopenia, drug-induced, 766
Leukotrienes, 357
Levamisole, 952
Levans, 158–159
Levopimaric acid, 272
Lewis antigen, 612, 616–620, 623
Life-span:
    lymphocytes, 48–49, 78
    macrophages, 107
Ligand, 285
Light chains, 170–174, *191*, 217–218, 860–861, 866
Limiting dilutions, 565
Linear Ig deposits, glomeruli, 830–832, 838–839, 842–846
Linkage disequilibrium, *656–658*, 661
Lipid, 155
Lipid A, 949–950
Lipodystrophy, partial, 850
Lipoid nephrosis, 841, 847, 852
Lipopolysaccharide (LPS), 54, 58, 76, 158–159, 544–545, 578, 584, 687, 948–950
Liver, fetal, 90, 93, 94, 100, 891
Liver antigen localization, 330–331
Local GvH reaction, 423
Local immunity, 344–345
Localization of antigen, 329–332

Long-acting thyroid stimulator (LATS), 918–920
Loop peptide, lysozyme, 143, 685, 690–691
Low (antigen) dose tolerance, *579–580*, 725
LPS, *see* Lipopolysaccharide
Lp system, 636
Lung disease, farmer's, 756–758
Lupus:
    antilymphocyte antibodies, 803–804
    antinuclear antibodies, 800–803
    cell-mediated immunity, 807
    complement in, 806–807
    defined, 797–798
    discoid, 800, 803, 804
    drug-induced, 810–812
    endocrine factors, 810
    etiology, 808–812
    genetic factors, 809
    glomerulonephritis, 798–799
    treatment, 812–813
    and virus, 808
    *see also* Systemic lupus erythematosus
Lutheran system, 612, 631, 643
LW, 624 628
Ly antigens, *65–68*, 92, 98, 412, 545, 552
Lymph, 24–25, 33, 404
Lymphatic organs, 15–36
Lymphatics, 24–25, 33
Lymph nodes, 24–28
    changes during immunization, 27–28, 332–333, 369, 370
    mesenteric, 33–34
    ontogenesis, 24
    structure, 24–28
Lymphoblastic transformation, *51–58*, 72, 76, 378–381, 394, 406–409
Lymphoblastoid cell lines, 69, 736
Lymphochoriomeningitis (LCM), 87, 477, 479, 481–485, 578, 579, *718–719*
Lymphocyte:
    activating factor (LAF), 533
    activation products, 385–389
    alloantigens, 65–69, 74
        *see also* Ly antigens; Theta antigen
    antigen receptors, 80–88
    B, *see* B cell
    circulation, 49–51, 77–78
    defined (LD) antigen, 647, *648–662*
    definition, 38
    dependent antibodies (LDA), *see* Antibody-dependent cell-mediated cytotoxicity
    differentiation, 39–40, 88–102
    interactions with macrophages, 530–533
    life-span, 48–49, 78
    markers, 64–77
    mediators, 385–389
    morphology, 40–47

origin, 39–40, 88–102
physical properties, 47–48, 78–79
separation, 47
T, see T cell
traffic, 49–51, 418, 959
transformation, 51–58, 72, 76, 378–381,
    394, 406–409
Lymphocytotoxicity, 405, 409–416, 439–441,
    481–482, 586–587, 666–668
Lymphocytotoxins, 713, 803–804, 893
Lymphoid cells, 38–58
Lymphoid organs, 15–38
Lymphoid stem cells, 39–40, 91, 99, 884–891
Lymphokines, 58, 349, 385–389, 396
    defined, 984
Lymphoma, 55, 877–878, 881–882
Lymphotoxin (LT), 388, 390
Lysosomes, 110, 120–124, 268, 731
Lysozyme, 143–144, 160, 450, 451, 471,
    537–538, 685, 690–691

MA, see Membrane antigen
MacKenzie's assay, LATS, 919
Macroglobulin, defined, 984
Macroglobulinemia, 819, 871–874
Macrophages:
    activating factor (MAF), 386, 415, 441,
        533–534
    adhesion, 116–117
    and adjuvants, 947, 950
    agglutinating factor (MAgF), 387
    arming, 387, 415, 533
    arming factor (MAF), 387, 441, 473
    and cellular cooperation, 530–533
    collection, 113–114
    cytotoxic, 415–416, 443
    and delayed hypersensitivity, 533–534
    evaluation, 111–112
    in graft rejection, 415–416
    and lymphocyte transformation, 57
    migration, 111–112
        inhibition test, 382–385, 394–396, 405,
            406, 439
        inhibitor factor (MIF), 383–385, 551,
            984
    morphology, 108–111
    spreading inhibitory factor (MSF), 387
    in tumor rejection, 441, 443
MAF, see Macrophage, arming factor
Major histocompatibility complex (MHC),
    647
Malaria antigens, glomeruli, 849
Male antigens, 654, 673
    sterility, 921–922
Malnutrition, 278, 396, 462, 910
Malpighi corpuscles, 29
Mancini immunodiffusion technique, 316
Maple bark pneumonitis, 757

Marek's virus, 433
Margination, leukocyte, 457
Markers, B and T cell, 64–77
    defined, 984
Marrow, see Bone marrow
Mastocyte (mast cell), 354–355, 459
    defined, 984
    see also Degranulation
Masugi's glomerulonephritis, 717–718,
    830–831
Maturation:
    B cells, 99–102
    T cells, 88–102
MBLA, see Mouse bone marrow leukocyte
    antigen
MDP, see Muramyl dipeptide
Measles, 73, 477, 480, 497–500, 808, 935
Mediators:
    of delayed hypersensitivity, 58, 358–389,
        390
    of immediate hypersensitivity, 356–358
Membrane antigen (MA), in Burkitt's
    lymphoma, 433, 438
Membrane immunoglobulins, 75, 81–84, 100
Membrano-proliferative glomerulonephritis,
    799, 838, 840, 850–851
    and complement, 276–277, 840–841,
        850–851
Membranous glomerulonephritis, 697, 799,
    838, 840
Memory, 337, 408, 412, 535–538
    defined, 984
Meningitis, vaccine, 497
MER, see Methanol extractable residue
6-Mercaptopurine (6-MP), 577, 955–957
Mesangium, 837
Messenger RNA, 239–243, 522–524
Metabolic studies:
    complement, 276
    immunoglobulin, 224–225
Methanol extractable residue (MER), 946
Methyldopa, 725, 765, 770, 810–811
Methylhydrazine, 586
α-Methyl-mannoside, 57
Methylxanthines, 359
MF, see Mitogenic factor
MHC, see Major histocompatibility complex
β₂-Microglobulin, 228–229, 665
Microsomal antigens, thyroid, 915
Migration inhibitory factor (MIF), 383–385
Milk allergy, 352, 747
Millipore chamber, 93, 102
Mineral salts, as adjuvants, 947–948
Minimal changes, nephrotic syndrome, 841,
    847
Minor histocompatibility antigens, 651–654
Mishell and Dutton's technique, 507
    defined, 984

Mitochondria, reactive antibody, 927, 937, 970
Mitogen:
  B cells, 76
  pokeweed, *52–54*, 58, 67, 76, 551, 887
  T cell, 72
Mitogenic factor (MF), 387
Mitomycin, 407
Mixed connective tissue disease, 803
Mixed cryoglobulins, *732–733*, 806, *876–877*, 968
Mixed lymphocyte reaction (MLR), *406–409*, 539–540, 545, 658–662, 672, 674
  cell origin, 72–73, 406–407
  defined, 984
MLC, *see* Mixed lymphocyte reaction
M locus, 661
MLR, *see* Mixed lymphocyte reaction
MNS system, 593, 612, 631
Modulation, antigenic, 84
  defined, 979
Moldy hay, 757–758
Moloney sarcoma virus (MSV), 441
Monoclonal antibodies, hybridome, 12, 66, 69, *169–170*
Monoclonal Ig, 169–170, 855–874
Monoclonal lymphocytic proliferation, 857–874
Monocytes, 75, 76, 107, 109
  in antibacterial defense, 474–475
  in antiviral defense, 481
Monogamous binding, 291, 311
Monokines, 533
Mosaics, 540
Mother-fetus relationships, 424–427, 752–753
Mouse bone marrow leukocyte antigen (MBLA), 74
6-MP, *see* 6-Mercaptopurine
MRL mice, 715
MSF, *see* Macrophage, spreading inhibitory factor
MSV, *see* Moloney sarcoma virus
Mucocutaneous candidiasis, 900–901
Mucoproteins, 450
Mucosal ulcers, 937
Mucous cells, 616–620
Multiparous women, 647, 752–756
Multiple sclerosis, 697, 934–935
  myeloma, *see* Myeloma
Mumps, 480, 497
Muramyl dipeptide (MDP), *945,* 947
Murine leukemia and sarcoma virus (MSV), 441
Muscle, reactive antibody, 927–929, 932, 937
Mutations, 244–246, 571–572
Myasthenia gravis, 697, 718, *926–929*

Mycobacterium tuberculosis, 365–366, 371–372, 471–472
Mycoplasma fermentans, 817
  pneumoniae, 725, 792
Mycosis fungoides, 879
Mycropolyspora faeni, 757–758
Myeloma, 168, 169, 525, 527, *859–867*, 907–908
  defined, 984
Myeloperoxidase, 121, 905
Myocardial infarction, 926
Myocardium, *see* Heart
Myositis, 823–825
Myxedema, 915–918, 924

$N_4$, 622
N-acetyl-galactosamine, 619–620
NADPH, 121, 905
Nasopharyngeal carcinoma, 433, 477
Native DNA, reactive antibodies, *see* Anti-DNA antibodies
Natural antibodies, *333–334*, 507, 598, 601–602, 620–622
Natural killer cells (NK cells), 416, 443–444
Natural selection, 560
NBT test, 904, 969
Necrotizing angiitis, 820–823
NeF, *see* Nephritic factor
Neonatal thymectomy, 61–63, 93, 483, 490, 540
Nephritic factor (NF, C3 NeF), 277, *850–851*
Nephrotic syndrome, 798, 837, 841, 847, 852
Network theory, 572–573
Neutralization:
  enzyme, 321
  phage, 322
  reactions, 322–323
  toxin, 322, 468–469
  viral, 323, 478–479
Neutropenias, 902–904, 925
Neutrophils, 107
Newborn hemolytic disease, 752–753
New Zealand Black (NZB) mice, 548, *712–715*, 820, 836–837
Nezelof's syndrome, 888
NF, *see* Nephritic factor
NIP (4-hydroxy-3-ido-5 nitrophenyl acetic acid), 535–536
Nippostrongylus Brasiliensis, 490, 491, 743
Nitroblue tetrazolium test (NBT), 969
NK cells, *see* Natural killer cells
Nocardia, 76
Nodules, 814, 821
Non A-Non B hepatitis virus, 933
Non-H-2 systems, 651, 653
Non-precipitating antibodies, 310–311, 322
Non-secretory myeloma, 861
Non-specific immunity, 459–463

Non-specific immunoglobulins, 489, 566–567
Norepinephrine, 359
Nuclear antigens, *800–803*, 817, 826, 932
Nucleic acids, 155
Nucleolar pattern, 801, 826
Nude mouse, 26, 27, 32, 34, 61, 66, 92
Null cells, 76–77, 881, 892
Nutritional factors, 462
NZB, *see* New Zealand Black mice

OAF, *see* Osteoclast activating factor
Obese chicken thyroiditis, 715–716
Octylamine, 355
Ontogeny:
    bursa of Fabricius, 20–21, 99–100
    immunoglobulins, 229–232
    spleen, 28
    T cells, 88–90
    thymus, 16–17, 89–92
Ophthalmia, sympathetic, *see* Sympathetic
    ophthalmia
Opsonic adherence, 781–782
Opsonins, 117, 330
Opsonization, 117, *268–269*, 323, 330,
    781–782
Optic neuritis, 697
Oral contraceptives, and lupus, 810
Organ:
    grafts, 402–404, 672–673
    specific antigens, 133, 673, 708
    specific autoimmune diseases, 708–711,
        914–929
Original antigenic sin, 131, *336–337*, 482,
    486
Origin of antibody diversity, 240–249,
    556–574
Osteoclast activating factor (OAF), 389
Outcherlony's technique, 315, 318
Ovarian insufficiency, 922–923
Oxazolone, 369, 551
Oxygen, 121–122
Oz factor, 191, 228

PAF-acether, *see* Platelets, activating factor
P antigen, 593, 631, 643, 774
Papain hydrolysis, 170–171, 178
Parabiosis, defined, 985
Paracortical area, of lymph nodes, 25–28,
    35–36, 369–370
Paralysis, immune, 575, 985
Parasite antigens, 488
Parathyroids, 17, 891–893, *921*
    reactive antibody, 921
Paratope, defined, 985
Partial lipodystrophy, 851
Passive cutaneous anaphylaxis (PCA), 324,
    346, *349–350*
Passive hemagglutination, 136, 321, 324

Passive immunization, 494–495
Patch formation, 82–83
Paternity exclusion, 608
Pattern, antigen, *see* Antigen, determinants
PBA, *see* Polyclonal B cell activator
PCA, *see* Passive cutaneous anaphylaxis
PCI antigen, 74
PEG, *see* Polyethylene glycol
Pemphigoid, bullous, 925–926
Pemphigus vulgaris, 697, 925
Penicillamine, 810, 811, 819, 822
Penicillin, 137, 336, 352, 762–767
Pepsin, 178
Periarteriolar zone, spleen, 30–31, 35–36
Peripheral pattern, 801
Pernicious anemia, 697, 923–924
Peroxidase, 46, 83, 321, 515–520
Persistent viral infection, 484–485
Pertussis, Bordetella, 950
Peyer's patches, 99–100
PFC, *see* Plaque forming cells
PG, *see* Prostaglandins
pH, and antigen-antibody dissociation, 293
PHA, *see* Phytohemagglutinin
Phacoanaphylaxis, 926
Phage neutralization, 322
Phagocytes, in antibacterial defense, 106,
    470–471
Phagocytic index, 111–112
Phagocytosis, *115–124*, 330–331, 470–471,
    532, 780–784
    defined, 985
Pharyngeal pouches, 16
Phenacetin, 766, 767
Phenotype:
    ABO, 613
    defined, 985
Phenoxybenzamine, 359
Phosphoglucomutase (PGM3), 672
Phospholipids, 358
    extract, adjuvant, 950–951
Phosphorycholine, 213, 215
Phylogenetically associated residues,
    207–208
Phylogeny:
    Ig, 225–232
    thymus, 226
Phytohemagglutinin (PHA), *51–58*, 73, 90,
    98
Picryl chloride, 369, 374, 551, 580
PIF, *see* Proliferation, inhibitory factor
Pigeon breeders' disease, 758–759
Pinocytosis, 82
    defined, 985
    reverse, 526
PK, *see* Prausnitz-Küstner reaction
PLA, 658
Placenta, 232, 424–427

Placental transfer, immunoglobulins, 232, 752–753
Plague, vaccine, 497
Planted antigen, 836
Plaque forming cells (PFC), 506–508, 517, 518, 578
defined, 985
Plasma cells:
cytology, 516–520
defined, 38
differentiation, 52, 99
fusion, hybridoma, 523
immunoglobulin synthesis, 521–528
myelomatous, 864
Plasmacytoma, murine, 169–170, 523, 859, 946
Plasmapheresis, 813, 852, 863, 873
Plasmin, 270
Plasmodium, 486–489, 493
Plate immunodiffusion, *see* Outcherlony's technique
Platelets, 268–270, 647, 764–765
activating factor (PAF-acether), 356–358, 730
agglutination, 764, 925
lysis, 864
Pleuropneumonia-like organisms (PPLO), 817
PLT, *see* Primed LD typing
Pneumococcal antigens (polysaccharides), 8, 152–153, 158–159, 290, 305–306, 324, 338, 540, 546–547, 578
Pneumococcus XIV, 616–620
Pneumocystis carnii, 889, 904
Podocytes, 837
Poison ivy, 760
Pokeweed mitogen, *52–54*, 58, 67, 76, 551, 887
Poliomyelitis, vaccine, 497, 498
Pollens, *351*, 742, 744
Poly (AU), 951
Polyagglutinability, 639, 776, 792
Polyarteritis nodosa, 485, *820–822*, 846
Polyclonal B cell activator (PBA), 58, 544
defined, 985
Polyethylene glycol (PEG), 169, 299, 734
Poly IC, 802
Polymerization, Ig, 523–524
*see also* IgA, dimeric; IgM, polymeric
Polymorph, 106, 121–122, 491
deficiency, 902–907
Polymorphism:
of complement factors, 271
genetic, 593, 607–609, 645
Polymyositis, 823–825
Polymyxin, 355
Polyoma virus, 433, 435, 482–483
Polyosidic antigens, 151–154, 617–620

Polypeptides, synthetic, 146–151, 679–683
Polypeptidyl proteins, 146
Polyribonucleotides, 408, 802, 951
Polyribosomes, 43, 52
Polysaccharides, 305–306
Polysomes, 523–524
Polyvinyl pyrrolidone (PVP), *158–159*, 160, 300, 545–547, 647, 687, 713
Population genetics, 597
Post capillary venules, 36, 48–50
Post-thymic cells, 91, 94–95
PPD, *see* Purified protein derivative
Pr antigens, 775
Prausnitz-Küstner reaction, 344, 349, 749
Pre B cells, 100
Precipitating antibodies, 305–319, 758
Precipitation reaction, 305–319, 324–325
Precursor cells, *see* Stem cells
Pregnancy, 232, 424–427, 647, 752–753, 911
and SLE, 810
Pre T cells, 89–90, 94–96, 692
Prick test, 748
Primary response, 334, 335
Primed LD typing (PLT), 661–662
Private antigens (specificities), 599, 651, 791
Proantigen, 130
Procainamide, 810–811
Proliferation:
glomerulus, 838, 840
inhibitory factor (PIF), 388
Promonocyte, 107
Properdin, 261–262
Propranolol, 359
Prostaglandins, 459, 460, 908
Provocation tests, 748–749, 758
Prozone phenomenon, 307, 320, 323
Pseudoalleles, 595
Pseudo-autoimmune hemolytic anemia, 776, 792
Psoriasis, 697
Public specificities, 651
Purification of Ig, 165–170
Purified protein derivative (PPD), 367, 370
Purpura:
Henoch Schönlein, 822, 841
thrombocytopenic, 764–765, 870, 897, 925
PVP, *see* Polyvinyl pyrrolidone
PWM, *see* Pokeweed mitogen
Pyroglobulin, 863
defined, 985
Pyroninophilic cells, 27, 332, 370
defined, 985

QA antigens, 68, 670

RA, *see* Rheumatoid arthritis
Rabies, 497, 499
RA cells, *see* Ragocytes

Radial immunodiffusion, *see* Mancini
    immunodiffusion technique
Radioallergosorbent test (RAST), 749–750
Radioautography, 36, 48, 83, 84, 330, 514,
    689
Radioimmunoadsorption test (RIST), 750
Radioimmunoassays, *302–304*, 324
    GBM, 843
    IgE, 749–750
Radioimmunoelectrophoresis, 317
Ragg (rheumatoid agglutinator), 632
Ragocytes (RA cells), 814
Ragweed, 351, 742
Raji cells, *736*, 806
Ramon's technique, 313
Rapidly progressive glomerulonephritis, 840,
    852
RAST, *see* Radioallergosorbent test
Reagins, defined, 985
    *see also* IgE
Rebuck's technique, 113
Receptors:
    antigenic recognition, 75, 81–89, 562–563
    B cell, 80–84
    lectins, *57–58*, 71–72
    T cell, 85–88
Reciprocal cross reaction, 132
Recirculation, 16, 48–51, 77–78
Recombinants mice, *see* Congenic mice
Recombinations, 222, 246–249, 569–570
Red blood cell, *see* Erythrocyte grouping
Redistribution, antigen receptors, 82–83
Red pulp, spleen, 29
Region:
    constant, 174, 191–199, 227–228
    H-2, 646–654, 670–671, 683–686
    thymus dependent, 26–27, 30, 35–36
    thymus independent, 26–27, 30, 35–36
    variable, 174, 199–207, 227
        defined, 987
Regional enteritis (Crohn's disease),
    935–936
Regular natural antibodies, 601
Regulation of antibody production, 340–342,
    530–552
Reiter's syndrome, 697
Rejection:
    crises, 402–404
    glomerulonephritis, 849
    hyperacute, 402, 404
    mechanisms, 416–422
Renal biopsies, 838–842
Renal failure, 910
Renal grafts, 402–404, 672–675, 849
RES, *see* Reticulo endothelial system
Responder animals, *vs.* non-responder,
    677–719

Restriction:
    allogeneic, 12, *87–88*, 446, 482, 690,
        691–692
    enzymes, 232
Reticular dysgenesis, 886
Reticulo endothelial system (RES), blockade,
    363
Reticulum cell sarcoma, 819
Reverse passive cutaneous anaphylaxis
        (RPCA), 349
    pinocytosis, 526
RF, *see* Rheumatoid factor
RFC, *see* Rosette-forming cells
Rg-V-1 factor, 670, 695
Rhesus (Rh), 593, 603, 612, 623–628,
        640–642
    alloimmunization, 751–756
    and autoantibodies, 765, 772–774,
        779–780
    erythroblastosis fetalis, 752–753
    grouping, 640–642
    null phenotype, 626–628
    sites, 603, 626
Rheumatic fever, 929–930
Rheumatoid arthritis (RA), 632, 697, 804,
        *814–819*, 826
    cell-mediated immunity, 817
    and complement, 816
    immune complexes, 816–817
Rheumatoid factor (RF), 423, 736, 805,
        *815–816*, 858, 868, 871, 876, 971
    defined, 985
Rhinitis, allergic, 744
RhLA, 658
Rhodamine, 304
Ribonuclease (RNase), 144, 183–184
Rickettsies, 337
Ring test, 305
Ripley serum, 815
RIST, *see* Radioimmunoadsorption test
RNA, 522–523
    antibodies, 801–802, 808
    messenger, 239–243, 522–524
    reactive antibody, *see* Anti-RNA antibody
    splicing, 239–240
RNase, *see* Ribonuclease
Rockett immuno-electrophoresis, 317
Rodgers, 671
Rosenfield's nomenclature, 626–627
Rose-Waaler reaction, 815
    defined, 986
    *see also* Rheumatoid factor
Rosette:
    active, 70
    defined, 986
    E, 69–70, 73, 509
    inhibition, 960, 962–963

in LE cell formation, 801
sheep erythrocytes spontaneous, 69
Rosette-forming cells (RFC), 83–85, 405, *508–513*, 518
Rough (lymphocytes), 46
Rouleau formation, 639, 863
Route of administration, antigen, 130–131
Rubella, vaccine, 497
Russel body, defined, 986
Ryegrass, 351

Salivary glands, 612, 617, 819–820
Sarcoidosis, 816, 819, 938
Scatchard's representation, 288
Schick's reaction, 327, 461, 469
Schistosomes, 486–488, 491–493
SCID, *see* Severe combined immunodeficiency
Scleroderma, 804, *825–826*
Scrapie, 484, 935
SD, *see* Sero-defined antigens
Secondary autoimmunization, 846
   response, 335–337
Secondary immunodeficiencies, 907–911
Second colloid antigen, thyroid, 915
Second set allografts, 402
Secretion, immunoglobulins, 526
Secretors, 612–620
Secretory component, 34, 195, 525
   defined, 850
Secretory granules, thymus, 18
Secretory IgA, 344–345, 525
Sedormid, 764–765
Selective theories of antibody formation, 560–564
Self antigens, 708–710, 722–727
   altered, *87–88*, 691–694
   tolerance, 722–727
Seminal antigens, 921–922
Sendai virus, 169
Separation:
   of B and T cells, 79
   of lymphocytes, 47
Septic familial granulomatosis, 124
Septic granulomatosis, 904–905
Sequence of immunoglobulins, 171–177
Sequestration, erythrocytes, 781–782
Sero-defined (SD) antigens, 647–658
Serotherapy, *494–495* 795–797
Serotonin, 266, *356–359*, 459, 460, 729
Serum sickness, 272, 273, 727–729, 795–797, 833–836, 848
   defined, 986
Serum thymic factor, 97
Se se, 613, 616
Severe combined immunodeficiency (SCID), 886–891

Sex hormones and immunity, 720, 810
Sex limited protein (Slp), 670, 685
Sex linked agammaglobulinemia, 551, 894–895
Sezary's syndrome, 879
Sheep cell rosettes, *see* Rosette
Sheep erythrocyte spontaneous rosettes, *69–70*, 73, 509, 512
Shock, anaphylactic, *347–348*, 743–744, 763–764
Shunt nephritis, 848–849
Shwartzman phenomenon, 273, *362–363*
   defined, 986
Sia test, 872
Sicca syndrome, 819–820
Silent antigens, 626
Silica, 947
Silk fibrillar protein, 142
Sin, original antigenic, 131, *336–337*, 482, 486
Sips' equation, 291
SIRS, *see* Soluble immune response suppression
Site:
   antibody, 184–190
   antigen, defined, 986
SJL mice, 715
Sjogren's syndrome, 804, 808, *819–820*, 824
Skin:
   as anatomical barrier, 450
   basement membrane, reactive antibody, 925–926
   grafts, 400–402, 648–658
   Ig deposits, 806
   lesions, SLE, 799–800
   reactive factor (SRF), 389, 390
   tests, 393–394, *748–749*, 761
SLA, 658
SLE, *see* Systemic lupus erythematosus
Slow reactive substance of anaphylaxis (SRS-A), 356–358, 745
Slow viruses, 484, 935
Slp, *see* Sex limited protein
Smallpox, vaccination, 497
Sm antigen, 803
Smooth lymphocytes, 46
Smooth muscle, reactive antibodies, 932, 937
SN Agg (serum normal agglutinator), 632
Snell's laws, 648
sNP (soluble nucleoprotein) antigen, 802
Sodium cromoglycate, 361, 745
Soluble immune response suppression (SIRS), 388, 542, 550–551
Somatic mutation theory, 244–246, 571–572
Somatic recombination theory, 234, 246–249, 569–570

Specificity:
  antibody, *see* Antibody, site
  antigen, *see* Antigen, determinants
Speckled pattern, 801
S peptide, 144
Spermagglutinins, 799, 921–922
Spermatozoa, 663, 921–922
Spike, 855, 860–862
Spleen, 28–31
  changes during immunization, 30–31, 332
  index, 423
  ontogenesis, 28
  structure, 28–30
Splenomegaly, 422–423
Split tolerance, 576
S protein, 144
S region, 650, 670–671
SRS-A, *see* Slow reactive substance of
  anaphylaxis
SSPE, *see* Subacute sclerosing panencephalitis
Steblay's glomerulonephritis, 832
Stem cells, 39–40, 91, 100, 884–891
Sterility, 921–923
Steroids:
  in glomerulonephritis, 852
  in lupus, 812–813
  in rheumatoid arthritis, 818
Still's disease, 815
Stomach, reactive antibody, 923–924
Streptococcal antigens, 86, 154, 167, 214, 550
  role in immunopathology, 833, 840, *848,*
    857–858
Streptolysin (anti), 848, 857–858, 929
Streptomycin, 763, 767
Striated muscle, reactive antibody, 926,
    929–930
Subacute bacterial endocarditis, 816, 849
Subacute sclerosing panencephalitis (SSPE),
    477, 484, 911, 935
Subclasses, Ig, 198–199
Substance A, 938–939
Suicide, antigen, 84, 563
Sulfonamides, 352, 760, 767, 810–811, 822
Super antigen, 532
Superoxide ions, 121–122
  dismutase, 122
Suppressor factors, 542, 547–548, 550–551
Suppressor T cells, 69, 71, 98, 160, 392–393,
    419, *546–552,* 583–584, 586, 588, 689,
    712–714, 726–727, 899, 958
  defined, 986
Surface Ig, 74, 81–83, 100, 857–859,
    868–870
Surveillance, immunologic, 443
  defined, 986
Susceptibility to diseases, 694–699
SV 40, 433, 435
Swan mice, 714–715

Switch (IgM/IgG), *237–238,* 337, 508, 522,
    687
Sympathetic ophthalmia, 926
Synergy, between T cells, 98, 545–546
Syngeneic, 400–401
  defined, 986
  restriction, 12, 87–88, 444, 482, 690,
    691–692
Synovectomy, 819
Synovial fluid, 799, 814, 816–817
Synthetic polypeptides, 146–151, 678–681
Syphilis:
  glomerulonephritis, 849
  reaction, false positive, 805, 808, 826, 934
Systemic lupus erythematosus (SLE),
    *797–813,* 820
  antinuclear antibodies, 800–803
  arthritis, 799
  clinical features, 797–800
  complement, 276–277, 283, *806–807,*
    809
  cutaneous lesions, 799–800
  defined, 797–798
  drug-induced, 810–812
  genetic factors, 697, 809
  glomerulonephritis, 798–799
  treatment, 812–813
Systemic sclerosis, *see* Scleroderma

T, or Tn, antigens, 776
Tachyphylaxy, 267
Takasugi and Klein's microcytotoxicity assay
    (MA), 410, 439–441, 586–587
Takayasu's arteritis, 823
TATA, *see* Tumor, associated transplantation
    antigen
T cell:
  and antibacterial defense, 471–475
  and antiviral defense, 480–483
  CLL, 879
  colonies, 40
  cytotoxic, 410–412, 439–441, 482,
    666–668
  defined, 986
  definitions, 60–64
  differentiation, 88–98
  growth factor, 538–539, 541–544, 590
    *see also* Interleukin 2; Lymphokines
  helper, 69, 71, 160, 420, *534–545,*
    687–689
  heteroantigens, 65–69
  immunodeficiency, 891–894, 899–902
  leukemias, 878–880
  receptor, *85–88,* 216
  replacing factor (TRF), 539–540, 542
  rosettes (E rosettes), 69–70, 77, 509
  specificity, 537, 666–668
  subsets, 97–98, 545

suppressor, 69, 71, 98, 160, 392–393, 419, *546–552*, 583–584, 586, 588, 689, 712–714, 726–727, 899, 958
TCGF, *see* T cell, growth factor
T6 chromosome, 72, 73, 93, 408, 535
Temperature, effect on antigen antibody complex, 294
Temporal arteritis, 822–823
Tensioactive substances, 948
Tetanus, 495–497, 622
   *see also* Anatoxins
Tetraparental mice, 587, 688
TF, *see* Transfer, factor
Tg cell, 70–71
Theory of antibody diversity, 240–249, 556–574
Theory of autoimmunity, 722–727, 788–792
Thermodynamics, of antigen-antibody interaction, 295, 603–607
Thermolability, *see* Bence-Jones proteins
Theta antigen (Thy-1), *65*, 91, 97, 681
   defined, 986
Thioglycollate, 113
Thiopurines, 812, 818, *955–957*, 962–966
Thiouracil, 822
Thorotrast, 363
Thrombocytopenia, 764–765, 870, 897
Thrombocytopenic purpura, 764–765, 822, 870, 897, 925
Thrombotic microangiopathy, 846
Thy-1 (θ), *see* Theta antigen
Thymectomy:
   adult, 61, 64, 98, 545
   man, 928
   neonatal, 61, 65, 77, 91
Thymic hormone, 95–96, 547, 712–713, 888, 893, 927, 951–952
   defined, 986–987
Thymidine uptake, 337–338, 359
Thymitis, 48, 51, 57, 65, 927
Thymocyte stimulating factor (TSF), 386, 388
Thymoma, 91, 551
Thymopoietin, 96, 927
   defined, 986–987
Thymosin, 96
   defined, 986–987
Thymus, 16–21
   atrophy, 20–21, 65, 77, 93, 97–98
   cortex *vs.* medulla, 19–21
   dependency, 61, 531–532
   dependent antigens, 61, 63, 158–159
      areas, 26–27, 30, 35–36
      defined, 987
   derived cells, *see* T cell
   epithelial cells, 17–19, 89–90, 93, 96–97, 691–692, 888
   germinal centers, 20, 927
   grafts, 91, 93–100, 893

hormone, 95–96, 547, 712–713, 888, 893, 927, 951–952
   defined, 986–987
independent antigen, 28, 61, 149, *158–159*, 338, 540, 544, 584
   areas, 35–36
   defined, 987
leukemia (TL), *see* TL antigen
ontogenesis, 16–17, 89–90
phylogeny, 226
structure, 18–20
Thyroglobulin, 715, 724, 849, *915–918*
Thyroid autoantigens, 915
Thyroiditis, 697, 715–716, *915–918*
Thyroid reactive antibodies, 715, 820, *915–920*, 924
Thyrotoxicosis, 697, 918–920
Till and MacCulloch's technique, 40
Timothy pollen, 351
TIP, *see* Translation inhibitory protein
TL antigen, 65, 91, 435, 670, 685
Tobacco mosaic virus, 143
Todd phenomenon, 218
Tolerance, 537, 562, *575–589*, 725
   defined, 575, 987
   and delayed hypersensitivity, 391
   *vs.* enhancement, allografts, 586–588
   high dose, 579
   low dose, 579–580
   suppressor cells in, 583, 585, 588
Tolerogens, 130, 577–579
Tomato bushy stunt virus, 143
Tonofilaments, thymus epithelial cells, 18
Tonsils, 31, 100
Topological model of immunoglobulins, 171, 188
Total lymphoid irradiation, 961
Toxin, 468–469, 497
   neutralization, 311, 322, 468–469
Toxoid, *see* Anatoxins
Transcobalamin deficiency, 901
Transfer:
   of delayed hypersensitivity, 366, 373–378
   factor (TF), *376–378*, 390, 897
      defined, 987
   of graft immunity, 416
   of tolerance, 581
   of tumor immunity, 437
Transformation of lymphocytes, 51–58, 72, 76, 378–381, 394, 406–409
Transfusion, 636–643, 753–756
Translation inhibitory protein (TIP), 452
Translocation groups, 207–208, 219, 221
Transplantation:
   antigens, 228, 572, *594–610, 648–653*, 692–694
   bone marrow, 887
   defined, 400

immunity, 399–429
   renal, 402–404, 672–673
   tolerance, 422, 586–588
Transport, immunoglobulins, 526
Tr cell, 70–71
Tread mill mechanism, 578
TRF, see T cell, replacing factor
Tributylamine, 137
Trophoblast, 424–427
Trypan blue, 647
Trypanosomes, 487–490, 493
TSA, see Tumor, specific antigen
TSTA, see Tumor, specific transplantation
      antigen
T/t locus, 671
Tuberculin, 76, 367, 370–372, 376, 382
   defined, 987
   fever, 372
   shock, 330, 371–372
   see also Purified protein derivative
Tuberculosis, see Mycobacterium tuberculosis
Tubular acidosis in Sjogren's syndrome, 819
Tubular antigen, 836, 849
Tumor:
   antigens, 430–436
   associated transplantation antigen (TATA),
      431, 434–436, 445
   chemically induced, 435
   immunity, 430–448, 908
   immunotherapy, 446–447
   specific antigen (TSA), 431
   specific transplantation antigen (TSTA),
      431, 434, 436
   vaccination, 436–437
Typhoid, vaccine, 497, 499
Typhus, 497

Ulcerative colitis, 936
Unidirectional MLR, 407
Unitary hypothesis, 324–325
Uropod, 44, 82
Urticaria, 746
Uterus, site, 426
Uvea, reactive antibody, 926
Uveitis, 926

Vaccination, 2, 469, 494–500
   anti-parasite, 494
   anti-tumor, 436–437
Vaccinia, generalized, 889
Valence:
   antibody, 286
   antigens, 143, 296, 307
   defined, 987
   haptens, 139–141, 307
Van der Waals forces, 293
Variability subgroups, 183–206
Variable regions, immunoglobulin, 174,
      199–207, 227
   defined, 987

Varicella, 477–480
Vasculitis, 796, 820–823
Vasectomy, 922
Vasoactive amines, 459
   see also Histamine
Vasopressin, 146
VCA, see Virus, capsid antigen
Velocity sedimentation, 46, 78
V gene, 233–237, 240–249, 567–573
Virus, 433–434, 476–486, 497–500
   antigens, 578–579
   capsid antigen (VCA), 438
   factor in autoimmunity, 714, 716, 718–719,
      721
   hemagglutination, 320–321
   hepatitis, see HBs antigen
   inclusions, 715, 808
   in lupus, 808
   neutralization, 323, 478–479
   replication test, 381–382
Virus-induced immunosuppression, 909
Visna, 484, 935
Vitamin B 12, 901
Vitamin B and C, 462
Vitamin K1, 189
V region, 174, 199–224

Waldenstrom's macroglobulinemia, 819,
      871–874
Waldeyer tonsillar ring, 31
Wasting disease, 422–423
Water soluble adjuvant (WSA), 945
Wax D, 945
Weak A groups, 637–638
Weber-Christian disease, 939
Wegener's granulomatosis, 822
White grafts, 402
White pulp, spleen, 30
Whooping cough, vaccine, 497, 909
Wiskott-Aldrich syndrome, 378, 897
WSA, see Water soluble adjuvant

Xenogeneic, 400–407
   defined, 987
Xenografts, 404
Xenotropic viruses, 714
Xerostomia, 819
Xg antigen, 609
X-linked agammaglobulinemia, 551,
      894–895
X-ray analysis, immunoglobulins, 179–181

Yellow fever, 481, 497
Yolk sac, 17, 21, 90, 94

Zeta potential, 606–607, 642
Zipp assay, 514
Zoster, 477–484
Zymosan, 261